D1576429

Oxford Textbook of
Sleep Disorders

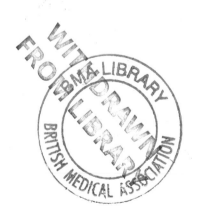

Oxford Textbooks in Clinical Neurology

PUBLISHED

Oxford Textbook of Epilepsy and Epileptic Seizures
Edited by Simon Shorvon, Renzo Guerrini, Mark Cook, and Samden Lhatoo

Oxford Textbook of Vertigo and Imbalance
Edited by Adolfo Bronstein

Oxford Textbook of Movement Disorders
Edited by David Burn

Oxford Textbook of Stroke and Cerebrovascular Disease
Edited by Bo Norrving

Oxford Textbook of Neuromuscular Disorders
Edited by David Hilton-Jones and Martin Turner

Oxford Textbook of Neurorehabilitation
Edited by Volker Dietz and Nick Ward

Oxford Textbook of Neuroimaging
Edited by Massimo Filippi

Oxford Textbook of Cognitive Neurology and Dementia
Edited by Masud Husain and Jonathan M. Schott

Oxford Textbook of Clinical Neurophysiology
Edited by Kerry R. Mills

Oxford Textbook of Sleep Disorders
Edited by Sudhansu Chokroverty and Luigi Ferini-Strambi

FORTHCOMING

Oxford Textbook of Neuro-oncology
Edited by Tracy Batchelor, Michael Weller, Nancy Tarbell, and Ryo Nishikawa

Oxford Textbook of Headache Syndromes
Edited by Michel Ferrari, Joost Haan, Andrew Charles, David Dodick, and Fumihiko Sakai

Oxford Textbook of Neuro-ophthalmology
Edited by Fion Bremner

Oxford Textbook of Clinical Neuropathology
Edited by Sebastian Brandner and Tamas Revesz

Oxford Textbook of
Sleep Disorders

Edited by

Sudhansu Chokroverty

Professor and Director of Sleep Research, Co-Chair Emeritus of Neurology,
JFK Neuroscience Institute, Edison, NJ, USA; Professor of Neuroscience,
Seton Hall University, South Orange, NJ, USA; Clinical Professor of Neurology,
Rutgers Robert Wood Johnson Medical School, New Brunswick, NJ, USA

Luigi Ferini-Strambi

Professor of Neurology, Vita-Salute San Raffaele University; Director of Sleep Disorder
Center, Division of Neuroscience, San Raffaele Scientific Institute, Milan, Italy

Series Editor

Christopher Kennard

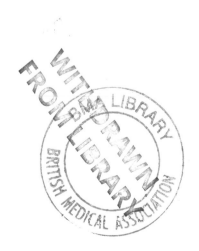

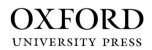

OXFORD
UNIVERSITY PRESS

OXFORD

UNIVERSITY PRESS

Great Clarendon Street, Oxford, OX2 6DP,
United Kingdom

Oxford University Press is a department of the University of Oxford.
It furthers the University's objective of excellence in research, scholarship,
and education by publishing worldwide. Oxford is a registered trade mark of
Oxford University Press in the UK and in certain other countries

Published in the United States of America by Oxford University Press
198 Madison Avenue, New York, NY 10016, United States of America

British Library Cataloguing in Publication Data
Data available

Library of Congress Control Number: 2016954561

ISBN 978–0–19–968200–3

Printed and bound in China by
C&C Offset Printing Co., Ltd.

Oxford University Press makes no representation, express or implied, that the
drug dosages in this book are correct. Readers must therefore always check
the product information and clinical procedures with the most up-to-date
published product information and data sheets provided by the manufacturers
and the most recent codes of conduct and safety regulations. The authors and
the publishers do not accept responsibility or legal liability for any errors in the
text or for the misuse or misapplication of material in this work. Except where
otherwise stated, drug dosages and recommendations are for the non-pregnant
adult who is not breast-feeding

Links to third party websites are provided by Oxford in good faith and
for information only. Oxford disclaims any responsibility for the materials
contained in any third party website referenced in this work.

Preface

There have been rapid advances recently in basic science, technical, clinical, and therapeutic aspects of sleep medicine that have captivated sleep scientists and clinicians. Concomitantly, there has been a rapid increase in the number of individuals involved in clinical sleep medicine and sleep research, in addition to an explosive growth in the number of sleep centers, laboratories, and programs and an increasing number of sleep societies (national and international) and sleep medicine journals worldwide. There is an eagerness and increasing desire to absorb this evolving knowledge about sleep and its disorders. Therefore, there is a need for new books encompassing all this new knowledge. Despite the publication of a number of sleep-related books in the last few years, gaps remain in many areas. It is obvious that there is a distinct lack of adequate knowledge and awareness of sleep disorders within the neurological community, and thus sleep disorders are not dealt with adequately by most practicing neurologists. There are a few neurologically oriented short books available, but these do not give in-depth coverage of the topic. It is therefore an opportune moment to produce a volume in a succinct and lucid manner, covering the topic in a logical and orderly way and emphasizing the practical aspects with an underlying basic science component. Peter Stevenson, Senior Commissioning Editor of Medicine, Neurology, Neurosurgery, Psychiatry, and Oxford Medical Libraries at Oxford University Press (OUP), Oxford, United Kingdom contacted the Senior Editor (SC) to consider compiling such a book to fill these gaps, in collaboration with a co-editor from the European continent. Professor Luigi Ferini-Strambi from Milan, Italy agreed to be co-editor. We then proceeded to produce a comprehensive,

balanced, and easily readable book emphasizing sleep neurology as part of the Oxford Textbooks in Clinical Neurology (OTCN) series in conformity with the wishes of Professor Chris Kennard, editor of the new OTCN series.

Most of the recent advances in sleep medicine have been captured in this monograph, with special emphasis on sleep neurology. The volume is essentially a clinical compendium, but also provides a background to the underlying basic science and techniques. The book is divided into 12 sections and several subsections: (1) Basic science; (2) Laboratory evaluation; (3) Clinical science: general introduction; (4) Hypersomnias; (5) Insomnias; (6) Circadian rhythm disorders; (7) Sleep neurology; (8) Parasomnias; (9) Sleep and medical disorders; (10) Sleep and psychiatric disorders; (11) Sleep in children, older adults, and women; (12) Miscellaneous sleep-related topics.

This book is directed primarily at neurologists and senior trainees, as well as internists (especially those specializing in pulmonary, cardiovascular, gastrointestinal, renal, and endocrine medicine), general practitioners/family physicians, psychiatrists, psychologists, pediatricians, otolaryngologists, dentists, neurosurgeons, and neuroscientists, and others interested in understanding sleep (eg, technologists, nurses, and other healthcare professionals). The book should be useful to both beginners and those advanced in the field.

Sudhansu Chokroverty
Luigi Ferini-Strambi

Acknowledgements

We must first thank all the contributors for their scholarly writings and their patience in waiting to see the volume finally in production after a long and protracted period (beyond our control). We also wish to thank all the authors, editors, and publishers for granting us permission to reproduce illustrations, boxes, and tables that have previously been published in other books and journals. We must thank Peter Stevenson, the Senior Commissioning Editor of the Oxford Textbooks in Clinical Neurology series for his dedication, patience, and professionalism, and the editorial and production staff at the Oxford University Press. The Senior Editor (SC) wishes to thank Toni Bacala, the editorial assistant to the *Sleep Medicine* journal, for her tremendous support in organizing the table of contents, making corrections, typing, and editing, in addition to her main function as editorial assistant to the journal. Since Ms. Bacala left, Ms. Jamie Winder, the current editorial assistant took care of these functions. Last but not least, the senior editor must express his love and gratitude to his wife, Manisha Chokroverty, MD for her unfailing and continued support, love, patience and tolerance throughout the long period of editing, writing, and proof-reading during the book's production.

Sudhansu Chokroverty
Luigi Ferini-Strambi

Contents

Abbreviations

5-HT	5-hydroxytryptamine (serotonin)		BIPN	bilateral isolated phrenic neuropathy
5-HT$_1$, ...	serotonin receptors		BMI	body mass index
5-HTT	serotonin transporter		BP	blood pressure
A	adrenaline (epinephrine)		BPAP	bilevel positive airway pressure
AAP	American Academy of Pediatrics		BPSD	behavioral and psychological signs of dementia
AASM	American Academy of Sleep Medicine		BRS	baroreflex sensitivity
ABG	arterial blood gas		BSMI	benign sleep myoclonus of infancy
ACE	angiotensin-converting enzyme		BZD	benzodiazepine
ACh	acetylcholine		BZDRA	benzodiazepine receptor agonist
AChR	acetylcholine receptor		CA	central apnea
ACTH	corticotropin (adrenocorticotropic hormone)		CA	confusional arousal
AD	Alzheimer disease		CAF	central activation failure
ADA	adenosine deaminase		CAP	cyclical alternating pattern
ADCADN	autosomal dominant cerebellar ataxia, deafness, and narcolepsy		CBF	cerebral blood flow
			CBT	cognitive–behavioral therapy
ADH	antidiuretic hormone		CBTI	cognitive–behavioral therapy for insomnia
ADHD	attention-deficit hyperactivity disorder		CBZ	carbamazepine
ADL	Activities of Daily Living		CCHS	congenital central alveolar hypoventilation syndrome
ADNFLE	autosomal dominant nocturnal frontal lobe epilepsy		CDR	Clinical Dementia Rating
AED	antiepileptic drug		CFS	chronic fatigue syndrome
AHI	apnea–hypopnea index		CGI	clinical global impression
AI	apnea index		CGRP	calcitonin gene-related peptide
AI	atonia index		CHF	chronic heart failure
AIDS	acquired immunodeficiency syndrome		CHF	congestive heart failure
ALMA	alternating leg muscle activation		CI	confidence interval
ALS	amyotrophic lateral sclerosis		CJD	Creutzfeldt–Jakob disease
ALTE	apparent life-threatening event		CKD	chronic kidney disease
AMD	acid maltase deficiency		CMD	congenital muscular dystrophy
AMS	acute mountain sickness		CMS	Centers Medicare and Medicaid Services
ANS	autonomic nervous system		CMS	chronic mountain sickness
APAP	autotitrating continuous positive airway pressure		CMS	congenital myasthenic syndrome
ARAS	ascending reticular activating system		CMT	Charcot–Marie–Tooth disease
ArD	arousal disorder		CNS	central nervous system
ASD	autism spectrum disorder		CNZ	clonazepam
ASPD	advanced sleep phase disorder		COMT	catechol-O-methyltransferase
ASV	adaptive servo-ventilation		COPD	chronic obstructive pulmonary disease
ASV	assisted support ventilation		CPAP	continuous positive airway pressure
ASWPD	advanced sleep–wake phase disorder		CPG	central pattern generator
BALM	Basic Language Morningness Scale		CRC	central respiratory chemoreceptor
BDNF	brain-derived neurotrophic factor		CRH	corticotropin-releasing hormone
BF	basal forebrain		CRP	C-reactive protein
Bic	bicuculline		CRSD	circadian rhythm sleep disorder

CRSWD	circadian rhythm sleep–wake disorder
CSB	Cheyne–Stokes breathing
CSF	cerebrospinal fluid
CSWS	electrical status epilepticus during slow-wave sleep (continuous spike and wave during slow-wave sleep)
CTb	cholera toxin b subunit
CV	cardiovascular
CVD	cardiovascular disease
CWP	chronic widespread pain
$D_1, …$	dopamine receptors
DA	disorder of arousal
DA	dopamine
DAT	dopamine transporter
dDpMe	dorsal deep mesencephalic reticular nucleus
DHE	dihydroergotamine
DLB	dementia with Lewy bodies
DLCO	diffusion capacity of carbon monoxide
DLMO	dim light melatonin onset
DM	dermatomyositis
DM	myotonic dystrophy (dystrophia myotonica)
DMD	Duchenne muscular dystrophy
DORA	dual orexin receptor antagonist
DPGi	dorsal paragigantocellular nucleus
DPS	diaphragm pacing stimulation
DR	dorsal raphe
DRG	dorsal respiratory group
DSM	Diagnostic and Statistical Manual of Mental Disorders
DSPD	delayed sleep phase disorder
DSPS	delayed sleep phase syndrome
DSWPD	delayed sleep–wake phase disorder
DU	duodenal ulcer
DZ	dizygotic
EA	epileptic activity
EAE	experimental autoimmune encephalomyelitis
EDS	excessive daytime sleepiness
EDSS	Expanded Disability Status Scale
EEG	electroencephalography
EFM	excessive fragmentary myoclonus
EHS	exploding head syndrome
EMG	electromyography
EOG	electrooculography
EPAP	expiratory positive airway pressure
EPSP	excitatory postsynaptic potential
EQS	excessive quantity of sleep
ERP	event-related potential
ESES	electrical status epilepticus during sleep
ESRD	end-stage renal disease
ESS	Epworth Sleepiness Scale
FAP	fixed action pattern
FASPD	familial advanced sleep disorder
FASPS	familial advanced sleep phase syndrome
FCD	focal cortical dysplasia
FDG	[^{18}F]fluorodeoxyglucose
FFI	fatal familial insomnia
FiO_2	fraction of inspired oxygen
FLEPS	Frontal Lobe Epilepsy and Parasomnias Scale
fMRI	functional magnetic resonance imaging
FOSQ	Functional Outcomes of Sleep Questionnaire
FOT	forced oscillation technique
FRC	functional residual capacity
FRSD	free-running (non-24-hour) sleep disorder
FSH	follicle-stimulating hormone
FSHD	facioscapulohumeral muscular dystrophy
FTD	frontotemporal dementia
FVC	forced vital capacity
GABA	γ-aminobutyric acid
GAD	glutamate decarboxylase
GBP	gabapentin
GBS	Guillain–Barré syndrome
GER	gastroesophageal reflux
GERD	gastro-esophageal reflux disease
GH	growth hormone
GHRH	growth hormone-releasing hormone
GI	gastrointestinal
Gia	alpha gigantocellular nucleus
GiV	ventral gigantocellular nucleus
Glu	glutamate
Gly	glycine
GnRH	gonadotropin-releasing hormone
GTCS	generalized tonic–clonic seizure
HA	histamine
HACE	high-altitude cerebral edema
HAPE	high-altitude pulmonary edema
HAPH	high-altitude pulmonary hypertension
Hcrt, hcrt	hypocretin (orexin)
HCSB	Hunter–Cheyne–Stokes breathing
HD	hemodialysis
HD	Huntington disease
HF	high-frequency
HFLM	high-frequency leg movements
HFpEF	heart failure with preserved ejection fraction
HFT	hypnagogic foot tremor
HH	hypnagogic hallucination
HHV	human herpesvirus
HIV	human immunodeficiency virus
HLA	human leukocyte antigen
HMSN	hereditary motor and sensory neuropathy
HPA	hypothalamic–pituitary–adrenal
HPS	hypothalamic–pituitary–somatotropic
HR	hazard ratio
HR	heart rate
HRQoL	health-related quality of life
HRV	heart rate variability
HUTT	head-up tilt test
HV	hippocampal volume
IBS	irritable bowel syndrome
ICD	International Classification of Diseases
ICHD	International Classification of Headache Disorders
ICSD	International Classification of Sleep Disorders
ICU	intensive care unit
IED	interictal epileptiform discharge
IFN	interferon
Ig	immunoglobulin
IH	idiopathic hypersomnia
IL	interleukin
ILD	interstitial lung disease

IPAP	inspiratory positive airway pressure	NDRI	norepinephrine (noradrenaline)–dopamine reuptake inhibitor
IPN	isolated phrenic neuropathy	NFLE	nocturnal frontal lobe epilepsy
ipRGC	intrinsically photoreceptive ganglion cell	NIV	noninvasive positive pressure ventilation
IPSP	inhibitory postsynaptic potential	NLP	no conscious light perception
iRBD	idiopathic REM sleep behavior disorder	NM	nucleus basalis of Meynert
IRLSSG	International Restless Leg Syndrome Study Group	NMDA	N-methyl-D-aspartate
ISI	Insomnia Severity Index	NMO	neuromyelitis optica
ISWRD	irregular sleep–wake rhythm disorder	NMS	non-motor symptoms
IVIg	intravenous immunoglobulin	NMSQuest	Non-Motor Symptoms Questionnaire
JLD	jet lag disorder	NMSS	Non-Motor Symptoms Scale
JME	juvenile myoclonic epilepsy	NO	nitric oxide
KLS	Kleine–Levin syndrome	NOA	number of awakenings
KSS	Karolinska Sleepiness Scale	NOS	not otherwise specified
LC	locus coeruleus	NPARM	non-polyalanine repeat mutation
LDT	laterodorsal tegmental nucleus	NPs	nasal prongs
LEMS	Lambert–Eaton myasthenic syndrome	NREM	non-rapid-eye-movement
LES	lower esophageal sphincter	NRS	nonrestorative sleep
LEV	levetiracetam	NSAID	nonsteroidal anti-inflammatory drug
LF	low-frequency	NTS	nucleus tractus solitarius
LGMD	limb-girdle muscular dystrophy	NYHA	New York Heart Association
LH	lateral hypothalamus	OA	obstructive apnea
LH	luteinizing hormone	OAHI	obstructive apnea–hypopnea index
LKS	Landau–Kleffner syndrome	OCD	obsessive–compulsive disorder
LTG	lamotrigine	OCST	out-of-center sleep studies
LV	left-ventricular	OHS	obesity–hypoventilation syndrome
LVEF	left-ventricular ejection fraction	ONS	occipital nerve stimulation
LVIDd	left-ventricular internal diameter in diastole	OR	odds ratio
MA	monoamine	OSA	obstructive sleep apnea
MAD	mandibular advancement device	OSAS	obstructive sleep apnea syndrome
MAO	monoamine oxidase	OXC	oxcarbazepine
MAOI	monoamine oxidase inhibitor	PA	paroxysmal arousal
MCH	melanin-concentrating hormone	$P_{A}CO_2$	alveolar partial pressure of carbon dioxide
MCI	mild cognitive impairment	$PaCO_2$	arterial partial pressure of carbon dioxide
MDD	major depressive disorder	PaO_2	arterial partial pressure of oxygen
MDMA	3,4-methylenedioxymethamphetamine	PAP	positive airway pressure
MEMA	middle ear muscle activity	PARM	polyalanine repeat mutation
MEP	maximum expiratory pressure	PB	phenobarbital
MEP	motor evoked potential	PCO_2	partial pressure of carbon dioxide
MG	myasthenia gravis	P_{crit}	critical closing pressure
MHA	morning headache	PD	Parkinson disease
MIBG	*meta*-iodobenzylguanidine	PDSS	Parkinson's Disease Sleep Scale
MIP	maximal inspiratory pressure	PE	pulmonary embolism
MMC	migrating motor complex	PeF	perifornical area
MMSE	Mini Mental State Examination	peri-LCα	peri-locus coeruleus alpha nucleus
MnPN	median preoptic nucleus	PET	positron emission tomography
MRI	magnetic resonance imaging	PFC	prefrontal cortex
MRS	magnetic resonance spectroscopy	PFT	pulmonary function tests
MS	multiple sclerosis	PGO	pontine–geniculate–occipital
MSA	multiple system atrophy	PH	posterior hypothalamus
MSLT	multiple sleep latency test	PHT	phenytoin
MT_1, MT_2	melatonin receptors	PIA	pontine inhibitory area
mTBI	minor traumatic brain injury	PIM/AIE	psychobiological inhibition/attention–intention–effort
MVC	maximum voluntary contraction	PIP	periorbital integrated potential
MWT	maintenance of wakefulness test	PLM	periodic leg/limb movements
MZ	monozygotic	PLMD	periodic limb movement disorder
NA	noradrenaline (norepinephrine)	PLMS	periodic leg/limb movements during sleep
nAChR	neuronal nicotinic acetylcholine receptor	PLMSI	PLMS index
NAVA	neurally adjusted ventilatory assist		
NC	narcolepsy with cataplexy		

PLMW	periodic leg/limb movements during wakefulness	SCN	suprachiasmatic nucleus
PM	polymyositis	SD	sleep deprivation
PMR	progressive muscle relaxation	SDB	sleep disordered breathing
PMS	propriospinal myoclonus	SE	sleep efficiency
PnC	pontis caudalis	SEP	somatosensory cortical evoked potential
PNE	primary nocturnal enuresis	Ser	serotonin
PnO	pontis oralis	SF-36	36-Item Short Form Health Survey
PNS	peripheral nervous system	SFMM	sleep-related faciomandibular myoclonus
PO_2	partial pressure of oxygen	sIBM	sporadic inclusion-body myositis
POA	preoptic area	SIDS	sudden infant death syndrome
POAH	proptic nucleus of the anterior hypothalamus	SLD	sublaterodorsal nucleus
PPS	postpoliomyelitis syndrome	SLE	systemic lupus erythematosus
PPT	pedunculopontine	SMA	spinal muscular atrophy
PRM	primidone	SMR	sensorimotor rhythm
PROM	proximal myotonic myopathy	SN	substantia nigra
PrP	prion protein	SNA	sympathetic neural activity
PS	paradoxical sleep	SNIP	supine vital capacity nasal inspiratory pressure
PSG	polysomnography	SNP	single nucleotide polymorphism
PSM	propriospinal myoclonus	SNRI	serotonin and norepinephrine (noradrenaline) reuptake inhibitor
PSP	progressive supranuclear palsy		
PSQI	Pittsburgh Sleep Quality Index	SOL	sleep onset latency
PST	problem-solving therapy	SooS	sudden onset of sleepiness
PTSD	post-traumatic stress disorder	SOREMP	sleep onset REM period
PTT	pulse transit time	SOREMS	sleep onset REM sleep
PVDF	polyvinylidene fluoride	SPECT	single-photon emission computed tomography
PVR	peripheral vascular resistance	SRBD	sleep-related breathing disorder
PWS	Prader–Willi syndrome	SRED	sleep-related eating disorder
QoL	quality of life	SRMD	sleep-related movement disorder
R&K	Rechtschaffen & Kales	SSI	Standard Shiftwork Index
rACC	rostral anterior cingulate cortex	SSRI	selective serotonin reuptake inhibitor
RAM	reward activation model	SubC	subcoeruleus nucleus
RBD	REM sleep behavior disorder	SUDEP	sudden unexpected death in epilepsy
RBDSS	RBD Severity Scale	SUNCT	short-lasting unilateral neuralgiform headache with conjunctival injection and tearing
rCBF	regional cerebral blood flow		
RCT	randomized controlled trial	SW	sleepwalking
RDI	respiratory disturbance index	SWA	slow-wave activity
REM	rapid eye movement	SWD	shift work sleep disorder
RERA	respiratory-effort-related arousal	SWD	sleep–wake disorder
RF	reticular formation	SWS	slow-wave sleep
RFM	rhythmic foot movement	SXB	sodium oxybate
RIA	radioimmunoassay	t-MHA	tele-methylhistamine
RIP	respiratory inductive plethysmography	T&A	tonsillectomy/adenoidectomy
RISP	recurrent isolated sleep paralysis	T2DM	type 2 diabetes mellitus
RLP	reduced light perception	TAC	trigeminal autonomic cephalalgia
RLS	restless legs syndrome	TBI	traumatic brain injury
RMD	rhythmic movement disorder	Th	thalamocortical
RMg	nucleus raphe magnus	TH	tyrosine hydroxylase
RMMA	rhythmic masticatory muscle activity	THC	Δ^9-tetrahydrocannabinol
RSWA	REM sleep without atonia	TIA	transient ischemic attack
rtPCR	real-time polymerase chain reaction	TLC	total lung capacity
RV	residual volume	TMD	temporomandibular disorder
RWA	REM sleep without atonia	TMN	tuberomammillary nucleus
SAHS	sleep apnea–hypopnea syndrome	TMS	transcranial magnetic stimulation
SaO_2	arterial oxygen saturation	TNF	tumor necrosis factor
SB	sleep bruxism	TPM	topiramate
SBD	sleep-related breathing disorder	TSH	thyroid-stimulating hormone
SCA	spinocerebellar ataxia	TST	total sleep time
SCD	sickle cell disease	TST	total sleep time

TTH	tension-type headache		VNS	vagus nerve stimulation
UA	upper airway		VNTR	variable number tandem repeat
UARS	upper airway resistance syndrome		VPA	valproate
UES	upper esophageal sphincter		VPSG	video-polysomnography
UPPP	uvulopalatopharyngoplasty		VRG	ventral respiratory group
VBM	voxel-based morphometry		VTA	ventral tegmental area
VC	vital capacity		W	wake
vGlut2	vesicular glutamate transporter 2		WASM	World Association of Sleep Medicine
vlPAG	ventrolateral part of the periaqueductal gray matter		WASO	wake after sleep onset
			WED	Willis–Ekbom disease
VLPO	ventrolateral preoptic nucleus		ZI	zona incerta

Contributors

Mark S. Aloia, National Jewish Health, Department of Medicine, Denver, CO, USA

Caroline Arbour, Center for Advanced Research in Sleep Medicine and Surgery Department—Trauma, Hospital of the Sacred Heart of Montreal, Montreal University, Montreal, QC, Canada

Josephine Arendt, Professor Emeritus Endocrinology, Faculty of Health and Medical Sciences, University of Surrey, Guildford, Surrey, UK

Julie M. Baughn, Pediatric Pulmonary and Sleep Medicine, Department of Pediatrics, Sleep Disorders Center, Mayo Clinic, Rochester, MN, USA

Christian R. Baumann, Department of Sleep Medicine, Department of Neurology, University Hospital Zurich, Switzerland

Francesco Benedetti, Department of Psychiatry and Clinical Neurosciences, Scientific Institute Ospedale San Raffaele, Milan, Italy

Sushanth Bhat, JFK Neuroscience Institute/Seton Hall University, Edison, NJ, USA

Michel Billiard, Sleep Disorders Center, Department of Neurology, Gui de Chauliac Hospital, Montpellier, France

Konrad E. Bloch, Pulmonary Division and Sleep Disorders Center, University Hospital of Zurich, Zurich, Switzerland

Nic Butkov, Education Coordinator, Asante Sleep Center, Medford, OR, USA

Giovanna Calandra-Buonaura, IRCCS, Institute of Neurological Sciences of Bologna,Bellaria Hospital, Bologna, Italy; Department of Biomedical and Neuromotor Sciences (DIBINEM), University of Bologna, Bologna, Italy

Maria Turchese Caletti, Department of Biomedical and Neuromotor Sciences, University of Bologna, Bologna, Italy

K. Ray Chaudhuri, Professor of Movement Disorders, Lead, National Parkinson Foundation Centre of Excellence, King's College London, UK

Sudhansu Chokroverty, Professor and Director of Sleep Research, Co-Chair Emeritus of Neurology, JFK Neuroscience Institute, Edison, NJ, USA; Professor of Neuroscience, Seton Hall University, South Orange, NJ, USA; Clinical Professor of Neurology, Rutgers Robert Wood Johnson Medical School, New Brunswick, NJ, USA

Carlo Cipolli, Department of Experimental, Diagnostic and Specialty Medicine (DIMES), University of Bologna, Bologna, Italy

Olivier Clément, Centre for Research in Neuroscience Lyon (CRNL), Universitè Claude Bernard Lyon 1, RTH Laennec Faculty of Medicine, Lyon, France

Pietro Cortelli, IRCCS, Institute of Neurological Sciences of Bologna, Bellaria Hospital, Bologna, Italy; Department of Biomedical and Neuromotor Sciences (DIBINEM), University of Bologna, Bologna, Italy

Michel A. Cramer Bornemann, Lead Investigator, Sleep Forensics Associates, Minneapolis/Saint Paul, MN, USA; Director, Sleep Medicine Services, Olmsted Medical Center, Rochester, MN, USA; Visiting Professor, Sleep Medicine Fellowship, Minnesota Regional Sleep Disorders Center, Hennepin County Medical Center, Minneapolis, MN, USA

Sara Dallaspezia, Department of Psychiatry and Clinical Neurosciences, Scientific Institute Ospedale San Raffaele, Milan, Italy

Yves Dauvilliers, National Reference Center for Orphan Diseases (Narcolepsy, Idiopathic Hypersomnia, Kleine–Levin Syndrome), Sleep Disorders Center, Department of Neurology, Gui de Chauliac Hospital, Montpellier, France

Marco De Los Santos, Sleep Medicine Chief Fellow, Baylor College of Medicine, Houston, TX, USA

Christopher L. Drake, Sleep Disorders and Research Center, Henry Ford Health System, Detroit, MI, USA

Mark Eric Dyken, Professor of Neurology, Director, Sleep Disorders Center and Sleep Medicine and Clinical Neurophysiology Fellowship Programs, University of Iowa Carver College of Medicine, Iowa City, IA, USA

Cristina Embid, Sleep Unit, Respiratory Department Hospital Clinic, Barcelon, Spain; IDIBAPS. University of Barcelona, CIBERES, Spain

Colin A. Espie, Sleep and Circadian Neuroscience Institute, Nuffield Department of Clinical Neurosciences, University of Oxford, UK

Julien Fanielle, Cyclotron Research Centre and CHU Liège, Department of Neurology, University of Liège, Belgium

Luigi Ferini-Strambi, Professor of Neurology, Chair, Department of Neurology OSR-Turro, Director, Sleep Disorders Center, Università Vita-Salute San Raffaele, Milan, Italy

Caterina Ferri, Department of Biomedical and Neuromotor Sciences, University of Bologna, Bologna, Italy

Raffaele Ferri, President, Italian Association of Sleep Medicine, Department of Neurology IC, Oasi Institute for Research on Mental Retardation and Brain Aging (IRCCS), Troina, Italy

Michela Figorilli, Sleep Disorder Center, Department of Medical Sciences and Public Health, University of Cagliari, Monserrato (CA), Italy

Patrice Fort, Centre for Research in Neuroscience Lyon (CRNL), Universitè Claude Bernard Lyon 1, RTH Laennec Faculty of Medicine, Lyon, France

Sergio Garbarino, Centre of Sleep Medicine, Department of Neuroscience, Rehabilitation, Ophthalmology, Genetics, Maternal and Child Health, University of Genoa, Genoa, Italy

Peter Gay, Mayo Center for Sleep Medicine, Department of Medicine, Mayo Clinic and Foundation, Rochester, MN, USA

Christoforos D. Giannaki, Department of Life and Health Sciences, University of Nicosia, Cyprus

Steve Gibbs, C. Munari Center of Epilepsy Surgery, Centre of Sleep Medicine, Department of Neuroscience, Niguarda Hospital, Milan, Italy

Nadia Gosselin, Center for Advanced Research in Sleep Medicine and Surgery Department—Trauma, Hospital of the Sacred Heart of Montreal, Montreal University, Montreal, QC, Canada

Alessandro Gradassi, Department of Biomedical and Neuromotor Sciences, University of Bologna, Bologna, Italy

Christian Guilleminault, Stanford University Sleep Medicine Division, Stanford, CA, USA

Elisabeth Hertenstein, Department of Clinical Psychology and Psychophysiology, Center for Mental Disorders, Freiburg University Medical Center, Germany

Max Hirshkowitz, Professor (emeritus), Department of Medicine, Baylor College of Medicine, Houston, TX, USA; Consulting Professor, Stanford University, School of Medicine, Division of Public Mental Health and Population Sciences, Stanford, CA

Kyoung Bin Im, Assistant Professor of Neurology in the Department of Neurology Sleep Disorders Center, University of Iowa Roy J. and Lucille A. Carver College of Medicine, Iowa City, IA, USA

Shahrokh Javaheri, Sleep Physician, Sleep Center, Bethesda North Hospital, Professor Emeritus of Medicine, Pulmonary Diseases and Sleep, University of Cincinnati, Cincinnati, Ohio, USA

Barbara E. Jones, Professor, Department of Neurology and Neurosurgery, Montreal Neurological Institute, McGill University, Montreal, QC, Canada

Mithri R. Junna, Assistant Professor in Neurology, Mayo Clinic Center for Sleep Medicine, Department of Neurology, Mayo Clinic, Rochester, MN, USA

Samar Khoury, Center for Advanced Research in Sleep Medicine and Surgery Department—Trauma, Hospital of the Sacred Heart of Montreal, Montreal University, Montreal, QC, Canada

Suresh Kotagal, Division of Child and Adolescent Neurology, Sleep Disorders Center, Mayo Clinic, Rochester, MN, USA

Simon D. Kyle, Sleep and Circadian Neuroscience Institute, Nuffield Department of Clinical Neurosciences, University of Oxford, UK

Gert Jan Lammers, Neurologist and Clinical Neurophysiologist, Somnologist, Department of Neurology, Leiden University Medical Center, Leiden, The Netherlands; Sleep Wake Center SEIN, Stichting Epilepsie Instellingen Nederland, The Netherlands

Sandrine H. Launois, Somnology and Pulmonary Function Unit, University Hospital Saint-Antoine, Paris, France

Gilles J. Lavigne, Center for Advance Research in Sleep Medicine and Surgery Department—Trauma, Hospital of the Sacred Heart of Montreal, Montreal University, Montreal, QC, Canada

Patrick Lévy, Grenoble Alpes University, Grenoble, France; Grenoble Alpes University Hospital, Department of Physiology and Sleep, Grenoble, France

Jennifer A. Liebenthal, Stanford University Sleep Medicine Division, Stanford, CA, USA

Deborah C. Lin-Dyken, Clinical Associate Professor of Pediatrics, Stead Family Department of Pediatrics, University of Iowa Roy J. and Lucille A. Carver College of Medicine, Iowa City, IA, USA

Pierre-Hervé Luppi, Centre for Research in Neuroscience Lyon (CRNL), Universitè Claude Bernard Lyon 1, RTH Laennec Faculty of Medicine, Lyon, France

Susan Mackie, Department of Internal Medicine, Brigham and Women's Hospital, Harvard Medical School, Boston, MA, USA; Massachusetts General Hospital, Department of Psychiatry, Boston, MA, USA; Instructor in Medicine, Harvard Medical School, Boston, MA, USA

Raffaele Manni, Unit of Sleep Medicine and Epilepsy, C. Mondino, National Neurological Institute, Pavia, Italy

Pierre Maquet, Cyclotron Research Centre and CHU Liège, Department of Neurology, University of Liège, Belgium

Sara Marelli, Department of Neurology OSR-Turro, Sleep Disorders Center, Università Vita-Salute San Raffaele, Milan, Italy

Robert W. McCarley, Veterans Affairs Boston Healthcare System/Harvard Medical School, Department of Psychiatry, Brockton, MA, USA

James T. McKenna, Veterans Affairs Boston Healthcare System/Harvard Medical School, Department of Psychiatry, West Roxbury, MA, USA

Josep M. Montserrat, Sleep Unit, Respiratory Department, Hospital Clinic, Barcelona, Spain; IDIBAPS, University of Barcelona, Spain; CIBERES, Spain

Timothy I. Morgenthaler, Chief Patient Safety Officer, Professor of Medicine, Co-Director of the Mayo Clinic Center for Sleep Medicine, Division of Pulmonary and Critical Care Medicine, Mayo Clinic, Rochester, MN, USA

Christoph Nissen, Department of Clinical Psychology and Psychophysiology, Center for Mental Disorders, Freiburg University Medical Center, Germany

Lino Nobili, C. Munari Center of Epilepsy Surgery, Centre of Sleep Medicine, Department of Neuroscience, Niguarda Hospital, Milan, Italy

Yvonne Nussbaumer-Ochsner, Pulmonary Division and Sleep Disorders Center, University Hospital of Zurich, Zurich, Switzerland

William C. Orr, President Emeritus, Lynn Health Science Institute, Clinical Professor of Medicine, University of Oklahoma Health Sciences Center, Oklahoma City, OK, USA

Milena Pavlova, Assistant Professor of Neurology, Harvard Medical School Medical Director, BWFH Sleep and EEG Testing Center, Department of Neurology, Brigham Health, Boston, MA, USA

Dirk Pevernagie, Sleep Medicine Centre, Kempenhaeghe Foundation, Heeze, the Netherlands; Department of Internal Medicine, Faculty of Medicine and Health Sciences, University of Ghent, Ghent, Belgium

Christelle Peyron, Centre for Research in Neuroscience Lyon (CRNL), Universitè Claude Bernard Lyon 1, RTH Laennec Faculty of Medicine, Lyon, France

Vivek Pillai[†], Sleep Disorders & Research Center, Henry Ford Health System, Detroit, MI, USA

Fabio Pizza, Department of Biomedical and Neuromotor Sciences (DIBINEM), University of Bologna, Bologna, Italy; IRCCS Istituto delle Scienze Neurologiche di Bologna, ASL di Bologna, Bologna, Italy

Giuseppe Plazzi, DIBINEM, Alma Mater Studiorum University of Bologna, Bologna, Italy; IRCCS, Istituto delle Scienze Neurologiche, Bologna, Italy

Ronald B. Postuma, Associate Professor, Department of Neurology, McGill University, Montreal General Hospital, Montreal, QC, Canada

[†] It is with regret that we report the death of Vivek Pillai during the preparation of this edition of the textbook

Mark R. Pressman, Sleep Medicine Services, Clinical Professor, Lankenau Institute for Medical Research, Wynnewood, PA, USA; Clinical Professor of Medicine, Jefferson Medical College, Philadelphia, PA, USA; Adjunct Professor of Law, Villanova University, Philadelphia, PA, USA

Paola Proserpio, C. Munari Center of Epilepsy Surgery, Centre of Sleep Medicine, Department of Neuroscience, Niguarda Hospital, Milan, Italy

Federica Provini, Department of Biomedical and Neuromotor Sciences, University of Bologna, Bologna, Italy; IRCCS, Institute of Neurological Sciences, Bellaria Hospital, Bologna, Italy

Monica Puligheddu, Sleep Disorder Center, Department of Medical Sciences and Public Health, University of Cagliari, Monserrato (CA), Italy

Winfried J. Randerath, Professor of Medicine, University of Cologne, Clinic of Pneumology and Allergology, Center for Sleep Medicine and Respiratory Care, Bethanien Hospital, Solingen, Germany

Paul J. Reading, Consultant Neurologist, Department of Sleep Medicine, The James Cook University Hospital, Middlesbrough, UK

George B. Richerson, Professor and Chairman, Neurology; Professor, Molecular Physiology and Biophysics, The Roy J. Carver Chair in Neuroscience, University of Iowa Roy J. and Lucille A. Carver College of Medicine, Iowa City, IA, USA

Dieter Riemann, Department of Clinical Psychology and Psychophysiology, Center for Mental Disorders, Freiburg University Medical Center, Germany

Pradeep Sahota, Professor and Chairman, Department of Neurology, Director, Sleep Disorders Center, University of Missouri—School of Medicine, University of Missouri Health Care, Columbia, MO, USA

Katerina Sajgalikova, Sleeping Laboratory, International Clinical Research Center of St Anne's University Hospital Brno (FNUSA-ICRC), Czech Republic

Giorgos K. Sakkas, Faculty of Sports and Health Sciences, University of St Mark and St John, Plymouth, UK

Bernardo J. Selim, Assistant Professor in Medicine, Mayo Clinic Center for Sleep Medicine, Division of Pulmonary and Critical Care Medicine, Mayo Clinic, Rochester, MN, USA

Rosalia Silvestri, Associate Professor of Neurology, Sleep Medicine Center, Department of Clinical and Experimental Medicine, Messina University, Italy

Niranjan N. Singh, Associate Professor of Clinical Neurology, University of Missouri—School of Medicine, Columbia, MO, USA

Elisaveta Sokolov, Specialist doctor of neurophysiology, Kings College Hospital, London

Mark Solms, Department of Psychology, University of Cape Town, Rondebosch, South Africa

Alexandra Sousek, Department of Physiology, Faculty of Biology and Medicine, University of Lausanne, Lausanne, Switzerland

Erik K. St. Louis, Mayo Center for Sleep Medicine, Departments of Medicine and Neurology, Mayo Clinic and Foundation, Rochester, MN, USA

Axel Steiger, Max Planck Institute of Psychiatry, Munich, Germany

Mehdi Tafti, Department of Physiology, Faculty of Biology and Medicine, University of Lausanne, Lausanne, Switzerland

Michele Terzaghi, Unit of Sleep Medicine and Epilepsy, C. Mondino, National Neurological Institute, Pavia, Italy

Michael Thorpy, Director, Sleep–Wake Disorders Center, Montefiore Medical Center, and Professor of Neurology, Albert Einstein College of Medicine, Bronx, NY, USA

Guy Warman, Associate Professor, Department of Anaesthesiology, School of Medicine, Faculty of Medical and Health Sciences, University of Auckland, Auckland, New Zealand

Gerald L. Weinhouse, The Division of Pulmonary and Critical Care Medicine, Brigham and Women's Hospital, Boston, MA, USA

John W. Winkelman, Massachusetts General Hospital, Department of Psychiatry, Boston, MA, USA; Associate Professor of Psychiatry, Harvard Medical School, Boston, MA, USA

Molly E. Zimmerman, Fordham University, Department of Psychology, Bronx, NY, USA

SECTION 1

Basic science

CHAPTER 1

Introduction to basic science

James T. McKenna and Robert W. McCarley

Sleep disorders are increasingly recognized as a major public health issue [1,2]. Sleep disorders of primary etiology include narcolepsy, insomnia, sleep apnea, and restless leg syndrome. Recent clinical attention has focused on sleep disturbance concomitant to psychiatric and neurological disease [3,4]. Furthermore, sleep loss due to vocational demands may attenuate attentional and cognitive processing, as well as producing dysfunctional physiological sequelae. Correspondingly, understanding of neural vigilance state regulation—wake, rapid eye movement (REM) sleep, and non-REM (NREM) sleep—has increased tremendously in the last half-century owing to advances in basic research employing lesioning, pharmacological, electrophysiological, molecular, optogenetic, chemogenetic, and calcium imaging techniques. The practitioner should have a sound understanding of the neurobiology involved in sleep–wake regulation in order to effectively treat sleep-related disorders. For example, understanding of the mechanism of action of the recently introduced hypnotic suvorexant depends on a knowledge of the orexin system and its projections and receptors. This section of this volume, on basic science, therefore provides an overview of the neurocircuitry and physiology involved and cites key references. For a comprehensive review, see Brown et al. [5].

As first described in the 1930s, vigilance states are defined by the neuronal field activity recorded in the cortex by means of electroencephalography (EEG). [6–8]. In animal research, invasive cortical and subcortical electrophysiological recordings may also be utilized, such as single-unit and local field potential electrode recordings. During wake, the cortical EEG exhibits low-amplitude activity with a prevalence of high frequency (theta, alpha, and gamma/beta). This electrical activity, indicative of arousal, is produced by the various components of the ascending reticular activating system (ARAS), as neural activity initiated in the brainstem traverses the thalamus (dorsal node) and basal forebrain (ventral node) to eventually promote cortical activation [9]. These subcortical ARAS nodes are largely responsible for the phasic oscillatory activity evident during wake; for example, basal forebrain GABAergic parvalbumin neurons play a major role in promoting cortical gamma-band oscillatory activity important in cognition and memory [10]. Numerous brain regions are involved in the ARAS, utilizing a number of neurotransmitters, including acetylcholine, serotonin, norepinephrine (noradrenaline), histamine, γ-aminobutyric acid (GABA), and glutamate (see Fig. 1.1) [5,11,12]. In addition, neurons containing the neuropeptide orexin (also known as hypocretin) and residing in the lateral hypothalamus are anatomically connected to both wake- and sleep-active neurons, and play a central role in the maintenance of wakefulness (reviewed below).

NREM sleep electrographic characteristics are strikingly different than those of wake, since the cortical EEG slows in frequency (to predominantly delta) as the overall amplitude increases. Although early studies assumed that sleep states were simply due to cessation of activity in arousal systems, more recent findings now indicate that there are specific sleep-active brain regions. For example, the reticular nucleus of the thalamus is active during NREM sleep, exhibiting phasic spindle activity (8–14 Hz) [13]. Also, select GABAergic hypothalamic preoptic nuclei inhibit components of the ARAS, allowing transitions into NREM sleep [14,15] In the "flip-flop switch" model of sleep–wake systems (see Fig. 1.2) [14], histaminergic tuberomammillary nucleus (TMN), serotonergic dorsal raphe (DR), and noradrenergic locus coeruleus (LC) neurons are wake-active, and inhibit sleep-active ventrolateral preoptic (VLPO) GABAergic/galaninergic neurons during wake. During sleep, VLPO neurons are active, inhibiting TMN, DR, and LC neurons. Furthermore, lateral hypothalamic orexinergic neurons stabilize the wake state by excitatory projections to the TMN, DR and LC, and during sleep they are inhibited by VLPO neurons.

REM sleep is also termed paradoxical sleep, since the cortical EEG exhibits low-amplitude, high-frequency activity similar to that of wake. Unlike wake, though, little muscle tone or movement occurs during this state. Other defining REM sleep characteristics beyond the EEG profile include brainstem neuronal spiking activity, muscle atonia, pontine–geniculate–occipital (PGO) waves, hippocampal theta-wave oscillations, and REMs. McCarley and colleagues initially proposed the "reciprocal interaction" model of the brain circuitry and neurotransmitters involved in the transition to and maintenance of the REM sleep state [16]. This model includes reactivation of cholinergic neurons that are largely silent during NREM sleep, although serotonergic and noradrenergic populations remain inactive. More recent investigations have defined specific REM sleep-active brain regions, including GABAergic neurons of the extended region of the ventrolateral preoptic nuclei [17], GABAergic and glutamatergic neurons of the subcoeruleus (also termed the sublaterodorsal nucleus) and nucleus pontine oralis [18–20], as well as neurons containing melanin-concentrating hormone (MCH) that reside in the lateral hypothalamus [21]. Narcolepsy is a unique sleep disorder in which orexinergic neuronal dysfunction leads to symptoms including cataplexy, excessive daytime sleepiness, sleep paralysis, and sleep-onset REM periods [22]. Investigations have concluded that disruption of orexinergic systems produces abnormal transitions between vigilance states, particularly from wake to REM sleep.

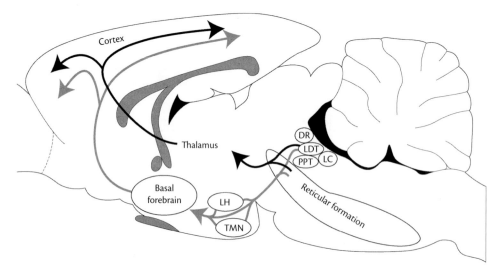

Fig. 1.1 The ascending reticular activating system (ARAS) is responsible for the cortical activation indicative of wake. In the dorsal pathway (black), brainstem glutamatergic reticular formation neurons, as well as serotonergic dorsal raphe (DR), noradrenergic locus coeruleus (LC), and cholinergic laterodorsal tegmental (LDT) and pedunculopontine tegmental (PPT) neurons, project to the thalamus, which in turn innervates the cortex. In the ventral pathway (gray), these same brainstem regions innervate the basal forebrain directly, or indirectly by means of projections to the GABAergic/histaminergic tuberomammillary nucleus (TMN) or orexinergic lateral hypothalamus (LH). The basal forebrain in turn innervates widespread cortical regions. For a comprehensive review, see Brown et al. [5].

Reproduced from Physiol Rev, 92(3), Brown RE, Basheer R, McKenna JT, Strecker RE, McCarley RW, Control of sleep and wakefulness, pp. 1087–187, Copyright (2012), with permission from The American Physiological Society.

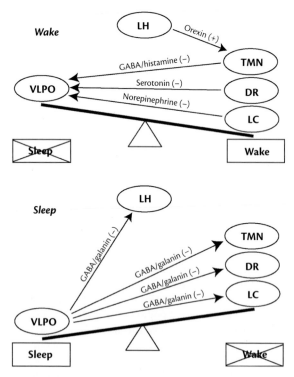

Fig. 1.2 In the "flip-flop switch" model of sleep–wake transitions [14], GABAergic/histaminergic tuberomammillary (TMN), serotonergic dorsal raphe (DR), and noradrenergic locus coeruleus (LC) neurons are wake-active, and inhibit sleep-active ventrolateral preoptic (VLPO) neurons. VLPO neurons are active during sleep, and inhibit TMN, DR, and LC neurons by means of GABAergic/galaninergic inhibitory projections. Orexinergic lateral hypothalamic neurons (LH) provide stabilization of wake by means of projections to the TMN, DR, and LC, and are inhibited by VLPO neurons during sleep.

Reproduced from Trends Neurosci., 24(12), Saper CB, Chou TC, Scammell TE, The sleep switch: hypothalamic control of sleep and wakefulness, pp. 726–31, Copyright (2001), with permission from Elsevier.

As described by Borbély, sleep is modeled by the homeostatic (process S) and circadian (process C) drives to sleep [23]. Process S can be understood as the drive to sleep that is produced by the amount of time spent awake; that is, the more an organism stays awake, the more it needs to sleep. Process C, the circadian drive, consists of rhythms of behavior and physiology of an approximately 24-hour periodicity. Circadian rhythms are controlled by environmental cues (zeitgebers), as well as endogenous neural oscillators including the suprachiasmatic nucleus (SCN) of the hypothalamus. Melanopsin is a photosensitive molecule found in retinal ganglion cells that project to the SCN, allowing direct input from zeitgebers (eg, light) to endogenous oscillatory systems [24]. The SCN exhibits rhythmicity, driven by autoregulatory loops involving period gene products (PER1 and PER2), cryptochrome gene products (CRY1 and CRY2), and transcription factors (CLOCK and BMAL1) [25,26]. Furthermore, the circadian oscillation of BMAL1 is regulated by the orphan nuclear receptors Rev-Erbα and the retinoid-related orphan receptor α (Rora). Mutations in clock-related genes may contribute to circadian rhythm sleep disorders (eg, advanced- and delayed-phase disorders) [27–28].

Basic research studies have begun to describe the possible functions of sleep, including consolidation of learning and memory. Consequences of sleep loss include attenuated attention, as well as dysfunctions in mood, memory formation, and executive function [29]. Some investigators have suggested that a function of sleep is to allow a reversal of learning-related synaptic potentiation that occurs during wake [30]. Others, though, argue that memory consolidation occurs during both NREM and REM sleep by means of synaptic potentiation that accompanies fast oscillatory wave activity. For example, hippocampal theta activity during REM sleep may promote synaptic potentiation integral for memory formation [31]. Also, hippocampal slow-wave/spindle/ripple coupling during NREM sleep may allow consolidation of memory and promote subsequent transfer of short-term memories to longer-term storage in cortical regions [32]. Sleep may also provide a mechanism by which cellular metabolism is re-established following the neural demands during wake [5], since wake-active brain regions are inhibited by sleep factors, including adenosine and nitric oxide [33,34], as well as by GABAergic inhibition [35] There is also new evidence that sleep may aid in the clearance of neurotoxins that accumulate during wake [36].

Recent technological advances have allowed description of the molecular mechanisms involved in sleep–wake regulation, as well as the consequences of sleep disruption for genetic signaling [37,38]. Early twin studies suggested that genetic expression influences vigilance state regulation, since many aspects of sleep were correlated in monozygotic twins [39]. More recent genetic studies have employed techniques such as hybridization, real-time polymerase chain reaction (rtPCR) analysis, and transgenic animal models in which gene function is knocked in or out. Gene expression is associated with electrographic hallmarks of sleep–wake states, as well as up- and down-regulation of various neurotransmitters and receptors involved in vigilance state regulation. Genetic studies have further indicated that adenosine, nitric oxide, and cytokines are all sleep factors that influence vigilance state-regulatory neurocircuitry. Various genetic signaling pathways involved in learning and memory have also been implicated in vigilance state regulation, further suggesting a possible function of sleep [5]. Recently, proteomic techniques have allowed investigation of vigilance state-related translation of mRNA into protein and subsequent post-translational processing [40].

An exemplary use of genetic techniques in basic sleep research is the description of orexinergic neuronal dysfunction in narcolepsy. A deficit in the orexin type II receptor was described in dogs that exhibited narcolepsy [41] and mice with a knockout of the prepro-orexin gene also exhibited narcolepsy-like characteristics [42]. Lesioning and knockdown studies also concluded that orexinergic neurons play a key role in stabilizing vigilance states, and dysfunction of this system leads to narcolepsy [22]. Knowledge of the orexin system led to development of a single neurotransmitter-based hypnotic, the dual orexin receptor antagonist (DORA) suvorexant, which antagonizes orexinergic neurotransmission at both type I and type II orexin receptors [43]. It is of note that while it might be thought that such an effect would not only inhibit wakefulness but also produce the side effects of narcoleptic-like symptoms, such major side effects have not been observed in clinical studies. This suggests a complexity of orexin effects and interactions with other brain systems that remain to be investigated.

The concordance of sleep disorders with psychiatric and neurological disease has been increasingly recognized in recent years [44,45]. For example, post-traumatic stress disorder (PTSD), drug withdrawal, and depression are all accompanied by drastic sleep disturbance, including insomnia. Alzheimer patients may suffer from disturbed vigilance state regulation due to circadian abnormalities (eg, sundowning syndrome). Notably, the dysfunctional neurocircuitry involved in such pathologies is inter-related to the sleep–wake regulatory circuitry reviewed here. Therefore, further understanding of vigilance state regulation will allow the clinician to make well-informed decisions in the treatment of primary sleep disorders as well as related psychiatric and neurological disease.

References

1. Mitler ME, Dement WC, Dinges DF. Sleep medicine, public policy, and public health. In: Kryger MH, Roth T, Dement WC, eds. Principles and practice in sleep medicine. Philadelphia, PA: WB Saunders, 2000:580–8.
2. Colten HR, Altevogt BM, eds. Committee on Sleep Medicine and Research, Institute of the National Academies. Sleep disorders and sleep deprivation: an unmet public health problem. Washington, DC: National Academies Press, 2006.
3. Chokroverty S. Sleep and neurodegenerative diseases. Semin Neurol 2009;29:446–67.
4. Saper CB, Scammell TE. Emerging therapeutics in sleep. Ann Neurol 2013;74:435–40.
5. Brown RE, Basheer R, McKenna JT, et al. Control of sleep and wakefulness. Physiol Rev 2012;92:1087–187.
6. Berger H. [Ueber das elektroenkelogramm des Menchen]. J Psychol Neurol 1930;40:160–79.
7. Loomis AL, Harvey EN, Hobart G. Potential rhythms of the cerebral cortex during sleep. Science 1935;81:597–8.
8. Davis H, Davis PA, Loomis AL, et al. Changes in human brain potentials during the onset of sleep. Science 1937;86:448–50.
9. Moruzzi G, Magoun HW. Brain stem reticular formation and activation of the EEG. Electroencephalogr Clin Neurophysiol 1949;1:455–73.
10. Kim T, Thankachan S, McKenna JT, et al. Cortically projecting basal forebrain parvalbumin neurons regulate cortical gamma band oscillations. Proc Natl Acad Sci U S A 2015;112:3535–40.
11. Jones BE. Modulation of cortical activation and behavioral arousal by cholinergic and orexinergic systems. Ann N Y Acad Sci 2008;1129:26–34.
12. Jones BE. Neurobiology of waking and sleeping. Handb Clin Neurol 2011;98:131–49.
13. Fuentealba P, Steriade M. The reticular nucleus revisited: intrinsic and network properties of a thalamic pacemaker. Prog Neurobiol 2005;75:125–41.
14. Saper CB, Chou TC, Scammell TE. The sleep switch: hypothalamic control of sleep and wakefulness. Trends Neurosci 2001;24:726–31.
15. Szymusiak R, McGinty D. Hypothalamic regulation of sleep and arousal. Ann N Y Acad Sci 2008;1129:275–86.
16. McCarley RW, Massaquoi SG. A limit cycle mathematical model of the REM sleep oscillator system. Am J Physiol 1986;251:R1011–29.
17. Lu J, Bjorkum AA, Xu M, Gaus SE, et al. Selective activation of the extended ventrolateral preoptic nucleus during rapid eye movement sleep. J Neurosci 2002;22:4568–76.
18. Lu J, Sherman D, Devor M, Saper CB. A putative flip-flop switch for control of REM sleep. Nature 2006;441:589–94.
19. Luppi PH, Gervasoni D, Verret L, et al. Paradoxical (REM) sleep genesis: the switch from an aminergic–cholinergic to a GABAergic–glutamatergic hypothesis. J Physiol Paris 2006;100:271–83.
20. Brown RE, McKenna JT, Winston S, et al. Characterization of GABAergic neurons in rapid-eye-movement sleep controlling regions of the brainstem reticular formation in GAD67–green fluorescent protein knock-in mice. Eur J Neurosci 2008;27:352–63.
21. Verret L, Goutagny R, Fort P, et al. A role of melanin-concentrating hormone producing neurons in the central regulation of paradoxical sleep. BMC Neurosci 2003;4:19.
22. Liblau RS, Vassalli A, Seifinejad A, Tafti M. Hypocretin (orexin) biology and the pathophysiology of narcolepsy with cataplexy. Lancet Neurol 2015;14:318–28.
23. Borbély AA. A two process model of sleep regulation. Hum Neurobiol 1982;1:195–204.
24. Hattar S, Liao HW, Takao M, et al. Melanopsin-containing retinal ganglion cells: architecture, projections, and intrinsic photosensitivity. Science 2002;295:1065–70.
25. Franken P, Dijk DJ. Circadian clock genes and sleep homeostasis. Eur J Neurosci. 2009;29:1820–9.

26. Franken P. A role for clock genes in sleep homeostasis. Curr Opin Neurobiol 2013;23:864–72.

27. Sack RL, Auckley D, Auger RR, et al. Circadian rhythm sleep disorders: Part I, basic principles, shift work and jet lag disorders. An American Academy of Sleep Medicine review. Sleep 2007;30:1460–83.

28. Sack RL, Auckley D, Auger RR, et al. Circadian rhythm sleep disorders: Part II, advanced sleep phase disorder, delayed sleep phase disorder, free-running disorder, and irregular sleep–wake rhythm. An American Academy of Sleep Medicine review. Sleep 2007;30:1484–501.

29. Jackson ML, Gunzelmann G, Whitney P, et al. Deconstructing and reconstructing cognitive performance in sleep deprivation. Sleep Med Rev 2013;17:215–25.

30. Tononi G, Cirelli C. Sleep and the price of plasticity: from synaptic and cellular homeostasis to memory consolidation and integration. Neuron 2014;81:12–34.

31. Vorster AP, Born J. Sleep and memory in mammals, birds and invertebrates. Neurosci Biobehav Rev 2015;50:103–19.

32. Staresina BP, Bergmann TO, Bonnefond M, et al. Hierarchical nesting of slow oscillations, spindles and ripples in the human hippocampus during sleep. Nat Neurosci 2015;18:1679–86.

33. Porkka-Heiskanen T, Strecker RE, Thakkar M, et al. Adenosine: a mediator of the sleep-inducing effects of prolonged wakefulness. Science 1997;276:1265–8.

34. Kalinchuk AV, McCarley RW, Porkka-Heiskanen T, Basheer R. Sleep deprivation triggers inducible nitric oxide-dependent nitric oxide production in wake-active basal forebrain neurons. J Neurosci 2010;30:13254–64.

35. Fort P, Bassetti CL, Luppi PH. Alternating vigilance states: new insights regarding neuronal networks and mechanisms. Eur J Neurosci 2009;29:1741–53.

36. Xie L, Kang H, Xu Q, et al. Sleep drives metabolite clearance from the adult brain. Science 2013;342:373–7.

37. Tafti M, Franken P. Molecular analysis of sleep. Cold Spring Harb Symp Quant Biol 2007;72:573–8.

38. Tafti M. Genetic aspects of normal and disturbed sleep. Sleep Med 2009;10(Suppl 1):S17–21.

39. Dauvilliers Y, Maret S, Tafti M. Genetics of normal and pathological sleep in humans. Sleep Med Rev 2005;9:91–100.

40. Naidoo N. Potential of proteomics as a bioanalytic technique for quantifying sleepiness. J Clin Sleep Med 2011;7(5 Suppl):S28–30.

41. Lin L, Faraco J, Li R, et al. The sleep disorder canine narcolepsy is caused by a mutation in the hypocretin (orexin) receptor 2 gene. Cell 1999;98:365–76.

42. Chemelli RM, Willie JT, Sinton CM, et al. Narcolepsy in orexin knockout mice: molecular genetics of sleep regulation. Cell 1999;98:437–51.

43. Winrow CJ, Renger JJ. Discovery and development of orexin receptor antagonists as therapeutics for insomnia. Br J Pharmacol 2014;171:283–93.

44. España RA, Scammell TE. Sleep neurobiology from a clinical perspective. Sleep 2011;34:845–58.

45. Bassetti CL, Ferini-Strambi L, Brown S, et al. Neurology and psychiatry: waking up to opportunities of sleep: state of the art and clinical/research priorities for the next decade. Eur J Neurol 2015;22:1337–54.

CHAPTER 2

An overview of sleep medicine
History, definition, sleep patterns, and architecture

Sudhansu Chokroverty and Sushanth Bhat

A brief history of sleep medicine

The importance of sleep is well recognized today, among both the academic and clinical communities. Advancements and refinement of functional neuroimaging have led to the ability to map various areas of the brain in different stages of sleep, and neurophysiological techniques have allowed researchers to study changes at the cellular level. However, the history of research into the mechanisms of sleep is one of fits and starts. The dawn of modern sleep medicine can be traced back to the identification of the different electroencephalography (EEG) stages of sleep by Loomis and colleagues in 1937 [1]. Rapid eye movement (REM) sleep was described in 1953 by Aserinsky and Kleitman [2], and the first identification of loss of muscle tone in REM sleep, or REM atonia, soon followed [3]. The standardization of what would become the science of polysomnography (PSG) began when Rechtschaffen and Kales (4) produced the standard sleep scoring technique monograph in 1968 (the R-K scoring technique), which for several decades remained the gold standard. Today, the scoring rules published in the American Academy of Sleep Medicine (AASM) Manual for the Scoring of Sleep and Associated Events [5] are universally accepted in clinical sleep medicine and in sleep research (see Chapter 11). The clinical community began to take notice of sleep medicine when obstructive sleep apnea (OSA) was found to be a common cause of cardiovascular morbidity and mortality, as well as a significant cause of impairment of quality of life [6,7]. The identification of continuous positive airway pressure (CPAP) devices as safe, effective, noninvasive means to dramatically relieve OSA-related symptoms [8] jump-started modern sleep medicine practice and led to the proliferation of sleep laboratories throughout the world. Since then, several new intervention techniques, including dental appliances, tongue-retaining devices, surgical procedures, nasal end-expiratory devices, and hypoglossal nerve stimulators have become available as alternatives to CPAP treatment in selected populations, making the field of sleep medicine truly multidisciplinary. Another seminal moment in the history of sleep medicine occurred when two independent groups of researchers contemporaneously identified a pair of neuropeptides, hypocretin 1 and 2 (orexin A and B) in the lateral hypothalamus and perifornical regions [9,10]. In the years that followed, the mechanisms underlying narcolepsy were better defined by pivotal research that showed that a canine model of the human narcolepsy

phenotype could be created by mutation of hypocretin 2 receptors (HCTR$_2$) [11] and that a similar phenotype could be created in prepro-hypocretin knockout and transgenic mice [12,13]. The documentation of decreased hypocretin 1 in cerebrospinal fluid in humans [14] and of decreased hypocretin neurons in the lateral hypothalamus at autopsy [15–17] in human narcolepsy patients added clinical significance to previous research.

Definition of sleep

Research has led to the realization that sleep is not simply an absence of wakefulness and perception, nor is it just a suspension of sensorial processes, but is a result of a combination of a passive withdrawal of afferent stimuli to the brain and functional activation of certain neurons in selective brain areas.

Distinguishing normal physiological sleep from pathological states of decreased or absent consciousness, such as coma, minimally conscious state, and persistent vegetative state (unresponsive wakefulness syndrome), is instructive in determining the underlying mechanisms of sleep. Pathological states of decreased consciousness all differ significantly from sleep in a number of ways. Consciousness requires two components: awareness (a function of the cerebral cortex) and arousal (a function of the ascending reticular activating system). Sleep is always reversible, whereas, depending on the underlying cause, this is not the case with pathological states of decreased consciousness. Brain metabolism and circulation, which show marked depression and impairment in pathological states of decreased consciousness, show only slight alterations in sleep. Indeed, in some stages of sleep, particularly REM sleep, the brain is as metabolically active as it is in wakefulness, which is not so in pathological states of decreased consciousness. The EEG in sleep shows an orderly progression from wakefulness to light sleep, deep sleep, and REM sleep, cycling throughout the night, whereas patients in pathological states of decreased consciousness almost always have slow disorganized abnormal backgrounds with lack of well-organized sleep architecture or progression of stages. Ultimately, the distinction between sleep and pathological states of decreased consciousness is made on both neurophysiological (i.e, EEG, electrooculography (EOG), and electromyography (EMG}) and clinical (i.e, behavioral) grounds. Table 2.1 and Table 2.2 list the behavioral and physiological criteria for wakefulness and various stages of sleep.

Table 2.1 Behavioral criteria for wakefulness and sleep

Criterion	Awake	NREM sleep	REM sleep
Posture	Erect, sitting, or recumbent	Recumbent	Recumbent
Mobility	Normal	Slightly reduced or immobile; postural shifts	Moderately reduced or immobile; myoclonic jerks
Response to stimulation	Normal	Mildly to moderately reduced	Moderately reduced to no response
Level of alertness	Alert	Unconscious but reversible	Unconscious but reversible
Eyelids	Open	Closed	Closed
Eye movements	Waking eye movements	Slow rolling eye movements	Rapid eye movements

Theories of the function of sleep

Sleep is an essential biological function, but its exact function remains unclear. Despite great strides in research into sleep, the answers to fundamental questions such as what sleep is and why it occurs remain tantalizingly elusive. Sleep deprivation is clearly detrimental; it has been experimentally demonstrated that sleep deprivation causes daytime sleepiness and impairment of performance, vigilance, attention, mood, concentration, and memory [18], as well as metabolic, hormonal, and immunological effects, as discussed in later sections of this chapter.

Sleep appears to engender an anabolic state; there is increased secretion of anabolic hormones (eg, growth hormone, prolactin, testosterone, and luteinizing hormone) and decreased levels of catabolic hormones (eg, cortisol) during sleep. Cerebral protein and nucleic acid synthesis is enhanced by sleep [19]. During non-REM (NREM) sleep, brain metabolism and cerebral blood flow decrease, whereas during REM sleep, the level of metabolism is similar to that of wakefulness and the cerebral blood flow increases. Nevertheless, sleep may represent an energy-saving process; overall reductions in general metabolism, including metabolic heat production, lowering of core body temperature, and certain behavioral signs (eg, immobile posture minimizing heat exchange), conserve energy.

Some researchers have suggested that a primary function of sleep is the maintenance of synaptic and neuronal network integrity and synaptic reorganization [20–22]. While it is generally held that sleep

Table 2.2 Physiological criteria for wakefulness and sleep

Criterion	Awake	NREM sleep	REM sleep
Electroencephalography	Alpha waves; desynchronized	Synchronized	Theta or sawtooth waves; desynchronized
Electromyography (muscle tone)	Normal	Mildly reduced	Moderately to severely reduced or absent
Electrooculography	Waking eye movements	Slow rolling eye movements	Rapid eye movements

is essential for optimal cognitive functioning, research data have provided discordant findings. Memory reinforcement with consolidation has been demonstrated to take place during REM sleep [23], and hippocampus-dependent memories (declarative memories) benefit primarily from slow-wave sleep [24]. Sleep spindle activity has been demonstrated to correlate with cognitive abilities and learning [25]. Yet, some studies have shown that individuals with brainstem lesions with elimination of REM sleep or those on antidepressant medications suppressing REM sleep exhibit no apparent cognitive deficits [26,27].

Thermoregulation also appears to be an important function of sleep; thermoregulatory homeostasis is maintained during sleep, whereas severe thermoregulatory abnormalities follow total sleep deprivation [28]. The preoptic anterior hypothalamic neurons participate in thermoregulation and NREM sleep. These two processes are closely linked by preoptic anterior hypothalamic neurons, but are clearly separate. Thermoregulation is maintained during NREM sleep but suspended during REM sleep, when, owing to a loss of thermosensitivity in the preoptic anterior hypothalamic neurons, thermoregulatory responses such as shivering, piloerection, panting, and sweating are impaired.

The glymphatic system

A recent discovery in the CNS of mice of a new metabolic waste-clearing pathway (equivalent to the lymphatic system in the body), termed the "glymphatic system" because of its dependence on glial cells (astrocytes) performing a "lymphatic"-like cleansing of the brain interstitial fluid in the perivascular space between the brain blood vessels and leptomeningeal sheaths surrounding these vessels. In sleep, the glial cells shrink and the extracellular pace expands, promoting clearance of interstitial waste products (Fig. 2.1). Furthermore, it appears that the ability of this system to remove misfolded or aggregated proteins (demonstrated experimentally by injection of labeled β-amyloid proteins into the brains

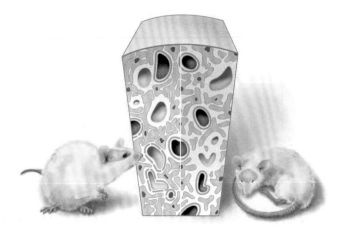

Fig. 2.1 An illustration of the glymphatic system, depicting the physiological differences in cerebrospinal fluid (CSF) flow between the awake and the sleeping brain of mice. The tissue perfused by CSF is correlated with CSF influx. and blood vessels are indicated in shaded (arteries) and white (veins). The extracellular (interstitial) space in the cortex of the mouse brain, through which CSF moves, increases from 14% in the awake animal to 23% in the sleeping animal, an increase that allows the faster clearance of metabolic waste products.

Table 2.3 Summary of NREM and REM sleep states

Sleep state	% sleep time
NREM sleep	75–80
N1	3–8
N2	45–55
N3	15–23
REM sleep	20–25
Tonic stage	—
Phasic stage	—

of sleeping and awake mice) is hampered. Although these findings have yet to be replicated in humans, they may play a role in drug development to prevent or halt the progression of these neurodegenerative diseases such as Alzheimer disease, Parkinson disease, and others [29–33].

Normal sleep architecture

Sleep is divided into NREM and REM sleep (Table 2.3). During a night of normal sleep, NREM and REM sleep alternate in a cyclic manner, with 4–6 cycles occurring per night, each cycle lasting on an average from 90–110 minutes. The first two cycles are dominated by slow-wave sleep (SWS) (stage N3 sleep, see below); subsequent cycles contain less or no SWS. In contrast, REM increases as the night progresses, with each REM sleep episode becoming longer than the one preceding it; the longest REM sleep episode toward the end of the night may last for an hour. Thus, in normal human adult sleep, the first third is dominated by SWS and the last third by

REM sleep. It is important to be aware of these facts because certain abnormal motor activities (NREM parasomnias like sleepwalking, night terrors, and confusional arousals) are characteristically associated with SWS and therefore occur in the first third of the night, and others (REM parasomnias like REM behavior disorder) occur in the last third of the night, i.e, early morning.

A hypnogram (Fig. 2.2) is a graphical representation of the events that occur during a sleep session as recorded during PSG. In addition to sleep stages, it typically depicts respiratory events, motor events, arousals, and position, and allows for a quick screening for abnormalities.

Sleep stages

The scoring criteria for wakefulness and various stages of sleep depend on EEG, EMG, and EOG recordings, and are described in detail in Chapter 10. The following subsections provide only a brief overview of normal sleep architecture.

NREM sleep

NREM sleep accounts for 75–80% of sleep time in an adult human. According to the AASM Scoring Manual [5], NREM sleep is further subdivided into three stages (N1, N2, and N3), primarily on the basis of EEG criteria. Stages N1 and N2 are generally referred to as "light sleep," and stage N3 as "deep sleep" or slow-wave sleep (SWS). Stage N1 sleep occupies 3–8% of total sleep time, N2 45–55%, and N3 15–23%. As a subject passes from wakefulness to stage N1, which is essentially a transitory phase into deeper stages of sleep, the posterior dominant rhythm (usually in the alpha range of 8–13 Hz) slows, becomes less well defined, and ultimately disappears to be replaced by poorly organized low-voltage mixed frequencies, predominantly theta rhythms (4–7 Hz) and beta waves. EMG activity decreases slightly, slow lateral eye movements (SLEMs) appear, and vertex sharp waves are noted. Stage

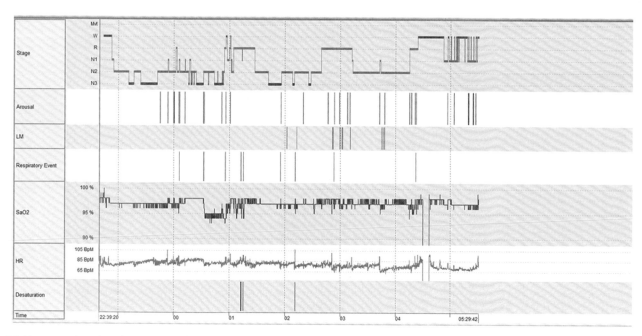

Fig. 2.2 Hypnogram from the polysomnogram of a 35-year-old male patient referred to the sleep laboratory for possible sleep apnea. The hypnogram is a graphical representation of the night's events. From top to bottom, this hypnogram represents sleep stages, arousals, leg movements, respiratory events, pulse oximetry, heart rate, and oxygen desaturations over time. Hypnograms provide quick, informative snapshots of the entire sleep study that aid in clinical decision making.

N2 begins approximately 10–12 minutes after stage N1. Sleep spindles and K-complexes herald the onset of stage N2 sleep. Towards the end of each cycle of stage N2 sleep, the EEG may show theta waves and slow waves (0.5–2 Hz) that occupy less than 20% of the epoch. Stage N3 sleep begins about 30–60 minutes after the onset of stage N2. Slow waves comprise 20–100% of each epoch of stage N3. Both eye and body movements normally decrease and nearly disappear as a subject progresses from light sleep to deep sleep. However, with the use of certain antidepressant medications (tricyclic antidepressants, selective serotonin reuptake inhibitors, and monoamine oxidase inhibitors), mixtures of slow lateral eye movements and rapid eye movements may occur late into stage N2 and sometimes N3 sleep; these are colloquially known as "Prozac eyes" (Fig. 2.3).

REM sleep

REM sleep accounts for 20–25% of total sleep time. The EEG in REM sleep is desynchronized and consists of low-voltage, mixed-frequency activity similar to that seen in stage N1 sleep. The EMG channels show hypotonia or atonia of antigravity muscles, with the exception of the diaphragm and the oculomotor muscles. While this "tonic" stage persists throughout REM sleep, there is a superimposed intermittent "phasic" stage characterized by bursts of REMs in all directions, in singlets or clusters (noted on EOG channels). Phasic swings in blood pressure and heart rate, irregular respiration, spontaneous middle ear muscle activity (MEMA), periorbital integrated potentials (PIPs) [34], myoclonic twitching of the facial and limb muscles, and tongue movements [35] are all characteristics of phasic REM sleep. Breathing tends to become irregular, especially in phasic REM

sleep, and scattered apneas and hypopneas are not uncommon. Sawtooth waves are EEG trains of sharply contoured, often serrated, 2–6 Hz waves, usually with rapid ascent and slow descent, seen maximally over the central regions, and are thought to be the gateway to REM sleep, often preceding a burst of REMs. PIPs are seen during REMs (Fig. 2.4), but not all REMs are accompanied by PIPs.

Sleep macrostructure (eg, sleep states and stages, sleep cycles, sleep latency and efficiency, and wakefulness after sleep onset) may be modified by a number of endogenous and exogenous factors (Box 2.1).

Cyclical alternating pattern

The cyclical alternating pattern (CAP) (Fig. 2.5) is an EEG pattern seen in NREM sleep that indicates sleep instability [36]. A CAP cycle [37] consists of an unstable phase (phase A) and a relatively stable phase (phase B), each lasting between 2 and 60 s. Phase A of CAP is marked by an increase in EEG potentials, with contributions from both synchronous high-amplitude slow activity and desynchronized fast rhythms in the EEG recording, standing out from a relatively low-amplitude slow background. The A phase is associated with increases in heart rate, respiration, blood pressure, and muscle tone. CAP rate (total CAP time during NREM sleep) and arousals both increase in older individuals and in a variety of sleep disorders, including both diurnal and nocturnal movement disorders. Non-CAP (sleep periods without CAP for at least 60 s) is thought to indicate a state of sustained stability. CAP is considered part of the sleep microstructure, which also includes sleep spindles, K-complexes, and arousals.

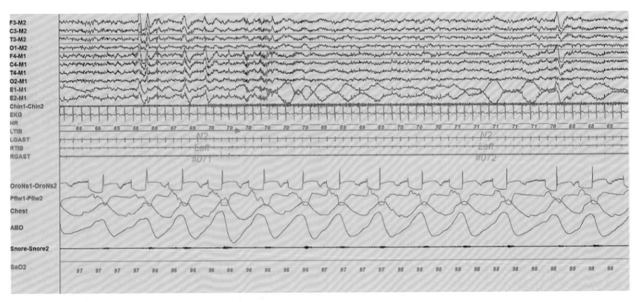

Fig. 2.3 A 60-second epoch from the overnight polysomnogram of a 35-year-old man complaining of excessive daytime sleepiness and with a prior diagnosis of obstructive sleep apnea. He also has a history of depression and is on citalopram, a selective serotonin reuptake inhibitor (SSRI). This epoch represents stage N2 sleep, as evidenced by the presence of K-complexes and sleep spindles. Note the presence of excessive eye movements, representing a combination of slow and rapid eye movements. Eye movements generally do not persist into stage N2 and beyond, but are often seen in patients on SSRIs (colloquially referred to as "Prozac eyes"). Top eight channels: EEG recording with electrodes placed according to the 10-20 international electrode placement system; Chin1-Chin2: submental electromyogram (EMG); EKG: electrocardiogram; HR: heart rate; LTIB, RTIB: left and right tibialis anterior EMG; LGAST, RGAST: left and right gastrocnemius EMG; OroNs1-OroNs2: oronasal airflow; Pflw1-Pflw2: nasal pressure transducer recording; Chest and ABD: effort belts; SaO2: arterial oxygen saturation by finger oximetry. Also included is a snore channel.
Reproduced from S. Chokroverty & R. Thomas [eds.], Atlas of Sleep medicine [2nd ed.], Copyright (2014), with permission from Elsevier.

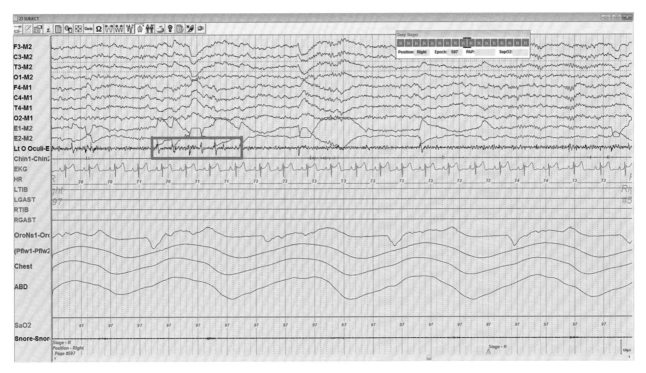

Fig. 2.4 A 20-second epoch of rapid eye movement (REM) from the overnight polysomnogram of a 54-year-old woman referred to the sleep laboratory with possible sleep apnea. Note the sharp periorbital integrated potentials (PIPs) in the left orbicularis oculi muscle channel (Lt O Oculi), co-occurring with rapid eye movements, as noted in the electrooculography channels (E1-M2, E2-M2). Top eight channels: EEG recording with electrodes placed according to the 10-20 international electrode placement system; Chin1-Chin2: submental electromyogram (EMG); EKG: electrocardiogram; HR: heart rate; LTIB, RTIB: left and right tibialis anterior EMG; LGAST, RGAST: left and right gastrocnemius EMG; OroNs1-OroNS2: oronasal airflow; Pflw1-Pflw2: nasal pressure transducer recording; Chest and ABD: effort belts; SaO2: arterial oxygen saturation by finger oximetry. Also included is a snore channel.

Box 2.1 Factors modifying sleep macrostructure

♦ **Exogenous**
- Noise
- Exercise
- Ambient temperature
- Drugs and alcohol

♦ **Endogenous**
- Age
- Prior sleep-wakefulness
- Circadian phase
- Sleep pathologies

Evolution of sleep with age

Sleep from birth through adolescence

Sleep patterns, sleep architectures, sleep habits, and sleep requirements evolve throughout the lifetime of an individual. Newborns sleep up to 16 hours in a 24-hour cycle, and their sleep occurs in the form of short scattered naps throughout the day, not consolidating into longer sleep periods until about 6 months of age [38]. The napping frequency continues to decline after 1.5 months, and

there is usually nocturnal sleep consolidation by the age of 1 year. By age 4–6 years, most children stop daytime napping; at this age, total sleep decreases to about 10 hours [39]. Sleep duration falls precipitously from childhood to adolescence; one recent large study showed decreases across the adolescent period from 8.5 hours per night at age 13 years to 7.3 hours at age 18 years [40], and there seems to have been a historical trend of a fall in adolescent sleep over the past few decades [41]. Several factors seem to be responsible for this, including a combination of natural phase delay at this age (see below), early school start times [42] and the impact of bedtime use of electronic media [43].

NREM–REM cycles also evolve with age. Newborn babies may enter sleep directly through REM sleep, or active sleep, almost half the time, which is accompanied by twitching of the limbs and face, irregular breathing, and brief central apneas. By 3 months of age, the NREM–REM cyclic pattern of adult sleep is better established, but is shorter in infants, lasting for approximately 45–50 minutes and increasing to 60–70 minutes between 5 and 10 years and reaching the normal adult cyclic pattern of 90–100 minutes by 10 years. REM sleep progressively declines with age, occupying 50% of total sleep time in newborns, about 30–35% by the end of the first year, and decreasing to adult levels of 20–25% by 5–6 years. A weak circadian rhythm is probably present at birth, but by 6–8 weeks it is established.

Sleep spindles appear from 6–8 weeks and are well formed by 3 months (they may be asynchronous during the first year, but by age 2 are synchronous). K-complexes are seen at 6 months, but

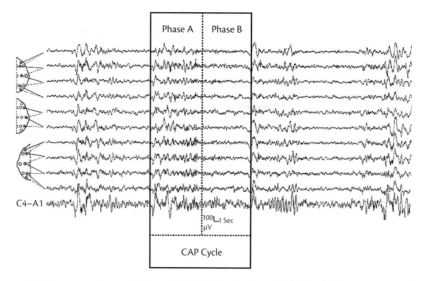

Fig. 2.5 A cyclical alternating pattern (CAP) sequence in stage N2 sleep with a highlighted CAP cycle (black box). The CAP cycle is defined by a phase A (aggregate of phasic events) and phase B (interval between two successive A phases). EEG recording with electrodes placed according to the 10-20 international electrode placement system.

Reproduced from S. Chokroverty & R. Thomas [eds.], Atlas of Sleep medicine [2nd ed.], Copyright (2014), with permission from Elsevier.

begin to appear at ages over 4 months. Hypnogogic hypersynchrony characterized by transient bursts of high-amplitude waves in the slower frequencies appears at 5–6 months and is prominent at 1 year. Pre-adolescents are highly alert during the day, with the multiple sleep latency test (MSLT) showing a mean sleep latency of 17–18 minutes.

Sleep in adults

Adults sleep an average duration of 7.5–8 hours per night, although this may be more a reflection of the exigencies of day-to-day living than of actual sleep requirements. Indeed, it has generally been held that we are chronically sleep-deprived in modern society [44]. However, the question of the "normal" amount of sleep that an adult needs is far from a settled issue. Chronic short sleep duration has been linked to a variety of health concerns, such as hypertension, obesity, insulin resistance and diabetes, and overall increased mortality [45,46], as well as cognitive issues and poor daytime functioning [47]. On the other hand, long sleep duration has also been associated with increased cardiovascular mortality [48,49]. Clinicians recognize the existence of short-sleepers (who sleep less than 6 hours a day) and long-sleepers (who sleep more than 10 hours a day) [50], suggesting that the need for sleep may vary considerably among normal individuals and may be genetically determined. Multiple studies evaluating differences between short- and long-sleepers in various physiological, psychological, and health-related spheres have not found consistent differences [51–53].

As adults age, sleep quality is generally thought to deteriorate. PSG analysis shows that older subjects spend more time awake and have repeated awakenings, resulting in low sleep efficiency and sleep maintenance. There is also an advancement of sleep phase (see the next section), resulting in early morning awakenings that prematurely terminate the night sleep. A marked reduction in the amplitude of the slow waves occurs, resulting in a decreased percentage of SWS in this age group [54]. The percentage of REM sleep

in normal elderly individuals remains relatively constant and the total duration of sleep time within 24 hours is also no different from that of young adults; however, elderly individuals often nap during the daytime compensating for lost sleep during the night. Patients with neurodegenerative conditions such as Alzheimer disease, however, may experience sleep fragmentation due to lesions of the suprachiasmatic nucleus, resulting in irregular sleep–wake cycles [55].

Figure 2.6 schematically represents the evolution of sleep step distribution in newborns, infants, children, adults, and elderly adults. Night sleep histograms of children, young adults, and of elderly adults are shown in Fig. 2.7.

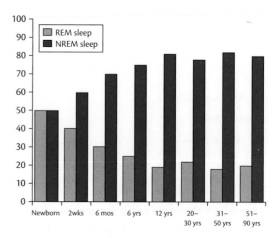

Fig. 2.6 Graphic representation of percentages of REM and NREM sleep at different ages. Note the dramatic changes in REM sleep in the early years.
Reproduced from Chokroverty S [ed], Sleep Disorders Medicine: Basic Science, Technical Considerations, and Clinical Aspects [3rd ed], Copyright (2009), with permission from Elsevier; Source data from Science, 152(3722), Roffwarg HP, Muzzio JN, Dement WC, Ontogenic development of the human sleep-dream cycle, pp. 604–619, Copyright (1966), AAAS.

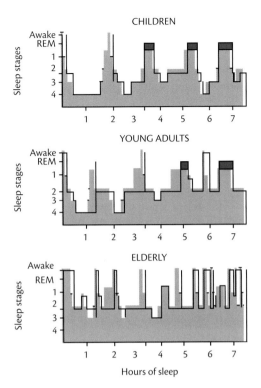

Fig. 2.7 Night sleep histograms from children, young adults, and elderly persons. Note the significant reduction of stage 4 NREM sleep with age.
Reproduced from Chokroverty S [ed], Sleep Disorders Medicine: Basic Science, Technical Considerations, and Clinical Aspects [3rd ed], Copyright (2009), with permission from Elsevier; Source data from N Engl J Med, 290, Kales A, Kales JD, Sleep disorders: recent findings in the diagnosis and treatment of disturbed sleep, pp. 487–99, Copyright (1974), Massachusetts Medical Society.

Circadian sleep–wake rhythm

Circadian rhythm disorders are discussed in detail in Chapters 21 and 22. This section provides a brief introduction to the underlying concepts.

In clinical sleep medicine, the term circadian rhythm refers to the internal clock in humans that regulates sleep–wake cycles. The circadian rhythm is exquisitely sensitive to external entraining agents, particularly light (as well as, to a much lesser extent, melatonin), that prime it for a 24-hour cycle, but in the absence of these environmental cues, the human body exhibits a free-running rhythm that runs slightly longer than 24 hours (approximately 24.2 hours). The paired suprachiasmatic nucleus (SCN) in the hypothalamus, above the optic chiasm, has been identified as the seat of the circadian rhythm, and experimental stimulation, ablation, and lesion of these nuclei alters circadian rhythms. The master circadian clock in the SCN receives afferent information from the retinohypothalamic tract, which sends signals through multiple synaptic pathways to other parts of the hypothalamus, plus the superior cervical ganglion and the pineal gland, where melatonin is released. The SCN contains melatonin receptors, so there is a feedback loop from the pineal gland to the SCN. Several neurotransmitters have been located within terminals of the SCN afferents and interneurons, including serotonin, neuropeptide Y, vasopressin, vasoactive intestinal peptide, and γ-aminobutyric acid [56]. At the molecular level, the paired SCN are controlled by at least eight genes (eg, *CLOCK, BMAL, PER, CRY*, and *TIM*), and their protein products and regulatory enzymes (eg, casein

kinase 1 epsilon and casein kinase 2 delta), but this field of research is in its embryonic stage and much work remains to be done [57].

The circadian rhythm, which regulates sleep–wake cycles, also coordinates with several other independent but synchronized biological rhythms, including those of body temperature and neuroendocrine secretion (see Chapter 6). Sleep decreases body temperature, whereas activity and wakefulness increase it. Body temperature rhythm is sinusoidal, and cortisol and growth hormone secretion rhythms are pulsatile. Cortisol has its own circadian rhythm, independent of sleep, whereas growth hormone secretion is coupled to SWS. It is also well known that plasma levels of prolactin and testosterone are all increased during sleep at night. The secretion of melatonin, the hormone synthesized by the pineal gland, has its own circadian rhythm, but is suppressed by light and thus may be an important modulator of human circadian rhythm entrainment by the light–dark cycle.

From a clinical perspective, circadian rhythm disorders are important when they affect the day-to-day functioning of patients. For example, there is a natural tendency toward a delayed sleep phase (going to bed late, usually after 3 AM and awakening well after noon) in adolescents and young adults; similarly, in older adults, there is a shift in circadian rhythms in the opposite direction (advanced sleep phase), with a tendency toward earlier bedtimes and early morning awakenings. While not pathological in themselves, they are labeled as "delayed sleep phase syndrome" and "advanced sleep phase syndrome," respectively, when they affect quality of life, such as school, work, or time with family. Additionally, there are environmentally induced circadian rhythm disorders, such as jet lag and shiftwork disorder, and those caused by underlying neurological disorders, such as non-24-hour rhythms (irregular rhythm and free-running rhythm). Treatment of these conditions involves various combinations of timed light exposure and avoidance (phototherapy), alerting and sedating medications (pharmacotherapy), and changes in sleep hours (chronotherapy) as appropriate for any given disorder. These are discussed in more detail in Chapters 21 and 22.

References

1. Loomis AL, Harvey EN, Hobart GA, Cerebral states during sleep, as studied by human brain potentials. J Exp Physiol 1937;21:127–44.
2. Aserinsky E, Kleitman N. Regularly occurring periods of eye motility and concomitant phenomena during sleep. Science 1953;118:273–4.
3. Berger RJ. Tonus of extrinsic laryngeal muscles during sleep and dreaming. Science 1961;134(3482):840.
4. Rechtschaffen A, Kales A. A manual of standardized terminology, techniques and scoring systems for sleep stages of human subjects. Los Angeles: UCLA Brain Information Service/Brain Research Institute, 1968.
5. Berry RB, Brooks R, Gamaldo CE, et al. The AASM manual for the scoring of sleep and associated events: rules, terminology, and technical specifications, version 2.0.3. Darien, IL: American Academy of Sleep Medicine, 2014.
6. Spicuzza L, Caruso D, Di Maria G. Obstructive sleep apnoea syndrome and its management. Ther Adv Chronic Dis. 2015;6:273–85.
7. Young T, Finn L, Peppard P, et al. Sleep disordered breathing and mortality: eighteen-year follow up of the Wisconsin Sleep Cohort. Sleep 2008;31:1071–8.
8. Sullivan CE, Issa FG, Berthon-Jones M, et al. Reversal of obstructive sleep apnoea by continuous positive airway pressure applied through the nares. Lancet 1981;1:862–5.
9. DeLecea L, Kilduff TS, Peyron C, et al. The hypocretins: hypothalamus-specific peptides with neuroexcitatory activity. Proc Natl Acad Sci USA 1998;95:322–7.

10. Sakurai T, Amemiya A, Ishii M, et al. Orexins and orexin receptors: a family of hypothalamic neuropeptides and G protein-coupled receptors that regulate feeding behavior. Cell 1998;92:573–85.

11. Lin L, Faraco J, Li R, et al. The sleep disorder canine narcolepsy is caused by a mutation in the hypocretin (orexin) receptor 2 gene. Cell 1999;98:365–76.

12. Chemelly RM, Willie JT, Sinton CM, et al. Narcolepsy in orexin knockout mice: molecular genetics of sleep regulation. Cell 1999;98:437–51.

13. Hara J, Beuckmann CT, Nambu T, et al. Genetic ablation of orexin neurons in mice results in narcolepsy, hypophagia, and obesity. Neuron 2001;30:345–54.

14. Nishino S, Ripley B, Overeem S, et al. Hypocretin (orexin) deficiency in human narcolepsy. Lancet 2000;355:39–40.

15. Thannical TC, Moore RY, Nienhuis R, et al. Reduced number of hypocretin neurons in human narcolepsy. Neuron 2000;27:469–74.

16. Guilleminault C, Abad VC. Narcolepsy. In: Chokroverty S, ed. Sleep disorders medicine: basic science, technical considerations, and clinical aspects, 3rd ed. Philadelphia: Saunders/Elsevier, 2009:377–96.

17. Peyron C, Faraco J, Rogers W, et al. A mutation in a case of early onset narcolepsy and a generalized absence of hypocretin peptides in human narcoleptic brains. Nat Med 2000;6:991–7.

18. Pilcher JJ, Huffcutt AJ. Effects of sleep deprivation on performance: a meta-analysis. Sleep 1996;19:318–26.

19. Nakanishi H, Sun Y, Nakamura RK, et al. Positive correlation between cerebral protein synthesis rates and deep sleep in *Macaca mulatta*. Eur J Neurosci 1997;9:271–9

20. Krueger JM, Obal F Jr, Kapas L, Fang J. Brain organization and sleep function. Behav Brain Res 1995;69:177–85.

21. Kavanau JL. Memory, sleep and the evolution of mechanisms of synaptic efficacy maintenance. Neuroscience 1997;79:7–44.

22. Kavanau JL. Origin and evolution of sleep: roles of vision and endothermy. Brain Res Bull 1997;42:245–64.

23. Karni A, Tanne D, Rubenstein BS, et al. Dependence on REM sleep of overnight improvement of a perceptual skill. Science 1994;265:679–82.

24. Born J, Rasch B, Cais S. Sleep to remember. Neuroscientist 2006;12:410–24.

25. Hoedlmoser K, Heib DP, Roell J, et al. Slow sleep spindle activity, declarative memory, and general cognitive abilities in children. Sleep 2014;37:1501–12.

26. Vertes R, JM Siegel JM. Time for the sleep community to take a critical look at the purported role of sleep in memory processing. Sleep 2005;28:1228–9.

27. Lavie P, Pratt H, Scharf B, et al. Localized pontine lesion: nearly total absence of REM sleep. Neurology 1984;34:118–20.

28. Bach V, Telliez F, Chardon K, et al. Thermoregulation in wakefulness and sleep in humans. Handb Clin Neurol 2011;98:215–27.

29. Xie L, Kang H, Xu Q, et al. Sleep drives metabolic clearance from the adult brain. Science 2013;342:373–7.

30. Nedergaard M. Neuroscience: garbage truck of the brain. Science 2013;340:1529–30.

31. Iliff JJ, Nedergaard M. Is there a cerebral lymphatic system? Stroke 2013;44:S93–5.

32. Iliff JJ, Wang M, Zeppenfeld DM, et al. Cerebral arterial pulsation drives paravascular CSF–interstitial fluid exchange in the murine brain. J Neurosci 2013;33:18190–9.

33. Iliff JJ, Wang M, Liao Y, et al. A paravascular pathway facilitates CSF flow through the brain parenchyma and the clearance of interstitial solutes, including amyloid β. Sci Transl Med 2012;4:147ra111.

34. Benson K, Zarcone VP Jr. Phasic events of REM sleep: phenomenology of middle ear muscle activity and periorbital integrated potentials in the same normal population. Sleep 1979;2:199–213.

35. Chokroverty S. Phasic tongue movements in human rapid-eye movement in sleep. Neurology 1980;30:665–8.

36. Terzano MG, Parrino L. Origin and significance of the cyclic alternating pattern (CAP). Sleep Med Rev 2000;4:10123

37. Terzano MG, Parrino L, Smeriari A, et al. Atlas, rules and recording techniques for the scoring of cyclic alternating pattern (CAP) in human sleep. Sleep Med 2002;3:187–99.

38. Parmelee AH. Sleep patterns in infancy a study of one infant from birth to eight months of age. Acta Paediatr 1961;50:160–70.

39. Iglowstein I, Jenni OG, Molinari L, Largo RH. Sleep duration from infancy to adolescence: reference values and generational trends. Pediatrics 2003;111:302–7.

40. Maslowsky J, Ozer EJ. Developmental trends in sleep duration in adolescence and young adulthood: evidence from a national United States sample. J Adolesc Health 2014;54:691–7.

41. Keyes KM, Maslowsky J, Hamilton A, Schulenberg J. The great sleep recession: changes in sleep duration among US adolescents, 1991–2012. Pediatrics 2015;135:460–8.

42. Owens J; Adolescent Sleep Working Group; Committee on Adolescence. Insufficient sleep in adolescents and young adults: an update on causes and consequences. Pediatrics 2014;134:e921–32.

43. Polos PG, Bhat S, Gupta D, et al. The impact of sleep time-related information and communication technology (STRICT) on sleep patterns and daytime functioning in American adolescents. J Adolesc 2015;44:232–44.

44. Bonnet MH, Arand DL. We are chronically sleep deprived. Sleep 1995;18:908–11.

45. Mullington JM1, Haack M, Toth M, et al. Cardiovascular, inflammatory, and metabolic consequences of sleep deprivation. Prog Cardiovasc Dis 2009;51:294–302.

46. Spiegel K, Knutson K, Leproult R, et al. Sleep loss: a novel risk factor for insulin resistance and type 2 diabetes. J Appl Physiol 2005;99:2008–19.

47. Van Dongen HP, Maislin G, Mullington JM, Dinges DF. The cumulative cost of additional wakefulness: dose-response effects on neurobehavioral functions and sleep physiology from chronic sleep restriction and total sleep deprivation. Sleep 2003;26:117–26.

48. Cappuccio FP, Cooper D, D'Elia L, et al. Sleep duration predicts cardiovascular outcomes: a systematic review and meta-analysis of prospective studies. Eur Heart J 2011;32:1484–92.

49. Tsai TC, Wu JS, Yang YC, et al. Long sleep duration associated with a higher risk of increased arterial stiffness in males. Sleep 2014;37:1315–20.

50. Hartmann E. Sleep requirement: long sleepers, short sleepers, variable sleepers, and insomniacs. Psychosomatics 1972;14:95–103.

51. Hao YL1, Zhang B2, Jia FJ2, Li XL2, Tang Y2, Ren YZ3, Liu WH2. A three-phase epidemiological study of short and long sleepers in a middle-aged Chinese population: prevalence and characteristics. Braz J Med Biol Res. 2014;47:157–65.

52. Webb WB. Are short and long sleepers different? Psychol Rep 1979;44:259–64.

53. Webb WB, Agnew HW Jr. Sleep stage characteristics of long and short sleepers. Science 1970;168:146–7.

54. Ehlers CL, Kupfer DJ. Effects of age on delta and REM sleep parameters. Electroencephalogra Clin Neurophysiol 1989;72:118–25.

55. Moran M, Lynch CA, Walsh C, et al. Sleep disturbance in mild to moderate Alzheimer's disease. Sleep Med 2005;6:347–52.

56. Saper CB, Scammell TE, Lu J. Hypothalamic regulation of sleep and circadian rhythms. Nature 2005;437:1257–63.

57. Turek FW, Vitaterna MH. Molecular neurobiology of circadian rhythms. Handb Clin Neurol 2011;99:951–61.

CHAPTER 3

Neurobiology of REM sleep

Pierre-Hervé Luppi, Olivier Clément,
Christelle Peyron, and Patrice Fort

Network generating paradoxical (REM) sleep

Glutamatergic neurons located in the SLD trigger REM sleep

REM sleep characterized by EEG activation and rapid eye movements (REMs) was discovered in 1953 by Aserinsky and Kleitman. It was shown to correlate in humans with dream activity [1,2]. In 1959, Jouvet and Michel discovered in cats that REM sleep is also characterized by a complete disappearance of muscle tone, paradoxically associated with a cortical activation and REMs, and named this state paradoxical sleep (PS) [3,4]. Soon after, they demonstrated that the brainstem is necessary and sufficient to trigger and maintain REM sleep in cats. Using electrolytic and chemical lesions, it was then shown that the dorsal part of the pontis oralis (PnO) and caudalis (PnC) nuclei contain the neurons responsible for REM sleep onset [5]. Furthermore, bilateral injections of a cholinergic agonist, carbachol, into these structures promote REM sleep in cats. The dorsal part, where carbachol injection induces REM sleep with the shortest latency, was termed the peri-locus coeruleus alpha nucleus (peri-LCα), the pontine inhibitory area (PIA), or the subcoeruleus nucleus (SubC) [6]. In contrast to the data from cats, carbachol iontophoresis into the rat sublaterodorsal tegmental nucleus (SLD), the equivalent of the cat peri-LCα, induces waking (W) with increased muscle activity [7]. Further, in rats, only a few of the numerous c-Fos-labeled cells located in the laterodorsal tegmental nucleus (Ldt) and SLD after REM sleep hypersomnia were cholinergic [8]. Moreover, it has been shown that injection of scopolamine, a cholinergic muscarinic antagonist, into the SLD has nearly no effect on REM sleep [9]. In addition, it has been shown that cholinergic neurons of the Ldt and SLD are active during both W and REM sleep and therefore should play a role in cortical activation during both W and REM sleep rather than a specific role in REM sleep genesis [10]. However, it has also been shown that optogenetic activation of Ldt and pedunculopontine (PPTg) cholinergic neurons increases the probability of REM sleep occurrence [11]. Altogether, these results strongly suggest that the pontine cholinergic neurons play a modulatory role in REM sleep genesis and a more central role in cortical activation during both W and REM sleep.

In addition, we have shown that SLD REM sleep-on neurons are not GABAergic. Indeed, the small number of c-Fos-positive neurons expressing a specific marker of GABAergic neurons (glutamate decarboxylase, GAD, the enzyme responsible for synthesis of GABA) in the SLD did not increase in rats displaying an REM sleep rebound compared with control or REM sleep-deprived animals [12]. In contrast, our results have shown that most of the c-Fos-labeled neurons localized in the SLD after REM sleep hypersomnia express a specific marker of glutamatergic neurons (vesicular glutamate transporter 2, vGlut2) [13] and are therefore glutamatergic. Further, a large number of the REM sleep-on neurons recorded in the SLD have been found to be glutamatergic [10].

A number of results further indicate that SLD REM sleep-on glutamatergic neurons generate muscle atonia via descending medullary projections to GABA/glycinergic neurons. Indeed, it has been shown that the SLD sends direct efferent projections to glycinergic neurons in the ventral (GiV) and alpha (Gia) gigantocellular nuclei (corresponding to the cat magnocellular reticular nucleus, Mc) and the nucleus raphe magnus (RMg). In addition, glycinergic neurons of the Gia, GiV and RMg express c-Fos after induction of REM sleep by bicuculline (Bic, a GABA$_A$ antagonist) injection in the SLD [7]. Further, glycinergic neurons of these structures project monosynaptically to lumbar spinal motoneurons [14]. These results suggest that Gia, GiV, and RMg glycinergic neurons hyperpolarize motoneurons. It is likely that these neurons are also GABAergic, since a large majority of the c-Fos-labeled neurons localized in these nuclei after 3 hours of REM sleep recovery following 72 hours of REM sleep deprivation express GAD [12]. Further, it has been shown that combined microdialysis of bicuculline, strychnine and phaclofen (a GABA$_B$ antagonist) in the trigeminal nucleus restored muscle tone during REM sleep [15,16]. Altogether, these results indicate that the premotoneurons responsible for muscle atonia of REM sleep are localized in the GiV and co-release GABA and glycine.

SLD glutamatergic neurons are inhibited by GABAergic neurons during wake and SWS

A long-lasting REM sleep-like episode can be pharmacologically induced with a short latency in head-restrained unanesthetized rats by iontophoretic applications of bicuculline or gabazine, two GABA$_A$ receptor antagonists, specifically to the SLD. Further, neurons within the SLD specifically active during REM sleep are activated following bicuculline or gabazine iontophoresis [7]. Taken together, these data indicate that the onset of SLD REM sleep-on neurons is mainly due to the removal during REM sleep of a tonic GABAergic tone present during W and slow-wave sleep (SWS). It is likely that such a strong tonic GABAergic inhibition is necessary to preclude in healthy subjects the occurrence of sleep onset REM sleep (SOREMS) and cataplexy. Combining retrograde tracing with cholera toxin b subunit (CTb) injected in the SLD and GAD immunostaining, we then identified neurons at the origin of the GABAergic innervation. These neurons were localized within the pontine (including the SLD itself) and the dorsal deep mesencephalic reticular nuclei (dDpMe) [17]. Further, the ventrolateral part of the periaqueductal gray (vlPAG) and the dDpMe are the only pontomedullary structures containing a large number of c-Fos-positive neurons expressing GAD67mRNA after 72 hours of REM sleep deprivation [12]. In addition, injection of muscimol in the vlPAG and/or the dDpMe induces a strong increase in REM sleep quantities [12]. These congruent experimental data lead us to propose that GABAergic neurons within the vlPAG and the dDpMe are gating REM sleep during W and SWS by tonically inhibiting REM sleep-on neurons from the SLD.

Role of monoaminergic neurons in the control of REM sleep

A major achievement in the identification of the mechanisms controlling REM sleep was the finding that serotonergic neurons from the raphe nuclei and noradrenergic neurons from the LC cease firing specifically during REM sleep, i.e, show a REM sleep-off firing activity, reciprocal to that of REM sleep-on neurons [18]. Later, it was shown that histaminergic neurons from the tuberomammillary nucleus and hypocretinergic neurons from the periformical hypothalamic area also exhibit REM sleep-off firing activity [19]. These electrophysiological data were the basis for a well-accepted hypothesis suggesting that REM sleep onset is gated by reciprocal inhibitory interactions between REM sleep-on and REM sleep-off monoaminergic neurons [18]. Supporting this neuronal model, drugs enhancing serotonergic and noradrenergic transmission—monoamine oxidase inhibitors (MAOs) and serotonin and norepinephrine (noradrenaline) reuptake inhibitors (SNRIs)—specifically suppress REM sleep [20]. Further, applications of norepinephrine, epinephrine (adrenaline), or benoxathian (an α_2 adrenergic agonist) to the peri-LCα inhibit REM sleep, but application of serotonin has no effect [21]. It is of note that our data combining a marker of noradrenergic neurons (tyrosine hydroxylase, TH) and c-Fos staining after REM sleep deprivation and recovery suggest that it is unlikely that the LC noradrenergic neurons are involved in the inhibition of REM sleep, particularly during its deprivation. Indeed, the LC noradrenergic neurons do not display c-Fos after 72 hours of REM sleep deprivation. Furthermore, no projection has been observed from the LC to the SLD [17]. Nevertheless, a substantial number of noradrenergic neurons from A1 and A2 cell groups display c-Fos after REM sleep deprivation, indicating that noradrenergic neurons from these medullary cell groups might contribute to REM sleep inhibition [22]. In summary, it is clear that norepinephrine and serotonin inhibit REM sleep, but the targeted neurons remain to be identified. We propose that rather than inhibiting SLD REM sleep-on neurons, norepinephrine and serotonin might inhibit REM sleep by means of a tonic excitation of the dDpMe and vlPAG REM sleep-off GABAergic neurons.

GABAergic neurons are responsible for the inactivation of monoaminergic neurons during REM sleep

The application of bicuculline to monoaminergic neurons during SWS or REM sleep induces a tonic firing in both types of neurons [23,24]. These results indicate the existence of a tonic GABA input to the LC and DRN that is active during sleep and strongly suggest that an increased GABA release is responsible for the REM sleep-selective inactivation of monoaminergic neurons. By combining retrograde tracing with CTb and GAD immunohistochemistry in rats, we found that the LC and DRN receive GABAergic inputs from neurons located in a large number of distant regions from the forebrain to medulla [24]. Two brainstem areas contained numerous GABAergic neurons projecting both to the DRN and LC, and were thus candidates for mediating the REM sleep-related inhibition of monoaminergic neurons: the vlPAG and the dorsal paragigantocellular nucleus (DPGi) [24]. We then demonstrated by using c-Fos that both nuclei contain numerous LC-projecting neurons selectively activated during REM sleep rebound following REM sleep deprivation [25]. Since the DPGi has not previously been considered in sleep mechanisms, we studied the firing activity of the DPGi neurons across the sleep–wake cycle in head-restrained rats [26]. In full agreement with our functional data using c-Fos, we found that the DPGi contains numerous REM sleep-on neurons that are silent during W and SWS and fire tonically during REM sleep. The REM sleep-on neurons start discharging approximately 15 s before REM sleep onset and become silent around 10 s before EEG signs of arousal. Taken together, these data highly suggest that the DPGi contains the neurons responsible for the inactivation of LC noradrenergic neurons during REM sleep [26]. A contribution from the vlPAG to this inhibitory mechanism is also likely. Indeed, an increase in c-Fos/GAD immunoreactive neurons has been reported in the vlPAG after a REM sleep rebound induced by deprivation in rats [12]. In summary, a large body of data indicates that GABAergic REM sleep-on neurons localized in the vlPAG and the DPGi hyperpolarize monoaminergic neurons during REM sleep.

Role of the hypothalamus in REM sleep control

Surprisingly, a very large number of c-Fos-positive cells were observed in the posterior hypothalamus (PH), including the zona incerta (ZI), the periformical area (PeF), and the lateral hypothalamic area (LH), after REM sleep hypersomnia [27]. By using double-immunostaining, it has been further shown that around 75% of PH cells labeled for c-Fos after REM sleep rebound express GAD67mRNA and are therefore GABAergic [28]. One-third of these GABAergic neurons were also immunoreactive for two neuropeptides, melanin-concentrating hormone (MCH) [27] and nesfatin [29]. In support of these data, it has been shown in head-restrained rats that MCH neurons fire exclusively during REM sleep [30]. Rats receiving intracerebroventricular (icv) administration of MCH showed a strong dose-dependent increase in quantities of REM sleep and, to a minor extent, SWS [27]. Such a sleep increase has been obtained using chronic (24-hour) optogenetic activation of MCH neurons [31]. Finally, it was shown that optogenetic activation of MCH neurons specifically at the onset of SWS epoch did not increase SWS duration but increased the probability of SWS-to-REM sleep transition. More important, optogenetic stimulation of MCH neurons at the REM sleep onset significantly prolonged the duration of REM sleep episodes [32]. In agreement with our results showing that MCH neurons constitute only one-third of the GABAergic neurons activated during REM sleep hypersomnia, it has been shown that a large population of GABAergic neurons not expressing MCH localized in the LH area also discharge maximally during REM sleep [33]. Since these neurons anticipate REM sleep onset, they could play a role in triggering REM sleep.

To determine the function of the LH MCH$^+$/GABA$^+$ and MCH$^-$/GABA$^+$ neurons in REM sleep control, either all LH neurons were inactivated with muscimol (a GABA$_A$ agonist) or only those bearing α_2-adrenergic receptors were inactivated using clonidine. It was found that muscimol and to a lesser degree, clonidine after bilateral injections in the LH induced an inhibition of REM sleep with or without an increase in SWS quantities, respectively. It has been further shown that after muscimol injection in the LH, the vlPAG/dDpMe region contains a large number of c-Fos/GAD67$^+$ and of c-Fos/CTb$^+$ neurons in animals with a CTb injection in the SLD. Our results indicate that the activation of REM sleep-on MCH/GABAergic neurons localized in the LH is a necessary step for REM sleep to occur. They further suggest that MCH/GABAergic REM sleep-on neurons localized in the LH control REM sleep onset and maintenance by means of a direct inhibitory projection to vlPAG/dDpMe REM sleep-off GABAergic neurons. On the basis of our results, it can be proposed that MCH/GABAergic neurons of the LH constitute a "master" generator of REM sleep that controls a "slave" generator located in the brainstem. To reconcile the Jouvet hypothesis (i.e, that the brainstem is necessary and sufficient to generate a state characterized by muscle atonia and REM [5]) with our results, it can therefore be proposed that after removal of the forebrain, the brainstem generator is sufficient to induce a state with muscle atonia and REM by means of a reorganization of the brainstem systems generating REM sleep. However, the brainstem generator would be under control of the LH generator in intact animals.

In addition to the descending pathway to the REM sleep-off GABAergic neurons, the MCH/GABAergic REM sleep-on neurons might also promote REM sleep by means of other pathways to the histaminergic neurons, the monoaminergic REM sleep-off neurons and the hypocretinergic neurons [7,32]. Indeed, Jego et al [32] have shown that optogenetic activation of MCH neurons inhibit other postsynaptic targets, such as histaminergic cells in the TMN and neurons of the medial septum, through activation of the GABA$_A$ receptor.

The mechanisms at the origin of the activation of the MCH/GABAergic neurons of the LH at the entrance to REM sleep remain to be identified. A large number of studies indicate that MCH neurons also play a key role in metabolic control [34]. Therefore, the activation of these neurons at the onset of and during REM sleep could be influenced by the metabolic state. In addition, it is likely that yet undiscovered endogenous cellular or molecular clock-like mechanisms may play a role in their activation.

The cessation of activity of the MCH/GABAergic REM sleep-on neurons and, more widely, of all the REM sleep-on neurons at the end of REM sleep episodes may be due to a different mechanism than the entrance into the state, possibly the reactivation of the arousal circuits, which are known to silence MCH neurons in vitro [35]. Indeed, animals enter REM sleep slowly from SWS, whereas they exit it abruptly by a microarousal. This indicates that the end of REM sleep episodes is induced by the activation of the wake systems like the monoaminergic, hypocretinergic, or histaminergic neurons. However, the precise mechanisms responsible for their activation remain to be identified.

A network model for REM sleep onset and maintenance

As described above, most of the populations of neurons responsible for REM sleep control were identified by means of c-Fos labeling induced by REM sleep deprivation and REM sleep hypersomnia. In the future, it will be important to employ additional experimental approaches to fully determine the role of these neurons, including tract-tracing, single-unit recordings, and inactivations and activations by genetic or pharmacological tools. Furthermore, several regions that contain a large number of c-Fos-labeled neurons require additional studies, including the lateral paragigantocellular nucleus, the lateral parabrachial nucleus, the nucleus raphe obscurus, and the dorsal PAG [8].

The observation that REM sleep episodes in the rat start from SWS after a relatively long intermediate state during which the EEG displays a mix of spindles and theta activity, and then terminate abruptly by a short microarousal, deserves further attention. These findings suggest that different mechanisms are responsible for the entrance to and exit from REM sleep. Altogether, these characteristics, as well as our current knowledge of the neuronal network, lead us to propose an updated model of the mechanisms controlling REM sleep onset and maintenance.

REM sleep onset would be due to the activation of glutamatergic REM sleep-on neurons in the SLD (Fig. 3.1). During W and SWS, the activity of these REM sleep-on neurons would be suppressed by a tonic inhibitory GABAergic tone originating from REM sleep-off neurons localized in the vlPAG and the dDpMe (Fig. 3.2). These REM sleep-off neurons would be activated during W by the Hcrt and the aminergic neurons. The onset of REM sleep would be due to the activation by intrinsic "clock-like" mechanisms of REM sleep-on MCH/GABAergic hypothalamic neurons and REM sleep-on GABAergic neurons localized in the DPGi and vlPAG. These neurons would inactivate the REM sleep-off GABAergic neurons and the aminergic and Hcrt waking neurons. The disinhibited ascending SLD REM sleep-on neurons would in turn induce cortical activation via their projections to intralaminar thalamic relay neurons in collaboration with W/REM sleep-on cholinergic and glutamatergic neurons from the laterodorsal (Ldt) and pedunculopontine (PPT), mesencephalic, and pontine reticular nuclei and the basal forebrain. Descending REM sleep-on SLD neurons would induce muscle atonia via their excitatory projections to glycinergic neurons localized in the Gia and GiV reticular nuclei and the nucleus raphe magnus (RMg) (Fig. 3.2). The exit from REM sleep would be due to the activation of waking systems. The waking systems would inhibit the hypothalamic MCH/GABAergic and the brainstem GABAergic REM sleep-on neurons.

Dysfunctions of the network that are responsible for REM sleep behavior disorder

REM sleep behavior disorder (RBD) is characterized by the acting out of dreams that are vivid, intense, and violent. Dream-enacting behaviors include talking, yelling, punching, kicking, sitting, jumping from bed, arm flailing, and grabbing. The person may be awakened or may wake up spontaneously during the acting and vividly recall the dream that corresponds to the physical activity. RBD is usually seen in middle-aged to elderly men. The disorder may occur in association with various degenerative neurological conditions such as Parkinson disease (PD), multiple system atrophy (MSA), and dementia with Lewy bodies (DLB) [36].

Several studies indicate that it is unlikely that RBD is due to a dysfunction of the dopaminergic nigrostriatal system. The strongest arguments are that RBD does not occur in about half of PD patients and that the use of dopaminergic agents usually does not improve

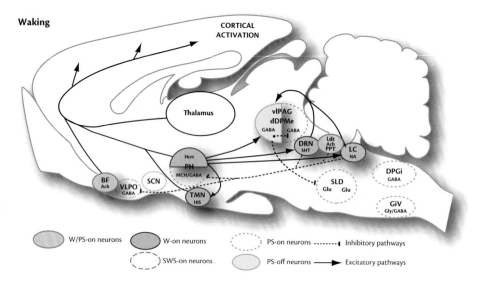

Fig. 3.1 State of the network responsible for REM sleep during wake and at the end of a REM sleep episode. During wake, REM sleep-off GABAergic neurons located in the vlPAG and dDpMe tonically inhibit SLD glutamatergic neurons. These REM sleep-off GABAergic neurons are excited by monoaminergic and hypocretin inputs. Wake-on neurons activate the cortex either directly or by means of a relay in the intralaminar thalamic nuclei. Direct pathways from the noradrenergic and serotonergic neurons to the cortex contributing to wake are not shown here for clarity. 5HT: serotonin; Ach: acetylcholine; BF: basal forebrain, DPGi: dorsal paragigantocellular reticular nucleus; dDpMe: dorsal deep mesencephalic reticular nucleus; DRN: dorsal raphe nucleus; GiV: ventral gigantocellular reticular nucleus; Glu: glutamate; Gly: glycine; Hcrt: hypocretin (orexin)-containing neurons; His: histamine; LC: locus coeruleus; Ldt: laterodorsal tegmental nucleus; LPGi: lateral paragigantocellular reticular nucleus; MCH: melanin-concentrating hormone; PH: posterior hypothalamus; PPT: pedunculopontine nucleus; vlPAG: ventrolateral periaqueductal gray; VLPO: ventrolateral preoptic nucleus; SCN: suprachiasmatic nucleus; SLD: sublaterodorsal nucleus.

RBD. In neurodegenerative diseases, where RBD is frequent, neuronal cell loss has been observed in the brainstem structures modulating REM sleep, such as the locus subcoeruleus, the pedunculopontine nucleus, and the gigantocellular reticular nucleus, and also in their rostral afferents, especially the amygdala [36]. In cats and rats, electrolytic and neurochemical lesions limited to the SLD eliminate the tonic muscle atonia and induce phasic muscle activity during REM sleep. The phasic events include large limb twitches, locomotion, fear, and attack and defensive behaviors [37]. Notably, larger lesions induce a decrease in the total quantities of REM sleep [5], whereas RBD patients display normal quantities of REM sleep. Selective experimental lesions in the ventromedial medullary reticular nuclei have been also reported to induce a decrease of atonia during REM sleep with an increase of phasic events [38].

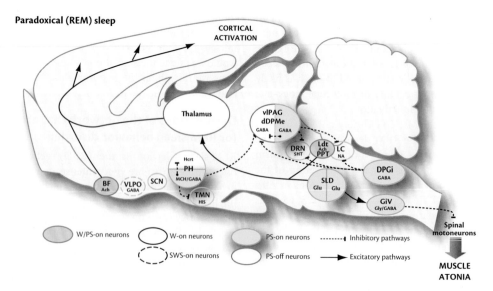

Fig. 3.2 State of the REM sleep-generating network during a REM sleep episode. The onset and maintenance of REM sleep is due to the intrinsic "clock-like" activation of GABAergic neurons localized in the posterior hypothalamus (some of them also containing MCH), the vlPAG/dDpMe, and the DPGi. These neurons inhibit all W neurons and the REM sleep-off GABAergic neurons of the vlPAG and dDpMe. SLD glutamatergic neurons are disinhibited and start to generate muscle atonia and cortical activation by means of their descending and ascending projections, respectively. They excite glycinergic/GABAergic neurons of the GiV, which in turn hyperpolarize spinal and cranial motoneurons.

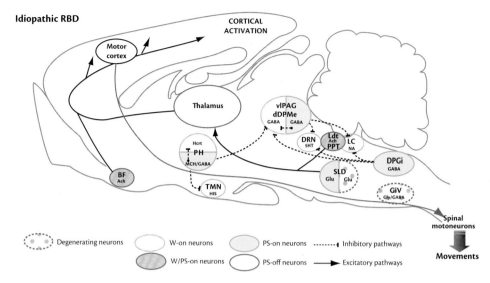

Fig. 3.3 State of the network responsible for REM sleep during idiopathic RBD. In idiopathic RBD patients, the descending but not the ascending SLD glutamatergic neurons have degenerated. Another possibility is that only the GiV glycinergic/GABAergic neurons have degenerated. Movements are induced during REM sleep by direct or indirect glutamatergic projections from the motor cortex to spinal and cranial motoneurons.

On the basis of these and our own experimental data, we propose that RBD in patients without atonia during REM sleep could be due to a lesion of a subpopulation of REM sleep-on glutamatergic neurons of the SLD responsible for inducing muscle atonia via their descending projections to the premotor GABA/glycinergic neurons of the GiV. This implies that REM sleep-on neurons of the SLD are divided into at least two subpopulations: one descending and responsible for muscle atonia, and the other inducing the state of REM sleep itself and EEG activation (Fig. 3.3). Data obtained in cats supports the existence of these two populations of SLD REM sleep-on cells (see above), but they have not been identified in rats. If these two populations exist, it remains to be discovered why only the descending SLD neurons would be destroyed in RBD patients. In any case, RBD patients should not have a large lesion of the SLD and surrounding nuclei, since they do not display a decrease in REM sleep amount. Another possibility is that SLD neurons are intact and the premotor GABA/glycinergic neurons of the GiV are damaged. This better fits with the fact that only the atonia is lost in RBD, and not the state of REM sleep per se (Fig. 3.3).

The RBD reported in narcoleptic patients is likely due to the absence of hypocretin, although it cannot be completely ruled out that the SLD–GiV atonia pathway is lesioned in these patients. One possibility is that, under normal conditions, Hcrt neurons excite the SLD–GiV atonia pathway during REM sleep, in particular during the muscle twitches induced by a phasic glutamatergic excitation of the motoneurons (Fig. 3.4). Two results support this hypothesis. First, although Hcrt neurons are mainly active during active waking, they display bursts of activity during the twitches of REM sleep [19]. Second, application of hypocretin in the SLD region induces REM sleep with atonia [39].

Dysfunctions of the network that are responsible for cataplexy in narcoleptic patients

Narcolepsy–cataplexy is characterized by two major symptoms, excessive daytime sleepiness (EDS) and cataplexy, and two auxiliary symptoms, hypnagogic hallucinations and sleep paralysis.

EDS occurs daily and is characterized by sleep episodes with a premature onset of REM sleep. A sudden decrease in muscle tone triggered by emotional factors, most often positive, characterizes cataplexy. It can affect all striated muscles or can be limited to facial muscles or to the upper or lower limbs. The monosynaptic H-reflex is suppressed, as during REM sleep. Patients remain fully conscious during cataplexy [40]. All these symptoms suggest that REM sleep is disinhibited in narcoleptic patients. It has been shown that disruption of the type 2 hypocretin receptor induces narcolepsy in dogs and mice [41,42]. No mutation has been found in human narcoleptics [43]. Instead, a marked reduction in the quantities of the peptide Hcrt 1 was found in their cerebrospinal fluid and a disappearance of Hcrt staining was observed in the hypothalamus of post-mortem brain tissues [43]. It is notable that Hcrt neurons are specifically active during W and increase their activity during muscle activation [19]. They are silent during SWS or REM sleep, except during phasic twitches, when they can fire in bursts. It is of interest that they start to fire several seconds before the onset of W at the end of REM sleep episodes [33]. Hcrt neurons, like aminergic neurons, send projections throughout the brain, from the olfactory bulb, cerebral cortex, and thalamus to the brainstem and the spinal cord [44]. It is therefore difficult to determine, solely on the basis of the projections of the Hcrt neurons, which missing pathway(s) are responsible for the four symptoms of narcolepsy. It has been proposed that the absence of dense Hcrt projections to the histaminergic and noradrenergic LC neurons might be responsible for narcolepsy symptoms. Indeed, icv administration or local injection of Hcrt in the noradrenergic LC or the histaminergic TMN neurons induces W and inhibits REM sleep [45,46]. Further, administration of selective norepinephrine reuptake inhibitors and α_1-adrenergic agonists specifically suppress cataplexy [40]. Besides, the absence of the hypocretin input on serotonin neurons could also play a role, since serotonin reuptake inhibitors are effective in treating cataplexy, at least in humans [40]. Strongly supporting this hypothesis, it has been shown that targeted restoration of orexin receptor expression in the dorsal raphe (DR) and in the locus coeruleus (LC) of

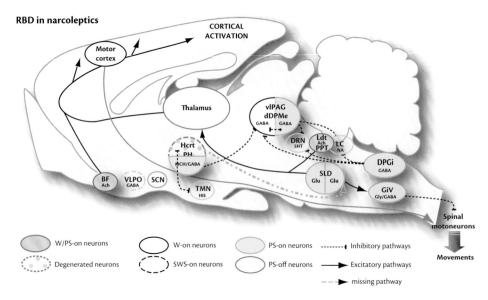

Fig. 3.4 State of the network responsible for REM sleep during RBD in narcoleptic patients. In narcolepsy, the network responsible for muscle atonia is intact. Phasic movements during REM sleep are induced by a phasic activation of motoneurons due to the absence of an excitatory projection of the Hcrt neurons specifically to the descending SLD REM sleep-on neurons.

mice lacking orexin receptors inhibited cataplexy-like episodes and pathological fragmentation of wakefulness (i.e, sleepiness), respectively [47]. Finally, a missing hypocretin projection to GABAergic REM sleep-off neurons might be implicated, since the most recent treatment for cataplexy, namely γ-hydroxybutyrate (GHB), may act through increased GABA$_B$ transmission [48]. This is an attractive hypothesis in view of our finding that GABAergic REM sleep-off neurons localized in the vlPAG/dDpMe region gate the onset of REM sleep by means of their tonic inhibition of the SLD neurons during W and SWS. Further, we have found that inactivating neurons in the vlPAG/dDpMe region by means of muscimol induces not only an increase in REM sleep quantities but also an increase

in SOREMS [12]. It thus can be hypothesized that during emotions in healthy subjects, there is a phasic increase in hypocretin release on GABAergic REM sleep-off neurons. Since the hypocretiner-gic neurons also project to aminergic neurons, they would excite these neurons, which in turn would reinforce the activation of the GABAergic REM sleep-off neurons via direct projections (Fig. 3.1). The phasic increase in inhibition by GABAergic REM sleep-off neurons would counterbalance an increased glutamatergic excitation of SLD neurons arising in the central amygdala (Fig. 3.5). We have indeed demonstrated that non-GABAergic neurons of the central amygdala project to the SLD [17]. Further, neurons increasing their activity during W and/or REM sleep or prior to and during

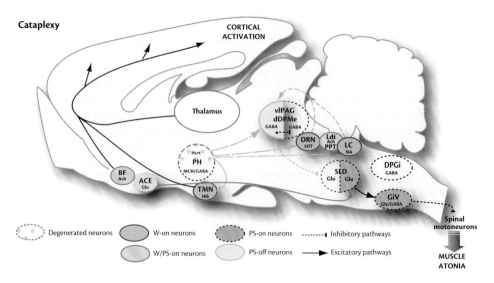

Fig. 3.5 State of the network responsible for REM sleep during cataplexy. Cataplexy is induced by activation of a glutamatergic pathway from the emotionally driven central amygdala (ACE) to the descending SLD glutamatergic neurons. In healthy subjects, the hypocretin neurons would be excited. They would excite GABAergic REM sleep-off neurons located in the vlPAG/dDpMe and thereby increase the inhibition of SLD glutamatergic neurons and counteract the excitation coming from the central amygdala.

cataplexy were recorded in the central amygdala [49]. In addition, bilateral, excitotoxic lesions of the amygdala markedly reduced cataplexy in orexin knockout mice [50]. In short, cataplexy could be due to a phasic activation of SLD neurons by central amygdala neurons, normally counterbalanced by an increased phasic GABAergic inhibition from vlPAG/dDpMe neurons. Notably, our hypothesis implies that the projection from central amygdala neurons specific to the REM sleep-on SLD neurons is responsible for muscle atonia projecting to GABA/glycinergic premotoneurons and not to those responsible for REM sleep itself or the EEG activation. Indeed, in such a case, a full REM sleep episode would be induced. Cataplexy would be inhibited in narcoleptic patients treated with SNRIs or α_1-adrenergic agonists by means of an increased excitation of the GABAergic REM sleep-off neurons. EDS, sleep paralysis, and hypnagogic hallucinations suggest that the Hcrt neurons might inhibit and delay the onset of REM sleep and strongly contribute to the abrupt cessation of REM sleep episodes, in line with the increase in their firing before the end of a REM sleep episode [30]. In their absence, the onset of REM sleep could occur more quickly and the end of REM sleep might take more time, leading to hypnagogic hallucinations and sleep paralysis, respectively. The inhibition of REM sleep by hypocretinergic neurons would be directly by means of excitation of the REM sleep-off GABAergic and aminergic neurons.

Acknowledgements

This work was supported by CNRS and University Claude Bernard of Lyon.

References

1. Aserinsky E, Kleitman N. Regularly occurring periods of eye motility and concomitant phenomena during sleep. Science 1953;118:273–4.
2. Dement W, Kleitman N. The relation of eye movements during sleep to dream activity: an objective method for the study of dreaming. J Exp Psychol 1957;53:339–46.
3. Jouvet M, Michel, F. Corrélations électromyographiques du sommeil chez le chat décortiqué et mésencéphalique chronique. C R Seances Soc Biol Fil 1959;153:422–5.
4. Jouvet M, Michel F, Courjon J. Sur un stade d'activité électrique cérébrale rapide au cours du sommeil physiologique. C R Seances Soc Biol Fil 1959;153:1024–8.
5. Jouvet M. Recherches sur les structures nerveuses et les mécanismes responsables des différentes phases du sommeil physiologique. Arch Ital Biol 1962;100:125–206.
6. Sakai K, Sastre JP, et al. State-specific neurones in the ponto-medullary reticular formation with special reference to the postural atonia during paradoxical sleep in the cat. In: Pompeiano O, Aimone Marsan C, eds. Brain mechanisms of perceptual awareness and purposeful behavior. New York: Raven Press, 1981:405–29.
7. Boissard R, Gervasoni D, Schmidt MH, et al. The rat ponto-medullary network responsible for paradoxical sleep onset and maintenance: a combined microinjection and functional neuroanatomical study. Eur J Neurosci 2002;16:1959–73.
8. Verret L, Leger L, Fort P, Luppi PH. Cholinergic and noncholinergic brainstem neurons expressing Fos after paradoxical (REM) sleep deprivation and recovery. Eur J Neurosci 2005;21:2488–504.
9. Grace KP, Vanstone LE, Horner RL. Endogenous cholinergic input to the pontine REM sleep generator is not required for REM sleep to occur. J Neurosci 2014;34:14198–209.
10. Boucetta S, Cisse Y, Mainville L, et al. Discharge profiles across the sleep–waking cycle of identified cholinergic, GABAergic, and glutamatergic neurons in the pontomesencephalic tegmentum of the rat. J Neurosci 2014;34:4708–27.
11. Van Dort CJ, Zachs DP, Kenny JD, et al. Optogenetic activation of cholinergic neurons in the PPT or LDT induces REM sleep. Proc Natl Acad Sci U S A 2015;112:584–9.
12. Sapin., Lapray D, Berod A, et al. Localization of the brainstem GABAergic neurons controlling paradoxical (REM) sleep. PLoS One 2009;4:e4272.
13. Clement O, Sapin E, Berod A, et al. Evidence that neurons of the sublaterodorsal tegmental nucleus triggering paradoxical (REM) sleep are glutamatergic. Sleep 2011;34:419–23.
14. Holstege JC, Bongers CM. A glycinergic projection from the ventromedial lower brainstem to spinal motoneurons. An ultrastructural double labeling study in rat. Brain Res 1991;566:308–15.
15. Brooks P, Peever J. Role for GABAB-mediated inhibition in the control of somatic motoneurons during REM sleep. Society for Neuroscience Meeting, SFN (Abstract) 2009.
16. Brooks PL, Peever JH. Identification of the transmitter and receptor mechanisms responsible for REM sleep paralysis. J Neurosci 2012;32:9785–95.
17. Boissard R, Fort P, Gervasoni D, et al. Localization of the GABAergic and non-GABAergic neurons projecting to the sublaterodorsal nucleus and potentially gating paradoxical sleep onset. Eur J Neurosci 2003;18:1627–39.
18. Hobson JA, Mccarley RW, Wyzinski PW. Sleep cycle oscillation: reciprocal discharge by two brainstem neuronal groups. Science 1975;189:55–8.
19. Lee MG, Hassani OK, Jones BE. Discharge of identified orexin/hypocretin neurons across the sleep–waking cycle. J Neurosci 2005;25:6716–20.
20. Luppi PH, Clement O, Sapin E, et al. The neuronal network responsible for paradoxical sleep and its dysfunctions causing narcolepsy and rapid eye movement (REM) behavior disorder. Sleep Med Rev 2011;15:153–63.
21. Crochet S, Sakai K. Alpha-2 adrenoceptor mediated paradoxical (REM) sleep inhibition in the cat. Neuroreport 1999;10:2199–204.
22. Leger L, Goutagny R, Sapin E, et al. Noradrenergic neurons expressing Fos during waking and paradoxical sleep deprivation in the rat. J Chem Neuroanat 2009;37:149–57.
23. Gervasoni D, Darracq L, Fort P, et al. Electrophysiological evidence that noradrenergic neurons of the rat locus coeruleus are tonically inhibited by GABA during sleep. Eur J Neurosci 1998;10:964–70.
24. Gervasoni D, Peyron C, Rampon C, et al. Role and origin of the GABAergic innervation of dorsal raphe serotonergic neurons. J Neurosci 2000;20:4217–25.
25. Verret L, Fort P, Gervasoni D, et al. Localization of the neurons active during paradoxical (REM) sleep and projecting to the locus coeruleus noradrenergic neurons in the rat. J Comp Neurol 2006;495:573–86.
26. Goutagny R, Luppi PH, Salvert D, et al. Role of the dorsal paragigantocellular reticular nucleus in paradoxical (rapid eye movement) sleep generation: a combined electrophysiological and anatomical study in the rat. Neuroscience 2008;152:849–57.
27. Verret L, Goutagny R, Fort P, et al. A role of melanin-concentrating hormone producing neurons in the central regulation of paradoxical sleep. BMC Neurosci 2003;4:19.
28. Sapin E, Berod A, Leger L, et al. A very large number of GABAergic neurons are activated in the tuberal hypothalamus during paradoxical (REM) sleep hypersomnia. PLoS One 2010;5:e11766.
29. Jego S, Salvert D, Renouard L, et al. tuberal hypothalamic neurons secreting the satiety molecule nesfatin-1 are critically involved in paradoxical (REM) sleep homeostasis. PLoS One 2012;7:e52525.
30. Hassani OK, Lee MG, Jones BE. Melanin-concentrating hormone neurons discharge in a reciprocal manner to orexin neurons across the sleep–wake cycle. Proc Natl Acad Sci U S A 2009;106:2418–22.
31. Konadhode RR, Pelluru D, Blanco-Centurion C, et al. Optogenetic stimulation of MCH neurons increases sleep. J Neurosci 2013;33:10257–63.

32. Jego S, Glasgow SD, Herrera CG, et al. Optogenetic identification of a rapid eye movement sleep modulatory circuit in the hypothalamus. Nat Neurosci 2013;16:1637–43.

33. Hassani OK, Henny P, Lee MG, Jones BE. GABAergic neurons intermingled with orexin and MCH neurons in the lateral hypothalamus discharge maximally during sleep. Eur J Neurosci 2010;32:448–57.

34. Qu D, Ludwig DS, Gammeltoft S, et al. A role for melanin-concentrating hormone in the central regulation of feeding behaviour. Nature 1996;380:243–7.

35. Van Den Pol AN, Acuna-Goycolea C, Clark KR, Ghosh PK. Physiological properties of hypothalamic MCH neurons identified with selective expression of reporter gene after recombinant virus infection. Neuron 2004;42:635–52.

36. Iranzo A, Santamaria J, Tolosa E. The clinical and pathophysiological relevance of REM sleep behavior disorder in neurodegenerative diseases. Sleep Med Rev 2009;13:385–401.

37. Sastre JP, Jouvet M. Le comportement onirique du chat [Oneiric behavior in cats]. Physiol Behav 1979;22:979–89.

38. Holmes CJ, Jones BE. Importance of cholinergic, GABAergic, serotonergic and other neurons in the medial medullary reticular formation for sleep-wake states studied by cytotoxic lesions in the cat. Neuroscience 1994;62:1179–200.

39. Xi MC, Fung SJ, Yamuy J, et al. Induction of active (REM) sleep and motor inhibition by hypocretin in the nucleus pontis oralis of the cat. J Neurophysiol 2002;87:2880–8.

40. Dauvilliers Y, Billiard M, Montplaisir J. Clinical aspects and pathophysiology of narcolepsy. Clin Neurophysiol 2003;114:2000–17.

41. Lin L, Faraco J, Li R, et al. The sleep disorder canine narcolepsy is caused by a mutation in the hypocretin (orexin) receptor 2 gene. Cell 1999;98:365–76.

42. Chemelli RM, Willie JT, Sinton CM, et al. Narcolepsy in orexin knockout mice: molecular genetics of sleep regulation. Cell 1999;98:437–51.

43. Peyron C, Faraco J, Rogers W, et al. A mutation in a case of early onset narcolepsy and a generalized absence of hypocretin peptides in human narcoleptic brains. Nat Med 2000;6:991–7.

44. Peyron C, Tighe DK, Van Den Pol AN, et al. Neurons containing hypocretin (orexin) project to multiple neuronal systems. J Neurosci 1998;18:9996–10015.

45. Huang ZL, Qu WM, Li WD, et al. Arousal effect of orexin A depends on activation of the histaminergic system. Proc Natl Acad Sci U S A 2001;98:9965–70.

46. Hagan JJ, Leslie RA, Patel S, et al. Orexin A activates locus coeruleus cell firing and increases arousal in the rat. Proc Natl Acad Sci U S A 1999;96:10911–6.

47. Hasegawa E, Yanagisawa M, Sakurai T, Mieda M. Orexin neurons suppress narcolepsy via 2 distinct efferent pathways. J Clin Invest 2014;124:604–16.

48. Van Nieuwenhuijzen PS, Mcgregor IS, Hunt GE. The distribution of gamma-hydroxybutyrate-induced Fos expression in rat brain: comparison with baclofen. Neuroscience 2009;158:441–55.

49. Jha SK, Ross RJ, Morrison AR. Sleep-related neurons in the central nucleus of the amygdala of rats and their modulation by the dorsal raphe nucleus. Physiol Behav 2005;86:415–26.

50. Burgess CR, Oishi Y, Mochizuki T, et al. Amygdala lesions reduce cataplexy in orexin knock-out mice. J Neurosci 2013;33:9734–42.

CHAPTER 4

Neuroanatomical, neurochemical, and neurophysiological bases of waking and sleeping

Barbara E. Jones

Introduction

Over the past century, studying the basic mechanisms of sleep–wake states has evolved from dissecting the principal neuroanatomical structures to identifying the important chemical neurotransmitters and revealing the precise physiological discharge by which specific neural systems influence the brain and body for execution of waking or sleeping (Fig. 4.1).

In both animals and humans, the sleep–wake cycle is actually composed of three distinct states: waking (W); non-REM (NREM) sleep, including slow-wave sleep (SWS); and REM sleep. W is characterized by prominent fast activity recorded on the cerebral cortex (EEG, upper left in Fig. 4.1), particularly in a gamma frequency range (30–60 Hz and up to 120 Hz), together with continuous postural muscle tone (on the EMG, lower right in Fig. 4.1). SWS is characterized by attenuated fast activity and prominent slow activity, particularly in a delta frequency range (0.5–<4 Hz), together with a decrease in postural muscle tone. REM sleep is characterized by moderate fast EEG activity, paradoxically occurring during behavioral sleep with the total absence of postural muscle tone on the EMG, or muscle atonia, which was originally discovered by Jouvet [1], who thus called this state paradoxical sleep (PS, a name still used today) in animals.

Neuroanatomical substrates of sleep–wake state systems

Since the early work of Moruzzi and Magoun [2,3], it has been known that the neurons distributed through the core of the brainstem in the mesencephalic, pontine, and medullary reticular formation (RF) are essential for maintaining a waking state with cortical activation and postural muscle tone along with behavioral arousal and responsiveness (Fig. 4.1). Within this core, the neurons in the oral pontine and mesencephalic RF are most important for cortical activation and form the ascending reticular activating system. They project rostrally along a dorsal course to the thalamus, where neurons of the nonspecific thalamocortical projection system project in turn in a widespread manner to the cerebral cortex to stimulate cortical activation. They also project ventrally into and through the hypothalamus up to the basal forebrain, where neurons of the basalocortical system also project in turn in a widespread manner to the cerebral cortex to stimulate cortical activation. Some neurons in the medullary RF also give rise to ascending projections by which they can influence other neurons in the rostral brainstem. By certain of these, SWS can be promoted. But the medullary RF neurons are most prominently involved in the modulation of movement and muscle tone, some enhancing during waking, others inhibiting muscle tone to induce muscle atonia of REM sleep via descending projections to the spinal cord.

Also in early work, von Economo [4] revealed the important role of the hypothalamus in controlling sleep–wake states (Fig. 4.1). From neuropathological analysis of brains from patients with encephalitis lethargica, he associated symptoms of insomnia with lesions of the anterior hypothalamus and those of coma with lesions of the posterior hypothalamus (PH) and thus proposed the existence in the hypothalamus of opponent sleep and wake centers, a notion later confirmed experimentally in animals by Nauta [5]. Later work indicated the additional importance of the more anterior preoptic area (POA), including the ventrolateral preoptic nucleus (VLPO), in the promotion of sleep (Fig. 4.1) [6,7].

These early studies and their later pursuit have revealed a continuous reticular core through the brainstem, diencephalon, and basal telencephalon where neurons promoting cortical activation and/or behavioral arousal with waking appear to be concentrated at certain levels and those promoting cortical deactivation and/or behavioral quiescence at other levels. These different neuronal clusters could effect their state alterations through local projections to other levels of the reticular core and long projections ascending to the cerebral cortex or descending to the spinal cord (Fig. 4.1).

Neurochemical identity and neurophysiological properties of sleep–wake neural systems

First through pharmacological evidence, then through histochemical studies, the important roles of particular chemical neurotransmitters and their neurons in sleep–wake state control became evident, pioneered in large part by Jouvet [8].

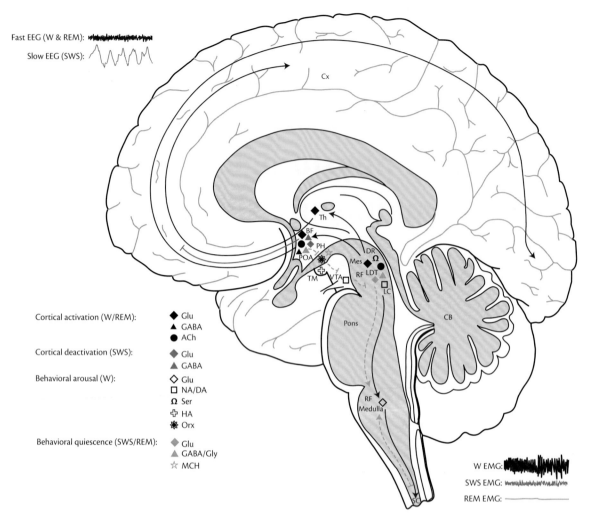

Fast EEG (W & REM):
Slow EEG (SWS):

Cortical activation (W/REM):
◆ Glu
▲ GABA
● ACh

Cortical deactivation (SWS):
◆ Glu
▲ GABA

Behavioral arousal (W):
◇ Glu
☐ NA/DA
Ω Ser
✚ HA
✳ Orx

Behavioral quiescence (SWS/REM):
◆ Glu
▲ GABA/Gly
☆ MCH

W EMG:
SWS EMG:
REM EMG:

Fig. 4.1 (See colour plate section) Sleep–wake state substrates. Sagittal schematic view of the human brain depicting neurons with their chemical neurotransmitters and pathways by which they influence cortical activity or behavior across the sleep-wake cycle. Neurons that are active during waking (red symbols) include cells with ascending projections toward the cortex, which stimulate cortical activation, and cells with descending projections toward the spinal cord, which stimulate behavioral arousal with postural muscle tone. Those with predominantly ascending projections discharge in association with fast, gamma EEG activity and cease firing with slow, delta activity to be active during both W and REM sleep (W/REM or W/PS, filled red symbols); they include neurons that release glutamate (Glu, diamonds), GABA (triangles) or acetylcholine (ACh, circles) (W/PS-max active, Fig. 4.2). Those with more diffuse or descending projections discharge in association with behavioral arousal and EMG activity and cease firing with muscle atonia to be active during W and silent during REM (W, empty red symbols); they include neurons that release glutamate (Glu, diamonds), noradrenaline (NA, square), serotonin (Ser, omega), histamine (HA, cross) or orexin (Orx, asterisk) (W-max active, Figs. 4.4 and 4.7). Neurons that are active during sleep (blue or aqua symbols) include cells with ascending projections toward the cortex, which dampen fast cortical activity, and those with descending projections toward the hypothalamus, brainstem or spinal cord, which diminish behavioral arousal and muscle tone. Those sleep-active neurons with ascending projections to the cortex or local relay neurons discharge in association with slow EEG activity during SWS (SWS, blue triangle; SWS-max active, Fig. 4.3). They include GABAergic neurons that can inhibit other W/REM cortical or subcortical neurons. Those sleep-active neurons with descending projections to the spinal cord or local relay neurons discharge in association with decreasing muscle tone and EMG (SWS/REM, aqua diamonds and triangles; PS-max active see Figs. 4.5 and 4.6). They include GABAergic neurons in the basal forebrain, preoptic area, hypothalamus and brainstem that can inhibit other W neurons, including Glu, MA or Orx neurons. They also include MCH neurons (aqua star, PS-max active, Fig. 4.7), which have more diffuse projections but can exert an inhibitory influence upon other neurons of the arousal systems including the MA, HA and Orx neurons. SWS/REM GABAergic neurons, which can also contain glycine (GABA/Gly), in the ventral medullary RF can inhibit motor neurons in the brainstem and spinal cord, particularly during REM sleep. BF, basal forebrain; CB, cerebellum; Cx, cortex; DR, dorsal raphe; LC, locus coeruleus nucleus; LDT, laterodorsal tegmental nucleus; Mes, mesencephalon; PH, posterior hypothalamus; POA, preoptic area; RF, reticular formation; SC, spinal cord; Th, thalamus; TM, tuberomammillary nucleus; VTA, ventral tegmental area.

Adapted from Jones BE, "Neurobiology of waking and sleeping" from Vinken PJ and Bruyn GW (eds), Handbook of clinical neurology, pp. 131–49, Copyright (2011), with permission from Elsevier.

Catecholamine systems

Through the actions of drugs associated with enhanced synaptic levels of catecholamines, such as amphetamine, it is clear that dopamine (DA), noradrenaline (norepinephrine) (NA) and adrenaline (epinephrine) (A) have the capacity to promote both cortical activation and behavioral arousal. Containing different synthetic enzymes,

A-containing neurons are located within the medulla, concentrated in regions associated with cardiorespiratory regulation (not shown); NA-containing neurons are predominantly located within the pontine tegmentum and concentrated within the locus coeruleus (LC); and DA-containing neurons are located in the mesencephalic tegmentum in the substantia nigra (SN) and ventral tegmental area

(VTA) (Fig. 4.1). In early studies involving lesions of these neurons, it appeared that NA neurons are important for promoting cortical activation of W and DA neurons for behavioral arousal and movement during W [8,9]. The NA LC neurons give rise to diffuse projections locally into the RF and distally to the thalamus, hypothalamus, and basal forebrain, where they relay onto cortically projecting neurons, while also continuing directly to the cerebral cortex [10]. They also project to the spinal cord. Thus, through varicose fibers and extensive collateralization similar to peripheral sympathetic nerves, single NA LC neurons can simultaneously influence the entire brain and spinal cord. LC neurons discharge selectively during W and become silent during REM(PS) [11,12]. Through their actions upon different adrenergic receptors, they would accordingly have the capacity to simultaneously stimulate cortical activation and behavioral arousal with postural muscle tone. The role of DA SN and VTA neurons is more ambiguous, since they continue to discharge through the sleep–wake cycle, including REM(PS) sleep, when they may burst as during waking in association with emotive situations [13]. Their role in stimulating movement during waking, as evidenced in their absence in patients with Parkinson disease, is thus less direct than that of LC NA neurons and may be overridden by other inhibitory mechanisms during REM(PS) sleep. On the other hand, their role in emotive behavior may contribute during REM(PS) to the emotive content of dreams.

Serotonin neurons

Also located in the brainstem, serotonin (Ser)-containing neurons are situated in midline, raphe nuclei through the medulla, pons, and mesencephalon. These neurons give rise to different projections, such that those in the medulla project predominantly to the brainstem and spinal cord, whereas those in the pons and mesencephalon, such as in the dorsal raphe (DR), give rise to ascending projections to provide the major Ser innervation to the forebrain, including the cerebral cortex (Fig. 4.1). The latter projections are widespread, yet not diffuse like the NA ones. Ser neurons were once thought to play an important role in promoting sleep, since lesions of the raphe nuclei resulted in insomnia [8]. However, the presumed Ser raphe neurons were found to discharge during waking and actually be silent, like the NA neurons, during SWS and REM(PS) sleep (14). Ser also appears to have a facilitatory role in motor activity and muscle tone. However, there is evidence that Ser can dampen cortical activation through its actions upon other relay neurons [15]. Single-unit recording studies have indicated that Ser neurons may facilitate rhythmic motor activity, such as grooming [16], which could be associated with a more quiet behavioral waking stage.

Clustered in the PH within the tuberomammillary nucleus (TM), histamine (HA)-containing neurons also play a role in promoting waking. Like the NA LC neurons, HA neurons give rise to diffuse projections through the forebrain and brainstem. Their role in promoting waking is particularly known through the pharmacological effects of antihistamine drugs that produce sleepiness. From animal experimental work, HA appears to be particularly important for attentive waking [17]. Like other monoamine (MA) neurons, the HA TM neurons discharge selectively during waking, particularly vigilant waking, and are silent during SWS and REM(PS) sleep [18]. Their role appears to be more prominent in stimulating cortical activation than in affecting muscle tone [19].

These neuromodulatory MA systems function together in partially redundant arousal systems, since no one system has proven to be essential for the maintenance of waking [20,21]. They also appear to play slightly different roles in waking behaviors.

Acetylcholine neurons

Neurons utilizing acetylcholine (ACh) have long been known to play an important role in stimulating cortical activation [22]. Indeed, the ascending reticular activating system was once considered to be the cholinergic reticular activating system based upon early histochemical and pharmacological studies. With immunohistochemical studies, it became evident that ACh-containing neurons were distributed in clusters through the reticular core, in the medullary RF (not shown), in the pontomesencephalic tegmentum within the laterodorsal tegmental nucleus (LDT) and adjoining the SubLDT and pedunculopontine tegmental nuclei (SubLDT and PPT, not shown), and in the basal forebrain (BF) (Fig. 4.1). The ACh neurons in the medulla project locally into the RF and also to the spinal cord. Those in the LDT, SubLDT, and PPT project in parallel with other neurons of the RF, first locally into the brainstem RF and most prominently into the forebrain and distally into the thalamus onto the nonspecific thalamocortical projection system. They also send some fibers into the hypothalamus and BF and a few directly up to the prefrontal cortex. The ACh neurons in the BF project in a widespread, though also topographical, manner to the cerebral cortex, where, through muscarinic and nicotinic receptors on different target neurons, they promote cortical activation [23]. However, in contrast to the MA neurons, which can also promote cortical activation, ACh neurons do not appear to promote behavioral arousal with muscle tone. On the contrary, they appear to promote cortical activation with loss of muscle tone, as occurs during natural REM(PS) sleep and narcolepsy with cataplexy [24]. Indeed, it was established by unit recording studies that, in contrast to the MA neurons, ACh neurons in the BF and LDT/SubLDT/PPT discharge in association with cortical activation (with high gamma EEG activity) during both W and PS (Fig. 4.2) [25–27]. They are silent during SWS. Their discharge is thus positively correlated with gamma EEG activity and not correlated with EMG activity across the sleep–wake cycle. Likely dependent upon the simultaneous activity or inactivity of other arousal systems, such as the NA LC neurons (or Orx neurons, discussed later in this section), ACh can induce cortical activation with either behavioral arousal or muscle atonia and PS. This conditional role of ACh neurons is evident from the induction of REM(PS) pharmacologically with systemic or local enhancement of synaptic ACh (by, for example, cholinesterase inhibitors) or activation of ACh receptors (by, for example, carbachol) under conditions of MA depletion or loss of other arousal systems [22,28]. The importance of the ACh LDT/SubLDT/PPT neurons in the promotion of PS with muscle atonia was indicated by the loss of PS following their destruction [29]. However, these neurotoxic lesions also destroyed other non-ACh neurons situated in the same region.

GABA and glutamate neurons

Like other neurons through the reticular core, the ACh neurons lie intermingled with many other noncholinergic neurons. These include large populations of GABA-containing and Glutamate (Glu)-containing neurons (Fig. 4.1). Unlike the ACh and MA neurons, these cell populations are functionally heterogeneous. In each region, they include different functional subtypes and as such can modulate different parameters of waking or sleeping.

First of all, intermingled with the ACh neurons in both the BF and LDT/SubLDT/PPT, are both GABA and Glu neurons, which discharge in parallel with the ACh neurons during both W and

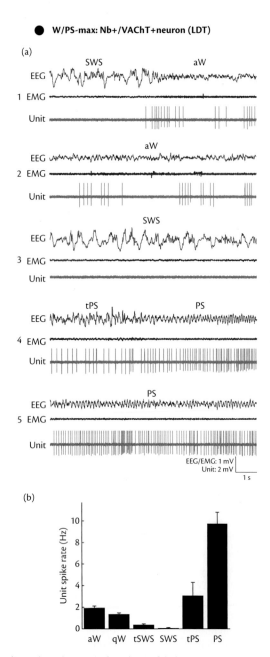

Fig. 4.2 (See colour plate section) Discharge of cholinergic W/PS-max active unit across sleep–wake states in rat. Data from a recorded, Neurobiotin (Nb)-labeled cell (#CBS28U03) that was identified as immunopositive for vesicular ACh transporter (VAChT) and located in the LDT. (a) Polygraphic records from 10 s epochs or periods of the unit together with EEG (from retrosplenial cortex) and EMG activity during a transition from SWS to aW (1), aW (2), SWS (3), a transition from tPS to PS (4), and PS (5). (b) Bar graph showing mean spike rate of the unit across sleep–wake stages. Note that during W (2), the unit discharged tonically at a slow rate (1.91 Hz) with prominence of fast EEG activity, ceased firing during SWS (3) (0.06 Hz) in association with slow EEG activity (~1–4 Hz), and discharged maximally and tonically to reach its highest rates during PS (5) (9.70 Hz) in association with prominent rhythmic theta (~6–8 Hz) along with fast EEG activity. It changed its rate of discharge prior to cortical activation in the transition from SWS to aW (1) and prior to PS during tPS (4) as EEG activity progresses to theta. The unit discharge was significantly positively correlated with EEG gamma ($r = 0.37$) along with theta activity ($r = 0.93$). aW: active wake; qW: quiet wake; tSWS: transition to slow-wave sleep; SWS: slow-wave sleep; tPS: transition to paradoxical sleep; PS: paradoxical sleep.

Reproduced from J Neurosci, 34(13), Boucetta S, Cisse Y, Mainville L, Morales M, Jones BE, Discharge Profiles across the Sleep–Waking Cycle of Identified Cholinergic, GABAergic, and Glutamatergic Neurons in the Pontomesencephalic Tegmentum of the Rat, pp. 4708–27, Copyright (2014), with permission from Society for Neuroscience.

PS and in association with cortical activation (Figs. 4.1 and 4.2) [26,27]. Such neurons are likely distributed through the RF in what is the large population of neurons contributing to the ascending reticular activating system (RF) and its relays in the nonspecific thalamocortical (Th) and basalocortical (BF) projection systems. Precisely why there are both GABA and Glu neurons with such an activity profile and projections remains to be understood, since GABA is the major inhibitory neurotransmitter and Glu the major excitatory neurotransmitter in the brain. Depending upon the target neurons in the cortex, however, as interneurons or projection neurons, both GABA and Glu neurons could produce increased excitability and activity of pyramidal neurons. In addition, GABA neurons, which are generally fast-spiking neurons, can also serve to pace activity in certain target neurons.

Second, there are GABA and Glu neurons that discharge in a reciprocal manner to the ACh neurons, being maximally active during SWS (Figs. 4.1 and 4.3). Though not very numerous, these SWS-max active neurons have been found in the BF and hypothalamus [26,30]. Chemically unidentified neurons with this discharge profile have also been identified in the preoptic area (POA) [31], including the ventrolateral preoptic area (VLPO) [32], where, as in the BF, GABA neurons that are active during sleep and inhibited by NA have been identified [33,34]. Here again, the fact that there are both GABA and Glu neurons with a sleep-active profile of discharge suggests that inhibition of one population of cells during excitation of another is integral to the sleep–wake cycle.

Third, there are Glu neurons that discharge during W and progressively decrease their discharge during sleep to become silent during PS with muscle atonia (Figs. 4.1 and 4.4). These W-max active Glu neurons have been recorded in the BF and LDT/SubLDT/PPT [26,27], though they are presumed to be present more widely through the RF. (Only two W-max active GABA neurons have yet to be identified, one in BF and one in LH (Hassani, Boucetta, and Jones, unpublished data).) The discharge of the W-max active Glu neurons is positively correlated with EMG activity. They are thus presumed to give rise to local and descending projections by which they may stimulate muscle tone and behavioral arousal.

Fourth, there are Glu and GABA neurons that discharge minimally during W and maximally during PS (Figs. 4.1, 4.5, and 4.6). Such identified Glu and GABA PS-max active neurons have been recorded in the BF, hypothalamus, and LDT/SubLDT/PPT, but are presumed to be distributed more widely through the reticular core [26,27,30]. Glu PS-max active neurons have been recorded in the BF and LDT/SubLDT/PPT regions, including the SubLDT (ventral to the LDT), a region that, together with the more caudal subcoeruleus (ventral to the LC), corresponds to an area where lesions produce a marked loss of PS and muscle atonia [35–37]. These Glu PS-max active neurons could exert an excitatory action upon other GABA or GABA/glycine (Gly) PS-max active neurons. The GABA PS-max active neurons likely correspond to those identified by c-Fos, an indicator of enhanced neural activity, in studies of PS rebound following deprivation [38–41]. They likely comprise GABAergic neurons in various regions that have the capacity to inhibit other W-active neurons, including the W-max active Glu neurons in BF, PH, and LDT/SubLDT/PPT or RF, the NA and Ser neurons in the brainstem, the HA neurons (and Orx neurons, discussed later in this section) in the PH. They would also likely comprise the GABA/Gly neurons in the medulla, which can inhibit motor neurons in the brainstem or spinal cord during PS (Fig. 4.1) [42,43].

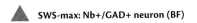

▲ SWS-max: Nb+/GAD+ neuron (BF)

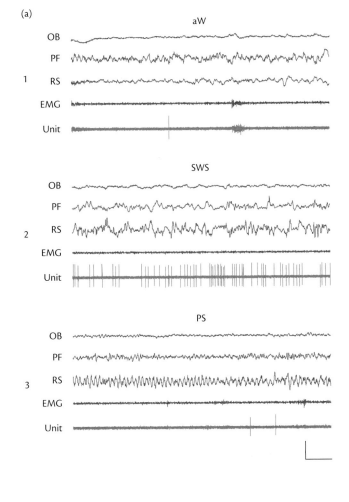

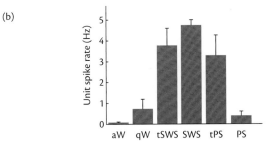

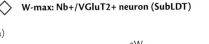

◇ W-max: Nb+/VGluT2+ neuron (SubLDT)

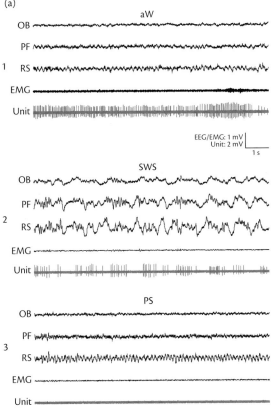

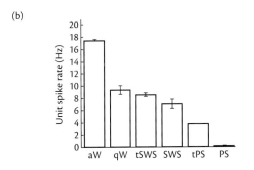

According to these neurochemical and neurophysiological findings, it appears that the major effector neurons of waking and sleeping and their cortical and peripheral variables are Glu and GABA neurons distributed through the reticular core of the brainstem

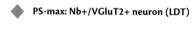 **PS-max: Nb+/VGluT2+ neuron (LDT)**

(a)

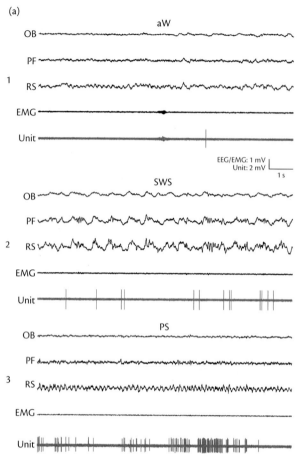

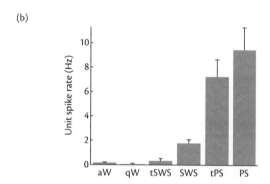

(b)

PS-max: Nb+/GAD+ neuron (SubLDT)

(a)

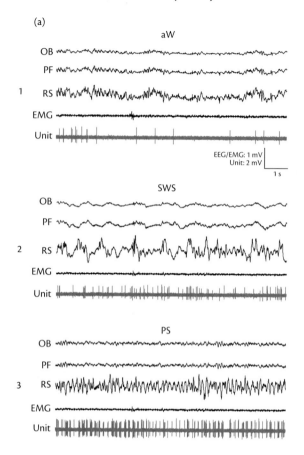

(b)

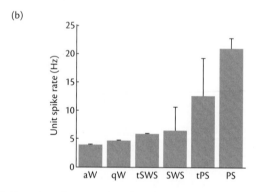

Fig. 4.5 (See colour plate section) Discharge of glutamatergic PS-max active unit across sleep–wake states in rat. Data from a recorded, Nb-labeled cell (#CBS46U02) that that was identified by in situ hybridization as expressing VGluT2 and was located in the LDT. (a, b) Note that this VGluT2+ cell discharged at its lowest rates during aW (1) (0.13 Hz) with fast EEG activity and high neck muscle tone, increased its firing during SWS (2) (1.77 Hz) in association with slow EEG activity and low muscle tone, and discharged maximally to reach its highest rate during PS (3) (9.42 Hz) in association with theta EEG activity and muscle atonia. It increased its rate most markedly preceding PS during tPS.

Reproduced from J Neurosci, 34(13), Boucetta S, Cisse Y, Mainville L, Morales M, Jones BE, Discharge Profiles across the Sleep-Waking Cycle of Identified Cholinergic, GABAergic, and Glutamatergic Neurons in the Pontomesencephalic Tegmentum of the Rat, pp. 4708–27, Copyright (2014), with permission from Society for Neuroscience.

Fig. 4.6 (See colour plate section) Discharge of GABAergic PS-max active unit across sleep–wake states in rat. Data from recorded, Nb-labeled cell (#CBS28U04) that was immunopositive for GAD and located in the SubLDT. (a, b) Note that this GAD+ cell discharged at relatively low rates during aW (1) (3.90 Hz) with fast EEG activity and high EMG amplitude, increased firing during SWS (2) (6.05 Hz) in association with slow delta EEG activity and low muscle EMG, and discharged maximally during PS (3) (20.98 Hz) with theta and fast EEG activity accompanied by muscle atonia. It increased its discharge most markedly immediately preceding PS during tPS. The unit discharge was positively correlated with EEG theta activity ($r = 0.53$) and negatively correlated with EMG amplitude ($r = -0.45$).

Reproduced from J Neurosci, 34(13), Boucetta S, Cisse Y, Mainville L, Morales M, Jones BE, Discharge Profiles across the Sleep-Waking Cycle of Identified Cholinergic, GABAergic, and Glutamatergic Neurons in the Pontomesencephalic Tegmentum of the Rat, pp. 4708–27, Copyright (2014), with permission from Society for Neuroscience.

and subcortical forebrain. The alternating activity of different W/PS-max active versus SWS-max active and W-max active versus PS-max active neurons would determine the cyclic changes in EEG activity from fast to slow and EMG activity from tonic to atonic, corresponding to cortical activation to deactivation and behavioral arousal to quiescence (Fig. 4.1). Owing to oscillations in these reciprocally active and interacting cell groups, a sleep–wake cycle with three states can emerge. These oscillations and resulting states are modulated by MA and ACh, which act through their diverse receptors differentially upon the executive Glu and GABA neurons. Other important modulators of these systems are the neuropeptides, which have yet slower actions than the MA and ACh.

Orexin neurons

With the discovery that mice lacking orexin (Orx, also called hypocretin) and dogs lacking the receptor for Orx were afflicted with narcolepsy with cataplexy [44,45], it became evident that the Orx neuropeptide was essential for the maintenance of waking with muscle tone (Fig. 4.1). Orx-containing neurons are located in the PH in that region originally found to be important for the maintenance of waking. Like NA LC neurons, they give rise to highly diffuse projections through the entire brain and spinal cord, with one neuron able to reach the cortex and spinal cord [46,47]. Under normal conditions, they are excited by all other arousal systems and excite in turn all other arousal systems, including the NA, DA,

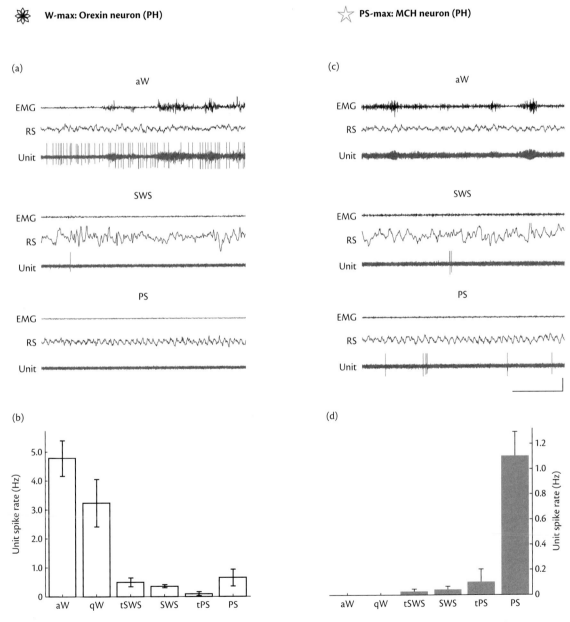

Fig. 4.7 (See colour plate section) Reciprocal discharge profile of Orx and MCH neurons across sleep-wake states in rat. (a, b) The mean spike rate per stage of Nb$^+$/Orx$^+$ units ($n = 6$; from [53]) varies in a reciprocal manner to that of Nb$^+$/MCH$^+$ units (c, d). The reciprocal firing profiles were not correlated with EEG gamma or delta activity, but were correlated in an inverse manner with EMG amplitude, positively for the wake-active Orx neurons and negatively for the MCH sleep-active neurons.

Reproduced from Proc Natl Acad Sci U S A, 106(7), Hassani OK, Lee MG, Jones BE, Melanin-concentrating hormone neurons discharge in a reciprocal manner to orexin neurons across the sleep–wake cycle, pp. 2418–22, Copyright (2009), with permission from National Academy of Sciences.

Ser, HA, ACh basalocortical, and Glu thalamocortical systems [48]. They can also directly excite neurons in the cerebral cortex [49] and motor neurons in the spinal cord [50]. Moreover, they release Glu in addition to Orx from certain terminals [51,52]. In unit recording studies, it was found that Orx neurons discharge during waking and become silent during sleep, as W-max active neurons (Fig. 4.7) [53,54]. When specifically activated by optogenetic stimulation during sleep, they promote awakening [55]. They can thus play a central role in stimulating and maintaining waking and do so by promoting both cortical activation and behavioral arousal with muscle tone, whereas, by their silence, they may permit the onset and maintenance of sleep, including REM(PS) sleep. Indeed, antagonists of the Orx receptors can facilitate the onset and progression of sleep along with loss of muscle tone [56].

Melanin concentrating hormone neurons

Melanin concentrating hormone (MCH) is contained in neurons that are partially overlapping in their distribution with Orx neurons in the PH (Fig. 4.1). When administered into the cerebral ventricles, MCH was found to promote sleep, including SWS and PS, and c-Fos, as an indicator of enhanced neural activity, was found in MCH neurons during SWS/PS rebound from total sleep or PS deprivation [57,58]. Most recently, specific optogenetic stimulation of MCH neurons has been shown to enhance sleep, both SWS and PS [59,60]. In unit recording studies, the MCH neurons were found to discharge in a reciprocal manner to the Orx neurons, being silent during W and discharging during sleep, minimally during SWS and maximally during PS as PS-max active neurons (Fig. 4.7) [61]. Given certain inhibitory actions of this peptide [62,63] and GABA, which is colocalized and released with MCH from certain terminals [64], MCH neurons can exert an inhibitory influence upon other arousal systems, including the NA LC and HA TM neurons. Moreover, the reciprocal profile of discharge between the W-active Orx neurons and the sleep-active MCH neurons may be mediated by reciprocal interactions between these cell groups [65].

Conclusion

The sleep–wake cycle is determined by populations of neurons that are distributed through the reticular core of the brainstem, hypothalamus, and basal forebrain. The principal effector neurons are functionally differentiated yet overlapping clusters of Glu and GABA neurons, which through different projections and profiles of discharge promote cortical activation versus deactivation or behavioral arousal versus quiescence in association with muscle tone versus atonia. The functionally different groups manifest reciprocal profiles of activity such as to suggest that through interlinked excitatory and inhibitory actions, accelerations in one group can lead to decelerations in another and thus reciprocal oscillations of activity that generate cyclic changes in cortical activity and behavior along with the three sleep–wake states. These Glu and GABA cell populations are influenced by other neuromodulatory systems that promote cortical activation by release of ACh selectively during W and REM(PS), promote behavioral arousal by release of NA, HA, or Orx selectively during W, or promote sleep by release of MCH during SWS/REM(PS).

Acknowledgements

I thank my colleagues and members of my laboratory, particularly Soufiane Boucetta, Oum Hassani and Maan Gee Lee, whose work (as cited) contributed greatly to the content of this chapter, and my sources of funding (the Canadian Institutes of Health Research (CIHR MOP-13458 and 82762) and the United States National Institutes of Health (NIH R01 MH-60119-01A)).

References

1. Jouvet M, Michel F, Courjon J. Sur un stade d'activité électrique cérébrale rapide au cours du sommeil physiologique. C R Seances Soc Biol Fil 1959;153:1024–8.
2. Moruzzi G, Magoun HW. Brain stem reticular formation and activation of the EEG. Electroencephalogr Clin Neurophysiol 1949;1:455–73.
3. Moruzzi G. The sleep–waking cycle. Ergeb Physiol 1972;64:1–165.
4. von Economo C. Sleep as a problem of localization. J Nerv Ment Dis 1930;71:249–59.
5. Nauta WJH. Hypothalamic regulation of sleep in rats. An experimental study. J Neurophysiol 1946;9:285–316.
6. McGinty DJ, Sterman MB. Sleep suppression after basal forebrain lesions in the cat. Science 1968;160:1253–5.
7. Sherin JE, Shiromani PJ, McCarley RW, Saper CB. Activation of ventrolateral preoptic neurons during sleep. Science 1996;271:216–19.
8. Jouvet M. The role of monoamines and acetylcholine-containing neurons in the regulation of the sleep–waking cycle. Ergeb Physiol 1972;64:165–307.
9. Jones BE, Bobillier P, Pin C, Jouvet M. The effect of lesions of catecholamine-containing neurons upon monoamine content of the brain and EEG and behavioral waking in the cat. Brain Res 1973;58:157–77.
10. Jones BE, Yang T-Z. The efferent projections from the reticular formation and the locus coeruleus studied by anterograde and retrograde axonal transport in the rat. J Comp Neurol 1985;242:56–92.
11. Hobson JA, McCarley RW, Wyzinski PW. Sleep cycle oscillation: reciprocal discharge by two brainstem neuronal groups. Science 1975;189:55–8.
12. Aston-Jones G, Bloom FE. Activity of norepinephrine-containing locus coeruleus neurons in behaving rats anticipates fluctuations in the sleep–waking cycle. J Neurosci 1981;1:876–86.
13. Dahan L, Astier B, Vautrelle N, Urbain N, Kocsis B, Chouvet G. Prominent burst firing of dopaminergic neurons in the ventral tegmental area during paradoxical sleep. Neuropsychopharmacology 2007;32:1232–41.
14. McGinty D, Harper RM. Dorsal raphe neurons: depression of firing during sleep in cats. Brain Res 1976;101:569–75.
15. Cape EG, Jones BE. Differential modulation of high-frequency gamma-electroencephalogram activity and sleep–wake state by noradrenaline and serotonin microinjections into the region of cholinergic basalis neurons. J Neurosci 1998;18:2653–66.
16. Jacobs BL, Fornal CA. 5-HT and motor control: a hypothesis. Trends Neurosci 1993;16:346–52.
17. Parmentier R, Ohtsu H, Djebbara-Hannas Z, et al. Anatomical, physiological, and pharmacological characteristics of histidine decarboxylase knock-out mice: evidence for the role of brain histamine in behavioral and sleep–wake control. J Neurosci 2002;22:7695–711.
18. Takahashi K, Lin JS, Sakai K. Neuronal activity of histaminergic tuberomammillary neurons during wake-sleep states in the mouse. J Neurosci 2006;26:10292–8.
19. John J, Wu MF, Boehmer LN, Siegel JM. Cataplexy-active neurons in the hypothalamus: implications for the role of histamine in sleep and waking behavior. Neuron 2004;42:619–34.

20. Jones BE, Harper ST, Halaris AE. Effects of locus coeruleus lesions upon cerebral monoamine content, sleep–wakefulness states and the response to amphetamine in the cat. Brain Res 1977;124:473–96.

21. Blanco-Centurion C, Gerashchenko D, Shiromani PJ. Effects of saporin-induced lesions of three arousal populations on daily levels of sleep and wake. J Neurosci 2007;27:14041–8.

22. Jones BE. The organization of central cholinergic systems and their functional importance in sleep-waking states. Prog Brain Res 1993;98:61–71.

23. Jones BE. Activity, modulation and role of basal forebrain cholinergic neurons innervating the cerebral cortex. Progr Brain Res 2004;145:157–69.

24. Nishino S, Tafti M, Reid MS, et al. Muscle atonia is triggered by cholinergic stimulation of the basal forebrain: implication for the pathophysiology of canine narcolepsy. J Neurosci 1995;15:4806–14.

25. Lee MG, Hassani OK, Alonso A, Jones BE. Cholinergic basal forebrain neurons burst with theta during waking and paradoxical sleep. J Neurosci 2005;25:4365–9.

26. Hassani OK, Lee MG, Henny P, Jones BE. Discharge profiles of identified GABAergic in comparison to cholinergic and putative glutamatergic basal forebrain neurons across the sleep–wake cycle. J Neurosci 2009;29:11828–40.

27. Boucetta S, Cisse Y, Mainville L, Morales M, Jones BE. discharge profiles across the sleep-waking cycle of identified cholinergic, GABAergic, and glutamatergic neurons in the pontomesencephalic tegmentum of the rat. J Neurosci 2014;34:4708–27.

28. Nishino S, Mignot E. Pharmacological aspects of human and canine narcolepsy. Prog Neurobiol 1997;52:27–78.

29. Webster HH, Jones BE. Neurotoxic lesions of the dorsolateral pontomesencephalic tegmentum-cholinergic cell area in the cat. II. Effects upon sleep–waking states. Brain Res 1988;458:285–302.

30. Hassani OK, Henny P, Lee MG, Jones BE. GABAergic neurons intermingled with orexin and MCH neurons in the lateral hypothalamus discharge maximally during sleep. Eur J Neurosci 2010;32:448–57.

31. Takahashi K, Lin JS, Sakai K. Characterization and mapping of sleep–waking specific neurons in the basal forebrain and preoptic hypothalamus in mice. Neuroscience. 2009;161:269–92.

32. Szymusiak R, Alam N, Steininger TL, McGinty D. Sleep–waking discharge patterns of ventrolateral preoptic/anterior hypothalamic neurons in rats. Brain Res 1998;803:178–88.

33. Gallopin T, Fort P, Eggermann E, et al. Identification of sleep-promoting neurons in vitro. Nature 2000;404:992–5.

34. Modirrousta M, Mainville L, Jones BE. GABAergic neurons with alpha2-adrenergic receptors in basal forebrain and preoptic area express c-Fos during sleep. Neuroscience 2004;129:803–10.

35. Sakai K, Sastre J-P, Salvert D, et al. Tegmentoreticular projections with special reference to the muscular atonia during paradoxical sleep in the cat: an HRP study. Brain Res 1979;176:233–54.

36. Friedman L, Jones BE. Computer graphics analysis of sleep–wakefulness state changes after pontine lesions. Brain Res Bull 1984;13:53–68.

37. Lu J, Sherman D, Devor M, Saper CB. A putative flip-flop switch for control of REM sleep. Nature 2006;441:589–94.

38. Maloney KJ, Mainville L, Jones BE. Differential c-Fos expression in cholinergic, monoaminergic and GABAergic cell groups of the pontomesencephalic tegmentum after paradoxical sleep deprivation and recovery. J Neurosci 1999;19:3057–72.

39. Maloney KJ, Mainville L, Jones BE. c-Fos expression in GABAergic, serotonergic and other neurons of the pontomedullary reticular formation and raphe after paradoxical sleep deprivation and recovery. J Neurosci 2000;20:4669–79.

40. Sapin E, Lapray D, Berod A, et al. Localization of the brainstem GABAergic neurons controlling paradoxical (REM) sleep. PLoS One 2009;4(1):e4272.

41. Sapin E, Berod A, Leger L, et al. A very large number of GABAergic neurons are activated in the tuberal hypothalamus during paradoxical (REM) sleep hypersomnia. PLoS One 2010;5(7):e11766.

42. Holmes CJ, Jones BE. Importance of cholinergic, GABAergic, serotonergic and other neurons in the medullary reticular formation for sleep–wake states studied by cytotoxic lesions in the cat. Neuroscience 1994;62:1179–200.

43. Boissard R, Gervasoni D, Schmidt MH, et al. The rat ponto-medullary network responsible for paradoxical sleep onset and maintenance: a combined microinjection and functional neuroanatomical study. Eur J Neurosci 2002;16:1959–73.

44. Chemelli RM, Willie JT, Sinton CM, et al. Narcolepsy in orexin knockout mice: molecular genetics of sleep regulation. Cell 1999;98:437–51.

45. Lin L, Faraco J, Li R, et al. The sleep disorder canine narcolepsy is caused by a mutation in the hypocretin (orexin) receptor 2 gene. Cell. 1999;98:365–76.

46. Peyron C, Tighe DK, van den Pol AN, et al. Neurons containing hypocretin (orexin) project to multiple neuronal systems. J Neurosci. 1998;18:9996–10015.

47. Krout KE, Mettenleiter TC, Loewy AD. Single CNS neurons link both central motor and cardiosympathetic systems: a double-virus tracing study. Neuroscience 2003;118:853–66.

48. Jones BE, Muhlethaler M. Modulation of cortical activity and sleep–wake state by hypocretin/orexin. In: de Lecea L, Sutcliffe JG, eds. The hypocretins: integrators of physiological systems. New York: Springer, 2005:289–301.

49. Bayer L, Serafin M, Eggermann E, et al. Exclusive postsynaptic action of hypocretin–orexin on sublayer 6b cortical neurons. J Neurosci 2004;24:6760–4.

50. van den Pol AN. Hypothalamic hypocretin (orexin): robust innervation of the spinal cord. J Neurosci 1999;19:3171–82.

51. Henny P, Brischoux F, Mainville L, et al. Immunohistochemical evidence for synaptic release of glutamate from orexin terminals in the locus coeruleus. Neuroscience 2010;169:1150–7.

52. Schone C, Cao ZF, Apergis-Schoute J, et al. Optogenetic probing of fast glutamatergic transmission from hypocretin/orexin to histamine neurons in situ. J Neurosci 2012;32:12437–43.

53. Lee MG, Hassani OK, Jones BE. Discharge of identified orexin/hypocretin neurons across the sleep-waking cycle. J Neurosci 2005;25:6716–20.

54. Mileykovskiy BY, Kiyashchenko LI, Siegel JM. Behavioral correlates of activity in identified hypocretin/orexin neurons. Neuron 2005;46:787–98.

55. Adamantidis AR, Zhang F, Aravanis AM, et al. Neural substrates of awakening probed with optogenetic control of hypocretin neurons. Nature 2007;450:420–4.

56. Black SW, Morairty SR, Fisher SP, et al. Almorexant promotes sleep and exacerbates cataplexy in a murine model of narcolepsy. Sleep 2013;36:325–36.

57. Verret L, Goutagny R, Fort P, et al. A role of melanin-concentrating hormone producing neurons in the central regulation of paradoxical sleep. BMC Neurosci 2003;4:19.

58. Modirrousta M, Mainville L, Jones BE. Orexin and MCH neurons express c-Fos differently after sleep deprivation vs. recovery and bear different adrenergic receptors. Eur J Neurosci 2005;21:2807–16.

59. Konadhode RR, Pelluru D, Blanco-Centurion C, et al. Optogenetic stimulation of MCH neurons increases sleep. J Neurosci 2013;33:10257–63.

60. Jego S, Glasgow SD, Herrera CG, et al. Optogenetic identification of a rapid eye movement sleep modulatory circuit in the hypothalamus. Nat Neurosci 2013;16:1637–43.

61. Hassani OK, Lee MG, Jones BE. Melanin-concentrating hormone neurons discharge in a reciprocal manner to orexin neurons across the sleep–wake cycle. Proc Natl Acad Sci U S A 2009;106:2418–22.

62. Wu M, Dumalska I, Morozova E, et al Melanin-concentrating hormone directly inhibits GnRH neurons and blocks kisspeptin activation, linking energy balance to reproduction. Proc Natl Acad Sci U S A 2009;106:17217–22.

63. Gao XB, van den Pol AN. Melanin-concentrating hormone depresses L-, N-, and P/Q-type voltage-dependent calcium channels in rat lateral hypothalamic neurons. J Physiol 2002;542:273–86.

64. Del Cid-Pellitero E, Jones BE. Immunohistochemical evidence for synaptic release of GABA from melanin-concentrating hormone containing varicosities in the locus coeruleus. Neuroscience 2012;223:269–76.

65. Apergis-Schoute J, Iordanidou P, Faure C, et al. Optogenetic evidence for inhibitory signaling from orexin to MCH neurons via local micro-circuits. J Neurosci 2015;35:5435–41.

CHAPTER 5

The genetics of sleep

Alexandra Sousek and Mehdi Tafti

Why hunt for genes involved in sleep?

The obvious variation of sleep phenotypes within the human population and their intra-individual stability, as well as familial aggregation of certain sleep-related disorders, led to the hypothesis that sleep might be influenced by genetic background. A multitude of twin studies and familial analyses on the prevalence and transmission of sleep traits suggested a genetic contribution to various aspects of sleep and its disturbances. In particular, the human sleep EEG was found to be strongly influenced by genetic factors, which is consistent with the finding that the human EEG in general is a highly heritable trait [1,2]. However, modulations by age, gender, and environmental factors remain to be fully determined. For a summary of twin studies, see Table 5.1, and for findings drawn from familial studies, see Table 5.2.

Twin studies

Early twin studies already found a higher concordance of sleep habits, such as sleep duration and quality, in monozygotic (MZ) than in dizygotic (DZ) twins, even when they were living apart and thus exposed to different environments [3–5]. The first polysomnographic recordings revealed concordant temporal sleep patterns in terms of sleep stages in MZ [6]. Since then, many twin studies have been performed to untangle the impact of dominant or additive genetic influences and shared or nonshared environmental factors on the various aspects of sleep. Genetic background was proposed to contribute substantially to sleep duration, quality, onset latency and efficiency, diurnal preference, sleep structure, and characteristics of NREM sleep such as amount of sleep stages 2 and 4, delta/slow-wave sleep (SWS), and spindle density, as well as REM sleep and wake after sleep onset (see Table 5.1) [6–13]. While findings on REM sleep remain controversial, NREM sleep is found consistently to be under strong genetic control in humans and mice [1,8,14,15]. REM sleep amount was found to be significantly correlated in MZ twins, and REM density was estimated to be up to 95% heritable in some studies, although others found no such relation [6,8–11]. Genetic influence on NREM sleep is well established. Even a genetically determined "individual fingerprint" of NREM sleep structure has been proposed, according to which an individual can be reliably distinguished from others, irrespective of sleep pressure as assessed by sleep deprivation studies [16–18]. Further, theta, delta, alpha, and sigma frequency bands of the wake and NREM sleep EEG were more significantly correlated in MZ than DZ twins [19].

Different aspects of sleep homeostasis, as assessed by effects of sleep deprivation, were found to be under genetic control in humans and mice. Franken et al. were able to show in various inbred mouse stains that delta activity rebound after sleep deprivation, and thus that processes of sleep homeostasis are under strong genetic control [14]. Supporting Van Dongen's claim that human neurobehavioral response toward sleep loss was an inter-individual trait-like characteristic, the neurobehavioral reaction toward sleep deprivation was determined as a highly heritable trait, in that decline in vigilance is significantly more similar in MZ than in DZ twins [13,20]. Since increases in slow-wave activity (SWA) and delta power during NREM sleep of recovery after sleep loss are well-established markers for sleep homeostasis in humans, twin studies recording EEGs during and after sleep deprivation could further elucidate the heritability of these homeostatic processes [21].

Another important aspect of sleep that has been intensively investigated is subjective sleep quality, mainly assessed by the Pittsburgh Sleep Quality Index (PSQI). Substantial heritability of up to 44%

Table 5.1 Genetic contribution to sleep phenotypes

Sleep trait	Estimated heritability	References
Sleep duration	30–44%	[3–5]
Sleep quality	44–46%	[5,22,25]
Sleep efficiency and wake after sleep onset	50% and 42%, in males only	[10,13,33]
Sleep onset latency	High sign correlation in MZ only	[10]
Sleep architecture, stage changes, frequency profiles	Higher concordance in MZ than DZ, sign correlation in MZ 96%	[6,10,17,19]
NREM sleep characteristics (frequency profile, stage 2 amount, stage 3/4 amount (SWS), spindle density)	50–96%	[7,9,11,13,17,19]
REM sleep characteristics (patterns, amount, density)	50–95%	[6,7,10,11,13]
Diurnal preference	45–52%	[22,34,35]
Neurobehavioral reaction to sleep loss	83%	[13]
Insomnia	43–57%	[24–26]
RLS and related symptoms	48–69%	[28,36]
Sleep-talking, bruxism, enuresis	54–70% in children 48–53% in adults	[29–31]

Table 5.2 Familial and linkage studies

Disease	Mode of inheritance	Involved molecules or loci	References
Familial advanced sleep phase syndrome (FASPS)	Autosomal dominant	hPer2, CK1ε, and CK1δ	[37,38]
Restless legs syndrome (RLS)	Autosomal dominant	12q: RLS1	[43–49,54,59]
		14q: RLS2	
		9q: RLS3 and RLS3*	
		2q: RLS4	
		20p: RLS5	
		19p	
RLS	Autosomal recessive	12q: RLS1	[50]
RLS	Unclear	12q: RLS2	[52,55–58]
		14q: RLS2	
		MEIS1, BTBD9, MAP2K5, LBOXCOR1, DMT1	
Primary nocturnal enuresis (PNE)	Autosomal dominant	4q	[60,62–65]
		12q	
		13q: ENUR1	
		22q: ENUR3	

was estimated in several studies [5,22]. Further, with 94% association, a strong overlap of genetic influence on sleep quality and diurnal preference was determined, suggesting common underlying mechanisms [22].

In dyssomnias and parasomnias, higher concordance and thus estimated heritability rates were found in MZ compared with DZ twins (see Table 5.1). Parasomnias comprise atypical behavior or physiological events occurring during specific sleep periods, such as sleepwalking or enuresis, while dyssomnias are characterized by unusual amount, quality, or timing of sleep. A study on 100 MZ and 199 DZ 8-year-old twin pairs estimated 71% of genetic contribution to variability for dyssomnias and 50% for parasomnias [23]. Studies on insomnia revealed up to 57% estimated heritability, whereas distinctive symptoms such as "trouble staying asleep" were found to be differentially modulated by genetic background or gender [24–26]. Likewise, in sleepwalking, genetic effects were estimated to account for 80% of variability in males and 36% in females [27]. Sleep-related breathing disorders and their associated disabling symptoms such as excessive daytime sleepiness were found to be heritable in up to 52% of cases [28]. Other conditions with substantial genetic contribution are enuresis, bruxism, sleeptalking, and restless legs syndrome [28–32].

Familial studies and linkage analysis

Certain sleep-related diseases show high familial risk and specific modes of transmission (see Table 5.2). Linkage studies using microsatellite markers and phenotypes, testing for co-segregation and inheritance patterns, aim to define chromosomal regions conferring risk and susceptibility to the development of a disease, and thus provide help to find the underlying genetic factors. This

can contribute to the development of appropriate treatments, risk assessment, and prevention. In the following, the potential of such studies will be demonstrated on the examples of familial advanced sleep phase syndrome, restless legs syndrome, and primary nocturnal enuresis.

Familial advanced sleep phase syndrome

Familial advanced sleep phase syndrome (FASPS) shows an autosomal dominant pattern of inheritance with high penetrance. Since this disease is characterized by early bedtime and early morning awakening, it is not surprising that links to genes underlying circadian rhythmicity have been found. In a linkage analysis, a specific haplotype of the human period (*PER2*) gene was found co-segregating with FASPS [37]. Within this haplotype, an A-to-G transition leads to substitution of a conserved serine by glycine. This missense mutation alters binding of casein kinase 1ε (CK1ε) to the Per2 protein and thus its phosphorylation. Further, a mutation in the gene encoding CK1δ (*CSNK1D*) itself can be causal for the disease. Screening an FASPS kindred for mutations, a T-to-A transversion in a highly conserved sequence of *CSNK1D* was detected, which co-segregates with the disease [38]. This missense mutation entails a threonine-to-alanine substitution leading to a decrease in enzymatic activity and phosphorylation. Accordingly, animal models carrying this mutation showed similar affected circadian phenotypes.

Restless legs syndrome

Restless legs syndrome (RLS) is suggested to be a polygenetic disease, with high familial vulnerability and an estimated heritability of 50%, whereas the involved genetic regions and their mode of inheritance remain controversial, indicating high heterogeneity and complexity [39–41]. Linkage studies of affected families revealed six associated loci on chromosomes 12q, 14q, 9p, 2q, 20p, and 6p termed *RLS1–6*, but without characterization of the responsible genes [40,42–49]. Autosomal dominant transmission was mainly suggested for *RLS2* and *RLS3*, and in families with early onset of the disease, while *RLS1* was repeatedly found to be recessive [40,42,44,50,51].

Loci on chromosome 9 (*RLS3* and possibly *RLS3**) were consistently found important [8, 43–45], while for other loci findings remained more controversial. Bonati et al. reported linkage to a locus on 14q (*RLS2*) and co-segregation in an autosomal dominant manner, while others could not confirm this in several French-Canadian families [48,52]. Desautels et al. were able to define a 14.71 cM region on chromosome 12q (*RLS1*) conferring susceptibility to the disease in an autosomal recessive way in a large French-Canadian family. This is especially interesting, since neurotensin (NTS) is encoded in that region and acts as neuromodulator of dopaminergic transmission, which has repeatedly been associated with RLS [49]. This putative connection is strongly supported by the observed relief of symptoms upon treatment with dopamine agonists [42]. However, sequencing of this gene in four affected families revealed two polymorphisms in the intronic region and one in the 5′ UTR, but no co-segregation with the disease [53]. In contrast to the findings by Desautels et al. Kock et al. determined autosomal dominant transmission concerning the 12q locus in two South Tyrolean families [54]. Further analyses in 19 affected families confirmed autosomal recessive transmission in some, and thus the involvement of another crucial locus was suggested [50]. The complexity and heterogeneity of the etiology of this disease are also supported by findings of a study assessing linkage of *RLS1*, *RLS2*, and *RLS3* in 12 Bavarian families, where neither clear proof nor disproof of linkage could be determined using parametric linkage analysis [55].

Xiong in 2007 investigated the possible influence of divalent metal transporter 1 (*DMT1*), which is a good candidate, given the reduced iron levels in the brains of affected individuals, the association with anemia, and the location of the gene on chromosome 12q, close to the *RLS1* locus. Cell culture techniques showed no difference in protein levels in blood cells of patients and controls. Neither a linkage between the *DMT1* gene region and RLS nor any underlying mutations within the gene region were found. However, two single nucleotide polymorphisms (SNPs) in the intronic region were associated with the disease in patients with anemia [56].

More recently, further regions conferring susceptibility have been identified by applying genome-wide association analysis (GWAS). Winkelmann et al. determined highly significant associations between the disease and intronic variants of *MEIS1* (homeobox) on 2p, *BTBD9* (POZ domain) on 6p, and a locus containing the *MAP2K5* (kinase) and *LBOXCOR1* (transcription factor) genes on chromosome 15q [57]. Accordingly, Stefansson found a common intronic variant of the *BTBD9* gene significantly associated with the disease and responsible for 50% of risk in this population [58]. Intriguingly, this was accompanied by decreased serum ferritin levels, since RLS is considered to be associated with disturbed brain iron metabolism [42,58]. This region on chromosome 6p21 is also referred to as RLS6 [40]. Recently, in a genome-wide linkage analysis including affected families from eight European countries, a novel region significantly linked to RLS in an autosomal dominant manner was detected [59]. However, mutations in the genes of interest located in that area could not be found.

Primary nocturnal enuresis

Linkage analyses concerning primary nocturnal enuresis (PNE) have revealed involvement of regions on chromosomes 12q, 13q (*ENUR1*), and 22q (*ENUR3*) [60–63]. Intriguingly, within the confined region on chromosome 12q, the aquaporin-2 water channel is encoded, but the transitions found did not lead to functional alteration of the protein [62]. More recently, a new locus on chromosome 4 has been found to segregate with nocturnal enuresis and incontinence with high penetrance. This region on 4p16 contains the dopamine receptor genes *DRD5* and *D1B*, which might be good candidates [64].

Effects of genetic variation on sleep

To understand the contribution of genetic variation and involved molecular pathways to sleep phenotypes and the development of disease, association to, and thus assumed influence of, naturally occurring SNPs and variable number of tandem repeats (VNTRs) have been extensively studied. This has indeed led to a considerable amount of knowledge being obtained about the factors involved, but the picture is not complete, and the interaction and mutual influence of involved pathways remain unclear and require further study. For an overview of genetic variations affecting sleep phenotypes, see Table 5.3.

Table 5.3 Genetic variations affecting sleep phenotypes

Gene	Modification	Affected phenotype/trait	References
ADA	SNP, missense mutation	Sleep architecture, SWS and delta power, reaction to sleep deprivation	[67,68]
ADORA	SNPs	EEG frequencies in sleep and wake, sensitivity to caffeine, vigilance, reaction to sleep deprivation	[69,70]
MAOA	VNTR	Sleep quality, depression, RLS, narcolepsy controversial	[71–74]
COMT	Missense mutation	SWS, reaction to sleep deprivation, sensitivity to modafinil, narcolepsy symptoms	[74,78–80]
SLC6A3 (DAT)	VNTR	Reaction to sleep deprivation, sensitivity to caffeine	[83]
HTR2A (5-HT$_{2A}$ receptor)	SNP	Risk for OSA	[90,91]
SLC6A4 (5-HTT)	Insertion/deletion variant	Risk for primary insomnia and sleep quality	[92–95]
GABRA (GABA$_A$ receptors)	Missense mutation	Primary insomnia	[99]
BDNF	Missense mutation	NREM frequencies, SWS, reaction to sleep deprivation, working memory	[101]
TNFA	SNPs in promoter and coding region	Association with narcolepsy, partly dependent on HLA type	[107,112]
TNFR2	Missense mutation	Association with narcolepsy	[113]
PRNP	Missense mutations	Trigger of FFI/CJD and modulation of phenotype	[114,116]
HCRT	Missense mutation in signal peptide	Severe early onset narcolepsy with cataplexy	[119]
PER3	VNTR, SNPs in promoter region,	Diurnal preference, sleep latency, DSPS, reaction to sleep deprivation	[135,136,138–142]
PER2 and *CSNK1*	Missense mutations	DSPS	[37,38]
CLOCK	SNP in 5′ UTR	Diurnal preference	[143,144]

Adenosinergic neurotransmission

Adenosinergic neurotransmission is suspected to play a major role in the regulation of sleep and wakefulness and their homeostasis in mice and humans [14,66]. Common genetic variants affecting different aspects of sleep homeostasis in healthy humans support this hypothesis. A functional SNP on the human chromosome 20q13.11 changes a guanine (G) to adenine (A) in the adenosine deaminase (ADA) enzyme. Asparagine (in the ADA*1 variant) is changed into aspartic acid (in the ADA*2 variant), which results in lower enzymatic activity and thus less adenosine degradation in heterozygous G/A (ADA*1–2) carriers compared with G/G (ADA*1). Concerning sleep, Retey et al. found an increase in slow-wave sleep (SWS) during an undisturbed night in ADA*1–2 carriers resembling the effects of one night of sleep deprivation. This was further accompanied by higher delta power in NREM sleep, which is a marker of sleep need [67,68]. Also, the response to sleep deprivation was found to be modulated by this genotype, with elevated SWS and delta activity in NREM sleep of recovery nights after 40 hours of prolonged wakefulness in ADA*1–2 subjects [67]. Thus, it is assumed that reduced enzymatic activity due to genetic variability leads to enhanced build-up of sleep pressure.

Among adenosine receptors, it is mainly subtypes A_1 and A_{2A} that are considered important in sleep regulation [66]. The thymine (T)-to-cytosine (C) transition in the coding region of the A_{2A} receptor gene (ADORA2A) on chromosome 22q11.2 not only affects EEG activity, generally irrespective of sleep and wake, but also modulates the effects of its antagonist caffeine on sleep and sleep deprivation. Only C/C carriers show increases in high-frequency EEG after sleep deprivation. Further, the C-allele was found to confer sensitivity to caffeine-induced sleep disturbances [69]. Analysis of the effects of combinations of eight SNPs of the ADORA2A gene revealed that one haplotype (HT4) was associated with enhanced vigilance at the baseline, but resistance to caffeine-induced rescue of vigilance decline after sleep loss was observed in non-HT4 carriers. Likewise, caffeine had differential effects on SWS in recovery sleep that were dependent on genotype. While non-HT4 carriers showed reduced SWS upon caffeine administration, this effect was missing in HT4 individuals. The build-up of sleep pressure assessed by EEG and increase in subjective sleepiness were not affected [70].

Monoamine oxidase

Monoamine oxidase (MAO) A and B are encoded on the X-chromosome and catalyze the degradation of monoamines: the catecholamines dopamine, noradrenaline (norepinephrine), and adrenaline (epinephrine) and the tryptamines serotonin and melatonin. Thus, it is an important enzyme for the regulation of major neurotransmitters implicated in sleep. Females carrying an allele conferring higher activity due to a variable number tandem repeat (VNTR) polymorphism in the MAO-A promoter region are at higher risk of developing RLS [71]. Further, the less active allele seems to confer susceptibility to depression and poor sleep quality [72]. Koch et al. proposed an association of a VNTR in intron 1 of the MAOA gene and a dinucleotide repeat in intron 2 of the MAOB gene with the occurrence of narcolepsy with cataplexy [73]. This could not be confirmed by others, suggesting HLA type and gender as underlying causes for the difference [74]. However, MAO-A and -B inhibitors are capable of reducing symptoms of narcolepsy such as cataplexy and abnormal REM sleep [75,76].

Dopaminergic neurotransmission

A G-to-A transition in catechol-O-methyltransferase (COMT) entails a functional polymorphism resulting in a valine–methionine exchange. This leads to reduced activity of the dopamine-metabolizing enzyme and thus higher dopaminergic transmission. Indeed, Val/Val homozygous subjects show less dopaminergic signaling in their prefrontal cortex (PFC) than those carrying Met/Met [77]. Bodenmann et al. found no effects of this polymorphism on baseline sleep, while Goel observed differences in SWS decline [78,79]. In chronic partial sleep deprivation of five consecutive nights with 4 hours sleep, Val homozygotes showed smaller increase in SWS, while Met homozygotes had steeper SWS decline. This was accompanied by shorter REM sleep latency in Val/Val subjects [79]. Further, the commonly used stimulant modafinil, which promotes dopaminergic neurotransmission, was shown to be effective in terms of counteracting total sleep deprivation-induced impairments of attention and other cognitive functions in Val homozygotes only [80]. Val genotype enhanced certain NREM frequency bands during recovery sleep, but without changing slow-wave activity [78]. Thus, homeostatic processes as well as stimulant efficiency seem to be modulated by dopaminergic signaling, and this polymorphism might be of interest in stimulant treatments.

Dauvilliers et al. found no association between COMT genotype and narcolepsy, but an interaction of gender and genotype as well as a strong influence on severity of the disease independent of gender was observed [74]. Females homozygous for the less active allele as well as heterozygotes exhibit higher sleep latency than those homozygous for the highly active variant. The opposite effect was observed in males. Irrespective of gender, more sleep paralysis but less sleep onset REM periods were observed in heterozygous narcoleptic patients. HLA type was found not to interact with COMT genotype.

A crucial player in dopaminergic signaling is the dopamine transporter (DAT), whose blockage by modafinil results in elevated dopamine levels in the extracellular space. DAT knockout mice are insensitive to modafinil, but show increased consolidated wakefulness, less REM sleep, and hypersensitivity to caffeine [81]. In humans, a VNTR polymorphism in the 3′ UTR of the DAT-encoding gene SLC6A3 leads to less DAT in the striatum in individuals homozygous for the long 10-repeat allele as compared with carriers of the 9-repeat allele [82]. According to the animal data, 10/10 carriers are more sensitive to caffeine generally, as well as to its effect on reducing SWS rebound after sleep deprivation, which was found more pronounced in 10-repeat homozygotes [83].

Serotonergic neurotransmission

It is well established that serotonergic or 5-hydroxytryptamine (5-HT) activity promotes wakefulness and inhibits REM sleep. The serotonergic receptors 5-HT$_{1-7}$ exert different functions according to their associated second messengers. Thus, postsynaptic cells can either be inhibited (5-HT$_{1A}$ and 5-HT$_{1B}$) or depolarized (5-HT$_{2A/2C}$, 5-HT$_3$, and 5-HT$_7$) upon receptor activation. Further, the outcome of their activation depends on their localization. Activation of 5-HT$_{1A}$ and 5-HT$_{1B}$ receptors expressed by GABAergic and of 5-HT$_3$ receptors expressed by glutamatergic interneurons lead to disinhibtion and stimulation, respectively. On the other hand, activation of 5-HT$_{2A/2C}$ or 5-HT$_7$ expressed by GABAergic interneurons leads to inhibition, and the activation of all receptor types leads to inhibition of cholinergic neurons. Within this complex system, 5-HT_{1A}, 5-HT_{1B}, 5-HT_{2A}, 5-HT_{2C}, 5-HT_{3}, and 5-HT_{7} receptors have been shown to be involved in the regulation of wakefulness and REM sleep [84]. Mice lacking 5-HT_{1A} or 5-HT_{1B} receptors have more REM sleep than wild types, but unchanged wake and SWS [85,86]. 5-HT_{7} knockouts show lower amounts and fewer episodes of REM sleep [87]. 5-HT_{2} subunits were suspected to be implicated in NREM sleep regulation, and knockout of 5-HT_{2A} or 5-HT_{2C} leads to more wake, reduced NREM sleep, and abnormalities in REM sleep in mice [88,89].

In humans, polymorphisms in the gene *HTR2A* encoding the 5-HT_{2A} receptor have been suspected to confer risk of obstructive sleep apnea (OSA), and functional binding of serotonin to 5-HT_{2A} expressed on motor neurons of the upper airways is crucial to ensure proper respiration during sleep. Recent meta-analyses of studies investigating associations of a −1438G/A polymorphism in the promoter region of *HTR2A* and/or silent T102C polymorphisms with the risk of OSA found a significant association for the first only in that homozygosity for the A variant confers risk, especially in males [90,91].

Also, the serotonin transporter (5-HTT), which determines the amount of serotonin in the synaptic cleft, might be involved. A common 44 base-pair insertion/deletion variant in the regulatory 5′ region of the serotonin transporter gene *SLC6A4* affects its expression and thus the abundance of 5-HTT at the synapse. An association study revealed that the short variant of this polymorphism is significantly more common in patients suffering from insomnia than in healthy controls [92]. Further, this polymorphism was proposed to mediate environmental effects such as chronic stress and stressful life events on sleep quality and length, respectively [93,94]. Nevertheless, another study found homozygosity for the long allele to be associated with poor sleep [95].

GABAergic neurotransmission

Several lines of evidence point to involvement of the main inhibitory neurotransmitter γ-aminobutyric acid (GABA) in the initiation of sleep, as well as in the etiology and maintenance of primary insomnia. Studies applying magnetic resonance spectroscopy found reduced GABA levels globally or in the occipital cortex and anterior cingulate cortex but not the thalamus of patients with primary insomnia [96,97]. Others detected elevated occipital cortical GABA levels and proposed that this was a countermeasure to hyperarousal [98]. Consistently, they found levels of GABA to be negatively correlated with the amount of wake after sleep onset [96,98]. Screening for mutations in ligand-binding domains of the α_1, β_3, and γ_2 genes of the GABA_A receptor revealed a heterozygous missense mutation in one patient with chronic insomnia. The substitution of arginine for histidine presumably entails reduced GABAergic inhibition [99].

Brain-derived neurotrophic factor

Evidence for the involvement of brain-derived neurotrophic factor (BDNF) in sleep–wake regulation was found in animal studies [14,100]. In a sleep deprivation study on six inbred mouse strains, a chromosomal region containing the gene encoding the BDNF receptor tyrosine kinase B (TrkB) determined 49% of variance in the build-up of sleep pressure [14]. In rats, BDNF secretion was suggested to be a mediator of sleep homeostasis [100]. In humans, a common functional polymorphism, a G-to-A transition,

leads to amino acid substitution from valine to methionine and thus impaired activity-dependent secretion of the protein, which is implicated in synaptic plasticity and associated with cognitive performance [1]. Heterozygous carriers of the Met allele show decreased slow wave sleep and delta and theta power in NREM sleep during undisturbed nights, as well as after one night of sleep deprivation [101]. Likewise, in previous studies, impacts on cognitive function, i.e. working memory, were observed [101,102]. Thus, implication of this polymorphism in plasticity and regulation of sleep homeostasis is assumed.

Tumor necrosis factor

Tumor necrosis factor (TNF) α is a pro-inflammatory cytokine involved in many processes and also proposed to be involved in sleep regulation. Evidence comes from observations that injection of TNF-α in rodents dose-dependently increases NREM sleep and suppresses REM sleep [103–105]. Accordingly, disruption of its functionality by administration of anti-TNF-antibodies or creation of TNF receptor knockout mice lead to blockage of NREM sleep and sleep disturbances [105,106]. Since in humans several polymorphisms in the promoter region of the *TNFA* gene are known and linked to neurological and inflammatory diseases and the gene lies within the HLA class II cluster, it has become a target of interest in the pathophysiology of narcolepsy [107]. Indeed, narcoleptic patients show elevated plasma levels of TNF-α and soluble TNF-α receptor but no mutation either in *TNFA* or in TNF-α receptor genes was detected [108–111]. Results for the numerous SNPs are inconsistent, partly owing to HLA type or ethnicity. In association studies, Hohjoh et al. found a SNP in the promoter region of *TNFA* significantly associated with narcolepsy independent of HLA haplotype *DRB1*15:01* as well as an association of disease with a polymorphism in the TNF receptor 2 gene (*TNFR2*) that leads to exchange of a methionine with an arginine [112,113]. Wieczorek et al. found a C857T polymorphism in *TNFA* associated with narcolepsy, but only in *DRB1*15/16*-negative German patients, while no such link was detected in a Taiwanese study [107,108]. The SNPs C863A and G308A of *TNFA* and a microsatellite adjacent to the gene were not found to be linked to narcolepsy independent of HLA in a German sample [107]. Likewise T-1031C, C-863A, and a SNP leading to a missense mutation in *TNFR2* were found not to be associated in the Taiwanese population [108].

Prion protein

Fatal familial insomnia (FFI) is a highly penetrant hereditary disease transmitted in an autosomal dominant manner. FFI is characterized by disrupted sleep, i.e., loss of sleep spindles and SWS, and impaired sleep stage organization, as well as progressive reduction of sleep time. This goes along with reduced metabolism in thalamic and limbic regions and degeneration of thalamic nuclei. Investigation of two Italian affected kindred revealed an underlying point mutation in the prion protein (PrP) gene (*PRNP*) on chromosome 20. A missense mutation, a G-to-A transition at codon 178, leads to substitution of aspartate for asparagine [114,115]. Creutzfeldt–Jakob disease (CJD) is characterized by the same mutation and accumulation of protease-resistant prion protein plaques, but differs from FFI regarding a polymorphism at codon 129, which is common and leads to either incorporation of a methionine or valine, and further to protein isoforms differing in size and glycosylation pattern [116]. While in FFI-affected individuals the mutated allele encodes for methionine, those with CJD express valine on the mutated *PRNP* allele [117]. Studies on further kindred confirmed the influence of the 129 polymorphism on the expressed phenotypes of the different prion-related diseases [115].

Orexin/hypocretin

Neurons expressing the neuropeptides hypocretin-1 (HCRT-1) and -2 (HCRT-2), also termed orexin A and B, which are processed from their common precursor prepro-hypocretin (*HCRT*), are exclusively found in the lateral hypothalamus. They have widespread projections throughout the brain, such as the cortex and pons, and are involved in the arousal system. Two receptors (HCRTR-1 and HCRTR-2) have been defined up to now. Several lines of evidence point toward involvement of deficiency in this system in narcolepsy. In humans, reduced levels of HCRT-1 in cerebrospinal fluid (CSF) and several brain regions and deficiency of prepro-hypocretin mRNA in the hypothalamus, as well as loss of orexin-producing cells, have been documented [118–120]. In dogs, an autosomal recessive mutation in the *Hcrtr2* gene causes narcolepsy, and mice that lack prepro-hypocretin show symptoms of the disease [121,122]. Consequently, intensive screening for human mutations has been performed. Neither a common C-to-T polymorphism in HCRT nor a previously reported polymorphism in its 5′ UTR were found to be associated with narcolepsy in a study with 105 families [123]. This holds also for 14 defined polymorphisms in hypocretin receptors, although normal CSF levels of HCRT-1 found in some patients point toward receptor defects [119]. Similarly, there are families lacking HCRT-1 in the CSF without mutations in the *HCRT* gene and delayed onset of disease [119]. To date, only one functional polymorphism is known, found in a patient with severe cataplexy and unusually early onset of the disease. A G-to-T transversion leads to a change in the signal peptide of HCRT, where a highly charged arginine is introduced in a hydrophobic polyleucine stretch of the peptide, which alters trafficking and impairs cleavage. The attempt to assign this as a de novo mutation failed because DNA was only available from the unaffected mother but not the unaffected father [119].

The strong association of the disease with HLA allelic variants led to the hypothesis of autoimmune destruction of hypothalamic hypocretin neurons [124]. Enriched tribbles homologue 2 (TRIB2), which can serve as an autoantigen, in hypocretin-producing neurons of a transgenic mouse model, as well as elevated levels of TRIB2-specific antibodies in serum of narcoleptic patients corroborate this theory [125,126]. However, the exact underlying mechanism of the destruction of orexin-producing cells remains unknown.

A recent study showed that the re-expression of orexin receptors on noradrenergic neurons in the locus coeruleus and on serotonergic neurons in the dorsal raphe nuclei of orexin receptor knockout mice could rescue symptoms of narcolepsy [127]. Intriguingly, the amount of restored orexin signaling on serotonergic neurons correlated with the observed reduction in cataplexy, and that on noradrenergic neurons correlated with reduced fragmentation of wakefulness [127]. This suggests a crucial interaction of different neurotransmitter systems in the pathophysiology of narcolepsy.

Circadian "clock" genes

In mammals, a transcription–translation feedback loop serves as the basic mechanism for the clock machinery in the suprachiasmatic nucleus (SCN) to control circadian rhythmicity. Briefly, the basic helix–loop–helix PAS transcription factors CLOCK and BMAL1 form the heterodimer BMAL1/CLOCK (alternatively BMAL1/NPAS2), which binds to E-Box elements of promoters and induces transcription of, among others, the cryptochrome 1 and 2 (*CRY1* and *CRY2*) and period (*PER1–3*, *PER3* only in humans) genes and the gene encoding the nuclear receptor Rev-Erbα (*NR1D1*). The PER and CRY proteins, in turn, act as negative regulators of CLOCK/BMAL1 activity by forming a repressor complex with casein kinase (CK) 1ε (encoded by the *CSNK1E* gene) and CK1δ (*CSNK1D*). Rev-Erbα represses transcription of *CLOCK* and *BMAL1* [128–130]. Besides their function in circadian rhythmicity, clock genes have also been found to influence sleep variables. Supporting evidence comes from animal models showing that knockout of *BMAL1* and *NPAS2* and double knockout of *Cry1* and *Cry2* lead to abnormalities in sleep homeostasis in mice [131–134].

One of the most intensively studied "clock" genes is the human period 3 (*PER3*) gene on chromosome 1. *PER3* polymorphism has repeatedly been associated with diurnal preference and delayed sleep phase syndrome (DSPS) [135–138]. A VNTR in the coding region leads to either a short or a long allele; *PER3⁴* or *PER3⁵*, respectively. Homozygosity for the longer variant *PER3⁵/⁵* is consistently found to be associated with morningness, and homozygosity for *PER3⁴/⁴* with eveningness. This variation further influences sleep latency, amount of SWS, and differences in recovery from sleep deprivation. Individuals homozygous for the long allele (*PER3⁵*) show more SWS in NREM and more alpha activity in REM sleep, earlier wake and bed times, and less daytime sleepiness, as well as a more intense response to sleep deprivation regarding cognitive decline and reduced brain activation when performing executive tasks, especially in the early morning [138–140]. Other studies applying chronic partial sleep deprivation found an effect of the polymorphism on sleep homeostasis but not on cognitive performance [141]. Several further polymorphisms of *PER3* were defined and associated with DSPS [142]. Four haplotypes consisting of five polymorphisms in the coding region were investigated and one haplotype was found to be significantly associated with the disease. Functionally, the glycine incorporated into the protein instead of a valine in that haplotype was suggested to alter phosphorylation of the PER3 protein by CKIε. Further, the majority (75%) of patients suffering from DSPS were found to carry the *PER3⁴/⁴* variant, which is associated with eveningness [136]. A study investigating the promoter region of *PER3* revealed two SNPs that were more prevalent in DSPS patients compared with either morning or evening types of the healthy control subjects and thus could contribute to the disease by changing the expression levels [135]. As described in the section on FASPS earlier in this chapter, altered phosphorylation of PER2 due to a missense mutation of CK1 or its binding site is involved in FASPS [37,38].

In 1998 Katzenberg found a T3111C polymorphism in the 3′ UTR of *CLOCK* associated with diurnal preferences, in that carriers of the C allele are more often evening-type [143]. Since then, controversial replications of that finding have been reported. In a Japanese sample, the highest eveningness was likewise found in C/C homozygous subjects, together with significantly delayed sleep onset, shorter sleep duration, and higher daytime sleepiness compared with either heterozygous or homozygous T-allele carriers. [144]. On the contrary, studies performed in Caucasian and Brazilian subjects found no association with either diurnal preference or DSPS [145,146].

Concluding remarks

The genetics of sleep, as opposed to all other complex traits, is still at its inception. Although progress has been made in demonstrating that most sleep phenotypes and sleep disorders are controlled by genetic factors, very few causal genetic factors have been discovered. Sleep is controlled at too many levels, from molecular to organismic behavioral level. So far, almost all candidate genes have been shown to affect sleep, adding to the complexity of this behavior. Whether single genes play an essential role remains elusive. Sleep disorders represent ideal models to uncover the molecular pathways that are critically involved. Nevertheless, examples from other fields strongly indicate that the best way to gain further insight must include both basic research and translational research, linking disorder phenotypes to normal mechanisms regulating the most basic biological substrates.

References

1. Landolt HP. Genetic determination of sleep EEG profiles in healthy humans. Prog Brain Res 2011;193:51–61.
2. van Beijsterveldt CEM, Molenaar PCM, deGeus EJC, Boomsma DI. Heritability of human brain functioning as assessed by electroencephalography. Am J Hum Genet 1996;58:562–73.
3. Gedda L, Brenci G. Sleep and dream characteristics in twins. Acta Genet Med Gemellol (Roma) 1979;28:237–9.
4. Gedda L, Brenci G.Twins living apart test: progress report. Acta Genet Med Gemellol (Roma) 1983;32:17–22.
5. Partinen M, Kaprio J, Koskenvuo M, et al. Genetic and environmental determination of human sleep. Sleep 1983;6:179–85.
6. Zung WW, Wilson WP. Sleep and dream patterns in twins. Markov analysis of a genetic trait. Recent Adv Biol Psychiatry 1966;9:119–30.
7. Hori A. Sleep characteristics in twins. Jpn J Psychiatry Neurol 1986;40:35–46.
8. Linkowski P. EEG sleep patterns in twins. J Sleep Res 1999;8(Suppl 1): 11–13.
9. Linkowski P, Kerkhofs M, Hauspie R, et al. Genetic determinants of EEG sleep: a study in twins living apart. Electroencephalogr Clin Neurophysiol 1991;79.114–18.
10. Webb WB, Campbell SS. Relationships in sleep characteristics of identical and fraternal twins. Arch Gen Psychiatry 1983;40:1093–5.
11. Linkowski P, Kerkhofs M, Hauspie R, et al. EEG sleep patterns in man: a twin study. Electroencephalogr Clin Neurophysiol 1989;73:279–84.
12. Barclay NL, Gregory AM. Quantitative genetic research on sleep: a review of normal sleep, sleep disturbances and associated emotional, behavioural, and health-related difficulties. Sleep Med Rev 2013;17:29–40.
13. Kuna ST, Maislin G, Pack FM, et al. Heritability of performance deficit accumulation during acute sleep deprivation in twins. Sleep 2012;35:1223–33.
14. Franken P., Chollet D, Tafti M. The homeostatic regulation of sleep need is under genetic control. J Neurosci 2001;21:2610–21.
15. Tafti M, Franken P, Kitahama K, et al. Localization of candidate genomic regions influencing paradoxical sleep in mice. Neuroreport 1997;8:3755–8.
16. Finelli LA, Achermann P, Borbely AA Individual "fingerprints" in human sleep EEG topography. Neuropsychopharmacology 2001;25(5 Suppl):S57–62.
17. De Gennaro L, Ferrara M, Vecchio F, et al. An electroencephalographic fingerprint of human sleep. Neuroimage 2005;26:114–22.
18. De Gennaro L, Marzano C, Fratello F, et al. The electroencephalographic fingerprint of sleep is genetically determined: a twin study. Ann Neurol 2008:64:455–60.
19. Ambrosius U, Lietzenmaier S, Wehrle R, et al. Heritability of sleep electroencephalogram. Biol Psychiatry 2008;64:344–8.
20. Van Dongen HP, Baynard MD, Maislin G, Dinges DF. Systematic interindividual differences in neurobehavioral impairment from sleep loss: evidence of trait-like differential vulnerability. Sleep 2004;27:423–33.
21. Borbely AA, Baumann F, Brandeis D, Strauch I, et al. Sleep deprivation: effect on sleep stages and EEG power density in man. Electroencephalogr Clin Neurophysiol 1981;51:483–95.
22. Barclay NL, Eley TC, Buysse DJ, et al. Diurnal preference and sleep quality: same genes? A study of young adult twins. Chronobiol Int 2010;27:278–96.
23. Gregory AM, A genetic decomposition of the association between parasomnias and dyssomnias in 8-year-old twins. Arch Pediatr Adolesc Med 2008;162:299–304.
24. Drake CL, Friedman NP, Wright KP Jr, Roth T. Sleep reactivity and insomnia: genetic and environmental influences. Sleep 2011;34:1179–88.
25. Hublin C, Partinen M, Koskenvuo M, Kaprio J. Heritability and mortality risk of insomnia-related symptoms: a genetic epidemiologic study in a population-based twin cohort. Sleep 2011;34:957–64.
26. Watson NF, Goldberg J, Arguelles L, Buchwald D. Genetic and environmental influences on insomnia, daytime sleepiness, and obesity in twins. Sleep 2006;29:645–9.
27. Hublin C, Kaprio J, Partinen M, et al. Prevalence and genetics of sleepwalking: a population-based twin study. Neurology 1997;48:177–81.
28. Desai AV, Cherkas LF, Spector TD, Williams AJ. Genetic influences in self-reported symptoms of obstructive sleep apnoea and restless legs: a twin study. Twin Res 2004;7:589–95.
29. Hublin C, Kaprio J, Partinen M, Koskenvuo M. Sleeptalking in twins: epidemiology and psychiatric comorbidity. Behav Genet 1998;28:289–98.
30. Hublin C, Kaprio J, Partinen M, Koskenvuo M. Sleep bruxism based on self-report in a nationwide twin cohort. J Sleep Res 1998;7:61–7.
31. Hublin C, Kaprio J, Partinen M, Koskenvuo M. Nocturnal enuresis in a nationwide twin cohort. Sleep 1998;21:579–85.
32. Ondo WG, Vuong KD, Wang Q. Restless legs syndrome in monozygotic twins: clinical correlates. Neurology 2000;55:1404–6.
33. Boomsma DI, van Someren EJ, Beem AL, et al. Sleep during a regular week night: a twin-sibling study. Twin Res Hum Genet 2008;11:538–45.
34. Koskenvuo M, Hublin C, Partinen M, et al. Heritability of diurnal type: a nationwide study of 8753 adult twin pairs. J Sleep Res 2007;16:156–62.
35. Hur YM. Stability of genetic influence on morningness-eveningness: a cross-sectional examination of South Korean twins from preadolescence to young adulthood. J Sleep Res 2007;16:17–23.
36. Xiong L, Jang K, Montplaisir J, et al. Canadian restless legs syndrome twin study. Neurology 2007;68:1631–3.
37. Toh KL, Jones CR, He Y, et al. An hPer2 phosphorylation site mutation in familial advanced sleep phase syndrome. Science 2001;291:1040–3.
38. Xu Y, Padiath QS, Shapiro RE, et al. Functional consequences of a CKIδ mutation causing familial advanced sleep phase syndrome. Nature 2005;434:640–4.
39. Winkelmann J, Polo O, Provini F, et al. Genetics of restless legs syndrome (RLS): state-of-the-art and future directions. Mov Disord 2007;22 (Suppl 18):S449–58.
40. Caylak E. The genetics of sleep disorders in humans: narcolepsy, restless legs syndrome, and obstructive sleep apnea syndrome. Am J Med Genet A 2009;149A:2612–26.
41. Vogl FD, Pichler I, Adel S, et al. Restless legs syndrome: epidemiological and clinicogenetic study in a South Tyrolean population isolate. Mov Disord 2006;21:1189–95.
42. Winkelmann J, Muller-Myhsok B. Genetics of restless legs syndrome: a burning urge to move. Neurology 2008;70:664–5.
43. Chen S, Ondo WG, Rao S, et al. Genomewide linkage scan identifies a novel susceptibility locus for restless legs syndrome on chromosome 9p. Am J Hum Genet 2004;74:876–85.
44. Liebetanz KM, Winkelmann J, Trenkwalder C, et al. RLS3: fine-mapping of an autosomal dominant locus in a family with intrafamilial heterogeneity. Neurology 2006;67:320–1.
45. Lohmann-Hedrich K, Neumann A, Kleensang A, et al. Evidence for linkage of restless legs syndrome to chromosome 9p: are there two distinct loci? Neurology 2008;70:686–94.
46. Levchenko A, Provost S, Montplaisir JY, et al. A novel autosomal dominant restless legs syndrome locus maps to chromosome 20p13. Neurology 2006;67:900–1.
47. Pichler I, Marroni F, Volpato CB, et al. Linkage analysis identifies a novel locus for restless legs syndrome on chromosome 2q in a South Tyrolean population isolate. Am J Hum Genet 2006;79:716–23.
48. Bonati MT, Ferini-Strambi L, Aridon P, et al. Autosomal dominant restless legs syndrome maps on chromosome 14q. Brain 2003;126:1485–92.

49. Desautels A, Turecki G, Montplaisir J, et al. Identification of a major susceptibility locus for restless legs syndrome on chromosome 12q. Am J Hum Genet 2001;69:1266–70.

50. Desautels A, Turecki G, Montplaisir J, et al. Restless legs syndrome: confirmation of linkage to chromosome 12q, genetic heterogeneity, and evidence of complexity. Arch Neurol 2005;62:591–6.

51. Winkelmann J, Muller-Myhsok B, Wittchen HU, et al. Complex segregation analysis of restless legs syndrome provides evidence for an autosomal dominant mode of inheritance in early age at onset families. Ann Neurol 2002;52:297–302.

52. Levchenko A, Montplaisir JY, Dube MP, et al. The 14q restless legs syndrome locus in the French Canadian population. Ann Neurol 2004;55:887–91.

53. Desautels A, Turecki G, Xiong L, et al. Mutational analysis of neurotensin in familial restless legs syndrome. Mov Disord 2004;19:90–4.

54. Kock N, Culjkovic B, Maniak S, et al. Mode of inheritance and susceptibility locus for restless legs syndrome, on chromosome 12q. Am J Hum Genet 2002;71:205–8; author reply 208.

55. Winkelmann J, Lichtner P, Putz B, et al. Evidence for further genetic locus heterogeneity and confirmation of RLS-1 in restless legs syndrome. Mov Disord 2006;21:28–33.

56. Xiong L, Dion P, Montplaisir J, et al. Molecular genetic studies of DMT1 on 12q in French-Canadian restless legs syndrome patients and families. Am J Med Genet B Neuropsychiatr Genet 2007;144B:911–17.

57. Winkelmann J, Schormair B, Lichtner P, et al. Genome-wide association study of restless legs syndrome identifies common variants in three genomic regions. Nat Genet 2007;39:1000–6.

58. Stefansson H, Rye DB, Hicks A, et al. A genetic risk factor for periodic limb movements in sleep. N Engl J Med 2007;357:639–47.

59. Kemlink D, Plazzi G, Vetrugno R, et al. Suggestive evidence for linkage for restless legs syndrome on chromosome 19p13. Neurogenetics 2008;9:75–82.

60. Eiberg H, Berendt I, Mohr J. Assignment of dominant inherited nocturnal enuresis (ENUR1) to chromosome 13q. Nat Genet 1995;10:354–6.

61. Arnell H, Hjalmas K, Jagervall M, et al. The genetics of primary nocturnal enuresis: inheritance and suggestion of a second major gene on chromosome 12q. J Med Genet 1997;34:360–5.

62. Deen PM, Dahl N, Caplan MJ. The aquaporin-2 water channel in autosomal dominant primary nocturnal enuresis. J Urol 2002;167:1447–50.

63. Eiberg H. Total genome scan analysis in a single extended family for primary nocturnal enuresis: evidence for a new locus (ENUR3) for primary nocturnal enuresis on chromosome 22q11. Eur Urol 1998;33(Suppl 3):34–6.

64. Eiberg H, Shaumburg HL, Von Gontard A, Rittig S. Linkage study of a large Danish 4-generation family with urge incontinence and nocturnal enuresis. J Urol 2001;166:2401–3.

65. von Gontard A, Eiberg H, Hollmann E, et al. Molecular genetics of nocturnal enuresis: clinical and genetic heterogeneity. Acta Paediatr 1998;87:571–8.

66. Landolt HP. Sleep homeostasis: a role for adenosine in humans? Biochem Pharmacol 2008;75:2070–9.

67. Bachmann V, Klaus F, Bodenmann S, et al. Functional ADA polymorphism increases sleep depth and reduces vigilant attention in humans. Cereb Cortex 2012;22:962–70.

68. Retey JV, Adam M, Honegger E, et al. A functional genetic variation of adenosine deaminase affects the duration and intensity of deep sleep in humans. Proc Natl Acad Sci U S A 2005;102:15676–81.

69. Retey JV, Adam M, Khatami R, et al. A genetic variation in the adenosine A2A receptor gene (ADORA2A) contributes to individual sensitivity to caffeine effects on sleep. Clin Pharmacol Ther 2007;81:692–8.

70. Bodenmann S, Hohoff C, Freitag C, et al. Polymorphisms of ADORA2A modulate psychomotor vigilance and the effects of caffeine on neurobehavioural performance and sleep EEG after sleep deprivation. Br J Pharmacol 2012;165:1904–13.

71. Desautels A, Turecki G, Montplaisir J, et al. Evidence for a genetic association between monoamine oxidase A and restless legs syndrome. Neurology 2002;59:215–19.

72. Brummett BH, Krystal AD, Siegler IC, et al. Associations of a regulatory polymorphism of monoamine oxidase-A gene promoter (MAOA-uVNTR) with symptoms of depression and sleep quality. Psychosom Med 2007;69:396–401.

73. Koch H, Craig I, Dahlitz M, et al. Analysis of the monoamine oxidase genes and the Norrie disease gene locus in narcolepsy. Lancet 1999;353:645–6.

74. Dauvilliers Y, Neidhart E, Lecendreux M, et al. MAO-A and COMT polymorphisms and gene effects in narcolepsy. Mol Psychiatry 2001;6:367–72.

75. Nishino S, Mignot E. Pharmacological aspects of human and canine narcolepsy. Prog Neurobiol 1997;52:27–78.

76. Hohagen F, Mayer G, Menche A, et al. Treatment of narcolepsy–cataplexy syndrome with the new selective and reversible MAO-A inhibitor brofaromine—a pilot study. J Sleep Res 1993;2:250–6.

77. Akil M, Kolachana BS, Rothmond DA, et al. Catechol-O-methyltransferase genotype and dopamine regulation in the human brain. J Neurosci 2003;23:2008–13.

78. Bodenmann S, Landolt HP. Effects of modafinil on the sleep EEG depend on Val158Met genotype of COMT. Sleep 2010;33:1027–35.

79. Goel N, Banks S, Lin L, et al. Catechol-O-methyltransferase Val158Met polymorphism associates with individual differences in sleep physiologic responses to chronic sleep loss. PLoS One 2011;6(12):e29283.

80. Bodenmann S, Xu S, Luhmann UF, et al. Pharmacogenetics of modafinil after sleep loss: catechol-O-methyltransferase genotype modulates waking functions but not recovery sleep. Clin Pharmacol Ther 2009;85:296–304.

81. Wisor JP, Nishino S, Sora I, et al. Dopaminergic role in stimulant-induced wakefulness. J Neurosci 2001;21:1787–94.

82. Costa A, Riedel M, Muller U, et al. Relationship between SLC6A3 genotype and striatal dopamine transporter availability: a meta-analysis of human single photon emission computed tomography studies. Synapse 2011;65:998–1005.

83. Holst SC, Bersagliere A, Bachmann V, et al. Dopaminergic role in regulating neurophysiological markers of sleep homeostasis in humans. J Neurosci 2014;34:566–73.

84. Monti JM. The role of dorsal raphe nucleus serotonergic and non-serotonergic neurons, and of their receptors, in regulating waking and rapid eye movement (REM) sleep. Sleep Med Rev 2010;14:319–27.

85. Boutrel B, Franc B, Hen R, et al. Key role of 5-HT$_{1B}$ receptors in the regulation of paradoxical sleep as evidenced in 5-HT$_{1B}$ knock-out mice. J Neurosci 1999;19:3204–12.

86. Boutrel B, Monaca C, Hen R, et al. Involvement of 5-HT$_{1A}$ receptors in homeostatic and stress-induced adaptive regulations of paradoxical sleep: studies in 5-HT$_{1A}$ knock-out mice. J Neurosci,2002;22:4686–92.

87. Hedlund PB, Huitron-Resendiz S, Henriksen SJ, Sutcliffe JG. 5-HT$_7$ receptor inhibition and inactivation induce antidepressantlike behavior and sleep pattern. Biol Psychiatry 2005;58:831–7.

88. Frank MG, Stryker MP, Tecott LH. Sleep and sleep homeostasis in mice lacking the 5-HT$_{2C}$ receptor. Neuropsychopharmacology 2002;27:869–73.

89. Popa D, Lena C, Fabre V, et al. Contribution of 5-HT$_2$ receptor subtypes to sleep–wakefulness and respiratory control, and functional adaptations in knock-out mice lacking 5-HT$_{2A}$ receptors. J Neurosci 2005;25:11231–8.

90. Wu Y, Liu HB, Ding M, et al. Association between the −1438G/A and T102C polymorphisms of 5-HT$_{2A}$ receptor gene and obstructive sleep apnea: a meta-analysis. Mol Biol Rep 2013;40:6223–31.

91. Zhao Y, Tao L, Nie P, et al. Association between 5-HT$_{2A}$ receptor polymorphisms and risk of obstructive sleep apnea and hypopnea syndrome: a systematic review and meta-analysis. Gene 2013;530:287–94.

92. Deuschle M, Schredl M, Schilling C, et al. Association between a serotonin transporter length polymorphism and primary insomnia. Sleep 2010;33:343–7.

93. Brummett BH, Krystal AD, Ashley-Koch A, et al. Sleep quality varies as a function of 5-HTTLPR genotype and stress. Psychosom Med 2007;69:621–4.

94. Carskadon MA, Sharkey KM, Knopik VS, McGeary JE. Short sleep as an environmental exposure: a preliminary study associating 5-HTTLPR genotype to self-reported sleep duration and depressed mood in first-year university students. Sleep 2012;35:791–6.

95. Barclay NL, Eley TC, Mill J, et al. Sleep quality and diurnal preference in a sample of young adults: associations with 5HTTLPR, PER3, and CLOCK 3111. Am J Med Genet B Neuropsychiatr Genet 2011;156B:681–90.

96. Winkelman JW, Buxton OM, Jensen JE, et al. Reduced brain GABA in primary insomnia: preliminary data from 4 T proton magnetic resonance spectroscopy (^{1}H-MRS). Sleep 2008;31:1499–506.

97. Plante, DT, Jensen JE, Schoerning L, Winkelman JW. Reduced gamma-aminobutyric acid in occipital and anterior cingulate cortices in primary insomnia: a link to major depressive disorder? Neuropsychopharmacology 2012;37:1548–57.

98. Morgan PT, Pace-Schott EF, Mason GF, et al. Cortical GABA levels in primary insomnia. Sleep 2012;35:807–14.

99. Buhr A, Bianchi MT, Baur R, et al. Functional characterization of the new human $GABA_A$ receptor mutation β_3(R192H). Hum Genet 2002;111:154–60.

100. Huber R, Tononi G, Cirelli C. Exploratory behavior, cortical BDNF expression, and sleep homeostasis. Sleep 2007;30:129–39.

101. Bachmann V, Klein C, Bodenmann S, et al. The BDNF Val66Met polymorphism modulates sleep intensity: EEG frequency- and state-specificity. Sleep 2012;35:335–44.

102. Egan MF, Kojima M, Callicott JH, et al. The BDNF val66met polymorphism affects activity-dependent secretion of BDNF and human memory and hippocampal function. Cell 2003;112:257–69.

103. Kapas L, Hong L, Cady AB, et al. Somnogenic, pyrogenic, and anorectic activities of tumor necrosis factor-alpha and TNF-alpha fragments. Am J Physiol 1992;263:R708–15.

104. Shoham S, Davenne D, Cady AB, et al. Recombinant tumor necrosis factor and interleukin 1 enhance slow-wave sleep. Am J Physiol 1987;253: R142–9.

105. Fang J, Wang Y, Krueger JM. Mice lacking the TNF 55 kDa receptor fail to sleep more after TNFα treatment. J Neurosci 1997;17:5949–55.

106. Takahashi S, Kapas L, Fang J, Krueger JM. An anti-tumor necrosis factor antibody suppresses sleep in rats and rabbits. Brain Res 1995;690:241–4.

107. Wieczorek S, Gencik M, Rujescu D, et al. *TNFA* promoter polymorphisms and narcolepsy. Tissue Antigens 2003;61:437–42.

108. Chen YH, Huang YS, Chen CH. Increased plasma level of tumor necrosis factor alpha in patients with narcolepsy in Taiwan. Sleep Med 2013;14:1272–6.

109. Himmerich H, Beitinger PA, Fulda S, et al. Plasma levels of tumor necrosis factor alpha and soluble tumor necrosis factor receptors in patients with narcolepsy. Arch Intern Med 2006;166:1739–43.

110. Okun ML, Giese S, Lin L, et al. Exploring the cytokine and endocrine involvement in narcolepsy. Brain Behav Immun 2004;18:326–32.

111. Kato T, Honda M, Kuwata S, et al. A search for a mutation in the tumour necrosis factor-alpha gene in narcolepsy. Psychiatry Clin Neurosci 1999;53:421–3.

112. Hohjoh H, Nakayama T, Ohashi J, et al. Significant association of a single nucleotide polymorphism in the tumor necrosis factor-alpha (TNF-alpha) gene promoter with human narcolepsy. Tissue Antigens 1999;54:138–45.

113. Hohjoh H, Terada N, Kawashima M, et al. Significant association of the tumor necrosis factor receptor 2 (*TNFR2*) gene with human narcolepsy. Tissue Antigens 2000;56:446–8.

114. Medori R, Montagna P, Tritschler HJ, et al. Fatal familial insomnia: a second kindred with mutation of prion protein gene at codon 178. Neurology 1992;42:669–70.

115. Montagna P, Gambetti P, Cortelli P, Lugaresi E. Familial and sporadic fatal insomnia. Lancet Neurol 2003;2:167–76.

116. Monari L, Chen SG, Brown P, et al. Fatal familial insomnia and familial Creutzfeldt–Jakob disease: different prion proteins determined by a DNA polymorphism. Proc Natl Acad Sci U S A 1994;91:2839–42.

117. Goldfarb LG, Petersen RB, Tabaton M, et al. Fatal familial insomnia and familial Creutzfeldt–Jakob disease: disease phenotype determined by a DNA polymorphism. Science 1992;258:806–8.

118. Nishino S, Ripley B, Overeem S, et al. Hypocretin (orexin) deficiency in human narcolepsy. Lancet 2000;355:39–40.

119. Peyron C, Faraco J, Rogers W, et al. A mutation in a case of early onset narcolepsy and a generalized absence of hypocretin peptides in human narcoleptic brains. Nat Med 2000;6:991–7.

120. Thannickal TC, Moore RY, Nienhuis R, et al. Reduced number of hypocretin neurons in human narcolepsy. Neuron 2000;27:469–74.

121. Chemelli RM, Willie JT, Sinton CM, et al. Narcolepsy in orexin knockout mice: molecular genetics of sleep regulation. Cell 1999;98:437–51.

122. Lin L, Faraco J, Li R, et al. The sleep disorder canine narcolepsy is caused by a mutation in the hypocretin (orexin) receptor 2 gene. Cell 1999;98:365–76.

123. Hungs M, Lin L, Okun M, Mignot E. Polymorphisms in the vicinity of the hypocretin/orexin are not associated with human narcolepsy. Neurology 2001;57:1893–5.

124. Mignot E, Tafti M, Dement WC, Grumet FC. Narcolepsy and immunity. Adv Neuroimmunol 1995;5:23–37.

125. Cvetkovic-Lopes V, Bayer L, Dorsaz S, et al. Elevated tribbles homolog 2-specific antibody levels in narcolepsy patients. J Clin Invest 2010;120:713–19.

126. Deloumeau A, Bayard S, Coquerel Q, et al. Increased immune complexes of hypocretin autoantibodies in narcolepsy. PLoS One 2010;5(10):e13320.

127. Hasegawa E, Yanagisawa M, Sakurai T, Mieda M. Orexin neurons suppress narcolepsy via 2 distinct efferent pathways. J Clin Invest 2014;124:604–16.

128. Reppert SM, Weaver DR. Coordination of circadian timing in mammals. Nature 2002;418:935–41.

129. Gekakis N, Staknis D, Nguyen HB, et al. Role of the CLOCK protein in the mammalian circadian mechanism. Science 1998;280:1564–9.

130. Kume K, Zylka MJ, Sriram S, et al. mCRY1 and mCRY2 are essential components of the negative limb of the circadian clock feedback loop. Cell 1999;98:193–205.

131. Franken P, Dudley CA, Estill SJ, et al. NPAS2 as a transcriptional regulator of non-rapid eye movement sleep: genotype and sex interactions. Proc Natl Acad Sci U S A 2006;103:7118–23.

132. Wisor JP, O'Hara BF, Terao A, et al. A role for cryptochromes in sleep regulation. BMC Neurosci 2002;3:20.

133. Franken P. A role for clock genes in sleep homeostasis. Curr Opin Neurobiol 2013;23:864–72.

134. Laposky A, Easton A, Dugovic C, et al. Deletion of the mammalian circadian clock gene *BMAL1/Mop3* alters baseline sleep architecture and the response to sleep deprivation. Sleep 2005;28:395–409.

135. Archer SN, Carpen JD, Gibson M, et al. Polymorphism in the *PER3* promoter associates with diurnal preference and delayed sleep phase disorder. Sleep 2010;33:695–701.

136. Archer SN, Robilliard DL, Skene DJ, et al. A length polymorphism in the circadian clock gene *Per3* is linked to delayed sleep phase syndrome and extreme diurnal preference. Sleep 2003;26:413–15.

137. Dijk DJ, Archer SN. *PERIOD3*, circadian phenotypes, and sleep homeostasis. Sleep Med Rev 2010;14:151–60.

138. Lazar AS, Slak A, Lo JC, et al. Sleep, diurnal preference, health, and psychological well-being: a prospective single-allelic-variation study. Chronobiol Int 2012;29:131–46.

139. Viola AU, Archer SN, James LM, et al. *PER3* polymorphism predicts sleep structure and waking performance. Curr Biol 2007. 17(7):613–18.

140. Groeger JA, Viola AU, Lo JC, et al. Early morning executive functioning during sleep deprivation is compromised by a *PERIOD3* polymorphism. Sleep 2008;31:1159–67.

141. Goel N, Banks S, Mignot E, Dinges DF. *PER3* polymorphism predicts cumulative sleep homeostatic but not neurobehavioral changes to chronic partial sleep deprivation. PLoS One 2009;4(6):e5874.

142. Ebisawa T, Uchiyama M, Kajimura N, et al. Association of structural polymorphisms in the human *period3* gene with delayed sleep phase syndrome. EMBO Rep 2001;2:342–6.

143. Katzenberg D, Young T, Finn L, et al. A *CLOCK* polymorphism associated with human diurnal preference. Sleep 1998;21:569–76.

144. Mishima K, Tozawa T, Satoh K, et al. The 3111T/C polymorphism of *hClock* is associated with evening preference and delayed sleep timing in a Japanese population sample. Am J Med Genet B Neuropsychiatr Genet 2005;133B:101–4.

145. Robilliard DL, Archer SN, Arendt J, et al. The 3111 *Clock* gene polymorphism is not associated with sleep and circadian rhythmicity in phenotypically characterized human subjects. J Sleep Res 2002;11:305–12.

146. Pedrazzoli M, Louzada FM, Pereira DS, et al. *Clock* polymorphisms and circadian rhythms phenotypes in a sample of the Brazilian population. Chronobiol Int 2007;24:1–8.

CHAPTER 6

Physiological changes in sleep

Sudhansu Chokroverty and Sushanth Bhat

Sleep is not a passive state where physiological processes are simply suspended. Research has shown that several important, well-defined physiological changes occur during sleep, involving the central nervous system (CNS) and the autonomic nervous system (ANS), the neuromuscular, respiratory, and cardiovascular systems, the gastrointestinal tract, the endocrine system, and the systems controlling temperature regulation and immune regulation. An understanding of these changes is important for the clinical care of patients with sleep disorders and sleep deprivation from a number of causes. This chapter provides a brief overview of the physiological changes associated with sleep in the above systems.

Changes in the central nervous system

The brain is not quiescent during sleep. Various areas of the CNS are highly active during sleep, as demonstrated by electrophysiological, immunohistochemical, and functional imaging studies of the brain, such as positron emission tomography (PET) and functional magnetic resonance imaging (fMRI), showing activation and deactivation of specific regions of the brain (see Chapter 11). There is decreased intracortical facilitation in rapid eye movement (REM) sleep and increased intracortical inhibition of interneurons in non-REM (NREM) sleep. During NREM sleep, some regions (such as the ventrolateral preoptic and median preoptic neurons in the anterior hypothalamic nuclei, and, to a certain extent, also the lower brainstem nucleus tractus solitarius (NTS) and the medullary GABAergic parafacial zone) are activated, whereas the activity of other regions (wakefulness-promoting histaminergic, aminergic, serotoninergic, and orexinergic neurons, the ascending reticular activating system, and most of the cerebral cortical regions) is markedly reduced. During REM sleep, much of the cortical regions are activated, along with the generators of REM sleep in the pons (the pedunculopontine and laterodorsal tegmental nuclei, and the sublaterodorsal (SLD) nucleus in rats, which is equivalent to the peri-locus coeruleus alpha in cats and the subcoeruleus in humans); simultaneously, mechanisms that paralyze the body are brought into action to ensure REM atonia, preventing dream-enacting behavior. Both somatosensory cortical (SEP) and motor evoked potential (MEP) amplitudes attenuate in sleep. There is dampening of spinal and cranial motor reflexes because of motor neuron hyperpolarization, presynaptic inhibition, and dysfacilitation of brainstem aminergic and lateral hypothalamic orexinergic neurons projecting to brainstem motor neurons as well as to ventral horn cells of the spinal cord. The extensor plantar response (Babinski's response), which is absent in wakefulness in normal individuals, may be elicited in sleep [1].

Changes in cerebral blood flow and metabolism during sleep are discussed in detail later in the chapter.

Changes in the autonomic nervous system

The ANS receives input from, and has widespread effects on, several body systems and functions. Peripheral receptors in the cardiovascular and respiratory systems, as well as the gastrointestinal tract, relay to the medullary NTS, which, through its diffuse afferent and efferent projections, exerts autonomic control on cardiac rhythm and rate, circulation, respiration, and gastrointestinal motility and secretion. The efferents from the NTS also project to the hypothalamic and limbic regions and to the ventral medulla, which exert significant control over cardiovascular regulation. The final common pathways from the NTS are parasympathetic efferents arising in the nucleus ambiguus and traveling through the vagus nerve, and sympathetic fibers arising in the hypothalamic paraventricular nucleus to sympathetic preganglionic neurons in the spinal cord. Acting together, these autonomic mechanisms maintain internal homeostasis [2–4].

Changes in the ANS during sleep result in profound alterations in multiple systems [5]. The basic autonomic changes during sleep include increased parasympathetic tone and decreased sympathetic activity during NREM sleep, accompanied by a reduction of circulating levels of norepinephrine (noradrenaline) and epinephrine (adrenaline). These changes lead to pupillary constriction, a fall in blood pressure and bradycardia. During REM sleep, there is a further increase in parasympathetic tone and a further decrease in sympathetic activity; however, there is an intermittent increase of sympathetic activity during phasic REM sleep resulting in phasic pupillary dilatation and swings in blood pressure and heart rate, causing tachy–brady arrhythmias. Heart rate variability (HRV) studies [6] reflect these changes; during NREM sleep, the low-frequency (LF) component decreases, whereas the high-frequency (HF) component increases, reflecting increased vagal tone. In contrast, during REM sleep, extreme variation in LF and HF with increased LF and decreased HF components occurs. The HF component mainly reflects the respiration–vagal modulation of sinus rhythm, whereas the nonrespiratory LF component reflects the sympathetic modulation of the heart in addition to baroreflex responsiveness to beat-to-beat variations in blood pressure [7–10]. Power spectral analysis [11] suggests that the wake/sleep transition period represents a transitional process between two physiologically different states, with a decrease in LF power and unchanged HF power causing a decrease in the LF/HF ratio and reflecting a shift toward parasympathetic predominance. Thus, NREM sleep is a state of relative cardiorespiratory stability, whereas REM sleep is a state of profound instability with intense autonomic and respiratory dysregulation. Reduced HRV may be noted in patients with myocardial infarction, cardiac transplantation, or diabetic autonomic neuropathy. Reduced HRV is a strong and independent predictor of mortality after acute myocardial infarction [12]. Additionally, lethal arrhythmias are related to either increased sympathetic activity or decreased vagal activity.

Sleep disorders can affect the normal changes that occur in the ANS during sleep. For example, patients with OSA have chronic sympathetic hyperactivity, which is thought to predispose to daytime hypertension, cardiac ischemia, heart failure, and stroke [13]. Similarly, patients with sleep terror, REM sleep behavior disorder (RBD), and narcolepsy suffer from episodic disruptions of autonomic control during sleep, which may have implications for the control of the circulatory, respiratory, gastrointestinal, and urogenital systems.

Changes in the peripheral nervous system

Muscle hypotonia

One of the cardinal features of sleep is progressive loss of muscle tone as a subject transitions from wakefulness to NREM sleep and finally to REM sleep, where muscle hypotonia is most pronounced. In NREM sleep, several factors seem to contribute to the mild hypotonia; in particular, inhibition of noradrenergic locus coeruleus and serotonergic midline raphe neurons, as well as mild hyperpolarization of motor neurons in the brainstem and spinal cord [14]. Additionally, during REM sleep, the near-complete paralysis of most voluntary muscles (with the exception of the diaphragm, extraocular, and middle ear muscles) is thought to be due to activation of a specific group of neurons in the dorsal pontine tegmentum [15,16], particularly pathways from the peri-locus coeruleus alpha and the SLD causing disinhibition of cholinergic neurons, and inhibition of noradrenergic and serotonergic neurons in the pons. The cholinergic neurons, in turn, excite pontine glutamatergic neurons projecting to the glycinergic and GABAergic premotor neurons in the medullary reticular formation, causing hyperpolarization of the motor neurons and muscle paralysis during REM sleep [17]. The ventral SLD sends both direct and indirect projections via the ventromedial medulla that hyperpolarize motor neurons in the brainstem and spinal cord through inhibitory GABAergic and glycinergic pathways. Additional contribution to REM atonia comes from dysfacilitation of lateral hypothalamic hypocretinergic neurons. At the cellular level, the atonia of REM sleep is due to enhanced inhibitory postsynaptic potentials (IPSPs). The abrupt, jerky, purposeless movements seen intermittently during phasic REM sleep, manifested as muscle twitching seen on EMG channels in PSG recordings and sometimes clinically, are thought to be due to excitatory postsynaptic potentials (EPSPs) in the motor neurons [18,19] mediated by the reticulospinal and vestibulospinal rather than the corticospinal and corticobulbar tracts [20]. The IPSPs and EPSPs are kept balanced during REM sleep to ensure that voluntary muscles remain paralyzed as the brain is active and dreaming; failure of this system results in pathological dream-enacting behavior, as may occur with RBD [21].

Thermal regulation in sleep

Body temperature regulation follows a circadian rhythm that is closely linked to, but is independent of, the sleep–wake rhythm

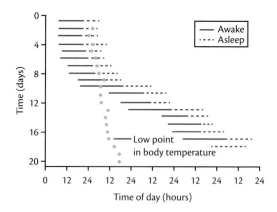

Fig. 6.1 Synchronized (light-entrained) and desynchronized (free-running) rhythms in a person showing dissociation between body temperature and sleep-activity cycles.
Reproduced from Aerospace Med, 40, Aschoff J, Desynchronization and resynchronization of human circadian rhythms, pp. 847, Copyright (1969), with permission from Aerospace Medical Association.

[22]. When sleep–wake cycles and temperature cycles are dissociated from each other, for example when environmental cues such as light are removed, the independent nature of the two becomes obvious (Fig. 6.1). Body temperature follows a sinusoidal rhythm with a peak around 9:00 pm and a minimum (nadir) around 3:00 am as a result of circadian rhythmicity (Fig. 6.2). Thus, the core temperature nadir occurs 2–3 hours before habitual wake time, a fact that is of crucial importance in the detection and treatment of circadian rhythm disorders (see Chapters 21 and 22).

As with the sleep–wake circadian rhythm (see Chapter 3), the master clock for the temperature regulation rhythm is in the suprachiasmatic nucleus (SCN) of the hypothalamus, through its projections to the thermosensitive neurons of the GABAergic median preoptic nucleus (MnPN) of the anterior hypothalamus (POAH). The MnPN and the ventrolateral preoptic (VLPO) nucleus of the POAH are also responsible for generation of NREM sleep [23]. Thus, the POAH region is responsible for both thermoregulation and NREM sleep, explaining the close association of the two rhythms. However, this arrangement is subject to external influences. Warmth-sensitive neurons of the POAH receive inputs from peripheral cutaneous receptors and increase firing rates at sleep onset while decreasing the rates at sleep offset [24]. Peripheral heat

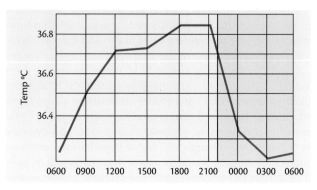

Fig. 6.2 Body temperature follows a sinusoidal rhythm with a peak around 9:00 pm and a minimum (nadir) around 3:00 am as a result of circadian rhythmicity.

loss, such as may occur with vasodilation after a hot bath, or even just warming the feet, results in shortened sleep onset latency and increased slow-wave sleep (SWS) [25–27]. Conversely, a rise in core body temperature, as occurs with vigorous exercise just before sleep, has traditionally been thought to hamper sleep onset [28], although this concept has been challenged recently [29]. Temperature control differs in NREM and REM sleep. The thermoregulatory responses that occur during NREM sleep, such as sweating and panting, are absent in REM sleep, where thermoregulation is impaired [30].

There has been interesting research into the role of thermoregulatory dysfunction or mismatch between thermoregulatory and sleep–wake cycles in patients with a number of sleep disorders. For example, patients with sleep onset insomnia have delayed core body temperature rhythms [31], suggesting that their sleep difficulties may be due to attempts to initiate sleep before the nocturnal dip in body temperature. Similarly, it has been suggested that age-related impairment of the heat loss mechanism or phase advance in body temperature rhythm may partly explain sleep initiation or maintenance difficulty in the elderly, and therefore behavior that enhances peripheral heat loss may improve sleep [32,33]. Jet lag and shift-work disorder may similarly be a result of environmentally induced disruption of thermoregulation and SWS, causing sleep initiation and maintenance problems, disorganization of sleep architecture, and poor daytime function [34]. Menopausal hot flashes may possibly also be a disorder of thermoregulation during sleep as a result of POAH dysfunction; hot flashes may be more common in the first than the second half of the night when REM sleep dominates, impairing the thermoregulatory mechanism [35,36].

Respiration and sleep

Control of respiration in wakefulness and sleep

The primary function of the respiratory system is to maintain arterial homeostasis of the partial pressures of carbon dioxide (pCO_2) and oxygen (pO_2). This requires adequate alveolar ventilation, which in turn is dependent on central controllers of respiration located in the medulla (with input from the cortex), peripheral chemoreceptors, and pulmonary and upper airway mechanoreceptors, the thoracic bellows (consisting of the ribcage, respiratory muscles, and their innervation), and the lungs (including the airways and the alveolar membrane where gas exchange occurs). Box 6.1 lists the respiratory muscles. The principal muscle of inspiration is the diaphragm (innervated by the phrenic nerve, formed by motor roots of C3, C4, and C5 anterior horn cells), assisted by the external intercostal muscles (innervated by the thoracic motor roots and nerves). Expiration is usually a passive process, resulting from elastic recoil of the lungs. However, during forced and effortful breathing (eg, dyspnea and orthopnea), accessory muscles of both inspiration and expiration are activated.

The "pacemaker" for breathing is the dorsal respiratory group (DRG) in the medulla, which mainly initiates inspiration and is responsible for the regularity, rhythmicity, and rate of breathing; the ventral respiratory group (VRG) lies in proximity and generally is activated when active expiration is required. These centers project to the anterior horn cells of spinal motor neurons innervating the diaphragm and the intercostal muscles. Two centers in the rostral pons, one in the region of the parabrachial and Kölliker–Fuse

---

Box 6.1 The respiratory muscles

Inspiratory muscles

- Diaphragm
- External intercostal

Accessory inspiratory muscles

- Sternocleidomastoideus
- Scalenus (anterior, middle, posterior)
- Pectoralis major
- Pectoralis minor
- Serratus anterior
- Serratus posterior superior
- Latissimus dorsi
- Alae nasi
- Trapezius

Expiratory muscles

(These are silent during quiet breathing, but contract during moderately severe airway obstruction or during forceful and increased rate of breathing)

- Internal intercostal
- Rectus abdominis
- External and internal oblique
- Transversus abdominis

Reproduced from Chokroverty S (ed.), Sleep Disorders Medicine: Basic Science, Technical Considerations, and Clinical Aspects (3rd ed), Copyright (2009), with permission from Elsevier.

---

nuclei (pneumotaxic center) and one in the dorsolateral region of the lower pons (apneustic center) [37,38] exert influences over these medullary centers (Fig. 6.3). The rate and rhythm of breathing are modulated by inputs to the medullary respiratory centers that arise from peripheral chemoreceptors (the carotid and aortic bodies that are sensitive to hypoxia, hypercapnia, and alterations in blood pH), the central chemoreceptors in the medulla (sensitive mainly to hypercapnia and increased blood pH), and pulmonary mechanoreceptors, sensitive to stretching of the lungs. Inputs from these receptors travel via the glossopharyngeal and vagus nerves and synapse in the NTS. This system works in concert to ensure homeostasis of blood gases, for example by increasing the rate and depth of respiration in response to hypoxia or hypercapnia, or by causing a cessation of breathing when pCO_2 falls below a certain level (the apneic threshold) [39]. This system is referred to as metabolic or autonomic control of breathing and is independent of volitional control. In wakefulness, the reticular activating system and the cortex exert an additional influence and allow for the voluntary control of breathing as well as for phonation. However, in sleep, this voluntary control is lost, and respiration is controlled purely by the metabolic system [40]. This situation explains the changes in respiration that occur in sleep.

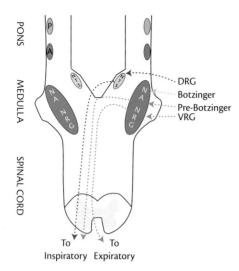

Fig. 6.3 Schematic representation of central respiratory neurons in the pons and medulla. DRG: dorsal respiratory group with projections to contralateral predominantly inspiratory muscles; VRG: ventral respiratory group with projections to contralateral inspiratory and expiratory muscles; P: pneumotaxic center; A: apneustic center.

Reproduced from Chokroverty S (ed.), Sleep Disorders Medicine: Basic Science, Technical Considerations, and Clinical Aspects (3rd ed), Copyright (2009), with permission from Elsevier.

Respiratory changes in sleep

There is a progressive fall in respiratory minute ventilation by approximately 0.5–1.5 L/min compared with wakefulness in NREM sleep and 1.6 L/min in REM sleep (with the biggest reduction being in phasic REM sleep). This is mainly due to a fall in tidal volume; respiratory rate does not decrease, although respiration becomes irregular in REM sleep, especially during phasic REM [41]. This fall in tidal volume in sleep is due to a number of factors, chief among which are hypotonia of all respiratory muscles except the diaphragm (leading to hypoventilation, reduced tone, and collapse of the upper airway dilators resulting in increased upper airway resistance) and reduced chemosensitivity; these are more marked in REM than NREM sleep. This fall in alveolar ventilation in sleep causes a rise in pCO_2 by 2–8 mmHg, a fall in pO_2 by 3–10 mmHg, and a decrease in arterial oxygen saturation (SaO_2) by less than 2% [42].

Sleep-related changes in the upper airway, in particular, play an important role in the pathogenesis of sleep-disordered breathing. In wakefulness, the activity of the upper airway inspiratory dilator muscles (Table 6.1) reflexively increases at the onset of inspiration due to the negative intrathoracic pressure; this is a protective mechanism guarding against upper airway narrowing. In sleep, this reflexive response is blunted, making the upper airway susceptible to collapse. This susceptibility is enhanced by agents that lower muscle tone, including alcohol and benzodiazepines, and worsens with aging and in the supine position [43]. The role of tongue muscles, particularly the genioglossus and geniohyoid muscles that protrude the tongue, in the pathogenesis of OSA is being increasingly recognized. EMG recordings have demonstrated that genioglossal muscle activity mildly decreases during NREM sleep, but markedly decreases during REM sleep [44]. The resulting backward displacement of the tongue partially or completely against the posterior pharyngeal wall restricts airflow and contributes to OSA. Several treatment modalities for OSA, including tongue-retaining devices [45] and hypoglossal nerve stimulation [46], target this phenomenon.

Table 6.1 Summary of physiological changes in the respiratory system occurring during sleep

Parameters	Wakefulness	NREM sleep	REM sleep
Respiratory rate	Normal	Decreases	Variable, apnea may occur
Minute ventilation	Normal	Decreases	Decreases further
Alveolar ventilation	Normal	Decreases	Decreases further
$PaCO_2$	Normal	Increases slightly	Increases further slightly
PaO_2	Normal	Decreases slightly	Decreases further slightly
SaO_2	Normal	Decreases slightly	Decreases further slightly
Hypoxic ventilatory response	Normal	Decreases	Decreases further
hypercapnic ventilatory response	Normal	Decreases	Decreases further
Upper airway muscle tone	Normal	Decreases slightly	Decreases markedly or is absent
Upper airway resistance	Normal	Increases	Increases further

Reproduced from Chokroverty S (ed.), Sleep Disorders Medicine: Basic Science, Technical Considerations, and Clinical Aspects (3rd ed), Copyright (2009), with permission from Elsevier.

Table 6.1 summarizes the physiological changes that occur in the respiratory system during sleep.

Cardiovascular system and sleep

Changes in cardiac and vascular function that occur in sleep are ultimately due to the control of the ANS (see the discussion earlier in this chapter). In phasic REM sleep, superimposed surges of sympathetic activity occur. Knowledge of these changes in ANS function aids in the understanding of hemodynamic changes that occur in sleep. These changes are summarized in Table 6.2.

Changes in cardiac function during sleep

Bradycardia during both NREM and REM sleep results from a tonic increase in parasympathetic activity (sympathectomy has little effect). The heart rate decreases by 5–8% during NREM sleep, but becomes more intense during REM sleep, with frequent upward and downward swings resulting in bradytachycardia occurring in phasic REM sleep due to superimposed spikes of sympathetic activity [47–49]. Similarly, cardiac output falls progressively during sleep, with the greatest decrease occurring during the last sleep cycle, particularly during the last REM sleep cycle early in the morning [50].

Changes in the circulatory system during sleep

Systemic blood pressure falls by approximately 10–20% during NREM sleep and swings up and down during REM sleep, with an overall increase by about 5% above that noted in NREM sleep. There is a sharp rise in blood pressure around the time of awakening [51].

Table 6.2 Summary of physiological changes in the heart and circulatory system occurring during sleep

Physiological characteristic	NREM	REM
Heart rate	↓	↑↓
Cardiac output	↓	↓↓
Systematic arterial BP:		
◆ Dippers	↓	↓↑
◆ Extreme dippers	↓↓	↓↑
◆ Non-dippers	↓–	↓↑
◆ Reverse dippers	↑	↓↑
Pulmonary arterial BP	↑	↑
Peripheral vascular resistance	–↓	↓
Systematic blood flow:		
◆ Cutaneous	–	↓
◆ Muscular	–	↓
◆ Mesenteric	–	↑
◆ Renal	–	↑
Cerebral blood flow	↓	↑

↓ = Decreased; ↑ = Increased; ↓↑ = Uncertain; – = Unchanged.

Reproduced from Chokroverty S (ed.), Sleep Disorders Medicine: Basic Science, Technical Considerations, and Clinical Aspects (3rd ed), Copyright (2009), with permission from Elsevier.

This circadian variation in blood pressure, with an overall reduction during sleep and increase on awakening, is referred to as "dipping." Normal dipping of systolic blood pressure, such that the night-wake ratio is between 0.8 but less than or equal to 0.9, is physiological, and these individuals are called "dippers" [52–54]. "Non-dippers" are subjects in whom the night-wake systolic blood pressure ratio is between 0.9 and 1, and "extreme dippers" are those in whom the ratio is less than 0.8. In "reverse dippers," the blood pressure actually increases during sleep (night-wake ratio greater than 1). Non-dippers, extreme dippers, and reverse dippers are at higher risk for cardiovascular or cerebrovascular events causing infarctions and periventricular hyperlucencies on brain MRI [55–57].

Pulmonary arterial pressure rises slightly during sleep. During wakefulness, the mean value is 18/8 mmHg; that during sleep is 23/12 mmHg. Cutaneous, muscular, and mesenteric vascular blood flow shows little change during NREM sleep, but during REM sleep, there is profound vasodilation in these splanchnic beds, resulting in increased blood flow in the mesenteric and renal vascular beds. As a result, peripheral vascular resistance (PVR) generally remains unchanged during NREM sleep, but falls significantly during REM sleep [58].

Changes in cerebral blood flow and metabolism during sleep

Cerebral blood flow (CBF) and metabolic rate are noted to be lower in NREM than in REM sleep, lower at the end of the night compared with at the beginning of the night, and lower in post-sleep wakefulness than in pre-sleep wakefulness [59,60]. CBF and metabolic rate for glucose and oxygen decrease by 5–23% during NREM sleep, whereas these values vary from 10% below up to 41% above waking levels during REM sleep [61–63]. Functional neuroimaging techniques, including PET scans, reveal significant differences in areas and levels of brain activation during wakefulness, NREM sleep, and REM sleep (see Chapter 13). During NREM sleep, there is a global decrease in CBF, with regional decreases in the dorsal pons, mesencephalon, thalami, basal ganglia, basal forebrain, anterior hypothalamus, prefrontal cortex, anterior cingulate cortex, and precuneus [64–66] and regionally specific increases in activities during SWS in the brainstem, cerebellum, ventral prefrontal cortex, posterior cingulate cortex/precuneus, and parahippocampal areas, in addition to areas generating fast and slow spindles. These findings suggest that during NREM sleep, the brain is actively involved in generating synchronized slow waves and spindles, which have important implications for memory processing [67]. In contrast, the brain in REM sleep is far more globally active, with increased blood flow and metabolism in the pontine tegmentum, thalamus, amygdala, anterior cingulate cortex, hippocampus, temporal and occipital regions, basal forebrain, cerebellum, and caudate nucleus, and regional deactivation in the dorsolateral prefrontal cortex, posterior cingulate gyrus, precuneus, and inferior parietal cortex [68]. REM sleep-related activation of the pontine tegmentum, thalamic nuclei, and basal forebrain supports the REM sleep-generating mechanisms in these regions [69].

The gastrointestinal tract and sleep

The activity of the gastrointestinal tract is controlled by both the ANS and the enteric nervous system, an intrinsic autonomic system within the walls of the visceral organs that works closely with the ANS. Changes that occur in the gastrointestinal tract during sleep are summarized in Table 6.3.

Changes in esophageal function and gastric acid secretion during sleep

There is a clear circadian rhythm to gastric acid secretion. During wakefulness, gastric acid secretion depends on food ingestion, increased salivation, and the activity of the vagus nerve. During the first 2 hours of sleep, there is a failure of inhibition of acid secretion, resulting in peak gastric acid secretion occurring between 10:00 pm and 2:00 am. Vagotomy abolishes this rhythm [70]. Studies have failed to demonstrate any difference in gastric acid secretion between NREM and REM sleep [71–73]. Esophageal motility and function are also affected by sleep. This is of particular importance for patients with gastro-esophageal reflux disease (GERD). There are two esophageal sphincters that act as barriers to reflux: the upper esophageal sphincter (UES) and the lower esophageal sphincter (LES). Although disputed by some authors [74], most studies have found that in normal individuals who experience episodes of GERD, there is generally a reduction in LES pressure during sleep [75,76]. Similarly, sleep-induced loss of UES pressure may promote reflux of esophageal contents into the pharynx and tracheobronchial tree. Also during sleep, reflux is cleared much slowly than during wakefulness, and salivary flow and swallowing are reduced, resulting in a longer acid–mucosa contact time. Proximal migration of gastric contents and decreased esophageal peristalsis in sleep (especially in SWS) also occur, and all of these factors predispose to development of esophagitis [77], Thus, patients with

Table 6.3 Summary of physiological changes in the gastrointestinal tract occurring during sleep

Physiological characteristics	Wakefulness	Sleep
Swallowing frequency	Normal	Decreased
Salivary flow	Normal	Decreased
Esophageal acid clearance time	Normal	Prolonged
Lower and upper esophageal sphincter pressure	Normal	Decreased
Esophageal peristaltic contractions	Normal	Decreased
Gastric motility	Normal	Decreased
Gastric acid secretion	Depends on food ingestion	Peak secretion between 10 pm and 2 am
Migrating motor complex (MMC) (recurs every 90 minutes)	Normal velocity	Reduced velocity
Colonic motility	Normal	Decreased
Rectal motor activity and anal canal pressure	Normal	Increased periodic activity with retrograde propagation and higher anal canal pressure

Reproduced from Chokroverty S (ed.), Sleep Disorders Medicine: Basic Science, Technical Considerations, and Clinical Aspects (3rd ed), Copyright (2009), with permission from Elsevier.

peptic ulcer disease and GERD may have repeated awakenings and arousals from nocturnal epigastric pain ("nightly heartburn"), particularly in the first few hours of the night. Concomitant OSA worsens GERD, although the mechanism is unclear, and treatment with continuous positive airway pressure (CPAP) improves symptoms [78]. Esophageal pH monitoring during polysomnography (PSG) may help in the evaluation and management of these patients.

Changes in gastrointestinal motility during sleep

There are contradictory reports in the literature about the effect of sleep on gastric motility, with both inhibition and enhancement of gastric motility having been described [79,80], and one group reporting that gastroduodenal motility during sleep was related to sleep-stage shifts and body movements [81]. In the stomach and small intestine, a cyclical pattern of motor activity, called the migrating motor complex (MMC), recurs every 90 minutes and has a circadian rhythm, with the lowest velocity occurring during sleep, although no consistent differences have been detected between NREM and REM sleep [82–86]. There is decreased colonic motility in the transverse, descending, and sigmoid colon, and there is retrograde periodic rectal motor activity during sleep, all of which serve to prevent passive escape of rectal contents during sleep [87].

Renal function and sleep

The volume of urine production generally decreases in sleep owing to decreased glomerular filtration, increased reabsorption of water, increased activation of the renin–angiotensin–aldosterone system (see the next section), decreased sympathetic activity and slightly higher plasma levels of antidiuretic hormone (ADH) [88]. In addition to lower ADH levels, patients with OSA have increased atrial natriuretic peptide, which suppresses plasma renin secretion; thus there is an increase in nocturnal urine output. This often results in patients with OSA complaining of nocturia and frequent awakenings for micturition [89].

Endocrine regulation and sleep

While the characteristic pattern of hormone secretion by most endocrine glands is an episodic or pulsatile secretion every 1–2 hours, suggesting an ultradian rhythmicity, the plasma concentrations of several hormones show circadian rhythms that in some cases are related to the sleep–wake cycle (Fig. 6.4). For example, adrenocorticotropic hormone (ACTH), cortisol, and melatonin rhythms are determined by the circadian clock, whereas growth hormone (GH), prolactin, thyroid-stimulating hormone (TSH), and renin rhythms are sleep-related. It is evident from Fig. 6.4 that during the first part of the night, the plasma GH level is high and the cortisol level low, whereas during the later part of the night, GH level is low and cortisol level high, suggesting a reciprocal interaction of the hypothalamic–pituitary–adrenocortical axis and the hypothalamic–pituitary–somatostatin system. Thus there are 24-hour oscillations of circulating levels of various endocrine secretions, showing a time-of-day dependence. These are driven not only by the endogenous circadian rhythms but also by sleep–wakefulness and behavioral or environmental factors.

Melatonin, the "hormone of darkness," is synthesized by the pineal gland and released directly into the bloodstream or cerebrospinal fluid. The maximum nocturnal secretion of melatonin has been observed in young children, aged 1–3 years; secretion then begins to fall around puberty and decreases significantly in the elderly [90]. Melatonin levels follow a circadian rhythm that is heavily influenced by environmental light, which suppresses its production. In the absence of light as a major influence, melatonin begins to rise in the evening, attaining maximum values between 3:00 am and 5:00 am and then decreasing to low levels during the day (Fig. 6.4). A negative feedback mechanism exists to regulate melatonin production; impulses from the retinal ganglion cells that perceive light are transmitted via the retinohypothalamic tract to the SCN, which then sends efferent fibers to the paraventricular nucleus of the hypothalamus and then to the intermediolateral horn cells of the upper thoracic spinal cord, and subsequently to the superior cervical ganglia, which in turn transmit impulses via the postganglionic efferent fibers to the pineal gland [91]. The SCN has two melatonin receptors (MT_1 and MT_2). MT_1 receptors inhibit SCN neuronal activity and MT_2 receptors phase-shift circadian firing rhythms in the SCN. Because of its hypnotic and chronobiological properties, melatonin has found application in the treatment of insomnia and circadian rhythm disorders. Melatonin administered in the evenings has a phase-advancing effect, and when administered in the mornings has a phase-delaying effect. Thus, it has been used in the treatment of jet lag, shiftwork disorder, and non-24-hour sleep–wake syndrome. The use of melatonin in the treatment of insomnia is described in Chapter 20, and its use in the treatment of circadian rhythm disorders in Chapters 21 and 22.

The secretion of GH, an anabolic hormone whose function is mediated through hepatic insulin-like growth factor 1, is closely linked to SWS [92,93]. In addition to the secretion of GH itself by the anterior pituitary gland, SWS enhances the release of GH-stimulating factors

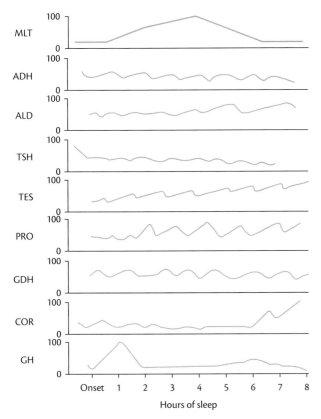

Fig. 6.4 Schematic representation of the plasma levels of hormones in an adult during 8 hours of sleep. Zero indicates lowest secretory episode and 100 indicates peak. MLT: melatonin; ADH: antidiuretic hormone; ALD: aldosterone; TSH: thyroid-stimulating hormone; TES: testosterone; PRO: prolactin; GDH: gonadotropic hormone; COR: cortisol; GH: growth hormone. Reproduced from Chokroverty S (ed.), Sleep Disorders Medicine: Basic Science, Technical Considerations, and Clinical Aspects (3rd ed), Copyright (2009), with permission from Elsevier.

such as hypothalamic GH-releasing hormone (GHRH) and ghrelin, an appetite-stimulant gastric peptide. It is notable that stimulation of the GABAergic hypothalamic GHRH neurons promotes both the onset of SWS and the peak GH levels, and agents promoting SWS (eg, γ-hydroxybutyrate) enhance GH secretion, suggesting a reciprocal link between SWS and GH secretion [94]. GH secretion occurs shortly after sleep onset during SWS and is inhibited by awakenings and sleep fragmentation. Conditions that fragment sleep, such as OSA and narcolepsy, cause diminished sleep-related GH secretion. In OSA patients, CPAP treatment increases GH secretion in sleep [95]. There is a natural decrease in sleep-related GH production in elderly populations, possibly related to the reduction of SWS and increased fragmentation of sleep with age. In acromegaly, a disorder of unregulated GH synthesis, the relationship between sleep and hormone secretion is lost [96].

The 24-hour secretion pattern of the ACTH–cortisol system has its own circadian rhythm, but one that is also modulated by the sleep–wake cycle. Cortisol secretion rapidly falls with sleep onset, most markedly with SWS, but then quickly rises in the later part of the night, being highest at awakening and subsequently declining throughout the day. However, this rhythmicity is absent during sleep deprivation, and only occurs during nocturnal sleep [97,98]. Awakenings causing sleep interruption will increase the pulsatile cortisol secretion [99] and some [100,101], but not all [102], studies have shown higher mean cortisol levels in patients with

primary insomnia. In patients with depression, the lowest point of cortisol level is advanced and cortisol secretion is not suppressed by dexamethasone, although the latter is a nonspecific finding that also occurs in healthy sleep-deprived individuals [103,104]. With sleep deprivation and sleep fragmentation (as may occur in OSA), evening cortisol concentrations and sympathetic nervous system activity are increased, resulting in impaired glucose tolerance and negative cardiovascular consequences [105].

Prolactin is a hormone that mainly promotes lactation in women and is synthesized by the anterior pituitary gland. It is tightly linked to sleep, with the highest levels occurring during sleep and the lowest during wakefulness. The prolactin level begins to rise approximately 60–90 minutes after sleep onset and peaks in the early morning hours from approximately 5:00 to 7:00 am. Prolactin secretion does not appear to have an independent circadian rhythm but vary in its secretion by sleep stage [106–109], although some authors have suggested that an independent circadian rhythm becomes evident during sleep deprivation [110].

Gonadotropin-releasing hormone (GnRH) produced by the hypothalamus stimulates the anterior pituitary gland to secrete the gonadotropins: luteinizing hormone (LH) and follicle-stimulating hormone (FSH). In men, LH is the stimulus for the secretion of testosterone by the testes, and FSH stimulates spermatogenesis. In women, the ovarian hormones estrogen and progesterone are secreted by the ovaries in response to LH and FSH, which are also responsible for ovarian changes during the menstrual cycle. The gonadotropins are secreted in a pulsatile pattern throughout the 24-hour cycle, and no relationship to the sleep–wake cycle has been demonstrated [111]. However, in both late pre-pubertal and pubertal boys and girls, gonadotropin levels appear to increase during sleep [112–116]. Plasma testosterone levels do not appear to correlate with the pulsatile secretion of FSH and LH. Testosterone levels rise at sleep onset and continue to rise during sleep at night, possibly related to REM sleep; this sleep-related rise in testosterone levels attenuates with age [117–120]. In women, sleep appears to inhibit LH secretion in the early parts of the follicular and luteal phases of the menstrual cycle, although the data are contradictory [121,122]. There is a suggestion that the shiftwork-related increased incidence of infertility in women may be related to a sleep-related inhibitory effect on gonadotropin release during the follicular phase of the menstrual cycle [123].

TSH secretion has a well-defined sleep-dependent circadian rhythm. Sleep has an inhibitory effect on TSH secretion that appears to be related to SWS; TSH levels are low during the daytime, increase rapidly in the early evening, peak shortly before sleep onset, and are followed by a progressive decline during sleep [124]. Sleep deprivation is associated with nocturnal increase of TSH, but TSH is not inhibited by daytime sleep. TSH is thus controlled by both circadian clock and sleep homeostasis.

The renin–angiotensin–aldosterone system plays a major role in maintaining hemodynamic stability in the face of decreased systemic blood pressure. The juxtaglomerular cells in the kidney sense decreasing renal perfusion and secrete renin, which converts angiotensinogen first to angiotensin I and then angiotensin II, which in turn stimulates aldosterone production in the zona glomerulosa of the adrenal cortex. The end result is increased blood pressure and blood volumes, increased sodium reabsorption, and increased potassium secretion. With the fall in blood pressure that occurs in NREM sleep as a result of decreased sympathetic activity, plasma renin levels rise; in contrast, during REM sleep, which is associated with fluctuating BP and intermittently increased sympathetic activity, there is a significant decrease in renin levels [125]. Sleep-related aldosterone levels are higher than those found in wakefulness, and do not appear to depend on fluctuations in plasma renin levels [126]. Some studies have shown that in addition to sleep-dependent changes, plasma renin and aldosterone levels have their own circadian rhythms [127,128].

The immune system and sleep

There has been a lot of research into the immunological changes brought about by sleep and sleep deprivation and into the changes in sleep that occur in the context of systemic infections. Sleep appears to act as a host defense against infection, and sleep deprivation may increase vulnerability to infection by altering immune function [129]. Cytokines are proteins produced by leukocytes and other cells that functioning as intercellular immunological mediators. Several cytokines, such as interleukins (IL), interferon alpha (IFN-α), and tumor necrosis factor (TNF) have been shown to promote sleep and play a role in cellular and immune changes noted during sleep deprivation, although their exact role remains to be clearly elucidated [130]. Pro-inflammatory cytokines such as IL-6 and TNF-α may also play an important role in the pathogenesis of excessive daytime sleepiness in sleep deprivation, as well as a variety of sleep disorders such as OSA, narcolepsy, and idiopathic hypersomnolence [131]. Other sleep-promoting agents that are secreted during infection include delta sleep-inducing peptides, muramyl peptides, cholecystokinin, arginine vasotocin, vasoactive intestinal peptide, growth hormone-releasing hormone (GHRH), somatostatin, prostaglandin D_2, nitric oxide (NO), and adenosine [132]. It has been shown that adenosine in the basal forebrain can fulfill the major criteria for the neural sleep factor that mediates these somnogenic effects of prolonged wakefulness by acting through adenosine-binding A1 and A2a receptors [133].

References

1. Chokroverty S, ed. Sleep disorders medicine: basic science, technical considerations, and clinical aspects, 3rd ed. Philadelphia: Saunders-Elsevier, 2009.
2. Lowey AD. Central autonomic pathways. In: Low PA, ed. Clinical autonomic disorders. Boston: Little, Brown, 1993: 88.
3. Barron KD, Chokroverty S. Anatomy of the autonomic nervous system: brain and brainstem. In: Low PA, ed. Clinical autonomic disorders. Boston: Little, Brown, 1993:3–15.
4. Spyer KM. The central nervous organization of reflex circulatory control. In: Lowey AD, Spyer KM, eds. Central regulation of autonomic functions. New York: Oxford University Press, 1990: 168.
5. Parmeggiani PL, Morrison AR. 1990 Alterations of autonomic functions during sleep. In: Lowey AD, Spyer KM, eds. Central regulation of autonomic functions. New York: Oxford University Press, 1990: 367.
6. Malik M. Writing Committee of the Task Force of the European Society of Cardiology and the North American Society of Pacing and Electrophysiology. Heart rate variability: standards of measurements, physiological interpretation and clinical use. Circulation 1996;93:1043–65.
7. Saul JP, Berger RD, Albrecht P, et al. Transfer function analysis of the circulation: unique insights into cardiovascular regulation. Am J Physiol 1991;26:H1231.
8. Pagani M, Lombardi F, Guzzetti S, et al. Power spectral analysis of heart rate and arterial pressure variabilities as a marker of sympatho-vagal interaction in man and conscious dog. Circ Res 1986;59:178–93.
9. Malliani A, Pagani M, Lombardi F, Ceruti S. Cardiovascular neural regulation explored in the frequency domain. Circulation 1991;84:482–92.
10. Sleight P, La Rovere MT, Mortara A, et al. Physiology and pathophysiology of heart rate and blood pressure variability in humans: is power spectral analysis largely an index of baroreflex gain? Clin Sci (Lond) 1995;88:103–9.
11. Shinar Z, Akselrod S, Dagan Y, Baharav A. Autonomic changes during wake–sleep transition: a heart rate variability based approach. Auton Neurosci 2006;130:17–27.
12. Malik M, Camm AJ. Heart rate variability and clinical cardiology. Br Heart J 1994;71:3.
13. Somers VK, White DP, Amin R, et al. Sleep apnea and cardiovascular disease: an American Heart Association/American College of Cardiology Foundation Scientific Statement from the American Heart Association Council for High Blood Pressure Research Professional Education Committee, Council on Clinical Cardiology, Stroke Council, and Council on Cardiovascular Nursing. J Am Coll Cardiol 2008;52:686–717.
14. Chase MH, Morales FR. Control of motoneurons during sleep. In: Kryger, MH, Roth T, Dement WC, eds. Principles and practice of sleep medicine. Philadelphia: Elsevier Saunders, 2005: 154.
15. Sakai K, Sastre JP, Salvert D, et al. Tegmentoreticular projections with special reference to the muscular atonia during paradoxical sleep in the cat: an HRP study. Brain Res 1979;176:233.
16. Ohta Y, Mori S, Kimura H. Neuronal structures of the brainstem participating in postural suppression in cats. Neurosci Res 1988;5:181–202.
17. Chase MH. Synaptic mechanisms and circuitry involved in motoneuron control during sleep. Int Rev Neurobiol 1983;24:213–58.
18. Takakusaki K, Ohta Y, Mori S. Single medullary reticulospinal neurons exert postsynaptic inhibitory effects via inhibitory interneurons upon alphamotoneurons innervating cat hindlimb muscles. Exp Brain Res 1989;74:11.
19. Pompeiano O. The neurophysiological mechanisms of the postural and motor events during desynchronized sleep. Res Publ Assoc Nerv Ment Dis 1967;45:351–423.
20. Morrison A. Motor control in sleep. Handb Clin Neurol 2011;99:835–49.
21. Montplaisir J, Gagnon JF, Postuma RB, Vendette M. REM sleep parasomnias. Handb Clin Neurol. 2011;99:869–82.
22. Aschoff J. 1983 Circadian control of body temperature. J Therm Biol 1983;8:14347.
23. Van Someren EJ, Raymann RJ, Scherder EJ, et al. Circadian and age-related modulation of thermoreception and temperature regulation: mechanisms and functional implications. Ageing Res Rev 2002;1:721–78.
24. Alam MN, McGinty D, Szymusiak R. Preoptic/anterior hypothalamic neurons: thermosensitivity in wakefulness and non rapid eye movement sleep. Brain Res 1996;718:76–82.
25. Kanda K, Tochilara Y, Ohnaka T. Bathing before sleep in the young and in the elderly. Eur J Appl Physiol Occup Physiol 1999;80:71–5.
26. Sung EJ, Tochihara Y. Effects of bathing and hot footbath on sleep in winter. J Physiol Anthropol Appl Human Sci 2000;19:21–7.
27. Krauchi K, Cajochen C, Werth E, Wirz-Justice A. Warm feet promote the rapid onset of sleep. Nature 1999;401:36–7.
28. O'Connor PJ, Youngstedt SD. Influence of exercise on human sleep. Exerc Sport Sci Rev 1995;23:105–34.
29. Cain SW, Rimmer DW, Duffy JF, Czeisler CA. Exercise distributed across day and night does not alter circadian period in humans. J Biol Rhythms 2007;22:534–41.
30. Bach V, Telliez F, Chardon K, et al. Thermoregulation in wakefulness and sleep in humans. Handb Clin Neurol 2011;98:215–27.
31. Morris M, Lack L, Dawson D. Sleep-onset insomniacs have delayed temperature rhythms. Sleep 1990;13:1–14.
32. Lushington K, Dawson D, Lack L. Core body temperature is elevated during constant wakefulness in elderly poor sleepers. Sleep 2000;23:504–10.
33. Raymann, RJ, Swaab DF, Van Someren EJ. Cutaneous warming promotes sleep onset. Am J Physiol Regul Interg Comp Physiol 2005;288:R1589–97.

34. Heller HC, Glotzback S, Grahn D, et al. Sleep-dependent changes in the thermoregulatory system. In: Lydic R, Biebuyck JF, eds. Clinical physiology of sleep. Bethesda, MD: American Physiological Society, 1988:145.

35. Woodward S, Freedman RR. The thermoregulatory effects of menopausal hot flashes on sleep. Sleep 1994;17:497–501.

36. Freedman RR. Postmenopausal physiological changes. Curr Top Behav Neurosci 2014;21:245–56.

37. Mitchell RA, Berger AJ. Neural regulation of respiration. Am Rev Respir Dis 1975;111:206–24.

38. Benarroch E. Brainstem respiratory chemosensitivity: new insights and clinical implications. Neurology 2007;68:2140–3.

39. White DP. Ventilation and the control of respiration during sleep: normal mechanisms, pathologic nocturnal hypoventilation, and central sleep apnea. In: Martin RJ, eds. Cardiorespiratory disorders during sleep. Futura: Mount Kisco, NY: Futura, 1990:53.

40. Phillipson EA. Control of breathing during sleep. Am Rev Respir Dis 1978;18:909–39.

41. Robin ED, Whaley RD, Crump CH, et al. Alveolar gas tensions, pulmonary ventilation, and blood pH during physiologic sleep in normal subjects. J Clin Invest 1958;37:981–9.

42. Horner RL. Respiratory motor activity: influence of neuromodulators and implications for sleep disordered breathing. Can J Physiol Pharmacol 2007;85:155–65.

43. Pontoppidan H, Bleecher HK. Progressive loss of protective reflexes in the airway with the advance of age. JAMA 1960;174:2209–13.

44. Sauerland EK, Harper RM. The human tongue during sleep: electromyographic activity of the genioglossus muscle. Exp Neurol 1976;51:160–70.

45. Dort L, Brant R. A randomized, controlled, crossover study of a noncustomized tongue retaining device for sleep disordered breathing. Sleep Breath 2008;12:369–73.

46. Mwenge GB, Rombaux P, Lengele B, Rodenstein D. Hypoglossal nerve stimulation for obstructive sleep apnea. Prog Neurol Surg 2015;29:94–105.

47. Baust W, Bohnert B. The regulation of heart rate during sleep. Exp Brain Res 1969;7:169.

48. Khatri IM, Freis ED. Hemodynamic changes during sleep. J Appl Physiol 1967;22:867–73.

49. Miller JC, Horvath SM. Cardiac output during human sleep. Aviat Space Environ Med 1976;47:1046–51.

50. Coccagna G, Mantovani M, Brignani F, et al. Arterial pressure changes during spontaneous sleep in man. Electroencephalogr Clin Neurophysiol 1971;31:277–81.

51. Lugaresi E, Coccagna G, Mantovani M, Lebrun R. Some periodic phenomena arising during drowsiness and sleep in man. Electroencephalogr Clin Neurophysiol 1972;32:701–5.

52. Fabbian F, Smolensky MH, Tiseo R, et al. Dipper and non-dipper blood pressure 24-hour patterns: circadian rhythm-dependent physiologic and pathophysiologic mechanisms. Chronobiol Int 2013;30:17–30.

53. Larochelle P. Circadian variation in blood pressure: dipper or nondipper. J Clin Hypertens (Greenwich) 2002;4(4 Suppl 1):3–8.

54. Fagard RH. Dipping pattern of nocturnal blood pressure in patients with hypertension. Expert Rev Cardiovasc Ther 2009;7:599–605.

55. Brotman DJ, Davidson MB, Boumitri B, Vidt DG. Impaired diurnal blood pressure variation and all-cause mortality. Am J Hypertens 2008;21:92–7.

56. Cohen MC, Rohtla KM, Lavery CE, et al. Meta-analysis of the morning excess of acute myocardial infarction and sudden cardiac death. Am J Cardiol 1997;79:1512–16.

57. Otto ME, Svatikova A, Barretto RB, et al. Early morning attenuation of endothelial function in healthy humans. Circulation 2004;109:2507–10.

58. Watson WE. Distensibility of the capacitance blood vessels of the human hand during sleep. J Physiol (Lond) 1962;161:392–8.

59. Zoccoli G, Walker AM, Lenzi P, Franzini C. The cerebral circulation during sleep: regulation mechanisms and functional implications. Sleep Med Rev 2002;6:443.

60. Hajak G, Klingelhofer J, Schulz-Varszegi M, et al. Relationship between cerebral blood flow velocities and cerebral electrical activity in sleep. Sleep 1994;17:11–19.

61. Buchsbaum MS, Gaillin JC, Wu J, et al. Regional cerebral glucose metabolic rate in human sleep assessed by positron emission tomography. Life Sci 1989;45:1349–56.

62. Heiss WD, Pawlik G, Herholz K. Regional cerebral glucose metabolism in man during wakefulness, sleep and dreaming. Brain Res 1985;327:362–6.

63. Madsen PL, Schmidt JF, Wildschiodtz G, et al. Cerebral oxygen metabolism and cerebral blood flow in humans during deep and rapid eye movement in sleep. J Appl Physiol 1991;70:2597–601.

64. Maquet P, Div D, Salmon E, et al. Cerebral glucose utilization during sleep–wake cycle in man determined by positron emission tomography and [^{18}F]2- fluoro-deoxy-D-glucose method. Brain Res 1997;513:136.

65. Braun AR, Belkin TJ, Wesenten NJ, et al. Regional cerebral blood flow throughout the sleep–wake cycle: an H$_2$^{15}O PET study. Brain 1997;120:1173.

66. Hofle N, Paus T, Reutens D, et al. 1997 Regional cerebral blood flow changes as a function of delta and spindle activity during slow wave sleep in humans. J Neurosci 1997;17:4800–8.

67. Maquet P. Understanding non rapid eye movement sleep through neuroimaging. World J Biol Psychiatry 2010;11(Suppl 1):9–15.

68. Desseilles M, Dang-Vu T, Maquet P. Functional neuroimaging in sleep, sleep deprivation and sleep disorders. Handb Clin Neurol 2011;98:71–94.

69. Maquet P, Smith C, Stickgold R. Sleep and brain plasticity. Oxford: Oxford University Press, 2003.

70. McCloy RF, Girvan DP, Baron JH. Twenty-four-hour gastric acidity after vagotomy. Gut 1978;19:664–8.

71. Stacher G, Presslich B, Starker H. Gastric acid secretion and sleep stages during natural night sleep. Gastroenterology 1975;68:1449–55.

72. Orr WC, Hall WH, Stahl ML, et al. Sleep patterns and gastric acid secretion in duodenal ulcer disease. Arch Intern Med 1976;136:655–60.

73. Orr WC, Dubois A, Stah MLl, et al. Gastric function during sleep. Sleep Res 1978;7:72.

74. Eastwood PR, Katagiri S, Shepherd KL, Hillman DR. Modulation of upper and lower esophageal tone during sleep. Sleep Med 2007;8:135–43.

75. Orr WC, Bollinger C, Stahl M. Measurement of gastroesophageal reflux during sleep by esophageal pH monitoring. In: Guilleminault S, ed. Sleeping and waking disorders: indications and techniques. Menlo Park, CA: Addison-Wesley, 1982:331.

76. Orr WC. Esophageal function during sleep: another danger in the night [Editorial]. Sleep Med 2007;8:1056.

77. Orr WC. Alterations in gastrointestinal functioning during sleep. Handb Clin Neurol 2011;98:347–54.

78. Green BT, Broughton WA, O'Connor B. Marked improvement in nocturnal gastroesophageal reflux in a large cohort of patients with obstructive sleep apnea treated with continuous positive airway pressure. Arch Intern Med 2003;163:41–5.

79. Bloom PB, Ross DL, Stunkard AJ, et al. Gastric and duodenal motility, food intake and hunger measured in man during a 24-hour period. Dig Dis Sci 1970;15:719–25.

80. Yaryura-Tobias HA, Hutcheson JS, White L. Relationship between stages of sleep and gastric motility. Behav Neuropsychiatry 1970;2:22–4.

81. Finch P, Ingram D, Henstridge J, et al. Relationship of fasting gastroduodenal motility to the sleep cycle. Gastroenterology 1982;83:605–12.

82. Kumar D, Idzikowski C, Wingate DL, et al. Relationship between enteric migrating motor complex and the sleep cycle. Am J Physiol 1990;259:G983–90.

83. Gorard DA, Vesselinova-Jenkins CK, Libby GW, Ferthing MJ. Migrating motor complex and sleep in health and irritable bowel syndrome. Dig Dis Sci 1995;40:2383

84. Kumar D, Wingate D, Ruckebusch Y. Circadian variation in the propagation velocity of the migrating motor complex. Gastroenterology 1986;91:926–30.

85. Kellow JE, Borody TJ, Phillips SF, et al. Human interdigestive motility: variations in patterns from esophagus to colon. Gastroenterology 1986;91:386.

86. David D, Mertz H, Fefer L, et al. Sleep and duodenal motor activity in patients with severe non-ulcer dyspepsia. Gut 1994;35:916–25.

87. Rao SS, Welcher K. Periodic rectal motor activity: the instrisic colonic gatekeeper?. Am J Gastroenterol 1996;91:890–7.

88. Rubin RT, Poland RE, Gouin PR, et al. Secretion of hormones influencing water and electrolyte balance (antidiuretic hormone, aldosterone, prolactin) during sleep in normal adult men. Psychosom Med 1978;40:44–59.

89. Krieger, J, Laks, L, Wilcox I, et al. Atrial natriuretic peptide release during sleep in patients during treatment with nasal continuous positive airway pressure. Clin Sci (Lond) 1989;77:407.

90. Sack RL, Lewy AJ, Erb DL, et al. Human melatonin production decreases with age. J Pineal Res 1986;3:379–88.

91. Zhdanova IV, Lynch HJ, Wurtman RJ. Melatonin: a sleep-promoting hormone. Sleep 1997;20:899–907.

92. Honda Y, Takahashi K,Takahashi S, et al. Growth hormone secretion during nocturnal sleep in normal subjects. J Clin Endocrinol Metab 1969;29:20–29.

93. Parker D, Sassin J, Mace J, et al. Human growth hormone release during sleep: electroencephalographic correlation. J Clin Endocrinol Metab 1969;29:871.

94. Obal F, Krueger JM. GHRH and sleep. Sleep Med Rev 2004;8:367.

95. Clark RW, Schmidt HS, Malarkey WB. Disordered growth hormone and prolactin secretion in primary disorders of sleep. Neurology 1979;29:855–61.

96. Carlson HE, JC Gillin JC, Gorden P, et al. Absence of sleep related growth hormone peaks in aged normal subjects and in acromegaly. J Clin Endocrinol Metab 1972;34:1102–7.

97. Weibal L, Follenius M, Spiegel K, et al. Comparative effective of night and daytime sleep on the 24-hour cortisol secretory profile. Sleep 1995;18:549–56.

98. Pietrowsky R, Meyrer R, Kern W, et al. Effects of diurnal sleep on secretion of cortisol, luteinizing hormone and growth hormone in man. J Clin Endocrinol Metab 1994;78:683–7.

99. Van Cauter E, Spiegel K. Hormones and metabolism during sleep. In: Schwartz WJ, ed. Sleep science: integrating basic research and clinical practice. Basel: Karger, 1997:144.

100. Vgontzas AN, Tsigos C, Bixler EO, et al. Chronic insomnia and activity of the stress system: a preliminary study. J Psychosom Res 1998;45:21–31.

101. Rodenbeck A, Huether G, Ruther E, Hajak G. Interactions between evening and nocturnal cortisol secretion and sleep parameters in patients with severe chronic primary insomnia. Neurosci Lett 2002;324:159–63.

102. Reimann D, Klein T, Rodenbeck A, et al. Nocturnal cortisol and melatonin secretion in primary insomnia. Psychiatry Res 2002;113:17.

103. Rush AJ, Giles DE, Roffwarg HP, et al. Sleep EEG and dexamethasone suppression test findings in outpatients with unipolar major depressive disorders. Biol Psychiatry 1982;17:327.

104. Klein HB, Seibold B. DST in healthy volunteers and after sleep deprivation. Acta Psychiatr Scand 1985;72:16.

105. Spiegel K, Leproult R, Van Cauter E. Impact of sleep debt on metabolic and endocrine function. Lancet 1999;354:1435–9.

106. Sassin JF, Frantz AG, Kepen S, et al. 1973 The nocturnal rise of human prolactin is dependent on sleep. J Clin Endocrinol Metab 1973;37:436.

107. Parker D, Rossman L, Vanderhaan E. Sleep-related nyctohemeral and briefly episodic variation in human prolactin concentration. J Clin Endocrinol Metab 1973;36:1119–24.

108. Spiegel K, Luthringer R, Follenius M, et al. Temporal relationship between prolactin secretion and slow wave electroencephalic activity during sleep. Sleep 1995;18:543–8.

109. Sassin J, Frantz A, Weitzman E, et al. Human prolactin: 24 hour patterns with increased release during sleep. Science 1972;177:1205–7

110. Waldstreicher J, Duffy JF, Brown EN, et al. Gender differences in the temporal organizations of prolactin (PRL) secretion: evidence for a sleep-independent circadian rhythm of circulating PRL levels—a clinical research center study. J Clin Endocrinol Metab 1996;81:1483–7.

111. Leproult R, Spiegel K, van Cauter E. Sleep and endocrinology. In: Amlaner CJ, Fuller PM, eds. Basics of sleep guide, 2nd ed. Darien, IL: Sleep Research Society, 2009:157–67.

112. Boyar R, Finkelstein J, Roffwarg H, et al. Synchronization of augmented luteinizing hormone secretion with sleep during puberty. N Engl J Med 1972;287:582–6.

113. Boyar RM, Rosenfeld RS, Kapen S, et al. Human puberty: simultaneous augmented secretion of luteinizing hormone and testosterone during sleep. J Clin Invest 1974;54:609–18.

114. Kapen S, Boyar RM, Finkelstein J, et al. Effect of sleep–wake cycle reversal on LH secretory pattern in puberty. J Clin Endocrinol Metab 1974;39:283.

115. Rosenfield RL, Bordini B, Yu C. Comparison of detection of normal puberty in girls by a hormonal sleep test and a gonadotropin-releasing hormone agonist test. J Clin Endocrinol Metab 2013;98:1591–601.

116. Rosenfield RL, Bordini B, Yu C. Comparison of detection of normal puberty in boys by a hormonal sleep test and a gonadotropin-releasing hormone agonist test. J Clin Endocrinol Metab 2012;97:4596–604.

117. Wu FC, Butler GE, Kelnar CJ, et al. Ontogeny of pulsatile gonadotropin releasing hormone secretion from mid-childhood, through puberty, to adulthood in the human male: a study using deconvolution analysis and then the ultrasensitive immunofluorometric assay. J Clin Endocrinol Metab 1996;81:1798–805.

118. Evans JI, MacLean AM, Ismail AAA, et al. Concentration of plasma testosterone in normal men during sleep. Nature 1971;229:261–2.

119. Luboshitzky R, Herer P, Levi M, et al. Relationship between rapid eye movement sleep and testosterone secretion in normal men. J Androl 1999;20:731–7.

120. Luboshitzky R, Shen-Orr Z, Herer P. Middle-aged men secrete less testosterone at night than young healthy men. J Clin Endocrinol Metab 2003;88:3160–6.

121. Soules M, Steiner R, Cohen N, et al. Nocturnal slowing of pulsatile luteinizing hormone secretion in women during the follicular phase of the menstrual cycle. J Clin Endocrinol Metab 1985;61:43–9.

122. Klingman KM, Marsh EE, Klerman EB, et al. Absence of circadian rhythms of gonadotropin secretion in women. J Clin Endocrinol Metab 2011;96:1456–61.

123. Turek FW, Van Cauter E. Rhythms in reproduction. In: Knobil E, Neill J, eds. The physiology of reproduction. New York: Raven, 1993:1789.

124. Lucke C, Hehrmann R, von Mayersbach K, et al. 1976 Studies in circadian variations of plasma TSH, thyroxine and triiodothyronine in man. Acta Endocrinol 1976;86:81–8.

125. Charloux A, Piquard F, Ehrhart J, et al. Time-courses in rennin and blood pressure during sleep in humans. J Sleep Res 2002;11:73–9.

126. Charloux A, Gronfier C, Chapotot F, et al. Sleep deprivation blunts the night time increase in aldosterone release in humans. J Sleep Res 2001;10:27–33.

127. Cugini P, Lucia P. Circadian rhythm of the renin–angiotensin–aldosterone system: a summary of our research studies. Clin Ter 2004;155:287–91.

128. Naito Y, Tsujino T, Masuyama T. Circadian variations of the renin–angiotensin–aldosterone system. Nihon Rinsho 2014;72:1381–5.

129. Everson CA, Toth LA. Systemic bacterial invasion induced by sleep deprivation. Am J Physiol Regul Integr Comp Physiol 2000;278:R905.

130. Krueger JM, Majde JA, Rector DM. Cytokines in immune function and sleep regulation. Handb Clin Neurol 2011;98:229–40.

131. Kapsimalis F, Basta M, Varouchakis G, et al. Cytokines and pathological sleep. Sleep Med 2008;9:603–14.

132. Dinges DF, Douglas SD, Hamarman S, et al. Sleep deprivation and human immune function. Adv Neuroimmunol 1995;5:97–110.

133. Porkka-Heiskanen T, Strecker E, Thakkar M, et al. Adenosine: a mediator of the sleep-inducing effects of prolonged wakefulness. Science 1997;276:1265–8.

SECTION 2

Laboratory evaluation

CHAPTER 7

Polysomnography
Technique and indications

Nic Butkov

Introduction

Polysomnography (PSG) is defined as the recording, analysis, and interpretation of multiple physiological parameters during sleep. The development of PSG began in the early 1970s, when a team of researchers at Stanford University led by William C. Dement, Jerome W. Holland, and David M. Raynal combined tracings from respiratory and cardiac sensors together with the electroencephalogram (EEG), electromyogram (EMG), and electrooculogram (EOG) in a simultaneous multichannel study. The concept was subsequently presented by the team in a 1974 publication titled "Polysomnography: a response to a need for improved communication," which helped establish PSG as the standard testing procedure for patients with suspected sleep disorders [1]. Since then, PSG has become a worldwide gold standard in both clinical and research applications, and it continues to enhance our understanding of sleep and its disorders to the present day.

From a practical perspective, the main attribute of PSG is the inclusion of physiological sleep measures that allow the reader to evaluate any suspected anomalies within the context of sleep and wake physiology. This is especially important when studying patients with complicated histories and comorbidities, where careful analysis of all recorded parameters becomes essential for accurate and complete diagnosis.

From a technological standpoint, PSG has undergone many changes over the past several decades, most notably in the 1990s, when analog polysomnographs were replaced with digital PSG recording systems. The transition to digital PSG has opened the doors to many possibilities and has dramatically changed the way in which PSG data are processed, stored, and analyzed. At the same time, the development of digital PSG has increased the complexity of the recording process. Technologists who perform the studies must not only be thoroughly familiar with the basic principles of biophysiological signal recording, but also understand the effects of any digitally based signal manipulation on the quality and accuracy of the data.

Understanding the recording process is equally important for those who score and interpret digital PSG. When reading a polysomnogram, it is essential to keep in mind that any form of biophysiological data collection includes the potential for recording artifacts. This holds especially true when recorded subjects are unrestricted in movement and are monitored for extended periods of time. Artifacts can stem from dislodged sensors, patient movement, postural changes, perspiration, electrical interference, poor connections, or malfunctioning equipment. Artifacts can affect bio-electrical signals, as well as signals derived from respiratory transducers, oximetry, or any other devices applied to the patient. Paradoxically, recording artifacts were often easier to recognize in the past when analog PSG systems were used, because these systems had less capability of altering the data. With the advent of digital PSG, there has been a tendency to "clean up" the record by selective filtering or by other forms of digital manipulation, which can make it more difficult for the reader to discern between real physiological data and artifacts that resemble physiological activity.

This chapter provides an overview of the PSG recording process, with emphasis on obtaining accurate data with appropriate, but not excessive, signal manipulation. The latter segment of the chapter describes and illustrates some of the more common recording artifacts, with practical strategies for minimizing their impact on the recording.

Indications for PSG

The following clinical indications for PSG are based on guidelines published by the American Academy of Sleep Medicine (AASM) in 2005 [2], which state that attended PSG is considered the standard of practice for

- diagnosis of sleep-related breathing disorders (SRBD);

- positive airway pressure titration;

- preoperative assessment for snoring or obstructive sleep apnea (OSA);

- evaluating results of treatment for moderate to severe OSA with oral appliances, surgery, or dental procedures;

- treatment results requiring follow-up PSG for substantial weight gain or loss;

- treatment results when clinical response is insufficient or when symptoms return;

- patients with systolic or diastolic heart failure and nocturnal symptoms of SRBD;

- patients whose symptoms continue despite optimal management of congestive heart failure;

- neuromuscular disorders with sleep-related symptoms;

- narcolepsy (for which PSG is followed by the multiple sleep latency test, MSLT);

+ periodic limb movement disorder in cases secondary to complaints by the patient or by an observer.

According to the AASM, PSG is not required to diagnose

+ parasomnias;

+ seizure disorders;

+ restless legs syndrome;

+ common, uncomplicated noninjurious events such as nightmares, enuresis, sleep-talking or bruxism;

+ circadian rhythm disorders.

In recent times, PSG has increasingly been used for diagnosing and treating patients with complicated forms of SRBD requiring the use of advanced positive airway pressure (PAP) modalities that deliver nocturnal noninvasive ventilation. PSG is essential for these studies, because it provides critical information regarding the patient's physiological responses to therapy during all phases of titration.

PSG recording parameters

In routine clinical practice, PSG includes (but is not limited to) the following parameters:

+ central, frontal and occipital EEG;

+ recording of eye movements (EOG);

+ recording of chin muscle activity (chin EMG);

+ recording of leg muscle activity (right and left anterior tibialis EMG);

+ the electrocardiogram (ECG);

+ nasal and oral airflow;

+ respiratory effort (based on chest and abdomen excursion);

+ pulse oximetry.

Depending on the intent of the study, or as indicated by individual laboratory protocols, additional PSG parameters may include

+ expanded number of EEG channels;

+ additional EOG leads (recommended for multiple sleep latency testing);

+ snoring sensors;

+ body position sensors;

+ esophageal pressure measurements;

+ esophageal pH measurements;

+ recording of arm muscle activity;

+ end-tidal or transcutaneous carbon dioxide (CO_2) recordings;

+ other parameters as indicated by individual protocols.

When interfacing PSG with PAP equipment, the recording should include all relevant PAP data, such as pressure levels, leak values, estimated tidal volumes, and inspiratory-to-expiratory ratios. Contemporary PAP equipment designed for in-laboratory titration provides this information by direct link to the computer that is used to collect the PSG data.

An important adjunct to PSG is audio/video monitoring combined with direct behavioral observation by a trained technologist.

This is particularly useful for documenting and/or verifying information that might otherwise be undetected or inaccurately represented by body sensor tracings. This may include verification of body position, description of breathing or snoring sounds, documentation of atypical behaviors, etc.

The patient/equipment interface

The application of electrodes and sensors to the patient represents the most essential, yet most vulnerable link in the entire chain of connections between the patient and the data output. Despite advances in technology, the old adage: "garbage in = garbage out" still stands, meaning that without a proper application technique, the accuracy of the recorded data becomes questionable. Consequently, the best insurance against faulty data collection is to pay close attention to the integrity of the electrode and sensor application. After the application has been completed, it is equally important to maintain signal quality for the duration of the study.

EEG, EOG, EMG, and ECG data are obtained by applying surface electrodes to the patient. EEG electrodes are applied according to the International 10/20 System of electrode placement (Figs. 7.1 and 7.2) [3], typically using gold-plated cup electrodes that are adhered to the scalp using either collodion or EEG paste. The AASM recommends using F_4/M_1 for recording frontal EEG activity (with F_3/M_2 as back-up), C_4/M_1 for recording central EEG activity (with C_3/M_2 as back-up), and O_2/M_1 for recording occipital EEG activity (with O_1/M_2 as back-up) [4].

EOG electrodes are placed in the proximity of the right and left outer canthus, offset vertically to detect both vertical and horizontal eye movements. The AASM recommends placing the right EOG electrode (E_2) 1 cm directly above the right outer canthus and the left EOG electrode (E_1) 1 cm directly below the left outer canthus. EOG recordings are based on the electrical potential difference between the cornea and retina of the eye. The cornea has a positive potential relative to the retina. When the eyes move, voltage shifts occur in relation to electrodes placed in the vicinity of each eye, generating corresponding deflections on the data display. Following conventional EOG electrode placements, when the eyes move to the right or upward, a positive (downward) deflection occurs in the right EOG channel and a negative (upward) deflection occurs in the left EOG channel. The opposite effect is seen when the eyes move to the left or downward. The distinct out-of-phase deflections produced by this configuration should be easily distinguishable from background frontal EEG activity recorded by the EOG channels. EOG electrodes (and other facial electrodes) are usually attached with tape. A skin-tight connection is obtained by using a double-sided adhesive electrode collar underneath the electrode cup and then covering the electrode with a small piece of paper tape to firmly secure it in place.

Chin EMG recordings are obtained from electrodes placed over the mentalis and submental muscles. The AASM recommends placing one electrode on the midline, 1 cm above the inferior edge of the mandible, and two electrodes 2 cm below the inferior edge of the mandible, offset 2 cm to the right and left of the midline, respectively. Two of the electrodes are referenced to each other in a bipolar derivation, while the third serves as a back-up. Some practitioners place the third electrode over a masseter muscle, to better detect bursts of bruxism. Chin EMG electrodes can be attached

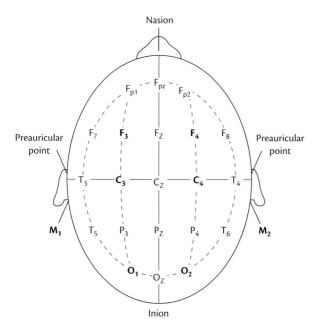

Fig. 7.1 The International 10/20 System of electrode placement (top view). Reproduced from Butkov N, Atlas of Clinical Polysomnography, Second Edition, Copyright (2010), with permission from Synapse Media.

with double-sided electrode collars and paper tape, or they can be glued in place if the patient has a beard. Recordings of the chin EMG should produce sufficient visible activity in the EMG channel even when the subject is relaxed in order to better detect the onset of REM sleep, when the chin EMG is expected to fall to the lowest level of the recording.

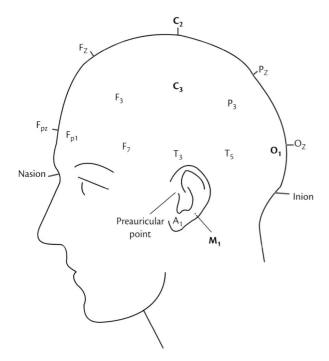

Fig. 7.2 The International 10/20 System of electrode placement (side view). Reproduced from Butkov N, Atlas of Clinical Polysomnography, Second Edition, Copyright (2010), with permission from Synapse Media.

ECG recordings in polysomnography are generally limited to a single modified lead II configuration, with additional leads used as back-up or according to individual protocols. To record a modified lead II ECG, one electrode is placed slightly below the right clavicle and the other over the lower left thorax. An additional electrode placed slightly below the left clavicle allows for recording a modified lead I and lead III ECG.

Leg EMG recordings are obtained by applying a pair of electrodes over the anterior tibialis muscle of each leg. The electrodes are spaced approximately 2–3 cm apart and referenced to each other in a bipolar derivation. In the absence of leg muscle activity, leg EMG channels generally display a flat line, with bursts of EMG activity seen when leg movements occur.

A single patient ground electrode is applied, typically on the patient's forehead, just below the hairline. The purpose of a patient ground is to divert excessive 50 or 60 Hz line frequency interference from the patient's body. To avoid the possibility of stray current passing through the patient, the ground input in the electrode jack box must be isolated, and to avoid the possibility of a ground loop, only a single ground electrode should be used on the patient.

Electrode site preparation and measuring electrode impedances

Before applying any surface electrode, the electrode site must be cleaned and lightly scrubbed with a gel-based prepping solution. The reason for this is because the skin acts as a natural barrier to the passage of the extremely low, rapidly fluctuating voltages generated by the patient. The rate of opposition to these voltages is described as impedance, technically defined as a combined measure of resistance and reactance (the reactance can be inductive or capacitive or both). Scrubbing the skin with the prepping solution is intended to lower impedance to an acceptable level, so as to preserve signal fidelity. For optimal results, all electrode impedance readings should be below 5000 Ω (5 kΩ). Impedance checks can be made either with a separate hand-held meter or by using an impedance measuring option provided by the digital recording system.

When scrubbing the skin with a prepping solution, it is important to only scrub an area no larger than the diameter of the electrode cup. Scrubbing large areas of the skin and/or spreading excessive amounts of any conductive substance (including skin-preparation material) can cause electrical bridging and increase the probability of artifacts.

After the electrode sites have been adequately prepared, the electrodes are carefully adhered to the skin directly over the scrubbed area. The electrode cups are filled with conductive gel, cream, or EEG paste, which serves as the interface between the skin and the electrode. After completing the application, the electrode leads are bundled and neatly secured in a way that provides maximum mobility for the patient, yet minimizes the chances of tangled wires or dislodged electrodes. A final impedance check should be made before initiating the study.

Application of respiratory sensors

One of the challenges of any form of sleep testing that includes respiratory parameters is that precise respiratory measurements during sleep are difficult to obtain. Pneumotachometry and esophageal pressure measurements are considered to be reference standards for detecting respiratory airflow and effort, respectively; however, both methods are intrusive and generally impractical for routine clinical use. Instead, recordings of respiratory airflow are usually obtained with thermal sensors and/or nasal air pressure transducers, while recordings of respiratory effort are usually obtained with piezoelectric or inductance plethysmography belts.

The two commonly used thermal sensors for recording airflow are thermistors and thermocouples. A thermistor is a temperature-sensitive variable resistor that requires an external power source, either from a battery or from the electrode jack box interface with the recording system. In contrast, a thermocouple generates its own voltage, based on the use of dissimilar metals within the sensor. Of the two, thermocouples tend to provide a more stable signal and are more sensitive to fluctuations in airflow. Both types of thermal sensors are available in a three-prong configuration, with two prongs positioned under the nares and one over the mouth. It is important to position the sensors in such a way as to avoid direct contact with skin; otherwise the signal can be dampened by the skin temperature.

A nasal air pressure transducer generates waveforms based on pressure changes at the nares, detected by a nasal cannula connected to a pressure sensor. Nasal air pressure transducers are more sensitive to minor changes in airflow than thermal sensors (especially when compared with thermistors); however, they are susceptible to signal loss when mouth breathing occurs. For this reason, nasal air pressure transducers are usually combined with thermal sensors, with the two derived signals recorded on separate channels.

An alternative method of recording airflow is with polyvinylidene fluoride (PVDF) sensors. This is a patented technology that uses a specially processed flexible film that detects both pressure and temperature changes at the nares and mouth.

Piezoelectric belts have been commonly used to record respiratory effort, based on fluctuating voltages generated by a piezocrystal film in response to chest and abdomen movement. Essentially motion sensors, piezoelectric belts can only be expected to provide a surrogate representation of respiratory effort, but otherwise they are easy to use and often provide a more reliable signal than other forms of respiratory effort monitoring. An alternative to piezoelectric belts are PVDF belts, which have recently been approved by the AASM as an acceptable method for recording respiratory effort.

Inductance plethysmography belts are used for recording respiratory effort based on changes in body circumference associated with breathing. A small electrical current is applied to wires woven in a sinusoidal pattern within the belts, generating an oscillating signal in response to resistance variations associated with body circumference changes. Inductance plethysmography has often been promoted as a means for obtaining semiquantitative measures of ventilation during sleep, based on calculations of the sum of the thoracic and abdominal signals. However, from a practical perspective, such measurements are unrealistic, because they rely on calibrated values that are difficult to maintain during a sleep study. Changes in body position and any displacement of the belts render the calibrations inaccurate. In addition, inductance plethysmography belts are generally less forgiving of belt displacement or deformation than piezoelectric belts and often require readjustments by the attending technologist during the course of the study to maintain an adequate signal.

When applying respiratory effort belts, the thoracic belt is positioned at the level of the nipples and the abdominal belt is placed over the umbilicus. The belts should be comfortably snug, but not over-tightened. Proper adjustment of the belts should be made when the patient initially settles into bed, and further adjustments should be made if signal distortion occurs later in the study due to body position changes and/or belt slippage.

Oximetry

Oximetry recordings are typically obtained by using either disposable or nondisposable finger probes. Alternatively, an earlobe probe can be used, and may be preferable in some instances, particularly if the signal from the finger probe proves to be faulty. Oximetry measurements rely on partial absorption of light waves by the patient's hemoglobin from a light-emitting diode (LED) aimed at a receptor diode opposite the LED. Erroneous readings can result if the LED is not properly positioned over the nail bed, if the light path is blocked by nail polish or artificial nails, or if blood flow is impeded by over-tightening the finger probe. Any questionable oximetry readings should be checked and corrected by the attending technologist. Problems often occur following body position changes if a probe becomes partially or completely dislodged.

Additional recording parameters

Additional recording parameters may be added to the study as deemed necessary by the ordering clinician. Most commonly, these include measures obtained from PAP therapy equipment. When applying PAP therapy, the airflow signal is obtained from the PAP flow sensor, which is generally superior to signals derived from thermocouples or nasal air cannulas. An added benefit of using the PAP flow sensor is that it can provide other essential PAP data, such as estimated air leak and estimated tidal volumes.

Signal processing

The electrical signals obtained from the patient are extremely low in voltage and must be greatly amplified before they are converted into visible tracings. The main challenge in the amplification process is to separate physiological signals of interest from unwanted electrical interference, which can originate from the patient, from devices used on the patient, or from the surrounding environment. The most pervasive interfering signal in any recording environment is 50 or 60 Hz power line frequency, stemming from electrical equipment or wiring in the vicinity of the study. The primary method of eliminating 50/60 Hz interference, or other extraneous signals, is by a process known as common mode rejection. This requires the use of two inputs for each channel, with signals from two sources applied to the two inputs and referenced to each other.

For example, when recording EEG activity, signals derived from the C_4 electrode are referenced to signals derived from the M_1 electrode. The output from this derivation represents only those signals that are dissimilar in voltage or polarity between the two inputs, while any identical, in-phase signals are rejected (these would include 50 or 60 Hz, or any other extraneous signals that are identical in both inputs). Common mode rejection is a function provided by the use of differential amplifiers, which are specifically designed to amplify only dissimilar signals from their two inputs (Fig. 7.3). In the past, these amplifiers were relatively large in size and constituted a major part of the polysomnograph, located in the laboratory

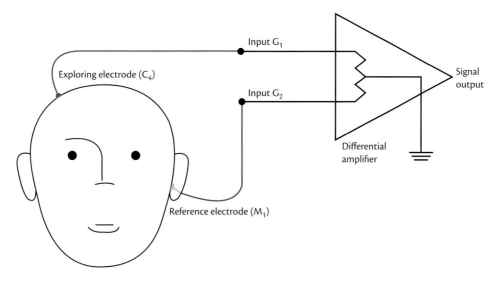

Fig. 7.3 Diagram of input signals processed by a differential amplifier.
Reproduced from Butkov N, Atlas of Clinical Polysomnography, Second Edition, Copyright (2010), with permission from Synapse Media.

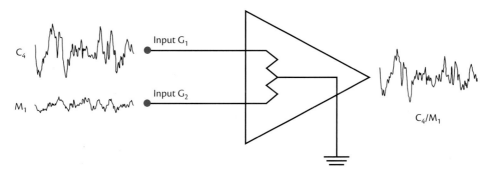

Fig. 7.4 Referential EEG recording (graphic simulation). By comparing an active EEG site with a relatively inactive reference (M_1), the output signal amplitudes are maximized.
Reproduced from Butkov N, Atlas of Clinical Polysomnography, Second Edition, Copyright (2010), with permission from Synapse Media.

control room. In the present day, the amplifiers have been miniaturized and are typically integrated with the electrode jack box in the patient's room.

The two inputs to the differential amplifier are commonly identified as G_1 and G_2. By international agreement, EEG and PSG equipment is configured to produce an upward deflection (as viewed on a computer screen or on paper) when a negative voltage is applied to the G_1 input, with respect to G_2. Because this configuration can be changed within the system software, it is important to verify correct polarity when viewing the PSG data. This can be accomplished during standard calibration procedures, by applying a negative DC calibration voltage to all channels and documenting appropriate signal response.

Signal derivations

The previously mentioned example of C_4 referenced to M_1 is described as a referential derivation. This means that EEG signals of specific interest (C_4) are compared with a relatively inactive EEG site (M_1). This arrangement provides maximum amplification of the signals of interest, by subtracting the relatively inactive (low-voltage) M_1 signals from the more active (higher-voltage) C_4

signals (Fig. 7.4). In this example, C_4 is described as the exploring electrode, whereas M_1 is the reference electrode.

An EEG derivation can be bipolar, in which case both inputs are relatively active. An example of a bipolar EEG derivation is F_4 referenced to C_4. Because of the close proximity of these two electrodes, the signals applied to the two inputs of the differential amplifier are very similar, resulting in tracings that are significantly attenuated (Fig. 7.5).

In PSG, referential derivations are used to record EEG data relevant to sleep stage and arousal scoring. By using a distant and relatively inactive reference site (M_1 or M_2), the signals of interest are optimally amplified while undesirable interfering signals are rejected. EOG recordings are likewise referential, with each EOG electrode referenced to an opposite mastoid.[1] Bipolar EEG derivations are primarily used in seizure montage recordings, for

---

[1] The AASM recommends referencing both EOG electrodes to the right mastoid (M_2). However, referencing the right EOG electrode (E_2) to the mastoid on the same side of the head can significantly attenuate the EOG. Consequently, some sleep centers prefer using a contralateral reference to equalize the out-of-phase signal deflections seen with conjugate eye movements.

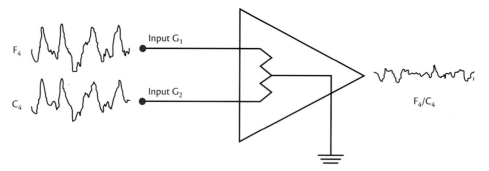

Fig. 7.5 Bipolar EEG recording (graphic simulation). When both input signals are similar, the output signal amplitudes are significantly attenuated.
Reproduced from Butkov N, Atlas of Clinical Polysomnography, Second Edition, Copyright (2010), with permission from Synapse Media.

the purpose of detecting dissimilar aberrant voltages between the two electrode sites and to localize their origin by comparing multiple derivations with one another. Other examples of bipolar derivations used in PSG include the recordings of EMG and ECG signals.

Gain, sensitivity, and digital data display

The term "gain" refers to the ratio of output signal level to input signal level, based on the number of times the raw signal from the subject is amplified. On most contemporary recording systems, the gain is a fixed value. Sensitivity refers more specifically to the ratio of input voltage to the vertical height of the signal display. This is a variable value that can be adjusted by the user. In PSG recordings, the sensitivity settings of the EEG, EOG and EMG channels are usually set to either 50 or 70 µV/cm, depending on individual laboratory protocols. Lower sensitivity settings (such as 100 µV/cm) are generally used for pediatric studies, because of the considerably higher EEG amplitudes seen in children.

Whereas in the past PSG tracings were presented in uniform size on grid paper, contemporary PSG systems allow for infinite variability in terms of the actual dimensions and aspect ratio of the data display. Although this can be useful in many ways, it can also lead to potential problems, particularly when the data display is excessively attenuated. It is possible, however, to calibrate a computer screen to produce a visual display that approximates a paper-based recording and allows for precise signal amplitude measurements. It is also helpful to develop a standard workspace within a laboratory, so that all who are involved in recording, scoring, or interpreting the PSG are viewing the data in the same way.

Filters

Filters are used to isolate specific frequency bandwidths relevant to each recording parameter. This prevents localized signal interference from obscuring the signals of interest. For example, when recording EEG, localized signal interference may stem from DC voltages generated by the skin or from fast frequencies generated by muscle activity. By limiting the frequency bandwidth, these extraneous signals are eliminated from the data display. The extent to which these signal are eliminated depends on the design and configuration of the applied filters. Whereas in the past, analog filters were designed to attenuate undesirable frequencies according to a specific frequency response curve during data collection, contemporary digital filters use software algorithms to delete selected

bandwidths after the amplified signals have been converted into digital form.

The use of digital filters has opened new possibilities, whereby raw data can be collected and stored with minimal filtering, while the data display can later be selectively filtered as deemed appropriate by the user. A cautionary note regarding any form of filtering is to avoid using filters as a means of "cleaning up" the study. Excessive signal filtering, whether by system design or by incorrect filter settings, can lead to loss of detail in the recording and prevent the operator from recognizing possible signal degradation. A common problem with excessive signal filtering is the absence of clearly identifiable artifacts (which are actually useful for identifying problems with loose electrodes, high impedances, etc.). With excessive filtering, outside signal interference may take on the *appearance* of physiological data instead of artifact, effectively resembling the EEG, EMG, ECG, etc., and consequently be misinterpreted by the reader. For example, a poor-quality, over-filtered ECG recording can produce signals that resemble ectopy within a normal sinus rhythm. Without the excessive filtering, a poor-quality signal can instead be recognized by the presence of 50 or 60 Hz artifact, or by other obvious signs of signal distortion.

The choice of filter settings for each recorded parameter is based on the information sought within that parameter. For example, when scoring sleep stages, the EEG is generally read within a frequency range of 0.5–25 Hz. To preserve each end of the frequency spectrum, the low- and high-frequency filters are set to a slightly wider range (0.3 Hz and 30 or 35 Hz, respectively). Table 7.1 displays filter settings for various PSG parameters based on recommendations by the AASM.

In addition to low- and high-frequency filters, PSG recording systems provide a 50 or 60 Hz filter to eliminate line frequency interference from the recording. It is recommended that each channel have an individual on–off setting for this filter and that the filter only be applied when other means of correcting the problem have failed. The reason for this is the same as described previously, i.e., these filters should not be used routinely to "clean up" the signal. This especially holds true for the EEG and EOG channels, which already employ a high-frequency filter setting below the 50–60 Hz range. It is reasonable, however, to use 50 or 60 Hz filters in the leg EMG channels (if necessary), because these channels are more likely to be affected by line frequency interference due to the extra-long electrode leads, and because it is sometimes difficult to obtain optimal impedance levels when recording leg EMGs.

Table 7.1 Examples of filter and sampling rate settings for various PSG parameters based on recommendations by the AASM

Derivation	Low-frequency filter (Hz)	High-frequency filter (Hz)	Minimal sampling rate (Hz)	Desirable sampling rate (Hz)
EEG–F_4/M_1 (or F_3/M_2)	0.3	30–35	200	500
EEG–C_4/M_1 (or C_3/M_2)	0.3	30–35	200	500
EEG–O_2/M_1 (or O_1/M_2)	0.3	30–35	200	500
R. EOG–E_2/M_2	0.3	30–35	200	500
L. EOG–E_1/M_2	0.3	30–35	200	500
Chin EMG	10	100	200	500
Right leg EMG	10	100	200	500
Left leg EMG	10	100	200	500
ECG	0.3	70	200	500
Airflow	0.1	15	25	100
Nasal pressure	DC or ≤0.03	100	25	100
Chest movement	0.1	15	25	100
Abdomen movement	0.1	15	25	100
Oximetry	DC	Not listed	10	25

Analog-to-digital conversion

Unlike paper-based recording systems of the past that transformed the continuous analog signals directly into mechanical pen movements, contemporary recording systems rely on analog-to-digital converters (ADC) to convert the analog physiological signals into digital form. The ADC converts the signals by assigning a numeric value to the amplitude of the analog waveforms at predetermined intervals.

The number of binary units (bits) used to represent the numeric value of each sampled interval determines the amplitude resolution of the digital recording. For optimal amplitude resolution, a 12-bit or higher system is recommended.

The number of sampled intervals obtained in the span of one second is defined as the sampling rate, which determines the frequency resolution of the signal. Different sampling rates can be applied to each individual channel; the choice being dependent on the range of frequencies recorded by the channel. According to the Nyquist theorem, basic frequency resolution requires a sampling rate that is twice the frequency sampled. Sampling rates less than the Nyquist rate result in signal distortion known as aliasing.

While the Nyquist theorem defines minimum sampling rates for basic frequency resolution, significantly higher sampling rates (5–10 times the frequency rate or higher) are necessary to obtain an adequate graphic representation of the individual waves [5]. The choice of an appropriate sampling rate for each channel is based on the highest frequency expected within that channel and according to how important it is to obtain full graphic resolution of the signal of interest. For example, full graphic resolution is desirable for EEG

recordings, using higher sampling rates to preserve all essential detail of the individual EEG waves; whereas EMG recordings can be adequately sampled at the Nyquist rate, because EMG analysis is largely based on relative amplitude changes, not individual wave scrutiny.

System referencing

System referencing is a feature offered by digital PSG recording systems for selecting and changing input derivations. System referencing relies on a common reference electrode, which is usually placed on the midline of the scalp (C_z). During data collection, signals from all the applied electrodes (including the standard reference electrodes M_2 and M_1) are initially referenced to the C_z electrode. This configuration is not seen by the operator, but instead it serves as a framework for viewing any derivation of interest, either during data collection or during playback. For each derivation selected by the operator, the computer subtracts the common reference (C_z) from the chosen pair of input signals. For example, if the operator chooses to view the derivation of C_4/M_1, the computer subtracts C_z from both C_4 and M_1 and combines the two input signals to produce the C_4/M_1 derivation. By using a common reference, virtually any combination of input signals can be selected to create the desired output derivation.

System referencing is a valuable tool that provides maximum flexibility for reviewing the PSG data. It is especially suitable for viewing full-montage EEG recordings, allowing the selection of any desired EEG derivation either during or after the study. In routine PSG, system referencing is primarily used to change derivations when recording artifacts occur. For example, if both C_4/M_1 and C_3/M_2 are displaying artifacts, a combination of either C_4/M_2 or C_3/M_1 can be used. Or, if one of the ECG electrodes becomes disconnected during the study, an alternate ECG derivation can be obtained by re-referencing the remaining ECG electrode to a leg electrode, or to any other distant electrode on the body.

The only drawback to system referencing is that all of the recorded data are dependent on a single common reference. If the reference electrode (C_z) becomes disconnected, or becomes the source of artifact, then all of the channels linked to C_z become affected. It is, therefore, important to pay attention to the integrity of the system electrode connection and to be able to recognize when a recording becomes compromised by a faulty system electrode.

Timescale

Historically, the timescale used in PSG was based on the paper speed of the recording instrument, which was most commonly set to 10 mm/s, establishing an epoch length (amount of time per page) of 30 s. Alternatively, a 20 s epoch length was used in conjunction with a paper speed of 15 mm/s. In the present day, the use of digital technology allows for multiple timescale settings, which can be applied either during recording or during playback (Figs. 7.6 and 7.7). For the purpose of sleep stage scoring, the 30 s epoch is the established standard; however, alternative timescales can be used for analyzing sleep-related events. For example, an epoch length of 10–15 s can be useful for more closely examining suspected EEG or ECG abnormalities, whereas epoch lengths of 2–5 minutes are useful for examining respiratory patterns, periodic limb movements and oximetry trends.

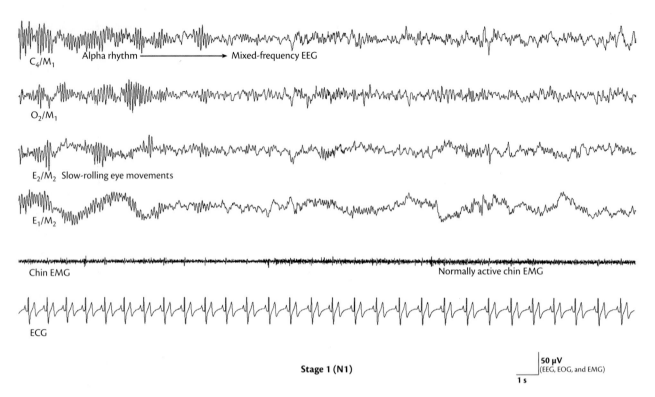

Fig. 7.6 PSG recording viewed in a 30 s epoch window. A timescale of 30 s per epoch provides a high level of detail in the EEG and EOG channels and is the standard scale for scoring sleep stages and arousals.

Reproduced from Butkov N, Atlas of Clinical Polysomnography, Second Edition, Copyright (2010), with permission from Synapse Media.

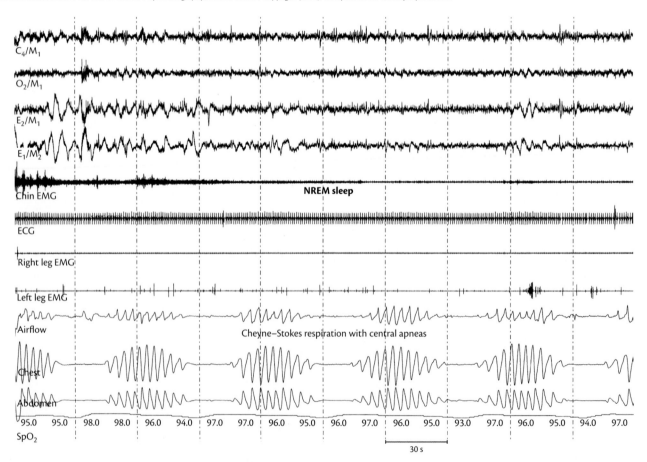

Fig. 7.7 PSG recording viewed in a 5 min epoch window. After scoring sleep stages and arousals in 30 s epochs, the timescale can be compressed into 2–5 min epochs, in order to better discern the respiratory patterns while correlating them to the patient's sleep and wake physiology.

Reproduced from Butkov N, Atlas of Clinical Polysomnography, Second Edition, Copyright (2010), with permission from Synapse Media.

Electrical safety

Because the patient is connected by conductive leads to electrical instrumentation, there is always a potential hazard of stray electrical current passing through the patient. To minimize this hazard, contemporary medical devices, including PSG recording systems, provide isolated inputs that meet strict patient safety guidelines. These inputs isolate the patient from ground, eliminating the possibility of leakage current reaching the patient from external sources and from devices connected to the patient. Nonetheless, technologists working with these devices must be adequately trained in electrical safety and recognize any potential problems stemming from improper use of equipment or improper wiring in the vicinity of the study.

Patient monitoring

Regardless of how well the electrodes and sensors are initially applied to the patient, recording problems occurring during the course of an overnight sleep study are common. While monitoring the patient, part of the job of a sleep technologist is to recognize and correct these problems in order to preserve the integrity of the recording for its duration. The other aspect of patient monitoring is to directly observe the patient, both for safety purposes and to document any information that can potentially enhance the interpretation of the PSG.

Artifact recognition

PSG artifacts are defined as extraneous signals appearing within any of the recorded parameters of the sleep study. Most recording artifacts can be readily identified by their exaggerated or distorted appearance. However, in some cases, it may be difficult to discern between artifacts and physiological signals of interest. One of the advantages of a multichannel recording is the ability to cross-examine the recording to see if the signals in question correlate with other parameters. For example, if questionable wave patterns are seen in an EEG channel but are not appropriately reflected in adjacent EEG or EOG channels, they are likely to be artifacts. By comparing adjacent channel tracings, one can also determine the origin of the artifact. For example, if an identical artifact is seen in two or more channels sharing the same reference (eg, C_4/M_1 and E_2/M_1), it can be assumed that the source of artifact is the reference electrode. However, if an artifact appears in only one channel (sharing a common reference with other channels), then the problem can be traced to the exploring electrode.

Because PSG recordings are conducted over an extended period of time (typically 7–8 hours) on patients who are unrestricted in movement, some degree of artifact can be expected in nearly every study. Part of the job of a sleep technologist is to minimize the occurrence of undesirable artifacts by utilizing proper electrode application techniques and by making appropriate corrections or adjustments to the study when artifacts occur.

In some instances, corrections can be made by re-referencing a channel to a back-up electrode (if available) or by using a back-up derivation (eg, C_3/M_2 instead of C_4/M_1). In other instances, correcting a faulty signal requires entering the patient's room to replace or reposition a sensor (eg, a loose respiratory belt or dislodged oximetry probe).

It is important to note that not all artifacts are undesirable. Certain physiological artifacts can be useful in the interpretation of the study and should not be arbitrarily removed. For example, "snoring artifact," recorded by the chin EMG, is useful for confirming that the patient snores. Muscle-generated artifacts occurring with body movements helps confirm that the patient moved. It is also important to understand that even undesirable artifacts serve a purpose, because they alert the operator that a faulty signal is present and needs correction.

50/60 Hz artifact

The presence of 50 or 60 Hz artifact in PSG stems from power-line frequency in the vicinity of the study.* The primary method of eliminating line frequency interference is by common mode rejection, as described earlier in this chapter. In addition, the patient ground electrode is used to divert stray electrical interference from the patient. Consequently, the presence of 50 or 60 Hz artifact in the recording generally indicates that either impedance levels are too high or the ground connection has degraded, or there is a combination of both. Excessive electromagnetic fields within the laboratory environment can further aggravate 50 or 60 Hz interference, as can excessive leakage current, which can originate from extension cords, power strips, lamps, televisions, electric beds, fans, or any other electrical devices in the vicinity of the study.

It is easy to recognize 50 or 60 Hz artifact, because it is a fast, uniform frequency that obscures the underlying tracings (Fig. 7.8). It can be diminished or removed by the use of a 50/60 Hz filter; however, this should not be standard practice. Instead, the source of the problem should be identified and corrected, either by re-referencing the channel or by reattaching the offending electrode.

High-frequency artifacts generated by electronic devices

High-frequency interference from electronic devices (commonly described as "noise") can resemble 50 or 60 Hz artifact, but does not respond to a 50/60 Hz filter. Although common mode rejection and the patient ground help minimize the presence of electronic noise, in some instances it might be necessary to identify the source of interference and either turn it off or move it to another location.

Muscle artifact

Muscle artifact appearing in the EEG or EOG is another high-frequency artifact that somewhat resembles 50 or 60 Hz artifact. However, unlike power line or electronic interference, muscle artifact is not uniform but irregular, and it may wax and wane with increased or decreased muscle tension (Fig. 7.9). Muscle artifact is caused by localized muscle activity in the vicinity of the exploring or reference electrode. When seen in the EEG or EOG channels, the artifact often stems from a reference electrode that was placed too low or too far from the ear flap (pinna), and is in close proximity to the muscles of the neck. Repositioning the electrode over a firm bony area close to the pinna can correct the problem. When muscle artifact is only limited to one or two EEG or EOG channels, it can

---

* Most European and Australasian countries use 50 Hz, while 60 Hz is used in the United States, Canada, and many South American countries.

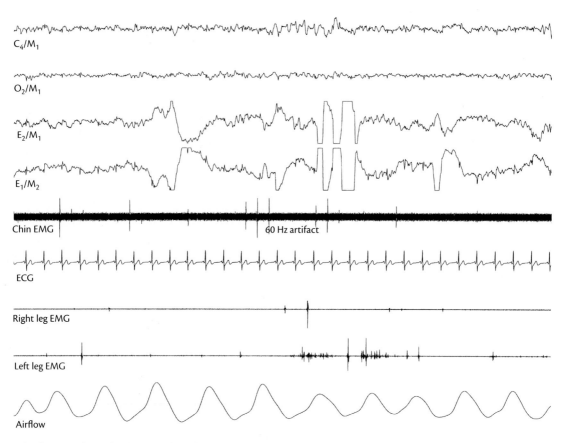

Fig. 7.8 An example of 60 Hz artifact in the chin EMG channel caused by faulty electrode connection.

Reproduced from Butkov N, Atlas of Clinical Polysomnography, Second Edition, Copyright (2010), with permission from Synapse Media.

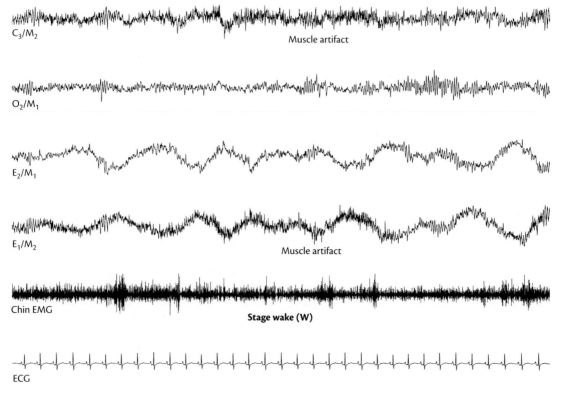

Fig. 7.9 Muscle artifact in the EEG and EOG. This is an example of muscle artifact appearing in the C_3/M_2 and E_1/M_2 channels. Because the artifact is identical in both channels sharing the same reference, it is evident that the artifact originates from the M_2 electrode.

Reproduced from Butkov N, Atlas of Clinical Polysomnography, Second Edition, Copyright (2010), with permission from Synapse Media.

usually be eliminated by re-referencing to a back-up derivation. Muscle artifact also often disappears without any intervention as the patient relaxes and falls asleep.

ECG artifact

Unlike localized low-voltage EEG waves, strong ECG signals can be detected from virtually any location on the body, including the scalp. Based on the principle of differential amplification, the probability of ECG artifact in the EEG or EOG channels increases in proportion to the distance between the exploring and reference electrodes. Because of the relatively long inter-electrode distances used in standard PSG referential recordings (such as C_4 referenced to M_1), it is not unusual to see a small amount of ECG artifact in the EEG and/or EOG channels.

While a small amount of ECG artifact in the EEG or EOG channels is usually not problematic, excessive amounts of ECG artifact can make it difficult to read the study. In addition, excessive amounts of ECG artifact generally indicate problems with the electrode application, such as improper placement or high impedance levels (Fig. 7.10). ECG artifact is especially common when studying obese patients, who may have increased body fluids or fatty tissue in the vicinity of the neck and scalp. ECG voltages are also seen more prominently when the electrode placement follows the electrical orientation (axis) of the heart, which may be horizontally deviated in massively obese individuals.

To reduce the possibility of ECG artifacts in the EEG and EOG, the reference electrodes (M_1 and M_2) should be placed over a firm bony area behind the ear, away from the soft fatty tissues of the neck. In some instances, it may be advantageous to place these electrodes slightly above the conventional mastoid process site, making sure not to place them too high. It is also possible to reduce or eliminate ECG artifact in the EEG or EOG channels by linking the two reference electrodes M_1 and M_2. This can be accomplished if the recording system has re-referencing capabilities. When the EEG and EOG channels are double-referenced, this essentially creates three divergent ECG signals that cancel each other, thereby reducing the artifact. However, it is important to note that double-referencing may attenuate the signals of interest, and that it opens up the possibility of other forms of artifact stemming from either of the combined reference electrodes to contaminate the recording. Therefore, double-referencing should only be used when absolutely necessary, and not as general practice.

ECG artifact should not be expected in the EMG channels, because the distance between any pair of EMG electrodes is minimal. The presence of ECG artifact in an EMG channel invariably indicates improper electrode placement or unequal impedance levels.

Slow-frequency artifacts

Slow-frequency artifacts in the EEG or EOG channels can be caused by perspiration or by direct pressure against an electrode. Perspiration induces chemical changes in the electrolyte interface between the electrode and the patient's skin, causing the appearance of slowly oscillating waves in the EEG and/or EOG, commonly described as "sweat artifact" (Fig. 7.11). A similar pattern,

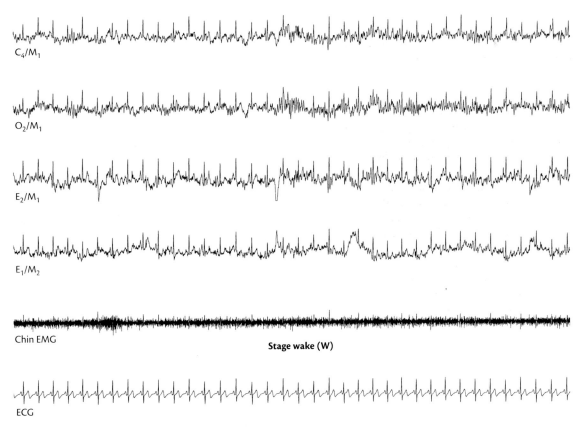

Fig. 7.10 An example of excessive ECG artifact in the EEG and EOG channels. Although small amounts of ECG artifact are sometimes unavoidable, ECG artifacts can be exacerbated by impedance imbalances between the EEG and EOG electrode connections or by poor placement of the mastoid reference electrode.

Reproduced from Butkov N, Atlas of Clinical Polysomnography, Second Edition, Copyright (2010), with permission from Synapse Media.

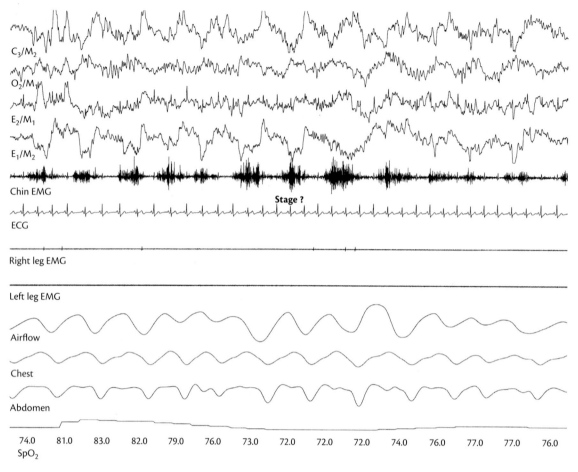

Fig. 7.11 Slow-frequency artifacts in the EEG and EOG. The slow-frequency artifacts in this example are most likely caused by a combination of sweat and slight rhythmic head motion associated with breathing. The artifacts are limited to the C_3/M_2 and E_1/M_2 channels. They are identified by their exaggerated appearance and by lack of correlation with the O_2/M_1 and E_2/M_1 derivations.
Reproduced from Butkov N, Atlas of Clinical Polysomnography, Second Edition, Copyright (2010), with permission from Synapse Media.

although more pronounced and abrupt, can be caused by intermittent pressure against an electrode or by tugging an electrode lead. This is commonly described as "popping artifact." Popping artifact can also be caused by dirty or faulty electrodes or by electrodes that are loosely attached to the skin.

Any body movement can further aggravate the presence of slow-frequency artifacts. A common phenomenon in PSG recordings is the appearance of slow artifacts in the EEG and EOG channels that appear synchronous with the patient's respiratory patterns. This is most likely due to the slight movement of the head associated with each breath. Slow-frequency artifacts that appear synchronous with breathing are often labeled as "respiration artifacts." This term may be misleading, because the source of the artifact is not really respiration, but rather a combination of chemical and mechanical instability of the EEG and EOG electrode/patient interface, which can be further affected by *any* motion, including slight head motion associated with breathing.

As with all artifacts, proper electrode application technique helps minimize the potential for slow-wave artifacts in the EEG and EOG. More specifically, it is important to make sure that all electrodes are well adhered, with a tight seal between the electrode and the patient's skin. This prevents the electrodes from "floating" over the electrode sites, which can cause signal disruption from

even the slightest movement. It is also important not to spread conductive substances (including skin prepping materials) beyond the boundary of the electrode cup when preparing the electrode site and when applying the electrodes.

Even with proper electrode application technique, slow-wave artifacts can be problematic when a patient perspires heavily or moves frequently during the study. When slow-wave artifacts are limited to the side of the head on which the patient is lying, they can be eliminated by re-referencing all the derivations to the opposite side of the head. Another strategy (especially when slow-wave artifacts appear in all EEG and EOG channels) is to attempt to cool the patient with a fan or air conditioning. As a last resort, slow-frequency artifacts can be eliminated from the recording by changing the low-frequency filter to a higher setting. This will effectively attenuate any slow frequencies within the channel, including sweat or popping artifacts. At the same time, however, any physiological slow-wave activity, including slow EEG waves and slow eye movements, will also be attenuated; therefore, this technique should be used sparingly, and not as routine practice. It is also important to note that using filters to remove slow-wave artifacts is only appropriate if the underlying EEG and EOG signals are intact and have not been degraded by high impedance levels or faulty electrode connections.

In the past, low-frequency filter settings in PSG recordings were typically limited to 0.03, 0.3, 1, and 10 Hz. Contemporary digital filters on some of the more advanced PSG systems can be set to almost any configuration. This is advantageous, because the operator of the equipment can select an appropriate filter setting that reduces the artifact but has less impact on the physiological data. For example, in the past, slow-wave artifacts were eliminated by changing the low-frequency filter from 0.3 to 1 Hz, which eliminated the artifact, but also significantly altered the EEG. A more conservative filter change to a setting of 0.5 or 0.6 Hz can be made with contemporary digital filtering, which effectively reduces the artifact, but at the same time preserves most of the underlying EEG data.

Movement artifacts

Movement artifact is a general term that describes any data distortion caused by body movement. When major body movements occur, often a combination of slow and fast artifacts, as well as generalized signal blocking, can be seen in the recording. To some extent, movement artifacts are expected and are useful for confirming that the patient moved. However, excessive signal distortion occurring with every movement makes it difficult to interpret the study, and is usually an indication of poor electrode application. To minimize the effects of body movement, it is important to practice proper application technique, and to use strategies that prevent patients from excessively pulling or tugging at the electrode wires.

Artifacts in the ECG channel

As with all bioelectrical recordings, the ECG relies on proper electrode application technique to ensure signal quality. Although much higher in voltage than the EEG, EOG, or EMG, the ECG is nonetheless susceptible to artifacts caused by high electrode impedances, faulty connections, pressure against an electrode, sweat, and patient movement. In some instances, artifacts in the ECG can resemble ectopic beats. To avoid misinterpreting the ECG, it is useful to compare any questionable tracings to alternative ECG derivations. If the recording equipment provides system referencing, an alternative ECG signal can be obtained from any two electrodes that are sufficiently distant from each other, such as the C4 electrode referenced to one of the left leg electrodes (Fig. 7.12).

Artifacts stemming from a faulty system reference

As noted earlier in this chapter, the use of a system reference opens up many possibilities for reconfiguring input signal derivations.

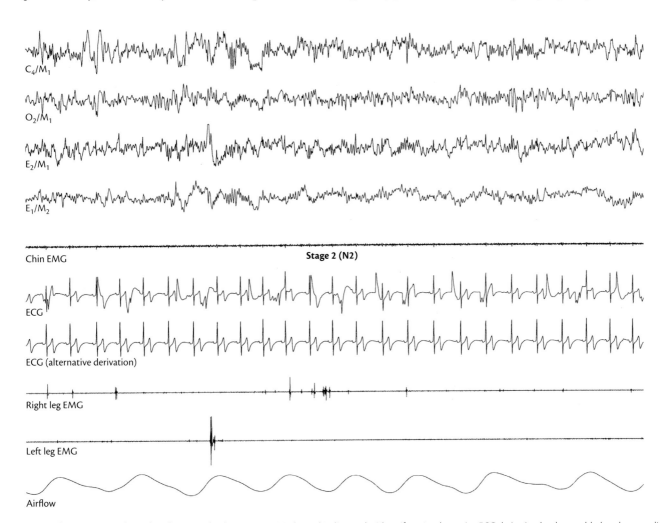

Fig. 7.12 Artifacts in an ECG channel. In this example, the primary ECG channel is distorted with artifact. An alternative ECG derivation has been added to the recording and demonstrates a normal sinus rhythm. The alternative derivation was obtained by referencing an ECG electrode to one of the left leg electrodes.

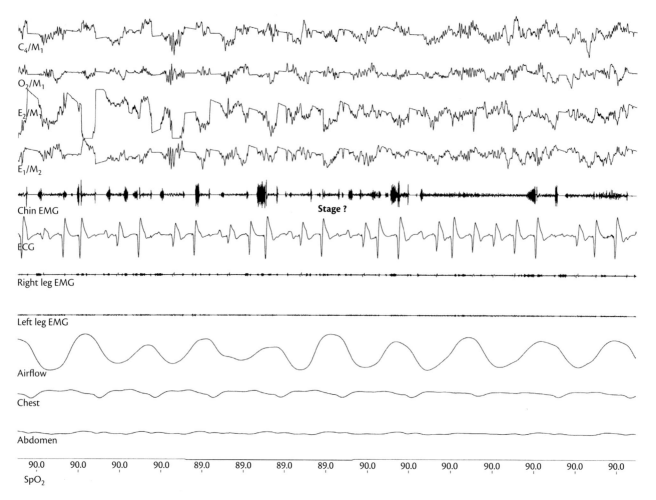

Fig. 7.13 Artifacts originating from the system reference electrode. In this example, a faulty system electrode connection is causing artifacts to appear in all of the channels that are linked to the system reference.

Reproduced from Butkov N, Atlas of Clinical Polysomnography, Second Edition, Copyright (2010), with permission from Synapse Media.

However, if the system reference electrode becomes detached or the signal is degraded, all of the channels that rely upon the system reference are affected (Fig. 7.13). The only solution to this problem is to properly reattach the system reference electrode.

Artifacts in the respiratory channels

As noted before, it is important to recognize that for practical reasons, most forms of respiratory monitoring during sleep rely on sensors that provide nonquantitative, indirect representations of respiratory airflow and effort. As such, these representations are often imprecise and subject to many forms of signal distortion. However, unlike bio-electrical recordings, inaccurate respiratory tracings do not necessarily demonstrate obvious signs of signal distortion; consequently, it can be easy to misinterpret the data, especially if one attempts to over-scrutinize each wave pattern individually without correlating the tracings with other PSG parameters. In many instances, artifacts in the respiratory channels can resemble physiological respiratory events. Although every attempt should be made to maintain adequate respiratory tracings throughout the duration of the sleep study, it is equally important for those who read the PSG data to be aware of the characteristics and limitations of respiratory sensors and interpret the study accordingly. A distinct advantage of multichannel PSG recordings is that all respiratory data can be evaluated within the context of sleep and wake physiology, and the various channels can be cross-examined to confirm or refute the validity and/or etiology of any suspected event (Fig. 7.14).

Artifacts in the oximetry channel

Inaccurate oximetry tracings can be caused by probe displacement, by over-tightening the probe on a patient's finger, by poor perfusion, by motion artifact, or by placing a probe over painted or artificial nails. Although most contemporary recording systems provide some form of signal quality verification, none of these systems is foolproof; therefore, it is essential for sleep technologists to be able to recognize a questionable signal and make the necessary corrections. Likewise, it is essential for the reader of the study to identify potentially false oximetry data, especially when interpreting unattended sleep studies or overnight oximetry screens (Fig. 7.15).

Summary

PSG is a complex procedure that requires extensive and systematic training for those who perform, score, and interpret the studies. When properly performed and accurately interpreted, PSG yields a wealth of information that is unattainable by other form of sleep testing. PSG provides an essential window into the physiology of

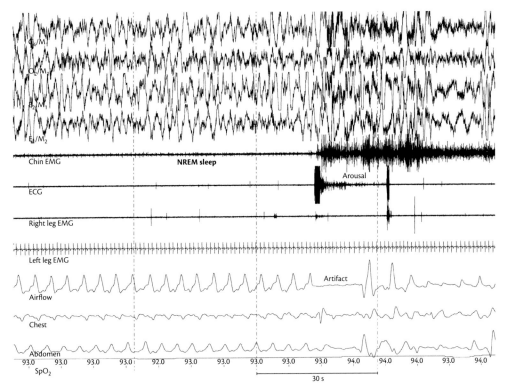

Fig. 7.14 Artifact in the airflow channel resembling an apnea. By examining the respiratory channels within the context of the patient's sleep and wake physiology (as documented by the top channels), it is evident that the apparent "absence of airflow" is actually an artifact caused by patient movement during an arousal. The flattening of the airflow signal may have been caused by the patient's mouth dropping open or by a dislodged airflow sensor. Note the continued attenuation of the airflow signal following the arousal. This is an example of an artifact that could be erroneously scored as an apneic event.

Reproduced from Butkov N, Atlas of Clinical Polysomnography, Second Edition, Copyright (2010), with permission from Synapse Media.

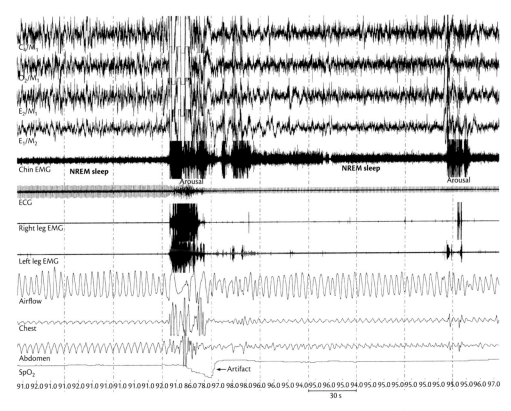

Fig. 7.15 Artifact in the oximetry channel. Artifacts in the oximetry channel are common, and may be caused by a number of factors, including patient movement or sensor displacement. It is important to identify and delete these artifacts during the scoring and interpretation process, to prevent false oximetry data from appearing on the final report.

Reproduced from Butkov N, Atlas of Clinical Polysomnography, Second Edition, Copyright (2010), with permission from Synapse Media.

sleep, offering optimal diagnostic capabilities for patients with sleep disordered breathing, narcolepsy, movement disorders, seizure disorders, medication effects on sleep, parasomnias, and other disorders that are undetectable during a person's waking hours.

In recent years, the scope of sleep medicine has expanded toward treating increasingly complicated patients, many of whom require nocturnal noninvasive ventilation. Advances in bilevel positive airway pressure (PAP) technology have made it possible to treat conditions that were previously refractory to conventional PAP therapy. Combining this technology with digital PSG has greatly enhanced our ability to effectively diagnose and treat complex forms of sleep disordered breathing, as seen in patients with congestive heart failure, COPD, neuromuscular disease, or obesity hypoventilation, patients who develop central apneas as a result of opioid use, and various other conditions that warrant a specialized approach to diagnosis and treatment.

References

1. Holland JV, Dement WC, Raynal DM. Polysomnography: a response to a need for improved communication. Presented at the 14th Annual Meeting of the Association for the Psychophysiological Study of Sleep, Jackson Hole, WY, June 1974.
2. Kushida CA, Littner MR, Morgenthaler T, et al. Practice parameters for the indications for polysomnography and related procedures: an update for 2005. Sleep 2005;28:499–521.
3. Jasper HH. The ten twenty electrode system of the International Federation. Electroencephalogr Clin Neurophysiol 1958;10:371–5.
4. Berry RB, Brooks R, Gamaldo CE, Harding SM, Marcus CL, and Vaughn BV for the American Academy of Sleep Medicine. The AASM Manual for the Scoring of Sleep and Associated Events: Rules, Terminology and Technical Specifications, Version 2.0. Darien Illinois: American Academy of Sleep Medicine, 2012.
5. Hirshkowitz M. R&K manual update. Sleep Review, March 6, 2005. http://www.sleepreviewmag.com/2005/03/rampk-manual-update/.

CHAPTER 8

Scoring of sleep stages, breathing, and arousals

Marco De Los Santos and Max Hirshkowitz

Introduction

Behavioral and measurable bioelectrical correlates characterizing sleep provide metrics for determining whether an individual is asleep or awake. Thus, in a real sense, the question "what is sleep" serves to determine "when is sleep?" Behavioral approaches for detecting sleep onset have involved monitored involuntary object dropping or releasing contact switches. Alternatively, the subject might lapse during a signal detection task (eg, pressing a button in response to sound or a visual target), and researchers have assumed that response cessation marks sleep onset. Armed with the assumption that sleep is a brain process, research breakthroughs followed from recording brain electrical activity. Hans Berger, a German physiologist and psychiatrist, and the inventor of electroencephalography (EEG), paired brainwave patterns with subject reports about sleep status. He described alpha-wave disappearance during relaxed wakefulness as a marker for when sleep occurred [1].

Less than a decade later and some 4000 miles away in Tuxedo Park, New York, Alfred Lee Loomis and colleagues made the first continuous, all-night EEG recordings in sleeping humans [2]. They described sleep spindles, slow waves, K complexes (at that time called random waves), and devised a scoring system to describe the sleep process. Sleep involved multiple processes; "sleep" was no longer a single entity. These processes appeared to proceed in an orderly fashion and were basically similar in all healthy, young adults.

Equipped with EEG technology, scientists began exploring other physiological processes and their alterations associated with sleep. Sleep's biological portrait became more complete when Aserinsky and Kleitman [3] described periodic ocular motility episodes during sleep correlated with dreaming. A sleep stage scoring system evolved to include what ultimately became known as rapid eye movement (REM) sleep [4,5]. An ad hoc committee established standardized methods in 1968 for classifying sleep stages in human adults [6].

Sleep medicine began to emerge as a subspecialty, and during the next decade and a half, techniques to detect, characterize, and summarize breathing and movement pathophysiologies emerged. The resulting EEG, eye movement, respiratory, electromyographic (EMG), snore sound, oxyhemoglobin saturation, and electrocardiographic (ECG) recording array constitutes what is now called polysomnography (PSG). Most laboratories also include simultaneous video recording to capture the patient's behavior during the sleep period. Chapters by various clinician-scientists in Guilleminault's (1982) *Sleeping and Waking Disorders: Indications and Techniques* [7] became the de facto manual for recording and scoring sleep-disordered breathing, periodic leg movements, gastroesophageal reflux, chronobiological rhythms, and sleep in infants. In the 1990,s several American Sleep Disorders Association task forces developed and published standardized rules (eg, [8]), but information and sources remained fragmented. It was not until 2007 that the American Academy of Sleep Medicine (AASM) published rules, terminology, and technical specifications for scoring sleep and its associated physiological events relevant to sleep medicine [9,10]. Techniques outlined in this "cookbook" for clinical polysomnography will be the main subject matter of this chapter.

This chapter's aim is to summarize and clarify the main technical and procedural aspects of performing and reading PSG. The principles adopted in this chapter are based on the AASM guidelines for scoring and staging sleep studies.

Sleep, wake, and central nervous system arousal

Recording montage

Attended polysomnography serves as the diagnostic test at the core of traditional sleep medicine. The term originates from both Latin and Greek roots: the Greek *polus* meaning "many," the Latin *somnus* referring to sleep, and the Greek *graphein* meaning "to write." The sleep study, as it is commonly known, is without debate a costly, labor-intensive, and time-consuming test. It requires skilled technicians and specialty-trained physicians to interpret the results. But even as the more affordable home sleep testing gains ground, in-laboratory PSG remains the gold standard. The vast majority of medically ordered sleep studies are used to diagnose or determine treatment for patients with sleep disordered breathing. Other medically approved PSG indications include narcolepsy assessment and differentiating parasomnias from nocturnal seizure disorder.

Frontal, central, and occipital lobe EEG, electrooculography (EOG), and submentalis (chin) EMG serve as core parameters used to (a) differentiate sleep from wakefulness, (b) classify the type of sleep, and (c) detect awakenings. Figure 8.1(a) illustrates recommended electrode placements. Other signals recorded for specific diagnoses include: oxygen saturation, body position, ECG, anterior tibialis (leg) EMG, nasal–oral airflow, and respiratory effort. These

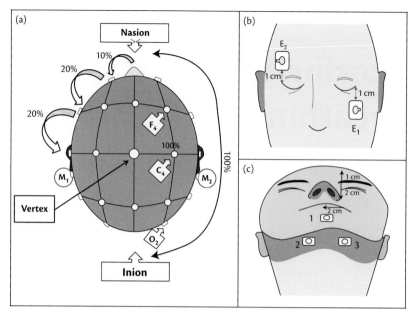

Fig. 8.1 EEG, EOG, and EMG electrode placements. (a) AASM recommended electrode positions based on the international 10-20 System. These include left mastoid referenced (M_1) right frontal lobe (F_4–M_1), central lobe (C_4–M_1), and occipital lobe (O_2–M_1) scalp derivations. Backup electrodes are place on the left frontal, central, and occipital scalp positions referenced contralaterally (i.e, F_3–M_2, C_3–M_2, and O_1–M_2, respectively). (b) Electrode placements for EOG recordings. (c) Placements recommended for recording submentalis EMG needed to classify REM sleep and detect CNS arousals from REM sleep.

parameters, when combined, recount the uninterrupted story of a sleeping patient.

EEG recording

EEG electrode placement accords with the 10-20 System, an internationally recognized standard for placing electrodes on the human scalp. This method landmarks scalp placement of 21 electrodes. To determine specific sites, the method uses four reference points; the nasion, inion, and auricular openings of left and right ears. The nasion, anatomically, is the point where the nasal and frontal bones merge. The inion is the most prominent protuberance of the occipital bone. With reference points well demarcated, the skull is measured in the transverse and median planes with electrodes placed by dividing these perimeters into 10% and 20% segments. Per recommendations, PSGs involve continuous recording of central (C), frontal (F), and occipital (O) EEG leads. The suggested EEG derivations are F_4–M_1, C_4–M_1, and O_2–M_1 (with backups at F_3–M_2, C_3–M_2, and O_1–M_2), where M_1 and M_2 refer to the left and right mastoid processes.

EOG recording

Electrodes placed near each eye's outer canthus (E_2 and E_1, for right and left eyes, respectively) will detect eye movement. Using a neutral reference site (M_1 or M_2) provides the basis for recording positive corneal potentials moving toward and/or away from these electrodes. This recording arrangement produces robust out-of-phase (E_1 versus E_2) activity when horizontal eye movements occur. Being out of phase, eye movements are easily differentiated from frontal EEG activity inadvertently recorded by EOG electrodes (which appears as an in-phase signal). The manual recommends E_2 placed 1 cm above and E_1 placed 1 cm below the outer canthus of the respective eyes. Staggering the electrode placements slightly above and below each eye's horizontal plane allows some appreciation of vertical eye movement. Better visualization of

vertical eye movements can be attained by placing the E_1 and E_2 electrodes 1 cm below the outer canthi and using a forehead placement as a reference site (Fig. 8.1b). However, this sacrifices easy eye movement differentiation from frontal EEG activity using the in- versus out-of-phase paradigm).

EMG

Three chin EMG electrodes are placed. The first is placed midline and 1 cm above the mandible's inferior edge. The second is attached 2 cm to the right of the midline and 2 cm below the mandible's inferior edge. The third placement is 2 cm to the left of the midline and 2 cm below the mandible's inferior edge (Fig. 8.1c). These chin EMG electrodes provide an uncalibrated muscle tone index used to appreciate REM-related atonia. Chin EMG activity increases also serve as part of the criteria for scoring CNS arousals during REM sleep.

Scoring

Sleep and wake

We designate each successive 30 s snapshot of a sleep study as an epoch. Each epoch is classified as either sleep or wakefulness. Sleep epochs are further classified as rapid eye movement (REM) sleep or non-rapid eye movement (NREM) sleep. Finally, NREM epochs are also further categorized as stage N1, stage N2, and stage N3. Staging proceeds from the start of the study (lights out) to the end of the study (lights on), and each epoch is exclusively assigned a single stage. When features characteristic of more than one stage coexist within a particular epoch, the stage is designated according to which sleep process (identified by specific waveforms) occupies the majority of the time. Although scoring is systematic and generally reproducible, ambiguities exist. Inter-rater reliability for sleep staging (and scoring of respiratory events), varies somewhat with a scorer's skill and experience level.

Table 8.1 Principal EEG waveforms and events for categorizing sleep stages and wakefulness

Term	Definition
Alpha activity	Rhythmic, sinusoidal-like EEG activity in the 8–13 Hz frequency range. When recognizably present, alpha EEG activity is the primary waveform used to differentiate sleep from wakefulness. On the scalp, alpha activity usually appears most prominently over the occipital region and predominates during relaxed wakefulness with eyes closed.
Theta activity	Groups of contoured or triangular EEG waves in the 4–7 Hz frequency range. Theta activity usually has greater amplitude when recorded from central derivations. Although theta activity is not part of formal delineation rule criteria for sleep stage scoring, it serves as a general confirmatory marker that sleep is present. Also, a special type of theta, called sawtooth theta, can help verify the presence of REM sleep. Sawtooth theta has a notched appearance resembling the serrated edge of a saw's cutting blade—hence the name.
Delta activity	Rhythmic EEG activity with a frequency below 4 Hz. A subcategory of delta activity falling in the 0.5–2 Hz frequency range called "slow waves" are important in sleep. Slow waves are high-amplitude EEG waves (peak-to-trough amplitude >75 µV on monopolar central or frontally derived recordings). Slow-wave activity duration within the 30 s time domain considered an "epoch" is used as a criterion to differentiated N3 from N2 sleep.
Sleep spindle	A greater than 0.5 s train of spindle-shaped waves with a center frequency of 11–16 Hz (or most commonly 12–14 Hz). Sleep spindles are usually most prominent in recordings from central EEG derivations. Sleep spindles are used to differentiate stage N2 from stage N1 sleep and stage R sleep.
K-complex	A greater than 0.5 s, high-amplitude, negative-going, EEG sharp wave that is immediately followed by a positive component. K-complex waves stand out from the background EEG activity and are most prominent in central and frontal EEG derivations. K-complex waves are used to differentiate stage N2 from stage N1 sleep and stage R sleep.

Five main EEG waveforms direct classification of an epoch as sleep or wakefulness or sleep and then subclassify sleep into one stage or another (see Table 8.1). Alpha activity, theta activity, delta activity (also known as slow waves), K-complexes and sleep spindles form sleep's basic central nervous system (CNS) microarchitecture. Staging is considerably easier when the microarchitectural waveforms are clearly present, are well formed, and readily stand out from background activity. It is worth remembering that sleep staging rules were developed as bioelectrical correlates in normal healthy subjects. In clinical practice, patients are very often older and infirm. Therefore, poorly formed and ambiguous features make it more difficult to score sleep and may reduce inter-rater reliability. While some problems may stem from poor recording technique, a sleep disorder itself often erodes the quality of EEG patterns and events. Sometimes, successful treatment improves sleep's basic microarchitecture and returns EEG quality to normal, a far more impressive accomplishment than increasing one or another specific sleep stage percentage.

Sleep staging rules

Stage W (wakefulness)

This is scored when alpha EEG activity occupies more than 50% of a given epoch; that is, more than 15 s duration. At first glance, this would appear to be a simple, easy-to-follow, and straightforward rule, and in patients with well-formed alpha EEG activity, it is (Fig. 8.2). However, EEG quality in many patients with sleep disorders is poor, and alpha activity can be indistinct. To complicate matters further, approximately 10% of individuals lack a discernable alpha rhythm on eye closure. In such cases, differentiating sleep from wakefulness presents greater difficulty, and scoring must rely on other characteristics. Conjugate REMs and blinking help identify wakefulness. The appearance of vertex sharp waves, generalized EEG flattening with some slowing into the theta bandwidth, sleep spindle or K-complex emergence, and delta activity indicate sleep.

Stage N1 sleep

This is established by the gradual waning of alpha activity to the point where it occupies less than 50% of the 30 s epoch (see fig. 8.3, top panel). The alpha rhythm is replaced by low-voltage, mixed-frequency (theta and beta rhythms) activity. In the absence of REMs, when this low-voltage, mixed-frequency activity does not contain sleep spindle, K-complex, or delta activity, the epoch is scored as stage N1 sleep. The presence of slow rolling eye movements and vertex waves is characteristic of but not essential to N1 sleep scoring criteria. As previously discussed, alpha EEG presence and/or integrity can be compromised in some patients, making stage N1 scoring difficult. Furthermore, because stage N1 sleep criteria essentially represent "rules of exclusion" and N1 occupies so little of overall sleep time, inter-rater reliability is quite low (18–42%).

Stage N2 sleep

This is defined by the presence of sleep spindles and/or K-complexes (see fig. 8.3, middle panel). In contrast to stage W and N1 scoring, stage N2 is easily identified, and scoring reliability is very high. Once a patient enters N2, the subsequent epochs are scored as N2 as long as there is evidence of K-complexes or sleep spindle activity. Stage N2 scoring terminates when sufficient slow-wave activity appears indicating a transition to N3, when the sleeper ascends to stages N1 or W, or at the onset of a REM sleep episode (see below).

Stage N3 sleep

This is scored when an epoch contains 6 s (or more) (i.e, ≥20%) of slow waves (>75 µV waves in the 0.5–2 Hz bandwidth) (see fig. 8.3, bottom panel). Stage N3 sleep is also called slow-wave sleep (SWS) or delta sleep. The older R&K Manual previously divided stage N3 sleep into NREM stage 3 and stage 4 sleep based on whether there was 20–50% or >50% slow-wave activity, respectively; some sleep specialists still make this distinction. Sleep spindles occur during stage N3 sleep, but eye movements are absent.

Stage R sleep

The background EEG for this stage is similar to that for stage N1 sleep; however, REM activity is also present. REMs appear as sharply peaked EOG channel deflections with an initial rise-time lasting less than 0.5 s. Stage R sleep was originally called JEM sleep (jerky eye movement sleep) by its discoverer. Subsequently, this sleep process became most commonly known as REM sleep (named for the accompanying REMs). However REM sleep possesses

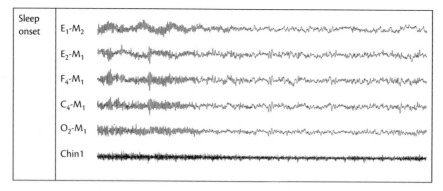

Fig. 8.2 Sleep onset. This figure represents a clear transition from wakefulness to sleep. The subject had well-defined alpha EEG activity that completely attenuates after the first third of this epoch, giving way to low-voltage, mixed-frequency EEG activity.

multiple alternative monikers, including D-sleep (dreaming sleep), paradoxical sleep (because there is awake-like EEG activity and eye movements), desynchronized sleep, active sleep, and, most recently, stage R sleep. Dreaming occurs during stage R sleep, and the eye movements appear to be changes in direction of gaze associated with dream content. Middle ear muscle activity, facial grimacing, twitching, penile erections, and sudden heart-rate alterations can also accompany REM sleep. Sawtooth theta waves and muscle atonia are also characteristic of the stage. Skeletal muscle atonia prevents the sleeper from enacting dreams or behaviorally reacting to the dream sensorium. Stage R sleep is easily recognizable during epochs in which eye movements are present; however, a REM sleep episode may continue for several minutes with ocular quiescence, only to be followed by subsequent bursts of REM activity. Once stage R has commenced, REM scoring continues until a K-complex, sleep spindle, chin EMG tone increase, or another scorable sleep or wake stage occur. In the past, many sleep specialists distinguished

between phasic REM (epochs with REM or other activity bursts) and tonic REM (quiescent periods). Figure 8.4 illustrates phasic and tonic REM sleep.

CNS arousal

CNS arousal scoring provides a sensitive index for sleep disturbance. This microarchitectural feature differs from awakening with respect to its duration. An awakening involves transition from any sleep stage to stage W (wakefulness). Such a transition requires an epoch to contain 15 s (or more) of alpha activity. Consequently, briefer sleep interruptions are not appreciated by sleep stage scoring. It was for this reason that CNS arousal scoring rules were developed.

CNS arousals include sleep interruptions ranging from 3 s up to, but not including, 15 s. The lower limit was established on the basis of how brief an event could be reliably detected visually by the original task force members developing the rules. CNS arousals can be evoked by external events (eg, noise), can be provoked

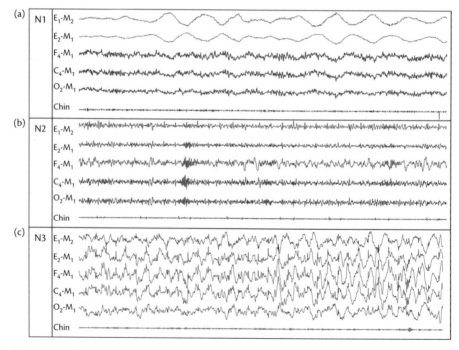

Fig. 8.3 NREM sleep stages. (a) An epoch of stage N1 with low-voltage, mixed-frequency activity and slow rolling eye movements. (b) Stage N2 with clear well-defined sleep spindle activity. (c) An archetypal example of slow-wave sleep in which slow-wave variants of delta EEG activity dominate the entire epoch.

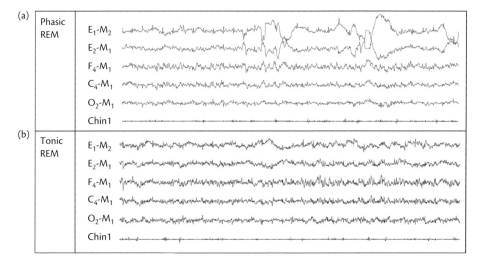

Fig. 8.4 REM sleep. (a) An epoch of REM sleep during which phasic events (in the form of rapid eye movements) accompany low-voltage, mixed-frequency EEG background activity with observable sawtooth theta waves. Additionally, submentalis EMG (chin) is virtually absent. (b) A quiescent epoch of REM sleep during which no rapid eye movements are seen. EEG background remains low-voltage with mixed frequencies, and EMG activity remains absent.

by pathophysiologies (eg, apnea episodes), or can occur spontaneously (which can mean either that they were caused by an undetected event or that they were truly spontaneous).

In adults, arousal scoring proceeds from EEG and chin EMG signals. In children, digital video and audio recording are also used. Arousal-associated EEG changes are typically most prominent in occipital leads. Although it seems obvious, it should be emphasized that the patient must be asleep for a CNS arousal to be scored. Preceding sleep must be 10 s or more. Arousals involve an abrupt increase in EEG frequency to bandwidths associated with alpha or theta (but not spindle) activity. The shift (sometimes referred to as EEG speeding) must persist for a minimum of 3 s. The above criteria hold for all NREM sleep stages (see fig. 8.5, top pane). In contrast, CNS arousals from stage R sleep also require a concurrent brief increase in chin EMG activity (see fig. 8.5, bottom panel).

Breathing

Recording

Diagnosing sleep-related breathing disorders and titrating positive airway pressure constitute the most common applications for PSG. Basically, the clinician must review airflow, respiratory effort, and the effect on oxyhemoglobin saturation. Information about carbon dioxide levels, while often very helpful, is not required in routine practice for adults. In the following paragraphs, we will review the essentials for recording and scoring sleep-related respiration.

Airflow

Airflow monitoring during sleep studies involves placing thermistors, thermocouples, and/or pressure transducers at the nares and near the mouth. Strictly speaking, thermistors and thermocouples

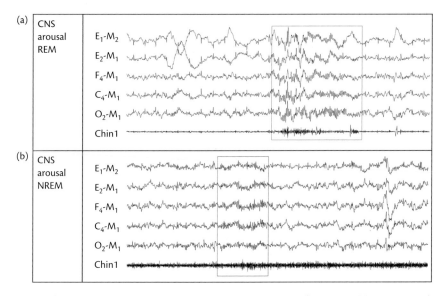

Fig. 8.5 CNS arousals. (a) A CNS arousal (boxed) from REM sleep. Note the sudden, prominent, and brief increase in alpha EEG activity, how it subsides after a few seconds, and how sleep returns. Also note that a submentalis EMG (Chin1) increase accompanies the EEG change. (b) A CNS arousal from REM sleep, also marked by a burst of alpha EEG activity but with little or no change in submentalis EMG.

do not measure airflow but rather sense changes in temperature. Comparatively cooler inspired ambient gases are warmed by the corporal blood flow before they are exhaled. That variance in temperature is calculable and can therefore be used as a surrogate to determine airflow over this thermally sensitive resistor (i.e, thermistor). These subtle fluctuations in temperature are measured at the nares and in front of the mouth. The sensors are advantageous in that they are low current and relatively small, but have an adequate sensing area to provide reliable information. Thermocouples achieve similar endpoints as thermistors by employing the differential expanding properties of different metals in response to thermal change. Both thermocouples and thermistors are commonly used in sleep study because of their ease of use and comfort for patients. Similarly, nasal pressure transducers are used to index airflow. The measurable difference between atmospheric pressure and the relatively positive pressure on exhalation or negative pressure on inhalation produces a waveform that can be accurately recorded. As opposed to the thermal changes of thermistors, pressure transducers measure a different consequence of airflow. Moreover, the pressure signal changes are more sensitive than thermal changes.

Airflow can also be estimated from differential chest and abdominal movement. When calibrated, some manufacturers boast the ability to quantitatively measure tidal volume. Finally, the most accurate, quantitative, and reliable technique for measuring airflow requires a pneumotachometer or a body box. Neither of these latter two approaches are routinely used in clinical PSG.

Respiratory effort

Chest and abdominal movements provide evidence for respiratory effort. Monitoring these movements may employ piezoelectric transducers, inductance plethysmography, or strain gauges. The downward contraction of the diaphragm creates a negative pressure that pulls air into the lungs. This process creates measureable differences in volumes by the expansion of the thoracic wall and increases in abdominal girth. An alternative approach for simply detecting an effort to breath involves measuring muscle activity. EMG activity recorded on or near intercostal muscles can provide a primitive but adequate indication of breathing effort. Because the electrodes are placed in the anterior chest, they tend to also contain ECG artifact, sometimes making the results difficult to interpret. Newer techniques using accelerometers hold promise.

Gases

Key to understanding sleep disordered breathing's pathophysiology is knowing oxyhemoglobin saturation level. Pulse oximetry provides information concerning the consequence of reduced ventilation. Typically recorded from earlobe or finger, spectrographic analysis determines blood oxygen content by taking advantage of hemoglobin's reddening when bound with O_2. Recording from the earlobe (rather than the finger) shortens circulatory delay and is preferred by many clinicians for laboratory studies. Pulse oximeters provide a readily available, affordable, and noninvasive method for uninterrupted oxygen saturation (SaO_2) monitoring. SaO_2 is required for scoring hypopnea, determining oxyhemoglobin nadir, and indexing the time spent at or below 88% saturation (i.e, respiratory insufficiency).

Carbon dioxide (CO_2) monitoring can also be helpful, but is not required for adult PSG according to current standards of practice. In children, it is more important because SaO_2 is not as sensitive. In adults, CO_2 represents the primary stimulus for ventilatory drive. Thus, it informs the clinician more about the cause and dynamics of sleep disordered breathing than the consequences. It can be especially helpful in patients with lung disease, central sleep apnea, and/or morbid obesity.

Scoring

The main terms used in sleep study reports are: obstructive apnea (OA), central apnea (CA), obstructive hypopnea (OA), and respiratory effort related arousal (RERA). Each term has a specific operational definition based on objective measurements. Accurate scoring of these events, however, ironically depends greatly on the PSG technologist's experience and skill. Computerized scoring, although promising, cannot be relied upon.

Apnea

An apnea event is the quantifiable temporal interruption of perceptible airflow. The time-based cutoff for an apnea in the adult is 10 s. In pediatrics, apnea minimum duration criteria are set at a two-breath equivalent. We can further classify each apnea episode as obstructive, central, or mixed, based on respiratory effort. Obstructive apnea involves breathing cessation notwithstanding continuing (and often increasing) respiratory effort. In contrast, when breathing stops because no effort to breathe is present, we call this a central apnea. As the name suggests, mixed apneas have a period without respiratory effort (usually at the episode's initiation) followed by unsuccessful attempts to breathe (because the airway is obstructed) indicated by respiratory effort. See Fig. 8.6 for illustrations of obstructive and central apnea events. The AASM Manual endorses the use of thermal sensors to detect apnea-related airflow cessations. Table 8.1 provides apnea event operational definitions according to current guidelines.

Hypopnea

AASM standards require nasal pressure sensors recordings to score hypopnea. These sensors are more sensitive to flow changes than thermistors or thermocouples. However, in its most literal sense, a hypopnea is merely a shallow breath. It is also worth emphasizing that tidal volume reductions are not intrinsically pathophysiological during wakefulness. They occur naturally while eating and speaking. However, when an airflow reduction during sleep induces a significant oxyhemoglobin desaturation, there may be reason for concern. Furthermore, if the event provokes a CNS arousal, thereby disrupting sleep continuity, it qualifies as pathophysiological. In the early 1980s, sleep clinicians began focusing more on sleep disordered breathing events, and hypopneas were generally regarded as airflow reductions associated with a 3% (or greater) oxygen saturation decline, a CNS arousal (or awakening), or both. Oxyhemoglobin desaturation threshold was typically set at 3% because many oximeters had up to 2% variation (due to "noise," i.e, error variability). Consequently, 3% represented the detectability threshold. In contrast, no real quantitative justification could be spun for how much airflow reduction was meaningful. Some clinicians used 50%, some used 30%, and still others used even less. Part of the problem revolves around the fact that percentage declines in the temperature-change-derived airflow sensors are not proportional to tidal volume changes. Additionally, other factors alter percentage change.[1] Thus, sleep specialists used

---

[1] To make this point, M.H. used to be fond of asking new sleep fellows what they would expect an airflow signal to look like if the bedroom temperature was 37°C?

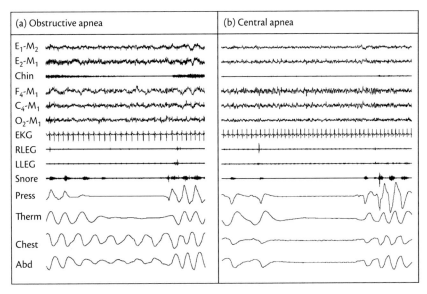

Fig. 8.6 Sleep apnea episodes. (a) An obstructive sleep apnea. Note how the airflow ceases according to nasal pressure (Press) and thermistor (Therm) recording channels, while respiratory effort recorded with chest and abdominal (Abd) movements continues. (b) In contrast, in the central sleep apnea illustrated here, the cessation of breathing is accompanied by cessation of respiratory effort.

to quibble about what percentage a PSG airflow tracing needed to drop in order score a hypopnea. The more pressing (and related) issue, however, was scoring reliability. Without a standard to reign in the wide variation in criteria, scoring reliability suffered. At one point, a group of sleep researchers attempted to create a standard; however, their work was accepted as research but not as providing clinical criteria [11]. As sleep medicine became more mainstream, a standardized definition was forced on the clinical sleep community by Centers Medicare and Medicaid Services (CMS) [12]. Unfortunately the CMS definition for hypopnea required 4% (or

more) oxyhemoglobin desaturation but paid no attention to sleep disruption. Thus, to a large extent, hypopneas became desaturation events (Fig. 8.7). Subsequently, the AASM attempted to restore the "sleep disruption" part of the hypopnea criteria—first by having more than one definition for hypopnea included in the AASM Scoring Manual and later by revising the scoring manual's definitions. To date, however, such attempts have been futile because not using CMS criteria (when they exist) for Medicare and Medicaid patients is considered fraud. Furthermore, to prevent a two-tiered medical system in the United States, CMS requires clinicians to use

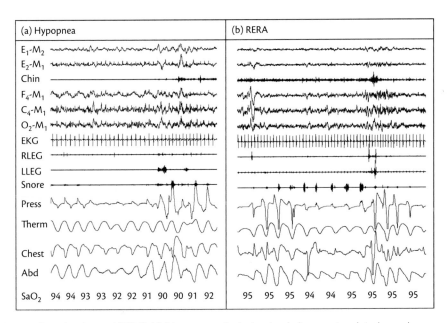

Fig. 8.7 Hypopnea and respiratory effort related arousal (RERA). (a) A hypopnea episode showing decline prominently in the nasal pressure recording (Press) but less clear in the thermistor (Therm) channel. The episode is also associated with a 4% decline in oxyhemoglobin saturation (SaO$_2$). (b) In contrast, the RERA event illustrated here shows decreased airflow accompanied by increased snoring sounds (presumably from increased airway resistance). The event is terminated by an arousal; however, no significant change occurs in oxyhemoglobin saturation.

CMS criteria for all patients if even a single Medicare or Medicaid patient is serviced by their practice. To do otherwise is also considered Medicare fraud. See Table 8.2 for both CMS and AASM definitions for hypopnea.

Respiratory-effort-related arousal

The concept of respiratory effort related arousal (RERA) originated because clinical researchers observed CNS arousals terminating very subtle respiratory perturbations. These events included extended inspiratory phase, paradoxical movement of the chest wall and abdomen, and/or overall signal flattening. These sleep-related breathing disorder events were not accompanied by obvious airflow reductions when standard clinical recording techniques were used. However, when esophageal pressure recordings were made, intrathoracic pressure increased until an arousal terminated the event. It appeared that increased airway resistance led to increased respiratory effort, and this sequence of events ultimately provoked sleep fragmentation. Because these patients typically suffered from moderate to severe sleepiness, the condition was dubbed "upper airway resistance syndrome" [13].

This conceptualization of RERA was short-lived. When CMS designated the term hypopnea to mean, to all intents and purposes, a sleep-related desaturation event, the term RERA was commandeered to identify nondesaturating hypopnea episodes. RERA became a way to identify and count those events that no longer met CMS hypopnea criteria—specifically, sleep disordered breathing events failing to provoke a 4% (or greater) oxyhemoglobin desaturation but were nonetheless terminated by a CNS arousal. See Table 8.2 for the operational definition for RERA.

Data processing

Over the past half-century, technological advances have extensively changed the methods used to record sleep. Older analog sleep recorders have given way to newer multichannel digital devices, with scoring now exclusively performed while viewing computer-generated displays rather than paper. Modern technology has reduced data storage requirements from rooms filled with paper PSGs to a few file cabinet drawers for DVD backup disks. Computerization and widespread server technology have greatly improved remote data accessibility.

Once a sleep study has been completed and data have been archived, sleep staging, sleep disordered breathing, arousal scoring, and leg movements can be identified and tabulated by a trained technologist (who can access data from anywhere in the world). Sleep parameters of interest usually include sleep efficiency (total sleep time as a percentage of time in bed), latency to sleep onset, latency from sleep onset to the first REM sleep episode, and the number of CNS arousals per hour of sleep. Sleep stages are typically summarized as percentages of total sleep time. Sleep-related respiratory parameters include the number of apnea episodes per hour of sleep (i.e, the apnea index, AI), the ratio of obstructive plus mixed apnea to central apnea, the number of apnea and hypopnea episodes per hour of sleep (i.e, the apnea–hypopnea index, AHI), and the number of apneas plus hypopneas plus RERAs per hour of sleep (i.e, the respiratory disturbance index, RDI). AI, AHI, and RDI are also usually sorted according

Table 8.2 Respiratory event criteria: definitions for the major sleep-disordered breathing events

Event	Definition and/or criteria
Obstructive apnea	An obstructive apnea is a 10 s decrease in the peak signal excursion by ≥90% of baseline. Measurement is ensured according to the type of study: via oronasal thermal sensor (diagnostic study) or PAP device flow (titration study). The OA need not be associated with an arousal or desaturation.
Central apnea	The definition is similar to that of an obstructive apnea except that a central apnea has a cessation of respiratory effort during the decrease in airflow.
Mixed apnea	Mixed apneas are scored when a sleep disordered breathing event meeting criteria for apnea occurs but during which the initial portion shows no respiratory effort but is followed by resumed inspiratory effort but still no airflow. Overall, a mixed apnea is considered an obstructive-type event.
CMS hypopnea	Hypopnea is defined as an abnormal respiratory event lasting at least 10 s with at least a 30% reduction in thoraco-abdominal movement or airflow as compared with baseline, and with at least a 4% oxygen desaturation.[1]
AASM hypopnea	The 2013 version of the American Academy of Sleep Medicine definition for hypopnea has three parts as follows:[2] (a) During diagnostic evaluation, airflow diminishes by 30% (or more) on nasal pressure (preferred) or other airflow sensor. During positive airway pressure (PAP) titration, machine flow oscillation declines by 30% (or more). (b) This 30% (or more) airflow decline persists for at least 10 s. (c) A 3% (or greater) oxyhemoglobin desaturation is provoked by the event or the event is terminated by a CNS arousal.
RERA	A respiratory effort related arousal or RERA is characterized by either an increase in respiratory or attenuation of airflow associated with arousal from sleep.
Cheyne–Stokes breathing	A breathing pattern exhibiting a crescendo and decrescendo amplitude in successive breaths. During sleep, if the decrescendo phase is extended to the point of constituting a 10 s (or longer) respiratory pause, the pattern becomes Cheyne–Stokes breathing and central sleep apnea (CSB–CSA). This pattern is characteristic of patients with decompensated congestive heart failure. A diagnosis of CSB–CSA requires that the events must have a total of 5 or more per hour of sleep.

[1] This definition was taken verbatim from the CMS website; however, we assume (although it was not explicitly stated) that to score an event as a hypopnea, it must as a prerequisite not qualify as an apnea.

[2] Although not explicitly stated, we assume that to qualify as a hypopnea, the event must first not qualify as an apnea.

to REM versus NREM stages and by supine versus nonsupine position. Arousals related to snoring can also be useful. To gauge hypoxemia, the SaO_2 nadir and the time spent below 88% or 85% saturation are calculated. According to the AASM, an adult AHI of 0–5 is normal, 5–15 is mild sleep apnea, 15–30 is moderate sleep apnea, and >30 is severe sleep apnea.[2] The sleep specialist is also able to remotely access the PSG tracing and tabulated information in order to evaluate the patient's sleep. During PSG review, the clinician also should identify significant abnormal EEG activity, cardiac arrhythmias, and other PSG events not routinely quantified by standard scoring rules.

References

1. Berger H. Ueber das elektrenkephalogramm des menschen. J Psychol Neurol 1930;40:160–79.
2. Loomis AL, Harvey N, Hobart GA. Cerebral states during sleep, as studied by human brain potentials. J Exp Psychol 1937;21:127–44.
3. Aserinsky E, Kleitman N. Regularly occurring periods of eye motility, and concomitant phenomena. Science 1953;118:273–4.
4. Dement W, Kleitman N. The relation of eye movements during sleep to dream activity: an objective method for the study of dreaming. J Exp Psychol 1957;53:339–46.
5. Williams RL, Agnew HW, Webb WB. Sleep patterns in young adults: an EEG study. Electroenceph Clin Neurophysiol 1964;17:376–81.
6. Rechtschaffen A, Kales A, eds. A manual of standardized terminology, techniques and scoring system for sleep stages of human subjects. NIH publication 204. Washington DC: US Government Printing Office, 1968.
7. Guilleminault C. Sleeping and waking disorders: indications and techniques. Menlo Park, CA: Addison-Wesley, 1982.
8. ASDA. Sleep Disorders Atlas Task Force. EEG arousals: scoring rules and examples: a preliminary report from the Sleep Disorders Atlas Task Force of the American Sleep Disorders Association. Sleep 1992;15:173–84.
9. Iber C, Ancoli-Israel S, Chesson A, Quan SF; American Academy of Sleep Medicine. The AASM manual for the scoring of sleep and associated events: rules, terminology and technical specifications. Westchester, IL: American Academy of Sleep Medicine, 2007.
10. Silber MH, Ancoli-Israel S, Bonnet MH et al. The visual scoring of sleep in adults. J Clin Sleep Med 2007;3:121–31.
11. AASM. The Report of an American Academy of Sleep Medicine Task Force. Sleep-related breathing disorders in adults: recommendations for syndrome definition and measurement techniques in clinical research. Sleep 1999;22:667–89.
12. Centers for Medicare and Medicaid Services. National coverage determination for continuous positive airway pressure (CPAP) therapy for obstructive sleep apnea (OSA) NCD #240.4. 2005. Available from: http://www.cms.hhs.gov.
13. Guilleminault C, Stoohs R, Clerk A, et al. A cause of excessive daytime sleepiness: the upper airway resistance syndrome. Chest 1993;104:781–7.

---

[2] AHI, however, is not an ideal index for severity. The duration of sleep disordered breathing events and their consequences on oxyhemoglobin saturation are also important. A patient with an AHI of 25 who never desaturates below 88% is arguably less severely afflicted than a patient with an AHI of 12 who spends 28 minutes at or below 85% SaO_2 level.

CHAPTER 9

Other sleep laboratory procedures (MSLT, MWT, and actigraphy)

Fabio Pizza and Carlo Cipolli

Introduction

Polysomnography (PSG) has long been considered the gold standard for the measurement of sleep because it provides objective measures not only of wake and sleep time, but also (and above all) of sleep architecture coupled with muscular and respiratory parameters. However, PSG is limited by cost and inconvenience as a method for long-term, continuous sleep monitoring, and is not able to provide any measure of the daytime sleepiness which is a frequent and cardinal symptom of a number of sleep disorders. These two main limitations have prompted researchers and sleep clinicians to set up, tune, and apply other tools to obtain objective measures for the evaluation of sleep architecture, sleep habits and sleepiness for longer periods (from days to weeks) and/or the diagnosis of specific sleep disorders. These tools, which have different costs and practical limitations compared with PSG, appear complementary, rather than alternative, to both PSG and subjective measures of sleepiness and sleep duration and quality, given the different types of information they provide.

Objective measures of sleep and sleepiness can be obtained mainly by using actigraphy, the multiple sleep latency test (MSLT), and the maintenance of wakefulness test (MWT), which are recording techniques and standardized laboratory-based procedures with different functions compared with PSG. In this chapter, we will describe these techniques and their clinical applications in the light of current recommendations.

Sleep laboratory procedures to objectively assess sleepiness: MSLT and MWT

Overview

The MSLT and MWT are two laboratory procedures aimed at quantifying sleepiness objectively, but the use of either is also recommended in specific clinical situations. Physiological sleepiness, which is a subjective feeling expressing the inner desire to sleep and is thus indicative of the biological need for sleep, differs substantially from hypersomnolence, which is a pathological individual trait resulting in an inability to stay awake during the major waking period of the day and leading to unintended lapses into drowsiness or sleep in inappropriate (and often potentially dangerous) situations [1].

To properly use the MSLT and MWT and interpret their results, the clinician first has to evaluate the features of the sleepiness complaint, namely to ascertain, by means of an accurate history, not only the subjective feeling, but also the potential occurrence and characteristics of sleep episodes (eg, refreshing and/or associated with dream content). In particular, the clinician should consider the time of day (i.e, circadian timing) of sleep episodes, the individual sleep habits (eg, misalignment of major sleep period from night–day cycle, chronic sleep deprivation, suggested by a significant difference between sleep time during working days and that during holidays/weekends, and individual chronotype), as well as other concomitant daytime and nocturnal symptoms suggesting the presence of sleep disorders (eg, cataplexy, restless legs, sleep disordered breathing, and nocturnal awakenings). Finally, the clinician should ascertain the possible concomitance of other (psychiatric, neurological, and/or medical) disturbances that can mimic or cause hypersomnolence and of the chronic use of treatments potentially affecting sleep or vigilance. Indeed, hypersomnolence can be either the cardinal symptom of several sleep disorders (eg, obstructive sleep apnea syndrome, central disorders of hypersomnolence), or the result of a wide range of medical disorders and medication use, but can be also frequently confused with other conditions characterized by "decreased energy" or fatigue, such as insomnia and depression. Fatigue differs from sleepiness as it refers to a cumulative disinclination toward a sustained effort that can lead to reduced performance efficiency and resolves with rest, whereas sleepiness resolves with sleep [2].

Sleepiness can be measured also by means of subjective scales, which evaluate sleepiness as a state (i.e, a contingent individual condition) [3,4] or a trait (i.e, as a stable individual characteristic) [5]. The subjective scales are commonly used to help the clinician in the preliminary evaluation, by minimizing inter-individual differences in introspection, awareness, and, finally, ability to report sleepiness. State sleepiness refers to the subjective feeling in a specific moment of the day: the subject rates his/her own feeling on an ordinal scale where numbers are associated with a list of verbal descriptors ordered from the lowest level of sleepiness to that of imminent sleep. The Stanford Sleepiness Scale includes seven items ranging from "feeling active, vital, alert, or wide awake" (score = 1) to "no longer fighting sleep, sleep onset soon; having dreamlike thoughts" (score = 7) [3]. The Karolinska Sleepiness Scale encompasses 10 items ranging from "extremely alert" (score = 1) to "extremely sleepy, falls asleep all the time" (score = 10) [4]. Both these scales, as well as the Visual Analogue Scale, where the subject has to indicate the subjective sleepiness (or the alertness) level on a 10 cm line [6], are useful in conjunction with sleep logs and/or actigraphy to track circadian fluctuations of sleepiness. They can also be administered before each MSLT or MWT trial (see below) to evaluate the subjective awareness of sleepiness in parallel with its objective measure.

Conversely, subjective trait sleepiness refers to a stable individual characteristic over a prolonged period of time, lasting at least some weeks. To identify subjects with hypersomnolence, the most frequently used tool is the Epworth Sleepiness Scale [1,5]. This is a self-administered questionnaire in which subjects rate the probability of dozing off or falling asleep in eight common situations encountered in daily life with a score ranging from 0 ("would never doze off") to 3 ("high chance of dozing"). The final score ranges from 0 to 24; 11 is considered the threshold to identify pathological sleepiness [5].

To overcome the intrinsic limits of all subjective measures, the MSLT and MWT have been standardized and validated to quantify different aspects of sleepiness. These tests, which require a sleep laboratory with a professional technician available for execution across the day, are based on the common assumption that the time needed to fall asleep reflects sleepiness. However, they have clear differences and specific clinical uses: the MSLT measures "sleep propensity," while the MWT quantifies the individual "ability to maintain wakefulness" (or to resist sleep) [1,7].

The MSLT

The MSLT was developed at the University of Stanford by Carskadon and Dement, who evaluated the impact of sleep deprivation on daytime sleep latency across pubertal development. In 1986, the procedures to perform the MSLT were published, and sleep laboratories worldwide de facto used the test as the gold standard measure of daytime sleepiness for both clinical and research purposes [8]. The huge amount of published data on MSLT findings in different clinical contexts made apparent the need for an extensive literature review [9], and this was followed by the release of new guidelines for MSLT execution and interpretation by the American Academy of Sleep Medicine in 2005 [7]. These guidelines are reflected in the third edition of the International Classification of Sleep Disorders [1]. In brief, the test should start in the morning between 8 and 10 am, 1.5–3 hours after awakening from the major sleep period documented by nocturnal PSG in the laboratory, with at least six hours of total sleep time, and possibly after one-week assessment of sleep–wake schedules carried out using sleep logs and/or actigraphy. Drugs potentially affecting sleep should ideally be stopped two weeks before; alternatively, their administration should be considered in the interpretation of MSLT results. A drug screening in the morning of the test may be useful to rule out pharmacologically-induced sleepiness. During the day, the subject should avoid stimulating substances (eg, coffee) or vigorous activities, including exposure to bright sunlight.

The MSLT requires the execution of five (or four) naps at two-hour intervals. The subject is not allowed to sleep between the nap opportunities, and the laboratory staff should control patient's activities (or continuously record them with ambulatory PSG) between naps. A light breakfast is recommended at least one hour before the first trial, and a light lunch is recommended immediately after the termination of the second noon trial. The MSLT montage includes two electroencephalographic (including central and occipital derivations: C3-A2, C4-A1, O1-A2, O2-A1), two electrooculographic (right and left eyes recorded by a lead referenced to the same mastoid), and one electromyographic (mental/submental muscle) channels together with electrocardiography according to technical requirements of sleep medicine [10]. Before undergoing each scheduled nap opportunity, the subject should not smoke for at least 30 minutes, should avoid activities for 15 minutes, and should prepare to go to bed (including going to the toilet if necessary) 10 minutes before the trial start. Then, five minutes before the start of the recording, the technician performs the biocalibration, and, in the minute before the lights are turned off, the subject rates his/her subjective state sleepiness. During each nap opportunity, the subject is recumbent in the sleep laboratory bed and is invited to "lie quietly, assume a comfortable position, keep your eyes closed, and try to fall asleep." Then, the lights are turned off (start of the trial), and the subject has 20 minutes to fall into sleep, defined as a 30 s epoch of any sleep stage, including non-REM sleep stage 1 (sleep onset). If the subject falls asleep, the technician should continue the recording for 15 minutes in order to document the potential early occurrence of REM sleep (sleep onset REM period, SOREMP). If the subject does not fall asleep, the nap opportunity is interrupted after 20 minutes. For the MSLT trials without evidence of sleep onset, the sleep latency is by convention considered to be 20 minutes. Events that represent deviations from the normal protocol should be reported by the technician in order to correctly interpret the results of the test. The MSLT report should include the start and end times of each nap opportunity, latency from lights-off to the first epoch of sleep, mean sleep latency (arithmetic mean of all nap opportunities), and number of SOREMPs. MSLT interpretation is thus based on two key objective measures: the mean sleep latency and the number of SOREMPs (Table 9.1). A mean sleep latency below eight minutes is considered pathological, although 30% of the general population may fall below this limit, and two or more SOREMPs (including any SOREMP present during the nocturnal PSG performed the night before the MSLT) are required to confirm the diagnosis of narcolepsy (with and without cataplexy, now defined as type 1 and type 2 narcolepsy, respectively): according to this criterion, the execution of the fifth nap is mandatory in specific clinical situations (eg, single SOREMP documented during the first four naps unless a SOREMP was observed in the previous night's PSG recording) [1,7]. A modified MSLT protocol to measure sleep propensity for research purposes requires awakening the subject after the onset of sustained sleep (i.e, at least three consecutive epochs of sleep stage 1 or one epoch of any other sleep stage) in order to avoid any influence of sleep on subsequent naps, and thus provides only a mean sleep latency as result [8].

Table 9.1 Overview of the MSLT procedure

Timing	Procedure	Recommendation
−2 weeks	Withdrawal of medications with stimulant or REM-suppressing effect	Recommended
−1 week	Regular sleep–wake schedules monitored by sleep logs/actigraphy	Suggested
−1 day	Nocturnal polysomnography documenting a total sleep time > 6 h and excluding significant sleep disorders. Split-night sleep studies are not allowed	Recommended
Not defined	Withdrawal of other usual medications (antihypertensives, insulin, etc.) with sedating or stimulating properties	Clinician decision
At awakening	Drug screening	Clinician decision
All day	Avoid vigorous activities, exposure to bright sunlight, and caffeinated beverages. Between MSLT scheduled naps, the patient is out of bed and prevented from sleeping (staff observation)	Recommended
1.5–3 h from awakening	Start of the test with five trials scheduled every 2 h (four-nap version is reliable for narcolepsy diagnosis only if two SOREMPs occurred)	Recommended
Meals	Light breakfast at least 1 h before the first trial, light lunch after the second trial	Recommended
Trials		
−30 min	Stop smoking	Recommended
−15 min	Stop any stimulating activity	Recommended
−10 min	Comfort adjustments, including restroom visit	Recommended
−5 min	Biocalibration*	Recommended
−1 min	Subjective state sleepiness evaluation	Suggested
−30 s	Assume a comfortable position for sleep	Recommended
−10 s	"Please lie quietly, assume a comfortable position, keep your eyes closed, and try to fall asleep"	Recommended
Time 0 (T0)	Lights-off	Recommended
T0 + 20 min	Trial interruption (if no sleep occurs)	Recommended
Sleep onset (SO)	SO is defined as the first epoch greater than 15 s of cumulative sleep in a 30 s epoch of any stage of sleep, including stage 1 NREM sleep	Recommended
SO + 15 min	Trial interruption (if sleep occurs)	Recommended
Scoring		
Sleep latency	Time elapsed between T0 and SO. If no sleep is recorded, the conventional sleep latency is 20 min	Recommended
REM latency	Time elapsed between SO and the first epoch of REM sleep, within the first 15 min of sleep onset	Recommended
Report		
	Start and stop times of each nap	Recommended
	Sleep latency of each nap and mean sleep latency across trials. A mean sleep latency < 8 min is considered pathological	Recommended
	Number of SOREMPs. A number of SOREMPs ≥ 2 is highly specific for narcolepsy	Recommended
	Events/conditions representing deviations from the protocol	Recommended

Recommendation Level rated as: recommended, suggested, or optional. *Instruction for biocalibration before each MSLT trial: "(1) Lie quietly with your eyes open for 30 seconds, (2) close both eyes for 30 seconds, (3) without moving your head, look to the right, then left, then right, then left, right and then left, (4) blink eyes slowly for 5 times, and (5) clench or grit your teeth tightly together."

Source data from Sleep, 28(1), Littner MR, Kushida C, Wise M, et al. Practice parameters for clinical use of the multiple sleep latency test and the maintenance of wakefulness test, pp. 113–21, Copyright (2005), Associated Professional Sleep Societies, LLC.

The MWT

Along with the routine use of the MSLT in sleep laboratories worldwide, the test showed limitations in documenting the treatment effect in severely sleepy patients whose MSLT changes seemed minimal compared with what was expected on the basis of patients' self-reports. The MSLT was also criticized because its laboratory setting may not reliably reproduce the workplace conditions where sleep tendency usually manifests. Therefore, the individual ability to resist sleep was proposed as an alternative objective measure of sleepiness.

The first proposed procedure required the subject, sitting in a comfortable chair in a quiet and dimly lit room, to stay awake in four (or five) 20-minute trials performed every two hours across daytime [11]. Only in 1997 a normative study standardized different test procedures (i.e, four naps lasting 20 or 40 minutes) and interpretation methods (sleep onset defined as first epoch of any sleep stage, or as three consecutive epochs of non-REM sleep stage 1 or a single epoch of any other sleep stage) leading to four different MWT protocols [12]. Therefore the MWT could be performed with four 20 minutes trials and interpreted considering either the sleep latency to the first epoch of sleep or that to the occurrence of sustained sleep (two protocols). Alternatively, the procedure could be based on four 40-minute trials interpreted considering either the sleep latency to the first epoch of sleep or that to the occurrence of sustained sleep (two protocols). Accordingly, a sleep latency cut-off was provided for each of the four procedures; however, this heterogeneity prevented the widespread use of the test. After few years, and in parallel to the MSLT, the available data were extensively reviewed [9], and unambiguous guidelines for MWT execution and interpretation were published [7]. The current version of the MWT requires four 40-minute trials at two-hour intervals. The first session should begin after 1.5–3 hours from the usual wake-up time (approximately between 9 and 10 am), without, however, a formal need to either objectively document sleep time in the night before the test by means of PSG or verify sleep patterns in the weeks before the test by means of sleep logs or actigraphy. At each trial, the subject sits in bed with the back and head supported by the bedrest (many laboratories, however, prefer the use of a comfortable armchair), in a sound-attenuated laboratory, which is also insulated from external light and has low illuminance (with the light placed out of the patient's field of vision, with 0.10–0.13 lux at the corneal level) and a temperature regulated to maximize patient comfort. The use or withdrawal of drugs, tobacco and caffeine is decided by the clinician, while a light breakfast and lunch should be administered one hour before the first nap and immediately after the second one, respectively. The recording montage is the same as for the MSLT [10]. Before each nap, the subject is asked about the need to go to the toilet or to have other adjustments for comfort. At the beginning of each trial, the technician performs the biocalibration, including a period of at least 30 seconds with eyes opened followed by another one with eyes closed. Then, the subject is instructed to "sit still and remain awake for as long as possible, to look directly ahead of you and not at the light." Extraordinary measures (eg, singing) to stay awake are forbidden. However, the technician is not allowed to enter the room during the trial. The trial is interrupted after 40 minutes if the subject stays awake, or after the occurrence of unequivocal/sustained sleep (i.e, three consecutive epochs of sleep stage 1 or an epoch of any other sleep stage). The sleep latency is calculated from lights-off to the first epoch of any sleep stage defined as a period greater than 15 seconds of cumulative sleep within a 30 second epoch. The MWT report should include start and stop times for each trial, sleep latency, total sleep time, stages of sleep achieved for each trial, and the mean sleep latency (the arithmetic mean of the four trials), together with events or conditions that may represent deviations from the normal protocol (Table 9.2). The definition of normal values is even more controversial than in the MSLT: a mean sleep latency below eight minutes has been conventionally established as the cut-off for impaired vigilance, whereas a mean value of 30 minutes or above is the cut-off established for normal alertness (7).

Comparison of and recommendations on the MSLT and MWT

Even though both the MSLT and MWT measure sleepiness by means of sleep latency, they are based on different conceptualizations: in the MSLT, sleepiness is viewed as sleep propensity, but in the MWT as a difficulty in maintaining wakefulness (and thus similar to alertness). When used in parallel on patient populations, the two tests provide data that are correlated, but this correlation can explain only a low percentage of the observed variability, thus confirming that the tests measure different aspects of the sleepiness phenomenon [13]. Individual motivation during the tests is also crucial and should be taken into account when interpreting results, as well as potential deviation from the established protocols. The same subject can appear more sleepy during the MWT (trying to fall asleep instead of remaining awake) or more alert during the MSLT (trying to remain awake instead of falling asleep), but the opposite attitudes do not affect the test results. Therefore, the MSLT is a better measure of sleepiness (rather than alertness), and the MWT one of alertness [14]. Finally, the two tests also show different relations with performance measures, as suggested by the stronger correlations between simulated driving performance and alertness (during the MWT) versus sleep propensity (during the MSLT) in patients with severe obstructive sleep apnea syndrome [15].

In the clinical practice of sleep medicine, the MSLT is a diagnostic tool recommended to characterize the central disorders of hypersomnolence (especially to document SOREMPs). Diagnostic criteria require a sleep latency below eight minutes with two or more SOREMPs (including any SOREMP noted in the nocturnal PSG performed the night before the test) in both type 1 and type 2 narcolepsy, and a sleep latency below eight minutes with fewer than two or no SOREMPs in idiopathic hypersomnia [1]. Conversely, the MSLT should not be used to quantify sleepiness in any other sleep disorder (eg, insomnia, circadian rhythm sleep disorders, and sleep disordered breathing), given the frequent occurrence of short sleep latencies in the general population [1,7] and the existence of conditions with high sleep ability in the absence of any sleepiness complaint [16]. However, despite the fact that MSLT is not indicated for quantifying sleepiness in the initial assessment of obstructive sleep apnea syndrome or to assess treatment response, it can be performed in patients whose sleepiness level remains pathological after adequate treatment with continuous positive airway pressure. The test can also be repeated in ambiguous cases of suspected narcolepsy with negative MSLT findings, as well as when the initial test execution was influenced by extraneous circumstances or when it provided ambiguous results [1,7].

Conversely, the MWT is not a diagnostic tool, and current guidelines recommend its use to test alertness in individuals such as professional drivers in whom the inability to maintain wakefulness can constitute a personal or public safety issue and in patients with hypersomnolence to assess treatment response [1,7]. The mean sleep latency values of normal subjects are 30.4 ± 11.2 minutes, and thus the pathological threshold is considered 8 minutes (two standard deviations below the mean). Indeed, considering as normal a sleep latency of 30 or 40 minutes leaves to the clinician a huge "gray area" of uncertain results that cannot be interpreted either as normal or as pathological.

Table 9.2 Overview of the MWT procedure

Timing	Procedure	Recommendation
Not defined	Withdrawal of medications	Clinician decision
Not defined	Regular sleep–wake schedules monitored by sleep logs/actigraphy	No consensus reached
−1 day	Nocturnal polysomnography prior to MWT	Clinician decision
Not defined	Withdrawal of other usual medications (eg, antihypertensives, insulin, etc.) with sedating or stimulating properties	Clinician decision
At awakening	Drug screening	Clinician decision
All day	Avoid caffeinated beverages	Clinician decision
1.3–3 h from awakening	Start of the test with four 40 min trials scheduled every 2 h starting between 9 and 10 am	Recommended
Meals	Light breakfast at least 1 h before the first trial, light lunch after the second trial	Recommended
Trials		
Not defined	Stop smoking	Clinician decision
Not defined	Stop any stimulating activity	Clinician decision
Not defined	Comfort adjustments, including restroom visit	Recommended
Not defined	Biocalibration*	Recommended
Not defined		
Not defined	Assume a comfortable position. The subject should be seated in bed with the back and the head supported by a bedrest (bolster pillow) so that the neck is not uncomfortably flexed or extended	Recommended
Not defined	"Please sit still and remain awake for as long as possible. Look directly ahead of you, and do not look directly at the light"	Recommended
Time 0 (T0)	Lights-off	Recommended
T0 + 40 min	Trial interruption (if no sleep occurs)	Recommended
Sleep onset (SO)	First epoch of greater than 15 s of cumulative sleep in a 30 s epoch	Recommended
Unequivocal sleep	Trial interruption, after the recording of three consecutive epochs of stage 1 sleep, or one epoch of any other stage of sleep	Recommended
Scoring		
Sleep latency	Time elapsed between T0 and SO. If no sleep is recorded, the conventional sleep latency is 40 min	Recommended
Report		
	Start and stop times of each nap	Recommended
	Sleep latency of each nap and mean sleep latency across trials. A mean sleep latency < 8 min is considered pathological. Values greater than this but less than 40 min are of uncertain significance	Recommended
	Stages of sleep achieved for each trial	Recommended
	Events/conditions representing deviations from the protocol	Recommended

Recommendation Level rated as: recommended, suggested, or optional. *Instruction for biocalibration before each MSLT trial: "(1) sit quietly with your eyes open for 30 seconds, (2) close both eyes for 30 seconds, (3) without moving your head, look to the right, then left, then right, then left, right and then left, (4) blink eyes slowly for 5 times, and (5) clench or grit your teeth tightly together."

Source data from Sleep, 28(1), Littner MR, Kushida C, Wise M, et al. Practice parameters for clinical use of the multiple sleep latency test and the maintenance of wakefulness test, pp. 113–21, Copyright (2005), Associated Professional Sleep Societies, LLC.

Actigraphy

Overview of the technique

Actigraphy is a minimally invasive objective monitoring technique that is able to record the occurrence of movements for prolonged periods of time. Its rationale is based on the fact that few movements occur during sleep, while active wakefulness is normally characterized by high motor activity. The actigraphic assessment of motor activity can provide a fairly accurate evaluation of sleep–wakefulness patterns with the key advantage of cost-effective limited equipment (modern devices are as invasive as wristwatches) allowing prolonged recordings (from days to weeks) in the natural environment, barely interfering with daily activities. It is thus optimal to examine sleep patterns of those subjects who do not tolerate the laboratory setting (eg, insomniacs, elderly demented patients, and children) and to accurately estimate their habitual sleep patterns across the 24 hours. However, it should be kept in mind that actigraphy does not record sleep per se, but provides an indirect evaluation of sleep quality and duration based on activity/inactivity as equivalent of wakefulness/sleep. Therefore, the interpretation of the collected data can be misleading in clinical situations where high motor activity occurs during the night (eg, patients with REM sleep behavior disorder) or low motor activity is noted during the day (eg, hypersomnia), respectively. Conversely, actigraphy provides good estimates of sleep–wake patterns in healthy subjects.

The first pioneering studies in which activity monitoring was applied to document sleep and wakefulness date back to the 1970s and were conducted by the groups of Kupfer [17] and Colburn [18]. Soon thereafter, sleep parameters provided by actigraphy were validated in comparison with PSG-defined sleep, and showed good reliability for the quantification of minutes spent in sleep and wakefulness during the sleep period [19].

While the first devices required a connection with a recorder to store the data, modern tools have miniaturized accelerometers and solid memories able to record for long periods and are included in an apparatus the size of a wristwatch. Several hardware and software methods have been developed to derive activity, and most of the currently available actigraphs analogically sample physical activity several times per second and digitize the signal in a user-defined time interval, with one minute being the most widely used epoch duration. Although the actigraph is mostly applied to the nondominant hand, the clinician can decide to apply the device to other body segments (eg, dominant hand, trunk, or legs), and tailor both sampling and epoch rates, or choose the digitizing approach if necessary, according to the specific clinical application or research purpose. Three different strategies to digitize the analog signal are currently available, and some devices utilize more than one method in parallel to increase data quality: (a) the "time above the threshold" mode counts the times per epoch when the motion signal is above a specific threshold (disregarding signal acceleration and amplitude); (b) the "zero-crossing" approach counts the times per epoch when the motion signal crosses zero (disregarding signal acceleration and amplitude); and (c) "digital integration" calculates the area under the curve of the signal, thus reflecting its amplitude and acceleration, but not its duration or frequency [20]. Some devices can also record light exposure and cutaneous temperature; moreover, most devices have an event button to be pushed in specific situations, for example when the light is turned off. Although the newest actigraphs can be water-resistant and some have software able to estimate metabolic measures from motor activity, the subject is generally instructed to remove the device while bathing as well as when engaged in strong physical activity (eg, sport). To properly interpret the recording, it is crucial to ask the subject to keep a daily sleep/actigraphy log with times of device removal, an overview of the activities performed across the 24 hours, and a self-evaluation of sleep quality. Downloading the data every week is also prudent to minimize data loss, especially when recording at high sampling frequency and across more weeks. Once data are downloaded on a personal computer, they should be manually edited using the information provided by the daily log (or event-marked points). This procedure is crucial to correctly attribute periods of actigraphy removal to sleep, wakefulness, or "missing data," and also to set lights-off and lights-on times into the scoring software. After the visual editing, several software packages, by applying different algorithms to interpret the rest–activity data, provide several quantitative parameters on the sleep–wake cycle (namely, daytime and nocturnal total sleep times, number of sleep episodes, sleep latency, and efficiency) [19,21,22].

Apart from using actigraphy to evaluate sleep and wakefulness measures, raw motor activity data can be directly analyzed to assess the circadian rhythm of motor activity. Indeed, data collected over prolonged periods of time lasting for multiple circadian periods can also give chronobiological information by directly analyzing the raw activity data as a rest–activity rhythm. The most popular method is the cosinor analysis, which allows computing the circadian rhythm quantified by the acrophase (time of peak activity), amplitude (peak-to-nadir difference) and mesor (mean) of the fitted curve of motor activity [23,24]. More sophisticated approaches (such as the five-parameter extended cosinor analysis) have also been developed to better fit the mathematical function to the activity data when they are poorly represented by the shape of a cosine curve [25]. However, also given the frequent nonsinusoidal waveform of rest–activity data, other nonparametric procedures such as 24-hour autocorrelations can be applied to describe the circadian rest–activity rhythm [26,27].

Actigraphy simply measures the motor activity of a limb, thus showing potential discrepancies when compared with objective sleep recording (by PSG) or subjective perception (by sleep logs or questionnaires). In more detail, actigraphy shows a strong reliability in distinguishing consolidated periods of sleep from wakefulness [28], but generally underestimates sleep latency for the typical immobility at the transition between wakefulness and sleep [29,30], and also suffers from a systematic tendency to underestimate short periods of wakefulness within nocturnal sleep. Actigraphy thus overestimates sleep time and efficiency [31]. Accordingly, actigraphic measurements of sleep and wakefulness are less accurate when sleep becomes more fragmented during nighttime, as well as when individuals spend prolonged motionless periods during daytime. Finally, the reliability of the sleep estimates increases in parallel with the number of recorded days, with seven nyctohemeral cycles being considered the minimal acceptable recording time [32].

Applications in the assessment of sleep and sleep disorders

Over the last decades the technical evolution of actigraphy devices has led to a progressive increase in its use for research and clinical purposes in both normal subjects and patients with sleep disorders (Fig. 9.1). Accordingly, each subsequent systematic literature review promoted by the American Academy of Sleep Medicine produced guidelines that continuously expanded the potential applications of actigraphy from a research tool for the study of sleep, which is reliable in normal subjects [33], to an objective monitoring technique increasingly useful for clinical diagnosis and management of several sleep disorders [34,35]. The latest guidelines stated that actigraphy should be used in the following circumstances with different levels of recommendation (namely, standard, guideline, and option) [35]: (1) to determine sleep patterns in healthy adults (standard), as well as to monitor sleep time and treatment response in insomnia patients (guideline option) [36]; (2) to evaluate patients with circadian sleep disorders, especially advanced and delayed sleep phase syndromes, shift work disorder (guideline) [37,38], as well as jet lag and non-24-hour sleep–wake syndrome (option) ([39,40]; (3) to estimate total sleep time in the absence of PSG in obstructive sleep apnea syndrome, also in association with cardiorespiratory monitoring, to improve the accuracy of respiratory indices when normalized for sleep time instead of time in bed (standard) [41]; (4) to characterize the circadian rhythms in patients with insomnia complaints [42], also when associated with mood disorders (option) [43]; (5) to determine the circadian patterns and estimate

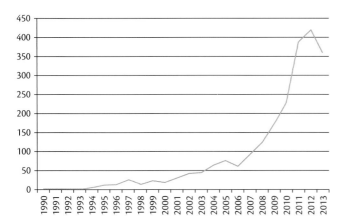

Fig. 9.1 Number of scientific publications per year retrieved by PubMed using the search term "actigraphy."

daily sleep time in patients with hypersomnolence complaint (option) [44]; (6) to assess, together with sleep logs, sleep–wake schedules for at least seven days before the execution of the MSLT, in order to better interpret its results (option) [1,7]; (7) to assess treatment response (guideline) in patients with circadian rhythm sleep disorders [45] and in insomniacs [46]; (8) to characterize sleep, circadian rhythm patterns, and treatment outcome in older adults (guideline) either living in the community [47]) or chronically hospitalized [48], the former in association with other measures and the latter being typically difficult to be studied by means of PSG; and (9) to delineate sleep patterns and treatment responses in normal infants, children, and special pediatric populations (guideline) [49].

In line with the above recommendations, actigraphy is listed within the available techniques to measure sleep duration and sleep patterns in the diagnostic criteria for several specific sleep disorders in the International Classification of Sleep Disorders, third edition [1]. Actigraphy (or sleep logs) is indeed primarily recommended when sleep patterns must be assessed over time, making PSG impractical, in the diagnostic approach to all circadian rhythm sleep disorders except the jet lag syndrome, in order to document the abnormal timing of the habitual sleep pattern. Similarly, actigraphy can be useful in patients with suspected paradoxical insomnia (a subtype of chronic insomnia), for the need to objectively document the mismatch between subjectively perceived and objectively documented nocturnal sleep time. Regarding central disorders of hypersomnolence, actigraphy is considered a useful tool before the execution of the MSLT in association with sleep logs, given the recommended stabilization of the habitual sleep pattern for one or two weeks before the test [7], and it is also deemed to aid in documenting a habitual nocturnal sleep shorter than expected from age-adjusted normative data in insufficient sleep syndrome.

Finally, several studies have also tested the reliability of actigraphy for the assessment of periodic leg movements during sleep (PLMs); however, its use has not yet reached a level of evidence adequate for the inclusion in the current guidelines [35]. To detect PLMs, actigraphy should be placed in the legs and used in a high-resolution mode (i.e, with shorter epochs, such as 5 seconds). When compared with the electromyographic assessment in the PSG setting, different actigraphs provide well-correlated measures of PLMs, which, however, show a systematic bias of over- or under-estimation depending on the specific device used [50]. Bilateral assessment of PLMs by means of actigraphy may provide a convenient alternative to PSG for epidemiological studies (51).

Conclusion

The MSLT, the MWT, and actigraphy are objective techniques complementary to clinical evaluation, PSG, and subjective reports. They provide quantitative measures of sleep propensity, alertness, and circadian patterns of motor activity, with specific clinical applications in the field of sleep medicine. Also, the application of these techniques for research purposes has proved capable of gathering items of evidence that are mirrored by their extended utilization in clinical practice.

Among recent research findings, it seems worth mentioning that other measures apart from MSLT sleep latencies have led to promising results for the characterization of the sleep onset period in the differential diagnosis of central disorders of hypersomnolence. For example, the order of sleep stages at sleep onset (sleep stage sequence analysis) disclosed that SOREMPs in patients with narcolepsy are more frequently preceded by non-REM sleep stage 1, whereas other forms of hypersomnia, such as insufficient sleep syndrome, reached also non-REM sleep stage two [52,53]. On the other hand, the wake-to-sleep transition has been shown to be longer in patients with idiopathic hypersomnia than in patients with narcolepsy, as measured by the combined application of two different sleep onset definitions (i.e, single epoch of sleep stage one versus sustained sleep) [54]. This sleep onset profile is similar to that of patients with obstructive sleep apnea syndrome [55]. To date, this additional information, and the potential utility of documenting the features of daytime sleepiness in settings closer to daily life by means of data obtained from continuous PSG monitoring across 24 hours [56] or by analyzing the circadian rhythm of motor activity and immobility [57], have been tested only in selected populations of sleep disorder patients. These data thus require further validation before being applicable to the clinical practice of sleep medicine. Future studies using techniques different from PSG are expected to provide specific evidence to refine the current objective measures for differential diagnosis of sleep disorders and predicting sleepiness-related risks.

References

1. American Academy of Sleep Medicine. International classification of sleep disorders, 3rd ed. Darien, IL: American Academy of Sleep Medicine, 2014.
2. Lal SK, Craig A. A critical review of the psychophysiology of driver fatigue. Biol Psychol 2001;55:173–94.
3. Hoddes E, Zarcone V, Smythe H, et al. Quantification of sleepiness: a new approach. Psychophysiology 1973;10:431–6.
4. Akerstedt T, Gillberg M. Subjective and objective sleepiness in the active individual. Int J Neurosci 1990;5:29–37.
5. Johns MW. A new method for measuring daytime sleepiness: the Epworth sleepiness scale. Sleep 1991;14:540–5.
6. Monk TH. A Visual Analogue Scale technique to measure global vigor and affect. Psychiatry Res 1989;27:89–99.
7. Littner MR, Kushida C, Wise M, et al. Standards of Practice Committee of the American Academy of Sleep Medicine. Practice parameters for clinical use of the multiple sleep latency test and the maintenance of wakefulness test. Sleep 2005;28:113–21.
8. Carskadon MA, Dement WC, Mitler MM, et al. Guidelines for the multiple sleep latency test (MSLT): a standard measure of sleepiness. Sleep 1986;9:519–24.
9. Arand D, Bonnet M, Hurwitz T, et al. The clinical use of the MSLT and MWT. Sleep 2005;28:123–44.
10. Iber C, Ancoli-Israel S, Chesson A, Quan S. The AASM manual for the scoring of sleep and associated events: rules, terminology and technical

specifications, 1st ed. Westchester, Illinois: American Academy of Sleep Medicine, 2007.

11. Mitler MM, Gujavarty KS, Sampson MG, Browman CP. Multiple daytime nap approaches to evaluating the sleepy patient. Sleep 1982;5 Suppl 2:S119–27.

12. Doghramji K, Mitler M, Sangal RB, et al. A normative study of the maintenance of wakefulness test (MWT). Electroencephal Clin Neurophysiol 1997;103:554–62.

13. Sangal RB, Thomas L, Mitler MM. Maintenance of wakefulness test and multiple sleep latency test. Measurement of different abilities in patients with sleep disorders. Chest 1992;101:898–902.

14. Bonnet MH, Arand DL. Impact of motivation on multiple sleep latency test and maintenance of wakefulness test measurements. J Clin Sleep Med 2005;1:386–90.

15. Pizza F, Contardi S, Mondini S, et al. Daytime sleepiness and driving performance in patients with obstructive sleep apnea: comparison of the MSLT, the MWT, and a simulated driving task. Sleep 2009;32:382–91.

16. Harrison Y, Horne JA. "High sleepability without sleepiness." The ability to fall asleep rapidly without other signs of sleepiness. Neurophysiol Clin 1996;26:15–20.

17. Kupfer DJ, Weiss BL, Foster G, et al. Psychomotor activity in affective states. Arch Gen Psychiatry 1974;30:765–8.

18. Colburn TR, Smith BM, Guarini JJ, Simmons NN. An ambulatory activity monitor with solid state memory. Biomed Sci Instrum 1976;12:117–22.

19. Kripke DF, Mullaney DJ, Messin S, Wyborney VG. Wrist actigraphic measures of sleep and rhythms. Electroencephalogr Clin Neurophysiol 1978;44:674–6.

20. Ancoli-Israel S, Cole R, Alessi C, et al. The role of actigraphy in the study of sleep and circadian rhythms. Sleep 2003;26:342–92.

21. Cole RJ, Kripke DF, Gruen W, et al. Automatic sleep/wake identification from wrist activity. Sleep 1992;15:461–69.

22. Sadeh A, Sharkey KM, Carskadon MA. Activity-based sleep–wake identification: An empirical test of methodological issues. Sleep 1994; 17:201–207.

23. Brown AC, Smolensky MH, D'Alonzo GE, Redman DP. Actigraphy: a means of assessing circadian patterns in human activity. Chronobiol Int 1990;7:125–33.

24. Youngstedt SD, Kripke DF, Elliott JA, Klauber MR. Circadian abnormalities in older adults. J Pineal Res 2001; 31:264–72.

25. Martin J, Marler M, Shochat T, Ancoli-Israel S. Circadian rhythms of agitation in institutionalized patients with Alzheimer's disease. Chronobiol Int 2000;17:405–18.

26. Dowse HB, Ringo JM. The search for hidden periodicities in biological time series revisited. J Theor Biol 1989;139:487–515.

27. Van Someren E, Swaab DF, Colenda CC, et al. Bright light therapy: improved sensitivity to its effects on rest–activity rhythms in Alzheimer's patients by application of nonparametric methods. Chronobiol Int 1999; 16:505–18.

28. Kushida CA, Chang A, Gadkary C, et al. Comparison of actigraphic, polysomnographic, and subjective assessment of sleep parameters in sleep-disordered patients. Sleep Med 2001;2:389–96.

29. Blood ML, Sack RL, Percy DC, Pen JC. A comparison of sleep detection by wrist actigraphy, behavioral response, and polysomnography. Sleep 1997;20:388–95.

30. Lichstein KL, Stone KC, Donaldson J, et al. Actigraphy validation with insomnia. Sleep 2006;29:232–9.

31. Pollak CP, Tryon WW, Nagaraja H, Dzwonczyk R. How accurately does wrist actigraphy identify the states of sleep and wakefulness? Sleep 2001;24:957–65.

32 Van Someren EJ. Improving actigraphic sleep estimates in insomnia and dementia: how many nights? J Sleep Res 2007;16:269–75.

33. American Sleep Disorders Association. Practice parameters for the use of actigraphy in the clinical assessment of sleep disorders. Sleep 1995;18:285–7.

34. Littner M, Kushida CA, Anderson WM, et al; Standards of Practice Committee of the American Academy of Sleep Medicine. Practice

35. Morgenthaler T, Alessi C, Friedman L, et al. Standards of Practice Committee; American Academy of Sleep Medicine. Practice parameters for the use of actigraphy in the assessment of sleep and sleep disorders: an update for 2007. Sleep 2007;30:519–29.

36. Vallières A, Morin CM. Actigraphy in the assessment of insomnia. Sleep 2003;26:902–6.

37. Ando K, Kripke DF, Ancoli-Israel S. Delayed and advanced sleep phase symptoms. Isr J Psychiatry Relat Sci 2002;39:11–18.

38. Borges FN, Fischer FM. Twelve-hour night shifts of healthcare workers: a risk to the patients? Chronobiol Int 2003;20:351–60.

39. Carvalho Bos S, Waterhouse J, Edwards B, et al. The use of actimetry to assess changes to the rest–activity cycle. Chronobiol Int 2003;20:1039–59.

40. Uchiyama M, Shibui K, Hayakawa T, et al. Larger phase angle between sleep propensity and melatonin rhythms in sighted humans with non 24-hour sleep–wake syndrome. Sleep 2002;25:83–8.

41. Elbaz M, Roue GM, Lofaso F, Quera Salva MA. Utility of actigraphy in the diagnosis of obstructive sleep apnea. Sleep 2002;25:527–31.

42. Natale V, Plazzi G, Martoni M. Actigraphy in the assessment of insomnia: a quantitative approach. Sleep 2009;32:767–71.

43. Harvey AG, Schmidt DA, Scarnà A, et al. Sleep-related functioning in euthymic patients with bipolar disorder, patients with insomnia, and subjects without sleep problems. Am J Psychiatry 2005;162:50–7.

44. Bassetti C, Gugger M, Bischof M, et al The narcoleptic borderland: a multimodal diagnostic approach including cerebrospinal fluid levels of hypocretin-1 (orexin A). Sleep Med 2003;4:7–12.

45. Beaumont M, Batéjat D, Piérard C, et al. Caffeine or melatonin effects on sleep and sleepiness after rapid eastward transmeridian travel. J Appl Physiol 2004;96:50–8.

46. Wilson SJ, Rich AS, Rich NC, et al. Evaluation of actigraphy and automated telephoned questionnaires to assess hypnotic effects in in-somnia. Int Clin Psychopharmacol 2004;19:77–84.

47. Ceolim MF, Menna-Barreto L. Sleep/wake cycle and physical activity in healthy elderly people. Sleep Res Online 2000;3:87–95.

48. Harper DG, Stopa EG, McKee AC, et al. Differential circadian rhythm disturbances in men with Alzheimer disease and frontotemporal de-generation. Arch Gen Psychiatry 2001;58:353–60.

49. Gnidovec B, Neubauer D, Zidar J. Actigraphic assessment of sleep–wake rhythm during the first 6 months of life. Clin Neurophysiol 2002;113:1815–21.

50. Gschliesser V, Frauscher B, Brandauer E, et al. PLM detection by actigraphy compared to polysomnography: a validation and comparison of two actigraphs. Sleep 2009;10:306–11.

51. King MA, Jaffre MO, Morrish E, et al. The validation of a new actigraphy system for the measurement of periodic leg movements in sleep. Sleep Med 2005;6:507–13.

52. Marti I, Valko PO, Khatami R, et al. Multiple sleep latency measures in narcolepsy and behaviourally induced insufficient sleep syndrome. Sleep Med 2009;10:1146–50.

53. Drakatos P, Suri A, Higgins SE, et al. Sleep stage sequence analysis of sleep onset REM periods in the hypersomnias. J Neurol Neurosurg Psychiatry 2013;84:223–7.

54. Pizza F, Vandi S, Detto S, et al. Different sleep onset criteria at the multiple sleep latency test (MSLT): an additional marker to differentiate central nervous system (CNS) hypersomnias. J Sleep Res 2011;20:250–6.

55. Fabbri M, Pizza F, Magosso E, et al. Automatic slow eye movement (SEM) detection of sleep onset in patients with obstructive sleep apnea syndrome (OSAS): comparison between multiple sleep latency test (MSLT) and maintenance of wakefulness test (MWT). Sleep Med 2010;11:253–7.

56. Pizza F, Moghadam KK, Vandi S, et al. Daytime continuous polysomnography predicts MSLT results in hypersomnias of central origin. J Sleep Res 2013;22:32–40.

57. Filardi M, Pizza F, Martoni M, et al. Actigraphic assessment of sleep/wake behavior in central disorders of hypersomnolence. Sleep Med 2015;16:126–30.

CHAPTER 10

Scoring guidelines for sleep-related movements

Michela Figorilli, Monica Puligheddu, and Raffaele Ferri

Leg movement activity during sleep

Sleep-related movement disorders are characterized by usually stereotyped and simple movements, disturbing sleep or its onset [1]. Movements involving the lower limbs are most frequently studied. Leg movement activity during sleep has been analyzed by recording of the surface electromyographic (EMG) activity of the tibialis anterior muscles. Recently, actigraphy has been proposed as an alternative diagnostic tool [2] in specific situations. The following sections describe several lower limb activities recorded during sleep.

Periodic limb movements

Periodic limb movements (PLM) are repetitive and somewhat stereotyped movements occurring in sleep (PLMS) or wakefulness (PLMW). PLM involve most frequently the lower extremities, and are manifested by an extension of the big toe, often in combination with partial flexion of the ankle, the knee, and sometimes the hip [1]. Lugaresi et al. [3] described for the first time in 1965 the features of PLM in patients suffering from restless legs syndrome/Willis–Ekbom disease (RLS/WED), characterizing their presence during both wakefulness and sleep. Originally, the quantification of PLM was based on the EMG recording of the tibialis anterior muscles [3]. In 1980, Coleman [4] laid the foundations for the scoring criteria of PLM, describing them in terms of duration, amplitude, and periodicity. Later, the criteria proposed by Coleman [4] were accepted by the American Sleep Disorders Association [5] and used for more than 20 years. Currently, rules for scoring PLM have been suggested based on algorithms for the automatic detection of leg movements during polysomnography (PSG), including analysis of several parameters, such as thresholds, intervals, amplitude, and periodicity [6–8]. The scoring guidelines for PLM were proposed first by a task force of the International Restless Leg Syndrome Study Group (IRLSSG)/World Association of Sleep Medicine (WASM) [9] and then incorporated by the American Academy of Sleep Medicine (AASM) [10] in its guidelines. Separate clinical and research criteria were initially described. The first step in the scoring of PLM should be a calibration of the EMG channel with relaxed anterior tibialis muscles, in order to obtain a non-rectified signal lower than ±5 μV (or 10 μV peak-to-peak) in clinical practice and ±3 μV (or 6 μV peak-to-peak) for research purposes. PLM are identified on the EMG signal, obtained from the anterior tibialis muscles, showing repetitive contractions characterized by the following features: the onset of each limb movement event is defined by an increase of the EMG signal ≥8 μV above resting baseline, and the end of each event is identified by a decrease to ≤2 μV above the resting EMG signal, lasting for at least 0.5 s. This duration cutoff has been introduced because an event may have one or more periods where the EMG signal drops below the offset criteria for less than 0.5 s. The duration of a limb movement is from to 0.5 to 10 s (15 s for research purposes). Leg movements are considered bilateral but counted as one event when these occur simultaneously or are separated from each other (offset-to-onset) by less than 0.5 s. An arousal and leg movement should be considered to be associated when there is <0.5 s interval between the end of one event and the onset of the other event, regardless of which is first. A leg movement should not be computed as a PLM if it occurs at the termination of an apnea or hypopnea, or the offset of the earlier event precedes the onset of the other by less than to 0.5 s. The interval between each event is measured from onset to onset, and the interval between two consecutive periodic events has to be from 5 to 90 s. A PLM sequence is represented by a series of at least four leg movements separated from each other by an interval lasting from 5 to 90 s. PLM can occur both during sleep and during wakefulness, particularly during any stage of sleep, and a single sequence may continue across changes in sleep–wake state. The basic analysis of PLM activity should always include the PLM index (number of PLM divided by number of hours of sleep), PLMS with arousal index (number of PLMS associated with arousals divided by number of hours of sleep), and PLMW index (number of PLMW divided by number of hours of wake). Moreover, it is recommended to differentiate the PLMS index during NREM sleep and that during REM sleep; the duration of PLMS (total, NREM, and REM) and that of PLMW; and the inter-movement interval of PLMS (total, NREM, and REM) and that of PLMW. Optionally, PLMS could be reported by sleep stages and isolated leg movements.

Time structure and periodicity of limb movements during sleep

Non-periodic leg movements, during sleep or wakefulness, are present in patients suffering from RLS/WED, PLMD, or other conditions, as well as in normal controls [8,11]. Moreover, PLMS are usually combined with cortical and autonomic changes, which can be present also in non-periodic leg movements [12–14]. Therefore, the standard scoring features seem to be inadequate to better discriminate PLMS from non-periodic leg movements [15]. Three additional indices are useful: the total LM index, the periodicity index (PI), and the time distribution of PLM throughout the night, not counting PLMS related to respiratory events [15]. The first

---

Box 10.1 Limb movements

- Onset: increase of electromyographic (EMG) signal ≥8 μV above resting baseline

- Offset: decrease of EMG signal ≤2 μV above resting baseline (lasting at least 0.5 s)

- Duration: 0.5–10 s

- Bilateral limb movements to be considered as single event if overlapping or the interval between movements (offset-to-onset) is <0.5 s

- Limb movements and arousal are associated when the interval from offset to onset is <0.5 s

---

indicates the total amount of limb movement activity recorded. The PI represents the degree of periodicity, that is the ratio of the inter-movement interval lasting from 10 to 90 s (at least three consecutive intervals) divided by the total number of intervals [8,15]. This index can vary from 0, representing the absence of periodicity with none of the intervals having a length between 10 and 90 s, to 1, representing complete periodicity, with all intervals lasting from 10 to 90 s and included in sequences of consecutive intervals all within this range. The third essential feature of PLMS is the nighttime hourly distribution, showing in the majority of RLS patients a decrease of PLM from sleep onset to the morning awakening [15,16].

These three main parameters show clear age-related changes, with particular features in children and in the elderly [13,17]. The elderly population shows a high degree of periodicity, and high total numbers of PLM, compared with children. Thus, normative values should be specific for different age groups [18].

These three parameters (total LM index, PI, and time structure) help to distinguish "true" PLM, typical of RLS, from other clinical conditions associated with PLMS, such as narcolepsy [16] and REM sleep behavior disorder (RBD) [19,20]. Finally, based on the evidence accumulated in the last decade, very recently, a joint task force of the International and European Restless Legs Syndrome Study Groups and World Association of Sleep Medicine revised and updated the prior standards [9] for recording and scoring leg

---

Box 10.2 Periodic limb movements (PLM)

- PLM sequences are identified by at least four limb movements

- Interval between two consecutive PLM (onset-to-onset) is 90 s

- Periodic limb movements in sleep (PLMS) index: number of PLMS divided by number of hours of sleep

- Total LM index

- PLMS with arousal index: number of PLMS associated with arousal divided by number of hours of sleep

- Periodic limb movements in wakefulness (PLMW) index: number of PLMW divided by number of hours of wake

- Periodicity index: ratio of consecutive inter-movement intervals, all separated by 10–90 s (at least three intervals) divided by total number of movements

- Time distribution of PLMS throughout the night

---

movements in polysomnographic recordings, published in 2006. Each new standard rule has been classified with a level of evidence [21]. The rules to detected leg movements have been substantially confirmed and only a new criterion for the morphology of leg movements, that applies only to computerized leg movement detection to better match expert visual detection, has been added. There have been two main changes introduced by these new rules: 1) Candidate leg movements (CLM), are any monolateral leg movement 0.5–10 s long or bilateral leg movements 0.5–15 s long; 2) PLM are now defined by runs of at least 4 consecutive CLM with an intermovement interval ≥10 and ≤90 s without any CLM preceded by an interval <10 s, interrupting the PLM series. There are also new options defining leg movements associated with respiratory events; the scorer can choose one of two different options: the first is essentially the same as in the previous standards [9] (leg movements overlapping within ±0.5 s the end of a respiratory event) while the second, more inclusive, is based on recent empirical data indicating that leg movements might be considered to be associated with a respiratory event when any part of the leg movement is between 2.0 s before and 10.25 s after the end of respiratory events [22]. PLMS should first be quantified by ignoring all possible associations including respiratory events and then determined after removing all leg movements associated with respiratory events. Reports and publications should explicitly state which of these rules are used. Finally, special considerations for pediatric studies have been included. With these new rules, the expert visual scoring of leg movements has only been altered by the new standards to require accepting all leg movements >0.5 s regardless of their duration, otherwise the technician scores the leg movements as for the old standards.

Box 10.1 summarizes the features of CLM. Box 10.2 reports the basic rules defining PLM.

Actigraphy

Actigraphy has been used to examine the sleep–wake rhythm and movements during sleep, especially using the shorter-term monitoring of rest–activity rhythm combined with PLM measurements [23,24]. However, actigraphy has several limitations, including an inability to distinguish wakefulness and sleep from each other because of the lack of EEG recording. Also, without a channel recording body position, PLM cannot be identified correctly. Therefore, PLM may be both under- and over-estimated using actigraphy. Some validation studies for actigraphy have been conducted [24–26], but only small samples of PSG results have been compared with actigraphy [24]. The filter settings of some actigraphic systems have a substantial impact on the PLM index [25]; thus, it would be important to choose a model of actigraphy that allows modification of its settings, such as duration of movement. Actigraphy essentially uses an accelerometer to measure mechanically generated movements. This can be worn on the big toe, the dorsum of the foot, or the ankle [27]. Conversely, in standard PSG, PLM are evaluated as EMG activity of the tibialis anterior muscle, not necessarily leading to any visible movement. Actigraphy may overestimate PLM because it can produce an output also in the case of passive movements. Nevertheless, actigraphy is more convenient and cheaper than standard PSG [2], and it can be carried out easily even in some populations, such as demented patients, dependent or frail seniors, and children, who are otherwise difficult to monitor. Further research studies are needed to find a more convenient and reliable tool to monitor movements during sleep, such as PLM.

Table 10.1 PSG features of alternating leg muscle activation (ALMA), hypnagogic foot tremor (HFT), and high-frequency leg movement (HFLM)

	Frequency (Hz)	Length of single event (ms)	Number of events in one series	Sleep stages	Burst series duration (s)
ALMA	0.5–3	100–500	4	Arousal, NREM, REM	20–30
HFT	0.3–4	250–1000	4	Transition wake/sleep, NREM stage N1 and N2	10–15
HFLM	0.3–4	100–700	4	Wakefulness, NREM, REM	15–30

Other leg motor activities during sleep

This section illustrates three sleep-related motor phenomena, which are very similar to each other, represented by small motor activations of lower limbs, short-lasting bilateral alternating or unilateral activations (agonist/antagonist), occurring during sleep or wakefulness, often associated with arousals, usually in trains. These movements can be so small that they can be seen only when filming without any covering, such as a blanket, on the legs.

Alternating leg muscle activation

Alternating leg muscle activation (ALMA) consists of brief alternating activation of the anterior tibialis muscles during sleep or arousal from sleep [1]. The frequency of the alternating EMG bursts is from 0.5 to 3.0 Hz, usually lasting for 100–500 ms; the minimum number of discrete and alternating bursts of leg muscle activity needed to score an ALMA series is four [28] and a sequence of ALMAs lasts up to 20–30 s. This motor activity can arise from all sleep stages, but especially during arousals [28,29]. ALMA may represent a benign phenomenon without clinical impact, but it is not clear if it represents one of the nocturnal motor activities related to RLS/WED.

Hypnagogic foot tremor

Hypnagogic foot tremor (HFT) is represented by a rhythmic movement of the feet or toes occurring at the transition between wake and sleep or during NREM sleep stage N1 and/or N [23]. This phenomenon is characterized by at least four recurrent EMG bursts, at 1–2 Hz (range 0.5–4 Hz) in one or both feet, lasting 250–1000 ms and with a duration of one train at least of 10 s [10].

High-frequency leg movements

High-frequency leg movements (HFLM) are identified as at least four leg movements occurring with a frequency of 0.3–4 Hz, mostly unilateral, rather than bilateral [30]. HFLM can occur in all sleep stages and also, frequently, during wakefulness [1]. The sequences of HFLM are in general longer than those of ALMA [1]. However, scoring criteria are not yet available, and further studies are needed to establish any possible relationship with RLS and their clinical relevance.

Do ALMA, HFT, and HFLM constitute a continuum?

The three sleep-related leg activities that have been mentioned may represent different manifestations of the same phenomenon along a spectrum, since they have many common features.

Furthermore, their clinical impact and their association with RLS/WED are not clear. Further studies are needed to better outline differences and similarities among these phenomena, and whether it would be possible to group them together in one entity. They might be gathered together as HFLM [30], because this seems a more descriptive and neutral term. Table 10.1 synthesizes the characteristics of the three sleep-related leg activities.

Excessive fragmentary myoclonus

Excessive fragmentary myoclonus (EFM) is characterized by brief, even invisible, muscle twitches that occur asynchronously, symmetrically, and bilaterally [31,32]. These movements involve distal muscles, like fingers, toes, and corners of the mouth, and occur at the sleep–wake transition or during sleep. The EMG activities typical of EFM can be recurrent and persistent, lasting from 75 to 150 ms, without any clear clustering. A sequence of EFM is defined by at least five potentials per minute for at least 20 minutes of stage N2 or N3 [32]. Another parameter to quantify EFM is the myoclonus index [33], identified as the number of 3 s mini-epochs containing at least one fragmentary myoclonus potential, included within each 30 s epoch; the myoclonus index can vary between 0 and 10. EFM is more common in males and increases with age. It should be mentioned that EFM can be found in patients suffering from other sleep disorders, including sleep-related breathing disorders [1]. Box 10.3 shows the main features of EFM. The definition of EFM will probably be revised in the near future [34].

Propriospinal myoclonus at sleep onset

Propriospinal myoclonus (PMS) at sleep onset is a rare motor disorder, characterized by generalized and symmetric jerks, arising first in spinal axial muscles of the trunk, neck, or abdomen and then propagating at low velocity to more rostral and caudal muscles, by means of slow propriospinal polysynaptic pathways [1,35–37]. PMS occurs during relaxed wakefulness or drowsiness, with diffuse EEG alpha activity, and is typically inhibited by mental activation and sleep onset [1]. For these reasons, it can cause insomnia [38], because the jerks appear several times during relaxed wakefulness or drowsiness and the patient cannot achieve stable sleep. PSM may resemble PLMW, longer and less periodic than PLMS; however, generally during PSM, there is no urge to move or other

---

Box 10.3 Excessive fragmentary myoclonus (EFM)

- Burst duration: 75–150 ms
- Sequence of EFM: at least 5 bursts per minute
- Minimum duration of a sequence: 20 minutes
- Occurrence during NREM stage N2 or N3
- Myoclonus index: number of 3 s mini-epochs containing at least one fragmentary myoclonus potential, included within each 30 s epoch

---

Box 10.4 Propriospinal myoclonus at sleep onset (PMS)

- Generalized and symmetric jerks, arising first in spinal axial muscles of trunk, neck, or abdomen and then propagating slowly to more rostral and caudal muscles
- Occurrence during relaxed wakefulness or during drowsiness
- Inhibited by mental activation and sleep onset

Box 10.5 Sleep bruxism (SB)

- Phasic or tonic increase of chin electromyographic (EMG) signal, at least twice the amplitude of the background EMG activity
- Tonic augmentation of the chin EMG signal lasting more than 2 s
- Phasic increases of chin EMG signal are also known as rhythmic masticatory muscle activity (RMMA)
- RMMA include at least three consecutive contractions, with a frequency of 1 Hz
- Burst duration: 0.25–2 s
- Interval between each episode of SB: 3 s of stable background chin EMG signal
- Polysomnographic (PSG) diagnosis: at least four episodes of SB per hour of sleep, or at least 25 individual masticatory muscle bursts per hour of sleep associated with at least two audible episodes of tooth-grinding

---

symptoms commonly seen during PLMW and RLS/WED. There are no available quantitative PSG scoring criteria for PSM, and all the descriptions are mainly qualitative [10]. The main features of PSM are summarized in Box 10.4.

Neck myoclonus during sleep

Neck myoclonus during sleep, or head jerks, is a short "stripe-shaped" movement-induced artifact visible vertically over the EEG channels during REM sleep [39]. Frauscher et al. found this phenomenon in more than 50% of their patients, suffering from various sleep disorders, during routine PSG, with low frequency during the night (1.0 ± 2.8 episodes per hour of REM sleep), slightly more prevalent in patients with RBD, and showing an inverse relation with age, being more frequent in younger patients [39]. However, further studies are needed to define a pathological cut-off for this phenomenon, its prevalence in normal controls, and its relationship with RBD [39]. Another similar phenomenon is facio-mandibular myoclonus during REM sleep, which is more frequent in the elderly, and is characterized by episodes of one to three contractions leading to awakenings, following biting of the tongue and forceful jaw closings [40].

Sleep bruxism

Sleep bruxism (SB) is identified as a repetitive jaw muscle activity characterized by clenching or grinding of the teeth or by bracing or thrusting of the mandible, generally associated with arousal from sleep [1]. According to the International Classification of Sleep Disorders, Third Edition (ICSD-3), the diagnosis of SB is based on clinical features, such as reports of tooth grinding sounds during sleep, the presence of abnormal tooth wear, complaints of morning jaw muscle pain or fatigue, temporal headache, or jaw locking upon awakening [1]. PSG is indicated when the clinician suspects another sleep disorder, such as obstructive sleep apnea or RBD, epilepsy, or other orofacial–mandibular disorders. In PSG, SB is represented by EMG artifacts recorded by the surface EEG channels, especially if the reference is the ear or mastoid. The scoring manual of the AASM recommends placement of chin EMG electrodes for scoring SB; however, additional masseter or temporal electrodes should be included at the discretion of the investigator or the clinician [10]. An episode of SB is identified by phasic and/or tonic elevations of chin EMG activity, at least twice the amplitude of the background EMG [10]. To be scored as SB, sustained contractions have to last more than 2 s. Phasic augmentations of chin EMG activity, known as rhythmic masticatory muscle activity (RMMA), are scored as SB if they are composed by at least three contractions, with a frequency of 1 Hz and a duration from 0.25 to 2 s. Bursts of chin EMG activity shorter than 0.25 s are scored as myoclonus, and are observed in about 10% of SB cases. RMMA may occur also in

normal subjects [41], without any clinical implication. A new episode of SB is scored if there is a preceding interval of at least 3 s of stable background chin EMG signal [10]. According to the AASM Manual, SB can be scored by a combination of audio and PSG, with a minimum of two audible tooth grinding episodes per night in the absence of epilepsy [10]. PSG diagnosis of SB needs the presence of at least four episodes of SB per hour of sleep, or at least 25 individual masticatory muscle bursts per hour of sleep, associated with at least two audible episodes of tooth grinding [1,10]. Box 10.5 shows the PSG features of SB.

Rhythmic movement disorder

Sleep-related rhythmic movement disorder (RMD) is identified by repetitive, stereotyped, and rhythmic motor behavior that occurs mainly during drowsiness or sleep and may involve large muscle groups, such as those of the head, neck, trunk, or limbs [1]. RMD is differentiated from developmentally normal sleep-related movements when it leads to significant clinical consequences, such as interference with sleep, important impairment of daytime performance, or injuries caused by the behavior [1]. Episodes may last seconds or minutes, and may be present also during wakefulness preceding sleep or after sleep onset, with duration and features similar to the episodes arising from sleep. Most episodes of RMD occur during NREM sleep, stages N1 and N2, rarely SWS or REM sleep. Sometimes episodes have been associated with the cyclic alternating pattern [42,43] and respiratory arousal. There is a single case report indicating an epileptic etiology for RMD [44]. The suggested criteria for scoring RMD include (a) frequency ranging from 0.5 to 2 Hz, (b) presence of at least four rhythmic movements, and (c) an amplitude of EMG bursts at least two times the EMG background activity. A video-PSG is required to reach a correct diagnosis. Typically, RMD is seen in infants and children, but also in adults. The pattern of motor behavior may involve the head (headbanging or headrolling), but also the body (body rocking) or occasionally the legs (leg rolling or leg banging) [1,42]. The clinical diagnosis of RMD is based on the history and, if they are

---

Box 10.6 Rhythmic movement disorder (RMD)

◆ Occurrence mainly during drowsiness or sleep, or after sleep onset (mostly during stage N1 or N2)

◆ RMD may interfere with sleep, cause important impairment of daytime performance, or lead to injuries

◆ Episode duration variable: seconds or minutes

◆ Frequency: 0.5–2 Hz

◆ Series of RMD: at least four rhythmic movements

◆ Amplitude of electromyographic (EMG) burst at least twice the EMG background

◆ Video-polysomnography (video-PSG) is required to reach a correct diagnosis, especially in doubtful cases

---

available, home- and self-made video recordings. Video-PSG is useful in doubtful cases or to rule out other sleep disorders, such as PLMS, ALMA, or motor seizures. Box 10.6 includes the PSG features of RMD.

REM sleep behavior disorder

Visual scoring of REM sleep without atonia (RSWA)

According to the ICSD-3, video-PSG is mandatory to diagnose RBD as well for the demonstration of REM sleep without atonia (RSWA), as defined by the guidelines for scoring of RBD in the AASM Manual [1]. The latest ICSD-3 introduces for the first time a clear suggested cut-off value for RSWA as any (tonic/phasic) chin EMG activity combined with bilateral phasic activity of the flexor digitorum superficialis muscles in >27% of REM sleep, scored in 30 s epochs, based on the Sleep Innsbruck Barcelona (SINBAR) Group scoring method [1,45–47]. Several studies have proposed different methods to analyze and quantify EMG activity during REM sleep [47–51]. The most widely accepted scoring system was published by Lapierre and Montplaisir [48,49] and differentiates between tonic and phasic chin EMG activity, respectively assessed on 20 s sleep epochs, but also adapted to 30 s epochs and 2 s sleep mini-epochs. According to this method, a tonic REM epoch is defined by the presence of tonic chin EMG activity for >50% of the epoch, with an amplitude at least twice that of the background or greater than 10 μV; phasic chin EMG activity is identified by the presence of chin EMG bursts lasting 0.1–10 s, with an amplitude exceeding four times the background [49]. Lapierre and Montplaisir proposed a cut-off value ≥30% for the tonic chin EMG activity (correct classification of 81.9%) and ≥15% of 2 s mini-epochs containing phasic chin EMG activity (correct classification of 83.8%); when both cut-off values are satisfied, the correct classification is 85.6% [49]. The SINBAR Group has evaluated different muscle combinations with the highest rate of REM sleep phasic EMG activity in patients with RBD, finding the best combination in the simultaneous recording of the mentalis, flexor digitorum superficialis, and extensor digitorum brevis muscles [45]. More recently, the same group has published normative and cut-off values for EMG activity during REM sleep in 11 different body muscles, showing that adding the analysis of phasic EMG activity at the upper limb flexor digitorum superficialis muscles improves sensitivity and specificity for RBD diagnosis [46]. The SINBAR Group recommended the analysis of tonic and/or phasic EMG activity in the mentalis muscle

combined with bilateral phasic EMG activity in the flexor digitorum superficialis muscles, with a cut-off of 32% of 3 s mini-epochs (and 27% of 30 s epochs) [46]. Tonic chin EMG activity was scored similarly to the Lapierre and Montplaisir method. Phasic EMG activity is scored in 3 s mini-epochs as any burst of EMG activity lasting from 0.1 to 5 s with amplitude exceeding twice the background activity irrespective of its morphology [45]. The authors showed that these cut-off values provide reasonable sensitivity, specificity values, and correct classification of RBD [46,47].

Automatic scoring of RSWA in RBD

Recently, some authors have proposed some automatic scoring algorithms to quantify the amplitude of chin EMG activity [52–54]. According to these automatic algorithms, the REM sleep atonia index (RAI) can vary from 0 (complete absence of EMG atonia) to 1 (stable EMG atonia). Initially, the threshold of the RAI was chosen arbitrarily at 0.7, by Ferri and co-workers, because normal controls rarely have values of RAI lower than this threshold [53]. However, It should be kept in mind that normal controls may also have a RSWA without clinical RBD [55]. After a noise reduction, the threshold of the RAI was set at 0.8 (correct classification 82.6%), while values of RAI between 0.8 and 0.9 indicated a less evident (mild) alteration of atonia, and values above 0.9 are found in normal controls [56]. Furthermore, RAI was compared between patients with Parkinson disease (PD) with or without RBD, finding high sensitivity and specificity to detect the presence of RSWA and RBD in this population [57]. The REM sleep Atonia Index correlated considerably with the Lapierre and Montplaisir method to detect RSWA in RBD patients [58], with an agreement of 85% between the two methods. However, the RAI has been validated only in the submentalis muscle, and occasionally RBD patients may have normal REM atonia at the chin, while loss of atonia is observed in other muscle groups. Furthermore, this index has been assessed in normal young and elderly controls, idiopathic RBD patients, and subjects with multiple system atrophy, PD, obstructive sleep apnea syndrome, narcolepsy, and idiopathic hypersomnia [53,56,57]. These results suggest that RAI could be used as a valid support for the diagnosis of RBD—so far for the detection and quantification of RSWA. Table 10.2 summarizes visual and automatic scoring methods for RSWA.

Video scoring of RBD episodes

The analysis of video-recorded behaviors is crucial in the diagnosis of RBD [1]. Some studies have classified behaviors as simple or complex [59], and others have distinguished between different severity categories, like mild, moderate, and severe [60]. The severity has been based on the excursion amplitude of the limbs and volume of vocalization [60]. Also, Frauscher et al. have published an extended analysis of all movement and behaviors, from the smallest motor events and vocalization to the most complex and violent behaviors, including a detailed analysis about the relationship between abnormal behaviors and REM sleep microstructure [61,62]. The video scoring of RBD can be carried out in two ways: (a) a full analysis of the video in real time for all REM sleep epochs [61–64], which is time-consuming but necessary for research purposes, and (b) a selective screening of video and PSG recording epoch by epoch (30 s epoch), which is more useful in clinical practice [65]. The latter approach, the RBD Severity Scale (RBDSS) in particular, evaluates severity of motor behavior events during REM sleep on video-PSG recordings and grades them visually on an event-to-event basis.

Table 10.2 Scoring method for REM sleep without atonia

Muscle	Lapierre and Montplaisir	SINBAR	RAI
	Submental	Mental, FDS	Chin
EMG activity	*Tonic:* 50% tonic >2 × background amplitude (or >10 μV) *Phasic:* >4 × background amplitude 0.1–10 s	*Tonic:* 50% tonic >2 × background amplitude (or >10 μV) *Phasic:* >2 × background amplitude 0.1–5 s *Any:* >2 × background amplitude 0.1 sec	*Tonic:* ≥1 μV
Epoch duration	20/2 s mini-epochs	30/3 s mini-epochs	1 s
Cut-off and combination	Tonic: >30% Phasic: >15%	Phasic chin: 16.3% Any chin EMG (3 s): 18% Any chin EMG + phasic FDS EMG (3 s): 32% Any chin EMG + phasic FDS EMG (30 s): 27%	RAI < 0.8
Specificity	Tonic: 90% Phasic: 87.5% Both: 82.5%	Phasic chin: NP Any chin EMG (3 s): NP Any chin EMG + phasic FDS EMG (3 s): NP Any chin EMG + phasic FDS EMG (30 s): NP	81%
Sensitivity	Tonic: 73.8% Phasic: 80% Both: 88.9%	Phasic chin: NP Any chin EMG (3 s): NP Any chin EMG + phasic FDS EMG (3 s): NP Any chin EMG + phasic FDS EMG (30 s): NP	84%
Correct classification	Tonic: 81.9% Phasic: 83.8% Both: 85.6%	Phasic chin: AUC 0.981 Any chin EMG (3 s): AUC 0.990 Any chin EMG + phasic FDS EMG (3 s): AUC 0.998 Any chin EMG + phasic FDS EMG (30 s): AUC 0.999	82.6%

SINBAR: Sleep Innsbruck Barcelona Group; FDS: flexor digitorum superficialis; EMG: electromyography; RAI: REM sleep Atonia Index; NP: not provided; AUC: area under the curve.

According to this scale, the location of movements is categorized as follows: 0 = no visible movement; 1 = slight movements or jerks 2 = movements involving proximal extremities, including violent behavior; 3 = axial involvement, including bed falls. Vocalizations are rated as 1 for present or 0 for absent. The final RBDSS score is reported as a two-digit number, the first representing the location of the movement and the second the vocalizations; the two digits are separated by a full stop (eg, 3.1).

Conclusion

The current scoring guidelines comprise the analysis of several muscles characterized by different variables of their signal (eg, frequency and amplitude). Thus, it is crucial to identify and assess thresholds and measurements, which should be reliably set out with quantitative measurement of digitally stored signals. Moreover, automated scoring methods are available, at least for PLMS and RSWA, which are likely soon to meet the sensitivity and specificity requirements for use in clinical practice. The evaluation of more complex movements or behaviors should be done by visual analysis of synchronized video-PSG recordings. However, new automatic video analysis scoring methods are being tested, although these will need further refinement and validation before they can be considered for research and clinical applications.

References

1. International Classification of Sleep Disorders. American Academy of Sleep Medicine, 2014.
2. Cippà MAT, Baumann CR, Siccoli MM, et al. Actigraphic assessment of periodic leg movements in patients with restless legs syndrome. J Sleep Res 2013;22:589–92.
3. Lugaresi E, Coccagna G, Tassinari CA, Ambrosetto C. [Polygraphic data on motor phenomena in the restless legs syndrome.] Riv Neurol 1965;35:550–61.
4. Coleman RM, Pollak CP, Weitzman ED. Periodic movements in sleep (nocturnal myoclonus): relation to sleep disorders. Ann Neurol 1980;8:416–21.
5. The Atlas Task Force. Recording and scoring leg movements. Sleep 1993;16: 748–59.
6. Ferri R, Zucconi M, Manconi M, et al. Computer-assisted detection of nocturnal leg motor activity in patients with restless legs syndrome and periodic leg movements during sleep. Sleep 2005;28:998–1004.
7. Wetter TC, Dirlich G, Streit J, et al. An automatic method for scoring leg movements in polygraphic sleep recordings and its validity in comparison to visual scoring. Sleep 2004;27:324–8.

8. Ferri R, Zucconi M, Manconi M, et al. New approaches to the study of periodic leg movements during sleep in restless legs syndrome. Sleep 2006;29:759–69.

9. Zucconi M, Ferri R, Allen R, et al. The official World Association of Sleep Medicine (WASM) standards for recording and scoring periodic leg movements in sleep (PLMS) and wakefulness (PLMW) developed in collaboration with a task force from the International Restless Legs Syndrome Study Group (IRLSSG). Sleep Med 2006;7:175–83.

10. Iber C, Ancoli-Israel S, Chesson A, Quan S, for the American Academy of Sleep Medicine. The AASM manual for the scoring of sleep and associated events: rules, terminology and technical specifications. Westchester, IL: American Academy of Sleep Medicine, 2007.

11. Manconi M, Ferri R, Zucconi M, et al. First night efficacy of pramipexole in restless legs syndrome and periodic leg movements. Sleep Med 2007;8:491–7.

12. Ferri R, Zucconi M, Rundo F, et al. Heart rate and spectral EEG changes accompanying periodic and non-periodic leg movements during sleep. Clin Neurophysiol 2007;118:438–48.

13. Ferri R, Manconi M, Lanuzza B, et al. Age-related changes in periodic leg movements during sleep in patients with restless legs syndrome. Sleep Med 2008;9:790–8.

14. Winkelman JW, Shahar E, Sharief I, Gottlieb DJ. Association of restless legs syndrome and cardiovascular disease in the Sleep Heart Health Study. Neurology 2008;70:35–42.

15. Ferri R. The time structure of leg movement activity during sleep: the theory behind the practice. Sleep Med 2012;13:433–41.

16. Ferri R, Zucconi M, Manconi M, et al. Different periodicity and time structure of leg movements during sleep in narcolepsy/cataplexy and restless legs syndrome. Sleep 2006;29:1587–94.

17. Picchietti DL, Bruni O, de Weerd A, et al. Pediatric restless legs syndrome diagnostic criteria: an update by the International Restless Legs Syndrome Study Group. Sleep Med 2013;14:1253–9.

18. Allen RP, Picchietti DL, Garcia-Borreguero D, et al. Restless legs syndrome/Willis–Ekbom disease diagnostic criteria: updated International Restless Legs Syndrome Study Group (IRLSSG) consensus criteria—history, rationale, description, and significance. Sleep Med 2014;15:860–73.

19. Manconi M, Ferri R, Zucconi M, et al. Time structure analysis of leg movements during sleep in REM sleep behavior disorder. Sleep 2007;30:1779–85.

20. Puligheddu M, Figorilli M, Aricò D, et al. Time structure of leg movement activity during sleep in untreated Parkinson disease and effects of dopaminergic treatment. Sleep Med 2014;15:816–24.

21. Ferri R, Fulda S, Allen RP, et al. World Association of Sleep Medicine (WASM) 2016 standards for recording and scoring leg movements in polysomnograms developed by a joint task force from the International and the European Restless Legs Syndrome Study Groups (IRLSSG and EURLSSG) Sleep Med 2016;26C:86–95.

22. Manconi M, Zavalko I, Fanfulla F, Winkelman JW, et al. An evidence-based recommendation for a new definition of respiratory-related leg movements. Sleep 2015;38:295–304.

23. Kazenwadel J, Pollmächer T, Trenkwalder C, et al. New actigraphic assessment method for periodic leg movements (PLM). Sleep 1995;18:689–97.

24. King MA, Jaffre M-O, Morrish E, et al. The validation of a new actigraphy system for the measurement of periodic leg movements in sleep. Sleep Med 2005;6:507–13.

25. Gschliesser V, Frauscher B, Brandauer E, et al. PLM detection by actigraphy compared to polysomnography: a validation and comparison of two actigraphs. Sleep Med 2009;10:306–11.

26. Sforza E, Johannes M, Claudio B. The PAM-RL ambulatory device for detection of periodic leg movements: a validation study. Sleep Med 2005;6:407–13.

27. Kemlink D, Pretl M, Sonka K, Nevsimalova S. A comparison of polysomnographic and actigraphic evaluation of periodic limb movements in sleep. Neurol Res 2008;30:234–8.

28. Chervin RD, Consens FB, Kutluay E. Alternating leg muscle activation during sleep and arousals: a new sleep-related motor phenomenon? Mov Disord 2003;18:551–9.

29. Cosentino FII, Iero I, Lanuzza B, et al. The neurophysiology of the alternating leg muscle activation (ALMA) during sleep: study of one patient before and after treatment with pramipexole. Sleep Med 2006;7:63–71.

30. Yang C, Winkelman JW. Clinical and polysomnographic characteristics of high frequency leg movements. J Clin Sleep Med 2010;6:431–8.

31. Broughton R, Tolentino MA. Fragmentary pathological myoclonus in NREM sleep. Electroencephalogr Clin Neurophysiol 1984;57:303–9.

32. Broughton R, Tolentino MA, Krelina M. Excessive fragmentary myoclonus in NREM sleep: a report of 38 cases. Electroencephalogr Clin Neurophysiol 1985;61:123–33.

33. Lins O, Castonguay M, Dunham W, et al. Excessive fragmentary myoclonus: time of night and sleep stage distributions. Can J Neurol Sci 1993;20:142–6.

34. Frauscher B, Kunz A, Brandauer E, et al. Fragmentary myoclonus in sleep revisited: a polysomnographic study in 62 patients. Sleep Med 2011;12:410–15.

35. Brown P, Thompson PD, Rothwell JC, et al. Axial myoclonus of propriospinal origin. Brain J Neurol 1991;114(Pt 1A);197–214.

36. Chokroverty S. Propriospinal myoclonus. Clin Neurosci 1995;3:219–22.

37. Montagna P, Provini F, Vetrugno R. Propriospinal myoclonus at sleep onset. Neurophysiol Clin 2006;36:351–5.

38. Montagna P, Provini F, Plazzi G, et al. Propriospinal myoclonus upon relaxation and drowsiness: a cause of severe insomnia. Mov Disord 1997;12:66–72.

39. Frauscher B, Brandauer E, Gschliesser V, et al. A descriptive analysis of neck myoclonus during routine polysomnography. Sleep 2010:33:1091–6.

40. Wehrle R, Bartels A, Wetter TC. Facio-mandibular myoclonus specific during REM sleep. Sleep Med 2009;10:149–51.

41. Kato T, Thie NM, Montplaisir JY, Lavigne GJ. Bruxism and orofacial movements during sleep. Dent Clin North Am 2001;45:657–84.

42. Manni R, Terzaghi M, Sartori I, et al. Rhythmic movement disorder and cyclic alternating pattern during sleep: a video-polysomnographic study in a 9-year-old boy. Mov Disord 2004;19:1186–90.

43. Terzano MG, Parrino L, Smerieri A, et al. Atlas, rules, and recording techniques for the scoring of cyclic alternating pattern (CAP) in human sleep. Sleep Med 2002;3:187–99.

44. Hoban TF. Rhythmic movement disorder in children. CNS Spectr 2003;8:135–8.

45. Frauscher B, Iranzo A, Högl B, et al. Quantification of electromyographic activity during REM sleep in multiple muscles in REM sleep behavior disorder. Sleep 2008;31:724.

46. Frauscher B, Iranzo A, Gaig G, et al. Normative EMG values during REM sleep for the diagnosis of REM sleep behavior disorder. Sleep 2012;35:835–47.

47. Frauscher B, Ehrmann L, Högl B. Defining muscle activities for assessment of rapid eye movement sleep behavior disorder: from a qualitative to a quantitative diagnostic level. Sleep Med 2013;14:729–33.

48. Lapierre O, Montplaisir J. Polysomnographic features of REM sleep behavior disorder: development of a scoring method. Neurology 1992;42:1371–4.

49. Montplaisir J, Gagnon J-F, Fantini ML, et al. Polysomnographic diagnosis of idiopathic REM sleep behavior disorder. Mov Disord 2010;25:2044–51.

50. Bliwise DL, He L, Ansari FP, Rye DB. Quantification of electromyographic activity during sleep: a phasic electromyographic metric. J. Clin. Neurophysiol 2006;23:59–67.

51. Bliwise DL, Rye DB. Elevated PEM (phasic electromyographic metric) rates identify rapid eye movement behavior disorder patients on nights without behavioral abnormalities. Sleep 2008;31:853.

52. Burns JW, Consens FB, Little RJ, et al. EMG variance during polysomnography as an assessment for REM sleep behavior disorder. Sleep 2007;30:1771.

53. Ferri R, Manconi M, Plazzi G, et al. A quantitative statistical analysis of the submentalis muscle EMG amplitude during sleep in normal controls and patients with REM sleep behavior disorder. J Sleep Res 2008;17:89–100.

54. Mayer G, Kesper K, Ploch T, et al. Quantification of tonic and phasic muscle activity in REM sleep behavior disorder. J Clin Neurophysiol 2008;25:48–55.

55. Sasai-Sakuma T, Frauscher B, Mitterling T, et al. Quantitative assessment of isolated rapid eye movement (REM) sleep without atonia without clinical REM sleep behavior disorder: clinical and research implications. Sleep Med 2014;15:1009–15.

56. Ferri R, Rundo F, Manconi M, et al. Improved computation of the atonia index in normal controls and patients with REM sleep behavior disorder. Sleep Med 2010:11:947–9.

57. Ferri R, Fulda S, Cosentino FII, et al. A preliminary quantitative analysis of REM sleep chin EMG in Parkinson's disease with or without REM sleep behavior disorder. Sleep Med 2012;13:707–13.

58. Ferri R, Gagnon J-F, Postuma RB, et al. Comparison between an automatic and a visual scoring method of the chin muscle tone during rapid eye movement sleep. Sleep Med 2014;15:661–5.

59. Sforza E, Zucconi M, Petronelli R, et al. REM sleep behavioral disorders. Eur Neurol 1988;28:295–300.

60. Iranzo A, Santamaría J, Rye DB, et al. Characteristics of idiopathic REM sleep behavior disorder and that associated with MSA and PD. Neurology 2005;65:247–52.

61. Frauscher B, Gschliesser V, Brandauer E, et al. Video analysis of motor events in REM sleep behavior disorder. Mov Disord 2007;22:1464–70.

62. Frauscher B, Gschliesser V, Brandauer E, et al. The relation between abnormal behaviors and REM sleep microstructure in patients with REM sleep behavior disorder. Sleep Med 2009;10:174–81.

63. De Cock VC, Vidailhet M, Leu S, et al. Restoration of normal motor control in Parkinson's disease during REM sleep. Brain J Neurol 2007;130:450–6.

64. Cygan F, Oudiette D, Leclair-Visonneau L, et al. Night-to-night variability of muscle tone, movements, and vocalizations in patients with REM sleep behavior disorder. J Clin Sleep Med 2010;6:551–5.

65. Sixel-Döring F, Schweitzer M, Mollenhauer B, Trenkwalder C. Intraindividual variability of REM sleep behavior disorder in Parkinson's disease: a comparative assessment using a new REM sleep behavior disorder severity scale (RBDSS) for clinical routine. J Clin Sleep Med 2011;7:75–80.

CHAPTER 11

Neuroimaging in normal sleep and sleep disorders

Pierre Maquet and Julien Fanielle

Normal sleep

NREM sleep

Neuroimaging techniques have established that brain energy metabolism, as assessed by cerebral blood flow (CBF) as well as oxygen or glucose metabolic rates, is decreased during non-REM (NREM) sleep in comparison with wakefulness and REM sleep: by 5–10% during stage N2 and by 25–40% during slow-wave sleep (SWS) [1–3] (Fig. 11.1). In SWS, regional CBF (rCBF) decreases are particularly prominent in the basal ganglia, thalami, mesencephalon, dorsal pons, hypothalamus, precuneus, mesial part of the temporal lobe, and prefrontal and anterior cingulate cortices [1,2].

Regional brain activity during stages N1 and N2 (light NREM sleep) shows a similar pattern, but the midbrain tegmentum maintains an activity similar to wakefulness. Comparison of absolute rCBF between light NREM sleep and SWS revealed that rCBF in the pons, midbrain tegmentum, cerebellar vermis, caudate nucleus, and thalamus significantly decreased during SWS [4].

The spatial distribution of regional brain activity during SWS is usually thought to reflect the generation of sleep rhythms, especially slow waves during SWS [3,5]. With the advent of event-related functional magnetic resonance imaging (fMRI), it became possible to directly probe this hypothesis. Spindles were shown to be associated with responses in thalami, paralimbic areas (anterior cingulate and insular cortices), and superior temporal gyri [6]. Fast spindles (13–15 Hz) further recruited a set of cortical regions involved in sensorimotor processing, as well as the mesial frontal cortex and hippocampus, whereas slow spindles (11–13 Hz) were associated with increased activity in the superior frontal gyrus.

Neural correlates of the slow oscillation (<1 Hz) were also reported [7]. Significant decreases in activity were associated with these waves in several cortical areas, including the inferior frontal, medial prefrontal, precuneus, and posterior cingulate areas, all of which are considered as main hubs in the human brain [7,8]. These results were independently confirmed by source reconstruction of high-density EEG signals [9].

REM sleep

Brain energy metabolism during REM sleep is similar to that during wakefulness and higher than during NREM sleep [1]. However, there are differences in the regional distribution of brain activity between REM sleep and wakefulness. Activity has been repeatedly shown to be elevated in the pontine tegmentum, amygdala, thalamus, hippocampus, anterior cingulate cortex, temporo-occipital areas, cerebellum, caudate nucleus, and basal forebrain [2,10–12]. These data can be separated into areas that are implicated in the generation and the maintenance of REM sleep, such as the pontine tegmentum and thalamus, and areas linked to limbic or paralimbic structures (amygdala, hippocampus, anterior cingulate cortex, etc.). Conversely, the precuneus, parietal cortex, posterior cingulate cortex, and dorsolateral prefrontal cortex are the least active brain regions during REM sleep [2,10,13]. Currently, the cellular mechanisms underpinning this peculiar regional activity pattern remain elusive, although the activation of pontolimbic areas and the quiescence of heteromodal associative cortices was putatively related to oneiric activity [10,11,13,14].

Rapid eye movements are the hallmark of REM sleep, and their generation is deemed different from saccades during wakefulness. REMs are more strongly associated during REM sleep than during wakefulness with an increase in regional blood flow in the lateral geniculate bodies and striate cortex [15,16]. This finding suggested that REMs are generated through mechanisms reminiscent of the ponto-geniculo-occipital waves typically recorded in animals just before or during REM sleep.

Another characteristic of REM sleep consists of an autonomous instability. Heart rate variability was more strongly associated during REM sleep than during wakefulness with the activity in the right amygdala and less so with the activity in the right insula, an important cardiovascular regulator during wakefulness [17].

Sleep disorders

Obstructive sleep apnea syndrome

Obstructive sleep apnea syndrome (OSAS) is known as a leading cause of daytime sleepiness and results in variable degrees of cognitive and performance deficits. However, the respective contributions of sleep fragmentation and hypoxemia to the emergence of these cognitive deficits are not yet firmly established. It is also not yet known whether these deficits are reversible or whether OSAS results in permanent alteration in brain structure or function.

MRI voxel-based morphometry (VBM) or magnetic resonance spectroscopy (MRS) showed gray matter loss in the frontal, parietal, and anterior cingulate cortices, in the cerebellum, and in the temporal lobe concerning the parahippocampal gyrus and in particular the hippocampus [18–21], which might account for alterations in memory, attention and executive functioning. A significant

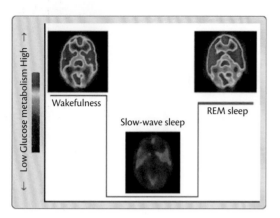

Fig. 11.1 (See colour plate section) Schematic representation of the variations in global cerebral glucose metabolism in resting wakefulness, slow-wave sleep, and REM sleep. The images represent the cerebral glucose metabolism measured in a single subject during three different sessions with [^{18}F]fluorodeoxyglucose positron emission tomography (FDG-PET). Functional images are displayed at the same brain level and using the same color scale. Similar rates of brain glucose metabolism are measured during wakefulness and REM sleep. Brain glucose metabolism is significantly decreased during slow-wave sleep relative to both wakefulness and REM sleep.
Adapted from Brain Res, 513(1), Maquet P, Dive D, Salmon E, et al, Cerebral glucose utilization during sleep–wake cycle in man determined by positron emission tomography and [^{18}F]2-fluoro-2-deoxy-D-glucose method, pp. 136–43, Copyright (1990) with permission from Elsevier.

correlation was observed between maximum apnea duration and cortical thinning in the dorsolateral prefrontal regions, pericentral gyri, and insula [22]. Furthermore, resting-state functional connectivity was shown to be altered in cognitive and sensorimotor-related brain networks in OSAS patients [23]. Some data suggest that continuous positive airway pressure (CPAP) treatment might result in both improved cognition and regional increases in gray matter in the hippocampus and frontal areas [24].

Intriguingly, unilateral gray matter alterations were reported in OSAS patients within the left ventrolateral prefrontal cortex and cerebellum (areas involved in upper airway motor regulation) and the anterior cingulate [21]. Likewise, neural response to the Valsalva maneuver is blunted in OSAS patients in regions with gray matter loss that are involved in upper airway and diaphragmatic motor control, breathing modulation, blood pressure regulation, and sensory input integration of the oropharynx, such as the left inferior parietal cortex, superior temporal gyrus, posterior insular cortex, cerebellar cortex, fastigial nucleus, and hippocampus [25].

Brain alterations in OSAS patients also involve white matter. Diffusion tensor imaging showed extensive white matter alteration in fibers of the limbic system, pons, frontal, temporal, and parietal regions, and projections to and from the cerebellum [26].

Restless legs syndrome

Restless legs syndrome (RLS) is a sleep disorder characterized by an urge to move the legs, usually associated with uncomfortable and unpleasant sensations in the legs that are relieved at least partially by movement. The symptoms are worse in the evening and are exacerbated by rest.

The physiopathology of RLS is not completely understood, but it is generally suspected that the dopaminergic circuits are involved, because there is clinical improvement with dopaminergic medications.

Imaging of the D_2 receptor using a selective antagonist (raclopride) and positron emission tomography (PET) showed a mild but significant decrease in D_2 receptor binding in the putamen in RLS patients in comparison with healthy subjects [27]. However, the decrease in binding was not related to symptom severity. Another study using the same technique found lower D_2 receptor binding in the nucleus accumbens and the caudate, but no significant differences in the putamen in an idiopathic RLS group of eight drug-naive patients compared with healthy controls. After a 2-week treatment with pramipexole, binding levels in the nucleus accumbens were negatively correlated with clinical severity scores and positively with the degree of post-treatment improvement in patients. These findings implicate alterations in mesolimbic D_2–D_3 receptors in RLS and show that baseline availability of these receptors is potentially predictive of clinical outcome after dopaminergic agonist treatment [28]. In contrast, there is no evidence for presynaptic dopaminergic transporter impairment in RLS patients according to a single-photon emission computed tomography (SPECT) study [29]. The decrease in D_2 receptor binding might be explained by a down-regulation or a dysfunction of the D_2 receptors or by a local augmentation in the levels of synaptic dopamine saturating binding sites, the latter suggestion being supported by recent data [30].

Iron deficiency has also been implicated in the pathophysiology of RLS. In fact, low ferritin levels and high transferrin levels were discovered in the cerebrospinal fluid (CSF) of idiopathic RLS patients [31]. Interestingly, tyrosine hydroxylase, the rate-limiting enzyme for dopamine synthesis, uses iron as cofactor, linking iron deficiency to dopamine dysregulation [32]. Using phase MRI, iron content was shown to be decreased in the thalamus, pallidum, substantia nigra, and putamen in a group of 15 RLS patients in comparison with 15 healthy subjects [33]. However, these findings remain contentious, since another study did not find any difference in brain iron content in RLS patients [34].

Likewise, for the time being, functional and structural brain abnormalities reported in RLS are inconsistent across magnetic resonance studies. Some VBM studies did not show any difference between patients and control subjects [35–37], whereas others found heterogeneous data such as gray matter increase in the pulvinar bilaterally [38], gray matter decrease in the middle orbitofrontal gyrus and left hippocampus [39], grey matter decrease in the primary somatosensory cortex bilaterally [40], or white matter volume reductions in small areas of the genu of the corpus callosum, the anterior cingulum, and the precentral gyrus [41]. Some argue that these discrepant results arise from sample heterogeneity and methodological differences (eg, statistical models) [37].

fMRI of RLS patients reported bilateral activation of the cerebellum and contralateral activation of the thalamus associated with unpleasant sensations in RLS [42]. In addition, there were also activations in the red nuclei and the brainstem close to the reticular formation during the symptomatic period, suggesting that subcortical cerebral generators are involved in the pathogenesis of RLS [43].

Narcolepsy

Several VBM studies have been conducted to characterize the alteration in gray matter in patients with narcolepsy, with variable results. Some studies reported a bilateral decrease in hypothalamic gray matter in narcoleptic patients [44–46], consistent with the known loss of hypocretin neurons in the lateral hypothalamus of such patients [47,48]. Other VBM studies found decreases in cortical gray matter of limbic-related areas: the inferior temporal and inferior frontal regions [46,49], the right prefrontal and frontomesial cortex [50], or the cingulate cortex [51–53]. Gray matter reduction was also observed in the right nucleus accumbens and in the cerebellar vermis [44] and, in narcoleptic patients with cataplexy, in both nuclei accumbentes [46]. Structural modifications in the limbic system are usually interpreted as a potential neural basis for altered emotional processing in narcoleptic patients.

REM sleep behavior disorder

REM sleep behavior disorder (RBD) is a disorder characterized by loss of skeletal muscle atonia during REM sleep while the patient is generally dreaming, a condition associated with unusual and often impressive motor behavior during sleep.

RBD predates clinical manifestations of alpha-synucleinopathies such as Parkinson disease (PD), dementia with Lewy bodies (DLB), and multiple system atrophy [54]. For this reason, neuroimaging features in RBD are variable, depending on the clinical context set by the underlying neurodegenerative disorder. Consequently, we will focus on neuroimaging features in idiopathic RBD (iRBD).

The mesopontine tegmentum (MT) was one of the first regions of interest to be considered with regard to RBD because of work on cats by Jouvet and his team since 1967, using a model of loss of skeletal muscle atonia during REM sleep as a result of MT impairment involving the sublaterodorsal nucleus [55,56]. Moreover, case reports illustrated secondary RBD due to brainstem lesions [57,58]. Actually, few MRI studies are available on iRBD, and these generally involve small samples and sometimes contradictory results. Nevertheless, two recent diffusion tensor imaging (DTI) studies identified subtle anomalies in brainstem white matter, especially in the pons and the midbrain, in iRBD patients versus control subjects [59,60] (Fig. 11.2).

Consistent with these results, gray matter density decreases in the pontine tegmentum [61], although a gray matter increase has also been reported in both hippocampi in iRBD patients, for reasons that remain unclear [60].

By contrast, a nigrostriatal dysfunction was consistently reported by SPECT and PET studies: dopaminergic innervation of the striatum is significantly decreased in iRBD patients, emphasizing the continuum between iRBD and alpha-synucleinopathies [62–64]. One of the difficulties with iRBD patients is then to identify who will eventually develop a neurodegenerative disorder. A SPECT study published in 2012 found that patients with iRBD who developed PD or DLB had an rCBF increase at baseline in the hippocampus in comparison with iRBD patients with a stable condition who did not develop PD or DLB, which is the first step in establishing a potential predictive biomarker for neurodegenerative evolution in iRBD [65]. In conclusion, actual data suggest that the etiopathogenesis of iRBD probably takes place in the brainstem and that associated neurodegenerative repercussions may be observed in hippocampal regions and the striatum.

Insomnia

Insomnia is a frequent disorder defined as a subjective perception of dissatisfaction with the amount and/or quality of sleep [66]. Major complaints are difficulty in falling asleep, impaired sleep maintenance, and early awakening. Insomnias are generally classified as comorbid insomnias, due to a medical or psychiatric disorder, and primary insomnias that are not explainable by a comorbid condition. Here, we will focus on primary insomnias because of the heterogeneity of comorbid insomnias.

Nofzinger et al. demonstrated in an FDG ([^{18}F]fluorodeoxyglucose)-PET scan study that, compared with control subjects, insomniac patients had a smaller decrease in relative metabolism between wakefulness and NREM sleep in the ascending reticular activating system, hypothalamus, insular cortex, amygdala, hippocampus, and cingulate and medial prefrontal cortices [67]. This observation is compatible with the hyperarousal theory of insomnia, which postulates that patients suffering from insomnia have inappropriate physiological arousal, with a diminution of the waking threshold and a sympathetic nervous system activation during sleep in comparison with normal subjects [68,69]. Moreover, in comparison

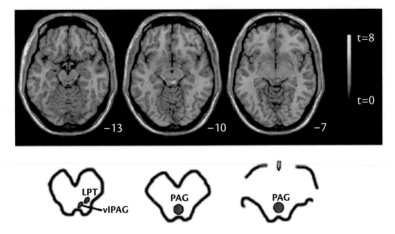

Fig. 11.2 (See colour plate section) Statistical parametric mapping (t) axial maximum intensity projection maps rendered onto a stereotactically normalized MRI scan, showing areas of significant decreases of fractional anisotropy values (color code, yellow to orange) in a cohort of patients with idiopathic REM sleep behavior disorder versus healthy control subjects. The number at the bottom right corner of each MRI scan corresponds to the z-coordinate in Talairach space. The schematic drawings below the scans correspond to the MRI and visualize proposed nuclei involved in REM sleep control (modified from Boeve et al. [94]). The REM-off region is represented by the ventrolateral part of the periaqueductal gray matter (vlPAG)/periaqueductal gray matter (PAG) and the lateral pontine tegmentum (LPT).

with healthy subjects, patients suffering from insomnia showed hypometabolism in a large part of the frontal cortex bilaterally, in the left hemisphere superior temporal, parietal, and occipital cortices, and in the thalamus, hypothalamus, and brainstem reticular formation [67] during wakefulness. Interestingly, the prefrontal hypometabolism seen in insomniac patients while awake is a feature that we also found in sleep-deprived subjects, and it might be related to inefficient sleep in insomniac patients [67,70].

Recently, executive function was probed using fMRI on a sample of 25 patients suffering from primary insomnia and 14 control subjects matched for age, sex, and education. Reduced recruitment of the head of the left caudate nucleus was found during executive functioning, with an association between caudate recruitment and hyperarousal severity [71]. A link was

also suggested between a decrease in gray matter density in the orbitofrontal area and altered caudate recruitment in insomniac patients due to attenuated input from orbitofrontal cortex projections to the caudate nucleus. Finally, persistence of altered caudate recruitment was observed even after successful treatment of insomnia, and, interestingly, attenuated caudate recruitment was obtained in healthy subjects by SWS fragmentation [71] (Fig. 11.3). In an fMRI study, during a verbal fluency task (letter fluency and category fluency), the left medial prefrontal and left inferior frontal cortices responded significantly less in elderly patients suffering from isolated chronic primary insomnia in comparison with control subjects. This reduced activation was partly restored after nonpharmacological sleep therapy (cognitive–behavioral therapy, CBT) [72].

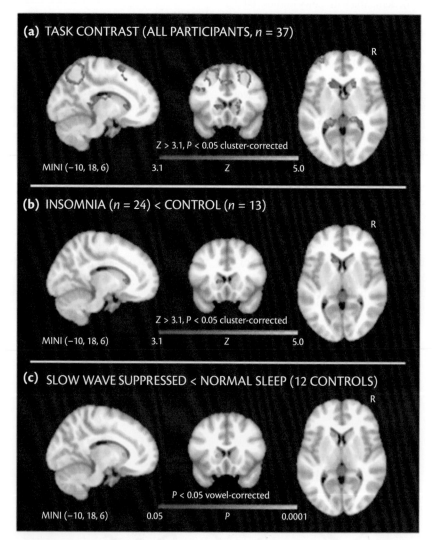

Fig. 11.3 (See colour plate section) Reduced caudate recruitment in insomnia and after slow-wave sleep fragmentation. (a) The head of the left caudate shows increased BOLD signal during executive functioning relative to baseline trials across all participants. (b) Patients with insomnia show an attenuated task-elicited BOLD response in the head of the left caudate nucleus when compared to controls (Z_{max} = 4.31 at MNI coordinates (−12, 18, 2); cluster size = 43 voxels = 344 mm³). (c) Controls show an attenuated task-elicited BOLD response in the head of the left caudate nucleus after a night of slow-wave sleep suppression relative to a night of normal sleep (Z_{max} = 3.32 at MNI coordinates (−12, 18, 4); 36 of 43 voxels in the region of interest = 84%). Significant clusters (a and b) or voxels (c) are shown in a gradient from red to yellow overlaid on the most informative orthogonal slices from the averaged MNI152 brain, displayed according to neurological convention (left = left). MNI coordinates for the orthogonal slices, statistical thresholds, and a color bar indicating Z-value or significance level are shown at the bottom.

Responses to a working memory task, as assessed by fMRI, were also reduced in insomnia patients, and their influence over default mode areas was decreased [73]. It is argued that these findings partly explain cognitive complaints reported by patients suffering from primary insomnia.

In a resting-state fMRI study, functional connectivity between the amygdala on the one hand and the thalamus, insula, and striatum on the other was reduced in insomniac patients. In contrast, functional connectivity was increased between the amygdala and the premotor and sensorimotor cortices in insomnia patients, suggesting a dysfunction in emotional pathways in primary insomnia [74].

In patients complaining about having difficulties in falling asleep but not fulfilling the criteria for primary insomnia, functional connectivity was increased between primary sensory regions and supplementary motor regions, suggesting a sustained sensory processing of environmental stimuli that potentially might delay sleep latency [75].

VBM in insomnia patients yielded contentious results. A study of 28 primary insomnia subjects and 38 good sleeper controls did not identify any difference between the groups in VBM analysis of gray and white matter volumes [76], whereas another study found a gray matter (decrease in the left orbitofrontal cortex correlated with subjective severity of insomnia and a gray matter decrease in the anterior and posterior precuneus [77].

Likewise, the hippocampal volume (HV) in chronic insomnia was found to be reduced in insomnia patients in one study [78], but not in another [79]. Interestingly, in the latter, actigraphic measures of poor sleep maintenance were still associated with smaller HV [79]. A third study did not observe any significant difference in HV or intracranial volume between primary insomnia patients and good sleepers, but in the patient group, bilateral HV was negatively correlated with duration of insomnia and arousal index and positively correlated with recognition rates of visual memory [80].

An enlargement of the bilateral rostral anterior cingulate cortex (rACC) was reported in patients with chronic primary insomnia in comparison with good sleeper controls. Moreover, there was a positive correlation between rACC volumes and self-reported and objective determinations of poor sleep quality. It was postulated that enlargement of rACC volumes might represent a compensatory response to repetitive sleep disturbance and be a sort of marker of resilience to developing a mood disorder [81].

Finally, a recent MRS study identified a reduction in γ-aminobutyric acid (GABA) levels in the anterior cingulate and occipital cortices of unmedicated primary insomnia patients by 33% and 21%, respectively, compared with age- and sex-matched healthy controls [82]. Similar phenomena were also described in major depressive disorder (MDD) [83–85], which is interesting because of the strong relationship between MDD and insomnia.

Kleine–Levin syndrome

Kleine–Levin syndrome (KLS) is a rare disorder occurring during the second and third decades of life and characterized by relapsing–remitting episodes of hypersomnia, behavioral disorders such as eating disorder (hyperphagia), thymic disorder (depressed mood), hypersexuality, feelings of derealization, or apathy. Patients also experience cognitive impairment during the episodes.

An FDG-PET scan study of two patients suffering from KLS reported significant metabolic decreases in the hypothalamus, the orbitofrontal and frontal parasagittal areas, and the bilateral occipital regions, contrasting with metabolic increases in the anterior caudate nuclei, the cingulate, and the premotor cortex [86]. Hypersomnia, hyperphagia, and hypersexuality were deemed to be related to the hypothalamic dysfunction, whereas frontal hypometabolism was thought to be involved in apathy and behavioral changes, including hyperphagia. No metabolic decrease was observed in the thalamus in these two patients, although previous studies had reported such a decrease in several cases of KLS [87,88]. This bilateral thalamic hypometabolism, observed with SPECT, was selectively seen during symptomatic episodes and disappeared during asymptomatic periods in all patients of a five-patient group [87]. Hypoperfusion in the temporal, frontal, and occipital cortices and in the basal ganglia was reported in some but not all patients [86,88,89]. Interestingly, some perfusion abnormalities persist in asymptomatic periods, especially after a long clinical evolution.

Concerning other SPECT imaging data, a reduction of striatal dopamine transporter availability was identified in KLS patients during the symptomatic period in a SPECT study with [^{99m}Tc] TRODAT-1 [90] and, in a case report, SPECT imaging with [^{123}I] iomazenil showed a decrease in benzodiazepine binding to $GABA_A$ receptors in the left mesial temporal lobe and the right frontal opercula [91].

Finally, MRS data are controversial. One study suggested an increase of glutamine metabolites in the left thalamus and in the basal ganglia in symptomatic compared with asymptomatic scans in a 20-year-old woman suffering from KLS [92], whereas a recent study with 14 KLS patients and 15 healthy controls using fMRI and MRS showed no difference in spectroscopic findings between patients and controls, but did identify a negative correlation between N-acetylaspartate levels and fMRI activity in the left thalamus in KLS patients, but not controls, while performing a working memory task [93].

Conclusion

Neuroimaging techniques, which are still in progress, contribute to the comprehension of sleep mechanisms and sleep disorders in a minimally invasive way. A combination of such techniques with electrophysiological devices provides great prospects for the future. But technical progress is not sufficient in the absence of a good methodology. In fact, real data from neuroimaging studies of sleep and its disorders are too often controversial because of the small size of the samples involved. That is why it is important to develop large-sample studies in the next few years with highly significant statistical power.

References

1. Maquet P, Dive D, Salmon E, et al. Cerebral glucose utilization during sleep–wake cycle in man determined by positron emission tomography and [18F]2-fluoro-2-deoxy-D-glucose method. Brain Res 1990;513:136–43.
2. Braun AR, Balkin TJ, Wesensten NJ, et al. Regional cerebral blood flow throughout the sleep–wake cycle. An H2(15)O PET study. Brain 1997;120(Pt 7):1173–97.
3. Maquet P. Functional neuroimaging of normal human sleep by positron emission tomography. J Sleep Res 2000;9:207–31.
4. Kajimura N, Uchiyama M, Takayama Y, et al. Activity of midbrain reticular formation and neocortex during the progression of human non-rapid eye movement sleep. J Neurosci 1999;19:10065–73.
5. Borbely AA. From slow waves to sleep homeostasis: new perspectives. Arch Ital Biol 2001;139:53–61.

6. Schabus M, Dang-Vu TT, Albouy G, et al. Hemodynamic cerebral correlates of sleep spindles during human non-rapid eye movement sleep. Proc Natl Acad Sci USA 2007;104:13164–9.

7. Dang-Vu TT, Desseilles M, Laureys S, et al. Cerebral correlates of delta waves during non-REM sleep revisited. NeuroImage 2005;28:14–21.

8. Hagmann P, Grant PE, Fair DA. MR connectomics: a conceptual framework for studying the developing brain. Frontier Syst Neurosci 2012;6:43.

9. Murphy M, Riedner BA, Huber R, et al. Source modeling sleep slow waves. Proc Natl Acad Sci USA 2009;106:1608–13.

10. Maquet P, Peters J, Aerts J, et al. Functional neuroanatomy of human rapid-eye-movement sleep and dreaming. Nature 1996;383:163–6.

11. Maquet P, Laureys S, Peigneux P, et al. Experience-dependent changes in cerebral activation during human REM sleep. Nat Neurosci 2000;3:831–6.

12. Nofzinger EA, Mintun MA, Wiseman M, Kupfer DJ, Moore RY. Forebrain activation in REM sleep: an FDG PET study. Brain Res 1997;770:192–201.

13. Maquet P, Ruby P, Maudoux A, et al. Human cognition during REM sleep and the activity profile within frontal and parietal cortices: a reappraisal of functional neuroimaging data. Progr Brain Res 2005;150:219–27.

14. Hobson JA. REM sleep and dreaming: towards a theory of protoconsciousness. Nat Rev Neurosci 2009;10:803–13.

15. Peigneux P, Laureys S, Fuchs S, et al. Generation of rapid eye movements during paradoxical sleep in humans. NeuroImage 2001;14:701–8.

16. Wehrle R, Czisch M, Kaufmann C, et al. Rapid eye movement-related brain activation in human sleep: a functional magnetic resonance imaging study. Neuroreport 2005;16:853–7.

17. Desseilles M, Vu TD, Laureys S, et al. A prominent role for amygdaloid complexes in the variability in heart rate (VHR) during rapid eye movement (REM) sleep relative to wakefulness. NeuroImage 2006;32:1008–15.

18. Alkan A, Sharifov R, Akkoyunlu ME, et al. MR spectroscopy features of brain in patients with mild and severe obstructive sleep apnea syndrome. Clin Imag 2013;37:989–92.

19. Morrell MJ, McRobbie DW, Quest RA, et al. Changes in brain morphology associated with obstructive sleep apnea. Sleep Med 2003;4:451–4.

20. O'Donoghue FJ, Wellard RM, Rochford PD, et al. Magnetic resonance spectroscopy and neurocognitive dysfunction in obstructive sleep apnea before and after CPAP treatment. Sleep 2012;35:41–8.

21. Macey PM, Henderson LA, Macey KE, et al. Brain morphology associated with obstructive sleep apnea. Am J Resp Crit Care Med 2002;166:1382–7.

22. Joo EY, Jeon S, Kim ST, Lee JM, Hong SB. Localized cortical thinning in patients with obstructive sleep apnea syndrome. Sleep 2013;36:1153–62.

23. Zhang Q, Wang D, Qin W, et al., Altered resting-state brain activity in obstructive sleep apnea. Sleep 2013;36:651–9.

24. Canessa N, Castronovo V, Cappa SF, et al. Obstructive sleep apnea: brain structural changes and neurocognitive function before and after treatment. Am J Resp Crit Care Med 2011;183:1419–26.

25. Henderson LA, Woo MA, Macey PM, et al. Neural responses during Valsalva maneuvers in obstructive sleep apnea syndrome. J Appl Physiol 1985;94:1063–74.

26. Macey PM, Kumar R, Woo MA, et al. Brain structural changes in obstructive sleep apnea. Sleep 2008;31:967–77.

27. Turjanski N, Lees AJ, Brooks DJ. Striatal dopaminergic function in restless legs syndrome: 18F-dopa and 11C-raclopride PET studies. Neurology 1999;52:932–7.

28. Oboshi Y, Ouchi Y, Yagi S, et al. In vivo mesolimbic D2/3 receptor binding predicts posttherapeutic clinical responses in restless legs syndrome: a positron emission tomography study. J Cerebral Blood Flow Metab 2012;32:654–62.

29. Linke R, Eisensehr I, Wetter TC, et al. Presynaptic dopaminergic function in patients with restless legs syndrome: are there common features with early Parkinson's disease? Mov Disord 2004;19:1158–62.

30. Earley CJ, Kuwabara H, Wong DF, et al. Increased synaptic dopamine in the putamen in restless legs syndrome. Sleep 2013;36:51–7.

31. Earley CJ, Connor JR, Beard JL, et al. Abnormalities in CSF concentrations of ferritin and transferrin in restless legs syndrome. Neurology 2000;54:1698–700.

32. Kaushik P, Gorin F, Vali S. Dynamics of tyrosine hydroxylase mediated regulation of dopamine synthesis. J Comput Neurosci 2007;22:147–60.

33. Rizzo G, Manners D, Testa C, et al. Low brain iron content in idiopathic restless legs syndrome patients detected by phase imaging. Mov Disord 2013;28:1886–90.

34. Knake S, Heverhagen JT, Menzler K, et al. Normal regional brain iron concentration in restless legs syndrome measured by MRI. Nat Sci Sleep 2010;2:19–22.

35. Celle S, Roche F, Peyron R, et al. Lack of specific gray matter alterations in restless legs syndrome in elderly subjects. J Neurol 2010;257:344–8.

36. Comley RA, Cervenka S, Palhagen SE, et al. A comparison of gray matter density in restless legs syndrome patients and matched controls using voxel-based morphometry. J Neuroimag 2012;22:28–32.

37. Rizzo G, Manners D, Vetrugno R, et al. Combined brain voxel-based morphometry and diffusion tensor imaging study in idiopathic restless legs syndrome patients. Eur J Neurol 2012;19:1045–9.

38. Etgen T, Draganski B, Ilg C, et al. Bilateral thalamic gray matter changes in patients with restless legs syndrome. NeuroImage 2005;24:1242–7.

39. Hornyak M, Ahrendts JC, Spiegelhalder K, et al. Voxel-based morphometry in unmedicated patients with restless legs syndrome. Sleep Med 2007;9:22–6.

40. Unrath A, Juengling FD, Schork M, Kassubek J. Cortical grey matter alterations in idiopathic restless legs syndrome: an optimized voxel-based morphometry study. Mov Disord 2007;22:1751–6.

41. Connor JR, Ponnuru P, Lee BY, et al. Postmortem and imaging based analyses reveal CNS decreased myelination in restless legs syndrome. Sleep Med 2011;12:614–19.

42. Bucher SF, Seelos KC, Oertel WH, Reiser M, Trenkwalder C. Cerebral generators involved in the pathogenesis of the restless legs syndrome. Ann Neurol 1997; 41:639–45.

43. Wetter TC, Eisensehr I, Trenkwalder C. Functional neuroimaging studies in restless legs syndrome. Sleep Med 2004;5:401–6.

44. Draganski B, Geisler P, Hajak G, et al. Hypothalamic gray matter changes in narcoleptic patients. Nat Med 2002;8:1186–8.

45. Buskova J, Vaneckova M, Sonka K, Seidl Z, Nevsimalova S. Reduced hypothalamic gray matter in narcolepsy with cataplexy. Neuro Endocrinol Lett 2006;27:769–72.

46. Joo EY, Tae WS, Kim ST, Hong SB. Gray matter concentration abnormality in brains of narcolepsy patients. Kor J Radiol 2009;10:552–8.

47. Nishino S, Ripley B, Overeem S, Lammers GJ, Mignot E. Hypocretin (orexin) deficiency in human narcolepsy. Lancet 2000;355:39–40.

48. Thannickal TC, Moore RY, Nienhuis R, et al. Reduced number of hypocretin neurons in human narcolepsy. Neuron 2000;27:469–74.

49. Kaufmann C, Schuld A, Pollmacher T, Auer DP. Reduced cortical gray matter in narcolepsy: preliminary findings with voxel-based morphometry. Neurology 2002;58:1852–5.

50. Brenneis C, Brandauer E, Frauscher B, et al. Voxel-based morphometry in narcolepsy. Sleep Med 2005;6:531–6.

51. Kim SJ, Lyoo IK, Lee YS, et al. Gray matter deficits in young adults with narcolepsy. Acta Neurol Scand 2009;119:61–7.

52. Joo EY, Jeon S, Lee M, et al. Analysis of cortical thickness in narcolepsy patients with cataplexy. Sleep 2011;34:1357–64.

53. Scherfler C, Frauscher B, Schocke M, et al. White and gray matter abnormalities in narcolepsy with cataplexy. Sleep 2012;35:345–51.

54. Schenck CH, Mahowald MW. REM sleep behavior disorder: clinical, developmental, and neuroscience perspectives 16 years after its formal identification in SLEEP. Sleep 2002;25:120–38.

55. Sakai K, Sastre JP, Salvert D, et al. Tegmentoreticular projections with special reference to the muscular atonia during paradoxical sleep in the cat: an HRP study. Brain Res 1979;176:233–54.

56. Boeve BF. REM sleep behavior disorder: updated review of the core features, the REM sleep behavior disorder–neurodegenerative disease association, evolving concepts, controversies, and future directions. Ann N Y Acad Sci 2010;1184:15–54.

57. Jianhua C, Xiuqin L, Quancai C, Heyang S, Yan H. Rapid eye movement sleep behavior disorder in a patient with brainstem lymphoma. Intern Med 2013;52:617–21.

58. Iranzo A, Aparicio J. A lesson from anatomy: focal brain lesions causing REM sleep behavior disorder. Sleep Med 2009;10:9–12.

59. Unger MM, Belke M, Menzler K, et al. Diffusion tensor imaging in idiopathic REM sleep behavior disorder reveals microstructural changes in the brainstem, substantia nigra, olfactory region, and other brain regions. Sleep 2010;33:767–73.

60. Scherfler C, Frauscher B, Schocke M, et al. White and gray matter abnormalities in idiopathic rapid eye movement sleep behavior disorder: a diffusion-tensor imaging and voxel-based morphometry study. Ann Neurol 2011;69:400–7.

61. Hanyu H, Inoue Y, Sakurai H, et al. Voxel-based magnetic resonance imaging study of structural brain changes in patients with idiopathic REM sleep behavior disorder. Parkinsonism Relat Disord 2012;18:136–9.

62. Iranzo A, Valldeoriola F, Lomena F, et al. Serial dopamine transporter imaging of nigrostriatal function in patients with idiopathic rapid-eye-movement sleep behaviour disorder: a prospective study. Lancet Neurol 2011;10:797–805.

63. Eisensehr I, Linke R, Noachtar S, et al. Reduced striatal dopamine transporters in idiopathic rapid eye movement sleep behaviour disorder. Comparison with Parkinson's disease and controls. Brain 2000;123(Pt 6):1155–60.

64. Albin RL, Koeppe RA, Chervin RD, et al. Decreased striatal dopaminergic innervation in REM sleep behavior disorder. Neurology 2000;55:1410–12.

65. Dang-Vu TT, Gagnon JF, Vendette M, et al. Hippocampal perfusion predicts impending neurodegeneration in REM sleep behavior disorder. Neurology 2012;79:2302–6.

66. American Academy of Sleep Medicine. The international classification of sleep disorders: diagnostic and coding manual, 2nd ed. Westchester, IL: American Academy of Sleep Medicine, 2005.

67. Nofzinger EA, Buysse DJ, Germain A, et al. Functional neuroimaging evidence for hyperarousal in insomnia. Am J Psychiatry 2004;161:2126–8.

68. Bonnet MH, Arand DL. Hyperarousal and insomnia. Sleep Med Rev 1997;1:97–108.

69. Bonnet MH, Arand DL. Hyperarousal and insomnia: state of the science. Sleep Med Rev 2010;14:9–15.

70. Thomas M, Sing H, Belenky G, et al. Neural basis of alertness and cognitive performance impairments during sleepiness. I. Effects of 24 h of sleep deprivation on waking human regional brain activity. J Sleep Res 2000;9:335–52.

71. Stoffers D, Altena E, van der Werf YD, et al. The caudate: a key node in the neuronal network imbalance of insomnia? Brain 2014;137(Pt 2): 610–20.

72. Altena E, Van Der Werf YD, Sanz-Arigita EJ, et al. Prefrontal hypoactivation and recovery in insomnia. Sleep 2008;31:1271–6.

73. Drummond SP, Walker M, Almklov E, et al. Neural correlates of working memory performance in primary insomnia. Sleep 2013;36:1307–16.

74. Huang Z, Liang P, Jia X, et al. Abnormal amygdala connectivity in patients with primary insomnia: evidence from resting state fMRI. Eur J Radiol 2012;81:1288–95.

75. Killgore WD, Schwab ZJ, Kipman M, Deldonno SR, Weber M. Insomnia-related complaints correlate with functional connectivity between sensory-motor regions. Neuroreport 2013;24:233–40.

76. Spiegelhalder K, Regen W, Baglioni C, et al. Insomnia does not appear to be associated with substantial structural brain changes. Sleep 2013;36:731–7.

77. Altena E, Vrenken H, Van Der Werf YD, van den Heuvel OA, Van Someren EJ. Reduced orbitofrontal and parietal gray matter in chronic insomnia: a voxel-based morphometric study. Biol Psychiatry 2010;67:182–5.

78. Riemann D, Voderholzer U, Spiegelhalder K, et al. Chronic insomnia and MRI-measured hippocampal volumes: a pilot study. Sleep 2007;30:955–8.

79. Winkelman JW, Benson KL, Buxton OM, et al. Lack of hippocampal volume differences in primary insomnia and good sleeper controls: an MRI volumetric study at 3 Tesla. Sleep Med 2010;11:576–82.

80. Noh HJ, Joo EY, Kim ST, et al. The relationship between hippocampal volume and cognition in patients with chronic primary insomnia. J Clin Neurol 2012;8:130–8.

81. Winkelman JW, Plante DT, Schoerning L, et al. Increased rostral anterior cingulate cortex volume in chronic primary insomnia. Sleep 2013;36:991–8.

82. Plante DT, Jensen JE, Schoerning L, Winkelman JW. Reduced gamma-aminobutyric acid in occipital and anterior cingulate cortices in primary insomnia: a link to major depressive disorder? Neuropsychopharmacology 2012;37:1548–57.

83. Sanacora G, Mason GF, Rothman DL, et al. Reduced cortical gamma-aminobutyric acid levels in depressed patients determined by proton magnetic resonance spectroscopy. Arch General Psychiatry 1999;56:1043–7.

84. Hasler G, van der Veen JW, Tumonis T, et al. Reduced prefrontal glutamate/glutamine and gamma-aminobutyric acid levels in major depression determined using proton magnetic resonance spectroscopy. Arch General Psychiatry 2007;64:193–200.

85. Price RB, Shungu DC, Mao X, et al. Amino acid neurotransmitters assessed by proton magnetic resonance spectroscopy: relationship to treatment resistance in major depressive disorder. Biol Psychiatry 2009;65:792–800.

86. Haba-Rubio J, Prior JO, Guedj E, et al. Kleine–Levin syndrome: functional imaging correlates of hypersomnia and behavioral symptoms. Neurology 2012;79:1927–9.

87. Huang YS, Guilleminault C, Kao PF, Liu FY. SPECT findings in the Kleine–Levin syndrome. Sleep 2005;28:955–60.

88. Hong SB, Joo EY, Tae WS, et al. Episodic diencephalic hypoperfusion in Kleine–Levin syndrome. Sleep 2006;29:1091–3.

89. Landtblom AM, Dige N, Schwerdt K, Safstrom P, Granerus G. Short-term memory dysfunction in Kleine–Levin syndrome. Acta Neurol Scand 2003;108: 363–7.

90. Hoexter MQ, Shih MC, Felicio AC, Tufik S, Bressan RA. Greater reduction of striatal dopamine transporter availability during the symptomatic than asymptomatic phase of Kleine–Levin syndrome. Sleep Med 2010;11:959.

91. Itokawa K, Fukui M, Ninomiya M, et al. Gabapentin for Kleine–Levin syndrome. Internal Med 2009;48:1183–5.

92. Billings ME, Watson NF, Keogh BP. Dynamic fMRI changes in Kleine–Levin syndrome. Sleep Med 2001;12:532.

93. Vigren P, Tisell A, Engstrom M, et al. Low thalamic NAA-concentration corresponds to strong neural activation in working memory in Kleine–Levin syndrome. PloS One 2013;8:e56279.

94. Boeve BF, Silber MH, Saper CB, et al. Pathophysiology of REM sleep behaviour disorder and relevance to neurodegenerative disease. Brain 2007;130:2770–88.

Clinical science: general introduction

CHAPTER 12

Clinical sleep medicine
An introduction

Jennifer A. Liebenthal and Christian Guilleminault

Sleep Medicine has now become a specialty in its own right, with many advances occurring over just a short time in recent years. Narcolepsy—now subdivided into type 1 with abnormally low cerebrospinal fluid (CSF) hypocretin levels (and usually cataplexy) and type 2, lacking this key sign—is considered today as a potential model autoimmune disorder of the brain. The demonstration of the association between HLA DQB1*0602 and a specific polymorphism of the T-cell receptor α in narcolepsy type 1, along with absent or pathologically low levels of hypocretin in the CSF, has led researchers in this direction. The finding of an abrupt and notably large increase in pediatric narcolepsy cases following a specific vaccination against the H1N1 virus in Nordic European countries, and the significant increase in the number of Chinese pediatric cases during the same H1N1 epidemic, have furthered our understanding of narcolepsy with cataplexy. Large-database studies from drug companies and general population surveys have clearly indicated the general health impact of narcolepsy, particularly on the childhood and adolescent populations. Increases in obesity, cardiovascular disease, psychiatric syndromes, and early mortality have been observed. Now that we better understand the impact of hypocretin (orexin) neuron destruction in the lateral hypothalamus, many types of knockout rodent models have explained the multiple health consequences of the neuronal destruction [1–3].

Obesity has become a significant health problem in recent decades, with a drastic impact on the regulation of metabolic function, particularly during sleep. Obesity has a direct impact on brain function during sleep, but also induces changes in breathing during sleep. However, it is difficult to distinguish between the consequences directly related to obesity and those occurring secondary to breathing impairment during sleep. Obesity per se is responsible for cardiovascular, metabolic, and neurological changes. Invasion by adipocytes of the abdominal walls, the base of the tongue, and the lateral pharyngeal walls may worsen the changes induced by obesity. Therefore, the many abnormal findings attributed to obstructive sleep apnea in an obese subject cannot be solely due to abnormal upper airway narrowing during sleep, but may be direct consequences of obesity. These developments in understanding have led to revisions of therapeutic recommendations, emphasizing weight loss programs and bariatric surgery in addition to positive airway pressure [4].

A clearer understanding of the growth and development of the orofacial region during early childhood has led to the recognition of factors that increase the collapsibility of the upper airway.

Orofacial growth is rapid early in life. By six years of age, 60% of the adult face is already formed, and many factors may negatively impact the width of the upper airway [5]. Today we also have a better understanding of nonsyndromic genetic mutations that lead to abnormal growth of bones supporting the upper airway. For example, in certain forms of Ehlers–Danlos syndrome associated with only minor laxity of limb articulations, there may be a congenital absence of teeth involved in the build-up of maxillary bone [6]. In addition to nonsyndromic genetic mutations, there are functional disorders related to abnormal suction, mastication, swallowing, and nasal breathing that may lead to mouth breathing and progress to abnormal orofacial growth and nasal disuse. Recognition of such functional changes has led to routine evaluation of premature infants and older individuals with such backgrounds, as well as systematic assessment for short lingual frenulum (leading to mandatory frenulum evaluation in the Federal State of Brazil). This recognition has also encouraged increasing involvement of pediatric dentists and orthodontists in the recognition and treatment of abnormal oral cavities using rapid maxillary expansion, not only in children but now also in adults (through the use of mini-palatal implants). Such recognition has also led to the worldwide development of orofacial myofunctional therapists and the creation of an international society [7]. The efficacy of this approach has been demonstrated in adults as well as in children.

Cardiologists have been reluctant to embrace the field of Sleep Medicine for many years, even though large studies have demonstrated the important association of sleep-disordered breathing with recurrence of atrial fibrillation, despite standard medical therapy. In patients with heart failure, a comparison of patients treated with adapt-servo-ventilation (ASV) during sleep [8] versus those treated without ASV shows improved cardiac function and prognosis in those treated with ASV, although recent SERVE-HF clinical trial results in Europe have led to some confusion in this regard [9]. Restless legs syndrome (RLS) is a pain syndrome that continues to be under-diagnosed and left untreated. This condition is particularly difficult to recognize in young children, who have difficulty expressing symptoms. All too often, such symptoms are attributed to "growing pains." There seems to be a variable ethnic risk for RLS, but new questionnaires have been constructed to help recognize the syndrome. Additionally, several new therapeutic avenues are being investigated, particularly those that avoid the risk of augmentation. The increasing number of medication options also means that the use of secondary drugs will become more widespread. However, one challenge involves the use of methadone and its potential impact on opioid neurons in the medulla, which are responsible for controlling inspiration. If such therapy turns out to be an important adjunct, particularly in medication-resistant older adults, then careful follow-up of breathing during sleep may be needed despite the usually low dosages (5–10 mg) commonly prescribed. Iron infusion has also been a successful approach in adults [10].

Sleep Medicine is also becoming increasingly involved in determining the role played in sleep and its disorders by the contemporary wide use of cellphones, computers, and other electronic devices. Among younger individuals, sleep is becoming more and more restricted, and sleep disruption related to these gadgets is becoming more common. The consequent poor sleep and reduced total sleep time lead to impaired daytime functioning [11]. While industrial accidents are a major concern in this regard, psychiatric well-being is also significantly affected. Sleep restriction and disturbance have been associated with increased suicide risk. Other medical consequences, including altered metabolism and even cancer, have been associated with restricted sleep. In this context, the technology industry has begun to collaborate with sleep researchers, even creating downloadable apps for dealing with these problems. The recent introduction of red light in cellphone and computer displays has the function of filtering out the blue–green frequencies that are known to stimulate receptors in the eye and to inhibit melatonin secretion in the evening.

The industrialized lifestyle, with its changing shift patterns, continuous time-zone changes, and poor sleep habits, has greatly increased the number of complaints of insomnia and the cohort of secondary medical complications. These include recent findings among large groups such as nurses or physicians participating in long-term follow-up studies, which have uncovered significantly increased risks of breast and prostate cancers. The importance of cognitive–behavioral therapy for insomnia (CBTI) has been emphasized year after year when the results of treatment comparisons between pharmacological and behavioral approaches have been presented. Basic research suggests an important role for the genes controlling our circadian and ultradian cycles. These genes are thought to be involved in the supervision of DNA–RNA exchange, with animal models showing increased numbers of erroneous base changes leading to the creation of abnormal cells.

Another large health problem in modern society is the increasing number of elderly people with cognitive impairment. While studies on Alzheimer's disease and sleep-related problems are still limited, the role of REM sleep behavior disorder as a prodromal marker of alpha synucleinopathies by years to decades is bringing more information [12]. Any drug trial aimed at slowing the progression of the neurodegenerative syndrome must include those individuals who may be the potential beneficiaries of any new finding.

In many parts of the world, Sleep Medicine has been allocated to different subspecialties, but such a division of labor is detrimental to patient care and the advancement of research. A multidisciplinary approach within a centralized location allows specialists to see the impact of a problem in its totality, such as the significance of sleep-disordered breathing on ophthalmological or otologic syndromes. The World Health Organization has recognized this need. If ICD-10 is still lacking an independent number for "Sleep/Wake Disorder," this should not be the case with ICD-11.

References

1. Black J, Reaven NL, Funk SE, et al. The Burden of Narcolepsy Disease (BOND) study: health-care utilization and cost findings. Sleep Med 2014;15:522–9.
2. Vijnans L, Lecomte C, de Vries C, et al. The incidence of narcolepsy in Europe, before, during, and after the influenza A (H1N1)pdm09 pandemic and vaccination campaigns. Vaccine 2013;3:1246–52.
3. Han F. Narcolepsy in China: when the east meets the west. Sleep Med 2014;15:605–6.
4. Bonsignore MR, McNicholas WT, Montserrat JM, et al. Adipose tissues in obesity and sleep apnea. Eur Respir J 2012;39:746–67.
5. Guilleminault C, Akhtar F. Pediatric sleep-disordered breathing: new evidence on its development. Sleep Med Rev 2015;24:46–56.
6. Guilleminault C, Primeau M, Chiu HY, et al. Sleep-disordered breathing in Ehlers–Danlos syndrome, a genetic model of OSA. Chest 2013;144:1503–11.
7. Camacho M, Certal V, Abdullatif J, et al. Myofunctional therapy to treat obstructive sleep apnea: a systematic review and meta-analysis. Sleep 2015;38:669–75.
8. Yoshihisa A, Shimizu T, Owada T, et al. Adaptive servo ventilation improves cardiac dysfunction and prognosis in chronic heart failure patients with Cheyne-Stokes respiration. Int Heart J 2011.
9. Cowie MR, Woehrle H, Wegscheider K, et al. Adaptive servo-ventilation for central sleep apnea in systolic heart failure. N Engl J Med 2015;373:1095–105.
10. Garcia-Borregueuero D, Kohnen R, Silber MH, et al. The long term treatment of restless leg syndrome/Willis–Ekbom disease: evidence based guidelines and clinical consensus best practice guidance: a report from the International RLS Study Group. Sleep Med 2013;14:675–84.
11. Nunten T, Ross E, Ray C, et al. Computer use, sleep duration and health symptoms: a cross sectional study of 15 years olds in three countries. Int J Public Health 2014;59:619–28.
12. Boeve BF, Silber MH, Saper CB, et al. Pathophysiology of REM sleep behaviour disorder and relevance to neurodegenerative disease. Brain 2007;130:2770–88.

CHAPTER 13

Classification of sleep disorders

Michael Thorpy

In 2013, the American Psychiatric Association published the revised version of the *Diagnostic and Statistical Manual of Mental Disorders, Fifth Edition* (DSM-V) [1], which includes a section entitled "Sleep Wake Disorders," an update of the DSM-IV section (Box 13.1). The intention of this classification system is to produce a classification for mental health and general medical clinicians who are not experts in sleep medicine. The result is a classification that differs from the *International Classification of Sleep Disorders* (ICSD-3) produced by the American Academy of Sleep Medicine, which was updated in 2014 [2]. The presence of two competing classifications produces some confusion, especially for health insurance companies and for epidemiological research. *The International Classification of Diseases, Modified Version* (ICD-10-CM) [3], adopted in the USA in 2014, contains a classification that more closely conforms to ICSD-3.

DSM-V

The first entry in the DSM-V is insomnia disorder; this diagnostic entry requires the presence of at least one sleep complaint, such as difficulty initiating sleep, that must be present at least three nights per week for at least 3 months. The diagnosis can be coded along with other mental, medical, and sleep disorders. It is a little confusing that the diagnosis can be specified as being episodic if it occurs for at least 1 month, but acute and short-term insomnia that has symptoms for less than 3 months should be coded as "other specified insomnia disorder."

Hypersomnolence disorder is a 3-month history of excessive sleepiness in the presence of significant distress or other impairment. Objective documentation is not required. This diagnosis can be coded along with other mental, medical, and sleep disorders. Narcolepsy is defined as recurrent episodes of sleep that occur for at least 3 months along with one of three additional features, such as cataplexy, hypocretin deficiency, or polysomnographic features, either a sleep onset REM period (SOREMP) on a nighttime polysomnogram (PSG) or a multiple sleep latency test (MSLT) showing a mean sleep latency less than 8 minutes and two or more SOREMPs. So narcolepsy can be diagnosed in DSM-V if just sleepiness occurs for 3 months and there is a SOREMP on the nocturnal PSG. This has the potential of leading to errors in diagnosis, since other disorders, including obstructive sleep apnea syndrome (OSA), can produce similar features. Five subtypes are specified according to the following criteria: the presence or absence of hypocretin deficiency; autosomal dominant cerebellar ataxia, deafness, and narcolepsy (ADCADN); autosomal dominant narcolepsy, obesity and type 2 diabetes (ADNOD); or secondary to another medical condition.

Obstructive sleep apnea syndrome (OSA) is defined as an apnea hypopnea index (AHI) of at least 5 per hour along with typical nocturnal respiratory symptoms, or daytime excessive sleepiness or fatigue. Alternatively the diagnosis requires an AHI of at least 15 regardless of accompanying symptoms. Mild OSA is regarded as an AHI of less than 15, moderate 15–30, and severe greater than 30. Central sleep apnea (CSA) requires the presence of 5 or more central apneas per hour of sleep. Sleep-related hypoventilation has PSG evidence of decreased ventilation with either elevated CO_2 levels or persistent oxygen desaturation unassociated with apneic/hypopneic events. Idiopathic hypoventilation, congenital central alveolar hypoventilation, and comorbid sleep-related hypoventilation can be specified.

Circadian rhythm sleep–wake disorders, with five subtypes, is defined as a persistent or recurrent pattern of sleep disruption due to an alteration or misalignment of the endogenous circadian rhythm and the individual's required sleep–wake schedule, along with symptoms of either insomnia or excessive sleepiness or both. The subtypes are delayed sleep phase type, advanced sleep phase type, irregular sleep–wake type, non-24-hour sleep–wake type, and shiftwork type, none of which has any specific diagnostic criteria.

The parasomnias are subdivided into five disorders; non-rapid eye movement (NREM) sleep arousal disorder, nightmare disorder, rapid eye movement (REM) sleep behavior disorder (RBD), restless legs syndrome (RLS), and substance/medication-induced sleep disorder. NREM sleep arousal disorder is divided into two types by the typical features of either sleepwalking or sleep terrors. Confusional arousals as defined in ICSD-3 are not included as a specific disorder. The sleepwalking type can have sleep-related eating or sleep-related sexual behavior (sexsomnia) specifications. Nightmare disorder is defined as repeated occurrences of extended, dysphoric, and well-remembered dreams that threaten the individual. Rapid orientation and alertness follows the episode and causes significant distress. RBD comprises recurrent episodes of arousal with vocalization and /or complex movements from REM sleep that is documented by either PSG or a history suggesting a synucleinopathy. RLS is an urge to move the legs accompanied by uncomfortable sensations in the legs with the typical features that occur at least three times per week for at least 3 months. It is unclear from where the definition of three times a week was derived. Sleep/medication-induced sleep disorder is a sleep disturbance either during or soon after substance intoxication or after withdrawal, or when the substance is known to cause sleep disturbance. The substance should be specified.

Other specified insomnia disorder is specified when the insomnia does not meet the criteria for insomnia disorder, and other

Box 13.1 DSM-V

Sleep–wake disorders

- ◆ Insomnia disorder
- ◆ Hypersomnolence disorder
- ◆ Narcolepsy
  - Subtypes:
    - Presence or absence of hypocretin deficiency
    - Autosomal dominant cerebellar ataxia
      Deafness and narcolepsy (ADCADN)
    - Autosomal dominant narcolepsy
      Obesity and type 2 diabetes (ADNOD)
    - Secondary to another medical condition
- ◆ Obstructive sleep apnea syndrome
- ◆ Central sleep apnea
- ◆ Sleep-related hypoventilation
  - Subtypes:
    - Idiopathic hyperventilation
    - Congenital central alveolar hypoventilation
    - Comorbid sleep-related hypoventilation
- ◆ **Circadian rhythm sleep disorder**
  - Delayed sleep phase type
  - Advanced sleep phase type
  - Irregular sleep–wake type
  - Non-24-hour sleep–wake type
  - Shiftwork disorder
  - Unspecified type
- ◆ **Parasomnias**
  - Non-rapid eye movement sleep arousal disorder
    - Subtypes:
      - Sleepwalking type
      - Sleep terror type
  - Nightmare disorder
  - Rapid eye movement sleep behavior disorder
- ◆ Restless legs syndrome
- ◆ Substance/medication-induced sleep disorder
- ◆ Other specified insomnia disorder
- ◆ Other specified hypersomnolence disorder
- ◆ Unspecified sleep–wake disorder
- ◆ Unspecified insomnia disorder
- ◆ Unspecified hypersomnolence disorder
- ◆ Unspecified sleep–wake disorder

Source data from American Psychiatric Association, Diagnostic and Statistical Manual of Mental Disorders, 5th Edition DSM-5, Copyright (2013), American Psychiatric Association.

hypersomnolence disorder when the excessive sleepiness does not meet the criteria for hypersomnolence disorder. Similarly, unspecified sleep–wake disorder is specified when the sleep–wake disorder does not meet the full criteria for the specified sleep–wake disorders. Unspecified forms of insomnia disorder, hypersomnolence disorder, and sleep–wake disorder exist.

ICSD-3

ICSD-3 is a major revision of ICSD-2 and was published in March 2014 (Table 13.1). The main change was the simplification of the insomnia disorders and an expansion of the sleep-related breathing disorders.

The organization of ICSD-3 produced a greater degree of standardization between disorder texts. It includes information in all the following categories where available:

- ◆ Alternate names
- ◆ Diagnostic criteria
- ◆ Essential features
- ◆ Associated features
- ◆ Clinical and pathophysiological subtypes
- ◆ Demographics: prevalence, gender bias, racial/ethnic bias, cultural issues
- ◆ Predisposing and precipitating factors: risk factors, familial pattern (genetics, familial clusters)
- ◆ Onset, course, and complications: medical, neurological, psychiatric/social
- ◆ Developmental issues: pediatric, geriatric
- ◆ Pathology and pathophysiology
- ◆ Objective findings: sleep logs, actigraphy, questionnaires, polysomnography, multiple sleep latency test (MSLT), neurological (electroencephalogram, cerebrospinal fluid (CSF), neuroimaging, electromyogram, autonomic), endocrine, genetic testing
- ◆ Physical findings: respiratory (arterial blood gas, pulmonary function, ventilatory response), cardiac (electrocardiogram, echocardiogram, cardiac catheterization), serum chemistry

Several disorders are now classified as isolated symptoms and normal variants, including excessive time in bed, short-sleeper, snoring, catathrenia, long-sleeper, sleep-talking, excessive fragmentary myoclonus, hypnagogic foot tremor and alternating leg muscle activation, and sleep starts (hypnic jerks).

Insomnia disorders

The insomnia disorders are characterized by one major disorder termed chronic insomnia disorder. This recognizes the fact that the clinical features of insomnia can be the result of a primary or secondary process, but the consequences are similar no matter what the etiology [4]. The diagnosis rests upon a sleep symptom such as difficulty initiating sleep that occurs three times per week for at least 3 months and has daytime consequences. Psychophysiological insomnia and insomnia disorders of ICSD-2 are mentioned as subtypes of chronic insomnia disorder. The inclusion of short-term insomnia disorder with similar diagnostic criteria applies to insomnia that is less than 3 months in duration. Excessive time in bed

Table 13.1 ICSD-3

	ICD-9-CM code	ICD-10-CM code
Insomnia disorders		
Chronic insomnia disorder	342	F51.01
Short-term insomnia disorder	307.41	F51.02
Other insomnia disorder	307.49	F51.09
Isolated symptoms and normal variants:		
Excessive time in bed		
Short sleeper		
Sleep-related breathing disorders		
Obstructive sleep apnea disorders:		
Obstructive Sleep apnea, adult	327.23	G47.33
Obstructive sleep apnea, pediatric	327.23	G47.33
Central sleep apnea syndromes:		
Central sleep apnea with Cheyne–Stokes breathing	786.04	R06.3
Central apnea due to a medical disorder without Cheyne–Stokes breathing	327.27	G47.37
Central sleep apnea due to high-altitude periodic breathing	327.22	G47.32
Central sleep apnea due to a medication or substance	327.29	G47.39
Primary central sleep apnea	327.21	G47.31
Primary central sleep apnea of infancy	770.81	P28.3
Primary central sleep apnea of prematurity	770.82	P28.4
Treatment-emergent central sleep apnea	327.29	G47.39
Sleep-related hypoventilation disorders:		
Obesity hypoventilation syndrome	278.03	E66.2
Congenital central alveolar hypoventilation syndrome	327.25	G47.35
Late-onset central hypoventilation with hypothalamic dysfunction	327.26	G47.36
Idiopathic central alveolar hypoventilation	327.24	G47.34
Sleep-related hypoventilation due to a medication or substance	327.26	G47.36
Sleep-related hypoventilation due to a medical disorder	327.26	G47.36
Sleep-related hypoxemia disorder:		
Sleep-related hypoxemia	327.26	G47.36
Isolated symptoms and normal variants:		
Snoring		
Catathrenia		

Table 13.1 Continued

	ICD-9-CM code	ICD-10-CM code
Central disorders of hypersomnolence		
Narcolepsy type 1	347.01	G47.411
Narcolepsy type 2	347.00	G47.419
Idiopathic hypersomnia	327.11	G47.11
Kleine–Levin syndrome	327.13	G47.13
Hypersomnia due to a medical disorder	327.14	G47.14
Hypersomnia due to a medication or substance	292.85 (drug-induced)	F11–F19
	291.82 (alcohol-induced)	
Hypersomnia associated with a psychiatric disorder	327.15	F51.13
Insufficient sleep syndrome	307.44	F51.12
Isolated symptoms and normal variants:		
Long sleeper		
Circadian rhythm sleep–wake disorders		
Delayed sleep–wake phase disorder	327.31	G47.21
Advanced sleep–wake phase disorder	327.32	G47.22
Irregular sleep–wake rhythm disorder	327.33	G47.23
Non-24-hour sleep–wake rhythm disorder	327.34	G47.24
Shiftwork disorder	327.36	G47.26
Jet lag disorder	327.35	G47.25
Circadian sleep–wake disorder not otherwise specified (NOS)	327.30	G47.20
Parasomnias		
NREM-related parasomnias:		
Disorders of arousal (from NREM sleep):		
Confusional arousals	327.41	G47.51
Sleepwalking	307.46	F51.3
Sleep terrors	307.46	F51.4
Sleep-related eating disorder	327.40	G47.59
REM-related parasomnias:		
REM sleep behavior disorder	327.42	G47.52
Recurrent isolated sleep paralysis	327.43	G47.51
Nightmare disorder	307.47	F51.5
Other parasomnias:		
Exploding head syndrome	327.49	G47.59
Sleep-related hallucinations	368.16	H53.16
Sleep enuresis	788.36	N39.44

(continued)

Table 13.1 Continued

	ICD-9-CM code	ICD-10-CM code
Parasomnia due to a medical disorder	327.44	G47.54
Parasomnia due to a medication or substance	292.85 (drug-induced)	F11–F19
	291.82 (alcohol-induced)	
Parasomnia, unspecified	327.40	G47.50
Isolated symptoms and normal variants:		
Sleep talking		
Sleep-related movement disorders		
Restless legs syndrome	333.94	G25.81
Periodic limb movement disorder	327.51	G47.61
Sleep-related leg cramps	327.52	G47.62
Sleep-related bruxism	327.53	G47.63
Sleep-related rhythmic movement disorder	327.59	G47.69
Benign sleep myoclonus of infancy	327.59	G47.69
Propriospinal myoclonus at sleep onset	327.59	G47.69
Sleep-related movement disorder due to a medical disorder	327.59	G47.69
Sleep-related movement disorder due to a medication or substance	292.85 (drug-induced)	F11–F19
	291.82 (alcohol-induced)	
Sleep-related movement disorder, unspecified	327.59	G47.69
Isolated symptoms and normal variants:		
Excessive fragmentary myoclonus		
Hypnagogic foot tremor and alternating leg muscle activation		
Sleep starts (hypnic jerks)		
Other sleep disorder	327.8	G47.8
Appendix A		
Fatal familial insomnia	046.8	A81.83
Sleep-related epilepsy	345	G40.5
Sleep-related headaches	784.0	R51
Sleep-related laryngospasm	787.2	J38.5
Sleep-related gastroesophageal reflux	530.1	K21.9
Sleep-related myocardial ischemia	411.8	I25.6
Appendix B		
ICD-10-CM coding for substance-induced sleep disorders		F10–F19

Source data from American Academy of Sleep Medicine, International classification of sleep disorders, 3rd ed., Copyright (2014) American Academy of Sleep Medicine.

and short-sleeper are included as isolated symptoms and normal variants, not as specific disorders.

Sleep-related breathing disorders

The sleep-related breathing disorders are organized into four main categories: obstructive sleep apnea (OSA) disorders, central sleep apnea (CSA) syndromes, sleep-related hypoventilation disorders, and sleep-related hypoxemia disorder. The CSA syndromes are divided into eight types: two related to Cheyne–Stokes breathing (CSB), namely, high altitude and substance, three primary CSA disorders of which one is infancy and the other prematurity, and a new entity entitled treatment-emergent CSA. The last category applies to central apnea that follows continuous positive airway pressure (CPAP) administration.

OSA syndrome maintains the criterion of 5 or more respiratory events per hour of sleep when studied in a sleep center or by out-of-center sleep studies (OCST), so long as typical symptoms are present; otherwise 15 or more predominantly obstructive respiratory events are sufficient to make the diagnosis. The OSA disorders are divided into adult and pediatric types. In the pediatric criteria, for those less than 18 years of age, only one obstructive event is required per hour of sleep, so long as respiratory symptoms or sleepiness are present; alternatively, obstructive hypoventilation along with symptoms is required.

CSA with CSB (CSA-CSB) is 5 or more central apnea or hypopneas per hour of sleep with a pattern that meets the criteria for CSB. CSA without CSB is diagnosed as CSA due to a medical disorder without CSB that occurs as a consequence of a medical or neurological disorder. CSA due to high-altitude periodic breathing is central apnea attributable to high altitude of at least 1500 m but usually above 2500 m. CSA due to a medicine or substance is most typically due to an opioid or respiratory depressant not associated with CSB. Primary CSA is 5 or more central apneas or central hypopneas per hour of sleep in the absence of CSB and of unknown etiology. Primary CSA of infancy occurs in an infant with greater than 37 weeks conceptional age with recurrent, prolonged (>20 s duration) central apneas and periodic breathing for more than 5% of total sleep time during sleep. Primary CSA of prematurity occurs in an infant of less than 37 weeks conceptional age with similar respiratory events.

Treatment-emergent CSA is diagnosed when 5 or more obstructive events during a PSG with CPAP that shows resolution of obstructive events and presence of central apneas or hypopneas [5].

Central disorders of hypersomnolence

There are eight central disorders of hypersomnolence. Narcolepsy has undergone a major revision with elimination of the disorder name terms "with cataplexy" and "without cataplexy." Type 1 narcolepsy is that presumed to be due to hypocretin loss with either measured reduction in CSF hypocretin or cataplexy with associated electrophysiological findings. Type 2 narcolepsy 2 is that which is confirmed by electrophysiological studies in the absence of cataplexy or with a normal CSF hypocretin level. A major change in the narcolepsy criteria is the inclusion of a SOREMP on the nocturnal PSG as one of the two requirements for meeting the MSLT criteria of two SOREMPs for diagnosis. This amendment was based upon a study indicating that the positive predictive value of a SOREMP on the nocturnal PSG for narcolepsy is 92% [6]. Approximately 50% of patients with narcolepsy will have a SOREMP of less than 15 minutes on the nocturnal PSG.

Idiopathic hypersomnia is now a single entity, with elimination of the two ICSD-2 hypersomnia disorders that had specific sleep duration criteria. The new idiopathic hypersomnia disorder requires either an MSLT mean sleep latency of 8 minutes or less or a total 24-hour sleep duration of at least 660 minutes. The ICSD-2 category of recurrent hypersomnia has been reduced to a single entry, namely, Kleine–Levin syndrome, with a subtype of menstrual-related Kleine–Levin syndrome [7]. The sleepiness must persist for 2 days to 5 weeks and occur at least once every 18 months. There can be only one symptom in addition to the sleepiness, namely, cognitive dysfunction, altered perception, eating disorder, or disinhibited behavior.

Insufficient sleep syndrome is the new term for the previous more cumbersome term of behaviorally induced insufficient sleep syndrome. The reduced sleep must be present most days for at least 3 months. Extension of sleep time must result in resolution of symptoms. The other three items in the hypersomnia disorders section are hypersomnia related to a medical disorder, to medication or substances, or to psychiatric disorder.

Long-sleeper is no longer regarded as a disorder but as a normal variant. There are no diagnostic criteria, but a total sleep time of 10 or more hours is suggested as being usually accepted.

Circadian rhythm sleep–wake disorders

The circadian rhythm sleep–wake disorders (CRSWDs) comprise six specific disorders: delayed sleep–wake phase disorder (DSWPD), advanced sleep–wake phase disorder (ASWPD), irregular sleep–wake rhythm disorder, non-24-hour sleep–wake rhythm disorder, shiftwork disorder, and jet lag disorder. These disorders arise when there is a substantial misalignment between the internal circadian rhythm and the desired sleep–wake schedule. Specific general diagnostic criteria are given for CRSWDs. A 3-month duration of symptoms is a requirement for diagnosing all these disorders except for jet lag disorder, which has a requirement of jet travel across at least two time zones. A circadian rhythm disorder not otherwise specified (NOS) is listed for patients who meet all the criteria for a CRSWD but not the specific types.

Parasomnias

The parasomnias are divided into three groups: NREM-related parasomnias, REM-related parasomnias, and other parasomnias. They are defined as undesirable physical events or experiences that occur during entry into sleep, within sleep, and during arousal from sleep.

The NREM-related parasomnias are defined based on general diagnostic criteria for the group heading of disorders of arousal (from NREM sleep). Specific general diagnostic criteria are given for disorders of arousal (DA), and the detailed text applies to all of the DAs, since no text is presented for each of the specific DAs except for diagnostic criteria. Sleep-related abnormal sexual behavior is listed as a subtype to be classified under confusional arousals. Diagnostic criteria are given for three disorders; confusional arousals, sleepwalking, and sleep terrors. The final NREM-related parasomnia, sleep-related eating disorder (SRED), requires an arousal from the main sleep period to distinguish it from night eating syndrome (NES) disorder, which is excessive eating between dinner and bedtime, and SRED requires an adverse health consequence from the disorder [8].

The REM-related parasomnias include REM sleep behavior disorder (RBD), recurrent isolated sleep paralysis (RISP) and nightmare disorder. RBD, which is repeated episodes of vocalizations and/or complex motor behaviors, requires PSG evidence of REM sleep without atonia (RWA) [9]. RISP is a recurrent inability to move the trunk and all of the limbs at sleep onset or upon awakening from sleep that causes distress or fear of sleep. Nightmare disorder is repeated occurrences of extended, extremely dysphoric, and well-remembered dreams that usually involve threats to survival, security, or physical integrity.

The section on other parasomnias includes three specific disorders: exploding head syndrome (EHS), sleep-related hallucinations, and sleep enuresis. EHS is a complaint of a sudden noise or sense of explosion in the head either at the wake–sleep transition or upon awakening during the night associated with abrupt arousal. Sleep-related hallucinations are predominantly visual hallucinations that are experienced just before sleep onset or upon awakening during the night or in the morning. Sleep enuresis is involuntary voiding during sleep at least twice a week in people older than 5 years of age. Parasomnias associated with medical disorders, and medication or substance and unspecific parasomnia, comprise the other entries in this category. Sleep talking is a normal variant that can occur in both NREM or REM sleep and can be associated with parasomnias such as RBD or DAs.

Sleep-related movement disorders

The sleep-related movement disorders (SRMDs) comprises seven specific disorders: restless legs syndrome (RLS), periodic limb movement disorder (PLMD), sleep-related leg cramps, sleep bruxism, sleep-related rhythmic disorder (RMD), benign sleep myoclonus of infancy (BSMI), and propriospinal myoclonus at sleep onset (PSM). SRMDs are relatively simple, usually stereotyped, movements that disturb sleep or its onset.

RLS (also known as Willis–Ekbom disease, WED) is an urge to move the legs, usually accompanied by or thought to be caused by uncomfortable and unpleasant sensations in the legs, and these symptoms begin or worsen during periods of rest or inactivity, are partially or totally relieved by movement, and occur exclusively or predominantly in the evening or night. In addition, these features are not solely accounted for as symptoms of another medical or behavioral condition. The ICSD-3 criteria do not include any frequency or duration criteria as is contained in the DSM-V criteria, but do include clinically significant RLS symptoms causing distress or impairment of function, in contrast to International Restless Legs Syndrome Study Group (IRLSSG) criteria.

PLMD is defined by the polysomnographic demonstration of periodic limb movements (PLMS) of >5 per hour in children and >15 per hour in adults that cause significant sleep disturbance or impairment of functioning. Sleep-related leg cramps are painful sensations that occur in the leg or foot with sudden, involuntary muscle hardness, or tightness. Sleep-related bruxism is tooth grinding during sleep that is associated with tooth wear or morning jaw muscle pain or fatigue. RMD is repetitive, stereotyped, and rhythmic motor behaviors involving large muscle groups that are sleep related. BSMI is repetitive myoclonic jerking that involves the limbs, trunk, or whole body and occurs from birth to 6 months of age during sleep. As PSM mainly occurs during relaxed wakefulness and drowsiness as the patient attempts to sleep, the term "at sleep onset" has been added to the propriospinal myoclonus name. The three final categories are related to a medical disorder, medication of substance, and an unspecified parasomnia.

Isolated symptoms and normal variants include excessive fragmentary myoclonus (EFM), hypnagogic foot tremor and alternating muscle activation, and sleep starts (hypnic jerks). EFM is now regarded as a normal variant found on PSG EMG recordings that are characterized by small movements of the corners of the mouth, fingers or toes or without visible movement. Hypnagogic foot tremor (HFT) is rhythmic movement of the feet or toes that occurs in the transition between wake and sleep or in light NREM sleep, and alternating muscle activation (ALMA) is brief activation of the anterior tibialis in one leg with alternation in the other leg. Sleep starts (hypnic jerks) are brief, simultaneous contractions of the body or one or more body segments occurring at sleep onset.

Other sleep disorder

The final category in the ICSD-3 is a general other sleep disorder category for disorders that cannot be classified elsewhere.

Appendices to ICDS-3

Appendix A lists several disorders that are coded in sections of ICD-10 other than the sleep sections, including fatal familial insomnia, sleep-related epilepsy, sleep-related headaches, sleep-related laryngospasm, sleep-related gastroesophageal reflux, and sleep-related myocardial ischemia (Box 13.2). Appendix B lists the ICD-10 sleep-related substance-induced sleep disorders.

Box 13.2 ICD-10-CM sleep disorders

F51 Sleep disorders not due to a substance or known physiological condition

  F51.0 Insomnia not due to a substance or known physiological condition

  F51.01 Primary insomnia

  F51.02 Adjustment insomnia

  F51.03 Paradoxical insomnia

  F51.04 Psychophysiological insomnia

  F51.05 Insomnia due to other mental disorder

  F51.09 Other insomnia not due to a substance or known physiological condition

  F51.1 Hypersomnia not due to a substance or know physiological condition

  F51.11 Primary hypersomnia

  F51.12 Insufficient sleep syndrome

  F51.13 Hypersomnia due to other mental disorder

  F51.19 Other hypersomnia not due to a substance or known physiological condition

  F51.3 Sleepwalking (somnambulism)

  F51.4 Sleep terrors (night terrors)

  F51.5 Nightmare disorder

  F51.8 Other sleep disorders not due to a substance or known physiological condition

  F51.9 Sleep disorder not due to a substance or known physiological condition, unspecified

---

Box 13.2 Continued

G47 Organic sleep disorders

  G47.0 Insomnia

    G47.00 Insomnia, unspecified

    G47.01 Insomnia due to medical condition

    G47.09 Other insomnia

  G47.1 Hypersomnia

    G47.10 Hypersomnia, unspecified

    G47.11 Idiopathic hypersomnia with long sleep time

    G47.12 Idiopathic hypersomnia without long sleep time

    G47.13 Recurrent hypersomnia

    G47.14 Hypersomnia due to medical condition

    G47.19 Other hypersomnia

  G47.2 Circadian rhythm sleep disorders

    G47.20 Circadian rhythm sleep disorder, unspecified type

    G47.21 Circadian rhythm sleep disorder, delayed sleep phase type

    G47.22 Circadian rhythm sleep disorder, advanced sleep phase type

    G47.23 Circadian rhythm sleep disorder, irregular sleep wake type

    G47.24 Circadian rhythm sleep disorder, free running type

    G47.25 Circadian rhythm sleep disorder, jet lag type

    G47.26 Circadian rhythm sleep disorder, shiftwork type

    G47.27 Circadian rhythm sleep disorder in conditions classified elsewhere

    G47.29 Other circadian rhythm sleep disorder

  G47.3 Sleep apnea

    G47.30 Sleep apnea, unspecified

    G47.31 Primary central sleep apnea

    G47.32 High-altitude periodic breathing

    G47.33 Obstructive sleep apnea (adult) (pediatric)

    G47.34 Idiopathic sleep related nonobstructive alveolar hypoventilation

    G47.35 Congenital central alveolar hypoventilation syndrome

    G47.36 Sleep related hypoventilation in conditions classified elsewhere

    G47.37 Central sleep apnea in conditions classified elsewhere

    G47.39 Other sleep apnea

  G47.4 Narcolepsy and cataplexy

    G47.41 Narcolepsy

      G47.411 Narcolepsy with cataplexy

      G47.419 Narcolepsy without cataplexy, NOS

(continued)

Box 13.2 Continued

G47.42 Narcolepsy in conditions classified elsewhere

G47.421 Narcolepsy in conditions classified elsewhere with cataplexy

G47.429 Narcolepsy in conditions classified elsewhere without cataplexy

G47.5 Parasomnia

G47.50 Parasomnia, unspecified

G47.51 Confusional arousals

G47.52 REM sleep behavior disorder

G47.53 Recurrent isolated sleep paralysis

G47.54 Parasomnia in conditions classified elsewhere

G47.59 Other parasomnia

G47.6 Sleep related movement disorders

G47.61 Periodic limb movement disorder

G47.62 Sleep-related leg cramps

G47.63 Sleep-related bruxism

G47.69 Other sleep-related movement disorders

G47.8 Other sleep disorders

G47.9 Sleep disorder, unspecified

Z72 Problems related to lifestyle

Z72.8 Other problems related to lifestyle

Z72.82 Problems related to sleep

Z72.820 Sleep deprivation

Z72.821 Inadequate sleep hygiene

Z73 Problems related to life management difficulty

Z73.8 Other problems related to life management difficulty

Z73.81 Behavioral insomnia of childhood

Z73.810 Behavioral insomnia of childhood, sleep onset association type

Z73.811 Behavioral insomnia of childhood, limit setting type

Z73.812 Behavioral insomnia of childhood, combined type

Z73.819 Behavioral insomnia of childhood, unspecified type

Source data from World Health Organization, International Classification of Diseases, Tenth Revision, Clinical Modification (ICD-10-CM), Copyright (2010), World Health Organization.

Conclusion

The new ICSD-3 is a major advance over previous versions, but it is unfortunate that some of the diagnostic criteria differ from those of DSM-V, for example, the criteria for narcolepsy. However, DSM-V serves as an entry level classification, mainly for psychiatrists, and it is to be hoped that in the future the two classifications will be merged into one that will cause less confusion not only for clinicians but also for agencies that reimburse for healthcare and provide for treatment options.

References

1. American Psychiatric Association. Diagnostic and statistical manual of mental disorders, 5th ed. (DSM-V). Washington DC: American Psychiatric Association, 2013.
2. American Academy of Sleep Medicine. International classification of sleep disorders, 3rd ed. Darien, IL: American Academy of Sleep Medicine, 2014.
3. International Classification of Diseases, Tenth revision, Clinical Modification (ICD-10-CM), National Center for Health Statistics. Centers for Disease Control and Prevention (CDC), December 20, 2010.
4. Edinger JD, Wyatt JK, Stepanski EJ, et al. Testing the reliability and validity of DSM-IV-TR and ICSD-2 insomnia diagnoses: results of a multi-method/multi-trait analysis. Arch Gen Psychiatry 2011;68:992–1002.
5. Westhoff M, Arzt M, Litterst P. Prevalence and treatment of central sleep apnoea emerging after initiation of continuous positive airway pressure in patients with obstructive sleep apnoea without evidence of heart failure. Sleep Breath 2012;16:71–8.
6. Andlauer O, Moore H, Jouhier L, et al. Nocturnal REM sleep latency for identifying patients with narcolepsy/hypocretin deficiency. JAMA Neurol 2013;6:1–12.
7. Arnulf I, Lin L, Gadoth N, et al. Kleine–Levin syndrome: a systematic study of 108 patients. Ann Neurol 2008;63:482–93.
8. Brion A, Flamand M, Oudiette D, et al. Sleep related eating disorder versus sleepwalking: a controlled study. Sleep Med 2012; 3:1094–101.
9. Schenck CH, Howell MJ. Spectrum of RBD (overlap between RBD and other parasomnias). Sleep Biol Rhythms 2013;11(Suppl 1):27–34.

SECTION 4

Hypersomnias

CHAPTER 14

Narcolepsy with cataplexy

Gert Jan Lammers

Introduction

Narcolepsy with cataplexy is usually described as a syndrome characterized by excessive daytime sleepiness (EDS), cataplexy, hypnagogic hallucinations, sleep paralysis, and disturbed nocturnal sleep. Although this is in itself correct, simply listing these symptoms does not convey what it means to suffer from narcolepsy. The key problem of these patients, relentlessly present each and every day of their lives, is their inability to remain fully alert or even awake during longer periods of the day, paradoxically accompanied by difficulty remaining asleep during the night. In addition, the strict physiological boundaries of specific components of wake and sleep stages are fluid. This leads to partial expressions, particularly of identifiable REM sleep, explaining such symptoms as cataplexy, hypnagogic hallucinations, and sleep paralysis. The loss of state boundaries leads to more symptoms that are not always emphasized in textbooks, such as automatic behavior, memory complaints, and dream delusions. Moreover, those who suffer from narcolepsy with cataplexy clearly bear a risk for obesity, fatigability, and psychiatric comorbidities such as anxiety, depression, and possibly also eating disorders. The disorder has a severe negative impact on daily functioning and quality of life. It is more detrimental when it starts during childhood than adulthood because of the additional negative impact on social development and achievements at school.

Narcolepsy can be divided into narcolepsy with and without cataplexy [1–4]. In the most recent International Classification of Sleep Disorders, these have been rephrased as narcolepsy type 1 and narcolepsy type 2, with the only difference being that if a patient who suffers from narcolepsy without cataplexy turns out to be hypocretin-deficient, that patient is labeled as suffering from narcolepsy type 1 [5]. Narcolepsy with cataplexy is considered to be a homogeneous disease entity, a "morbus sui generis," of which the pathophysiological hallmark is a loss of hypocretin (also called orexin) cells in the hypothalamus (Fig. 14.1). A very small percentage of these patients (less than 2%) suffer from a familial or symptomatic form. "Symptomatic" in this context means that that there is a known cause, in contrast to the majority who suffer from what is also called "idiopathic" narcolepsy (in fact, this chapter is about the 98% of idiopathic narcolepsy patients). Symptomatic cases may also be labeled as "narcolepsy with cataplexy due to medical condition". Possible causes are a tumor in the hypothalamic area, paraneoplastic or Niemann-Pick disease type C. The majority of these cases also show other symptoms beyond the known symptoms of narcolepsy. In some hypocretin cells may remain intact, and hypocretin-1 levels in the CSF may remain normal. In these cases a disturbance of hypocretin transmission on a different level is presumed.

Narcolepsy without cataplexy may be no more than a heterogeneous group of disorders characterized by EDS in combination with abnormal expressions of REM sleep on the multiple sleep latency test (MSLT) [6]. Some of this group will develop narcolepsy with cataplexy later on, and some may represent a "forme fruste" of narcolepsy with cataplexy. These patients may have a less severe hypocretin cell loss than narcolepsy with cataplexy patients. Post-mortem brain studies, performed in a very limited number of patients, support this view [7]. However, probably a larger percentage represents both patients with a real hypersomnia of undetermined cause (at least not caused by a deficient hypocretin transmission) and subjects with a lifestyle-induced hypersomnia. The existence of these last groups raises the question of whether the ICSD-3-required PSG/MSLT findings for narcolepsy type 2 are specific and consistent enough to be useful. There are indications that chronic sleep deprivation or shiftwork in otherwise healthy individuals may be enough to cause the MSLT abnormalities, and repeated testing may show occurrence and disappearance of sleep onset REM sleep on MSLT testing [8–10]. At any rate, most cases of narcolepsy without cataplexy do not develop cataplexy later on, so it is not simply an early stage of narcolepsy with cataplexy.

Epidemiology

Narcolepsy with cataplexy has an estimated prevalence of 25–50 per 100 000. The incidence is estimated to be 0.74–1.37 per 100 000 person-years [11–13]. There are no reliable prevalence or incidence estimations of narcolepsy without cataplexy.

Age of onset is usually between 15–35 years, but it may start at any age. EDS is the first symptom to occur in the vast majority of patients [14]. In less than 10%, the first symptom is cataplexy. In more than 40% of patients, cataplexy appears within weeks from the start of EDS, and in 85% within 3 years. Nevertheless, appearance many years or even decades after the first symptoms is possible. During the last few years, a growing number of childhood cases have been diagnosed.

The symptoms

Excessive daytime sleepiness

EDS is the leading symptom of narcolepsy (Fig. 14.2). It usually develops over weeks to months, but may also start more acutely. After its occurrence, it is relentlessly present daily [1–3,5].

EDS is characterized not just by an inability to stay awake, but also by a subjective feeling of sleepiness that is expressed in a difficulty in concentrating and in sustaining attention, leading to impaired performance while seemingly being awake [15]. Performance deficits and sleep(iness) typically occur during monotonous activities such as watching television, reading a book, attending a meeting, or

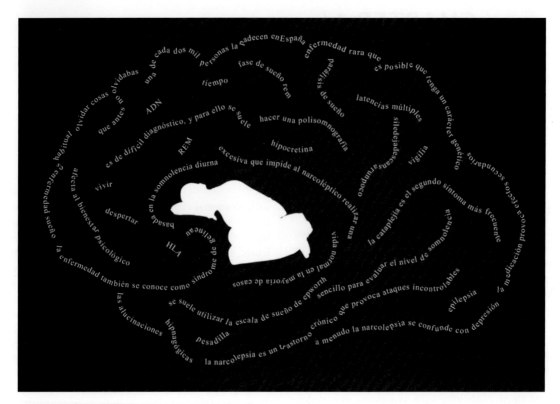

Fig. 14.1 Narcolepsy is caused by selective cell loss in the hypothalamus.
Illustration made by Guillermo Rodilla Marin.

being a passenger in a car. In more severe cases, sleep attacks may also occur when patients are more active, such as during dinner, while walking, or even when riding a bicycle. Sleep attacks tend to be short, usually less than 20 minutes, sometimes only several minutes, and refreshing for some time. However, longer sleep attacks do not exclude the diagnosis. The number may vary from one to over ten each day, depending not only on the severity of the narcolepsy but also on the circumstances. Physical activity reduces the chance to fall asleep. Although falling asleep during the day is labeled as "sleep attacks," the onset of sleep is typically insidious over at least seconds and often more than half a minute, and not very sudden/acute.

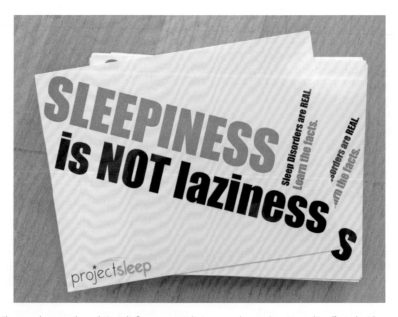

Fig. 14.2 Postcards made by Julie Flygare, who runs the website Julieflygare.com. Julie is a narcolepsy advocate and is affected with narcolepsy.
Julieflygare.com

Narcolepsy patients do not actually spend a greater portion of their time asleep across the 24 hours of the day when compared with people who do not have narcolepsy. This is mainly explained by recurring wake periods during their nocturnal sleep. There are some indications that if narcolepsy starts abruptly, there may be a significantly increased need for sleep in the early stage of the disease, disappearing over weeks to months.

EDS must be distinguished from tiredness or fatigue. The last two conceptions refer to an experience related to exhaustion. This may be a complaint of narcolepsy (as in many other chronic conditions, including depression), but is not a (core) symptoms of narcolepsy [16]. Fatigue without sleepiness is not compatible with narcolepsy. When fatigue is present, it may aggravate the complaint of EDS, because it is usually associated with less (physical) activity.

Automatic behavior is another expression of EDS: the performance of a semi-purposeful, inadequate daytime activity. A patient may for instance continue to write in a state of drowsiness, resulting in illegible handwriting, or put the laundry in the tumble dryer instead of the washing machine.

In childhood cases, behavioral abnormalities including hyperactive or aggressive behavior may accompany EDS and may even be more pronounced problems than EDS, at least for parents [17]. This behavior is not seen in adult cases, although in adulthood EDS may be accompanied by irritability.

Cataplexy

Cataplexy is the only specific symptom of narcolepsy. It is characterized by a sudden bilateral loss of skeletal muscle tone, with preserved consciousness, elicited by emotions [2,5,18]. All striated skeletal muscles can be involved, except the extraocular and respiratory muscles. Cataplexy may be complete, indicating complete loss of activity of all muscle groups. But more often it is partial, only affecting control over the knees, face, and neck. Neck weakness, producing head drop, is common, whereas facial weakness may lead to sagging of the jaw and dysarthria (Fig. 14.3). Although respiratory muscles are not involved, patients sometimes describe shortness of breath during an attack. Complete attacks may cause falls. Because it takes several seconds for a complete attack to build up, most patients are able to take countermeasures and prevent injury. Jerks and twitches may occur, usually in the face. Mirth is the most typical trigger, which usually involves laughter. Laughing out loud, telling a joke, and making a witty remark are typical triggers [18]. Although laughter is the strongest trigger, various emotions may induce an attack, including, for example, the unexpected meeting of an acquaintance and anger [18].

The cataplexy phenotype differs widely between patients, but usually is stereotypical within a patient. If complete attacks occur, they usually start as the typical partial attack of the individual. Also, the frequency of attacks varies widely from dozens a day to less than once a month. Most attacks last seconds to half a minute, sometimes up to 2 minutes, but only rarely longer. If longer, these are usually sequential attacks when the trigger remains. Partial attacks tend to be shorter than complete ones, the majority even (much) less than 10 seconds. Patients may avoid situations in which cataplexy may occur. A so-called "status cataplecticus" may be induced by acute withdrawal of medication, such as tricyclics and mazindol, or when initiating prazosin treatment for concomitant hypertension. It is characterized by an almost continuous succession of cataplectic attacks, in part without identifiable trigger, that may last from hours to days. Although cataplexy is the only truly specific feature of narcolepsy, it is the first symptom to appear in less than 10% of cases, and it may appear many years or even decades after developing EDS.

During childhood, a different phenotype may develop, characterized by prominent facial involvement with a droopy expression, eyelid ptosis, and paroxysmal episodes of mouth opening and tongue protrusion, also called "cataplectic facies." This predominant facial hypotonia may be accompanied by prolonged periods of hypotonia presenting as a paroxysmal gait disorder that may mimic cerebellar ataxia [17,19,20]. Frequently there are superimposed active motor phenomena that can be confused with tics, chorea, or dystonia. Typical triggers for children include watching a funny movie and playing (video) games. However, an emotional trigger may be hard to identify or may even be absent in young children, particularly close to disease onset.

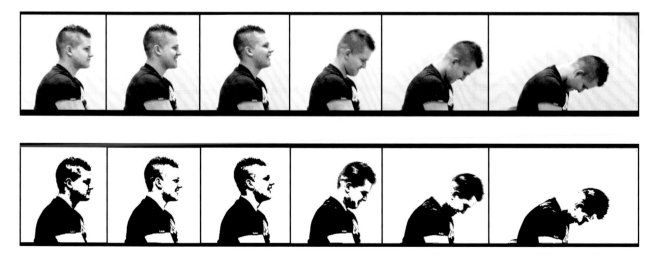

Fig. 14.3 A partial cataplectic attack in the face and neck (lateral view). Stills from a video footage. A family member is telling a joke. Laughter starts after approximately 5 s, the punchline is reached after 25 s. First image: neutral; second: start of laughter; third: start of attack about 1 s before reaching the punchline. Fourth to sixth images: 2, 3, and 3.5 s later, respectively.

Because patients rarely have attacks during consultation, the presence of cataplexy needs to be established based on the clinical interview alone. In the exceptional case that an attack is observed, it may be relevant to try to elicit the deep tendon reflexes, which will transiently disappear during an attack, including during a partial attack.

Hypnagogic hallucinations

Hypnagogic hallucinations (HH) are very vivid dreamlike experiences that occur during the transition from wakening to sleep, but may also occur on awakening (hypnopompic). The content varies, but often they are extremely unpleasant and frightening. In 85% of the hallucinations, multiple senses are simultaneously involved: visual, auditory, and tactile [21]. The hallucinations may be "pasted" over the actual environment, i.e, the room in which the patient is located—for example, someone they know seems to enter that room. Patients may see and feel animals walking on their skin or scratching it with their nails. However, people may also experience being in a totally different surrounding. Usually, narcolepsy patients recognize immediately after the event that the experience was not real, which helps distinguish HH from hallucinations in a psychiatric context. Their occurrence during the transition between wakefulness and sleep also helps the diagnosis, since hallucinations in psychiatric disorders can occur at any moment. There is no reason to think that HH point towards a psychotic disorder: psychotic disorders do not occur any more frequently in narcolepsy patients than in the general population [21].

HH are not specific for narcolepsy with cataplexy, since they are also present in the general population and in other sleep disorders [22]. However, the prevalence, and probably also the frequency, are higher in narcolepsy.

Dream delusions

Dream delusions are memories of a dream experience that are taken for a real event, forming sustained delusions, sometimes about significant events. This is a symptom of narcolepsy that has only recently been identified and that should be separated from HH [23]. As opposed to the fleeting characteristic of an HH during the sleep/wake transition, dream delusions are false memories induced by the experience of a vivid dream, which lead to counterfactual beliefs that may persist for days or weeks. For example, a man, after dreaming that a young girl had drowned in a nearby lake, asked his wife to turn on the local news in full expectation that the event would be covered. Or a woman who experienced sexual dreams of being unfaithful to her husband believed that this had actually happened and felt guilty about it until she had a chance to meet the "lover" from her dreams to realize they had not seen each other in years and had not been romantically involved.

Sleep paralysis

Sleep paralysis is the inability to move or speak on awakening or when falling asleep while being subjectively awake and conscious. The paralysis may be complete, so patients are unable to raise as much as a little finger. Attacks presumably last up to several minutes. Sleep paralysis has similarities with both cataplexy and HH: the timing resembles that of HH, whereas the pattern of affected muscles resembles that of complete attacks of cataplexy. Sleep paralysis may occur simultaneously with HH.

Sleep paralysis occurs as a symptom on its own and is therefore not specific for narcolepsy.

Disturbed nocturnal sleep

Sleep latency in narcolepsy is typically very short: patients usually fall asleep as soon as they lie down and their heads touch their pillow. They do not stay asleep, however, which is reflected in frequent awakening, which is often labeled as "sleep fragmentation" [24]. Most awakenings are brief, but some last for more than an hour. The first hours of nocturnal sleep are usually the most consolidated. Comorbid parasomnias and periodic leg movements are more frequent than in the normal population (see the next section). The total duration of nocturnal sleep is by and large comparable to the situation before the patient developed narcolepsy. In a minority of cases, nocturnal sleep time increases temporarily or structurally.

Comorbidity
Obesity

About 30% of patients have a BMI of at least 30 kg/m^2, which is about twice as much as in the general population [25]. The explanation is probably complex, and the pathways are not fully understood. Part of the explanation may be decreased activity or increased caloric intake, but, since it typically occurs in hypocretin-deficient patients, this seems to be a direct consequence of hypocretin deficiency and not part of the "sleep phenotype." There are no convincing indications that basal metabolism is changed in narcolepsy, although several studies point to a slightly lower (daytime) body temperature [26]. Probably diabetes type 2 is more frequent when compared with the normal population, but not when compared with age- and BMI-matched subjects [27].

Fatigue

Fatigue differs qualitatively from EDS and it is therefore important to differentiate between them. Fatigue is the experience of mental and physical exhaustion that does not disappear after a period of sleep. In can be found in up to 60% of patients and is usually more resistant to therapy than EDS [16]. Severe fatigue may increase the impact of EDS, since it impairs daytime activity, which is a major countermeasure to combat EDS.

Sleep apnea, periodic limb movements, and parasomnias

Obstructive sleep apnea (OSA) is reported in up to 30% patients diagnosed with narcolepsy with cataplexy [28,29]. Treatment of sleep apnea in these patients is problematic, and its necessity has been questioned. Patients often do not experience benefit or cannot endure the treatment [28,29]. Therefore, in general, it is recommended to treat the narcoleptic symptoms first. However, severe comorbid sleep apnea may be treated first. When treating the narcoleptic symptoms first, it must also be kept in mind that sodium oxybate treatment may aggravate the apneas [30].

Periodic limb movements in sleep have been described in up to two-thirds of the subjects with narcolepsy, although it is unclear whether they really contribute to the impaired quality of nocturnal sleep [29]. Patients usually only experience benefit from treatment of the periodic limb movements if there are coexisting RLS complaints.

Parasomnias

REM sleep behavior disorder (RBD) has a significantly higher prevalence compared with the general population, affecting 12–36% of patients [31,32]. Specific treatment is hardly ever necessary. Other parasomnias such as nightmares and sleepwalking are probably also more frequent.

Anxiety and depression

Anxiety disorders, especially panic attacks and social phobias, often affect patients with narcolepsy [33].

Since depression may cause complaints of EDS and lack of energy, as well as neurophysiological abnormalities that may resemble narcolepsy, it can be difficult to diagnose depression as a comorbid disorder. Nevertheless, depression is considered to have a higher prevalence than in the general population; 5–30% of patients are reported to fulfill the criteria for depression. Major depression is probably not more common [33].

Memory complaints

Many patients have memory complaints. It is not clear if these are due to impaired sustained attention and impaired executive function only, or if there is a dysfunction of the memory system itself or both. Standardized memory tests usually do not show abnormalities.

Diagnosis: criteria, classifications, and limitations of diagnostic tests

ICSD-2 versus ICSD-3

In the second edition of the International Classification of Sleep Disorders, ICSD-2, published in 2005, the criteria to diagnose narcolepsy with and without cataplexy are mainly based on clinical symptomatology [4]. Clinical criteria define cataplexy. If there is no cataplexy, the MSLT "decides." In the context of a complaint of EDS, either with or without the presence of cataplexy, an MSLT with a mean sleep latency < 8 minutes and two or more sleep onset REM periods (SOREMPs) is considered to be diagnostic for narcolepsy. In contrast, the ICSD-3 criteria, published in 2014, are mainly based on the presumed pathophysiology, i.e, the presence of hypocretin deficiency [5]. Narcolepsy types 1 and 2 are distinguished. A measured hypocretin deficiency, or, if no measurement has been performed, a very high a priori chance of hypocretin deficiency, defines type 1. All other cases without a clear other cause for EDS that show the typical MSLT abnormalities are labeled as type 2. Another difference is the calculation of the number of SOREMPs: if a SOREMP occurs during the night preceding the MSLT, it may be added to the number of SOREMPs found during the MSLT. So, if the MSLT shows a mean sleep latency < 8 minutes and only one SOREMP, it can still be diagnostic for narcolepsy if a SOREMP has been identified on the PSG during the night preceding the MSLT.

MSLT

Both ICSD-2 and ICSD-3 heavily rely on the MSLT. Unfortunately, the MSLT has significant limitations as a diagnostic test for narcolepsy. There are several recent studies that show that the specificity of the MSLT for narcolepsy is very low because up to several percent of people in the normal population, even in a substantial number of subjects without a complaint of EDS, may show the abnormalities that are considered to be diagnostic for narcolepsy [9,10]. Also the test–retest variation seems not to be high, at least in subjects without cataplexy [8]. Most likely, the majority of these MSLTs are false positives due to factors such as shiftwork, insufficient sleep, and, to a lesser extent, sleep apnea. Insufficient sleep as a cause of EDS is supported by published case reports showing sleep extension to "cure" the complaint and MSLT abnormalities [34]. The occurrence of sleep stage N2 before the occurrence of REM on MSLT testing may be a marker for insufficient sleep as a cause of the abnormal result.

The MSLT may also be falsely negative in subjects clinically suspected to have narcolepsy with cataplexy. In a recent study, 7% of patients with typical complaints of narcolepsy with cataplexy did not show the typical findings [35]. The false-negative rate for narcolepsy without cataplexy is unknown, since the MSLT results are part of the definition. Sometimes the MSLT may be negative owing to poor sleep induced by environmental factors, anxiety, older age, or medications that interfere with sleep.

Age influence the MSLT results in patients with narcolepsy. With advancing age, the number of SOREMPs decreases and the mean sleep latency increases [36]. For instance, mean sleep latency is lower in adolescents with narcolepsy (3.6 minutes) compared with narcolepsy patients above 65 years (5.2 minutes). Also, the use or discontinuation of medication, particularly antidepressants, may significantly impact the occurrence of REM sleep. How to deal with all these potential confounders is not discussed in any formal guidelines about the use of the MSLT.

Despite all these limitation, the MSLT is the best test we currently have to quantify sleepiness in a considered objective way.

Hypocretin-1 measurement

Hypocretin-1 deficiency, measured in cerebrospinal fluid (CSF), is the most specific and sensitive diagnostic test for narcolepsy with cataplexy [37] (Fig. 14.4). Additional advantages are the lack of influence of age, medication use or discontinuation, or lifestyle. In patients with typical cataplexy, who are positive for histocompatibility leukocyte antigen (HLA) *DQB1*06:02*, nonfamilial and asymptomatic (these are more than 95% of diagnosed patients), hypocretin-1 concentration in the CSF is low or undetectable in about 98% of cases [38]. The specificity of a low or undetectable hypocretin-1 is even higher than 98%.

For narcolepsy without cataplexy, the situation is more complex: the sensitivity of low or absent hypocretin-1 is low, 20–33%, depending on a cut-off of 110 or 200 pg/mL,* but remains very specific [5]. In ICSD-3, all patients with complaints of EDS and who show hypocretin-1 deficiency in their CSF, irrespective of the presence of cataplexy, are labeled as having type 1 narcolepsy. ICSD-3 defines values below 110 pg/mL as deficient, rather than the 200 pg/mL that has recently been advocated by the Stanford group [39].

---

* The currently available commercial kit for the hypocretin-1 radioimmunoassay (RIA) has a large inter-assay variation, and therefore reference samples must always be included. Many centers use reference samples from Stanford and convert their values to the Stanford values. The values mentioned in ICSD-3 and in this chapter are based on Stanford values. Levels below 40 pg/mL (in crude CSF) are usually below the detection limit of the RIA and therefore called "undetectable."

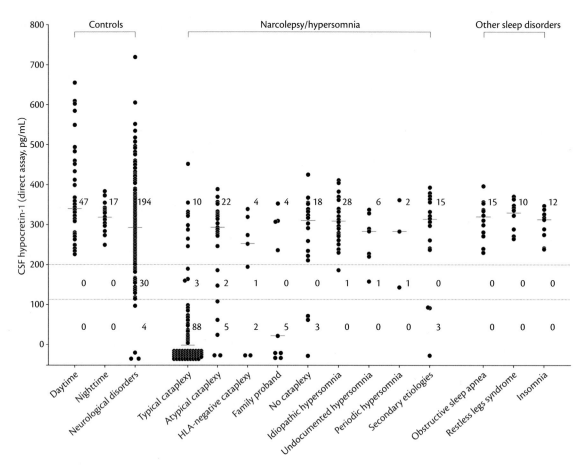

Fig. 14.4 Cerebrospinal fluid hypocretin-1 levels (direct assay) across various disease categories. Each dot represents a single patient. Diagnostic categories are as detailed in Box 14.1. Hypocretin-1 values of 110 pg/mL or less were determined as the best cut-off point to diagnose narcolepsy as defined by the International Classification of Sleep Disorders. A second cut-off point of 200 pg/mL best determines healthy control values. The number of subjects with hypocretin values below or equal to 110 pg/mL, above 200 pg/mL, and between these two values is indicated for each category.

Reproduced from Arch Neurol., 59(10), Mignot E, Lammers G J, Ripley B, Okun M, Nevsimalova S, Overeem S, Vankova J, Black J, Harsh J, Bassetti C, Schrader H, Nishino S, The Role of Cerebrospinal Fluid Hypocretin Measurement in the Diagnosis of Narcolepsy and Other Hypersomnias, pp. 1553–1562, Copyright (2002), with permission from the American Medical Association.

HLA

Narcolepsy is tightly associated with *HLA-DQB1*06:02*, which is in linkage disequilibrium with HLA-DQA1*01.02. Worldwide, about 85–95% of narcolepsy with cataplexy patients carry this *DQB1*06:02–DQA1*01:02* haplotype, compared with 12–38% of the general population. For nonfamilial cases and those with typical cataplexy, the association may exceed 95% [38]. Therefore, carrying this haplotype is thought to represent an almost certain risk factor for developing narcolepsy. Since the prevalence in the general population is relatively high, HLA typing is not of use in diagnosing narcolepsy. HLA positivity barely increases the likelihood of the diagnosis. It might be argued that HLA typing can be used to exclude narcolepsy as a diagnosis. However, this also is of limited usage, because cases with typical cataplexy are almost always *DQB1*06:02*-positive, but, in contrast, less typical and rare familial or symptomatic cases more often are HLA-negative, but may still be diagnosed as narcolepsy [5].

Current diagnostic criteria

See Box 14.1.

Differential diagnosis

Cataplexy must be differentiated from cataplexy-like episodes in normal subjects ("weak with laughter"), and from "drop attacks." Falls and sudden muscle weakness in the context of seizures, psychogenic attacks, and transient ischemic attacks are usually simple to be differentiated from cataplexy by history [40].

EDS and MSLT findings resembling narcolepsy can be seen particularly in patients with shiftwork, sleep deprivation, and sleep apnea [10].

Pathophysiology

State boundary control and the hypocretin system

All symptoms of narcolepsy can be explained by a state instability for which the term "loss of state boundary control" was introduced by Broughton in 1986 [41] . "Loss of state boundary control" results in two qualitatively different phenomena. The first is that no sleep or wake state can be maintained for a normal length of time: when awake, patients fall asleep easily, and when asleep, they awaken easily. The second is that various phenomena that normally occur together in a certain sleep stage now occur out of context. Muscle atonia that physiologically occurs during REM sleep is occurring during wakefulness in the form of cataplexy and sleep paralysis. HH are considered to be intrusions of dream imagery into wakefulness or drowsiness. Other findings in narcolepsy can be explained in a similar manner. Nowadays, the hypocretin system (also named the orexin system) is considered to represent the natural "glue" for state boundary control [42]. Its loss causes a loss of state boundary control and the symptoms of narcolepsy.

Hypocretin-producing cells are found solely in the lateral hypothalamus. The system consists of the peptides hypocretin 1 and 2 (orexin A and B), derived from the same precursor, preprohypocretin [43,44]. The cells project throughout the neuraxis, and hypocretin receptors (receptor 1 and 2) are found accordingly throughout the neuraxis [44]. These wide projections fit with the hypothesis that the hypocretin system has a "state control" function.

Risk factors and cause

Genetic and environmental factors

Narcolepsy with cataplexy is currently viewed as a disorder arising from the interaction of a genetic predisposition and environmental factors, causing an autoimmune response that leads to a selective destruction of hypothalamic hypocretin-producing cells. Although the cell loss has been proven, the autoimmune mechanisms proposed are still waiting for proof [46,47].

HLA *DQB1*06:02* is by far the most important genetic risk factor for hypocretin-deficient narcolepsy with cataplexy, among others that were identified in recent genomewide association studies [38,48,49]. All identified polymorphisms have a link to the immune system.

Many environmental triggers have been considered—most consistently, infections and head trauma. Based on the apparent increase in incidence of narcolepsy in 2009 and 2010 during the H1N1 pandemic and the vaccination campaign, the most convincing environmental factor is vaccination for or infection with influenza (particularly H1N1) [50–52]. *Streptococcus pyogenes* is another candidate, since patients show increased antigen titers close to disease onset [53].

Involvement of the immune system

The identified genetic and environmental risk factors point to an autoimmune cause for the loss of hypocretin cells. A T-cell-mediated destruction of hypocretin cells is likely. A mimicry between the identified hypocretin epitopes and HA epitopes of H1N1 influenza virus has been proposed as an explanation for the increased numbers of diagnosed new-onset narcolepsy cases in 2009 and 2010, but has not been proven up to now [51,52].

A role of B-cells and auto-antibodies in the proposed autoimmune mechanism is unclear. Anti-tribbles homolog 2 autoantibodies and IgG abnormalities were reported in narcolepsy; however, these antibodies may also be secondary to hypocretin cell loss [54].

Treatment

Unfortunately, we currently have only symptomatic treatment for narcolepsy. However, although symptomatic, it may lead to profound improvement. There are two known effective treatment modalities: behavioral modification and pharmacological therapy. As a rule, both are needed to achieve sufficient improvement.

Before starting treatment, it is of paramount important that patients and their relatives be informed about the consequences of this chronic disease and learn to accept the diagnosis. This greatly facilitates the implementation of the behavioral modifications and decreases the burden of the disease. A supportive social environment (eg, family members, friends, employer, colleagues, patient group organizations, and support groups) is also valuable.

Behavioral modification

Patients should be advised to live a regular life, go to bed at the same hour each night, and get up at the same time each morning, as much as possible. Scheduled daytime naps, usually less than 20 minutes, may temporarily alleviate and prevent daytime sleepiness, and a short nap just before certain activities demanding a high degree of attention may facilitate the proper completion. The optimal frequency, duration, and timing of these naps has to be established on an individual basis [55].

Because narcoleptic patients are probably more sensitive to the sleep-inducing properties of carbohydrates, they should not eat large carbohydrate-rich meals [56]. For similar reasons, alcohol consumption should preferably be avoided.

Pharmacological treatment

Despite these behavioral measures, the majority of patients will have residual complaints, requiring adjuvant pharmacological treatment.

A variety of substances may be used in the treatment of narcolepsy. This observation indicates that there is not one drug that is efficacious in all. As most drugs predominantly address either EDS or cataplexy, combinations are often needed to control both symptoms. The only available drug that may improve all major symptoms of narcolepsy is sodium oxybate (SXB). Combinations of SXB with, for example, stimulants may have a synergistic effect for the amelioration of EDS, and may therefore be preferred over monotherapy.

The following should be kept in mind when choosing a drug or drug combination for an individual patient and evaluating its efficacy:

- Sleepiness will never be completely alleviated in any patient, whereas cataplexy may completely disappear in some. Long-term improvement of nocturnal sleep can only be achieved with SXB. Patients must be made aware of this, and this knowledge must guide physicians in trying new drugs or combinations of drugs and in deciding on the right balance between efficacy and side effects.

- History taking from both patients and partners/relatives is the best way to guide therapy.

- Improvement of daytime performance is a much more important treatment goal than a reduction in the total amount of daytime sleep.

- Improvement of cataplexy is not simply defined by a reduction in the number of attacks. Its severity also depends on several other features: the duration, the number of muscles involved, and, very important, the threshold. The threshold may determine whether patients try to avoid situations in which attacks may occur. If patients feel that it is safe for them be involved in any upcoming daily activity, despite continuing attacks, this may indicate a huge improvement.

- Individual differences in efficacy, side-effects and tolerability appear to be large. Knowledge about the efficacy of a drug as assessed in groups is therefore of relative importance for individuals.

- Pharmacokinetic aspects, i.e, short- and fast-acting versus slow- and long-acting drugs, may be more important than the expected efficacy.

Treatment of EDS

Stimulants are the mainstay of treatment of EDS [57,58]. These include dextroamphetamine (5–60 mg/day, usually in one or two doses per day), methylphenidate (10–60 mg/day, usually in two to four doses per day), and mazindol (1–6 mg/day, usually in one or two doses per day, but not available in the USA). Side effects and tolerance are drawbacks to the use of stimulants. The most important side effects include irritability, agitation, headache, and peripheral sympathetic stimulation. These are usually dose-related. Although addiction does not seem to be a problem in narcolepsy, some patients tend to increase their dosage because they prefer high alertness [59]. Tolerance develops in about one-third of patients [59,60]. Mazindol has been withdrawn in most countries owing to observed uncommon, but severe, side effects in related drugs that suppress appetite, in particular fenfluramines. The side effects were pulmonary hypertension and valvular regurgitation [61]. However, as some patients respond better to mazindol than to any other drug, it may be considered, provided that treatment is closely monitored.

Modafinil (100–400 mg/day, usually in one or two doses) is usually grouped with the stimulants, but is chemically unrelated to amphetamine. Its efficacy is probably equal to that of the stimulants, although direct comparisons are lacking [62]. The clinical impression is that all the described side effects of stimulants, including tolerance, may occur during treatment with modafinil, but, in general, less frequent and less severe. More specific side effects of modafinil are headache and nausea; however, they usually disappear after 2–3 weeks of treatment. Armodafinil is the *R* enantiomer of modafinil and has very similar effects but also has sustained duration. It is not available in most European countries.

Long-acting agents (modafinil, armodafinil, dexamphetamine, and methylphenidate controlled release) are generally better tolerated than the short-acting ones. The quick- and short-acting ones, such as methylphenidate, can be used to good effect when "targeted" at social events or difficult periods during the day. For this reason, combinations of stimulants may be tailored to the circumstances. Unfortunately, there are no studies assessing the advantages or disadvantages of combinations of stimulants.

Sodium oxybate, the sodium salt of γ-hydroxybutyrate, has been shown to be effective in reducing EDS. The usual starting dose is 2.25 g twice a night. The dose must be gradually increased, keeping in mind that the optimal daytime effects are reached after weeks. A relevant improvement of EDS is in most patients achieved with higher dosages (6–9 g/night). The effect on EDS of higher doses is similar to that of modafinil, and side effects are, if present, usually mild [63]. The combination of both therapies is even more effective. The most frequent side effect is nausea, and the most disabling are enuresis and sleepwalking. Lowering the dose may solve these problems. Weight loss may occur [64].

In follow-up studies, there is no indication that tolerance develops, and abrupt cessation does not induce rebound cataplexy. However, long-term clinical experience shows that a substantial proportion of patients may develop tolerance for the sleep-promoting effects, although efficacy for the other symptoms remains.

SXB should not be used in conjunction with other sedatives or alcohol. If patients have consumed alcohol in the evening, they should omit one or both doses afterwards. In patients with comorbid OSA, treatment should be closely monitored, since SXB may worsen OSA. Co-treatment with continuous positive airway pressure (CPAP) may be indicated [30].

Unfortunately, there is concern for misuse. Although potential threats related to misuse may result in hesitation among patients to take, and physicians to prescribe, it is important to realize that when the drug is properly used, it is safe and bears no risk of dependence [65].

Caffeine may alleviate sleepiness, but has a weak effect: the alerting effect of six cups of strong coffee is comparable to that of 5 mg of dexamphetamine [59,60].

Treatment of REM sleep dissociation phenomena

Most studies concerning the treatment of REM dissociation phenomena have focused on cataplexy. Amelioration of cataplexy is generally associated with improvement of HH and sleep paralysis. SXB and tricyclic antidepressants are the most effective treatments. The different tricyclic antidepressants all inhibit the reuptake of norepinephrine and serotonin and are potent REM sleep inhibitors. The most commonly used are imipramine (10–100 mg/day) and clomipramine (10–150 mg/day) [2,57,58]. As with stimulants, side effects are a drawback. These are largely due to the anticholinergic properties; the most frequently reported are dry mouth, increased sweating, sexual dysfunction (impotence, delayed orgasm, and erectile and ejaculatory dysfunction), weight gain, tachycardia, constipation, blurred vision, and urinary retention. However, very low doses, up to 20 mg, may often be remarkably effective and are seldom accompanied by significant side effects. Therefore, many consider clomipramine to be the treatment of choice [66]. The most relevant drawback even with low dosages is the possible occurrence of tolerance. Tricyclic antidepressants should never be stopped abruptly, because of the risk of severe aggravation of cataplexy, which may even lead to a status cataplecticus.

Many alternative antidepressants have been studied, especially selective serotonin reuptake inhibitors (SSRIs) and more selective noradrenergic reuptake inhibitors such as fluoxetine, zimelidine, viloxazine, femoxitine, fluvoxamine, and paroxetine in a relatively higher dosage than the tricyclics [2,58,67]. They are usually not as effective in low doses as clomipramine is. The side effect of these higher dosages seems not to be favorable when compared with the side effects with low dosages of clomipramine. These substances seem to act mainly via less selective desmethyl metabolites [68]. In recent years, venlafaxine and atomoxetine have become very popular in the treatment of cataplexy, although there are no randomized placebo controlled studies available.

SXB is the best studied drug and is a very potent inhibitor of cataplexy [69]. It has never been compared with any antidepressant, so it is difficult to know whether it is really more effective than the antidepressants. However, its relatively mild side effect profile makes it a more favorable drug, even independent of the beneficial effect of SXB on other symptoms.

Several drugs may theoretically be expected to aggravate cataplexy, but the only one for which this is reliably documented is prazosin, an α_1 antagonist used to treat hypertension.

Treatment of disturbed nocturnal sleep

Disturbed nocturnal sleep can be a major complaint of patients. Unfortunately, treatment options are limited, since SXB is the only drug with a proven long-term effect on nocturnal sleep [70]. Short-term beneficial effects of benzodiazepines have been described [71]. Although nocturnal sleep may (temporarily) be improved with benzodiazepines, improvement of EDS is not the rule.

Treatment in children

Treatment of children suffering from narcolepsy does not differ significantly from treatment in adulthood, although hardly any treatment studies have focused on children. Behavioral problems only occur at a young age, and there are indications that treatment of EDS may have a positive impact on behavior as well, but studies focusing in this important symptom are urgently needed.

Treatment of associated symptoms and comorbidities

Obesity is an associated symptom, for which there is no treatment other than the usual advice for any obese person. However, some patients are happy to lose weight during treatment with SXB [64].

Fatigue or lack of energy may occasionally improve during treatment with stimulants or SXB. There is no other therapy with a proven effect for this complaint.

Treatment of sleep apnea usually does not improve the EDS, and compliance with CPAP and other treatments is a problem. Whether there is an indication for treatment is controversial [28,29]. Treatment with SXB may facilitate the acceptance of CPAP treatment. However, since SXB may worsen the course of sleep apnea, it is important in these cases that patients be compliant [30].

Treatment of periodic limb movements must be considered if there is coexistent RLS, otherwise only in very severe cases.

Treatment for RBD is rarely indicated, and in those cases clonazepam and melatonin may be effective.

Anxiety and depression should be treated separately if they are severe. Psychotherapy as well as pharmacological treatment may be considered.

Recommendations for the initiation of pharmacological treatment

The scheduled daytime naps should be continued. One should always start with a single medication at a time. It is usually best to treat the most incapacitating symptom(s) first. If this is clearly the EDS, then one should start with a stimulant; if it is clearly cataplexy or HH, then one should start with a low dose of clomipramine. If both disturbed nocturnal sleep and cataplexy are severe, then SXB may be considered as first choice. One should always start with a low dose, and increase the dose based on history taking, keeping in mind the trade-off between efficacy and side effects.

Future pharmacological treatments

Several histamine-3 receptor (H_3) antagonists are currently being studied for the treatment of EDS. Pitolisant, a selective H_3 antagonist, has recently been submitted to the EMA to become available in Europe. Published studies showed encouraging results particularly regarding improvement of EDS, but also, to a lesser extent, regarding improvement of cataplexy [72].

Immune-based therapies are controversial, and if used should be given close to disease onset. Although an autoimmune cause is very probable, there is no convincing evidence that immune modulating therapies improve symptoms or long-term outcome. A limiting factor for initiating trials with immune modulating therapies is the potential for serious side effects with many of them. The current available non-immunological treatments are relatively effective and safe, and narcolepsy does not reduce life expectancy, and therefore it is difficult from an ethical perspective to initiate studies with risk-bearing therapies. Moreover, since we can only speculate about autoimmune mechanisms, it is impossible to make a rational choice for a specific immune modulating therapy.

References

1. Daniels LE. Narcolepsy. Medicine 1934;13:1–122.
2. Overeem S, Mignot E, van Dijk JG, Lammers GJ. Narcolepsy: clinical features, new pathophysiologic insights, and future perspectives. J Clin Neurophysiol 2001;18:78–105.
3. Dauvilliers Y, Arnulf I, Mignot E. Narcolepsy with cataplexy. Lancet 2007;369:499–511.
4. American Academy of Sleep Medicine. International classification of sleep disorders, 2nd ed.: Diagnostic and coding manual. Westchester, IL: American Academy of Sleep Medicine, 2005.
5. American Academy of Sleep Medicine. The international classification of sleep disorders, 3rd ed. Darien, IL: American Academy of Sleep Medicine, 2014.
6. Baumann CR, Mignot E, Lammers GJ, et al. Challenges in diagnosing narcolepsy without cataplexy: a consensus statement. Sleep 2014;37:1035–42.
7. Thannickal TC, Nienhuis R, Siegel JM. Localized loss of hypocretin (orexin) cells in narcolepsy without cataplexy. Sleep 2009;32:993–8.
8. Trotti LM, Staab BA, Rye DB. Test–retest reliability of the multiple sleep latency test in narcolepsy without cataplexy and idiopathic hypersomnia. J Clin Sleep Med 2013;9:789–95.
9. Mignot E, Lin L, Finn L, et al. Correlates of sleep-onset REM periods during the multiple sleep latency test in community adults. Brain 2006;129:1609–23.
10. Goldbart A, Peppard P, Finn L, et al. Narcolepsy and predictors of positive MSLTs in the Wisconsin Sleep Cohort. Sleep 2014;37:1043–51.
11. Silber MH, Krahn LE, Olson EJ, Pankratz VS. The epidemiology of narcolepsy in Olmsted County, Minnesota: a population-based study. Sleep 2002;25:197–202.
12. Longstreth WT, Koepsell TD, Ton G, et al. The epidemiology of narcolepsy. Sleep 2007;30:13–26.
13. Wijnans L, Lecomte C, De Vries C, et al. The incidence of narcolepsy in Europe: before, during, and after the influenza A(H1N1) pandemic and vaccination campaigns. Vaccine 2013;31:1246–54.
14. Luca G, Haba-Rubio J, Dauvilliers Y, et al. European Narcolepsy Network. Clinical, polysomnographic and genome-wide association analyses of narcolepsy with cataplexy: a European Narcolepsy Network study. J Sleep Res 2013;22:482–95.
15. Fronczek R, Middelkoop HA, Van Dijk JG, Lammers GJ. Focusing on vigilance instead of sleepiness in the assessment of narcolepsy: high sensitivity of the sustained attention to response task (SART). Sleep 2006;29:187–91.
16. Droogleever Fortuyn HA, Fronczek R, et al. Severe fatigue in narcolepsy with cataplexy. J Sleep Res 2012;21:163–9.
17. Rocca FL, Pizza F, Ricci E, Plazzi G. Narcolepsy during childhood: an update. Neuropediatrics 2015;46:181–98.
18. Overeem S, van Nues SJ, Van der Zande WL, et al. The clinical features of cataplexy: a questionnaire study in narcolepsy patients with and without hypocretin-1 deficiency. Sleep Med 2011;12:12–18.
19. Serra L, Montagna P, Mignot E, et al. Cataplexy features in childhood narcolepsy. Mov Disord 2008;23:858–65.
20. Plazzi G, Pizza F, Palaia V. Complex movement disorders at disease onset in childhood narcolepsy with cataplexy. Brain 2011;134:3477–89.
21. Fortuyn HA, Lappenschaar GA, Nienhuis FJ, et al. Psychotic symptoms in narcolepsy: phenomenology and a comparison with schizophrenia. Gen Hosp Psychiatry 2009;31:146–54.
22. Ohayon MM, Priest RG, Zulley J, et al. Prevalence of narcolepsy symptomatology and diagnosis in the European general population. Neurology 2002;58:1826–33.
23. Wamsley E, Donjacour CE, Scammel TE, et al. Delusional confusion of dreaming and reality in narcolepsy. Sleep 2014;37:419–22.
24. Montplaisir J, Billiard M, Takahashi S, et al. Twenty-four-hour recording in REM-narcoleptics with special reference to nocturnal sleep disruption. Biol Psychiatry 1978;13:73–89.
25. Kok SW, Overeem S, Visscher TL, et al. Hypocretin deficiency in narcoleptic humans is associated with abdominal obesity. Obes Res 2003;11:1147–54.
26. van der Heide A, Donjacour CE, Pijl H, et al. The effects of sodium oxybate on core body and skin temperature regulation in narcolepsy. J Sleep Res 2015;24:566–75.
27. Donjacour CE, Aziz NA, Overeem S, et al. Glucose and fat metabolism in narcolepsy and the effect of sodium oxybate: a hyperinsulinemic–euglycemic clamp study. Sleep 2014;37:795–801.
28. Sansa G, Iranzo A, Santamaria J. Obstructive sleep apnea in narcolepsy. Sleep Med 2010;11:93–5.
29. Pizza F, Tartarotti S, Poryazova R, et al. Sleep-disordered breathing and periodic limb movements in narcolepsy with cataplexy: a systematic analysis of 35 consecutive patients. Eur Neurol 2013;70:22–6.
30. Feldman NT. Clinical perspective: monitoring sodium oxybate-treated narcolepsy patients for the development of sleep-disordered breathing. Sleep Breath 2010;14:77–9.
31. Nightingale S, Orgill JC, Ebrahim IO, et al. The association between narcolepsy and REM behavior disorder (RBD). Sleep Med 2005;6:253–58.
32. Billiard M. REM sleep behavior disorder and narcolepsy. CNS Neurol Disord Drug Targets 2009;8:264–70.
33. Fortuyn HA, Lappenschaar MA, Furer JW, et al. Anxiety and mood disorders in narcolepsy: a case–control study. Gen Hosp Psychiatry 2010;32:49–56.
34. Marti I, Valko PO, Khatami R, et al. Multiple sleep latency measures in narcolepsy and behaviourally induced insufficient sleep syndrome. Sleep Med 2009;10:1146–50.
35. Andlauer O, Moore H, Jouhier L, et al. Nocturnal REM sleep latency for identifying patients with narcolepsy/hypocretin deficiency. JAMA Neurol 2013;6:1–12.
36. Dauvilliers Y, Gosselin A, Paquet J, et al. Effect of age on MSLT results in patients with narcolepsy–cataplexy. Neurology 2004;62:46–50.
37. Mignot E, Lammers GJ, Ripley B, et al. The role of cerebrospinal fluid hypocretin measurement in the diagnosis of narcolepsy and other hypersomnias. Arch Neurol 2002;59:1553–62.
38. Tafti M, Hor H, Dauvilliers Y, et al. *DQB1* locus alone explains most of the risk and protection in narcolepsy with cataplexy in Europe. Sleep 2014;37:19–25.
39. Andlauer O, Moore H, Hong SC, et al. Predictors of hypocretin (orexin) deficiency in narcolepsy without cataplexy. Sleep 2012;35:1247–55F.
40. Bassetti CL, Lammers GJ. Hypersomnias of central origin: pathophysiology. In: Bassetti C, Dogas Z, Peigneux P, eds. Sleep medicine textbook. Regensburg: European Sleep Research Society, 2014:281–92.
41. Broughton R, Valley V, Aguirre M, et al. Excessive daytime sleepiness and the pathophysiology of narcolepsy–cataplexy: a laboratory perspective. Sleep 1986;9:205–15.
42. Mochizuki T, Crocker A, McCormack S, et al. Behavioral state instability in orexin knock-out mice. J Neurosci 2004;24:6291–300.
43. Sakurai T, Amemiya A, Ishii M, et al. Orexins and orexin receptors: a family of hypothalamic neuropeptides and G protein-coupled receptors that regulate feeding behavior. Cell 1998;92:573–85.

44. de Lecea L, Kilduff TS, Peyron C, et al. The hypocretins: hypothalamus-specific peptides with neuroexcitatory activity. Proc Natl Acad Sci U S A 1998;95:322–27.

45. Peyron C, Tighe DK, Van den Pol AN, et al. Neurons containing hypocretin (orexin) project to multiple neuronal systems. J Neurosci 1998;18:9996–10015.

46. Peyron C, Faraco J, Rogers W, et al. A mutation in a case of early onset narcolepsy and a generalized absence of hypocretin peptides in human narcoleptic brains. Nat Med 2000;6:991–7.

47. Thannickal TC, Moore R, Nienhuis R, et al. Reduced number of hypocretin neurons in human narcolepsy. Neuron 2000;27:469–74.

48. Hallmayer J, Faraco J, Lin L, et al. Narcolepsy is strongly associated with the T-cell receptor alpha locus. Nat Genet 2009;41:708–11.

49. Faraco J, Lin L, Kornum BR, et al. ImmunoChip study implicates antigen presentation to T cells in narcolepsy. PLoS Genet 2013;9(2):e1003270.

50. Han F, Lin L, Warby SC, et al. Narcolepsy onset is seasonal and increased following the 2009 H1N1 pandemic in China. Ann Neurol 2011;70:410–17.

51. Partinen M, Kornum BR, Plazzi G, et al. Narcolepsy as an autoimmune disease: the role of H1N1 infection and vaccination. Lancet Neurol 2014;13:600–13.

52. Partinen M, Kornum BR, Plazzi G, et al. Does autoreactivity have a role in narcolepsy? Lancet Neurol 2014 ;13:1072–3.

53. Aran A, Lin L, Nevsimalova S, et al. Elevated anti-streptococcal antibodies in patients with recent narcolepsy onset. Sleep 2009;32:979–83.

54. Cvetkovic-Lopes V, Bayer L, Dorsaz S, et al. Elevated tribbles homolog 2-specific antibody levels in narcolepsy patients. J Clin Invest 2010;120:713–19.

55. Mullington J, Broughton R. Scheduled naps in the management of daytime sleepiness in narcolepsy–cataplexy. Sleep 1993;16:444–56.

56. Bruck D, Armstrong S, Coleman G. Sleepiness after glucose in narcolepsy. J.Sleep Res.1994;3:171–9.

57. Wise MS, Arand DL, Auger RR, et al. Treatment of narcolepsy and other hypersomnias of central origin. Sleep 2007;30:1712–27.

58. Billiard M, Bassetti C, Dauvilliers Y, et al. EFNS guidelines on management of narcolepsy. Eur. J Neurol 2006;13:1035–48.

59. Parkes JD, Dahlitz M. Amphetamine prescription. Sleep 1993;16:201–03.

60. Mitler MM, Aldrich MS, Koob GF, Zarcone VP. Narcolepsy and its treatment with stimulants. ASDA standards of practice. Sleep 1994;17:352–71.

61. Ryan DH, Bray GA, Helmcke F, et al. Serial echocardiographic and clinical evaluation of valvular regurgitation before, during, and after treatment with fenfluramine or dexfenfluramine and mazindol or phentermine. Obes Res 1999;7:313–22.

62. Mitler MM, Harsh J, Hirshkowitz M, Guilleminault C. Long-term efficacy and safety of modafinil (PROVIGIL®) for the treatment of excessive daytime sleepiness associated with narcolepsy. Sleep Med 2000;1:231–43.

63. Black, J, Houghton, WC. Sodium oxybate improves excessive daytime sleepiness in narcolepsy. Sleep 2006;29:939–46.

64. Husain, AM, Ristanovic, RK, Bogan, RK. Weight loss in narcolepsy patients treated with sodium oxybate. Sleep Med 2009;10:661–3.

65. Lammers GJ, Bassetti C, Billiard M, et al. Sodium oxybate is an effective and safe treatment for narcolepsy. Sleep Med 2010;11:105–6.

66. Parkes, D. Introduction to the mechanism of action of different treatments of narcolepsy. Sleep 1994;17:S93–6.

67. Nishino, S, Mignot, E. Pharmacological aspects of human and canine narcolepsy. Prog Neurobiol 1997;52:27–78.

68. Nishino S, Arrigoni J, Shelton J, et al. Desmethyl metabolites of serotonergic uptake inhibitors are more potent for suppressing canine cataplexy than their parent compounds. Sleep 1993;16:706–12.

69. U.S. Xyrem Multicenter Study Group. Sodium oxybate demonstrates long-term efficacy for the treatment of cataplexy in patients with narcolepsy. Sleep Med 2004;5:119–23.

70. Xyrem Multicenter Study Group. A 12-month, open-label, multicenter extension trial of orally administered sodium oxybate for the treatment of narcolepsy. Sleep 2003;26:31–5.

71. Thorpy MJ, Snyder M, Aloe FS, et al. Short-term triazolam use improves nocturnal sleep of narcoleptics. Sleep 1992;15:212–16.

72. Dauvilliers Y, Bassetti C, Lammers CJ, et al. HARMONY I study group. Pitolisant versus placebo or modafinil in patients with narcolepsy: a double-blind, randomised trial. Lancet Neurol 2013;12:1068–75.

CHAPTER 15

Idiopathic hypersomnia, Kleine–Levin syndrome, and symptomatic hypersomnias

Michel Billiard and Yves Dauvilliers

Besides the most prevalent obstructive sleep apnea syndrome (OSAS) and the emblematic narcolepsy, which have been the topics of multiple articles and books, there are a number of other causes of excessive daytime sleepiness (EDS). They include idiopathic hypersomnia, Kleine–Levin syndrome (KLS), and several symptomatic hypersomnias. These conditions are less familiar to sleep specialists and are often neglected by internists and psychiatrists. Moreover, their less rich symptomatology may be the cause of delayed diagnosis, and their treatment is not as well standardized as in the case of sleep-related breathing disorders and narcolepsy. Yet, these sleep disorders may seriously impact the quality of life of patients. In this chapter, we will focus on idiopathic hypersomnia and KLS, reviewing clinical features, polysomnography (PSG) and other objective findings, differential diagnosis, pathophysiology, and treatment, and then mention the key points of symptomatic hypersomnias

Idiopathic hypersomnia

Historical background

Idiopathic hypersomnia was progressively identified, beginning with the description of sleep drunkenness by Roth in 1956 [1] and ending with the publication by the same Roth in 1976 of a series of 642 personally observed cases, including 368 patients with narcolepsy and 274 with hypersomnia, of which 103 had "idiopathic hypersomnia, polysymptomatic form," 71 "idiopathic hypersomnia, monosymptomatic form," 12 hypersomnia with disorders of breathing during sleep, and 5 neurotic hypersomnia [2]. Idiopathic hypersomnia polysymptomatic form was characterized by excessive diurnal sleep, prolonged night sleep of a duration of 12–18 hours, and great difficulty awakening in the morning, while idiopathic hypersomnia monosymptomatic form was characterized by the most prominent symptom of diurnal sleep of a duration of one to several hours, not as irresistible as in narcolepsy. In 1979, the Diagnostic Classification of Sleep and Arousal Disorders referred to idiopathic hypersomnia as one of the disorders of excessive somnolence [3], and in 1990, the first edition of the International Classification of Sleep Disorders (ICSD) referred to idiopathic hypersomnia as one of the intrinsic sleep disorders [4]. Neither classification retained the division into two forms. In 2005, the second edition (ICSD-2) reverted to a division into two forms, namely, idiopathic hypersomnia with and without long sleep time [5]. Finally, in March 2014, the third edition (ICSD-3) was released [6], and, in the absence of specific symptoms in idiopathic hypersomnia with and without long sleep time, the division into two forms was again abandoned, awaiting the discovery of consistent biological markers.

Epidemiology

Owing to uncertainty regarding the nosological limits of idiopathic hypersomnia, no prevalence study has ever been conducted. Instead, ratios of idiopathic hypersomnia to narcolepsy in cohorts of patients published by different sleep disorder centers are available (Table 15.1). These ratios span from 9.2% to 47.2%, obviously reflecting the lack of common diagnostic criteria. The onset of the condition is most often during adolescence or young adulthood. According to some cohorts, there is a higher prevalence of idiopathic hypersomnia in women [11,22,23].

Apart from these evaluations, a recent study has developed the concept of "excessive quantity of sleep" (EQS), defined as a main sleep period or 24-hour sleep duration ≥ 9 hours accompanied by complaints of impaired functioning or distress due to excessive sleep [24]. This study used the Sleep-EVAL expert system to ask questions on life and sleeping habits, health, and sleep, mental, and organic disorders, according to the Diagnostic and Statistical Manual of Mental Disorders, fourth edition, (DSM-IV-TR) [25], in a nonselected population sample of 15 929 individuals. EQS was observed in 1.6% of the sample, and the prevalence of DSM-IV hypersomnia disorder was 0.5%. These results are of major interest, even if DSM-IV hypersomnia based on subjective reports cannot be equated with idiopathic hypersomnia based on clinical, polysomnographic, and MSLT criteria.

Predisposing factors

A familial background has been found in up to 40% of idiopathic hypersomnia patients in an earlier study [26], but more rigorous studies with direct clinical interview and sleep studies in relatives are warranted. Precipitating factors like head trauma, viral illness, and general anesthesia have been reported, but are less convincing than in narcolepsy.

Table 15.1 Series of patients with narcolepsy and idiopathic hypersomnia published by various sleep disorder centers, and ratios of idiopathic hypersomnia to narcolepsy

Authors	Narcolepsy	Idiopathic hypersomnia	Idiopathic hypersomnia/ narcolepsy (%)
Roth [2]	104	64	47.2
Van den Hoed et al. [7]	41	17	41.4
Baker et al. [8]	257	74	28.7
Aldrich [9]	67	26	38.8
Bruck and Parkes [10]	50	18	36.0
Bassetti and Aldrich [11]	258	42	16.2
Billiard et al. [12]	380	35	9.2
Kanbayashi et al. [13]	67	26	38.8
Vignatelli et al. [14]	108	42	37.6
Heier et al. [15]	54	10	18.5
Martinez-Rodriguez et al. [16]	42	8	19.0
Kanbayashi et al. [17]	67	26	38.7
Coelho et al. [18]	54	14	25.9
Tanaka and Honda [19]	159	28	17.6
Pizza et al. [20]	51	16	31.3
Dauvilliers et al. [21]	83	11	13.2

Clinical features

EDS is the key symptom of idiopathic hypersomnia. It is generally considered as more continuous and less irresistible than in narcolepsy type 1. Naps tend to be long and nonrefreshing in half to three-quarters of patients [6]. Night sleep is abnormally long in at least a third of patients [6]. Waking up in the morning or at the end of naps may be difficult or even present itself as sleep drunkenness, consisting of difficulty in coming to complete wakefulness, accompanied by confusion, disorientation, poor motor coordination, slowness, and repeated returns to sleep [27]. Headache, orthostatic hypotension, and Raynaud-like symptoms are sometimes present. In addition, subjective symptoms such as being more alert in the evening than in the morning, difficulty in focusing more than one hour, complaints of attention and memory deficit, mental fatigability, and hyperactivity helping to resist sleepiness have also been reported [28]. Altogether, the phenotype of idiopathic hypersomnia is not unitary—hence the successive suggestions of nosological separation of the condition into two or three forms.

Diagnostic tests

PSG followed by a multiple sleep latency test (MSLT) is mandatory [6]. PSG generally demonstrates a normal architecture of sleep. Obstructive sleep apneas (OSA) should theoretically be fewer than 5 per hour and respiratory-effort-related arousals (RERAs) fewer than 10. Moreover, periodic limb movements should be fewer than 10 per hour.

An MSLT performed according to standard techniques shows fewer than two sleep onset REM periods (SOREMPs), or no SOREMP if the REM latency on the preceding PSG is 15 minutes or less [6].

Finally, one of the following should be present: a mean sleep latency of 8 minutes or less on the MSLT, or a total 24-hour sleep time of 660 minutes or more documented on a 24-hour PSG or on a 7-day wrist actigraphy performed in a period of unrestricted sleep (eg, holidays) in association with a sleep diary [6].

In addition, psychiatric evaluation should be performed in subjects suspected of having a psychiatric disorder, mainly bipolar disorder II, major depression disorder, or schizoaffective disorder, and neuroimaging in case of neurological signs.

Course

Once established, fluctuations in disease severity may be observed as documented by changes in MSLT results at several-year intervals [29]. Moreover, cases of spontaneous disappearance have been reported [10,11,30]. At first sight, the complications of idiopathic hypersomnia appear similar to those of narcolepsy, including poor performance at school or at work, sleeping during recreational activities, and car and work accidents. However, in the case of patients complaining of long sleep time and difficulty on awakening, complications have some peculiarities. These patients report arriving late at work, receiving negative comments from their employer, and often being dismissed as a consequence. Second, the lengthy time these patients spend in bed is hardly tolerated by family members over the long term. Third, in contrast to narcoleptic patients, idiopathic hypersomnia patients rarely benefit from extended night sleep, to the extent that they never feel refreshed. Finally, EDS is most often amenable to stimulant medications, whereas difficulty in awakening is often resistant to treatment [31].

Pathophysiology

Several non-mutually exclusive hypotheses have been proposed, but understanding is still limited.

Neurochemistry

More than 40 years ago, Petitjean and Jouvet reported hypersomnia with proportional increase of NREM and REM sleep suggestive of idiopathic hypersomnia, after destruction of noradrenergic neurons of the rostral third of the locus coeruleus complex or of the noradrenergic bundle at the level of the isthmus, in the cat [32]. Subsequently, in the 1980es, a series of studies measuring monoamine metabolites in the cerebrospinal fluid (CSF) of idiopathic hypersomnia patients were performed. However, biological methods for measuring monoamine metabolites have been criticized, and none of these studies has ever been replicated.

More recently, it has been shown that CSF hypocretin-1 concentrations are normal in patients with idiopathic hypersomnia [13,33,34]. Reduced CSF histamine levels have been observed in hypocretin-deficient narcolepsy with cataplexy, in hypocretin nondeficient narcolepsy and in idiopathic hypersomnia, but not in OSA syndrome [17]. These findings led to the suggestion that CSF histamine is a biomarker reflecting the degree of hypersomnia of central origin. However, using a new validated method of CSF histamine and tele-methylhistamine (t-MHA) measurement [35], Dauvilliers et al. did not find any CSF histamine or t-MHA level differences between the various etiologies of central disorders of hypersomnolence (narcolepsy type 1 and 2, idiopathic hypersomnia, and unspecified excessive daytime sleepiness) and neurological controls [21].

Another perspective comes from a recent experiment which showed that CSF from hypersomnolent subjects (excluding known causes of excessive sleepiness) contains a small (500–3000 Da), not yet identified, trypsin-sensitive substance that stimulates the in vitro function of selected γ-aminobutyric acid (GABA) receptors, only in the presence of GABA, relative to the stimulation obtained with CSF from control subjects [36]. Notably, flumazenil, a drug that is generally believed to antagonize the sedative–hypnotic action of benzodiazepines, reversed enhancement of $GABA_A$ signaling by hypersomnolent CSF in vitro. However, this recent discovery requires replication, since CSF alone from hypersomnolent patients had no effect on $GABA_A$ signaling. Furthermore, no differences were observed between different diagnostic categories, and no correlation was found between GABA potentiation and objective measures of sleepiness. In contrast, a recent study using the *Xenopus* oocyte assay found an absence of GABA-A receptor potentiation with CSF from patients with central hypersomnolence disorders, with no significant differences between hypocretin- and non-hypocretin-deficient patients compared to controls. The major discrepancies between these results may have arisen from differences in the phenotyping of patients affected with hypersomnolence, sample size, control group selection, lumbar puncture procedure, or treatment intake, as well as methodological issues in the GABA-A response assessment [37].

Genetics

Before the eventual identification of idiopathic hypersomnia in 1976, a series of 23 probands with "essential hypersomnia," with data from 190 family members of these probands, was published by Czech authors [27]. A familial occurrence was found in nine families (39.1%), and an autosomal dominant mode of inheritance was suggested. In 2001, in a series of 35 idiopathic hypersomnia patients, 25 with the polysymptomatic form and 10 with the monosymptomatic form, a familial history was found in 10 patients with the polysymptomatic form (40%), including 3 with several relatives, and in 3 subjects with the monosymptomatic form (30%), including 1 with several relatives [12]. Recently, a report of three adolescent-onset cases of idiopathic hypersomnia assessed clinically and by use of ad libitum PSG was published, arguing for a genetic origin in this family [38]. The pedigree was compatible with an autosomal dominant inheritance. Incidentally, no report of twins affected with idiopathic hypersomnia has ever been published. Given these observations, there has been an early interest in potential HLA markers in idiopathic hypersomnia, but no consistent findings have emerged so far.

Immunology

Tanaka and Honda assessed immunoglobulin G (IgG) profiles in Japanese narcolepsy–cataplexy patients positive for the *HLA-DQB1*0602* allele, idiopathic hypersomnia patients with long sleep time, and healthy controls [19]. The distribution of serum IgG was significantly different among healthy controls, narcolepsy patients, and idiopathic hypersomnia patients [19]. Decreases in IgG1 and IgG2 levels, a stable expression of IgG3, and an increase in the proportion of IgG4 were found in narcolepsy–cataplexy patients,

compared with increases in IgG3 and IgG4, a decrease in IgG2, and an IgG1/IgG2 imbalance in idiopathic hypersomnia patients, thus favoring immunological differences between narcolepsy and idiopathic hypersomnia. However, no other clinical or biological study has supported an immunopathological process in idiopathic hypersomnia.

Homeostatic and circadian regulation

In a study comparing the level of slow-wave activity (SWA) in the first two NREM–REM sleep cycles, this level was significantly lower in idiopathic hypersomnia patients than in controls [39]. Thus, patients with idiopathic hypersomnia may need prolonged sleep time because of a lower intensity of their NREM sleep. Two other studies compared the sleep spindle index in idiopathic hypersomnia and controls [40] and in idiopathic hypersomnia and narcolepsy [41]. They documented an increased spindle index predominating by the end of night sleep in idiopathic hypersomnia, which might explain the symptoms of difficulty waking up or of "sleep drunkenness."

In addition, a disturbed circadian rhythm has been hypothesized on the basis of a phase delay in the rhythm of melatonin and cortisol secretion in 15 patients with idiopathic hypersomnia with long sleep time [42]. In a more recent study, Horne and Östberg scores were lower in idiopathic hypersomnia subjects than in controls, consistent with a delayed sleep phase in idiopathic hypersomnia [43]. Moreover, investigations of the dynamics of the expression of circadian clock genes in dermal fibroblasts of idiopathic hypersomnia patients in comparison with those of healthy controls have shown that the amplitude of rhythmically expressed BMAL1, PER1, and PER2 was significantly dampened in dermal fibroblasts of idiopathic hypersomnia patients compared with healthy controls, suggesting an aberrant dynamics in the circadian clock of idiopathic hypersomnia patients [44].

Differential diagnosis

Differentiating idiopathic hypersomnia from other conditions is not always an easy task. This is reflected in the establishment in several countries of reference centers with specialized clinicians and access to long-term PSG or actigraphic monitoring.

OSAS

Idiopathic hypersomnia may be confused with OSAS, especially when RERAs rather than apneas/hypopneas are predominant. In case of any doubt, a continuous positive airway pressure (CPAP) trial should be proposed.

Narcolepsy type 2

This is not easy to distinguish from idiopathic hypersomnia. First, the ICSD-3 clinical criteria, A and C of narcolepsy type 2 and A and B of idiopathic hypersomnia, are similar [6]. Second, narcolepsy type 2 is supposed to differ from idiopathic hypersomnia by the presence of two or more SOREMPs on the MSLT, but the distinction between two SOREMPs or more for narcolepsy type 2 and fewer than two SOREMPs for idiopathic hypersomnia sounds both arbitrary and subtle, since the number of SOREMPs may vary from one MSLT to another in the same individual, depending on the disease process and age [29]. Third, a total sleep time of 660 minutes or more is not a compulsory PSG criterion for idiopathic hypersomnia but a criterion in balance with a mean sleep latency of 8 minutes or less. Thus, the distinction between the two conditions still awaits further clarification.

Delayed sleep phase syndrome

This is another diagnosis to consider, given the major difficulty waking up in the morning. However, these subjects do not complain of EDS in the afternoon and evening, and their total sleep time is usually normal.

Chronic fatigue syndrome

This is characterized by persistent or relapsing fatigue that does not resolve with sleep or rest. The disabling fatigue is accompanied by joint and muscle pain, headache, poor concentration, impaired short-term memory, disturbed sleep, recurrent subjective feverish feelings, and sore throat [45]. PSG shows reduced sleep efficiency and may include alpha intrusion into sleep EEG [46].

Long sleeper

A long sleeper is an individual who consistently sleeps more in 24 hours than the typical person of his or her age group. The main difference with idiopathic hypersomnia is the absence of any complaint of EDS or difficulty in awakening as long as sufficient sleep is obtained to fulfill the sleep need [6]. A consistent daily pattern, documented by a carefully kept sleep diary (preferably confirmed by actigraphy) showing 9 hours or more of sleep per night over a minimum of 7 days is desirable for the identification of the long sleeper.

Other differential diagnoses

These, which include hypersomnia due to a medical disorder, hypersomnia due to a medication or a substance, hypersomnia associated with a psychiatric disorder, and insufficient sleep disorder, will be considered later in this chapter.

Treatment

Behavioral treatment

Behavioral treatment of idiopathic hypersomnia is not as successful as for narcolepsy. Naps are nonrefreshing, and extension of sleep time for several days to saturate the patients' sleep need does not bring relief on the long term.

Conventional pharmacological options

Up to now, although EDS may not have the same character in narcolepsy and in idiopathic hypersomnia, the same pharmacological options, namely, stimulants, including amphetamines and methylphenidate, and eugregorics (from the Greek εν meaning "good" and γρηγοροσ meaning "which is watchful"), including modafinil and armodafinil, have been used in both conditions.

The first trial with modafinil in idiopathic hypersomnia was performed in an open-label study in 1988 [47]. Eighteen patients participated in the study. Modafinil was administered in the morning and at noon. The number of drowsiness and sleep episodes during daytime was significantly reduced in 15 patients. It then took 20 more years to have large observational studies and consecutive clinical cohorts available. Among the first are two studies, one by Anderson et al. [30] and one by Ali et al. [23], which showed that only 50–75% of patients remained on the prescribed drug, modafinil or methylphenidate, and only 60–70% of those remaining on the drug were good responders.

As for consecutive clinical cohorts, the first one tested the benefits and risks (habituation and adverse effects) of modafinil in 104 patients with idiopathic hypersomnia and 126 patients with narcolepsy with cataplexy [48]. Modafinil had an excellent benefit/risk ratio in idiopathic hypersomnia, similar to its effects on narcolepsy–cataplexy, as estimated by patients and clinicians. Loss of efficacy and habituation were rare in both groups. However, idiopathic hypersomnia patients reported more frequent adverse effects with modafinil than narcolepsy patients. The second study compared quality of life, Epworth Sleepiness Scale (ESS) scores, and items concerning psychosocial and environmental variables in patients with narcolepsy with cataplexy (83 on psychostimulants and 28 drug-naive), patients with narcolepsy without cataplexy (48 on psychostimulants and 27 drug-naive), patients with idiopathic hypersomnia without long sleep time (54 on psychostimulants and 82 drug-naive), with Japanese normative data [49]. All three diagnostic groups had significantly lower scores for most Short Form 36 (SF-36) domains compared with the Japanese normative data, and the ESS scores were significantly reduced with treatment.

Recently, two randomized, double-blind, placebo-controlled trials have been published. The first, a multicenter study, was performed in 31 adult patients with idiopathic hypersomnia without long sleep time, 14 of whom were on modafinil and 17 on placebo [50]. Modafinil 200 mg given in the morning improved ESS and clinical global impression (CGI) compared with placebo and led to a nonsignificant increase in the mean sleep latency on the maintenance of wakefulness test (MWT). The second, a crossover study, was conducted in 13 narcolepsy patients and 14 idiopathic hypersomnia patients receiving modafinil (400 mg) or placebo [51]. Modafinil improved driving performance judged on the mean number of inappropriate line crossings and standard deviation of lateral position of the vehicle compared with placebo, as well as the mean sleep latency on the MWT, equally in patients with narcolepsy and idiopathic hypersomnia.

Another treatment, mazindol, a tricyclic non-amphetamine stimulant, was evaluated in a retrospective analysis of the files of 37 idiopathic hypersomnia patients refractory to modafinil, methylphenidate, and sodium oxybate, in three different hospitals [52]. Patients received an average dose of 3.6 mg/day. The benefit on sleepiness, measured as the difference between the final ESS score and the one before starting treatment, was 4.8 ± 4.7 ($p < 0.0001$). Treatment was stopped in 5 patients (13.5%) owing to loss of efficacy, in 4 patients (11%) owing to adverse effects, and in 10 patients owing to other reasons (difficulties in obtaining the drug, pregnancy, unknown). Selective serotonin reuptake inhibitors and tricyclic antidepressants may have a positive effect.

Of note, in view of a possible alteration of circadian regulation, an improvement in half of 10 idiopathic hypersomnia patients treated with melatonin (2 mg of the slow-release form at bedtime) has been reported [53].

Finally, a recent chart review of 46 patients with idiopathic hypersomnia and 47 patients with narcolepsy type 1 treated with sodium oxybate, with smaller doses in idiopathic hypersomnia patients than in narcolepsy type 1 patients, showed similar changes in excessive daytime sleepiness in idiopathic hypersomnia and narcolepsy type 1, and an improvement of severe morning inertia in 24 of 34 patients with idiopathic hypersomnia [54].

Newer therapies

Levothyroxine, 25 µg/day, has been orally administered to nine patients with idiopathic hypersomnia with long sleep time [55]. Mean total sleep time was 12.9 ± 0.3 hours and ESS was 17.8 ± 1.4 before treatment. After treatment, mean total sleep times were 9.1 ± 0.7 and 8.5 ± 1 hours at 4 and 8 weeks, respectively, and mean ESS scores were 8.8 ± 2.3 and 7.4 ± 2.8, respectively. No adverse effects were noted. One patient dropped out during the second week owing to poor effect.

Flumazenil, an antagonist of the sedative–hypnotic action of benzodiazepines, was first used in idiopathic hypersomnia after the nearly complete reversal, even if controversial, of the effect of hypersomnolent CSF on $GABA_A$ receptor-mediated chloride currents in vitro by co-application of 10 µmol/L GABA [36,37]. Subsequently, flumazenil improved psychomotor vigilance and subjective alertness in seven hypersomnolent patients, two with a diagnosis of idiopathic hypersomnia, two with a diagnosis of narcolepsy type 2, and three habitually long sleepers [36]. However, flumazenil has a number of potential adverse effects, including dizziness, nausea, headache, anxiety, confusion, and hyperphagia.

To get round of these limitations, clarithromycin, a macrolide antibiotic acting through an endogenous enhancement of $GABA_A$ receptors, has been tested in a group of 39 "hypersomnolent patients" [56]. A subjective improvement was obtained in 34. Of these 34 patients, 23 chose to use clarithromycin on a long-term basis: 16 used it on a daily basis, 4 on an intermittent basis, while 3 discontinued it after a mean of 5 months. More recently, a 5-week, randomized, placebo-controlled, double-blind, crossover trial of clarithromycin conducted in 20 patients with hypersomnolence syndromes (excluding narcolepsy type 1), some of them already treated with psychostimulants, and evidence of abnormal CSF potentiation of $GABA_A$ receptors, showed a significant improvement of subjective measures of sleepiness (ESS and Stanford Sleepiness Scale), but not on an objective measurement of vigilance (a psychomotor vigilance test being the primary outcome measure) [57].

Pitolisant, an inverse agonist of H_3 histamine receptors, has been effective in patients with narcolepsy type 1 [58]. A recent retrospective analysis of 78 patients with idiopathic hypersomnia evaluated the benefits and risks of pitolisant. The median ESS score decreased from 17 (range 15.5–18.5) to 14 (range 12–17), and by more than 3 in 35.4% of patients [59]. Most frequent side-effects, in 16–12% of patients, included epigastralgia and abdominal pain, increased appetite, weight gain, headache, and insomnia.

Kleine–Levin syndrome

Historical background

The name KLS was coined in 1942 [60]. However, "a syndrome of periodic somnolence and morbid hunger" had been described in detail as early as 1936 [61], reports of patients with episodes of hypersomnia, gluttony, odd behaviors and cognitive symptoms had been published in the 1920s [62–64], and scattered reports of the condition were available even earlier, with one dating back to the eighteenth century [65].

In 1962, Critchley published a masterpiece article "Periodic hypersomnia and megaphagia in adolescent males," in which he collected 15 "genuine" instances from the literature and 11 cases of

his own, which he described in depth [66]. He gave the definition of "a syndrome composed of recurring episodes of undue sleepiness lasting some days, associated with an inordinate intake of food, and often with abnormal behavior." In addition, he emphasized four hallmarks: (1) sex incidence whereby males are preponderantly if not wholly affected; (2) onset in adolescence; (3) spontaneous eventual disappearance of the syndrome; (4) the possibility that the megaphagia is in the nature of compulsive eating, rather than bulimia. Following this publication, several reviews were published, with the emphasis being put on clinical features.

In 2005, the second edition of the ICSD published diagnostic criteria of recurring hypersomnia and gave a definition of KLS modifying Levin's and Critchley's views, in that hyperphagia was no longer necessary for the diagnosis, but only one of the possible symptoms of the syndrome [5].

Following this publication, several large reviews appeared, allowing quantitative evaluations of predisposing factors, circumstances at onset, symptoms, physical signs, and comparisons of symptoms in men and women [67–69]. One of these reviews was a most valuable cross-sectional, systematic evaluation of 108 new cases and comparison with matched control subjects [68]. Finally, the third edition of the ICSD changed the word "recurrent hypersomnia" to "KLS" [6].

Epidemiology

KLS is a rare disorder. No systematic prevalence study is available. Only large series of patients originating from single sleep disorder centers (Table 15.2) and comprehensive reviews of the world literature [67,69] have been published. The number of reported KLS patients is high in Israel [70] and, in one American series, there were six times more Jewish patients than expected, all Ashkenazi, suggesting a founder effect in this population [68].

Age of onset is predominantly adolescence and young adulthood, with only 10 patients (3.7%) starting their condition before the age of 10 years and 16 (5.4%) starting their condition after the age of 30, in a population of 293 patients [69]. Familial cases are not exceptional, with 5 of 104 patients (4.8%) in one series [68] and 9 of 297 patients (3%) in another [77]. Among these nine families, three included more than two affected relatives [78–80].

Predisposing and precipitating factors

An increased frequency of the *HLA-DQB1*02:01* allele had been reported in a multicenter group of 30 unrelated patients with KLS [81]. However, in a later American series of 108 patients and 108 matched controls, *HLA-DR* and *-DQ* alleles did not differ between patients and controls [68]. Factors precipitating the first episode are mentioned in all series, consisting most frequently of an upper airway infection or a flu-like illness and less frequently of an emotional stress, alcohol intake, head trauma, anesthesia, vaccination, or exhaustion.

Clinical features

KLS is characterized by relapsing–remitting episodes of severe hypersomnolence in association with cognitive, behavioral, and psychiatric disturbances. The episodes begin within a few hours, or gradually over a period of one to three days, with patients becoming extremely tired, muzzy and detached. Hypersomnia is the major symptom present in each episode. Patients lie in bed,

Table 15.2 Largest series of patients with Kleine–Levin syndrome originating from single sleep disorder centers

Authors	Country	Number of cases	Males	Females
Critchley [66]	England	11	11	0
Takahashi [71]	Japan	28	21	7
Roth [72]	Czechoslovakia	15	?	?
Smolik and Roth [73]	Czechoslovakia	14	5	9
Gadoth et al. [70]	Israel	34	28	6
Arnulf et al. [68]	USA	108	82	26
Huang et al. [74]	Taiwan	30	26	4
Li et al. [75]	China	42	?	?
Kas et al. [76]	France	41	23	8

sometimes with restlessness and untidiness. Vivid dreams may occur. Usual sleep duration ranges from 12 to 18 hours, especially during the first days. Patients wake up spontaneously to void. They may be irritable or even aggressive when awakened or prevented from sleeping.

Cognitive symptoms may be severe, such as altered perception (with people and objects appearing as distorted, distant, or unreal), confusion, delusions, or hallucinations, or less impressive, such as abnormal speech, impaired concentration, impaired memory, or apathy.

Behavioral symptoms include compulsive eating, disinhibited sexuality, and odd behaviors. Patients do not necessarily look for food, but cannot refrain from eating food within reach, in a compulsive manner, such as in the case of an 18-year-old ordinary seaman "who ate about a dozen large helpings of suet pudding (in addition to his own heavy meal), the pudding having been rejected by the majority of sailors as being underdone and too stodgy for consumption" [66]. A preference for sweets is common. Increased drinking is sometimes associated. In some cases or in some episodes, compulsive eating may be replaced by anorexia. Sexual disinhibition can take the form of overt masturbation, sexual advances, or shamelessly expressed sexual fantasies. Sexual disinhibition is apparently less frequent in women than in men, although it could assume a less visible expression such as fantasies of being "chatted up" by men or experiencing love affairs. Odd behaviors, also designated as compulsive behaviors, are very special to KLS. They include stereotyped behaviors (repetitive and excessive), disinhibited social behavior, childish behavior, aggression, loss of decency, bizarre postures, or imaginative actions.

Psychiatric symptoms include depression during the episodes, more often in women than in men, and, less frequently, anxiety, equally reported by men and women.

KLS is remarkable for the absence of any neurological sign. On the other hand, autonomic symptoms such as profuse sweating, reddish, congestive, or puffy face, low or high blood pressure, bradycardia or tachycardia, and intense body odor or nauseating urine are found in about 20% of men and women. In addition, weight gain of a few kilograms may be observed during the attacks and is much more frequent in women than in men [69].

The episodes of hypersomnia may end abruptly or insidiously over a few days. In up to a third of cases, the episode is followed by amnesia of the past events and elation with insomnia, as if the patient were trying to catch up for lost time, for one or two days.

Diagnostic tests

The diagnosis of KLS is purely clinical. Routine blood tests, including blood count, plasma electrolytes, urea, creatinine, and hepatic function, are normal. Static and dynamic hormonal tests (growth hormone, prolactin, thyroid-stimulating hormone, testosterone, and cortisol) are normal. Agents responsible for upper airway infection, flulike illness, or other infections are rarely identified. CSF white blood cell counts and protein levels are normal in all patients, ruling out infectious meningitis. Immunoelectrophoresis is also normal. Routine EEG is remarkable for a general slowing of background activity. Bursts of synchronous, generalized, moderate- to high-voltage, 5–7 Hz waves 0.5–2 sec in duration, mainly in the bilateral temporal or temporofrontal areas, are frequent and a cause of misdiagnosis with epilepsy. PSG is not easy to organize from one day to the next and is difficult to interpret, given the frequent evolution of sleep patterns throughout an attack. Altogether, the duration of recorded sleep is often shorter or much shorter than the behavioral sleep as observed by parents or nurses. Sleep efficiency is poor, while SOREMPs are frequent. MSLT is of questionable interest in view of the frequent limited cooperation of patients. Structural brain imaging (computerized tomography or magnetic resonance imaging) is normal in primary forms of KLS. Psychological interview and testing should be performed during and after the episode.

Course

KLS is characterized by episodes lasting a median of 9 days (range 1–180 days) in men and of 8 days (range 1–60 days) in women and a cycle length (time elapsed from onset of one episode to the onset of the next episode) lasting a median of 106 days (range 14–1095 days) in men and 60 days (range 15–1460 days) in women [69]. KLS vanishes spontaneously within months or years. However, the duration of the condition is variable, and in some patients may exceptionally last up to 20–30 years. It is commonly assumed that the episodes of KLS decrease in frequency, severity, and duration with time before fading out. However, this was clearly evidenced in a limited number of cases only in one series [69].

Clinical variant

Menstrual-related KLS is a very rare disease characterized by episodes of hypersomnia, plus or minus other symptoms and physical signs of KLS, which occur in association with the menstrual cycle and sometimes with puerperium [69]. The condition occurs for the first time within the first months after menarche or later.

Differential diagnosis

The most important differential diagnosis is a psychiatric condition, such as psychotic disorder, depressive disorder, bipolar disorder, somatic symptom, and related disorder, due to the cognitive, behavioral, and psychiatric symptoms. However, the onset and offset of symptoms are less abrupt than in KLS and the episodes of longer duration.

Another frequently evoked diagnosis is epilepsy, given the frequent bursts of synchronous, generalized, moderate- to high-voltage, 5–7 Hz waves on the EEG, but the symptomatology does not fit well with epileptic seizures.

Less common differential diagnoses are brain tumors developing inside the third ventricle (colloid cyst, epidermoid cyst, or choroid papilloma) responsible for paroxystic blockages to the drainage of CSF. In this case, the onset of sleep is generally preceded by sudden headaches, which may be associated with vomiting and vague sensory disorders. Other intraventricular tumors in the fourth ventricle, craniopharyngioma, or pinealoma may give rise to the same symptomatology. Diagnosis in all these cases is based on brain imaging.

Other possible diagnoses are encephalitis, head trauma, recurrent stupor, porphyria, and Lyme disease.

Pathophysiology

Neuropathological examinations have been performed in three cases of typical KLS [82–84] and in one case of KLS secondary to a presumptive brain tumor [85]. They have shown various abnormalities in different locations of the brain, but have not led to consistent conclusions.

Neuroimaging studies performed during symptomatic periods and asymptomatic intervals have documented modifications in tracer perfusion or metabolism in different regions of the brain, particularly in the thalamus, hypothalamus, basal ganglia, and frontotemporal areas [74,76,86–90]. However, conflicting results have been recorded concerning the topography and direction of changes, which may be due to the use of different imaging methods, small sample sizes, imaging at different stages of disease evolution, clinical symptoms during scanning, and delay from episode onset [91].

Based on the generally young age at onset, the recurrence of symptoms, the frequent infectious trigger, and a significant increased frequency of the *HLA-DQB1*02:01* allele in the multicenter group of 30 unrelated patients with KLS, an autoimmune origin of KLS has been suggested [81].

Similar to narcolepsy with cataplexy, 3% of cases are familial, suggesting that the familial risk of KLS is high, given the low prevalence of the disease [77]. Moreover, two cases of monozygotic twin pairs concordant for KLS have been published [92,94] supporting a strongly genetic basis for the condition. Finally, rare multiplex families suggest an autosomal Mendelian inheritance, indicating that single-gene mutations may cause KLS [77]. However, none has been identified up to now.

Given the role of hypocretin neuropeptides in both sleep–wake regulation and feeding, hypocretins seemed good candidates to be involved in KLS. Effectively, according to several investigations, CSF hypocretin-1 might be temporarily decreased during hypersomnia episodes at least in some patients [34,75,94–96].

Treatment

Most patients do not require any treatment when episodes are sufficiently spaced out and do not have major social impact.

A Cochrane Database Systematic Review did not find any randomized controlled trials of pharmacological treatments in KLS [97]. Therefore, one is left with individual cases or small series in which one or several drugs have been administered and clinically evaluated. There are two types of treatment: symptomatic and prophylactic. Symptomatic treatments are mainly based on stimulants (amphetamine or methylphenidate) and on the wake-promoting drug, modafinil. Proper evaluation of these drugs is rather unreliable because of the spontaneous eventual disappearance of the symptoms after a few days of evolution. In addition, psychostimulants are of poor efficacy in treating the symptomatic periods, since cognitive and behavioral problems will remain potentially poorly tolerated after normalization of the vigilance state. In contrast, prophylactic treatments based on mood stabilizers (lithium and antiepileptic drugs) are easier to evaluate, based on the recurrence (or not) of symptomatic episodes. Lithium is effective in some cases. A recent large, prospective, open-label study provides class IV evidence that for patients with KLS, lithium decreases the frequency and duration of KLS episodes [98]. Risks of thyroid and kidney insufficiency must be considered, however. Among antiepileptic drugs, valproic acid may be the most effective. Recently, two trials of clarithromycin have been carried out in patients with KLS: in the first, a short-term effect was noted in one patient [99], while the second showed a partial response in four patients, although the optimal timing of treatment was not determined [100].

Hypersomnia due to a medical disorder

A direct cause of EDS is a coexisting medical disorder. In most cases, EDS only stands as an associated symptom, to the extent that it is often neglected as far as it does not compromise the vital prognosis.

Neurological disorders

Brain tumors

Clinically, sleepiness tends to be continuous, interspersed with brief arousals, whether spontaneous or provoked. Sleepiness may occur in any intracranial hypertension syndrome, or more rarely result from tumors of the diencephalon or peduncular region with no associated intracranial hypertension. These tumors include gliomas or hamartomas affecting the posterior hypothalamus; posterior and superior suprasellar craniopharyngiomas compressing the floor of the third ventricle; and pinealomas or teratomas affecting the posterior part of the third ventricle. A fair number of cases of narcolepsy symptomatic of brain tumors affecting the hypothalamus or midbrain regions have been reported [101].

Stroke

EDS is often a transient state between confusional state, agitation, or even coma, marking the initial period of the stroke. Among the most typical causes of sleepiness of vascular origin are paramedian uni or bithalamic infarcts characterized by vertical ocular paresis, "skew deviation," paresis of the third cranial pair, dysarthria, and instability in walking; paramedian pedunculothalamic infarcts characterized by altered ocular motility due to paresis of the third or of the sixth cranial pair; and tegmental infarcts affecting the pontine tegmentum and the reticular formation of this region [102].

Neurodegenerative disorders

EDS affects 16–50% of Parkinson disease patients [103], a finding that is, however, rarely confirmed by the gold standard MSLT evaluation [104]. It may precede Parkinson disease by several years and often worsens after the introduction of dopaminergic treatment. A degeneration of hypocretinergic neurons and monoaminergic neurons may be involved. It is of concern that the occurrence of sudden irresistible sleep episodes is facilitated by the intake of dopaminergic agonists [105].

Multiple system atrophy gives rise to EDS in 25 –30% of patients [106]. However, the mechanism is not the same as in Parkinson disease. It often depends on OSAS, present in 15–37% of patients [107].

EDS is common in Alzheimer-type dementia. It is often a component of a more profound sleep–wake disturbance with frequent awakenings at night. The symptom of EDS is accounted for in several ways: sundowning syndrome, which affects roughly one-quarter of subjects with dementia, psychotropic medications, depression, and OSAS [108].

Neuromuscular diseases

Any neuromuscular disease—motoneuron disease, motor neuropathy, neuromuscular junction disorder, or muscular disease—is likely to be accompanied by sleep-related breathing impairment resulting in EDS. A typical example is myotonic dystrophy characterized by weakness of limb, facial, and respiratory muscles, myotonia, cardiomyopathy, endocrinopathy, frontal baldness, neuropsychological deficits, and cataract. Myotonic dystrophy is the chronic neuromuscular disease entailing the highest prevalence of self-reported EDS, with up to 70–80% of patients being affected with this condition [109]. Available clinical, neurophysiological, and histopathological evidence supports the hypothesis that EDS most often stems from a primary central nervous system (CNS) disturbance, and possibly from a central dysfunction of sleep regulation leading to REM sleep alteration.

Post-traumatic sleepiness

In addition to residual symptoms such as focal neurological deficit, post-traumatic epilepsy, movement disorder, hormonal disturbance, cognition deficit, and psychotic disorder, subjects with traumatic brain injury (TBI) may develop sleep–wake disturbances, including excessive daytime sleepiness. According to Baumann et al., subjective post-traumatic sleepiness (as assessed with the ESS) was found in 28% of 65 consecutive patients 6 months after traumatic brain injury and objective post-traumatic sleepiness (as assessed with the MSLT) in 25% [110]. Another prospective study conducted in 87 subjects, at least 3 months after TBI, found post-traumatic sleepiness in 25% of subjects [111]. Imaging studies may reveal various findings: lesions affecting the hypothalamic region, the midbrain, or the pontine tegmentum, or more often an absence of any significant lesion. The etiology of post-traumatic sleepiness has yet to be elucidated, and it is likely that multiple factors, both physical and psychological, may be involved.

Epilepsy

Although epilepsy can be the cause of sleepiness, the association of epilepsy and sleepiness is not straightforward. Some studies have demonstrated EDS in 17–28% of patients with epilepsy [112,113], while others have found no difference in ESS scores in patients with epilepsy and in controls [114,115]. The location of the ictal focus likely influences the expression of sleepiness; patients with frontal lobe epilepsy have increased sleep fragmentation, which may lead to EDS [116]. Moreover, many antiepileptic drugs (although not lamotrigine) are known to induce sleepiness.

Multiple sclerosis

There is conflicting evidence regarding sleepiness in multiple sclerosis (MS), with some study reporting sleep disturbances and EDS in MS patients compared with non-MS groups [117] and others revealing ESS scores in the upper normal range [118,119]. In the case of severe sleepiness in MS, the presence of hypothalamic lesions

and low CSF hypocretin levels need to be ruled out, since rare cases of narcolepsy with EDS and several SOREMPs, with or without cataplexy, secondary to bilateral hypothalamic lesions and hypocretin levels below 40 pg/mL have been reported [120,121].

Infectious and parasitic diseases

Infections caused by Epstein–Barr virus and other viruses

In the aftermath of infectious mononucleosis, most subjects feel intense asthenia and lengthening of total sleep time, difficulty awakening, and EDS, evoking idiopathic hypersomnia [122]. This type of transient hypersomnia also develops following viral pneumopathy, hepatitis B viral infection, and Guillain–Barré syndrome, probably through the same mechanism.

Encephalitis caused by viruses

Disorders of wakefulness and/or consciousness are found in virtually all patients affected by viral encephalitis. However, in the absence of PSG studies, it is very difficult to define the border between wakefulness disorders and disorders affecting consciousness. Two nosological entities are worthy of mention, arboviruses and epidemic encephalitis.

The arboviruses represent a heterogeneous group of viruses whose common characteristic is that they are transmitted by arthropod vectors. Infections by the various arboviruses share the same initial symptoms, evoking a fairly severe flu-like state with high fever, headache, and myalgias. Encephalitic signs then develop, which vary according to the agent responsible. Sleepiness is a fairly characteristic feature of European tick-borne encephalitis [123].

First appearing in Europe in 1917, epidemic encephalitis affected tens of thousands of subjects in the 10 years that followed. Its cause has never been fully identified, even though the pathological lesions and inflammatory sites located mainly in the gray matter of the diencephalon and basal ganglia strongly suggest a viral infection. The most common form, referred to as the lethargic form, consisted of a febrile flu-like condition, rapidly complicated by sleepiness culminating in a permanent state of sleep, stupor, and coma, associated with frequent oculogyric crises with nystagmus. This clinical picture corresponded to lesions in the posterior hypothalamus and midbrain tegmentum [124]. Sporadic cases are still exceptionally reported.

Acquired immunodeficiency syndrome (AIDS)

Subjects infected by the human immunodeficiency virus (HIV) sometimes complain of EDS. Darko et al. found that HIV-infected patients were significantly more likely to sleep more, nap more, and have diminished midmorning alertness in comparison with noninfected subjects [125]. More recently, poor nighttime sleep was significantly correlated with fatigue intensity and EDS in a sample of 128 individuals in a longitudinal study [126].

African trypanosomiasis (sleeping sickness)

African trypanosomiasis is a subacute or chronic parasitic disease caused by the inoculation of a protozoon, *Trypanosoma brucei*, transmitted by the tsetse fly. It is endemic to certain regions of tropical Africa. The form found in West and Central Africa is due to *T. brucei gambiense*. It causes over 98% of reported cases. The form found in East Africa is caused by *T. brucei rhodesiense*.

The West and Central African form is divided into three successive stages. Several hours after the fly's bite, a hot, edematous and erythematous tender nodule, referred to as the chancre, appears around the inoculation point. After a phase of inoculation varying from several days to several months, the invasion of the blood and lymphatic organs by multiple trypanosomes constitutes the hemo-lymphatic stage 1. This stage lasts until the appearance of the parasite in the CSF, referred to as the meningo-encephalitic stage 2, characterized by exacerbated headaches and fatigue, mental disturbances, and a wealth of neurological signs, including disorders of tone and mobility. Sleep and wake alterations consist of sleep episodes randomly spread over 24 hours, causing a loss of the circadian alternation of sleep and wakefulness and the occurrence of SOREMPs in several sleep episodes [127]. Demyelinating encephalitis ends the time course of the disease, along with apathy, dementia, epileptic seizures, incontinence, and death in a state of cachexia.

Multisystem diseases

Sarcoidosis, a chronic multisystem disease, most frequently affects the lungs. However, CNS involvement is thought to occur in about 10% of cases. Neurosarcoidosis can affect any part of the CNS, especially the hypothalamus and pituitary gland, and in that case includes symptoms of sleepiness, hyperphagia, polydipsia, and variations in body temperature.

Systemic lupus erythematosis is another chronic multisystem disorder that may be associated with EDS.

Endocrine disorders

EDS has been associated with several endocrine disorders, in part due to the co-occurrence of OSAS.

Hypothyroidism

Several studies have demonstrated that OSAS is more prevalent among patients with hypothyroidism than among control subjects [128]. However, a primary effect of hypothyroidism on sleep is also possible, with potential benefit from thyroid stimulants [129].

Acromegaly

Sleep-disordered breathing is common in acromegaly, and is connected with the insidious onset of facial features, bony proliferation, and soft tissue swelling. In a study involving 17 patients (11 women and 6 men) diagnosed with acromegaly, ten patients (58.8%) had an apnea–hypopnea index (AHI) greater than 10, nine had OSAS and one had central sleep apneas [130]. Seven (five with an AHI >10 and two with an AHI < 10) reported EDS with an ESS score greater than 10.

Diabetes

Diabetes and OSAS share a high prevalence in industrial nations. The presence of OSAS seems to promote the development of diabetes mellitus and vice versa.

There are limited data regarding EDS in type 2 diabetes patients, with huge a confounder in between, namely, obesity. In one study involving 614 type 2 diabetes patients, EDS, as measured by ESS, occurred in 8.5% of patients [131]. However, apneas were assessed by the Sleep Disorders Questionnaires using sleep apnea subscales only, and the relationship between apneas and EDS was not specifically assessed. In another study involving 110 patients with type 2 diabetes, EDS was found in 55.5% of patients, in association with depressive symptoms in 44.5% individuals [132].

Genetic disorders

EDS is highly prevalent in patients suffering from diverse genetic syndromes. It is often the consequence of nocturnal breathing disorder, most often OSAS, but it may also be due to a primary wakefulness dysfunction. A comprehensive review of these syndromes has been published [133] and the present subsection will review only the most common genetic disorders accompanied by EDS.

Chromosomal abnormalities

Autosomal abnormalities

Down syndrome is the most common autosomal abnormality. Most cases result from trisomy 21, although less commonly Down syndrome occurs when part of chromosome 21 becomes attached to another chromosome (translocation Down syndrome), and a very small percentage of patients with Down syndrome have an extra copy of chromosome 21 in only some of the body cells (mosaicism of trisomy 21). EDS is frequent. It is connected with OSAS, the prevalence of which is higher than 50%, or with sleep fragmentation and arousals, independently of respiratory events and periodic limb movements.

Chromosomal anomalies in various dystrophic syndromes

Prader–Willi syndrome is due to a lack of expression of the paternally active genes in the q11–13 region of chromosome 15. EDS is the most common sleep-related symptom in Prader–Willi syndrome. Although OSAS may have a role to play in some patients, the primary cause of EDS is thought to lie in hypothalamic dysfunction, with comorbid symptomatic narcolepsy in some cases.

Smith–Magenis syndrome is associated with a deletion of chromosome 17 (17p11.2). Most patients exhibit sleep attacks occurring at the end of the day, as the expression of an inversion of the melatonin circadian rhythm.

Norrie disease is a rare genetic form of blindness and variable mental retardation due to an Xp11.3–p11.4 microdeletion. Features of narcolepsy including irresistible episodes of sleep and attacks resembling cataplexy have been described in three related boys in North America [134].

Inherited neurometabolic disorders

These diseases result from a single mutant gene coding for an enzymatic protein mostly involved in the catabolic pathways. Most striking sleep disorders are found in lysosomal storage disorders including glycogenoses, mucopolysaccharidoses, and sphingolipidoses. Pompe disease results from an acid α-glucosidase deficiency. Diaphragm weakness responsible for respiratory insufficiency or sleep apnea may appear in any stage of the disease and be associated with EDS. Mucopolysaccharidoses are heterogeneous syndromes involving mental and physical retardation. OSAS is often associated with self-reported EDS. Niemann–Pick disease type C is a lysosomal storage sphingolipidosis with four main forms: early infantile, late infantile, juvenile, and adult. Cataplexy may be present in 25–50% of late infantile and juvenile forms, even in the absence of hypocretin deficiency. Total sleep time, sleep efficiency, REM sleep amount, and delta sleep amount are decreased on PSG in comparison with age-matched controls, and MSLT shows shortened mean sleep latency [135].

Hypersomnia due to a medication or substance

Patients with this disorder have excessive nocturnal sleep, daytime sleepiness, or excessive napping that is attributable to sedating medications, alcohol, or drugs of abuse, or to withdrawal from amphetamines and other drugs.

This sleep disorder has become a public heath concern, owing to the consequences of somnolence not only on driving, but also on occupational activities and thus on productivity.

Sedating medications

These medications lead to "a state of calm or reduced nervous activity" (Collins English Dictionary) which may eventually result in EDS. They cause sedation via effects on the neural systems involved in sleep–wake regulation, primarily by increasing GABA or inhibiting histamine, norepinephrine (noradrenaline), or serotonin. Important factors affecting the degree of sedation include receptor binding profile, dose, half-life, and time of administration, as well as age and association with multiple medication ingestion. These medications include benzodiazepine and non-benzodiazepine hypnotics, anti-anxiety drugs, some antidepressants, first-generation antihistamines, antipsychotics, antiepileptic drugs, opiates, anticholinergics, and skeletal muscle relaxants.

Another frequent source of excessive somnolence is the use of some dopamine agonists such as pramipexole and ropinirole. Excessive somnolence may less frequently be caused by various other medications, including antihypertensive drugs, mostly α_2 agonists, (eg, clonidine) and less frequently nonselective β-antagonists (eg, propranolol) and α_1 antagonists (eg, prazosin), nonsteroidal anti-inflammatory drugs, and antispasmodic drugs. Of note, this adverse effect occurs only in a fraction of patients using these drugs and its severity can vary considerably. In some cases, failure to provide treatment with the incriminated drug may be more disruptive than EDS.

Substance abuse

EDS can occur with abuse of alcohol, benzodiazepines, barbiturates, γ-hydroxybutyrate acid, opiates, and cannabis. Alcohol intoxication typically causes sedation for 3–4 hours and then insomnia, whereas intake of caffeine or cocaine causes insomnia, and their withdrawal sedation. Sedation is a common adverse effect of opioid medication. The degree of sedation may depend on the specific drug, dosage, and duration of use, as well as the severity of the underlying disease.

Cannabis use may be associated with EDS, sluggishness, giddiness, and inability to concentrate.

Stimulant withdrawal

EDS is common with abrupt discontinuation of stimulants. In chronically heavy amphetamine users, EDS peaks during the first week of withdrawal and can persist for up to several weeks. In people consuming caffeine daily, discontinuation can produce EDS and fatigue for several days.

Hypersomnia associated with a psychiatric disorder

EDS can be a symptom of psychiatric disorders belonging to different diagnostic classes of the Diagnostic and Statistical Manual of Mental Disorders, fifth edition (DSM-5) [136]: major depressive disorder, persistent depressive disorder, premenstrual dysphoric disorder, and other specified depression disorders in the class of depressive disorders; bipolar I and II disorders in the class of bipolar and related disorders; and schizoaffective disorder in the class of schizophrenia spectrum and other psychiatric disorders.

As a rule, EDS is not systematically present in these disorders. First, the accompanying sleep symptom is either insomnia or excessive daytime sleepiness; second, the sleep symptom is part of a list of symptoms, a certain number of which have to be present during the same 2-week period and represent a change from previous functioning; third, and above all, most psychiatric disorder studies addressing EDS have assessed daytime sleepiness using ESS or other subjective tests, but rarely objective sleepiness as measured by MSLT, actigraphy, or continuous PSG [137]. Moreover, the few studies using objective sleepiness tests have failed to demonstrate objective EDS. However, clinical experience shows that subjects with psychiatric disorders often spend hours in bed during the daytime. Thus, it is of the utmost importance that future studies measure both EDS and total sleep time per 24 hours outside of psychotropic medication use.

Insufficient sleep syndrome

"Insufficient sleep syndrome occurs when an individual persistently fails to obtain the amount of sleep required to maintain normal levels of alertness and wakefulness" [6]. As a consequence, the subject is abnormally sleepy, with daily periods of irrepressible need to sleep or daytime lapses into sleep. The patient's sleep time, established by personal or collateral history, sleep diary, and actigraphy, is usually shorter than expected for age. Sleep time is markedly extended on weekend nights or during holidays compared with weekday nights. Depending upon the extent of sleep loss, individuals are at risk for a range of neurobehavioral deficits, including lapses of attention, slowed working memory, reduced cognitive function, depressed mood, and fatigue.

This syndrome was systematically investigated for the first time in 1983, in a population of 59 adults (37 men and 22 women) with mean age 40.8 ± 12.2 years [138]. Since then, studies have been carried out mainly among adolescents [139,140], except for a Japanese study based on interviews with 1243 patients referred to a sleep disorder outpatient clinic for complaint of excessive daytime sleepiness: the combination of insufficient sleep and EDS was about 7.1% of the sample [141]. However, no differential diagnosis was applied.

Positive diagnosis is primarily based on interview, sleep diaries maintained for more than a week, and actigraphy. PSG and MSLT are not required to establish a diagnosis of insufficient sleep syndrome. Rather, sleep time is extended first and the patient is clinically reevaluated. If the symptoms disappear, insufficient sleep syndrome is confirmed.

If unchecked, insufficient sleep syndrome may predispose to depression and other psychological difficulties, as well as poor work performance or traffic accidents. Differential diagnosis includes mainly central disorders of hypersomnolence, mood disorders, and long sleepers. Treatment relies on a longer major sleep episode or, if the patient's professional life does not allow this, one or several daytime naps.

Conclusion

In addition to OSAS and narcolepsy, etiologies of EDS are numerous. Some of them, namely, idiopathic hypersomnia, Kleine–Levin syndrome, and insufficient sleep syndrome, are well known to sleep physicians, while others, mainly symptomatic causes, are familiar to some only. It is of the utmost importance that sleep physicians be aware of the possibility of EDS in a large variety of somatic and psychiatric conditions, and that specialists, including neurologists, cardiologists, chest physicians, endocrinologists, specialists in infectious diseases and internal medicine, and psychiatrists, learn to recognize EDS as an important symptom, in terms of both diagnosis and treatment.

References

1. Roth B. Spankova opilost a spankova obrna [Sleep drunkenness and sleep paralysis]. Ceskoslovenska Neurol 1956;19:48–58.
2. Roth B. Narcolepsy and hypersomnia; review and classification of 642 personally observed cases. Schweiz Arch Neurol Neurochir Psychiat 1976;119:31–41.
3. Association of Sleep Disorders Centers. Diagnostic classification of sleep and arousal disorders, first edition, prepared by the Sleep Disorders Classification Committee. Roffwarg HP, Chairman. Sleep 1979;2:1–137.
4. ICSD. International classification of sleep disorders: Diagnostic and coding manual. Diagnostic Classification Steering Committee. Thorpy MJ, Chairman. Rochester, MN: American Sleep Disorders Association, 1990.
5. American Academy of Sleep Medicine. International classification of sleep disorders. Diagnostic and coding manual, 2nd ed. Westchester, IL: American Academy of Sleep Medicine, 2005.
6. American Academy of Sleep Medicine. International classification of sleep disorders, 3rd ed. Darien, IL: American Academy of Sleep Medicine, 2014.
7. Van den Hoed J, Kraemer H, Guilleminault C, et al. Disorders of excessive daytime somnolence: polygraphic and clinical data for 100 patients. Sleep 1981:4:23–37.
8. Baker TL, Guilleminault C, Nino-Murcia G, et al. Comparative polysomnographic study of narcolepsy and idiopathic central nervous system hypersomnia. Sleep 1986;9:232–42.
9. Aldrich MS. The clinical spectrum of narcolepsy and idiopathic hypersomnia. Neurology 1996;46:393–401.
10. Bruck D, Parkes JD. A comparison of idiopathic hypersomnia using self report measures and sleep diary data. J Neurol Neurosurg Psychiatry 1996;60:576–8.
11. Bassetti C, Aldrich MS. Idiopathic hypersomnia. A series of 42 patients. Brain 1997;120:1423–35.
12. Billiard M, Dauvilliers Y. Idiopathic hypersomnia. Sleep Med Rev 2001;5:351–60.
13. Kanbayashi T, Inoue Y, Chiba S, et al. CSF hypocretin-1 (orexin-A) concentrations in narcolepsy with and without cataplexy and idiopathic hypersomnia. J Sleep Res 2002;11:91–3.
14. Vignatelli L, d'Alessandro R, Mosconi P et al. Health-related quality of life in Italian patients with narcolepsy: the SF-36 health survey. Sleep Med 2004;5:467–75.
15. Heier MS, Evsiukova T, Vilming S, et al. CSF hypocretin-1 levels and clinical profiles in narcolepsy and idiopathic CNS hypersomnia in Norway. Sleep 2007;30:969–73.
16. Martinez-Rodriguez JE, Iranzo A, Casamitjana R et al. Comparative analysis of patients with narcolepsy–cataplexy, narcolepsy without cataplexy and idiopathic hypersomnia. Med Clin (Barc) 2007;128:361–4.
17. Kanbayashi T, Kodama T, Kondo H et al. CSF histamine contents in narcolepsy, idiopathic hypersomnia and obstructive sleep apnea syndrome. Sleep 2009;32:181–7.
18. Coelho FM, Pradella-Hallinan M, Predazzoli Neto M et al. Prevalence of the *HLA-DQB1*0602* allele in narcolepsy and idiopathic hypersomnia patients seen at a sleep disorder outpatient unit in Sao Paulo. Rev Bras Psiquiatr 2009;31:10–14.
19. Tanaka S, Honda M. IgG abnormality in narcolepsy and idiopathic hypersomnia. PLoS One 2010;5:e9555.
20. Pizza F, Vandis S, Detto S, et al. Different sleep onset criteria at the multiple sleep latency test (MSLT): an additional marker to differentiate central nervous system (CNS) hypersomnias. J Sleep Res 2011;20:250–6.
21. Dauvilliers Y, Delallée N, Jaussent I, et al. Normal cerebrospinal fluid histamine and tele-methyl histamine levels in hypersomnia conditions. Sleep 2012;35:1359–66.
22. Dauvilliers Y, Paquereau J, Bastuji H, et al. Disorders of excessive daytime somnolence: the French Harmony Study. J Neurol Neurosurg Psychiatry 2009;80:636–41.
23. Ali M, Auger RR, Slocumb NL, et al. Idiopathic hypersomnia: clinical features and response to treatment. J Clin Sleep Med 2009;5:562–8.
24. Ohayon MM, Reynolds CF III, Dauvilliers Y. Excessive sleep duration and quality of life. Ann Neurol 2013;73:785–94.
25. American Psychiatric Association. Diagnostic and statistical manual of mental disorders, fourth edition (DSM-IV-TR). Washington DC: American Psychiatric Association, 2000.
26. Nevsimalova-Bruhova S, Roth B. Heredofamilial aspects of narcolepsy and hypersomnia. Schweiz Arch Neurol 1972;110:45–54.
27. Roth B, Nevsimalova S, Rechtschaffen A. Hypersomnia with "sleep drunkenness." Arch Gen Psychiatry 1972:26:456–62.
28. Vernet C, Leu-Semenescu S, Buzare MA, et al. Subjective symptoms in idiopathic hypersomnia: beyond excessive sleepiness. J Sleep Res 2010;19:525–34.
29. Trotti LM, Staab BA, Rye DB. Test–retest reliability of the multiple sleep latency test in narcolepsy without cataplexy and idiopathic hypersomnia. J Clin Sleep Med 2013;9:789–95.
30. Anderson KN, Pilsworth S, Sharples LD, et al. Idiopathic hypersomnia: a study of 77 cases. Sleep 2007;320:1274–81.
31. Billiard M. Narcolepsy and idiopathic hypersomnia. In: Léger D, Pandi-Perumal SR, eds. Sleep disorders: their impact on public health. Abingdon: Informa Healthcare, 2007:225–34.
32. Petitjean F, Jouvet M. Hypersomnie et augmentation de l'acide 5-hydroxy-indoleacétique cérébral par lésion isthmique chez le chat. C R Séances Soc Biol (Paris) 1970;164:2288–93.
33. Mignot E, Lammers GJ, Ripley B, et al. The role of cerebrospinal fluid hypocretin measurement in the diagnosis of narcolepsy and other hypersomnias. Arch Neurol 2002;59:1553–62.
34. Dauvilliers Y, Baumann CR, Carlander B, et al. CSF hypocretin-1 levels in narcolepsy, Kleine–Levin syndrome, and other hypersomnias and neurological conditions. J Neurol Neurosurg Psychiatry 2003;74:1667–73.
35. Croyal M, Dauvilliers Y, Labeeuw O, et al. Histamine and tele-methylhistamine quantification in cerebrospinal fluid from narcoleptic subjects by liquid tandem mass spectrometry with precolumn derivatization. Anal Biochem 2011;409:28–36.
36. Rye DB, Bliwise DL, Parker K, et al. Modulation of vigilance in the primary hypersomnias by endogenous enhancement of $GABA_A$ receptors. Sci Transl Med 2012;4:161ra151.
37. Dauvilliers Y, Evangelista E, Lopez R, et al. Absence of γ-aminobutyric acid—a receptor potentiation in central hypersomnolence disorders. Ann Neurol 2016;80(2):259–68.
38. Janackova S, Motte J, Bakchine S, et al. Idiopathic hypersomnia: a report of three adolescent-onset cases in a two-generation family. J Child Neurol 2011;26:522–5.
39. Sforza E, Gaudreau H, Petit D, et al. Homeostatic sleep regulation in patients with idiopathic hypersomnia. Clin Neurophysiol 2000;11:91–3.
40. Billiard M, Rondouin G, Espa F, et al. Pathophysiology of idiopathic hypersomnia. Rev Neurol (Paris) 2001;157:5S101–6.
41. DelRosso LM, Chesson AL, Hoque R. Manual characterization of sleep spindle index in patients with narcolepsy and idiopathic hypersomnia. Sleep Disord 2014;2014:271802.
42. Nevsimalova S, Blazejova K, Illnerova H, et al. A contribution to pathophysiology of idiopathic hypersomnia. Suppl Clin Neurophysiol 2000;53:366–70.
43. Vernet C, Arnulf I. Idiopathic hypersomnia with and without long sleep time: a controlled series of 75 patients. Sleep 2009;32:753–9.

44. Lippert J, Halfter H, Heidbreder A, et al. Altered dynamics in the circadian oscillation of clock genes in dermal fibroblasts of patients suffering from idiopathic hypersomnia. PLoS One 2014;9:e85255.

45. Fukuda D, Strauss SE, Hickie I, et al. The chronic fatigue syndrome: comprehensive approach to its definition and study. Ann Int Med 1994;121:953–9.

46. Manu P, Lane TJ, Matthews DA, et al. Alpha–delta sleep in patients with a chief complaint of chronic fatigue. South Med J 1994;87:465–70.

47. Bastuji H, Jouvet M. Successful treatment of idiopathic hypersomnia and narcolepsy with modafinil. Prog Neuropsychopharmacol Psychiatry 1988;12:695–700.

48. Lavault S, Dauvilliers Y, Drouot X, et al. Benefit and risk of modafinil in idiopathic hypersomnia vs narcolepsy with cataplexy. Sleep Med 2011;12:550–6.

49. Ozaki A, Inoue Y, Hayashida K, et al. Quality of life in patients with narcolepsy with cataplexy, narcolepsy without cataplexy, and idiopathic hypersomnia without long sleep time: comparison between patients on psychostimulants, drug-naive patients and the general Japanese population. Sleep Med 2012;13:200–6.

50. Mayer G, Benes H, Young P, et al. Modafinil in the treatment of idiopathic hypersomnia without long sleep time-a randomized, double-blind, placebo-controlled study. J Sleep Res 2015;24:74–81.

51. Philip P, Chauffon C, Taillard J, et al. Modafinil improves real driving performance in patients with hypersomnia: a randomized double-blind placebo-controlled crossover clinical trial. Sleep 2014;37:483–7.

52. Nittur N, Konofal E, Dauvilliers Y et al. Mazindol in narcolepsy and idiopathic and symptomatic hypersomnia refractory to stimulants: a long-term chart review. Sleep Med 2013;14:30–6.

53. Montplaisir J, Fantini L. Idiopathic hypersomnia: a diagnosis dilemma. Sleep Med Rev 2001;5:361–2.

54. Leu-Semenescu S, Louis P, Arnulf I. Benefits and risk of sodium oxybate in idiopathic hypersomnia versus narcolepsy type 1: a chart review. Sleep Med 2016;17:38–44.

55. Shinno H, Ishikawa I, Yamanaka M, et al. Effects of levothyroxine on prolonged nocturnal sleep and excessive daytime somnolence in patients with idiopathic hypersomnia. Sleep Med 2011;12:578–83.

56. Trotti LM, Saini P, Freeman AA, et al. Improvement in daytime sleepiness with clarithromycin in patients with GABA-related hypersomnia: clinical experience. J Psychopharmacol 2013; 28:697–702.

57. Trotti LM, Saini P, Bliwise DL, et al. Clarithromycin in γ-aminobutyric acid-related hypersomnolence: a randomized, crossover trial. Ann Neurol 2015;78:454–65.

58. Dauvilliers Y, Bassetti C, Lammers GI, et al. Pitolisant versus placebo or modafinil in patients with narcolepsy: a double-blind randomized study. Lancet Neurol 2013;12:1068–75.

59. Leu-Semenescu S, Nittur N, Golmard JL, et al. Effects of pitolisant, a histamine H3 inverse agonist, in drug-resistant idiopathic and symptomatic hypersomnia: a chart review. Sleep Med 2014;15:681–7.

60. Critchley M, Hoffman HL. The syndrome of periodic somnolence and morbid hunger (Kleine–Levin syndrome). Br Med J 1942;1:137–9.

61. Levin M. Periodic somnolence and morbid hunger. A new syndrome. Brain 1936;59:494–504.

62. Kleine W. Periodische Schlafsucht. Mschr Psychiat Neurol 1925;57:285–320.

63. Lewis NDC. The psychoanalytic approach to the problem of children under twelve years of age. Psychoanal Rev 1926;13:424–43.

64. Levin M. Narcolepsy (Gelineau's syndrome) and other varieties of morbid somnolence. Arch Neurol Psychiatr (Chicago) 1929;22:1172–200.

65. Oliver W. An account of an extraordinary sleepy person. Philos Trans R Soc Lond 1705;304:2177–82.

66. Critchley M. Periodic hypersomnia and megaphagia in adolescent males. Brain 1962;85:627–56.

67. Arnulf I, Zeitzer JM, File J, et al. Kleine–Levin syndrome: a systematic review of 186 cases in the literature. Brain 2005;128:2763–76.

68. Arnulf I, Lin L, Gadoth N, et al. Kleine–Levin syndrome: a systematic study of 108 patients. Ann Neurol 2008;63:482–92.

69. Billiard M, Jaussent I, Dauvilliers Y, et al. Recurrent hypersomnia: a review of 339 cases. Sleep Med Rev 2011;15:247–57.

70. Gadoth N, Kesler A, Vainstein G, et al. Clinical and polysomnographic characteristics of 34 patients with Kleine–Levin syndrome. J Sleep Res 2001;10:337–41.

71. Takahashi Y. Clinical studies of periodic somnolence. Analysis of 28 personal cases. Psychiat Neurol Jpn 1965;10:853–89.

72. Roth B. Narcolepsy and hypersomnia. Prague: Avicenum Czechoslovak Medical Press, 1980.

73. Smolik P, Roth B. Kleine–Levin syndrome. Etiopathogenesis and treatment. Acta Universitatis Carolinae. Monographia CXXVIII. Prague: Charles University, 1988.

74. Huang YS, Guilleminault C, Lin KL, et al. Relationship between Kleine–Levin syndrome and upper respiratory infection in Taiwan. Sleep 2012;35:123–9.

75. Li Q, Wang J, Dong X, et al. CSF hypocretin level in patients with Kleine–Levin syndrome. Sleep Med 2013;14 (Suppl 1):e47.

76. Kas A, Lavault S, Habert MO, et al. Feeling unreal: a functional imaging study in patients with Kleine–Levin syndrome. Brain 2014;137:2077–87.

77. Billiard M, Peraita-Adrados R, Tafti M. Genetics of recurrent hypersomnia. In: Shaw P, Tafti M, Thorpy M, eds. The genetic basis of sleep and sleep disorders. Cambridge: Cambridge University Press, 2013:272–7.

78. Suwa K, Toru M. A case of periodic somnolence whose sleep was induced by glucose. Folia Psychiatr Neurol Jpn 1969;23:253–62.

79. Popper JS, Hsia YE, Rogers T, et al. Familial hibernation (Kleine–Levin) syndrome [Abstract]. Am Hum Genet 1980;32:123A.

80. BaHammam AS, GadElRab MO, Owais SM et al. Clinical characteristics and HLA typing of a family with Kleine–Levin syndrome. Sleep Med 2008;9:575–8.

81. Dauvilliers Y, Mayer G, Lecendreux M, et al. An autoimmune hypothesis based on clinical and genetic analyses. Neurology 2002;59:1739–45.

82. Carpenter S, Yassa R, Ochs R. A pathological basis for Kleine–Levin syndrome. Arch Neurol 1982;39:25–8.

83. Koerber RK, Torkelson ER, Haven G, et al. Increased cerebrospinal fluid 5-hydroxytryptamine and 5-hydoxyindoleacetic acid in Kleine–Levin syndrome. Neurology 1984;34:1597–600.

84. Fenzi F, Simonati A, Crossato F, et al. Clinical features of Kleine–Levin syndrome with localized encephalitis. Neuropediatrics 1993;24:292–5.

85. Takrani LB, Cronin D. Kleine–Levin syndrome in a female patient. Can Psychiatr Assoc 1976;21:315–18.

86. Landtblom AM, Dige N, Schwerdt K, et al. Short-term memory dysfunction in Kleine–Levin syndrome. Acta Neurol Scand 2003;108:363–7.

87. Huang YS, Guilleminault C, Kao PF, et al. SPECT findings in the Kleine–Levin syndrome. Sleep 2005;28:955–60.

88. Hong SB, Joo EY, Tae WS, et al. Episodic diencephalic hypoperfusion in Kleine–Levin syndrome. Sleep 2006;29:1091–3.

89. Itokawa K, Fukui M, Nicomiya M, et al. Gabapentin in Kleine–Levin syndrome. Intern Med 2009;48:1183–5.

90. Haba-Rubio J, Prior JO, Guedj E, et al. Kleine–Levin syndrome: functional imaging correlates of hypersomnia and behavioral symptoms. Neurology 2012;79:1927–9.

91. Dauvilliers Y, Bayard S, Lopez R et al. Widespread hypermetabolism in symptomatic and asymptomatic episodes in Kleine–Levin syndrome. PLoS One 2014;9(4):e93813.

92. Peraita-Adrados R, Vicario JL, Tafti M, et al. Monozygotic twins affected with Kleine–Levin syndrome. Sleep 2012;35:595–96.

93. Ueno T, Fukuhara A, Ikegami A et al. Monozygotic twins concordant for Kleine–Levin syndrome. BMC Neurol 2012;12:31.

94. Podesta C, Ferreras M, Mozzi M et al. Kleine–Levin syndrome in a 14-year-old girl: CSF hypocretin-1 measurements. Sleep Med 2006;7:649–51.

95. Lopez R, Barateau L, Chenini S et al. Preliminary results on CSF and autonomic function biomarkers for hypothalamic dysfunction in Kleine–Levin syndrome. Sleep Med 2015;16:194–96.

96. Wang JY, Han F, Dong SX, et al. Cerebrospinal fluid orexin A levels and autonomic function in Kleine–Levin syndrome. Sleep 2016;39:855–60.

97. Oliveira MM, Conti C, Saconato H, et al. Pharmacological treatment for Kleine–Levin syndrome. Cochrane Database Syst Rev 2009;(15):1–12.

98. Leu-Semenescu S, Le Corvec T, Groos E et al. Lithium therapy in Kleine–Levin syndrome. An open-label study in 130 patients. Neurology 2015;85:1655–62.

99. Rezvanian E, Watson NF. Kleine–Levin syndrome treated with clarithromycin J Clin Sleep Med 2013;9:1211–12.

100. Trotti LM, Bliwise DL, Rye DB. Further experience using clarithromycin in patients with Kleine–Levin syndrome. J Clin Sleep Med 2014;10:457–8.

101. Nishino S, Kanbayashi T. Symptomatic narcolepsy, cataplexy and hypersomnia, and their implications in the hypothalamic hypocretin/orexin system. Sleep Med Rev 2005;9:269–310.

102. Bassetti CL, Valko P. Poststroke hypersomnia. Sleep Med Clin 2006;1:131–55.

103. Arnulf I. Excessive daytime sleepiness and parkinsonism. Sleep Med Rev 2005;9:185–200.

104. Cochen de Cock V, Bayard S, Jaussent I et al. Daytime sleepiness in Parkinson's disease: a reappraisal. PLoS One 2014;9(9):e107278.

105. Fabbrini G, Barbanti P, Aurilia C, et al. Excessive daytime somnolence in Parkinson's disease. Follow-up after 1 year of treatment. Neurol Sci 2003;24:178–9.

106. Moreno-Lopez C, Santamaria J, Salamero M, et al. Excessive daytime sleepiness in multiple system atrophy (SLEEMSA Study). Arch Neurol 2011;68:223–30.

107. Ferini-Strambi L, Marelli S. Sleep dysfunction in multiple system atrophy. Curr Treat Options Neurol 2012;14:464–73.

108. Rothman SM, Mattson MP. Sleep disturbances in Alzheimer's and Parkinson's diseases. Neuromol Med 2012;14:194–204.

109. Laberge L, Gagnon C, Dauvilliers Y. Daytime sleepiness and myotonic dystrophy. Curr Neurol Neurosci Rep 2013;13:340.

110. Baumann CR, Werth E, Stocker R, et al. Sleep–wake disturbances 6 months after traumatic brain injury: a prospective study. Brain 2007;130:1873–83.

111. Castriotta RJ, Wilde MC, Lai JM, et al. Prevalence and consequences of sleep disorders in traumatic brain injury. J Clin Sleep Med 2007;3:349–56.

112. Malow BA, Bowes RJ, Lin X. Predictors of sleepiness in epilepsy patients. Sleep 1997;20:1105–10.

113. Piperidou C, Karlovasitou A, Triantafyllou N, et al. Influence of sleep disturbance on quality of life of patients with epilepsy. Seizure 2008;17:588–94.

114. Manni R, Politini L, Sartori I, et al. Daytime sleepiness in epilepsy patients: evaluation by means of the Epworth sleepiness scale. J Neurol 2000;247:716–17.

115. Khatami R, Zutter D, Siegel A, et al. Sleep–wake habits and disorders in a series of 100 adult epilepsy patients—a prospective study. Seizure 2006;15:299–306.

116. Zucconi M, Oldani A, Smirne S, et al. The macrostructure and microstructure of sleep in patients with autosomal dominant nocturnal frontal lobe epilepsy. J Clin Neurophysiol 2000;17:77–86.

117. Bamer AM, Johnson KL, Amtmann D et al. Prevalence of sleep problems in individuals with multiple sclerosis. Mult Scler 2008;14:1127–30.

118. Rammohan KW, Rosenberg JH, Lynn DJ, et al. Efficacy and safety of modafinil (Provigil) for the treatment of fatigue in multiple sclerosis: a two center phase 2 study. J Neurol Neurosurg Psychiatry 2002;72:179–83.

119. Zifko UA, Rupp M, Schwarz S, et al. Modafinil in treatment of fatigue in multiple sclerosis. Results of an open-label study. J Neurol 2002;249:983–7.

120. Oka Y, Kanbayashi T, Mezaki T, et al. Low CSF hypocretin-1/orexin-A associated with hypersomnia secondary to hypothalamic lesion in a case of multiple sclerosis. J Neurol 2004;251:885–6.

121. Kanbayashi T, Abe M, Hishikawa Y, et al. Symptomatic narcolepsy with cataplexy and without cataplexy or hypersomnia, with and without hypocretin (orexin) deficiency. In: Bassetti CL, Billiard M, Mignot E, eds. Narcolepsy and hypersomnia. New York: Informa Healthcare, 2007:307–34.

122. Guilleminault C, Mondini S. Infectious mononucleosis and excessive daytime sleepiness. A long-term follow-up study. Arch Intern Med 1986;146:1333–35.

123. Krbkova L, Stroblova H, Bednarova J. Clinical course and sequelae for tick-borne encephalitis among children in South Moravia (Czech Republic). Eur J Pediatr 2015;174:449–58.

124. Berger JR, Vilensky JA. Encephalitis lethargica. Handbook Clin Neurol 2014;123:745–61.

125. Darko DF, McCutchan JA, Kripke DF, et al. Fatigue, sleep disturbance, disability, and indices of progression of HIV infection. Am J Psychiatry 1992;149:514–20.

126. Salahuddin N, Barroso J, Leserman J, et al. Daytime sleepiness, nighttime sleep quality, stressful life events, and HIV-related fatigue. J Assoc Nurses AIDS Care 2009;20:6–13.

127. Buguet A, Bourdon L, Bouteille B, et al. The duality of sleeping sickness: focusing on sleep. Sleep Med Rev 2001;5:139–53.

128. Misiolek M, Marek B, Namyslowski G, et al. Sleep apnea syndrome and snoring in patients with hypothyroidism with relation to overweight. J Physiol Pharmacol 2007;58(Suppl 1):77–85.

129. Ruiz-Primo E, Jurado JL, Solis H, et al. Polysomnographic effects of thyroid hormones in primary myxoedema. Electroencephalogr Clin Neurophysiol 1982;53:559–64.

130. Blanco-Perez JJ, Blanco-Ramos MA, Zamarron Sanz C, et al. Acromegaly and sleep apnea. Arch Bronconeumol 2004;40:355–9.

131. Cho EH, Lee H, Ryu OH et al. Sleep disturbances and glucoregulation in patients with type 2 diabetes. J Korean Med Sci 2014;29:243–7.

132. Medeiros C, Bruin V, Ferrer D, et al. Excessive daytime sleepiness in type 2 diabetes. Arq Bras Endocrinol Metabol 2013;57:425–30.

133. Nevsimalova S. Genetic disorders and sleepiness. In: Thorpy MJ, Billiard M, eds. Sleepiness, causes, consequences and treatment. Cambridge: Cambridge University Press, 2011:335–50.

134. Vossler DG, Wyler AR, Wilkus RJ et al. Cataplexy and monoamine oxidase deficiency in Norrie disease. Neurology 1996;46:1258–61.

135. Vankova J, Stepanova I, Jech R et al. Sleep disturbances and hypocretin deficiency in Niemann–Pick disease type C. Sleep 2003;26:427–30.

136. American Psychiatric Association. Diagnostic and statistical manual of mental disorders, fifth edition (DSM-V). Arlington, VA: American Psychiatric Association, 2013.

137. Dauvilliers Y, Lopez R, Ohayon M, et al. Hypersomnia and depressive symptoms: methodological and clinical aspects. BMC Med 2013;11:78.

138. Roehrs T, Zorick F, Sicklesteel J et al. Excessive daytime sleepiness associated with insufficient sleep. Sleep 1983;6:319–25.

139. Kang V, Shao J, Zhang K, et al. Sleep deficiency and sleep health problems in Chinese adolescents. Clin Med Insights Pediatr 2012;6:11–17.

140. Perez-Lloret S, Videla AJ, Richaudeau A, et al. A multi-step pathway connecting short sleep duration to daytime somnolence, reduced attention, and poor academic performance: an exploratory cross-sectional study in teenagers. J Clin Sleep Med 2013;9:469–73.

141. Komada Y, Inoue Y, Hayashida K, et al. Clinical significance and correlates of behaviorally induced insufficient sleep syndrome. Sleep Med 2008;9:851–6.

CHAPTER 16

Obstructive sleep apnea and upper airway resistance syndrome

Cristina Embid and Josep M. Montserrat

Introduction

In recent decades, the existence of sleep disordered breathing, its clinical consequences, and its high prevalence have been progressively recognized and have become to be considered a major health problem [1,2]. The apneas result in a number of different pathophysiological and biological changes, leading to a variety of clinical features (Fig. 16.1). Initially, attention focused just on sleep apnea, through studies of the classical picture of Pickwickian syndrome involving groups of obese patients who presented a large number of apneas during sleep. However, our concept of sleep disordered breathing has substantially changed since these early descriptions

of Pickwickian syndrome. The spectrum of sleep disordered breathing as presently understood is much broader, with different types of patients and patients with different characteristics involved, such as elderly people, children, non-obese patients, and the non-clinical population (Table 16.1).

On the other hand, in addition to apneic events, the study by the group led by Douglas of the airflow reduction or hypopnea due to partial upper airway (UA) collapse revealed the same disturbances as occur incomplete apnea [3], and both these events are now considered together. The apnea hypopnea index (AHI) has become the most appropriate measure to quantify events of sleep disordered breathing. Furthermore, upper airway resistance syndrome (UARS),

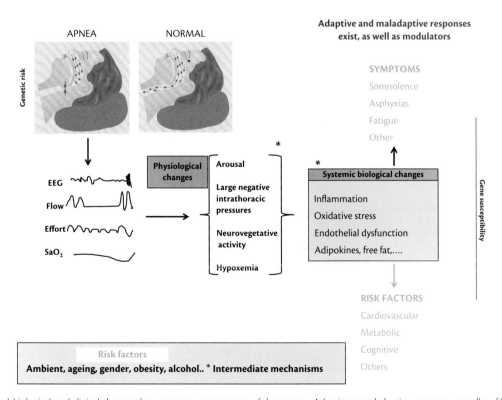

Fig. 16.1 Physiological, biological, and clinical changes that occur as a consequence of sleep apnea. Adaptive or maladaptive responses, as well as different risk factors, modulate the clinical consequences.

Table 16.1 Characteristics of the patients

Typical patients	Actual patients
Pickwickian syndrome	Elderly and children
Obesity	Pregnancy
Heavy snoring	Fibromyalgia
Breathing pauses	Uvulopalatopharyngoplasty (UPPP)
	Maxillomandibular problems
	Bariatric surgery
	Cardiovascular/resistant hypertension
	Non-clinic population
	Mild symptoms
	Neurological/psychiatric disease
	Myopathies and metabolic disorders

Table 16.2 Different definitions related to sleep apnea

Definitions
Apnea: Cessation of breathing flow for more than 10 s.
Hypopnea: Discernible reduction of flow for more than 10 s with arousal or a 3% decrease in oxygen saturation.
Other definitions of hypopnea: (1) Reduction in flow (30%) plus 3% decrease in oxygen saturation; (2) reduction in flow (50%) plus 4% decrease in oxygen saturation. However, sensors to analyze flow are not qualitative, and therefore these definitions are difficult to apply in practice.
RERA (or UARS event): Short period of flow limitation (but > 10 s), ending with an arousal (frequently scored as hypopnea).
Apnea and hypopnea index (AHI): number of apneas and hypopneas recorded per hour of sleep.
RDI: number of apneas and hypopneas plus RERAs recorded per hour of sleep.
Short period of flow limitation (but > 10 s) without consequences: This is not scored as an event.
Prolonged period of limitation without consequences: This is not scored as an event.

Severity of sleep apnea
Mild OSA: AHI 5–15/h; moderate OSA: AHI 15–30/h; severe OSA: AHI > 30/h.

Clinical entities that have to be treated (sleep apnea–hypopnea syndrome)
Sleep apnea–hypopnea syndrome with AHI > 5–15/h plus mild symptoms: General measures (Personalize).
Sleep apnea–hypopnea syndrome with AHI > 15–30/h plus symptoms: General measures before CPAP (Personalize).
Severe sleep apnea with AHI > 30/h plus minor symptoms: General measures and CPAP.*

*Some authors use a cut-off point of AHI >15/h instead of AHI > 30/h for more rigorous treatment (straight to CPAP).

also known as respiratory-effort-related arousal (RERA), has been described, with pathophysiology similar to that of hypopnea. In this case, the respiratory disturbance index (RDI), which is the sum of the numbers of apneas, hypopneas, and RERAs per hour, is used to express the total spectrum of sleep respiratory events (Fig. 16.2(a)). Table 16.2 summarizes different definitions related to sleep-related breathing disorders (SBDs). SBDs have been described as forming a continuous range of disorders, from snoring, through RERA and then hypopneas to sleep apneas. From the pathophysiological point of view, these correspond to UA vibration (snoring), dynamic obstruction (hypopnea and RERA) (see below), and finally static obstruction (apnea). Of course, depending on the phenotype of the patient, the continuity of this process is artificial, at least in part. Figure 16.2(b) illustrates the definition of the AHI, for events when RERAs and hypopneas are considered together, (frequently all obstructive respiratory events are scored in this way. We consider RERAs and hypopneas as the same respiratory event, scoring the obstructive load as the sum of apneas and hypopneas (i.e, the AHI) (Fig. 16.2(b)).

It should be mentioned that around 20% of the population have an AHI of around 5–10 events per hour but without symptoms. From 4% to 8% or more of the population have more than five events per hour with symptoms, which defines sleep apnea–hypopnea syndrome (SAHS) [1,2]. Repeated episodes of UA obstruction trigger cortical arousals, large negative intrathoracic pressures, an increased neurovegetative response, and finally a hemoglobin oxygen desaturation [4]. Intermittent hypoxia leading to increased oxidative stress, systemic inflammation, and sympathetic activity coupled with intrathoracic pressure changes leading to excessive mechanical stress on the heart and large artery walls, together with arousal-induced reflex sympathetic activation with resultant repetitive blood pressure rises, are responsible for the symptoms and the cardiovascular, neurocognitive, and metabolic effects [5–9] (Fig. 16.1). Other forms of sleep apnea include central and complex apneas.

Pathophysiology

As can be seen in Fig. 16.3, obstructive sleep apnea (OSA) occurs when there is an imbalance between the anatomical factors that tends to decrease the size of the pharyngeal airway lumen (craniofacial structure, UA body fat, and tongue disproportion between container and content) and the activity during sleep of the UA muscles that maintain airway patency. When these anatomical factors are not compensated by increased neuromuscular activity, an increase in UA collapsibility occurs that induces apneas or hypopneas (Fig. 16.3(b)). The absence of compensation occurs only during sleep, because these patients when awake have a normal or even an increased muscle activity that eliminates UA obstruction.

The critical closing pressure P_{crit} [10] is commonly used to quantify pharyngeal collapsibility, which depends on two factors: UA wall tissue compliance and UA muscle tone. P_{crit} is defined as the minimum pressure inside the airway that allows the airway to remain patent. Figure 16.4 shows three examples of the possible spectrum of P_{crit}: (a) a fully open airway; (b) total obstruction; and (c) partial obstruction. When the UA has normal compliance or when the activity of the UA tone is high, P_{crit} is negative, meaning that a very negative intraluminal pressure is required to close the UA. Very negative values of P_{crit} suggest a stable UA, and therefore normal breathing is allowed. In the apnea group, the high compliance of the low muscle tone of the UA tends to close it, thereby

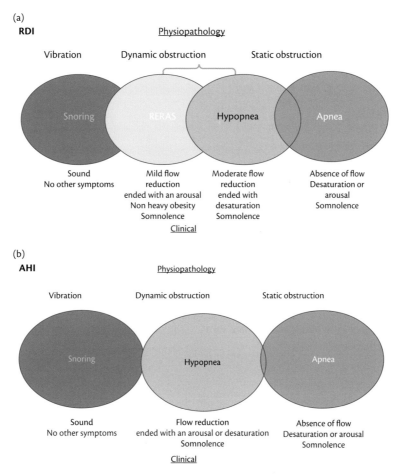

Fig. 16.2 (a) Definition of the respiratory disturbance index (RDI). (b) Definition of the apnea–hypopnea index (AHI). In the latter case, the upper airway resistance syndrome (UARS, or RERAs) and hypopneas are scored together.

inducing airway collapse and thus apnea (static occlusion). In Fig. 16.4(c), the intraluminal pressure is just above P_{crit}. In this situation, inspiratory flow itself decreases intraluminal pressure below P_{crit}, and then the UA partially collapses during inspiration. This situation is called dynamic occlusion, because the obstruction depends in part on the inspiratory flow [11]. Depending on the magnitude of this dynamic UA obstruction, among other effects, ventilation may be reduced substantially (hypopnea) or slightly (RERAS).

The Harvard group has recently described different traits such as the open loop or the arousability that contribute markedly to the upper airway collapsibility and even can open up different therapeutic options, as summarized in Fig. 16.5. This figure shows the basic pathophysiological abnormalities of SAHS, different phenomena that contribute to the upper airway collapsibility (open loop, low arousal threshold, and upper airway muscle response), as well different possible alternatives of treatment of these phenomena.

Sleep studies to measure respiratory events

Oronasal flow

The chapters in Section 2 of this volume describe various methods of sleep evaluation. However, some important aspects must be

considered here specifically in relation to respiratory events. Sleep disorder breathing changes may not be recognized if the devices used to analyze and quantify airflow are not sensitive enough. Guilleminault [12] clarified the relationship between increased respiratory resistance, snoring, and sleep fragmentation on the one hand and daytime sleepiness on the other, thereby providing further insight into this complex situation. In 1991, he produced an initial report on the effect of increased respiratory load during sleep in children with symptoms similar to those of sleep apnea. Along these lines, he identified heavy snoring as a cause of excessive daytime sleepiness [12]. Together with co-workers, Guilleminault reformulated the concept of sleep disordered breathing with a description of the UA resistance syndrome (UARS/RERA) [13]. They focused their attention on a group of subjects with complaints of excessive daytime sleepiness (EDS) presenting a trivial number of obstructive events as currently scored during full polysomnography (PSG). However, these events were measured using a thermistor, which has a very poor frequency response, and therefore it was not possible to measure the dynamic obstruction accurately. This is why Guilleminault had to measure esophageal pressure with a balloon. Sleep fragmentation with short repetitive arousals secondary to increased UA resistance in the absence of apnea and hypopnea was observed and was related to EDS. Some of the patients had maxillomandibular abnormalities. Reversal of sleep fragmentation

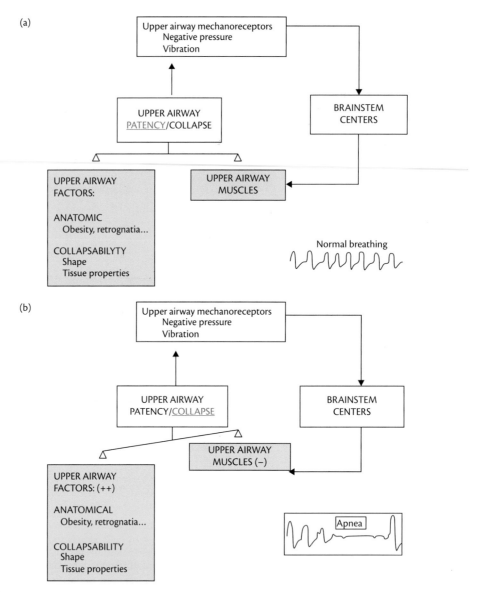

Fig. 16.3 Physiopathology of upper airway obstruction. (a) Normal balance between the anatomical factors that tend to decreases the size of the pharyngeal airway and the activity of the upper airway muscles during sleep. (b) An imbalance of the anatomical factors tends to decrease the size of the pharyngeal airway and the activity of the upper airway muscles during sleep, promoting respiratory events.

and sleepiness was achieved with nasal continuous positive airway pressure (CPAP), providing further evidence that abnormal UA resistance is responsible for the disorder. Therefore, it is credible that UARS is not an independent disorder from hypopneas but is perhaps a subgroup with particular identifiable traits in the spectrum of SAHS, which, like hypopneas, requires appropriate technology for its diagnosis. The gold standard device to measure flow is the pneumotachograph; however, its use during sleep requires the patient to wear a nasal or full-face mask, and for this reason it is not suitable for routine diagnostic sleep studies. Therefore, nonobtrusive sensors to detect breathing flow are especially suitable for this application. Two types of small and simple devices, placed close to the airway opening, are used to provide surrogate flow signals: thermistors/thermocouples and nasal prongs. The ventilation disturbances caused by obstructive sleep events are also monitored indirectly by means of thoraco-abdominal bands. In fact, the use

of thermistor-type flow-measuring devices for detecting hypopneas has been questioned [14]. Farré et al. [14] assessed the accuracy of thermistors/thermocouples as devices for detecting hypopneas in sleep studies (Fig. 16.6). They demonstrated that thermistors were only qualitative sensors, with strongly nonlinear characteristics, and greatly underestimated flow reductions: a 50% reduction in the real flow resulted in only an 18% reduction in the thermistor signal.

The example in Fig. 16.6 clearly shows that a thermistor is not able to accurately measure the real flow or reproduce the morphology of the inspiratory flow. Therefore, the use of thermistors to quantify hypopneas may lead to considerable underdetection of respiratory periods of increased UA resistance. Another technical aspect is the concept of the morphology of the inspiratory flow as a simple and easy way to detect increases in UA resistance. However, this cannot be determined by the thermistor. Therefore, to recognize dynamic obstruction, hypopneas, and UARS events,

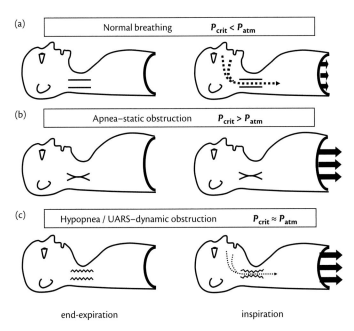

Fig. 16.4 Dynamic and static occlusion of the upper airway: (a) normal breathing; (b) apnea; (c) hypopnea. P_{crit}: critical pressure; P_{atm}: atmospheric pressure; UARS: upper airway resistance syndrome
Reproduced from Sleep Breath, 5(4), Montserrat JM, Farré R, Navajas D, New technologies to detect static and dynamic upper airway obstruction during sleep, pp. 193–206, Copyright (2001), with permission from Thieme.

other devices than thermistors are needed. Pneumotachography or esophageal pressure measurements would be ideal, except for the fact that they are inconvenient to use in clinical practice and are therefore confined to research studies. The use of nasal prongs (NPs) and measurement of total thoraco-abdominal movement are appropriate in most cases. Thermal devices measure both oral

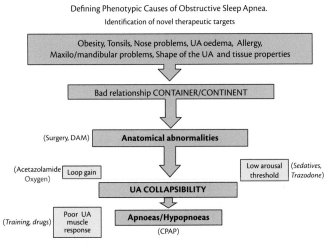

Fig. 16.5 Different anatomical elements that contribute to the upper airway collapsibility that, together with an absence of upper airway muscle response at night, results in apneas or hypopneas. Other traits such as changes in the open loop or the arousability also contribute markedly to increase the upper airway collapsibility and therefore increase the number of respiratory events. As can be seen in this Figure, these traits can open up different therapeutic options. Reproduced from Eckert.

and nasal flow, while nasal prongs only measure nasal flow. When conventional NPs similar to those designed for long-term oxygen therapy are inserted into the nostrils and connected to a pressure transducer, it is possible to measure the pressure fluctuations that occur during breathing. These oscillations are used as a surrogate for the nasal flow [15,16]. The set-up is simple and this method has an excellent dynamic response. NPs work as follows: the tip of the cannula is inside the nostril while the other side of the pressure transducer is open to the atmosphere, and so there is a drop in pressure between cannula tip and atmosphere during breathing, due to the resistance of the nostrils. As the flow is turbulent, the relationship between pressure changes, flow, and resistance is nonlinear, and so NPs provide only a qualitative estimate of the flow, although, in contrast to a thermistor, because of the quadratic pressure–flow relationship, they overestimate flow reduction [15,16] (Fig. 16.6) Nevertheless, the NP signal can be linearized [15,16] to obtain an excellent surrogate flow signal (Fig. 16.6).

However, even when linearized, the NP signal may not provide an absolutely accurate reading of total airflow over the entire night. Changes in the position of the cannula, periods of partial oral ventilation, and obstruction of the cannula by nasal secretions make the linearized NP signal a less accurate measure of flow over the entire night [14–16]. As with thermal sensors, the changes in breathing pattern detected in a given sleep event should be compared with the signal in the previous normal cycles. The major advantage of NPs is their fast response. This permits the detection of flow limitation, since the device can track the details of the inspiratory waveform contour, particularly if the signal is linearized. NPs have been used not just to detect reductions in the flow signal, like thermal devices, but also, more importantly, to detect and assess dynamic flow limitation. The American Academy of Sleep Medicine (AASM) scoring manual recommends nasal–oral thermal sensors for the detection of apnea and NP sensors (with or without square root transformation of the signal) for the detection of hypopnea [17]. The simultaneous use of both NPs and nasal–oral thermal sensors is recommended, providing the additional advantage of a backup sensor if one of the airflow detection devices fails. Tables 16.2 and 16.3 summarize the criteria and recommendations for detection of sleep disordered breathing.

Thoraco-abdominal motion

Thoraco-abdominal bands are used to analyze thoracic and abdominal excursions, although the magnitudes of these excursions are not proportional to swings in esophageal pressure. These bands are only semiquantitative and sometimes may even misclassify obstructive events as central. They analyze the amplitude of motion of the thoracic and abdominal compartments, as well as the synchrony between the movements of these compartments. Piezoelectric bands have frequently been used [18]. Currently, the AASM recommends the use of respiratory inductive plethysmograph (RIP) bands [17,19]. Other options are polyvinylidene fluoride (PVDF) sensors (excellent, but still not widely used) and pneumatic bands, which have been used in the past with acceptable and more economical results in many cases. However, discrepancies have been observed in the assessment of thoraco-abdominal asynchrony, depending on the choice of respiratory movement sensors. The literature contains a number of references to the RIP, but surprisingly, hardly any to other older systems. Figure 16.7 shows the correlations between the esophageal pressure and the inspiratory flow contour (representing the degree of flow limitation) and

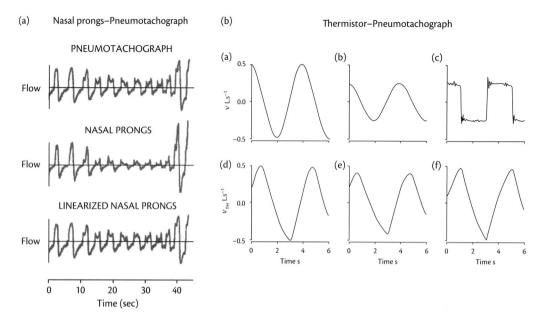

Fig. 16.6 Flow measurement. (a) Nasal prongs overestimate the reduction in the pneumotachograph flow signal but correctly analyze the shape of the flow. Taking the square root of the nasal prongs measurement provides an optimized result. (b) Comparison between a pneumotachograph and a thermistor. The thermistor does not respond properly when the pneumotachograph signal decreases to 50% (it underestimates the drop). The thermistor does not correctly analyze the shape of the flow signal. In summary, thermistors underestimate and nasal prongs overestimate the real reduction of flow.

Reproduced from Eur Respir J, 11(1), Farre R, Montserrat JM, Rotger M, Ballester E, Navajas D, Accuracy of thermistors and thermocouples as flow-measuring devices for detecting hypopnoeas, pp. 179–182, Copyright (1998), with permission from European Respiratory Society.

between the esophageal pressure and the degree of coordination of the thoracic bands. In both cases the correlation is acceptable, although it is better in the case of the inspiratory flow contour.

Other techniques

The forced oscillation technique (FOT) superimposes on spontaneous breathing a small pressure oscillation through a nasal mask attached to the patient. Respiratory impedance Z is derived online from pressure and flow signals recorded at the nasal mask. The potential application of FOT for the assessment of airway obstruction in SAHS has been confirmed in a model study[20]. Its clinical applicability to assess airflow obstruction in real time during CPAP treatment has also been demonstrated in a limited number of patients in comparison with measurements of esophageal pressure [21]. However, further research on FOT is needed to assess sensitivity and specificity in the detection of increased UA resistance before it can be introduced as a routine clinical procedure.

The pulse transit time (PTT) method [22] is capable of detecting increased respiratory effort and neurological activation (either arousal or autonomic arousal).

Clinical findings

Diagnosis of sleep apnea requires a combination of various clinical findings and the presence of an abnormal number of apneas and hypopneas per hour of sleep [4,6,17,23]. According to current diagnostic criteria, a large number of abnormal respiratory events with or without minor abnormal symptoms are necessary. The main points that have to be considered in the diagnosis and

assessment of sleep apnea are (a) the most common symptoms and the physical examination (Fig. 16.8 and Table 16.3), (b) the risk factors and the associated diseases that present a high risk for OSA (Table 16.4), and (c) the results of the sleep study (Tables 16.2 and 16.3) [17,23].

The diagnostic criteria for SBD have already been shown in Table 16.2, while Table 16.3 shows those specifically for SAHS. EDS, the most common SAHS symptom, may develop gradually, with the patient being unaware of the change. Other patients, especially women, complain of related fatigue instead of EDS, while

Table 16.3 Sleep apnea: definition criteria of the AASM

A patient with **obstructive sleep apnea–hypopnea syndrome** must fulfill criteria A and B or just criterion C:
A) At least one of the following complaints:
• Excessive daytime sleepiness that is not better explained by other factors, unrefreshing sleep, daytime, or fatigue.
• Awakenings with asphyxia, choking, or gasping.
• Bed partner reports louds snoring and apneas during sleep.
B) Sleep study:
Five* or more obstructed breathing events per hour during sleep.
C) AHÍ >15.**
The sleep disorder should not be explicable by another sleep entity such as central sleep apnea or hypoventilation.

*Some authors prefer 10 events/h.

**Some authors prefer 30 events/h.

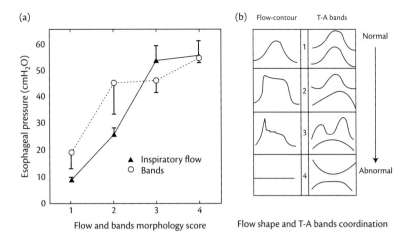

Fig. 16.7 (a) Evaluation of inspiratory flow and thoraco-abdominal (T-A) motion score characteristics related to esophageal pressure measurements. There is an acceptable correlation between the esophageal pressure and the T-A bands and between the esophageal pressure and the flow shape signals. (b) Definitions of qualitative variables and the score assigned to them. The inspiratory flow contour (upward direction) is classified as follows: 1 = well-contoured; 2 = partially limited; 3 = severely limited; 4 = no flow. The degree of thoraco-abdominal motion paradox is classified as: 1 = no paradox; 2 = slight partial paradox; 3 = partial paradox; and 4 = complete paradox. Reproduced from Am J Respir Crit Care Med, 155(1), Montserrat JM, Farre R, Ballester E, Felez MA, Pasto M, Navajas D, Evaluation of nasal prongs for estimating nasal flow, pp. 211–215, Copyright (1997), with permission from American Thoracic Society.

others experience an impairment in social functioning [24,25]. The clinical expression of the disease may differ from patient to patient, with some experiencing only snoring and respiratory pauses without EDS or other significant symptoms, while others are prone to sleepiness during driving [26]. Therefore, two patients with the same AHI can have different clinical phenotypes or arterial oxygen desaturation.

Typical symptoms are snoring, witnessed apneas, night asphyxias, and daytime somnolence or fatigue (Figs 16.8 and 16.9 and Table 16.3) not explained by other entities (Table 16.5). Sometimes, the symptoms are not as clear and specific. It is important to inquire about the patient's consumption of alcohol, sedatives, and other drugs. Gastroesophageal reflux should be ruled out. Moreover, it is essential to question the patient about other common causes of

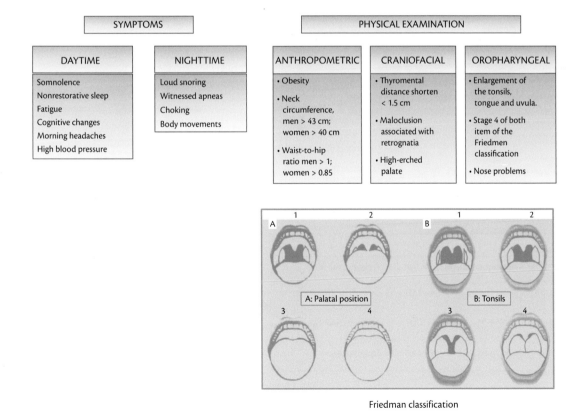

Fig. 16.8 Suggested initial basic clinical assessment of patients with sleep apnea.

Table 16.4 The three main clinical features of sleep apnea

Patients at risk	Risk factors	SAHS, high pretest (not so clear in females)
Obesity	Lack of exercise	*Heavy snorer*
Resistant hypertension	Male and elderly	*Witnessed apneas*
		Nocturnal choking
Pulmonary hypertension	Maxillomandibular and ENT abnormalities	Maxillomandibular alterations
		Retrognathia
Metabolic disturbances	Postmenopausal	ENT abnormalities
		Enlargement of the tonsils and adenoids and nasal obstruction
Arrhythmia	Alcohol	*Waist circumference* <102 cm (men), <88 cm (women)
Stroke and cardiac failure	Tobacco	*Enlarged neck* circumference (men: <43 cm; women: <37 cm)
Myopathies	Sedatives	Systemic hypertension
Hypothyroidism Acromegaly	Genetic	Daytime fatigue or *somnolence* that disturb life (no other cause found)

sleepiness, such as depression, insufficient sleeping time, and inadequate sleeping routines (Table 16.5).

Sleepiness can be assessed in different ways. The easiest is to ask the patient if EDS affects daily life in passive or active situations, including driving, in ways that cannot be explained by other diseases or circumstances. There are different questionnaires that attempt to quantify sleepiness and other sleep complaints, although there is no relationship with the physiological variables. There are three representative questionnaires: the Epworth Sleepiness Scale (ESS) [27], the Functional Outcomes of Sleep Questionnaire (FOSQ) [28] and the QUEBEC [29] questionnaire, which analyze different sleep complaints, and finally the EURO-COL, a very simple tool that assesses general quality of life [30]. The ESS, the most commonly used scale, is a subjective estimation of the propensity to doze off in eight situations.

A complete examination (Fig. 16.8) with especial attention to nasal problems, craniofacial abnormalities, macroglossia, dental malocclusion, enlarged tonsils, BMI, neck circumference, the waist-to-hip ratio, and cardiac, neurological, and metabolic features, has to be performed. Blood tests are needed if there is a clinical suspicion of hypothyroidism or significant metabolic or cardiac problems. SBDs are associated with an increased rate of road traffic accidents, although effective therapy is capable of reducing this risk [26]. Sleep apnea is a risk factor for significant cardiovascular disease and new onset of arterial hypertension [31,32], congestive cardiac failure, atrial flutter, and stroke [4–6]. SAHS is also related

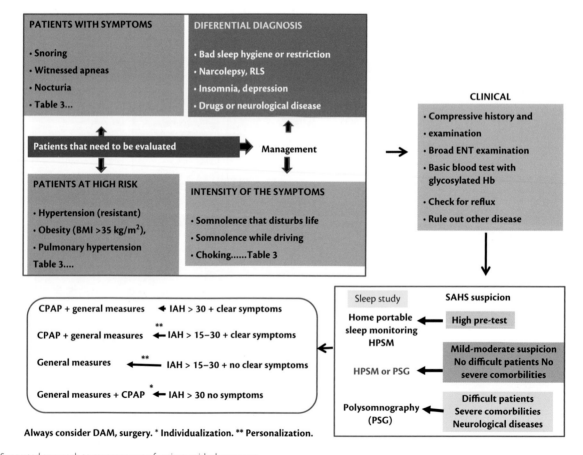

Fig. 16.9 Suggested approach to management of patients with sleep apnea.
It should be mentioned that the AHI taken in isolation is only a guide and the final therapeutic decision has to be made on the basis of overall evaluation (clinical features and cardiovascular comorbidities).

Table 16.5 Differential diagnosis and other sleep disorders

Daytime somnolence	Bad sleep hygiene, shiftwork, sleep apnea, depression, narcolepsy
Narcolepsy	Cataplexy: sudden and transient episodes of loss of muscle tone triggered by emotions
Restless legs syndrome (RLS)	Need to move the legs that improves on moving Can cause insomnia or somnolence
Depression	Lack of interest and pleasure in daily activities Negative thoughts
Insomnia	Difficulty in initiating (20 min) or maintaining sleep, with perception of poor quality Very stressful in some patients
Somnolence induced by drugs	Antianxiety agents, some antidepressants or antihistamines, narcotics, and pramipexole
Neurological diseases	Infections, tumors, Steinert disease (myotonic dystrophy type 1), stroke
REM behavior disorder	Singular, usually violent, behaviors during sleep In some cases, precedes degenerative brain diseases
Classical parasomnias	Somnambulism, nocturnal terrors, nightmares
Chronobiological diseases	Very important to be considered nowadays

to diabetes and the metabolic syndrome [8], independent of other cardiovascular risk factors such as obesity or lipid disorders, which are highly prevalent in these patients. CPAP treatment for SAHS has been shown to cause a risk reduction in fatal and nonfatal cardiovascular events [5] (Some controversies exist after the SAVE study). Table 16.4 shows the different groups of patients at risk for developing sleep apnea, in most of whom a sleep test has to be performed, especially if the complaint is snoring with respiratory

Table 16.6 Central sleep apnea (CSA)

Causes	Clinical features	Treatment

Hypercapnic:
  Idiopathic central hypoventilation
  Arnold–Chiari
  Neuromuscular disease
  Narcotics
	Somnolence
	Fatigue
	Headache
		Treatment of the underlying disease
		Noninvasive ventilation

CSA is also associated with obstructive sleep apnea at sleep onset, in which case CSA events are common		

Non-hypercapnic:
  Cheyne–Stokes (cardiac failure)
  High altitude
  Brain disorders
  Renal failure
	Insomnia
	Fatigue
	Dyspnea
	Asphyxias at night
		ASV
		BiPAP
		Oxygen
		Acetazolamide

pauses. At present, it is estimated that 50–90% of people with the condition remain undiagnosed. Heavy snoring, breathing pauses with asphyxia, and an increased neck or waist circumference point to the possibility of sleep apnea (Table 16.3, in bold).

After the clinical interview and examination, a sleep study will generally be performed. Depending on patient characteristics, a simplified study, normally carried out at home, or a full PSG will be performed (Fig. 16.9). Tables 16.2 and 16.3 summarize the different definitions of the respiratory events that can be identified in a sleep study and the recommended classification of SAHS severity as per the AASM recommendations [17]. SAHS is graded as mild when AHI is between 5 and 15 events per hour, moderate between 15 and 30 events per hour, and severe with more than 30 events per hour [23]. Table 16.3 presents the sleep apnea hypopnea syndrome as defined by clinical criteria and sleep study characteristics as per the AASM.

Central sleep apnea (CSA) is much less common than OSA [33]. It is caused by loss of ventilatory motor output. There is no flow or thoraco-abdominal motion. Common causes, clinical findings and treatment, are shown in Table 16.6.

An especially important cause is cardiac failure (crescendo–decrescendo pattern) because of its prognostic significance for cardiac disease and narcotics use. Patients who have obstructive apnea may also develop episodes of central apnea in the transition from awake to sleep. The pathophysiology is related to ventilatory instability (Cheyne–Stokes) or depression of the respiratory centers (by opiates or sedatives). Treatment requires an optimization of the disease, O_2 supplementation in the ventilatory instability group, and mechanical ventilation. Complex sleep apnea can appear during CPAP titration in patients with OSA [34]. Usually, this is transitory and is eliminated after 4–8 weeks of CPAP therapy. In some patients bilevel positive airway pressure (BiPAP) or assisted support ventilation (ASV) is needed. To use ASV it is necessary to have a heart ejection fraction of more than 45.

Management, including non-CPAP treatments

Management

SBD, as a common chronic condition, ideally requires a multidisciplinary approach for its management [35–38]. Figure 16.9 shows what should be the most appropriate approach to diagnosis and management.

Figure 16.10 shows the most appropriate sensors to detect the different SBD events. Figures 16.11 and 16.12 show a recommendation relationship between the primary care physician and sleep centers. Typical sleep apnea patients without severe associated disease can be managed by non-reference centers (Fig. 16.12) while more difficult patients must be managed at the sleep unit. An adequate follow-up to improve adherence (compliance) to CPAP treatment is a key point.

Non-CPAP treatment

Although CPAP is generally a very effective therapeutic modality, a significant percentage of patients cannot tolerate this treatment. In addition, in patients with mild to moderate SAHS, non-CPAP treatments can play an important role, although the degree of

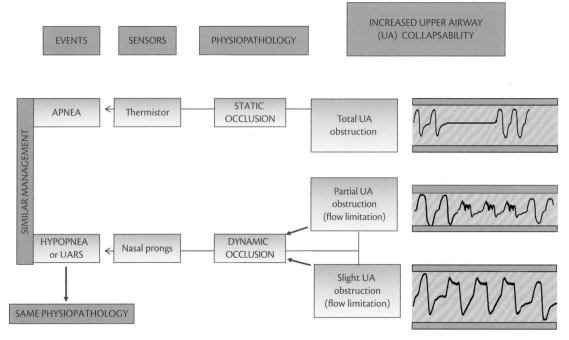

Fig. 16.10 Suggested sensors for use in understanding the physiology of respiratory events.

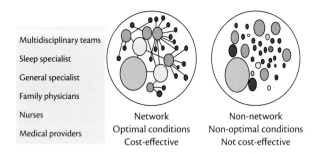

Fig. 16.11 The most appropriate approach for the management of SAHS, is the development of a network with different medical levels on.

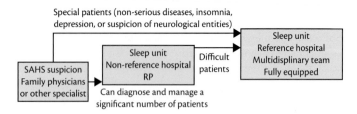

Fig. 16.12 Recommended algorithm for choosing between primary care physicians and sleep center. Tertiary hospitals can solve a significant number of patients, using simple devices in accordance with guidelines.

evidence for the effectiveness of each of these varies greatly [39] (Table 16.7).

Treatment of obesity and lifestyle modifications

Obesity is a major risk factor for SAHS. Weight loss increases the size of the pharynx and reduces collapsibility, which often results in an improvement of the SAHS [40]. The usual procedures for loss of weight in SAHS patients are dietary treatment

Table 16.7 Non-CPAP treatment of sleep apnea

♦ Weight reduction

♦ Positional therapy

♦ Lifestyle modification: exercise, increased sleep time

♦ Intraoral protrusion devices: mandibular advancement devices, tongue-retaining devices

♦ Surgical: nose, craniofacial structures and upper airway soft tissue (UPPP, tongue base and hypopharynx, multilevel)

♦ Others: drug therapy, training the upper airway muscles, neurostimulation, oxygen, measures to decrease upper airway edema and treatment of esophageal reflux

and bariatric surgery. The results are variable. The Task Force Committee of the AASM [41] concluded that effective dietary management may improve AHI in obese patients with OSA, with a few cases even achieving recovery, and therefore dietary management must be combined with a primary treatment (CPAP, intraoral devices, or surgery of the UA). Moreover, the AASM states that bariatric surgery may play a role in the treatment of patients with SAHS and morbid obesity, in combination with a primary treatment such as CPAP. Exercise, sufficient amount of sleep, avoidance of alcohol and sedatives, and treatment of gastroesophageal reflux are general measures that have to be implemented in all cases.

Postural treatment

It is well know that respiratory events are worse in the supine position. The term "postural treatment" usually refers to prevention of supine position during sleep, for which various methods have been used; the tennis ball technique, the use of vests and special pillows, or positional alarms. Postural treatment is used in patients with positional SAHS, which is generally defined as an AHI at least two times higher in the supine than the lateral position. Veasey et al. [41] and Oksenberg et al. [42] in their reviews mentioned several studies in which postural treatment produced clinical or PSG improvement in AHI, especially in young but not obese patients, with mild to moderate SAHS, but more studies are needed. The AASM [41] stated that postural treatment is an effective secondary treatment or may be a supplement to primary treatment in patients with positional OSA.

Intraoral devices

Intraoral devices together with surgery in selected cases are the main alternative to CPAP, but are currently underutilized. Mandibular advancement devices (MADs), which act by moving the jaw and tongue forward, are the types most commonly used [43,44]. Other intraoral devices, such as tongue-retaining devices that keep the tongue in a forward position by suction, are used very little. The AASM [41] recommend MADs in patients with mild to moderate OSA as an alternative to CPAP. Patients with severe SAHS should initially receive CPAP treatment. It is essential to carry out a process of re-evaluation and titrating MADs in a new sleep study performed with the intraoral device, since the improvement of symptoms does not predict accurately the degree of reduction in the AHI.

Drug treatment

There are many drugs that have been studied in clinical trials as potential treatments for SAHS, and this topic has been the subject of several reviews [41,45]. Most of these have concluded that evidence regarding the pharmacological treatment of SAHS is lacking. The AASM recommends modafinil in the treatment of patients with SAHS with residual sleepiness after adequate CPAP treatment and topical nasal steroids when the condition is associated with rhinitis. However, the reviews do not recommend the use of other drugs in the treatment of SAHS [41,45].

Surgical treatment

A wide variety of surgical techniques have been used in the treatment of SAHS as an alternative to CPAP and MADs, in order to reduce or eliminate the anatomical obstruction at the nose, the oropharynx, or hypopharynx or, in the case of tracheotomy, bypassing the pharyngeal part of the UA. The results are unpredictable and depend on various circumstances, particularly the criteria used for selection of patients, the type of technique used, and the experience of the surgeon. The main patient-related factors that influence the success of the intervention are the following: age, BMI, location of the obstruction, and severity of SAHS. For selection of the surgical technique and localization of the site of obstruction, a clinical examination and lateral cephalometric fiberoptic nasopharyngoscopy are needed. If patients are appropriately selected, surgery may have a clear role in sleep apnea treatment. There are different surgical procedures: maxillomandibular advancement, tonsillectomy in patients with tonsillar hypertrophy, radiofrequency procedures at different levels, or soft palate implants [46,47]. Regarding the uvulopalatopharyngoplasty (UPPP) as an isolated procedure, the guidelines are very restrictive, and it is only recommended in a few selected cases. Finally, multilevel surgery is considered an acceptable option in patients with multilevel obstruction of the UA as a last resort in cases where CPAP and other conservative measures do not have good results. An adequate selection process means satisfactory results.

SAHS as a chronic disease

Patients with SAHS often have multiple comorbidities, so a rational approach to disease management should include coordination with physicians treating the comorbidities, and in most cases through

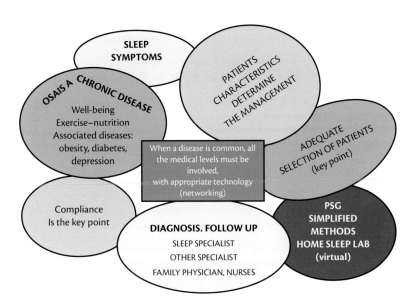

Fig. 16.13 SAHS has to be considered as a chronic disease and therefore is needed to treat all the associated comorbidities. This slide summarizes all the levels and strategies that may be involved in the appropriate management of SAHS patients.

the primary care physician. SAHS therapeutic strategies can be divided into three categories: general health measures and medical and surgical treatment. Considering that SAHS is a chronic disease, there are different elements that should all be included in the comprehensive strategic plan of SAHS management [48]. They can be summarized as follows:

◆ Patient education on healthy lifestyle. Counsel the patient to avoid factors, and explain potential benefits of SAHS treatment and potential complications if the disease is not treated. Patient education increases self-efficacy, commitment, and motivation for treatment.

◆ Choice and adaptation of specific treatment for each patient based on symptoms, associated comorbidities, and severity of illness. All patients with SAHS, which is a chronic disease, should have long-term monitoring. Patients on CPAP and MADs should have regular checkups to monitor treatment adherence, development of side effects or medical complications associated with SAHS, and resolution of symptoms. Patients who have had surgery or lost weight should be followed to monitor modification of risk factors and to evaluate possible recurrence of symptoms.

◆ Specifically, treatment with CPAP should be accompanied by behavioral therapy to promote adherence; this has proven to be very effective in terms of performance and achieving increased hours of nightly use (over at least 5 hours/night).

◆ Detection and early treatment of associated comorbidities: SAHS patients are often diagnosed with coexisting cardiovascular disorders that require different levels of medical attention to the patient, increasing the overall costs and patient's quality of life. The rational management of OSA therefore includes adopting a multidisciplinary management approach involving dietitians, psychologists, physiotherapists, cardiologists, surgeons, primary care physicians, trained sleep nurses, and sleep medicine specialists. Figure 16.13 summarizes all the levels and strategies that may be involved in the appropriate management of SAHS patients (telemedicine is useful).

References

1. Duran J, Esnaola S, Rubio R, Iztueta A. Obstructive sleep apnea–hypopnea and related clinical features in a population-based sample of subjects aged 30 to 70 yr. Am J Respir Crit Care Med 2001;163(3 Pt 1):685–9.
2. Young T, Palta M, Dempsey J, Skatrud J, Weber S, Badr S. The occurrence of sleep-disordered breathing among middle-aged adults. N Engl J Med 1993;328:1230–5.
3. Gould GA, Whyte KF, Rhind GB, et al. The sleep hypopnea syndrome. Am Rev Respir Dis 1988;137:895–8.
4. Dempsey JA, Veasey SC, Morgan BJ, O'Donnell CP. Pathophysiology of sleep apnea. Physiol Rev 2010;90:47–112.
5. Marin JM, Carrizo SJ, Vicente E, Agusti AG. Long-term cardiovascular outcomes in men with obstructive sleep apnoea–hypopnoea with or without treatment with continuous positive airway pressure: an observational study. Lancet 2005;365(9464):1046–53.
6. McNicholas WT, Bonsignore MR. Sleep apnoea as an independent risk factor for cardiovascular disease: current evidence, basic mechanisms and research priorities. Eur Respir J 2007;29:156–78.
7. Nieto FJ, Young TB, Lind BK, et al. Association of sleep-disordered breathing, sleep apnea, and hypertension in a large community-based study. Sleep Heart Health Study. JAMA 2000;283:1829–36.
8. Reichmuth KJ, Austin D, Skatrud JB, Young T. Association of sleep apnea and type II diabetes: a population-based study. Am J Respir Crit Care Med 2005;172:1590–5.
9. Barbé F, Durán-Cantolla J, Sánchez-de-la-Torre M, et al. Spanish sleep and breathing network. Effect of continuous positive airway pressure on the incidence of hypertension and cardiovascular events in nonsleepy patients with obstructive sleep apnea: a randomized controlled trial. JAMA 2012;307:2161–8.
10. Patil SP, Punjabi NM, Schneider H, et al. A simplified method for measuring critical pressures during sleep in the clinical setting. Am J Respir Crit Care Med 2004;170:86–93.
11. Farré R, Rigau J, Montserrat JM, et al. Static anddynamic upper airway obstruction in sleep apnea: role of the breathing gas properties. Am J Respir Crit Care Med 2003;168:659–63.
12. Guilleminault C, Stoohs R, Duncan S. Snoring (I). Daytime sleepiness in regular heavy snorers. Chest 1991;99:40–8.
13. Guilleminault C, Stoohs R, Clerk A, Simmons J, Labanowski M. From obstructive sleep apnea syndrome to upper airway resistance syndrome: consistency of daytime sleepiness. Sleep 1992;15(6 Suppl):S13–16.
14. Farre R, Montserrat JM, Rotger M, Ballester E, Navajas D. Accuracy of thermistors and thermocouples as flow-measuring devices for detecting hypopnoeas. Eur Respir J 1998;11:179–82.
15. Farre R, Montserrat JM, Navajas D. Noninvasive monitoring of respiratory mechanics during sleep. Eur Respir J 2004;24:1052–60.
16. Montserrat JM, Farre R, Ballester E, et al. Evaluation of nasal prongs for estimating nasal flow. Am J Respir Crit Care Med 1997;155:211–15.
17. Berry RB, Budhiraja R, Gottlieb DJ, et al. Rules for scoring respiratory events in sleep: update of the 2007 AASM Manual for the Scoring of Sleep and Associated Events. J Clin Sleep Med 2012;8:597–619.
18. Pennock BE. Rib cage and abdominal piezoelectric film belts to measure ventilatory airflow. J Clin Monit 1990;6:276–83.
19. Sackner MA, Adams JA. Piezoelectric sensor vs. respiratory inductive plethysmograph. J Appl Physiol (1985) 2001;901:403–4.
20. Farre R, Peslin R, Rotger M, Navajas D. Inspiratory dynamic obstruction detected by forced oscillation during CPAP. A model study. Am J Respir Crit Care Med 1997;155:952–6.
21. Navajas D, Farre R, Rotger M, et al. Assessment of airflow obstruction during CPAP by means of forced oscillation in patients with sleep apnea. Am J Respir Crit Care Med 1998;157:1526–30.
22. Pitson DJ, Sandell A, van den HR, Stradling JR. Use of pulse transit time as a measure of inspiratory effort in patients with obstructive sleep apnoea. Eur Respir J 1995;8:1669–74.
23. American Academy of Sleep Medicine Task Force. Sleep-related breathing disorders in adults: recommendations for syndrome definition and measurement techniques in clinical research. The report of an American Academy of Sleep Medicine Task Force. Sleep 1999;22:667–89.
24. Akashiba T, Kawahara S, Akahoshi T, et al. Relationship between quality of life and mood or depression in patients with severe obstructive sleep apnea syndrome. Chest 2002;122:861–5.
25. Engleman HM, Douglas NJ. Sleep. 4: Sleepiness, cognitive function, and quality of life in obstructive sleep apnoea/hypopnoea syndrome. Thorax 2004;59:618–22.
26. Teran-Santos J, Jimenez-Gomez A, Cordero-Guevara J. The association between sleep apnea and the risk of traffic accidents. Cooperative Group Burgos–Santander. N Engl J Med 1999;340:847–51.
27. Johns MW. A new method for measuring daytime sleepiness: the Epworth sleepiness scale. Sleep 1991;14: 540–5.
28. Chasens ER, Ratcliffe SJ, Weaver TE. Development of the FOSQ-10: a short version of the Functional Outcomes of Sleep Questionnaire. Sleep 2009;32:915–19.
29. Lacasse Y, Bureau MP, Sériès F. A new standardised and self-administered quality of life questionnaire specific to obstructive sleep apnoea. Thorax 2004;59:494–9.
30. The EuroQol Group (1990). EuroQol—a new facility for the measurement of health-related quality of life. Health Policy 1990;16:199–208.

31. Peppard PE, Young T, Palta M, Skatrud J. Prospective study of the association between sleep-disordered breathing and hypertension. N Engl J Med 2000;342:1378–84.

32. Martínez-García MA, Capote F, Campos-Rodríguez F, et al. Effect of CPAP on blood pressure in patients with obstructive sleep apnea and resistant hypertension: the HIPARCO randomized clinical trial. JAMA 2013;310:2407–15.

33. Javaheri S, Dempsey JA. Central sleep apnea. Compr Physiol 2013;3:141–63.

34. Khan MT, Franco RA. Complex sleep apnea syndrome. Sleep Disord 2014;2014:798487.

35. Chai-Coetzer CL, Antic NA, Rowland LS, et al. A simplified model of screening questionnaire and home monitoring for obstructive sleep apnoea in primary care. Thorax 2011;66:213–19.

36. Chamorro N, Sellarés J, Millán G, et al. An integrated model involving sleep units and primary care for the diagnosis of sleep apnoea. Eur Respir J 2013;42:1151–4.

37. Heatley EM, Harris M, Battersby M, et al. Obstructive sleep apnoea in adults: a common chronic condition in need of a comprehensive chronic condition management approach. Sleep Med Rev 2013;17:349–55.

38. Montserrat JM, Barbé F, Masa F. Diagnostic algorithms. In: Simonds AK, De Backer W, eds. ERS handbook of respiratory sleep medicine. Sheffield: European Respiratory Society, 2012.

39. Morgenthaler TI, Kapen S, Lee-Chiong T, et al. Practice parameters for the medical therapy of obstructive sleep apnea. Sleep 2006;29:1031–5.

40. Schwartz AR, Gold AR, Schubert N, et al. Effect of weight loss on upper airway collapsibility in obstructive sleep apnea. Rev Respir Dis 1991;144:494–8.

41. Veasey SC, Guilleminault C, Strohl KP, et al. Medical therapy for obstructive sleep apnea: a review by the Medical Therapy for Obstructive Sleep Apnea Task Force of the Standards of Practice Committee of the American Academy of Sleep Medicine. Sleep 2006;29:1036–44.

42. Oksenberg AS. Positional therapy for sleep apnea: a promising behavioral herapeutic option still waiting for qualified studies. Sleep Med Rev 2014;18:3–5.

43. Randerath WJ, Verbraecken J, Andreas S, et al. Non-CPAP therapies obstructive sleep apnoea. Eur Respir J 2011;37:1000–28.

44. Marklund M, Verbraecken J, Randerath W. Non-CPAP therapies in obstructive sleep apnoea: mandibular advancement device therapy. Eur Respir J 2012;39:1241–7.

45. Mason M, Welsh EJ, Smith I. Drug therapy for obstructive sleep apnoea in adults. Cochrane Database Syst Rev 2013;5:CD003002.

46. Kushida CA, Morgenthaler TI, Littner MR, et al. Practice parameters for the treatment of snoring and Obstructive Sleep Apnea with oral appliances: an update for 2005. Sleep 2006;29:240–3.

47. Aurora RN, Casey KR, Kristo D, et al. Practice parameters for the surgical modifications of the upper airway for obstructive sleep apnea in adults. Sleep 2010;33:1408–13.

48. Heatley EM, Harris M, Battersby M, et al. Obstructive sleep apnoea in adults: a common chronic condition in need of a comprehensive chronic condition management approach. Sleep Med Rev 2013;17:349–55.

CHAPTER 17

Positive airway pressure therapy

Dirk Pevernagie

Introduction

Medical conditions characterized by impaired breathing during sleep are collectively referred to as sleep disordered breathing (SDB). These disorders are heterogeneous and may result from different pathogenetic mechanisms. Inhibition of respiratory rhythm generation in the central nervous system underlies central sleep apnea (CSA), whereas obstruction of the upper airway (UA) due to muscle atonia in sleep is causal to obstructive sleep apnea (OSA). Disorders of impaired pulmonary ventilation, whether associated with lung diseases, obesity, or neuromuscular/skeletal diseases, are designated as alveolar hypoventilation. Typically, sleep is the time where alveolar hypoventilation emerges at first and deteriorates later on in the course of the respiratory disease. Combinations of these impaired breathing patterns are frequently observed in clinical practice. Yet, it is customary to decide in the individual patient whether SDB is mainly central, obstructive, or related to hypoventilation. A classification of SDB according to these pathophysiological conditions is presented in the International Classification of Sleep Disorders (ICSD-3) [1].

SDB may be associated with significant symptoms such as insomnia, unrefreshing sleep, excessive daytime sleepiness (EDS), fatigue and decreased neurocognitive performance [2]. These symptoms, as well as health-related quality of life, may improve significantly with effective therapy [3,4]. Moderate to severe OSA is causally related to arterial hypertension, cardiovascular comorbidity, and decreased life expectancy [5]. Again, appropriate treatment may redress these adverse outcomes, and therefore adequate medical management of SDB is paramount.

Given their heterogeneity, respiratory sleep disorders cannot be addressed by a generic approach. Some general principles are important, including advice on behavior and lifestyle and treatment of underlying or comorbid diseases. Pharmacological therapy, treatment with oral devices, or surgical interventions may be appropriate in individual patients. Those treatment modalities are outside the scope of this chapter: the interested reader should consult other literature sources for further reference. Treatment of SDB with positive airway pressure (PAP) devices has been around for more than three decades now. Continuous PAP (CPAP) is the cornerstone in the management of OSA and some types of CSA as well. Bilevel PAP is indicated for the treatment of alveolar hypoventilation. Adaptive servo-ventilation (ASV) is a sophisticated PAP treatment mode for Cheyne–Stokes respiratory pattern with CSA (CSR-CSA.) This chapter will focus on indications, physiological effects, modalities, and outcomes of PAP therapy. Since treatment must be tailored to the individual patient's requirements, combining different therapeutic options can be considered at any time in the course of treatment.

Treatment of SDB may aim at different outcomes. To achieve adequate symptomatic control is the principal goal, as it promotes the patient's quality of life. To reduce or normalize the apnea–hypopnea index (AHI) is a means to monitor treatment efficacy, but not necessarily a treatment objective. There is only a weak correlation between symptomatic control and reduction in AHI [6]. Additional objectives are to prevent comorbidities and to prolong life expectancy. Adequate therapeutic control of AHI improves cardiovascular outcomes in patients with severe OSA [5]. Whether the same holds true for patients with mild to moderate OSA, or CSA, has not been confirmed yet.

Physiological mechanisms of PAP treatment

The principal effect of CPAP is to increase intraluminal pressure in the UA. The results of CPAP application in patients with sleep-related UA obstruction were first published by Sullivan et al. in 1981 [7]. It was shown that with nasal pressure ranging from 4.5 to 10 cmH$_2$O, sleep-related collapse of the UA could be abolished in five OSA patients. There is empirical evidence to show that the elevated pressure acts as a pneumatic splint supporting the action of UA dilating muscles that becomes insufficient during sleep. Passive collapse of the UA during sleep is prevented when the intraluminal pressure exceeds the critical closing pressure of the UA [8,9] (Fig. 17.1). Imaging of the UA has shown that increasing nasal CPAP progressively enlarges the cross-sectional area of the pharyngeal airway and that this effect is most obvious in the lateral as compared with the anteroposterior dimension [10] (Fig. 17.2).

Besides stabilizing the UA on the basis of mechanical splinting, CPAP may exert other effects on the respiratory system. Elevated intrapulmonary pressure may increase lung volume [11], which in turn may decrease collapsibility of the UA through a caudal tug on the central airways [12,13]. Possible other effects of CPAP are improved stability of the central respiratory drive, decreased work of breathing, and improved cardiac function due to reductions in preload and afterload. These factors could play a role in the gradual attenuation of CSA that is observed in some patients with chronic heart failure (CHF) treated with fixed CPAP [14].

Bilevel PAP devices deliver a preset pressure support (inspiratory PAP: IPAP) on top of a preset positive end-expiratory pressure level (expiratory PAP: EPAP). As with CPAP, the EPAP should be sufficient to stabilize the UA. Setting IPAP at higher levels will increase tidal volume and minute ventilation, the aim of which is to compensate for hypoventilation. The pressure support is triggered by spontaneous breaths. Bilevel PAP machines also feature a timed mode that provides IPAP/EPAP cycles at a preset frequency when the patient stops breathing.

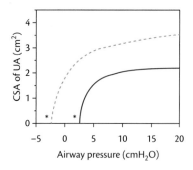

Fig. 17.1 Compliance of the upper airway (UA) in a subject with OSA (full line) and a normal control (dashed line) presented in a pressure–area plot. The cross-sectional area (CSA) of the upper airway is smaller in the OSA patient for any given intraluminal airway pressure, indicating that the UA is less compliant. The critical closing pressure (P_{close}, *) is the intraluminal airway pressure at which CSA is reduced to 0 cm^2. P_{close} is positive in the OSA patient, whereas negative suction pressure in needed in the normal subject to close the airway.

Source data from J Appl Physiol, 82(4), Isono S, Remmers JE, Tanaka A, Sho Y, Sato J, Nishino T, Anatomy of pharynx in patients with obstructive sleep apnea and in normal subjects, pp. 1319–26, Copyright (1997), The American Physiological Society; J Appl Physiol, 105(5), Younes M, Role of respiratory control mechanisms in the pathogenesis of obstructive sleep disorders, pp. 1389–405, Copyright (2008) The American Physiological Society.

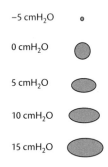

Fig. 17.2 Reconstruction of cross-sectional area (CSA) and shape of the velopharyngeal airway at different intraluminal pressures obtained by CT scan in an awake normal subject.

Adapted from Am J Respir Crit Care Med, 1996, 154(4), Schwab RJ, Pack AI, Gupta KB, Metzger LJ, Oh E, Getsy JE, et al, Upper airway and soft tissue structural changes induced by CPAP in normal subjects, pp. 1106–16, Copyright (1996), with permission from American Thoracic Society.

ASV is a special type of bilevel PAP therapy. ASV devices provide adaptive pressure support that is inversely proportional to the instant spontaneous tidal volume. The difference between IPAP and EPAP is minimal during normal breathing and particularly during hyperpneic periods, whereas it automatically and proportionally increases during the waning phases of respiration (Fig. 17.3). The aim is to counteract periodic breathing and to reduce overall minute ventilation.

PAP devices and interfaces

Treatment with PAP is based on delivery of pressurized airflow, generated with fan-driven or turbine systems, adjustable by varying valve diameter or turbine speed [15]. To this end, a blower device is used that is connected to the UA via a hose and an interface. The interface is a mask that transmits the pressure to the nasal or oronasal airways (Fig. 17.4).

Intentionally, PAP should be used every night, either at or away from home (eg, during trips). Therefore, PAP devices must be versatile with respect to power supply (eg, 110–230 V) and should be comfortable in terms of portability and ease of use. Contemporary PAP machines are lightweight and quite silent. With modern electronic technology, monitoring of compliance, air leakage, and effects on AHI has become a standard. Regular updates of this machine-derived information may assist the practitioner with ongoing patient education and fine-tuning of the PAP settings.

The available literature on the physiological effects of CPAP is based on the use of nasal masks. This is an important reality, because delivery of positive pressure via the nose exerts a direct stabilization of the velopharynx, i.e, the retropalatal segment of the UA, which has an important role in the pathogenesis of OSA. Application of CPAP via the oral or oronasal route may have less potent or even adverse effects on the stability of the velopharyngeal airway, which could lead to persistence of respiratory events, even in the presence of higher pressure levels [16,17].

Based on this evidence and because the nose is the default physiological route for tidal breathing, PAP should primarily be administered via the nasal airway [18]. The oronasal route may be considered in cases of impaired nasal breathing, but medical or surgical treatment of nasal obstruction should always be considered prior to switching from a nasal to an oronasal mask. There is no convincing argument to use oral masks. Interface technology has thrived in recent years. With the introduction of inflatable or moldable mask cushions, patients' comfort has improved a lot. A broad variety of nasal and oronasal interfaces is currently on the market. A venting mechanism to remove exhaled carbon dioxide is an integral part of the interface. A small hole or array of minuscule perforations in the mask is sufficient for this purpose.

The interface should be optimally adjusted to fit the anatomical configuration of nose (and also the mouth in the case of full-face masks). It is important to prevent air leakage from the edges while not strapping the interface too tightly to the facial structures. Sores, especially on the nasal bridge, may be caused by excessive clamping of the mask, and this may be a reason for PAP discontinuation. The final choice of the type of interface depends on anatomical characteristics, but also on personal preferences. It is not uncommon

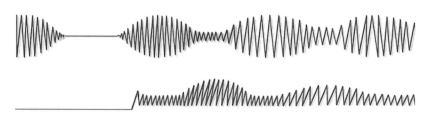

Fig. 17.3 The principle of adaptive servo-ventilation (ASV): effects of ASV on Cheyne–Stokes respiration with central sleep apnea (CSA-CSR). During the increasing phase of respiration, pressure support decreases to a minimum, whereas during the waning phase and especially during apneas pressure support reaches a maximum.

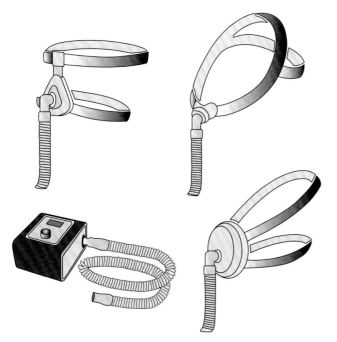

Fig. 17.4 PAP equipment. A blower device is connected to an interface via a tube. The interface is fixed to the external nasal or oronasal airway with headgear, consisting of adjustable straps. In this drawing, a classical nasal mask (top left), nasal pillows (top right), and full-face mask (bottom right) are shown.
Reproduced courtesy of http://www.fotosearch.com/CSP813/k8137593/

having to try several masks in the early phase of PAP treatment, but regular nasal masks or nasal pillows are suitable for most PAP indications in common practice.

Initiation of PAP treatment

Therapy with PAP can be initiated either in a clinical environment or at home. The former option ensures adequate supervision for purposes of education and dedicated nursing support. Remedying adverse side effects right from the start is favorable for better compliance in the long term (see the discussion further in this chapter). However, admission to the sleep laboratory or hospital ward is expensive and labor-intensive. Economic constraints have promoted alternative approaches requiring fewer staff or enabling commencement of PAP therapy at home. Which of these management strategies is superior in terms of medical outcomes is uncertain. Contemporary information and communications technology hold promise for telemonitoring of PAP utilization and may offer a compromise between these two methods for initiating PAP treatment [19].

The supervised setting offers the advantage of having the possibility to start up and titrate CPAP in the second half of an overnight polysomnographic (PSG) procedure. A so-called split-night study combines diagnosis of OSA and commencement of CPAP treatment in one session. The split-night approach seems feasible for patients with moderate to severe OSA. PSG all-night trends may show dramatic improvements of sleep architecture and cardiorespiratory variables (Fig. 17.5). Manual upward pressure titration is carried out as in full-night titration studies. However, insufficient time to assess the effective pressure level or issues with adaptation to the PAP equipment are salient limitations to this intervention [20].

As the aim of CPAP treatment in OSA patients is to ensure unimpeded breathing during sleep, the fixed pressure must warrant sufficient patency of the UA in all sleep stages and body postures. CPAP is effective when all apneas, hypopneas, respiratory effort-related arousals, and snoring events are controlled. The American Academy of Sleep Medicine (AASM) used to advocate in-lab manual pressure titration to determine the effective CPAP level [20]. However, methods based on autotitrating CPAP (APAP) [21] and CPAP prediction formulas [22,23] may also be effective in this respect. A comprehensive multicenter trial from the Spanish Sleep and Breathing Network nicely demonstrated that different titration techniques yield similar results [24]. Masa et al. randomized 360 CPAP-naive patients with severe OSA and EDS, into three parallel groups, characterized by different CPAP initiation modes: standard manual titration, APAP initiated at home or fixed CPAP assessed with a prediction formula. After 3 months, a comparable improvement in AHI, subjective sleepiness and compliance was found in all three groups. Obviously, effective CPAP can be determined in different ways, and there is increasing evidence for non-superiority of the different assessment strategies [25]. The preference for a certain method is linked with patient-related characteristics including severity of OSA, the presence of obesity or comorbid diseases, as well as social and psychological intricacies.

No guidelines exist for setting effective CPAP in CSA. Evidence for pressure-dependent control of central respiratory events is lacking, whereas it has been shown that the CSA index may diminish over time with continued CPAP use [14]. A short-term trial of CPAP may be insufficient to draw conclusions regarding its treatment efficacy in CSA. It is recommended to empirically start CPAP at low pressure levels and to reexamine the AHI after 6 and 12 weeks of treatment in this patient category.

Bilevel PAP and ASV must be started in a supervised setting. To elaborate on these procedures is outside the scope of this chapter.

Clinical results of PAP therapy

Nasal CPAP is the gold standard for the treatment of moderate to severe OSA [26]. Satisfactory clinical effects appear soon after commencement of therapy, often already following the first nights of successful CPAP use. Sleep quality is positively affected. Rebound of slow-wave sleep and REM sleep may be observed in the first nights of CPAP treatment. Moreover, this apparent change in sleep architecture seems to correlate with subjective improvement in sleep quality [27]. EDS may recover substantially, as has been shown in several randomized controlled trials [28,29]. Partial improvement in cognitive performance has been reported, and a significant effect on attention seems most noticeable [30]. Drowsy driving is a hazard in untreated OSA patients. They have a significantly elevated risk of motor vehicle accidents [31], which is reduced after successful treatment with CPAP [32].

CPAP therapy also has favorable effects on cardiovascular status and prognosis. Blood pressure may be significantly reduced in patients with moderate to severe OSA. A recent meta-analysis found a mean net reduction in systolic blood pressure of 2.6 ± 0.5 mmHg and in diastolic blood pressure of 2.0 ± 0.4 mmHg [33]. Moreover, a higher baseline AHI was associated with a greater mean net decrease in systolic blood pressure. In a recent study including patients with OSA and resistant hypertension, CPAP treatment for 12 weeks compared with control resulted in a decrease in 24-hour

Fig. 17.5 All-night trends from a split night study. This demonstrates all-night trends from a split-night study in a patient with severe OSA. From top to bottom are shown oxygen saturation from pulse oximetry (SpO$_2$, %), instantaneous heart rhythm derived from the ECG (bpm), and the hypnogram (showing stages wake, REM sleep, and NREM sleep 1, 2, and 3). The left part represents spontaneous breathing with untreated severe OSA. There are marked SpO$_2$ dips, cardiac arrhythmias, and severely disrupted sleep. At 02:00, CPAP was started with a pressure of 8 cmH$_2$O. As a consequence, SpO$_2$ and cardiac rhythm become remarkably stable and there is a rebound of slow-wave sleep and REM sleep.

mean and diastolic blood pressure and in an improvement of the nocturnal blood pressure pattern [34]. Untreated severe OSA has been shown to be a strong independent predictor for cardiovascular events and all-cause mortality. In a long term follow-up study, effective CPAP treatment was associated with markedly improved cardiovascular outcomes in this category of OSA severity [35]. To what extent CPAP may prevent cardiovascular complications in patients who are not somnolent or who have only mild disease remains equivocal [36,37].

Besides obesity and arterial hypertension, OSA is also associated with disturbed glucose metabolism, insulin resistance, diabetes mellitus and hyperlipidemia/hypercholesterolemia, and elevated serum markers of systemic inflammation. This cluster of symptoms and signs is commonly referred to as metabolic syndrome [38]. Several trials have studied the effects of OSA and CPAP treatment on glycemic control and insulin resistance. In non-diabetic patients, a significantly improved insulin resistance was found when patients with moderate to severe OSA were treated with CPAP [39]. In male patients with type 2 diabetes and OSA, therapeutic CPAP did not significantly improve measures of glycemic control or insulin resistance as compared with placebo [40]. Neither does CPAP seem to reduce hemoglobin A1c levels in patients with or without type 2 diabetes [41]. Effects of CPAP on markers of systemic inflammation are uncertain and as yet still controversial [42].

Data on effects of CPAP in CSA have predominantly been obtained in patients with CHF. In one large survey (the CANPAP

trial), CPAP attenuated CSR-CSA and improved CSA index, nocturnal oxygenation, ejection fraction, norepinephrine (noradrenaline) levels, and six-minutes-walking distance [43]. However, CPAP treatment was not associated with a better transplant-free survival. While these data did not support the use of CPAP to extend life in patients with CHF and CSA-CSR, a post hoc analysis demonstrated improvement of cardiac function and transplant-free survival rates in CHF patients in whom AHI was effectively reduced by CPAP as compared with CPAP-resistant controls [44].

The application of bilevel PAP seems to bring no advantage over CPAP treatment in patients with CSA and CHF [45]. In contrast, deterioration of SDB has been reported in CSA patients on bilevel PAP therapy, presumably because of excessive minute ventilation, which tends to worsen hypocapnia and the associated periodic breathing pattern [46]. With the introduction of ASV about a decade ago, a convenient treatment modality for CSR-CSA became available. ASV has been proven superior in reducing the CSA-index in CHF patients, as compared with other treatment options, including CPAP, bilevel PAP, and oxygen supplementation [47]. In addition, treatment compliance with ASV may be better than with CPAP [48]. Although it was observed that ASV may improve left-ventricular ejection fraction in patients with CHF and CSR-CSA [49], a large controlled trial with this therapeutic modality failed to show any significant effect on salient clinical outcomes (SERVE-HF study) [50]. There were no improvements regarding mortality, need for lifesaving cardiovascular interventions, or unplanned hospitalization for worsening heart failure. Moreover, there was evidence that all-cause and cardiovascular mortality were both increased with this therapy. As a consequence, it is advised not to prescribe ASV to patients with CSR-CSA and CHF if the ventricular ejection fraction is less than 45% [50].

Optimizing adherence and compliance with PAP therapy

Difficulties with acceptance and tolerance are commonly seen as the main disadvantages of PAP treatment. While adherence means continuing the treatment, and compliance refers to using PAP for a certain amount of time, both terms are used interchangeably in the literature. Although the definition of adequate compliance is arbitrary, between 46% and 83% of unselected OSA patients have been reported not to meet the requirement of using CPAP at least 4 hours per night for at least 70% of nights [51]. Certain measures can be taken to optimize PAP use, the goal of which should be to use PAP for at least 6 hours every night [52]. Indeed, in OSA patients, a dose–response relationship has been found between time used and improvement of EDS [53], as well as effects on arterial hypertension [54].

Factors determining adherence and compliance

Several factors are related to compliance with CPAP therapy in OSA patients. Improvement of sleep quality and REM rebound is predictive of adherence [55,56]. Socio-economic status, age, and gender have not been reported to be important, whereas OSA severity and daytime dysfunction are associated with better treatment outcomes [51]. Appropriate usage at the start of treatment is also a good indicator for adequate long-term adherence to CPAP [57]. Therefore, technical troubles and annoying side effects should be tackled early on.

Besides assuring optimal treatment comfort, appropriate patient education may enhance therapeutic results. Extensive information provided at the outset of CPAP treatment does not seem to increase compliance, whereas supportive interventions to continue CPAP therapy may be helpful [58]. Cognitive–behavioral therapy aiming at accepting and thinking positively about CPAP therapy may boost compliance when compared with care as usual [59].

Adverse side effects and their management

Because the PAP device is connected to the UA by an interface, side effects may arise from the physical impact of the mask and/or the insufflation of air into the respiratory tract (and sometimes the gastrointestinal tract). These side effects may be bothersome but are as a rule not serious or life-threatening. Any nuisance or complication of PAP therapy should be managed appropriately and promptly as to preserve optimal treatment compliance. Some hints to correct common side effects are detailed in Table 17.1.

Psychological problems with respect to accepting treatment may also adversely affect adherence and compliance. Table 17.2 lists some frequently reported psychosocial issues and how they can be managed.

Adaptations of PAP technology to improve compliance

In recent years, several adjustments have been made to commercial PAP machines in order to enhance versatility and comfort of use.

Table 17.1 Adverse side effects of PAP therapy and proposed remedies

Adverse side effect	Proposed remedies
Rhinitis and nasal congestion	Apply heated humidification; prescribe topical steroids; consult ENT surgeon
Sores (ulceration) of nasal bridge or other facial structures	Change mask type; loosen straps or headgear
Eczema, irritation of skin	Change mask type
Streaks on face (visible upon awakening in the morning)	Change type of mask and/or headgear
Ectopic insufflation of air (bloating, ructus, flatus)	Reduce pressure settings; change to non-PAP therapy
Air leaks at boundaries of interface	Tighten headgear or use other type of mask
Mouth leakage	Reduce pressure settings; use chin straps; change to non-PAP therapy
Noise of apparatus (machine and/or mask)	Check sealing of mask; check operational aspects of CPAP device
Water condensation in mask and circuit	Increase bedroom temperature; use heated CPAP hose

The manufacturing industry has made serious efforts to upgrade systems with air conditioning and adaptive pressure modalities.

To enhance the comfort of nasal breathing, heated humidification has been added to most commercially available PAP devices. Indeed, conditioning the inspired air with heat and moisture may prevent or relieve symptoms of rhinitis. While recent evidence confirms that CPAP-associated inflammation of the nasal mucosa may be alleviated with heated humidification [60], it is unclear whether this addition may improve long-term adherence.

To tackle complaints of pressure intolerance, modifiable pressure settings have been introduced. Most CPAP machines feature a ramp facility allowing a gentle increase of pressure to the preset level over 20 minutes or so. This mode may be helpful to allow the patient to get accustomed to the external pressure sensation, especially at the beginning of PAP treatment. Adapting the pressure profile in the course of the respiratory cycle is another means to enhance breathing comfort. Expiratory pressure relief (EPR) may improve tolerance to the administration of higher levels of inspiratory pressure,

Table 17.2 Psychosocial issues related to PAP therapy and suggestions for management

Psychosocial issues	Management
Unable to tolerate mask owing to claustrophobia	Carry out assisted training sessions during daytime; psychotherapy
Not fancying the idea of being dependent on a machine "for the rest of my life"	Increase educational efforts; cognitive–behavioral therapy; involve partner or relatives
Interference with talking and intimacy in bed	Schedule activities; do not put on mask except when preparing to go to sleep
Having to disclose PAP equipment from carry-on bags at security checks	Put equipment in luggage to be checked in

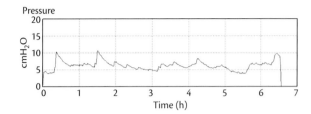

Fig. 17.6 Pressure profile downloaded from the electronic memory of an APAP machine, showing its pressure variation, with pressure ranging between 4 and 10 cmH$_2$O. The pressure rises presumably when obstructive respiratory events occur. In between pressure peaks, the pressure gradually drops to lower levels. There are no means to check the appropriateness of the pressure changes.

but there is no evidence that EPR improves compliance with CPAP treatment. Some OSA patients who restart CPAP therapy after previous treatment failure may benefit from this adaptive pressure mode [61].

Equipment for autotitrating CPAP (APAP) has been commercialized for about two decades now. These devices change the required CPAP level based on feedback from various variables such as airflow, pressure fluctuations, or measures of airway resistance. The algorithm drives the machine to increase the pressure when obstructive events are identified, and to lower the pressure when central apneas are detected or when obstructive events have disappeared for a while. APAP devices are geared to instantaneously adapt pressure to a certain degree of UA obstruction and to keep the pressure as low as possible at the same time (Fig. 17.6). Therefore, APAP could be a surrogate for manual CPAP titration or could even be a means for permanent use, replacing fixed CPAP treatment [21].

Appropriate detection of respiratory anomalies and adequate pressure response to these events is fundamental to APAP technology. However, both mechanisms may fail. Nonrespiratory artifacts such as movements and mouth leaks can be mistaken for respiratory events. In this case, inappropriate pressure responses may be triggered, resulting in over- or under-reacting of the APAP device. Event detection is the intellectual property of the manufacturing company and may not be disclosed for commercial reasons. Accordingly, the performance of APAP devices cannot be checked, and inadvertent operating deficiencies cannot be ruled out with certainty. Also, the assumption that APAP devices deliver the lowest effective pressure levels at all times is fallacious. In some patients, better results are obtained when the CPAP level is set according to a prediction formula than with the recommended use of the 95th percentile of the pressure range produced by APAP devices [62]. Nevertheless, APAP devices are being used on a large scale and offer convenient treatment to many OSA patients. Several trials have compared efficacy of APAP devices versus fixed CPAP therapy, but superiority of APAP technology has not been proven [63]. APAP is contraindicated in patients with CHF or chronic obstructive pulmonary disease (COPD) and is not useful in the treatment of CSA [21].

References

1. American Academy of Sleep Medicine. The international classification of sleep disorders, 3rd ed. Darien, IL: American Academy of Sleep Medicine, 2014.
2. Bucks RS, Olaithe M, Eastwood P. Neurocognitive function in obstructive sleep apnoea: a meta-review. Respirology 2013;18(1):61–70.
3. Jing J, Huang T, Cui W, Shen H. Effect on quality of life of continuous positive airway pressure in patients with obstructive sleep apnea syndrome: a meta-analysis. Lung 2008;186(3):131–44.
4. Sanchez AI, Martinez P, Miro E, Bardwell WA, Buela-Casal G. CPAP and behavioral therapies in patients with obstructive sleep apnea: effects on daytime sleepiness, mood, and cognitive function. Sleep Med Rev 2009;13(3):223–33.
5. Sanchez-de-la-Torre M, Campos-Rodriguez F, Barbe F. Obstructive sleep apnoea and cardiovascular disease. Lancet Respir Med 2013;1(1):61–72.
6. Kingshott RN, Vennelle M, Hoy CJ, et al. Predictors of improvements in daytime function outcomes with CPAP therapy. Am J Respir Crit Care Med 2000;161(3 Pt 1):866–71.
7. Sullivan CE, Issa FG, Berthon-Jones M, Eves L. Reversal of obstructive sleep apnoea by continuous positive airway pressure applied through the nares. Lancet 1981;18;1(8225):862–5.
8. Isono S, Remmers JE, Tanaka A, et al. Anatomy of pharynx in patients with obstructive sleep apnea and in normal subjects. J Appl Physiol (1985) 1997;82(4):1319–26.
9. Younes M. Role of respiratory control mechanisms in the pathogenesis of obstructive sleep disorders. J Appl Physiol (1985) 2008;105(5):1389–405.
10. Schwab RJ, Pack AI, Gupta KB, et al. Upper airway and soft tissue structural changes induced by CPAP in normal subjects. Am J Respir Crit Care Med 1996;154(4 Pt 1):1106–16.
11. Heinzer RC, Stanchina ML, Malhotra A, et al. Effect of increased lung volume on sleep disordered breathing in patients with sleep apnoea. Thorax 2006;61(5):435–9.
12. Van de Graaff WB. Thoracic influence on upper airway patency. J Appl Physiol 1988;65(5):2124–31.
13. Squier SB, Patil SP, Schneider H, et al. Effect of end-expiratory lung volume on upper airway collapsibility in sleeping men and women. J Appl Physiol 2010;109(4):977–85.
14. Arzt M, Schulz M, Schroll S, et al. Time course of continuous positive airway pressure effects on central sleep apnoea in patients with chronic heart failure. J Sleep Res 2009;18(1):20–5.
15. Kushida CA, Littner MR, Hirshkowitz M, et al. Practice parameters for the use of continuous and bilevel positive airway pressure devices to treat adult patients with sleep-related breathing disorders. Sleep 2006;29(3):375–80.
16. Ebben MR, Oyegbile T, Pollak CP. The efficacy of three different mask styles on a PAP titration night. Sleep Med 2012;13(6):645–9.
17. Borel JC, Tamisier R, Dias-Domingos S, et al. Type of mask may impact on continuous positive airway pressure adherence in apneic patients. PLoS One 2013;8(5):e64382.
18. Chai CL, Pathinathan A, Smith B. Continuous positive airway pressure delivery interfaces for obstructive sleep apnoea. Cochrane Database Syst Rev 2006;(4):CD005308.
19. Dellaca R, Montserrat JM, Govoni L, et al. Telemetric CPAP titration at home in patients with sleep apnea–hypopnea syndrome. Sleep Med 2011;12(2):153–7.
20. Kushida CA, Chediak A, Berry RB, et al. Clinical guidelines for the manual titration of positive airway pressure in patients with obstructive sleep apnea. J Clin Sleep Med 2008;4(2):157–71.
21. Morgenthaler TI, Aurora RN, Brown T, et al. Practice parameters for the use of autotitrating continuous positive airway pressure devices for titrating pressures and treating adult patients with obstructive sleep apnea syndrome: an update for 2007. An American Academy of Sleep Medicine report. Sleep 2008;31(1):141–7.
22. Miljeteig H, Hoffstein V. Determinants of continuous positive airway pressure level for treatment of obstructive sleep apnea. Am Rev Respir Dis 1993;147(6 Pt 1):1526–30.
23. Stradling JR, Hardinge M, Paxton J, Smith DM. Relative accuracy of algorithm-based prescription of nasal CPAP in OSA. Respir Med 2004;98(2):152–4.
24. Masa JF, Jimenez A, Duran J, et al. Alternative methods of titrating continuous positive airway pressure: a large multicenter study. Am J Respir Crit Care Med 2004;170(11):1218–24.

25. Gao W, Jin Y, Wang Y, et al. Is automatic CPAP titration as effective as manual CPAP titration in OSAHS patients? A meta-analysis. Sleep Breath 2012;16(2):329–40.

26. Epstein LJ, Kristo D, Strollo PJ Jr, et al. Clinical guideline for the evaluation, management and long-term care of obstructive sleep apnea in adults. J Clin Sleep Med 2009;5(3):263–76.

27. Verma A, Radtke RA, VanLandingham KE, King JH, Husain AM. Slow wave sleep rebound and REM rebound following the first night of treatment with CPAP for sleep apnea: correlation with subjective improvement in sleep quality. Sleep Med 2001;2(3):215–23.

28. Patel SR, White DP, Malhotra A, Stanchina ML, Ayas NT. Continuous positive airway pressure therapy for treating sleepiness in a diverse population with obstructive sleep apnea: results of a meta-analysis. Arch Intern Med 2003;163(5):565–71.

29. Giles TL, Lasserson TJ, Smith BH, et al. Continuous positive airways pressure for obstructive sleep apnoea in adults. Cochrane Database Syst Rev 2006;(3):CD001106.

30. Kylstra WA, Aaronson JA, Hofman WF, Schmand BA. Neuropsychological functioning after CPAP treatment in obstructive sleep apnea: a meta-analysis. Sleep Med Rev 2013;17(5):341–7.

31. Strohl KP, Brown DB, Collop N, et al. An official American Thoracic Society Clinical Practice Guideline: sleep apnea, sleepiness, and driving risk in noncommercial drivers. An update of a 1994 Statement. Am J Respir Crit Care Med 2013;187(11):1259–66.

32. Antonopoulos CN, Sergentanis TN, Daskalopoulou SS, Petridou ET. Nasal continuous positive airway pressure (nCPAP) treatment for obstructive sleep apnea, road traffic accidents and driving simulator performance: a meta-analysis. Sleep Med Rev 2011;15(5):301–10.

33. Fava C, Dorigoni S, Dalle VF, et al. Effect of continuous positive airway pressure (CPAP) on blood pressure in patients with obstructive sleep apnea/hypopnea. A systematic review and meta-analysis. Chest 2014;145(4):762–71.

34. Martinez-Garcia MA, Capote F, Campos-Rodriguez F, et al. Effect of CPAP on blood pressure in patients with obstructive sleep apnea and resistant hypertension: the HIPARCO randomized clinical trial. JAMA 2013;310(22):2407–15.

35. Marin JM, Carrizo SJ, Vicente E, Agusti AG. Long-term cardiovascular outcomes in men with obstructive sleep apnoea–hypopnoea with or without treatment with continuous positive airway pressure: an observational study. Lancet 2005;365(9464):1046–53.

36. Barbe F, Duran-Cantolla J, Sanchez-de-la-Torre M, et al. Effect of continuous positive airway pressure on the incidence of hypertension and cardiovascular events in nonsleepy patients with obstructive sleep apnea: a randomized controlled trial. JAMA 2012;307(20):2161–8.

37. Ge X, Han F, Huang Y, et al. Is obstructive sleep apnea associated with cardiovascular and all-cause mortality? PLoS One 2013;8(7):e69432.

38. Drager LF, Togeiro SM, Polotsky VY, Lorenzi-Filho G. Obstructive sleep apnea: a cardiometabolic risk in obesity and the metabolic syndrome. J Am Coll Cardiol 2013;62(7):569–76.

39. Iftikhar IH, Khan MF, Das A, Magalang UJ. Meta-analysis: continuous positive airway pressure improves insulin resistance in patients with sleep apnea without diabetes. Ann Am Thorac Soc 2013;10(2):115–20.

40. West SD, Nicoll DJ, Wallace TM, Matthews DR, Stradling JR. Effect of CPAP on insulin resistance and HbA1c in men with obstructive sleep apnoea and type 2 diabetes. Thorax 2007;62(11):969–74.

41. Iftikhar IH, Blankfield RP. Effect of continuous positive airway pressure on hemoglobin A(1c) in patients with obstructive sleep apnea: a systematic review and meta-analysis. Lung 2012;190(6):605–11.

42. Baessler A, Nadeem R, Harvey M, et al. Treatment for sleep apnea by continuous positive airway pressure improves levels of inflammatory markers—a meta-analysis. J Inflamm (Lond) 2013;10(1):13.

43. Bradley TD, Logan AG, Kimoff RJ, et al. Continuous positive airway pressure for central sleep apnea and heart failure. N Engl J Med 2005;353(19):2025–33.

44. Arzt M, Floras JS, Logan AG, et al. Suppression of central sleep apnea by continuous positive airway pressure and transplant-free survival in heart failure: a post hoc analysis of the Canadian Continuous Positive Airway Pressure for Patients with Central Sleep Apnea and Heart Failure Trial (CANPAP). Circulation 2007;115(25):3173–80.

45. Dohi T, Kasai T, Narui K, et al. Bi-level positive airway pressure ventilation for treating heart failure with central sleep apnea that is unresponsive to continuous positive airway pressure. Circ J 2008;72(7):1100–5.

46. Johnson KG, Johnson DC. Bilevel positive airway pressure worsens central apneas during sleep. Chest 2005;128(4):2141–50.

47. Teschler H, Dohring J, Wang YM, Berthon-Jones M. Adaptive pressure support servo-ventilation: a novel treatment for Cheyne–Stokes respiration in heart failure. Am J Respir Crit Care Med 2001;164(4):614–19.

48. Philippe C, Stoica-Herman M, Drouot X, et al. Compliance with and effectiveness of adaptive servoventilation versus continuous positive airway pressure in the treatment of Cheyne–Stokes respiration in heart failure over a six month period. Heart 2006;92(3):337–42.

49. Kasai T, Usui Y, Yoshioka T, et al. Effect of flow-triggered adaptive servo-ventilation compared with continuous positive airway pressure in patients with chronic heart failure with coexisting obstructive sleep apnea and Cheyne–Stokes respiration. Circ Heart Fail 2010;3(1):140–8.

50. Cowie MR, Woehrle H, Wegscheider K, et al. Adaptive servo-ventilation for central sleep apnea in systolic heart failure. N Engl J Med 2015;373(12):1095–105.

51. Weaver TE, Grunstein RR. Adherence to continuous positive airway pressure therapy: the challenge to effective treatment. Proc Am Thorac Soc 2008;5(2):173–8.

52. Sawyer AM, Gooneratne NS, Marcus CL, et al. A systematic review of CPAP adherence across age groups: clinical and empiric insights for developing CPAP adherence interventions. Sleep Med Rev 2011;15(6):343–56.

53. Weaver TE, Maislin G, Dinges DF, et al. Relationship between hours of CPAP use and achieving normal levels of sleepiness and daily functioning. Sleep 2007;30(6):711–19.

54. Barbe F, Duran-Cantolla J, Capote F, et al. Long-term effect of continuous positive airway pressure in hypertensive patients with sleep apnea. Am J Respir Crit Care Med 2010;181(7):718–26.

55. Somiah M, Taxin Z, Keating J, et al. Sleep quality, short-term and long-term CPAP adherence. J Clin Sleep Med 2012;8(5):489–500.

56. Koo BB, Wiggins R, Molina C. REM rebound and CPAP compliance. Sleep Med 2012;13(7):864–8.

57. McArdle N, Devereux G, Heidarnejad H, et al. Long-term use of CPAP therapy for sleep apnea/hypopnea syndrome. Am J Respir Crit Care Med 1999;159(4 Pt 1):1108–14.

58. Smith I, Nadig V, Lasserson TJ. Educational, supportive and behavioural interventions to improve usage of continuous positive airway pressure machines for adults with obstructive sleep apnoea. Cochrane Database Syst Rev 2009;(2):CD007736.

59. Richards D, Bartlett DJ, Wong K, Malouff J, Grunstein RR. Increased adherence to CPAP with a group cognitive behavioral treatment intervention: a randomized trial. Sleep 2007;30(5):635–40.

60. Koutsourelakis I, Vagiakis E, Perraki E, et al. Nasal inflammation in sleep apnoea patients using CPAP and effect of heated humidification. Eur Respir J 2011;37(3):587–94.

61. Pepin JL, Muir JF, Gentina T, et al. Pressure reduction during exhalation in sleep apnea patients treated by continuous positive airway pressure. Chest 2009;136(2):490–7.

62. Hertegonne KB, Volna J, Portier S, et al. Titration procedures for nasal CPAP: automatic CPAP or prediction formula? Sleep Med 2008;9(7):732–8.

63. Smith I, Lasserson TJ. Pressure modification for improving usage of continuous positive airway pressure machines in adults with obstructive sleep apnoea. Cochrane Database Syst Rev 2009;(4):CD003531.

CHAPTER 18

Central sleep apnea and hypoventilation syndromes

Mithri R. Junna, Bernardo J. Selim, and Timothy I. Morgenthaler

Pathophysiology

Normally, ventilation during sleep is carefully regulated to maintain homeostasis of blood pH and blood oxygen content by the central nervous system response to anatomic detectors of pH (most prominently chemoreceptors on the ventrolateral surface of the medulla oblongata) and oxygen content (detected predominantly in carotid and aortic bodies). These chemoreceptors, in proportion to higher $PaCO_2$ (lower serum pH) and low oxygen content, stimulate activity of the pontomedullary pacemaker, which in turn activates inspiratory thoracic muscles with augmentation of ventilation. The resultant increased ventilation tends to ameliorate the initially detected disturbance in homeostasis, re-establishing the desired pH and oxygen set points. [Recall that ventilation has an inverse relationship to $PaCO_2$ (and, to a lesser extent, the oxygen content of the blood), and that pH in turn has a reciprocal relationship to $PaCO_2$ (so that a higher $PaCO_2$ is associated with a lower pH)]. In general, the ventilatory response to $PaCO_2$ is thus proportional, and is blunted in NREM and REM sleep. Sudden changes from sleep to wake or vice versa can result in sudden changes in the desired $PaCO_2$ set point, with resultant instability in ventilatory patterns. Such instability is particularly notable when $PaCO_2$ is normal or low, and less likely to occur in conditions where it is high [1]. In central sleep apnea (CSA) syndromes, apnea events generally result from temporary cessation of pontomedullary pacemaker activity. Considering the mechanism(s) and the resulting tension of carbon dioxide in blood ($PaCO_2$), CSA may be grouped into (1) non-hypercapnic CSA (the most prevalent category) and (2) alveolar hypoventilation syndromes.

Non-hypercapnic CSA

The most prevalent forms of CSA fall into this category. If measured, the $PaCO_2$ is either normal (35 mmHg $\leq PaCO_2 \leq$ 45 mmHg) or low ($PaCO_2$ < 35 mmHg). In non-hypercapnic CSA, apneic events are most often the result of over-response or under-response of the respiratory control system to minimal changes in nocturnal $PaCO_2$ (high "loop gain") [2]. Loop gain is an engineering term that describes the degree of response, in this case, of the respiratory control system, after a ventilatory disturbance. The higher the loop gain, the higher the overventilation or underventilation response, resulting in respiratory instability. Loop gain comprises three components: (1) the controller gain, which is the chemoreceptor-driven

ventilatory response to changes in $PaCO_2$ and PaO_2; (2) the plant gain, which is the ventilatory response to changes in pulmonary capillary $PaCO_2$ and PO_2; and (3) the mixing gain, which is the circulatory time needed for changes in $PaCO_2$ and PO_2 in pulmonary capillaries to be detected by the chemoreceptors (effective circulatory time) [3]. Disorders such as idiopathic CSA, Cheyne–Stokes respiration (CSR), and high-altitude CSA are considered to be the result of high "loop gain" of the respiratory control system. Because of the dependency on a $PaCO_2$-driven ventilatory response, these breathing disorders are generally exclusive to NREM sleep, where the ventilatory pattern is particularly influenced by chemical drive. In REM sleep, ventilatory pattern is influenced by a combination of chemical and other nonmetabolic influences, producing lower ventilatory responsiveness to hypercapnia and hypoxia, and less tendency to over- or under-react to transient perturbations in ventilation.

Alveolar hypoventilation syndromes

This group of disorders are defined by an elevated nocturnal $PaCO_2$ level (>45 mmHg), which may extend into the daytime. The main respiratory abnormality resides anywhere along the brainstem respiratory control center (e.g., congenital central alveolar hypoventilation syndrome), throughout the respiratory motor output unit, from the motor neuron to the innervated respiratory muscle.

Because the causes of alveolar hypoventilation with or without central apneas are multiple, a clinical classification based upon the patient's pulmonary function can help to differentiate abnormalities of the ventilatory drive (autonomic/metabolic respiratory control system) associated with normal pulmonary function, versus abnormalities of pulmonary mechanics with subsequent abnormal pulmonary function. Pulmonary function is commonly evaluated based upon information obtained in a pulmonary function test (PFT), further narrowing the differential diagnosis in hypoventilation. Patterns of volume and flow changes observed via spirometry and lung volumes can support an obstructive (e.g., chronic obstructive pulmonary disease, COPD) or restrictive (eg, neuromuscular-skeletal diseases) physiology. Information from the diffusion capacity of carbon monoxide (DLCO) can point to changes in the surface of gas exchange (e.g., emphysema) or vasculature (e.g., pulmonary hypertension). When neuromuscular diseases are in question, maximal respiratory pressures can reflect

Table 18.1 Chronic alveolar hypoventilation syndromes and evaluations

Evaluation	Brainstem respiratory control center failure	Respiratory motor output unit failure*	Thoracic cage or pulmonary disease
$PaCO_2$	↑, or may be ↓ by voluntary hyperventilation	↑	↑
Chest X-ray	N, or signs of pulmonary hypertension	N, low lung volumes, or hemidiaphragm elevation	N or abnormal, depending on underlying disease
Diaphragmatic fluoroscopy ("sniff test")	N	N or paradoxical upward movement of hemidiaphragm	N
Nerve conduction study	N	↓ or absence of phrenic nerve action potential	N
Diaphragmatic EMG	N	Abnormal	N
Pulmonary function test (PFT)	N	Restrictive	Restrictive (e.g., kyphoscoliosis) or obstructive (e.g., COPD)
MIP/MEP or P_{dif}	N	↓	N
Ventilatory response to CO_2 and O_2	Abnormal	N or slightly blunted	N or slightly blunted
Polysomnography	Hypoventilation with sustained oxyhemoglobin desaturations, more severe during slow-wave sleep, less in REM. Variable presence of central apneas	Hypoventilation with sustained oxyhemoglobin desaturations, worse in REM. Presence of central or obstructive apneas	Hypoventilation with sustained oxyhemoglobin desaturations, worse in REM

*Respiratory motor neurons, spinal cord, phrenic nerves, respiratory muscles.

N: normal; EMG: electromyogram; MIP: maximal inspiratory pressure; MEP: maximal expiratory pressure; P_{dif}, transdiaphragmatic pressure; REM, rapid eye movement.

changes in inspiratory and expiratory respiratory muscle strength (Table 18.1).

CSA with Cheyne-Stokes breathing

Clinical presentation

This disorder tends to occur in older men, particularly those with atrial dysrhythmias, diastolic or systolic congestive heart failure (CHF), or stroke. Bed partners may report nocturnal snoring, gasping, and apneas. Patients may report sleep maintenance difficulties, with frequent nocturnal awakenings and consequent nonrestorative sleep and daytime sleepiness.

Diagnosis

During diagnostic polysomnography (PSG), five or more central apneas or hypopneas per hour of sleep must be demonstrated, and at least 50% of the total number of apneas and hypopneas seen during the diagnostic PSG must be central apneas or hypopneas. The pattern of ventilation should fulfill criteria for Cheyne–Stokes breathing defined as a crescendo–decrescendo pattern, typically of length 45–60 s (Fig. 18.1). The disorder should not be better explained by a concurrent sleep disorder or medication or substance use.

Treatment

If underlying heart failure is present, optimal medical management of this condition is recommended through diet, lifestyle, and pharmacological therapies. Assistive devices such as continuous positive airway pressure (CPAP) and adaptive servo-ventilation (ASV) devices remain the mainstay of treatment. Attended PSG is recommended to determine effectiveness for either device. Contradictory information exists regarding survival (transplant-free survival) and cardiac function with the use of CPAP. If used, it should be titrated to ensure control of sleep disordered breathing [4]. Retrospective studies, or subgroup analysis of prospective studies, show that patients with systolic heart failure on treatment with ASV have long-term improvements in respiratory events, cardiac NYHA functional class, and cardiopulmonary exercise tolerance parameters, and a decrease in the number of cardiac events (cardiac death and re-hospitalization) at 6-month follow-up. A similar profile of improvements has also been shown in patients with diastolic CHF-CSR on ASV [5], as well as CHF patients with obstructive and central sleep apnea occurring concurrently within the same night [6], independent of the severity of sleep disordered breathing [7]. However, prospective randomized control trials are needed to confirm the impact of ASV on mortality rates and transplantation-free survival rates [8]. A word of caution is needed regarding ASV treatment in systolic heart failure in view of the recent SERVE-HF clinical trial report [9] showing increased mortality in patients with ejection fraction ≤ 45%.

CSA due to drug or substance use

Clinical presentation

This disorder occurs in those using long-term opioid medications, most often methadone, although also others. Bed partners may report nocturnal snoring, gasping, and apneas. Patients may report sleep maintenance difficulties, with frequent nocturnal awakenings and consequent nonrestorative sleep and daytime sleepiness.

Diagnosis

During diagnostic PSG, five or more central apneas or hypopneas per hour of sleep must be demonstrated, and at least 50% of the total number of apneas and hypopneas seen during the diagnostic PSG must be central apneas or hypopneas. Cheyne–Stokes breathing pattern must be absent. The breathing pattern must be due to use of an opioid or other respiratory depressant. Other irregular patterns of ventilation such as ataxic or Biot's patterns may be noted (Fig. 18.2). The disorder should not be better explained by a concurrent sleep disorder.

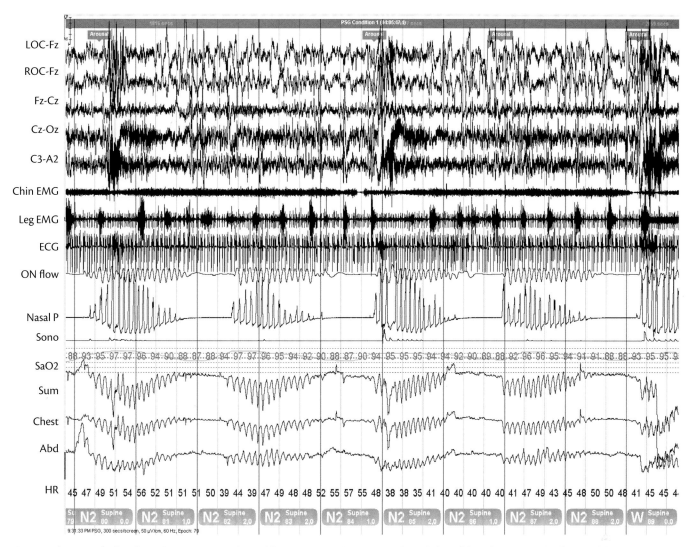

Fig. 18.1 Cheyne–Stokes breathing. This PSG segment obtained from a patient with compensated systolic heart failure shows 10 epochs of 30 s. Each heavy vertical line demarks 30 s. The thermal sensor channel (ON flow) shows the presence of apneic events as a drop of ≥ 90% of peak thermal sensor signal from baseline. The nasal pressure signal (Nasal P) denotes episodes of ≥ 3 consecutive central apneas separated by a crescendo and decrescendo change in breathing amplitude with a cycle length of ≥ 40 s. LOC-Fz and ROC-Fz are left and right electro-oculograms. Fz-Cz, Cz-Oz, and C3-A2 are frontal, occipital, and central EEG montages, respectively. Chin EMG and Leg EMG represent submental and pre-tibial EMGs. The electrocardiogram (ECG) shows sinus rhythm. Sono is a snoring microphone, and is unremarkable. Abd and Chest are abdominal and chest respiratory impedance plethysmography signals that demonstrate changes in circumference at those levels, usually taken to represent muscular effort. The Sum signal is the arithmetic summation of deflection of Abd and Chest signals, and parallels tidal volume when calibrated. HR is the pulse rate, as read.

Treatment

As the effect of opioids on central apneas is dose-dependent, discontinuation or reduction of the dose of opioid, as tolerated, is recommended [10].

There are limited data to support the use of assistive devices. Attended PSG is needed to determine effectiveness. CPAP may reduce the number of respiratory events, but frequently does not result in effective control of sleep disordered breathing. There are conflicting data about the role of ASV in this group of patients. One study that did not show ASV efficacy did not titrate therapy according to protocol. In two other studies with appropriate titrations, ASV was effective in the majority of cases. At this point, if efforts at reducing or eliminating opioids are not fruitful, the use of ASV is probably appropriate. However, caution must be used, as ASV is not designed

to provide ventilatory support in hypoventilation syndromes, but only a slight hypoventilatory target from baseline values.

Primary CSA

Clinical presentation

This rare disorder is considered to be idiopathic, or of unknown etiology, often occurring in middle-aged to older adults. Bed partners may report nocturnal snoring, gasping, and apneas. Patients may report sleep maintenance difficulties, with frequent nocturnal awakenings and consequent nonrestorative sleep and daytime sleepiness.

Diagnosis

During diagnostic PSG, five or more central apneas or hypopneas per hour of sleep must be demonstrated and at least 50% of the total

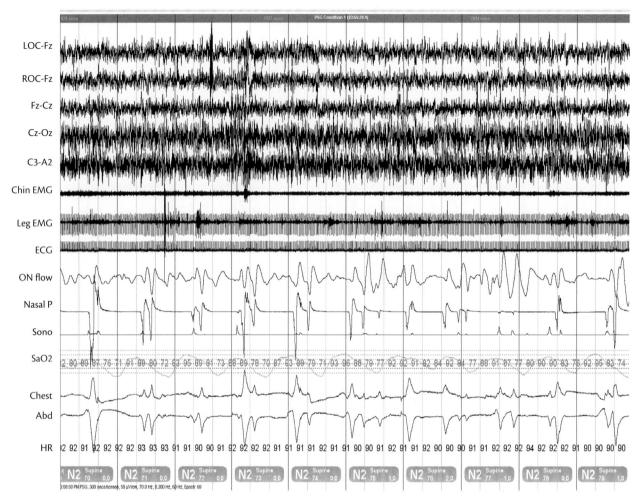

Fig. 18.2 Opioids and ataxic breathing. This PSG segment obtained from a patient on chronic opioid medications shows 10 epochs of 30 s. Each heavy vertical line demarks 30 s. The thermal sensor channel (ON flow) and the nasal pressure signal (Nasal P) denote an ataxic or irregular breathing pattern with clustering. Note that most apneas here are central, but there is no clear period. Not discernible from this level of scrutiny, most of these apneas are not associated with arousals, despite the clear oxyhemoglobin desaturation (see the signal labeled SaO$_2$). LOC-Fz and ROC-Fz are left and right electro-oculograms. Fz-Cz, Cz-Oz, and C3-A2 are frontal, occipital, and central EEG montages, respectively. Chin EMG and Leg EMG represent submental and pre-tibial EMGs. The electrocardiogram (ECG) shows sinus rhythm. Sono is a snoring microphone, and is unremarkable. Abd and Chest are abdominal and chest respiratory impedance plethysmography signals that demonstrate changes in circumference at those levels, usually taken to represent muscular effort. The Sum signal is the arithmetic summation of deflection of Abd and Chest signals, and parallels tidal volume when calibrated. HR is the pulse rate, as read.

number of apneas and hypopneas seen during the diagnostic PSG must be central apneas or hypopneas. Cheyne–Stokes breathing pattern must be absent. There should be no evidence for daytime or nocturnal hypoventilation. The disorder should not be better explained by a concurrent sleep disorder, medical or neurological disorder, or medication or substance use.

Treatment

There are limited data to support pharmacological use of acetazolamide, zolpidem, or triazolam.

There are limited data to support the use of assistive devices in the form of CPAP, bilevel PAP with a back-up respiratory rate (BPAP-ST), or ASV [4].

Oxygen supplementation may decrease respiratory controller gain and stabilize breathing, but may worsen respiratory acidosis associated with alveolar hypoventilation. Therefore, it should be tried first under monitored conditions, and an arterial blood gas

should be obtained to ensure that ventilation is not worsened with supplemental oxygen.

Treatment emergent central apnea (also called complex sleep apnea syndrome)

Clinical presentation

This disorder is thought to occur in 5–20% of individuals undergoing initial titration with positive airway pressure treatment for predominantly obstructive sleep apnea. Bed partners may report nocturnal snoring, gasping, and apneas. Patients may report sleep maintenance difficulties, with frequent nocturnal awakenings and consequent nonrestorative sleep and daytime sleepiness.

Diagnosis

During therapeutic PSG with the use of a positive airway pressure device without a back-up rate, (1) resolution of obstructive

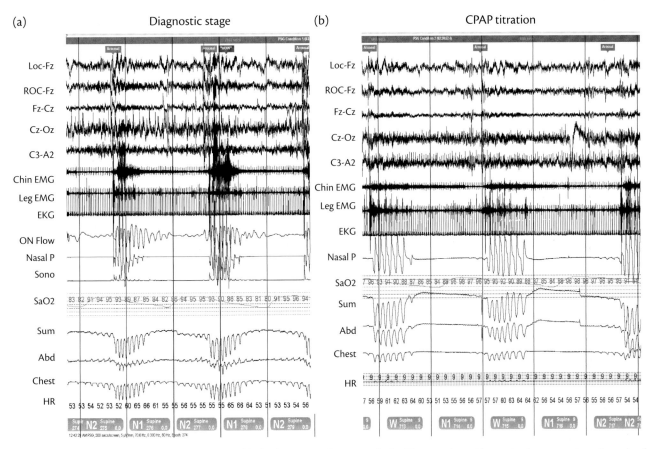

Fig. 18.3 Treatment emergent central (complex) sleep apnea. (a) This diagnostic PSG segment obtained from a patient with complex sleep apnea shows 5 epochs of 30 s with obstructive sleep apnea events. Each heavy vertical line demarks 30 s. The thermal sensor channel (ON flow) shows a drop of ≥ 90% of peak thermal sensor signal from baseline. LOC-Fz and ROC-Fz are left and right electro-oculograms. Fz-Cz, Cz-Oz, and C3-A2 are frontal, occipital, and central EEG montages, respectively. Chin EMG and Leg EMG represent submental and pre-tibial EMGs. The electrocardiogram (ECG) shows sinus rhythm. Sono is a snoring microphone showing reopening of the upper airway with reinstitution of airflow at the end of the apneic event. Abdominal (Abd) and chest (Chest) respiratory impedance plethysmography signals demonstrate paradoxical respiratory efforts. HR is the pulse rate, as read. (b) The CPAP titration trial shows elimination of obstructive apneas followed by emergence of central apneas. The thermal sensor channel (ON flow) shows a drop of ≥ 90% of peak thermal sensor signal from baseline. Abdominal (Abd) and chest (Chest) respiratory impedance plethysmography signals demonstrate absence of respiratory efforts during apneic events.

disordered breathing events must be demonstrated and (2) emergence of central apneas must be seen (Fig. 18.3). During this portion of the study, there must be five or more central apneas and hypopneas per hour of sleep, and at least 50% of the total number of apneas and hypopneas seen must be central in nature. The disorder should not be better explained by another CSA disorder.

Treatment

Treatment of complex sleep apnea syndrome is currently somewhat controversial. Even though the disorder most often becomes apparent during titration of CPAP, many advocate a more protracted trial of CPAP. Retrospective studies suggest that as many as 95% of patients will stabilize their breathing patterns on CPAP. These retrospective studies are potentially biased by significant drop-out rates. A prospective trial has shown that only two-thirds of such patients resolve, while over 90% of those treated with ASV show both initial and long-term control of sleep disordered breathing [11]. The data available up until now discourage the use of BPAP-S mode in complex sleep apnea syndrome. The BPAP-ST mode may offer an alternative to CPAP or ASV in controlling respiratory events, even though the consolidation of sleep may still be suboptimal in

certain patients [12]. Given the current limited data, patients with this disorder should probably be initially treated with ASV, or if good follow-up is assured, it may be reasonable to try CPAP for up to 30 days and reassess.

Obesity hypoventilation syndrome

Clinical presentation

This disorder is seen in obese individuals and often coexists with obstructive sleep apnea. Patients may complain of sleep maintenance difficulty and nonrestorative sleep, but, more consistently, they complain of early morning headaches, confusion, and daytime sleepiness, often correlating with their degree of nocturnal hypercapnia.

Diagnosis

Patients are noted to be obese, as defined by a body mass index (BMI) over 30 kg/m^2. During wakefulness, there is presence of hypoventilation, as measured by arterial PaCO$_2$, end-tidal CO$_2$, or transcutaneous PCO$_2$ > 45 mmHg. Diagnostic PSG demonstrates worsening of hypoventilation during sleep if PaCO$_2$ or other noninvasive estimates are used. The hypoventilation should not be due to underlying lung disease, chest wall disorder, neuromuscular disorder, medication use, or congenital central alveolar hypoventilation syndrome.

Treatment

Weight loss is an important long-term goal in the management of obesity hypoventilation syndrome and may be pursued by medical or surgical/bariatric means.

Assistive devices are considered first-line treatment modalities in this condition. CPAP may be effective in many patients, especially those associated with increased upper airway obstruction. A trial of CPAP is indicated before BPAP-S or -ST therapy is tried. If non-invasive mechanical ventilation fails, tracheostomy for mechanical ventilation may be required.

Congenital central alveolar hypoventilation syndrome

Clinical presentation

This is a rare genetic disorder of autonomic dyscontrol of breathing, due to a mutation in the *PHOX2B* gene, often presenting at birth, but sometimes not until adulthood, in the presence of a stressor such as anesthesia or respiratory illness. Patients may present with cyanosis, an apparent life-threatening event, cor pulmonale, or respiratory failure.

Diagnosis

Daytime hypoventilation may or may not be present. However, sleep-related hypoventilation is present as measured by arterial $PaCO_2$, end-tidal CO_2, or transcutaneous $PCO_2 > 45$ mmHg. Mutation of the *PHOX2B* gene is present.

Treatment

Most patients require ventilatory assistance during sleep.

Summary

Sleep disordered breathing may occur in a variety of ways. While obstructive sleep apnea is the most common, we have reviewed here the most common types of sleep disordered breathing that occur independently of upper airway obstruction. In many cases, there is concurrent upper airway obstruction and neurological respiratory dysregulation. Thus, along with attempts to correct the underlying etiologies (when present), stabilization of the upper airway is most often combined with flow generators (noninvasive positive pressure ventilation devices) that modulate the inadequate ventilatory pattern. Among these devices, when CPAP alone does not allow correction of sleep disordered breathing, ASV is increasingly used for non-hypercapnic CSA types, while BPAP-ST is more often reserved for hypercapnic CSA/alveolar hypoventilation syndromes (Table 18.2). Coordination of care among neurologists, cardiologists, and sleep specialists will often benefit such patients.

Table 18.2 Positive airway pressure (PAP) devices

Type	Indications	Set-up	Disadvantages
CPAP Continuous PAP Device that applies the same constant level of positive airway pressure during inhalation and exhalation	CSA with Cheyne–Stokes breathing CSA due to drug or substance Primary CSA Obesity hypoventilation syndrome	Single pressure setting, most often determined during attended polysomnography	No ventilatory support in hypoventilation syndromes
BPAP Bilevel PAP Device that delivers a higher inspiratory pressure (IPAP) and a lower expiratory pressure (EPAP), potentially increases tidal volumes, and hence alveolar ventilation	Primary CSA (BPAP-ST mode) Treatment emergent CSA (BPAP-ST mode) Obesity hypoventilation syndrome (BPAP-S or BPAP-ST)	Inspiratory pressure (IPAP), expiratory pressure (EPAP). Spontaneous (S) mode: no back-up rate Spontaneous-timed (ST) mode: back-up respiratory rate for patients with impaired respiratory drive or neuromuscular disease with insufficient triggering of IPAP	BPAP-S may generate central apneas in CSA with Cheyne–Stokes breathing and treatment emergent CSA
ASV Adaptive pressure support servo-ventilation Feedback control system with self-adjustable pressures that target an average ventilation or inspiratory flow	CSA with Cheyne–Stokes breathing (except symptomatic congestive heart failure patients with ejection fraction ≤ 45% [9]) CSA due to drug or substance Primary CSA Treatment emergent CSA	Maximum and minimum inspiratory pressures End-expiratory pressure Back-up ventilatory rate and flow characteristics may also be set, but default values are provided	Not designed to provide ventilatory support in hypoventilation syndromes; device designed to provide slight hypoventilatory target from baseline values

References

1. Nakayama H, Smith CA, Rodman JR, et al., Effect of ventilatory drive on carbon dioxide sensitivity below eupnea during sleep. Am J Respir Crit Care Med 2002;165:1251–60.
2. Khoo MC, Kronauer RE, Strohl KP, Slutsky AS. Factors inducing periodic breathing in humans: a general model. J Appl Physiol Respir Environ Exerc Physiol 1982;53:644–59.
3. Khoo MC. Determinants of ventilatory instability and variability. Respir Physiol 2000;122:167–82.
4. Aurora RN, Chowdhuri S, Ramar K, et al. The treatment of central sleep apnea syndromes in adults: practice parameters with an evidence-based literature review and meta-analyses. Sleep 2012;35:17–40.
5. Bitter T, Westerheide N, Faber L, et al. Adaptive servoventilation in diastolic heart failure and Cheyne–Stokes respiration. Eur Respir J 2010;36:385–92.
6. Koyama T, Watanabe H, Kobukai Y, et al. Beneficial effects of adaptive servo ventilation in patients with chronic heart failure. Circ J 2010;74:2118–24.
7. Takama N, Kurabayashi. M. Effectiveness of adaptive servo-ventilation for treating heart failure regardless of the severity of sleep-disordered breathing. Circ J 2011;75:1164–9.
8. Yoshihisa A, Shimizu T, Owada T, et al. Adaptive servo ventilation improves cardiac dysfunction and prognosis in chronic heart failure patients with Cheyne–Stokes respiration. Int Heart J 2011;52:218–23.
9. Cowie M, Woehrle H, Wegscheider K, et al. Adaptive servo-ventilation for central sleep apnea in systolic heart failure. N Engl J Med 2015;373:1095–105.
10. Ramar K. Reversal of sleep-disordered breathing with opioid withdrawal. Pain Pract 2009;9:394–8.
11. Morgenthaler T, Kuzniar TJ, Wolfw LF, et al. The Complex Sleep Apnea Resolution Study: a prospective randomized controlled trial of continuous positive airway pressure vs. adaptive servoventilation therapy. Sleep 2014;37:927–34.
12. Allam JS, Olsen EJ, Gay PC, Morgenthaler TI. Efficacy of adaptive servoventilation in treatment of complex and central sleep apnea syndromes. Chest 2007;132:1839–46.

SECTION 5

Insomnias

CHAPTER 19

Insomnias
Classification, evaluation, and pathophysiology

Simon D. Kyle and Colin A. Espie

"When you lose sleep, you lose the better part of yourself. You're *not all there*—as insomniacs know, as we say with the terms we use for ourselves: *zombies, the living dead, nobody home*. It seems ironic that sleep is feared as the loss or disappearance of the self, when it may actually be the way we become most fully ourselves, maintain the continuity of past and present selves, retain our identities through time and change, become our most creative, intelligent, and alive. Sleep is how we manage to be all there. You might even say, *I sleep, therefore I am*."

Greene (2008, p. 48)

Insomnia: defining features

The core symptoms of insomnia, specified in major disease and sleep disorder classification manuals (ICSD-2 in 2005 [2], ICSD-3 in 2014 [3], DSM-5 in 2013 [4], and ICD-10 in 1992 [5]), correspond to difficulties with initiating sleep, maintaining sleep, waking up early (with an inability to resume sleep) or nonrestorative sleep (i.e. poor quality, unrefreshing sleep). To achieve disorder "status," sleep disturbance must not be a function of restricted sleep opportunity (eg, voluntary curtailment) or environmental perturbation (bed-partner snoring, traffic noise, etc.). Notably, the diagnosis of *insomnia disorder* is made only when impairment to daytime function is present, which is linked attributionally to nighttime sleep difficulties. Daytime impairments may be measured with reference to isolated symptoms, such as fatigue, impaired concentration, poor memory, and low mood [6,7], but also more global dysfunction, for example, in areas of occupational, relationship, or social functioning [8]. It is often these daytime concerns that drive treatment-seeking in those with insomnia [9,10]. Additional markers of insomnia severity refer to the frequency and length (persistence) of insomnia symptoms, which, for an insomnia diagnosis, is usually set at greater than or equal to three nights per week [11,12], being present for at least a 1-month period [2,6,13,14]. Of note, the most recent editions of the Diagnostic and Statistical Manual of Mental Disorders (DSM-5) [4] and the International Classification of Sleep Disorders (ICSD-3) [3] have updated this duration criterion to a minimum of 3 days per week for 3 or more months (see Table 19.1 for DSM-5 and ICSD-3 criteria for insomnia disorder). DSM-5 and ICSD-3 have also eliminated the *nonrestorative sleep* subtype, owing to its lack of specificity for insomnia and poorly defined features.

Historically, the two main diagnostic manuals for categorizing insomnia (ICSD and DSM) varied with respect to level of symptomatic detail and subtype classification. In particular, the second edition of the ICSD identified several different subtypes of insomnia disorder, including four primary insomnia phenotypes (each with key defining features; see Table 19.2). However, thorough assessment, by three clinician pairs, of 352 adults reporting insomnia revealed low levels of reliability and validity for the *psychophysiological, paradoxical*, and *inadequate sleep hygiene* phenotypes [15]. Such data has influenced the latest revision of ICSD, published in 2014, which has dropped the primary insomnia subtypes and refined the number of insomnia categories to three: *chronic insomnia disorder, short-term insomnia disorder* and *other insomnia disorder* [3]. This refinement is also consistent with recent revisions to DSM-5. Previous editions, including DSM-IV [13,14], listed "primary insomnia," essentially an exclusionary diagnosis ruling out comorbidity, and "secondary insomnia," indicating that poor sleep is a consequence of a so-called primary condition. Taking heed of evidence that insomnia is involved in the onset, maintenance, and exacerbation of mental and physical illness and that causality is often difficult, if not impossible to determine in clinical practice [16], DSM-5 [4] replaces "primary" and "secondary" insomnia with the more encompassing term, "insomnia disorder." The American Psychiatric Association notes: "… *this change underscores that the individual has a sleep disorder warranting independent clinical attention, in addition to any medical and mental disorders that are also present, and acknowledges the bidirectional and interactive effect between sleep disorders and coexisting medical and mental disorders*" [4].

Insomnia prevalence, natural history, and associated risk factors

Numerous epidemiological studies have been conducted to assess insomnia symptom and disorder prevalence rates [17,18]. Estimates naturally depend on the definition used, but insomnia symptoms are estimated to affect one-third of the population, while

Table 19.1 Criteria for insomnia disorder according to the Diagnostic and Statistical Manual of Mental Disorders, Fifth Edition (DSM-5) [4] and the International Classification of Sleep Disorders, Third Edition (ICSD-3) [3]

	DSM-5: insomnia disorder	ICSD-3: chronic insomnia disorder
Sleep	A predominant complaint of dissatisfaction with sleep quantity or quality, associated with one (or more) of the following symptoms: 1. Difficulty initiating sleep 2. Difficulty maintaining sleep, characterized by frequent awakenings or problems returning to sleep after awakenings 3. Early morning awakening with inability to return to sleep	The patient reports (or the patient's parent or caregiver reports) marked concern about or dissatisfaction with sleep, comprising one or more of the following: 1. Difficulty initiating sleep 2. Difficulty maintaining sleep 3. Waking up earlier than desired 4. Resistance to going to bed on the appropriate schedule 5. Difficulty sleeping without the parent or caregiver present
Consequences	The sleep disturbance causes clinically significant distress or impairment in social, occupational, educational, academic, behavioral, or other important areas of functioning	The patient reports (or the patient's parent or caregiver reports) one or more of the following as being associated with the nighttime sleep difficulty: 1. Fatigue 2. Mood disturbance 3. Interpersonal problems 4. Reduced cognitive function 5. Reduced performance 6. Daytime sleepiness 7. Behavioral problems (eg, hyperactivity, impulsivity, aggression) 8. Reduced motivation/ initiative 9. Proneness to errors/accidents
Frequency	The sleep difficulty occurs at least 3 nights per week	The sleep disturbance and associated daytime symptoms occur at least 3 times per week
Chronicity	The sleep difficulty is present for at least 3 months	The sleep disturbance and associated daytime symptoms have been present for at least 3 months
Exclusions	The sleep difficulty occurs despite adequate opportunity for sleep The insomnia is not better explained by and does not occur exclusively during the course of another sleep/wake disorder The insomnia is not attributable to the physiological effects of a substance Coexisting mental disorders and medical conditions not adequately explain the predominant complaint of insomnia	The reported sleep/wake complaints cannot be explained purely by inadequate opportunity (i.e, enough time is allotted for sleep) or inadequate circumstances (i.e, the environment is safe, dark, quiet, and comfortable) for sleep The sleep/wake difficulty is not better explained by another primary sleep disorder

insomnia disorder (core sleep symptoms plus daytime impairment) affects between 5% and 15% [19,20]. This large variation reflects, in part, lack of standardized case definition and assessment procedures across studies [18]. Of note, few epidemiological studies have implemented strict diagnostic criteria in relation to both classification manuals (ICSD and DSM) or recorded data on whether the individual actually endorses a sleep problem/complaint. One study by Ohayon and Reynolds [12] employed both DSM-IV and ICSD-2 criteria to assess prevalence rates in a large sample of individuals (25 579), aged 15 years and over, residing in seven European countries. It was found that 34.5% of the sample reported at least one difficulty at the "symptom" level (i.e, sleep initiation and/or maintaining difficulties or nonrestorative sleep), and 9.8% were found to meet insomnia disorder at the criterion level, that is, reporting both nighttime symptoms and daytime consequences. After excluding those not scoring "positive" for the *complaint of insomnia*, it was found that 6.6% of the general population met criteria for DSM-IV insomnia disorder. When further broken down, based on DSM-IV criteria, 3.3% of the sample met classification for primary insomnia. These results reasonably approximate those of previous epidemiological studies (eg, [9,17,18]). An important issue, however, was the large number of individuals who, although reporting an insomnia complaint, failed to be categorized by the classification systems, suggesting that future refinement of criteria and measurement may be necessary. Of note, one recent epidemiological study [21], adopting putative DSM-5 criteria, reported a prevalence rate of 7.9% in The Norde-Trondelag region of Norway. However the applied daytime criterion (self-report of daytime sleepiness attributed to poor sleep) is not particularly characteristic of those with insomnia [8] and thus may represent an underestimate of insomnia disorder prevalence. Further prevalence studies adopting strict DSM-5/ICSD-3 criteria are required.

Table 19.2 Essential features of primary insomnia phenotypes listed in the International Classification of Sleep Disorders, Second Edition [2]

Disorder	Characteristic features
Psychophysiological insomnia	Learned sleep-preventing associations, racing mind, conditioned arousal
	Arousal may be conceptualized in physiological, cognitive, or emotional terms
	Excessive focus on sleep and consequences of sleep loss
Paradoxical insomnia	Complaint of little sleep, or total sleep loss, that greatly exceeds objective evidence of sleep disturbance
	Level of subjective sleep disturbance is not commensurate with the reported degree of daytime deficit
Idiopathic insomnia	Persistent complaint of insomnia typically initiating during childhood or from birth, with no or few extended periods of sustained remission
Inadequate sleep hygiene	Insomnia associated with daily living activities that are inconsistent with good sleep quality
	Practices and activities typically produce increased arousal or directly interfere with sleep, eg, use of caffeine, nicotine, or alcohol, irregular sleep scheduling, or engaging in non-sleep behaviors in the sleep environment

Adapted from Journal of Clinical Sleep Medicine, 4(5), Schutte-Rodin, S., Broch, L., Buysse, D., Dorsey, C. & Sateia, M, Clinical guideline for the evaluation and management of chronic insomnia in adults, pp. 487–504, Copyright (2008), with permission from American Academy of Sleep Medicine.

Several risk factors have been associated with increased insomnia prevalence. Among the most strongly supported are increasing age, being female, shift work, and comorbid medical and psychiatric disorders [20,22]. Psychiatric disorders are particularly pronounced in those with insomnia, with estimates suggesting 40% of all patients with insomnia experience a co-occurring psychiatric condition [23]. In particular, depression and anxiety have been found to be highly prevalent in those with an insomnia diagnosis compared with those without [24]. Moreover, those with insomnia syndrome, compared with both good sleepers and individuals with insomnia symptoms, demonstrate higher scores on questionnaire measures of depression, anxiety, neuroticism, arousal predisposition, and stress perception, as well as a tendency toward emotion-oriented coping [25]. Those with insomnia *symptoms* also tend to score higher than good sleepers on measures of depression, anxiety, and neuroticism, suggesting a possible linear trend with increasing insomnia "severity."

Clinically, patients often "anchor" the onset of sleep disturbance to significant life events. In support of this, Bastien and colleagues [26] systematically examined precipitating factors of insomnia in a sample of 345 patients presenting at a sleep disorders clinic. They found that events relating to family, health, work, or school were most frequently associated with the onset of sleep disturbance. Across all recorded events, the majority (65%) were considered to be negative in nature (eg, loss of job or bereavement). Longitudinal natural history studies are also beginning to shed light on factors involved in the development of insomnia, as well as the stability of poor sleep over time. An important prospective study of good sleepers ($n = 464$), measured at three time-points over the course of a 1-year period (0, 6, and 12 months), revealed that baseline assessments of elevated depressive and anxiety symptoms, higher arousability, lower extraversion and poorer mental and physical health were linked to the prospective onset of insomnia syndrome "incident" cases [27]. A recent small study of 54 adults with either acute insomnia (poor sleep in response to a stressor) or normal sleep revealed that baseline sleep architecture—namely decreased slow-wave sleep (SWS) and reduced latency to REM—was associated with greater likelihood of transitioning between acute and chronic insomnia, assessed 3 months later [28]. Once established, insomnia seems to be persistent in nature, with one prospective study showing that for a group of insomnia patients assessed at baseline, nearly 50% will continue to meet insomnia disorder criteria each year for the next 3 years [29]. According to another study, sampling over 5000 participants meeting DSM-5 insomnia disorder criteria, 46% of the sample reported sleeping poorly for more than 6 years, while 25% reported sleeping poorly since childhood [7]. Important new evidence, however, looking at micro-fluctuations from month to month over a 1-year period, reveals a high level of symptom fluctuation: 60% of those with insomnia syndrome and 93% of those with insomnia symptoms reported a change in sleep status at least once over the 12 monthly assessment points [30]. Such data suggest that prospective studies should be sampling more frequently than the typical annual assessments in order to understand the natural course of insomnia.

Several studies have reported increased familial susceptibility to developing insomnia. For example, Dauvilliers et al. [31] found that 73% of a sample of primary insomnia patients ($n = 77$) had a positive family history for familial insomnia, compared with just 24% in a normal-sleeping control group. A population-based study similarly found that those with a past or current history of insomnia had a greater likelihood of a positive family history for insomnia, relative to good sleepers who had never experienced insomnia before [32]. This pattern was also recently replicated in first-degree relatives of adolescents meeting criteria for insomnia disorder [33]. Further evidence of genetic influence comes from twin studies, where monozygotic twins have been found to have higher rates of insomnia concordance, within pairs, in comparison with dizygotic twin pairs (heritability estimate = 57%) [34].

Recent work has attempted to uncover potential genes involved in the expression of insomnia, through both candidate gene studies and genomewide association studies (GWAS) [35]. Although candidate genes have not yet been reliably identified, there are several possible targets relating to sleep homeostasis (eg, adenosine deaminase), circadian timing (eg, clock genes: *CLOCK, PER, BMAL, CRY*), and general arousal/de-arousal (eg, γ-aminobutyric acid (GABA) regulation) [35,36]. Such an approach may be particularly fruitful given the high heritability of sleep EEG power spectra (δ, θ, α, and σ bands) [37], as well as conventional polysomnographic (PSG) sleep parameters [38]. A study by a group in Germany [39] revealed an association between primary insomnia and a serotonin transporter length polymorphism (the *5HTTLPR* short allele). The association remained robust after controlling for those with a lifetime incidence of affective disorder. This finding requires replication but is intuitively appealing given the greater occurrence of this genotype within other stress-related psychiatric conditions (which are frequently related to insomnia) and observations of enhanced cortisol reactivity to experimental psychosocial stress in healthy individuals with this genotype [40]. Finally, recent GWAS data from the UK Biobank (n = 112 586) has identified several novel genetic loci associated with insomnia symptoms, meeting genomewide significance, including near *MEIS1* and *TMEM132E* [41]. These loci and related regions have been linked to restless legs syndrome/limb movements during sleep and anxiety sensitivity. Future work is required to replicate these observations and test for specific genetic associations with insomnia disorder rather than just insomnia symptoms.

Insomnia assessment and evaluation

Insomnia is typically diagnosed according to subjective report, through clinical interview, prospective sleep diary completion, and retrospective questionnaire assessments (see Table 19.3). Assessments probe history, frequency, and severity of sleep and daytime functioning symptoms, but also lifestyle factors, beliefs and attitudes about sleep, pre-sleep arousal, and applied sleep effort [49]. Thorough work-up involves investigation of other sleep-related symptoms and features (eg, snoring, leg twitches, and sleep-walking episodes), as well as the presence of, and relationship to, mental and physical health comorbidities. Similarly, the potential role of drug and substance (mis)use should also be interrogated.

PSG, the gold standard for objectively measuring sleep, is only indicated in circumstances where insomnia is suspected to be related to other sleep disorder pathology, such as periodic limb movements and sleep-related breathing disorders [50]. There are at least two main reasons for this conservative use of PSG. First, it has been known for several decades that individuals with insomnia tend (as a group) to misperceive sleep, significantly underestimating

Table 19.3 Domains to probe when assessing the complaint of insomnia and possible investigative tools

Domain/sub-domain	Possible assessment tool
Sleep history, pattern, and complaint Insomnia severity and impact on functioning	Clinical interview (input from partner/carer) Sleep disorders screen [122] Sleep diary [123] Actigraphy Insomnia Severity Index [124] Sleep Condition Indicator [125] Glasgow Sleep Impact Index [8]
Sleep psychology and lifestyle factors (including work pattern)	Clinical interview Dysfunctional beliefs and attitudes about sleep scale [126] Pre-Sleep Arousal Scale [127] Glasgow Sleep Effort Scale [128]
Physical and mental health comorbidities, including use of prescription drugs and substances	Clinical interview Psychiatric history and examination Physical history and examination
Occult sleep disorders (eg, sleep disordered breathing, or periodic limb movements)	Polysomnography

total sleep time and overestimating time taken to fall asleep compared with PSG recordings [51,52]. This notwithstanding, insomnia patients report *statistically significant* differences in sleep parameters compared with normal sleepers, specifically reduced total sleep time, lower sleep efficiency, increased latency to sleep, greater number of awakenings and less time spent in SWS and REM sleep [53]. Objective sleep continuity differences, however, are typically disproportionate to the subjective complaints of patients [54,55]. Indeed, the core defining feature of the paradoxical insomnia subtype (see Table 19.2) is gross sleep misperception, when a substantial mismatch occurs between subjective report and objective recordings (PSG or actigraphy). PSG is also an expensive procedure, and, given the high prevalence of insomnia disorder in the general population, coupled with limited clinical/treatment insight, overnight laboratory recording of sleep is not cost-effective. However, PSG is recommended in research as a screening tool and as an outcome measure in efficacy studies (though not as the primary dependent variable) [56].

A recent challenge to the view that classic PSG has limited utility in the clinical management of insomnia comes from the group of Alexondros Vgontzas, who have reliably demonstrated that reported insomnia combined with objective short sleep duration represents the most biologically severe insomnia "phenotype," being strongly connected with adverse health outcomes, including increased risk of cognitive impairment, hypertension, depression, diabetes, and early mortality [57]. These authors also suggest that this phenotype would be more likely to respond to pharmacological therapy (targeting physiological hyperarousal), while patients with reports of insomnia but with "normal" sleep duration may be more responsive to cognitive–behavioral therapy (CBT). This proposition awaits empirical testing and confirmation. A related observation from recent work is that sleep restriction therapy (part of CBT for insomnia) is associated with marked sleep loss and vigilance impairment during acute treatment, owing to restricted sleep schedules that are based on self-report (i.e, large baseline objective–subjective sleep discrepancies). This work raises the question of whether objective sleep recordings should be used to guide treatment implementation [58,59].

While PSG continues to play a limited role in the clinical management of insomnia, sleep recordings have advanced understanding of insomnia pathophysiology. For example, increased frequency of microarousals and shifts between sleep stages has been observed in insomnia relative to healthy controls [54]. Moreover, EEG power-spectral analysis during wake, NREM sleep, and REM sleep states can provide information on levels of cortical arousal/excitability. A number of studies (eg, [60–66]) have reported evidence for increased power, both relative and absolute, in fast EEG rhythms (sigma, beta, or gamma frequencies) during wakefulness and NREM and REM sleep, compared with normal sleepers. These alterations often occur in the absence of conventional PSG abnormalities (when compared with controls), and are thought to account, in part, for the subjective experience of being awake during objectively scored sleep (eg, [67]). Indeed, Perlis et al. [63] observed that increased beta power during NREM sleep was associated with greater subjective–objective sleep discrepancies. Similarly, slow-wave spectral power in the delta range (0.5–4 Hz), a marker of homeostatic drive for sleep (or sleep intensity), has been found to be both reduced [60,64] and increased [65] in primary insomnia patients relative to controls. One study also revealed that treatment of insomnia through CBT led to a more rapid decline in delta power (reflecting appropriate discharge of the sleep homeostat) across the sleep period, and that the magnitude of the decline was associated with improved perception of sleep post-treatment [68]. In general, variability in methods, small sample sizes, and findings concerning sex differences [65] suggest that further investigations of microstructural aspects of the sleep EEG are required.

Insomnia-related costs and morbidity

A handful of studies have estimated both direct (eg, healthcare utilization and physician consultations) and indirect costs (downstream consequences, eg, work productivity) of insomnia [69]. One of the most comprehensive studies to date on cost impact was carried out by Daley and colleagues [70] in the province of Quebec, Canada. A random sample (n = 948) of residents were classified, according to strict diagnostic criteria, into good sleepers, those with insomnia symptoms, and those with insomnia syndrome (disorder). Assessments were made for use of healthcare services, products to treat sleep disturbance, accidents, insomnia-related work absenteeism and productivity (*presenteeism*). Objective data were also obtained through a government register regarding recorded health-related consultations. The total estimated cost of insomnia for that particular region (when extrapolated) was 6.6 billion (Canadian) dollars. In particular, insomnia-related absenteeism, reduced work-related productivity, and use of alcohol as a sleep aid were the three biggest contributors. The average annual cost per person with insomnia syndrome was $5010, compared with $1431 for those with insomnia symptoms and just $421 for good sleepers. This study underscores the economic costs associated with both chronic and transient symptoms of sleep disturbance.

While insomnia manifests in the context of the sleep period, it is considered a 24-hour problem, affecting both sleep and daytime periods. Indeed, it is impairment in the daytime that often prompts people to seek help. Sleep-related daytime impairment can range from irritable mood to an inability to hold down a job. As a group, the most commonly endorsed domains of impairment reflect difficulties with energy and motivation, work performance, and cognitive function, and emotion (dys)regulation (see Table 19.4 for verbatim patient reports). The diffuse nature and persistence of daytime symptoms in insomnia is reflected in reduced ratings of overall health-related quality of life [71,72]. Perhaps contrary to expectation, sleepiness is not a commonly reported consequence of insomnia [8], suggesting that dysfunctional arousal or "hyperarousal," is present throughout the entire 24-hour period. The most comprehensive study on daytime sleepiness assessed objective sleep and next-day multiple sleep latency test (MSLT) performance across four scheduled naps [73]. Despite sleeping more than an hour less than healthy control subjects, patients with insomnia disorder took longer to fall asleep (by about 2 minutes, on average) during the day [73], supporting the notion of 24-hour hyperarousal.

Phenomenology of daytime insomnia complaints has also been probed at the level of neurobehavioral performance and neural activity. Despite many historical studies failing to observe reliable differences in neurobehavioral performance between insomnia patients and controls [74], a recent meta-analysis concluded that patients show reliable differences of small to moderate magnitude in tasks probing episodic memory, problem solving, and manipulation and retention in working memory [75]. Several large studies

Table 19.4 Domains of daytime impairment reported by patients with insomnia, supported by verbatim examples

Domains of impairment	Patient-generated examples
Energy/motivation	"feeling exhausted during the day"/"lack of energy and motivation"
Performance at work/school/daily activities	"quality of work/output"/"not able to do the amount of work I would like to"
Cognitive functioning	"memory, concentration, focus"/"sharpness"
Emotional regulation	"my ability to deal with unexpected situations-I panic easily"/"feeling down"
Health/well-being	"always not feeling quite well"/"I don't feel healthy"
Social functioning	"unwilling to arrange to go out to socialize at night"/"I don't look forward to social activities"
Relationships/family functioning	"quality of time with family"/"lack of desire for physical intimacy or sex"
Outlook	"ambition"/"attitude"
Frustration/concern/preoccupation with sleep loss	"worry about what the next night will bring"/"obsession with sleep"
Appearance	"eye appearance (dark circles)"/"people saying you look tired all the time"
Happiness	"general quality of life"/"happiness"
Daytime sleepiness	"always wanting to go to sleep"/"feeling sleepy during day at weekend"
Confidence	"confidence"/"low self-esteem"

Source data from Sleep Medicine, 14(6), Kyle, S.D., Crawford, M., Morgan, K., Spiegelhalder, K., Clark, A., Espie, C.A, The Glasgow Sleep Impact Index (GSII): a novel patient-centred measure for assessing sleep-related quality of life impairment in Insomnia Disorder, pp. 493–501, Copyright (2013), Elsevier.

have also now shown that switching-of-attention tasks (though not sustained attention) are sensitive to the complaint of insomnia [76,77].

With respect to neuroimaging, two task-related functional magnetic resonance imaging (fMRI) studies are particularly relevant to daytime dysfunction. Altena and colleagues [78] scanned patients during a verbal fluency task, observing hypoactivation of medial and inferior prefrontal cortical areas, a pattern that normalized post-CBT. Drummond et al. [79] compared 25 insomnia patients with 25 controls on a widely used working memory task (the N-back task). They observed an abnormal pattern of neural activity in the insomnia group, with failure to engage task-appropriate regions, including widespread areas within the frontoparietal working memory network, motor and visual processing regions, thalamus and cerebellum. They also observed reduced disengagement (lower deactivation) of regions within the default mode network (areas of the brain that are typically active when attention is not focused on the external world). Of note, both the Altena and Drummond studies found no evidence of *behavioral* impairment when comparing insomnia patients with controls.

Insomnia also appears to have general health costs. It has been nearly three decades since Ford and Kamerow [23] published their seminal finding that insomnia is a risk factor for the development of subsequent psychopathology, namely, depression. This relationship has been repeatedly found across several studies, suggesting that insomnia may be an independent risk factor for the onset of depression [80] and anxiety [81]. Mounting evidence also supports a role for insomnia in the perpetuation of depression. For example, Pigeon and colleagues [82] showed, in a large sample of elderly individuals undergoing treatment for major depression, that persistent insomnia at baseline was significantly associated with poorer (depression) treatment response. Similar results have now been documented in the context of social anxiety disorder [83]. Insomnia in addition to mood or anxiety disorder also significantly enhances disability over and above mood or anxiety disorder in isolation [84]. The potential causal role of poor sleep in mental ill-health is further supported by interventional research. Specifically, targeting insomnia within the context of standard treatment for depression, using both CBT [85,86] and eszopiclone [87], leads to improvements in sleep, but also potentiates the antidepressant effect beyond monotherapy.

Associations between insomnia and cardiovascular morbidity have similarly been reported for some time, but possible confounders have limited conclusions regarding causality [88,89]. An important study by Vgontzas et al. [90] has advanced the field in terms of identifying a robust link between insomnia and hypertension. Using PSG recordings (one night) in a large random population sample ($n = 1741$), it was found that those meeting criteria for insomnia disorder and who also (objectively) slept less than 5 hours had a greatly increased risk of experiencing hypertension. This was not the case for individuals without insomnia symptoms and who also slept less than 5 hours (short sleepers). Notably, this insomnia–hypertension relationship held after controlling for several major confounders, including depression and sleep apnea. Further work from the same group also revealed that insomnia and objective sleep duration were associated with incident hypertension over a 7.5-year period [91]. Experimental data showing attenuated systolic blood pressure (SBP) (i.e, wake-to-sleep "dipping,") and elevated nighttime SBP in normotensive primary insomnia patients compared with normal sleepers suggests a possible mechanistic pathway linking sleep disturbance and hypertension risk [92].

Prospective studies consistently identify insomnia as being associated with new-onset physical and mental ill-health [93]. The mechanisms are still unclear, but experimental studies with primary insomnia samples hint at putative pathways, including attenuated heart-rate "dipping" from wake to sleep [94], elevated secretion of inflammatory markers [95], lower levels of cellular immunity [96], increased activity of the hypothalamic–pituitary–adrenal (HPA) axis [97], and altered social–emotional processing [98]. Such modifications, over time, may influence cellular ageing [99] and increase vulnerability to a range of physical and mental health conditions and mortality.

Contemporary models of the development and maintenance of insomnia

Several hypotheses have been proposed to explain the etiology and maintenance of insomnia disorder. For example, *single-factor* accounts have tended to focus on specific sleep–wake abnormalities, psychological mechanisms, or general arousal explanations. These include altered sleep homeostasis [100], impaired circadian regulation of sleep [101], caudate nucleus dysfunction [102],

stimulus dyscontrol and instrumental conditioning [103], physiological hyperarousal [104–106], and dysfunctional cognitive processes relating to sleep and daytime functioning (eg, [107]). While these accounts are well formulated, it is likely that *multi-component* perspectives are required to capture the heterogeneity of insomnia symptoms, associated subtypes, clinical features, and insomnia development/trajectory. Although it is outwith the scope of this chapter to describe each multicomponent model in detail, it is worth outlining some of the main accounts, which are inclusive and encompassing with regard to associated characteristics of insomnia disorder.

The 3P (predisposing, precipitating, perpetuating) model: a general diathesis–stress framework

The main organizing framework for most working models of insomnia was laid out by Spielman et al. [108] in the *3-P model*. This classic stress–diathesis conceptualization outlines how chronic insomnia may develop over time, proposing, as a first step, that acute sleep disturbance occurs as a consequence of the interaction between predisposing factors (eg, altered neurotransmission, trait arousal, genetic susceptibility, and ruminative personality) and precipitating factors (eg, life-stressors such as occupational stress, and emotional and health problems). These precipitants push an individual over a hypothetical insomnia threshold (see Fig. 19.1), engendering insomnia symptoms. Perpetuating factors refer to maladaptive sleep practices, which interact with experienced insomnia symptoms and are aimed at coping with the consequences of poor sleep during the day (eg, drinking coffee to improve alertness) or directly trying to increase the probability of "achieving" sleep (eg, extending time in bed). After the precipitant resolves, most individuals will return to the default position of normal sleep, but in those with a predisposition for sleep disturbance, combined with the continued practice of maladaptive perpetuating behaviors, sleep disturbance may become chronic.

Thus a main assumption of this model is that sleep disturbance may, over time, become dislocated from the precipitating trigger

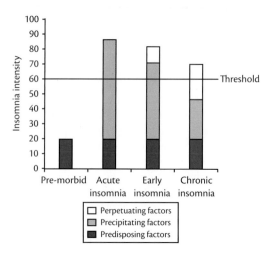

Fig. 19.1 Factors contributing to the development of insomnia, according to the "3-P" framework.

Reproduced from Espie CA, Kyle SD, Cognitive and behavioural psychological therapies for chronic insomnia, in: Barkoukis TJ, Matheson JK, Ferber R, Dohramji K (Ed.), Therapy in Sleep Medicine, pp. 161–171, Copyright (2012), with permission from Elsevier.

[109]. Such a model is intuitively appealing because it suggests that treatment should specifically target perpetuating factors involved in the maintenance of insomnia. This is exactly what CBT for insomnia attempts to do, with an emphasis on correcting maladaptive coping strategies, behaviors, and sleep-related dysfunctional beliefs and attitudes [49].

Neurocognitive model

Perlis and colleagues [110]extend this behavioral perspective, acknowledging that acute insomnia is initially triggered by stress, and is similarly maintained by maladaptive coping strategies (eg, extending time in bed), but that, notably, the associated wakefulness becomes classically conditioned in terms of arousal (somatic, cognitive, and cortical). It is argued that increased cortical arousal (as measured by fast rhythms (beta/gamma) in the EEG) at sleep onset, and during both sleep, and middle-of-the-night awakenings disrupts sleep initiation and maintenance through enhanced sensory/information processing and attenuated mesograde amnesia. These altered cognitive parameters may subsequently help explain "sleep-state misperception" or "paradoxical insomnia." A later addition to this model also includes the possibility that sleep-related objects (bed, pillow, etc.) become conditioned stimuli for cortical arousal [111] and hence contribute to the perpetuation of continued sleep disturbance. The implication of the neurocognitive account is that cortical arousal can act as the biological substrate that precipitates cognitive arousal (*racing mind*) in patients, rather than the notion that people are simply awake and aroused because they are engaged in worry and rumination.

Psychobiological inhibition/attention–intention–effort (PIM/AIE) model

Espie and colleagues [112,113] take a starting point of normal sleep for their model of insomnia. They acknowledge that normal sleep is tightly regulated by two oscillatory processes—an endogenous oscillating circadian rhythm and an "hourglass" sleep homeostat—which operate in concert with good stimulus control, rendering the (adaptive) sleep process automatic, involuntary, and, hence, not under direct control. Acute stressful life events can, however, create both physiological and psychological "over-arousal," which interacts negatively with normal sleep–wake regulation, leading to acute sleep disturbance. For most individuals, the "plasticity" of the sleep system accommodates such transient disruptions, without any lasting chronic modifications; remission of the stressor heralds the return to normal sleep. However, it is argued that the development of acute to chronic insomnia, where the defining feature is a fundamental difficulty in inhibiting wakefulness, is precipitated by three related cognitive processes [113] (see Fig. 19.2). Attending to sleep-related stimuli, explicitly intending to sleep, and applying voluntary effort to the sleep onset process all represent an attempt to control sleep, an otherwise automatic process. These attempts have the opposite effect: preventing de-arousal by failure to reach a level of inhibitory sufficiency. Factors relevant to this resultant "sleep effort syndrome" [114] include enhanced sleep preoccupation, affect dysregulation, sleep-incompatible conditioning, dysfunctional beliefs and expectations about sleep, and enhanced focus on the consequences of poor sleep. Rather than viewing insomnia as a problem of hyperarousal or excessive arousal, Espie and colleagues regard insomnia, particularly the psychophysiological phenotype, as a fundamental difficulty with the inhibition of wakefulness. While evidence exists to support some aspects of the model (eg, sleep-related attention bias) [115], further work is required to determine causal involvement of the aforementioned cognitive processes in the development and perpetuation of insomnia.

Beyond dualistic tendencies: toward an integrative psychobiological insomnia model

The psychological–behavioral models that we have outlined have considerable face validity and clinical value, and have formed the basis of effective cognitive–behavioral intervention. In the last decade, however, a *new perspective* has been put forward to explain insomnia across a number of different "levels"; with particular emphasis on underlying neurobiology. In this respect two recent contributions are noteworthy.

Riemann and colleagues [36] synthesize work on the hyperarousal concept of insomnia, focusing on empirical evidence of hyperarousal across autonomic (heart rate and heart-rate variability), neuroendocrine (HPA axis), neuroimmunological (interleukin-6), electrophysiological (event-related potentials, high-frequency EEG, and compound action potential), and neuroimaging (positron emission tomography data) parameters. They also draw on extensive theorizing by Perlis and colleagues [116–118] in relation to possible neurobiological abnormalities relevant to the features of insomnia, as well as rodent models of stress-induced insomnia [119]. The development of testable hypotheses has been aided largely by recent understandings on the neurobiology of normal sleep–wake regulation [120,121].

The perspective outlined is a further update of the neurocognitive account, originally set out by Perlis et al. [110]. Although at a speculative stage regarding possible mediators of insomnia etiology and development, it is proposed that a genetic arousal predisposition may render certain individuals at greater risk of developing insomnia via altered neurobiology and neurochemistry. Modified levels of several neurochemicals, including orexin (also known as hypocretin), monoamines (histamine, dopamine, norepinephrine (noradrenaline), and serotonin), adenosine, and the stress hormone cortisol, may, during acute periods of stress, disrupt arousal-related (ascending reticular activating system, ARAS) and/or sleep-promoting (ventrolateral preoptic nuclei, VLPO) components of the "flip-flop" sleep switch. Inputs to the VLPO from various limbic structures may also directly impact the capacity to de-arouse adequately, overcoming homeostatic sleep pressure [122]. This would normally represent a typical adaptive response to stress. However, the subsequent development of chronic "arousal," post-acute phase, which is possibly more likely in those with a genetic predisposition for arousability and/or increased stress responsivity [123], interacts with maladaptive sleep practices, resulting in both circadian and homeostatic dysregulation. This dysregulation may, over time, induce chronic changes in the sleep–wake system, reflected in cortical hyperarousal, arousal across other physiological parameters, and difficulties in inhibiting wakefulness. Work by Seugnet et al. [124] in which *Drosophila melanogaster* were artificially selected and bred over many generations to create insomnia-like characteristics (sleep initiation and maintenance difficulties and daytime impairment) helps one conceive of an inherited sleep system with reduced plasticity and/or an altered stress reactivity threshold [111].

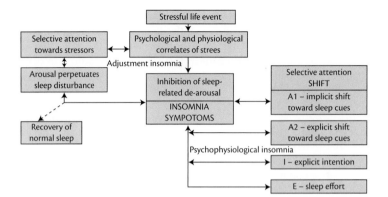

Fig. 19.2 The attention–intention–effort pathway to psychophysiological insomnia. Insomnia occurs in a persistent fashion when there is a sufficient level of attention, intention, and/or effort to outweigh good stimulus control and the intrinsic drives of sleep homeostatic and circadian regulation.
Reproduced from Sleep Medicine Reviews, 10(4), Espie, C.A, Broomfield, N.M., MacMahon, K.M., Macphee, L.M. & Taylor, L.M, The attention-intention-effort pathway in the development of psychophysiological insomnia: a theoretical review, pp. 215–245, Copyright (2006), with permission from Elsevier.

Although this perspective focuses predominantly on neurobiology, it clearly acknowledges that insomnia is a *psychobiological disorder*, with psychological and neurobiological abnormalities likely to be highly inter-related [117]. This seems to be a more convincing integrative account of insomnia and its associated features, rather than a pure physiological hyperarousal perspective in isolation [105]. Indeed, in an inclusive depiction, physiological changes are paralleled with cognitive–behavioral features, which are likely to interact at multiple levels, capturing maintenance and development factors relevant to the original neurocognitive model, Spielman's 3P framework, and Espie's PIM/AIE formulations. It will be important to investigate insomnia at each "level," and ultimately to understand how genetic, biological, and psychological factors interact to determine the course of sleep disturbance over time.

Buysse and colleagues [125] also outline a new framework in which to understand clinical features of insomnia, grounded in basic sleep–wake neuroscience. The main tenet of this hypothesis is that insomnia is characterized by heightened neural activity in wake-promoting brain structures (limbic and parietal cortices, thalamus, hypothalamic–brainstem arousal centers) during NREM sleep (cf. [126]). This wake-like activity, co-occurring alongside PSG recorded sleep, may explain several clinical features of insomnia, including (1) subjective–objective sleep discrepancies and (2) why a small change in objective sleep may be associated with large subjective sleep improvement, post-treatment. The model, consistent with the notion that sleep and wake are not global "all-or-nothing" phenomena [127], but rather an emergent property of individual neurons/neuronal assemblies, draws on evidence from human neuroimaging studies with insomnia patients [126,128] and animal models of acute insomnia [119]. Preliminary evidence points to the possibility of concurrent sleep- and wake-like neural activity. This abnormal pattern of neural activity may manifest as heightened psychophysiological arousal, across the 24-hour period, coupled with impaired circadian rhythmicity/amplitude and attenuated homeostatic sleep pressure. Treatments for insomnia may target different levels of dysfunction; that is, CBT may focus on homeostatic sleep pressure (sleep restriction), circadian timing (strict bed and rise times, standardization of light exposure/activity/meals), and cognitive arousal (relaxation training), with feedback onto corticolimbic cognitive-affective neural

systems, hypothalamic sleep–wake centers and brainstem arousal centers. On the other hand, pharmacotherapy approaches, including sleep-promoting hypnotics, may directly modify cognitive affective brain circuitry and dampen activity in arousal-promoting structures. Further empirical studies are required to test the main tenets of this neurobiological perspective and to elaborate on the development/acquisition of insomnia. Similar to the proposal by Riemann et al. [36], work is required to integrate sleep–wake neurobiology with psychological and behavioral constructs, from which the most effective treatment (CBT) modality has been derived (see Fig. 19.3).

Conclusion

Insomnia is highly prevalent, at both the symptom and syndromal levels. The consequences of insomnia disorder range from impaired day-to-day function and quality of life, through to significant socioeconomic burden and enhanced vulnerability to the development of physical and mental ill-health. Accumulating evidence for a bidirectional and interactive relationship between insomnia and health is changing how insomnia is viewed, classified, and subsequently treated. Contemporary models of insomnia emphasize impairments in down-regulating arousal, across

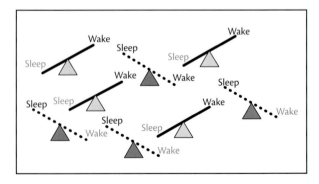

Fig. 19.3 "Local sleep" model of insomnia, proposing that different brain regions may simultaneously show sleep-like and wake-like activity in insomnia patients.
Reproduced from Drug Discovery Today: Disease Models, 8(4), Buysse, D.J., Germain, A., Hall, M., Monk, T.H., Nofzinger, E.A, A neurobiological model of insomnia, pp. 129–137, Copyright (2011), with permission from Elsevier.

cognitive and physiological parameters. Psychological–behavioral models have made important contributions in explaining the trajectory and maintenance of insomnia, emphasizing the role of maladaptive sleep practices and cognitions. Recent developments in basic sleep–wake neurobiology have paved the way for clear and testable hypotheses concerning the brain bases of insomnia disorder. The challenge, going forward, will be to integrate psychological constructs with fundamental sleep–wake neuroscience to enhance explanatory power when accounting for different expressions of insomnia disorder. Given the heterogeneity in insomnia symptom manifestation, history, phenomenological features, and degree of objective sleep disturbance/sleep perception, the field would benefit from detailed subgroup characterization across the multiple levels of brain–behavior explanation.

References

1. Greene G. Insomniac. Oakland, CA: University of California Press, 2008.
2. American Academy of Sleep Medicine. ICSD-2—international classification of sleep disorders: diagnostic and coding manual, 2nd ed. Westchester, IL: American Academy of Sleep Medicine, 2005.
3. American Academy of Sleep Medicine. ICSD-3—international classification of sleep disorders, 3rd ed. Darien, IL: American Academy of Sleep Medicine, 2014.
4. American Psychiatric Association. Diagnostic and statistical manual of mental disorders, 5th ed. Arlington, VA: American Psychiatric Association, 2013.
5. World Health Organization. The ICD-10 classification of mental and behavioural disorders. Clinical descriptions and diagnostic guidelines. Geneva: World Health Organization, 1992.
6. Edinger JD, Bonnet MH, Bootzin RR, et al. Derivation of research diagnostic criteria for insomnia: report of an American Academy of Sleep Medicine workgroup. Sleep 2004;27:1567–96.
7. Espie CA, Kyle SD, Hames P, Chylarova E, Benzeval M. The daytime impact of DSM-5 insomnia disorder: comparative analysis of insomnia subtype from the Great British Sleep Survey (n = 11,129). J Clin Psychiatry 2012;73: e1478–84.
8. Kyle SD, Crawford M, Morgan K, et al. The Glasgow Sleep Impact Index (GSII): a novel patient-centred measure for assessing sleep-related quality of life impairment in insomnia disorder. Sleep Med 2013;14:493–501.
9. Morin CM, LeBlanc M, Daley JP, Merette C. Epidemiology of insomnia: prevalence, self-help treatments, consultations, and determinants of help-seeking behaviors. Sleep Med 2006;7:123–30.
10. Cheung JMY, Bartlett DJ, Armour CL, Glozier N, Saini B. Insomnia patient's help-seeking experiences. Behav Sleep Med 2014;2:106–22.
11. Lichstein KL, Durrence HH, Taylor DJ, Bush AJ, Riedel BW. Quantitative criteria for insomnia. Behav Res Ther 2003;41:427–45.
12. Ohayon MM, Reynolds CF III. Epidemiological and clinical relevance of insomnia diagnosis algorithms according to the DSM-IV and the International Classification of Sleep Disorders (ICSD). Sleep Med 2009;10:952–60.
13. American Psychiatric Association. DSM-IV: diagnostic and statistical manual of mental disorders, 4th edn. Washington, DC: American Psychiatric Press, 1994.
14. American Psychiatric Association. Diagnostic and statistical manual of mental disorders, 4th edn, text revisions. Washington, DC: American Psychiatric Association, 2000.
15. Edinger JD, Wyatt JK, Stepanski EJ, et al. Testing the reliability and validity of DSM-IV-TR and ICSD-2 insomnia diagnoses: results of a multitrait–multimethod analysis. Arch General Psychiatry 2011;68(10):992–1002.
16. Lichstein KL. Secondary insomnia: a myth dismissed. Sleep Med Rev 2006;10:3–5.
17. Ohayon MM. Epidemiology of insomnia: what we know and what we still need to learn. Sleep Med Rev 2002;6:97–111.
18. Morin CM, Jarrin D. Epidemiology of insomnia: prevalence, course, risk factors and public health burden. Sleep Med Clinics 2013:281–97.
19. Roth T. Insomnia: definition, prevalence, etiology, and consequence. J Clin Sleep Med 2007;15:S7–10.
20. Morin CM, Benca R. Chronic insomnia. Lancet 2012;379:1129–41.
21. Uhlig BL, Sand T, Odegard SS, Hagen K. Prevalence and associated factors of DSM-V insomnia in Norway: the Nord-Trondelag Health Study (HUNT3). Sleep Med 2014;15:708–13.
22. Budhiraja R, Roth T, Hudgel DW, Budhiraja P, Drake C. Prevalence and polysomnographic correlates of insomnia comorbid with medical disorders. Sleep 2011;34:859–67.
23. Ford DE, Kamerow DB. Epidemiologic study of sleep disturbances and psychiatric disorders. An opportunity for prevention? JAMA 1989;262:1479–84.
24. Taylor DJ, Lichstein KL, Durrence HH, Riedel BW, Bush AJ. Epidemiology of insomnia, depression, and anxiety. Sleep 2005;28:1457–64.
25. Leblanc M, Beaulieu-Bonneau S, Merette C, et al. Psychological and health-related quality of life factors associated with insomnia in a population-based sample. J Psychosom Res 2007;63:157–66.
26. Bastien CH, Vallieres A, Morin CM. Precipitating factors of insomnia. Behav Sleep Med 2004;2:50–62.
27. Leblanc M, Merette C, Savard J, et al. Incidence and risk factors of insomnia in a population-based sample. Sleep 2009;32:540–8.
28. Ellis JG, Perlis ML, Bastien CH, Gardani M, Espie CA. The natural history of insomnia: acute insomnia and first-onset depression. Sleep 2014;37:97–106.
29. Morin CM, Belanger L, LeBlanc M, et al. The natural history of insomnia: a population-based 3-year longitudinal study. Arch Intern Med 2009;169:447–53.
30. Morin CM, Leblanc M, Ivers H, et al. Monthy fluctuations of insomnia symptoms in a population-based sample. Sleep 2014;37:319–26.
31. Dauvilliers Y, Morin C, Cervena K, et al. Family studies in insomnia. J Psychosomatic Res 2005;58:271–8.
32. Beaulieu-Bonneau S, LeBlanc M, Merette C, Dauviliers Y, Morin CM. Family history of insomnia in a population-based sample. Sleep 2007;30:1739–45.
33. Wing YK, Zhang J, Lam SP, et al. Familial aggregation and heritability of insomnia in a community-based study. Sleep Med 2012;13:985–90.
34. Watson NF, Goldberg J, Arguelles L, Buchwald D. Genetic and environmental influence on insomnia, daytime sleepiness, and obesity in twins. Sleep 2006;29: 645–9.
35. Gehrman PR, Pfeiffenberger C, Byrne EM. The role of genes in the insomnia phenotype. Sleep Med Clinic 2013;3:323–31.
36. Riemann D, Spiegelhalder K, Feige B, et al. The hyperarousal model of insomnia: a review of the concept and its evidence. Sleep Med Rev 2010;14:19–31.
37. Ambrosius U, Lietzenmaier S, Wehrle R, et al. Heritability of sleep electroencephalogram. Biol Psychiatry 2008;64:344–8.
38. Tafti M. Genetic aspects of normal and disturbed sleep. Sleep Med 2009;10:S17–21.
39. Deuschle M, Schredl M, Schilling C, et al. Association between a serotonin transporter length polymorphism and primary insomnia. Sleep 2010;33:343–7.
40. Way BM, Taylor SE. The serotonin transporter polymorphism is associated with cortisol response to psychosocial stress. Biol Psychiatry 2010;67:487–92.
41. Lane JM, Liang J, Vlasac I, et al. Genome-wide association analysis of sleep disturbance traits identify new loci and highlight shared genetics with neuropsychiatric and metabolic traits. Nature Genetics 2016; doi:10.1038/ng.3749.
42. Wilson SJ, Nutt DJ, Alford C, et al. British Association for Psychopharmacology consensus statement on evidence-based treatment of insomnia, parasomnias and circadian rhythm disorders. J Psychopharmacol 2010;24:1577–600.

43. Carney CE, Buysse DJ, Ancoli-Israel S, et al. The consensus sleep diary: standardizing prospective sleep self-monitoring. Sleep 2012;35:287–302.

44. Morin CM. Insomnia: psychological assessment and management. New York: Guildford Press, 1993.

45. Espie CA, Kyle SD, Hames P, et al. The sleep condition indicator: a clinical screening tool to evaluate insomnia disorder. BMJ Open 2014;4:e004183.

46. Morin CM, Vallieres A, Ivers H. Dysfunctional beliefs and attitudes about sleep (DBAS): validation of a brief version (DBAS-16). Sleep 2007;30:1547–54.

47. Nicassio PM, Mendlowitz DR, Fussell JJ, Petras L. The phenomenology of the pre-sleep state: the development of the pre-sleep arousal scale. Behav Res Ther 1985;23:263–71.

48. Broomfield NM, Espie CA. Towards a valid, reliable measure of sleep effort. J Sleep Res 2005;14:401–7.

49. Espie CA, Kyle SD. Primary insomnia: an overview of practical management using cognitive behavioural techniques. Sleep Med Clinic 2009;4:559–69.

50. Schutte-Rodin S, Broch L, Buysse D, Dorsey C, Sateia M. Clinical guideline for the evaluation and management of chronic insomnia in adults. J Clin Sleep Med 2008;4:487–504.

51. Carskadon MA, Dement WC, Mitler MM, et al. Self-reports versus sleep laboratory findings in 122 drug-free subjects with complaints of chronic insomnia. Am J Psychiatry 1976;133:1382–8.

52. Manconi M, Ferri R, Sagrada C, et al. Measuring the error in sleep estimation in normal subjects and patients with insomnia. J Sleep Res 2010;19:478–86.

53. Baglioni C, Regen W, Teghen A, et al. Sleep changes in the disorder of insomnia: a meta-analysis of polysomnographic studies. Sleep Med Rev 2014;3:195–213.

54. Feige B, Al-Shajlawi A, Nissen C, et al. Does REM sleep contribute to subjective wake time in primary insomnia? A comparison of polysomnographic and subjective sleep in 100 patients. J Sleep Res 2008;17:180–90.

55. Harvey AG, Tang NK. (Mis)perception of sleep in insomnia: a puzzle and a resolution. Psychol Bull 2012;138:77–101.

56. Buysse DJ, Ancoli-Israel S, Edinger JD, Lichstein KL, Morin CM. Recommendations for a standard research assessment of insomnia. Sleep 2006;29:1155–73.

57. Vgontzas AN, Fernandez-Mendoza J, Duanping L, Bixler EO. Insomnia with objective short sleep duration: the most biologically severe phenotype of the disorder. Sleep Med Rev 2013;17:241–54.

58. Kyle SD, Miller CB, Rogers Z, et al. Sleep restriction therapy for insomnia is associated with reduced total sleep time, increased daytime somnolence, and objectively-impaired vigilance: implications for the clinical management of insomnia disorder. Sleep 2014;37:229–37.

59. Kyle SD, Aquino MR, Miller CB, et al. Towards standardisation and improved understanding of sleep restriction therapy for insomnia disorder: a systematic examination of CBT-I trial content. Sleep Med Rev 2016;23:83–8.

60. Merica H, Blois R, Gaillard JM. Spectral characteristics of sleep EEG in chronic insomnia. Eur J Neurosci 1998;10:1826–34.

61. Freedman RR. EEG power spectra in sleep-onset insomnia. Electroencephalogr Clin Neurophysiol 1986;63:408–13.

62. Perlis ML, Kehr EL, Smith MT, et al. Temporal and stagewise distribution of high frequency EEG activity in patients with primary and secondary insomnia and good sleepers controls. J Sleep Res 2001;10:93–104.

63. Perlis ML, Smith MT, Andrews PJ, Orff H, Giles DE. Beta/gamma EEG activity in patients with primary and secondary insomnia and good sleeper controls. Sleep 2001;24:110–17.

64. Krystal AD, Edinger JD, Wohlgemuth WK, Marsh GR. NREM sleep EEG frequency spectral correlated of sleep complaint in primary insomnia subtypes. Sleep 2002;25:630–40.

65. Buysse DJ, Germain A, Hall ML, et al. EEG spectral analysis in primary insomnia: NREM period effects and sex differences. Sleep 2008;31:1673–82.

66. Spiegelhalder K, Regen W, Feige B, et al. Increased EEG sigma and beta power during NREM sleep in primary insomnia. Biol Psychol 2012;37:329–33.

67. Borkovec TD, Lane TW, VanOot PH. Phenomenology of sleep among insomniacs and good sleepers: wakefulness experience when cortically asleep. J Abnorm Psychol 1981;90:607–9.

68. Krystal AD, Edinger JD. Sleep EEG predictors and correlates of the response to cognitive behavioural therapy for insomnia. Sleep 2010;33:669–77.

69. Martin SA, Aikens JE, Chervin RD. Toward cost-effectiveness analysis in the diagnosis and treatment of insomnia. Sleep Med Rev 2004;8:63–72.

70. Daley M, Morin CM, LeBlanc M, Gregoire JP, Savard J. The economic burden of insomnia: direct and indirect costs for individuals with insomnia syndrome, insomnia symptoms, and good sleepers. Sleep 2009;32:55–64.

71. Kyle SD, Morgan K, Espie CA. Insomnia and health-related quality of life. Sleep Med Rev 2010;14:69–82.

72. Kyle SD, Espie CA, Morgan K. "… Not just a minor thing, it is something major, which stops you from functioning daily": quality of life and daytime functioning in insomnia. Behav Sleep Med 2010;8:123–40.

73. Roehrs TA, Randall S, Harris E, Maan R, Roth T. MSLT in primary insomnia: stability and relation to nocturnal sleep. Sleep 2011;34:1647–52.

74. Fulda S, Schulz H. Cognitive dysfunction in sleep disorders. Sleep Med Rev 2001;5:423–45.

75. Fortier-Brochu E, Bealieu-Bonneau S, Ivers H, Morin CM. Insomnia and daytime cognitive performance: a meta-analysis. Sleep Med Rev 2012;16:83–94.

76. Shekleton JA, Flynn-Evans EE, Miller B, et al. Neurobehavioural performance impairment in insomnia: relationships with self-reported sleep and daytime functioning. Sleep 2014;37:107–16.

77. Edinger JD, Means MK, Carney CE, Krystal AD. Psychomotor performance deficits and their relation to prior nights' sleep among individuals with primary insomnia. Sleep 2008;31:599–607.

78. Altena E, Van Der Werf YD, Sanz-Arigita EJ, et al. Prefrontal hypoactivation and recovery in insomnia. Sleep 2008;31:1271–6.

79. Drummond SPA, Walker M, Almklov E. Neural correlates of working memory performance in primary insomnia. Sleep 2013;36:1307–16.

80. Baglioni C, Battagliese G, Feige B, et al. Insomnia as a predictor of depression: a meta-analytic evaluation of longitudinal epidemiological studies. J Affect Disord 2011;135:10–19.

81. Neckelmann D, Mykletun A, Dahl AA. Chronic insomnia as a risk factor for developing anxiety and depression. Sleep 2007;30:873–80.

82. Pigeon WR, Hegel M, Unutzer J, et al. Is insomnia a perpetuating factor for late-life depression in the IMPACT cohort? Sleep 2008;31:481–8.

83. Zalta AK, Dowd S, Rosenfield D, et al. Sleep quality predicts outcome in CBT for social anxiety disorder. Depress Anxiety 2013;30:1114–20.

84. Soehner AM, Harvey AG. Prevalence and functional consequences of severe insomnia symptoms in mood and anxiety disorders: results from a nationally representative sample. Sleep 2012;35:1367–75.

85. Manber R, Edinger JD, Gress JL, et al. Cognitive behavioral therapy for insomnia enhances depression outcome in patients with comorbid major depressive disorder and insomnia. Sleep 2008;31:489–95.

86. Watanabe N, Furukawa TA, Shimodera S, et al. Brief behavioural therapy for refractory insomnia in residual depression: an assessor-blind, randomized controlled trial. J Clin Psychiatry 2011;72:1651–8.

87. Fava M, McCall WV, Krystal A, et al. Eszopiclone co-administered with fluoxetine in patients with insomnia coexisting with major depressive disorder. Biol Psychiatry 2006;59:1052–60.

88. Bonnet M, Arand DL. Cardiovascular implications of poor sleep. Sleep Med Clinic, 2007;2:529–38.

89. Spiegelhalder K, Scholtes C, Riemann D. The association between insomnia and cardiovascular diseases. Nat Sci Sleep 2010;4:71–8.

90. Vgontzas AN, Liao D, Bixler EO, Chrousos GP, Vela-Bueno A. Insomnia with objective short sleep duration is associated with a high risk for hypertension. Sleep 2009;32:491–7.

91. Fernandez-Mendoza J, Vgontzas AN, Liao D, et al. Insomnia with objective short sleep duration and incident hypertension: the Penn State cohort. Hypertension 2012;60:925–35.

92. Lanfranchi PA, Pennestri MH, Fradette L, et al. Nighttime blood pressure in normotensive subjects with chronic insomnia: implications for cardiovascular risk. Sleep 2009;32:760–6.

93. Sivertsen B, Lallukka T, Salo P, et al. Insomnia as a risk factor for ill health: results from the large population-based prospective HUNT study in Norway. J Sleep Res 2014;23:124–32.

94. Spiegelhalder K, Fuchs L, Ladwig J, et al. Heart rate and heart rate variability in primary insomnia. J Sleep Res 2011;20:137–45.

95. Burgos I, Richter L, Klein T, et al. Increased nocturnal interleukin-6 excretion in patients with primary insomnia: a pilot study. Brain Behav Immun 2006;20:246–53.

96. Savard J, Laroche L, Simard S, Ivers H, Morin CM. Chronic insomnia and immune functioning. Psychosom Med 2003;65:211–21.

97. Vgontzas AN, Bixler EO, Lin HM, et al. Chronic insomnia is associated with nyctohemeral activation of the hypothalamic–pituitary–adrenal axis: clinical implications. J Clin Endocrinol Metab 2001;86, 3787–94.

98. Kyle SD, Beattie L, Spiegelhalder K, Rogers Z, Espie CA. Altered emotion perception in insomnia disorder. Sleep 2014;37:775–83.

99. Carroll JE, Esquivel S, Goldberg A, et al. Insomnia and telomere length in older adults. Sleep 2016;39:559–64.

100. Pigeon WR, Perlis ML. Sleep homeostasis in primary insomnia. Sleep Med Rev 2006;10:247–54.

101. Lack LC, Wright HR. Treating chronobiological components of chronic insomnia. Sleep Med 2007;8:637–44.

102. Stoffers D, Altena E, van der Werf YD, et al. The caudate: a key node in the neuronal network imbalance of insomnia? Brain 2014;137:610–20.

103. Bootzin RR. Stimulus control treatment for insomnia. Proceedings of the 80th American Psychological Society Annual Convention, 1972:395–6.

104. Bonnet MH, Arand DL. Hyperarousal and insomnia. Sleep Med Rev 1997;1:97–108.

105. Bonnet MH, Arand DL. Hyperarousal and insomnia: state of the science. Sleep Med Rev 2010;14:9–15.

106. Richardson GS. Human physiological models of insomnia. Sleep Med 2007;8:S9–14.

107. Harvey AG. A cognitive model of insomnia. Behav Res Ther 2002;40:869–93.

108. Spielman A, Caruso L, Glovinsky P. A behavioral perspective on insomnia treatment. Psychiatric Clinic N Am 1987;10:541–53.

109. Ebben MR, Spielman AJ. Non-pharmacological treatment for insomnia. J Behav Med 2009;32:244–54.

110. Perlis ML, Giles DE, Mendelson WB, Bootzin RR, Wyatt JK. Psychophysiological insomnia: the behavioral model and a neurocognitive perspective. J Sleep Res 1997;6:179–88.

111. Perlis M, Shaw P, Cano G, Espie C. Models of insomnia. In: Kryger MH, Roth T, Dement W, eds. Principles and practices of sleep medicine, 5th edn. Philadelphia: Elsevier & Saunders Co., 2011.

112. Espie CA. Insomnia: conceptual issues in the development, persistence, and treatment of sleep disorders in adults. Annu Rev Psychol 2002;52:215–43.

113. Espie CA, Broomfield NM, MacMahon KM, Macphee LM, Taylor LM. The attention–intention–effort pathway in the development of psychophysiological insomnia: a theoretical review. Sleep Med Rev 2006;10:215–45.

114. Espie CA. Understanding insomnia through cognitive modelling. Sleep Med 2007;8:S3–8.

115. Harris K, Spiegelhalder K, Espie CA, et al. Sleep-related attentional bias in insomnia: a state-of-the-science review. Clin Psychol Rev 2015;42:16–27.

116. Perlis ML, Pigeon WR, Drummond SPA. Neurobiology of insomnia. In: Gilman S, ed. Neurobiology of disease. Cambridge, MA: Academic Press, 2007:735–44.

117. Perlis M, Gehrman P, Pigeon WR, Findley J, Drummond S. Neurobiologic mechanisms in chronic insomnia. Sleep Med Clinic 2009;4:549–58.

118. Pigeon WR, Perlis ML. Insomnia and depression: birds of a feather? Int J Sleep Disord 2007;1:82–91.

119. Cano G, Mochizuki T, Saper CB. Neural circuitry of stress-induced insomnia in rats. J Neurosci 2008;28:10167–84.

120. Saper CB, Scammell TE, Lu J. Hypothalamic regulation of sleep and circadian rhythms. Nature 2005;437:1257–63.

121. Schwartz JR, Roth T. Neurophysiology of sleep and wakefulness: basic science and clinical implications. Curr Neuropharmacol 2008;6:367–78.

122. Saper CB, Cano G, Scammell TE. Homeostatic, circadian, and emotional regulation of sleep. J Comp Neurol 2005;493:92–8.

123. Harvey CJ, Gehrman P, Espie CA. Who is predisposed to insomnia: a review of familial aggregation, stress reactivity, personality and coping style. Sleep Med Rev 2014;18:217–27.

124. Seugnet Suzuki Y, Thimgan M, Donlea J, et al. Identifying sleep regulatory genes using a *Drosophila* model of insomnia. J Neurosci 2009;22:7148–57.

125. Buysse DJ, Germanin A, Hall M, Monk TH, Nofzinger EA. A neurobiological model of insomnia. Drug Discov Today Dis Models 2011;8:129–37.

126. Nofzinger EA, Buysse DJ, Germain A, et al. Functional neuroimaging evidence for hyperarousal in insomnia. Am J Psychiatry 2004;161:332–42.

127. Krueger JM, Rector DM, Roy S, et al. Sleep as a fundamental property of neural assemblies. Nat Neurosci 2008;9:910–19.

128. Nofzinger EA, Nissen C, Germain A, et al. Regional cerebral metabolism correlates of WASO during NREM sleep in insomnia. J Clin Sleep Med 2006;2:316–22.

CHAPTER 20

Pharmacological and non-pharmacological treatments of insomnia

Elisabeth Hertenstein, Christoph Nissen, and Dieter Riemann

Introduction

Persistent insomnia is a disabling disorder accompanied by a reduced health-related quality of life [1], enhanced absenteeism, and reduced job performance [2]. This has been identified as a risk factor for the first onset of a major depressive episode [3]. Insomnia is defined as a subjective difficulty initiating sleep or maintaining sleep accompanied by subjective daytime impairments [4]. Frequent complaints during the day include fatigue, reduced motivation or energy, mood disturbances, impaired cognitive functioning, interpersonal difficulties, avoidance behavior, and a significant impact on comorbid conditions [5]. In this chapter, the term "insomnia" is used for both primary insomnia and comorbid insomnia associated with a somatic or mental disorder.

Psychological and pharmacological interventions are mainly offered to patients with chronic insomnia (>4 weeks). However, Morin has raised the issue whether treatment should be initiated earlier [6]. Offering therapy to individuals who present with acute (3–14 days) or transient (2–4 weeks) insomnia might have the potential to reduce subjective distress and to prevent a chronic course.

The first step toward successful treatment consists of a detailed diagnostic process, encompassing a thorough clinical evaluation of sleep, medical, psychiatric, and substance histories [5]. A patient who presents with a predominant complaint of insomnia and nonrestorative sleep and with daytime fatigue should always be screened for other sleep disorders that require different treatments (eg, restless legs syndrome, sleep apnea syndrome, or narcolepsy). Consideration should also be given to the possibility that insomnia might occur as a side effect of medication (eg, β-adrenoceptor antagonists, cortisone, or stimulating antidepressants [7]) or can be explained by a behavior that is incompatible with nighttime sleep (eg, excessive daytime naps). Insomnia is often associated with somatic disorders, depression and other mental disorders, or chronic pain [8]. In the case of comorbidities, it is essential to recognize and treat the comorbid disorder, because the latter might lead to the exacerbation of insomnia or vice versa.

Pharmacological treatment

Key points

There is reliable evidence for the effectiveness of benzodiazepines (BZDs) and benzodiazepine receptor agonists (BZDRAs) for the short-term treatment of insomnia. Effects on sleep variables are within the medium range [9]. The efficacy and safety of BZDs and BZDRAs for short-term treatment (approximately four weeks) has been demonstrated in high-quality randomized controlled trials (RCT) and meta-analyses, but data relating to the long-term efficacy and safety are sparse [9].

Low doses of sedating antidepressants are commonly prescribed for the treatment of chronic insomnia in clinical practice [10]. However, research on the short- and long-term efficacy and safety of these substances, compared with placebo and standard hypnotic treatment with BZs/BZRAs, is to date limited [11].

Other sedating substances, including antipsychotics and mood stabilizers that are sometimes used for the treatment of insomnia, are suitable exclusively for patients with insomnia who present with psychiatric comorbid conditions (eg, schizophrenia or bipolar disorder). They are not recommended for patients with primary insomnia, owing to the risk of severe side effects.

Some substances that are available for insomnia treatment without prescription, including valerian and melatonin, appear to be relatively safe without major adverse effects, but are of limited efficacy.

In the following section, the most relevant classes of hypnotic agents will be presented with regard to their assumed mode of action, their effects on insomnia, and their side effects based on current empirical evidence.

Benzodiazepines and benzodiazepine receptor agonists

Mode of action

BZDs and a group of newer BZDRAs commonly referred to as the z-drugs (zaleplon, zolpidem, zopiclone, and eszopiclone) are a class of agents that enhance the effect of γ-aminobutyric acid (GABA), the most important inhibitory neurotransmitter in the central nervous system [12]. Both groups of substances act at the GABA-A benzodiazepine receptor complex and enhance neuronal inhibition. Whereas BZDs bind to different subunits of the GABA-A receptor complex, the z-substances are structurally different and bind more selectively to the α₁ subunit. They have been developed to overcome side effects of the BZDs such as hangover, withdrawal syndrome, and tolerance/dependency. These z-drugs have reduced muscle-relaxing and anxiolytic effects compared with BZDs. However, they still have the potential to cause tolerance, dependence, and withdrawal symptoms, and their sedating effects may also persist into the next day.

Effects on insomnia

Choice of a specific substance

The UK National Institute for Clinical Excellence in 2004 carried out an investigation to determine the superiority of one BZD or BZDRA drug over another [13]. The assessment group reviewed data from 24 RCTs comparing the effects of BZDs and z-substances regarding sleep quality outcomes (sleep diaries and questionnaires). The authors concluded that there is no consistent pattern of superiority of one drug over another. Specifically, there were no significant differences in the rates of treatment-associated adverse events. This lack of consistency may in part be due to the limited quality of the studies.

In a meta-analysis, Duendar and colleagues [14] included 24 RCTs (data of $n = 3909$ patients with insomnia) comparing one of the z-drugs (zaleplon, zolpidem, or zopiclone) with classical BZDs (diazepam, alprazolam, lorazepam, lormetazepam, nitrazepam, and temazepam). They found only minor differences, but increased costs for the z-drugs. One minor difference was that zaleplon produced shorter sleep latencies than zolpidem and zopiclone.

In the absence of a clear overall superiority of one substance, the choice of a specific BZD or BZDRA should be guided by the subjective complaint of the patient, the treatment goals and the half-life of the substance. A BZD or BZDRA with a shorter half-life (a shorter duration of action) is suitable for patients with sleep onset insomnia. In contrast, substances with longer half-lives have the potential to reduce wake after sleep onset (WASO) and early morning awakening, but bear the risk of carry-over effects the next morning. Table 20.1 provides an overview of BZDs and BZDRAs, their half-lives, and their recommended dosages (based on [15]). As illustrated, zaleplon is a substance with a particularly short half-life, which is recommendable for patients who mainly suffer from difficulties falling asleep. Zaleplon usually does not produce carry-over effects on the next morning. However, it is less well suited for patients who mainly suffer from difficulties maintaining sleep or early morning awakenings [5]. Eszopiclone and temazepam, on the contrary, are well suited for patients who wish to reduce WASO. Flurazepam is a substance with a very long half-life, and is most often not recommendable because it frequently produces hangover effects.

Evidence

Several large meta-analyses demonstrated that BZDs and BZDRAs have a superior effect compared with placebo in improving sleep parameters in adults with insomnia.

In a first meta-analysis, Nowell and colleagues summarized 22 placebo-controlled RCTs ($n = 1894$) investigating the effects of

Table 20.1 Benzodiazepines and benzodiazepine receptor agonists with half-lives and recommended dosages

Drug name	Half-life (h)	Recommended dose (mg)	Trade name (examples)
BZD			
Triazolam	2–6	0.125–0.25	Halcion
Alprazolam	5–11	1–2	Sonin
Lormetazepam	8–11	1–2	Noctamid
Temazepam	8–20	15–30	Remestan
Flunitrazepam	10–20	0.5–1	Rohypnol
Estazolam	8–24	1–2	Eurodin
Nitrazepam	25–35	5–10	Mogadan
Flurazepam	48–120	15–30	Dalmadorm
Quazepam	48–120	7.5–15	Dormalin
BZDRA			
Zaleplon	1	5–10	Sonata
Zolpidem	1.5–2.5	10 (age < 65 yrs) 5–10 (age > 65 yrs)	Stilnox
Zopiclone	5–6	7.5 (age < 65 yrs) 3.75 (age > 65 yrs)	Ximovan
Eszopiclone	5–7	2–3 (age < 65 yrs) 1 (age > 65 yrs)	Lunesta

BZD, benzodiazepine; BZDRA, benzodiazepine receptor agonist.

BZDs (alprazolam, chlordiazepoxide, diazepam, estazolam, flurazepam, lorazepam, quazepam, temazepam, and triazolam) and zolpidem in adults with insomnia [16]. The duration of treatment was seven days on average. The authors found stable effects of medium size. The combined effect sizes were 0.6 for sleep onset latency (SOL), 0.7 for the number of awakenings (NOA), 0.7 for total sleep time (TST), and 0.6 for subjective sleep quality.

Holbrook et al. [17] included 45 studies ($n = 2672$) into their meta-analysis and investigated the effects of short-term (average seven days) BZD administration (triazolam, flurazepam, temazepam, midazolam, nitrazepam, estazolam, lorazepam, diazepam, brotizolam, quazepam, loprazolam, and flunitrazepam) and zopiclone on self-reported sleep parameters in patients with insomnia. Compared with placebo, they found a reduction in SOL of 14.3 minutes and an increase in TST of 48.4 minutes.

A subsequent meta-analysis by Glass and colleagues [18] included 24 studies ($n = 2417$) on patients aged over 60 years with insomnia. The analyzed substances were BZDs (loprazolam, nitrazepam, triazolam, chlormethiazole, quazepam, flunitrazepam, midazolam, brotizolam, flurazepam, temazepam, and lormetazepam), z-drugs (zolpidem, zopiclone, and zaleplon), and the antihistaminic agent diphenhydramine. The authors found only small improvements in sleep compared with placebo. The effect sizes were 0.1 for subjective sleep quality and 0.6 for NOA. TST increased by 25 minutes. However, in this sample of elderly individuals, adverse events were more common with sedating substances than with placebo. Adverse cognitive events were 4.8 times more common, adverse psychomotor events 2.6 times more common, and reports of daytime fatigue 3.8 times more common with medications than placebo. The authors concluded that the small positive effects do not outweigh the risks in older patients with insomnia.

Side effects

Barbiturates, which have been widely used as sedatives for many decades, bind to the β subunit of the GABA-A receptor and act as direct agonists at the receptor. Since the late twentieth century, barbiturates have rarely been used as hypnotics owing to their side effects, most important of which is the high risk of lethal overdose arising from the narrow span between the therapeutic and toxic dosages.

BZDs, on the contrary, are indirect GABA agonists and exert their modulating effect at the α subunit of the GABA-A receptor exclusively in the presence of GABA. Owing to their different mode of action, BZDs, in contrast to barbiturates, have a low risk of lethal overdose. They have thus largely replaced barbiturates as hypnotic medications.

However, within the last 20 years, many publications have demonstrated several critical side effects of BZDs and BZDRAs (see, eg, [17]). Adverse effects are primarily morning hangover (drowsiness and light-headedness), cognitive disturbances associated with performance deficits and a reduced learning and memory capacity, abuse, tolerance and dependency, parasomnia (eg, sleepwalking and nocturnal eating), nocturnal falls related to muscle relaxation, confusion, and ataxia, especially in the elderly. Besides, BZDs may enhance and prolong the effects of other substances, such as alcohol. Kripke and colleagues [19,20] even found an elevated mortality rate associated with the intake of hypnotics, including zolpidem, temazepam, eszopiclone, zaleplon, other BZDs, barbiturates, and sedative antihistamines. Thus, patients who receive a BZD or BZDRA should always be closely monitored by their health practitioner. For each individual patient, positive effects and undesired side effects must be examined and weighed against each other. Especially in individuals over the age of 60 years, the prescription is often not recommended in light of the small benefits and the risk of severe adverse events [18].

Although the z-drugs were initially praised for generating substantially fewer adverse effects than classical BZDs, recent research suggests that this assumption is not justified. Duendar et al. [14] concluded in their meta-analysis that, regarding benefits as well as adverse events, the z-substances (zaleplon, zolpidem, and zopiclone) do not offer convincing advantages compared with the investigated BZDs, but impose elevated costs on the healthcare system. Holbrook and colleagues [17] also found in their meta-analysis that zopiclone was not superior to BZDs on any of the investigated outcomes, including adverse events.

Mode of administration

Frequency

Concerning the frequency of administration, a study by Perlis et al. [21] supports the use of an intermittent dosing strategy, which is often adopted in clinical practice. In this study, patients with primary insomnia were instructed to take no fewer than three and no more than five doses of 10 mg zolpidem per week over a period of three months. The authors found significantly improved sleep compared with placebo, no decrease of the effect with time, no rebound insomnia, and no dose escalation with time.

Duration

Concerning the duration of the treatment, a sufficient data base supports the efficacy and safety of short-term treatment (up to four weeks) with BZDs or BZDRAs. However, research on the effects of long-term administration remains insufficient. In 2005, the State of the Science Conference of the American National Institutes of Health [22] pointed out that it is still unclear for which patients, if any, long-term medication with BZDs and BZDRAs is useful and sufficiently safe. However, insomnia is often chronic and thus is most often not satisfactorily treated with a short-term course (up to four weeks).

Several newer randomized, placebo-controlled studies have addressed the long-term efficacy and safety of the z-substances. Krystal et al. [23] investigated an extended use of eszopiclone versus placebo for six months. They included 788 patients with primary insomnia and reported a significantly reduced SOL (43 minutes), a significantly reduced WASO, a significantly increased TST (76 minutes), and improved ratings of daytime function, which were stable over six months. They found no evidence for clinically relevant changes in laboratory parameters or vital signs under eszopiclone versus placebo. The most common side effects under eszopiclone were a bitter taste, pain, nausea, and pharyngitis. No withdrawal symptoms and no rebound insomnia after discontinuation of eszopiclone were reported. Another study by Krystal and colleagues [24] investigated the effects of a retarded form of zolpidem over six months with an administration of three to seven nights per week in over 1000 patients with primary insomnia. Zolpidem, compared with placebo, produced significant and sustained improvements in sleep onset and maintenance, next-day concentration, and daytime sleepiness. No signs of rebound-insomnia were found during the first 3 nights of discontinuation. The most frequent adverse events associated with zolpidem, compared with placebo, were headache, somnolence, and anxiety. Ancoli-Israel et al. [25] published the results of a 12-month open-label study on the extended use of zaleplon in 260 older adults with primary insomnia. They reported statistically significant improvements in SOL, NOA, and TST over the one-year period. No rebound insomnia associated with discontinuation was observed.

BZDs and BZDRAs are not approved in Europe for the long-term treatment (longer than four weeks) of insomnia.

Discontinuation

Discontinuation of a BZD or BZDRA after more than a few days of use is often associated with a withdrawal syndrome including rebound insomnia, anxiety, loss of appetite, tremor, tinnitus, hallucinations, confusion, and convulsions [26]. In order to minimize withdrawal symptoms, guidelines recommend tapering of the frequency and dosage in small steps until the smallest possible dosage [5]. Tapering may require several weeks or even months.

Melatonin and melatonin agonists

Mode of action

Melatonin is an endogenous hormone released by the pineal gland that is involved in the regulation of circadian rhythms and sleep. Melatonin secretion is highest during the nighttime and is suppressed by dawn [27]. The hormone binds to MT1 and MT2 receptors in the suprachiasmatic nucleus. In the USA, melatonin is available as an over-the-counter medication. Melatonin receptor agonists are available on a prescription basis: ramelteon (Rozerem) in the USA and Circadin in Europe. Circadin is a prolonged-release form of melatonin. The half-life of ramelteon is 1.4 hours and that of Circadin is 2.5 hours. Both thus belong to the hypnotics with a rather short duration of effect, which are mostly recommended to patients with sleep onset, but not sleep maintenance, difficulties.

Effects on insomnia

Melatonin

A meta-analysis of the efficacy and safety of exogenous melatonin was performed by Buscemi and colleagues in 2005 [28]. They found that melatonin decreased SOL to a clinically relevant degree in patients with delayed sleep phase syndrome, but not in patients with insomnia. The weighted mean reduction of SOL was only seven minutes in patients with insomnia. The authors found no evidence of adverse effects of melatonin. They concluded that short-term treatment with melatonin is not effective in patients with primary insomnia.

Ramelteon

In a review of the literature, Sateia and colleagues [29] identified eight clinical trials on the efficacy and safety of ramelteon, all of them conducted or sponsored by the pharmaceutical company that synthesizes the agent, and five of them RCTs. They concluded that ramelteon is moderately effective in reducing SOL in adults of all ages with chronic insomnia, but produces negligible or no effects on WASO and TST. The effect on SOL was comparable to standard hypnotic agents. Safety data indicated a low side effect profile with no significant impairments of next-day performance.

A meta-analysis by Liu et al. [30] included eight RCTs (n = 4055) investigating the effects of ramelteon versus placebo. They found significant improvements with ramelteon in subjective and polysomnographic SOL, TST, and latency to REM sleep, but no effect on the percentage of REM sleep. In this meta-analysis, the effect on subjective SOL was only significant for the group of patients aged under 65 years. With a reduction in subjective SOL by 14.3 minutes in the younger age group and an increase in TST by 8.7 minutes, the effects of ramelteon appear to be small. Ramelteon was not associated with relevant adverse events compared with placebo.

Side effects

To date, the literature on melatonin and ramelteon has yielded no evidence for any severe side effects [28–30]. The most frequent adverse events reported after the use of ramelteon were headache, nasopharyngitis, and somnolence [30]. However, none of these occurred significantly more often after ramelteon than after placebo. In contrast to BZDs and BZDRAs, melatonin agonists do not carry risks of dose escalation, abuse, dependence, or rebound insomnia upon withdrawal.

Mode of administration

The recommended dose for ramelteon is 8–16 mg, and that for Circadin is 2 mg. However, the meta-analysis by Liu et al. suggests that for ramelteon, 16 mg is not more effective than 4 mg [30]. A study by Mayer and colleagues [31] in 451 patients with chronic primary insomnia found that ramelteon consistently reduced SOL over six months of nightly administration. The authors found no carry-over effects the next morning and no signs of

rebound insomnia or withdrawal syndrome upon discontinuation. However, the literature concerning the long-term administration of melatonin agonists does not yet allow for recommendations concerning the optimal duration of treatment. Additional studies on the long-term efficacy and safety of these substances are warranted.

Antidepressants

Mode of action

Antidepressants that are commonly used off-label for the treatment of insomnia include trazodone, doxepine, mirtazapine, trimipramine, and amitriptyline [10]. For the treatment of persistent insomnia, they are usually prescribed in low doses, below the therapeutic dosages for depression. Antidepressants influence several neurotransmitter systems in the central nervous system and thus exert various therapeutic and side effects. Their antidepressant effect is assigned to an inhibition of the reuptake of serotonin and noradrenaline into the synaptic cleft and subsequent neuronal remodeling. Their hypnotic effects, by contrast, relate to an antagonism to the H1 histamine receptor. Table 20.2 provides an overview of the most relevant sedating antidepressants, their half-lives, and their recommended dosages for antidepressant versus hypnotic treatment (based on [15]). The table shows that most sedating antidepressants have relatively long half-lives and may thus produce a morning hangover.

Effects on insomnia

Prescribing low-dose sedating antidepressants for the treatment of chronic primary and comorbid insomnia is common clinical practice in Europe and the USA [10]. Yet there is a gap between the widespread use of this practice and a scarcity of evidence for its efficacy and safety. Buscemi et al. investigated the efficacy and safety of drug treatments, including antidepressants, for chronic insomnia in a meta-analysis [32]. The weighted mean reduction in SOL measured by polysomnography after antidepressant treatment compared with placebo was 7 minutes. For SOL measured by sleep diaries, the reduction was 12 minutes. The weighted means were based on four studies for SOL measured by polysomnography and two studies for SOL measured by sleep diaries. Based on five studies, there was an increase in sleep efficiency (polysomnography) by 13% after antidepressant treatment versus placebo. Notably, the

Table 20.2 Sedating antidepressants with half-lives and recommended dosages

Drug name	Half-life (h)	Recommended dose (mg)		Trade name (examples)
		Antidepressant	Hypnotic	
Trazodone	3–14	150–600	25–150	Thombran
Doxepin	10–30	100–300	3–150	Aponal
Mirtazapine	13–40	15–45	3.75–30	Remergil
Trimipramine	15–40	100–300	10–150	Stangyl
Amitriptyline	5–45	100–300	25–150	Saroten, Equilibrin

increase in TST measured by polysomnography was large, at 79.4 minutes (based on four studies), but TST measured by sleep diaries decreased by 54.3 minutes (based on one study). Patients treated with antidepressants reported significantly more adverse events than patients who had received placebo, the relative risk difference being 0.09 (three studies). The most commonly reported adverse events were somnolence, headache, dizziness, and nausea. There were no reports of falls, injury, or death.

A study of the effects of doxepin on polysomnographically measured sleep was published by Hajak et al. in 2001 [33]. Forty-seven patients with primary insomnia were randomized to either 25–50 mg of doxepin or placebo for a treatment phase of four weeks. Doxepin, compared with placebo, was associated with a significantly better sleep efficiency, sleep quality, and ability to work over the treatment phase of four weeks. Subjective improvements were small to moderate in size. Sleep returned to its baseline level after discontinuation of doxepin. There were significantly more patients with severe rebound insomnia in the doxepin group, and two patients dropped out of the doxepin group due to severe side effects (increased liver enzymes, leukopenia, and thrombocytopenia). The second doxepin study was published by Roth et al. in 2007 [34]. In the crossover-study, 67 patients with primary insomnia were randomized to doxepin in three different low dosages (1, 3, and 6 mg) versus placebo for two nights with a drug-free interval of 5 or 12 days. The authors found significant improvements in WASO, TST, and sleep efficiency measured by polysomnography for doxepin in all dosages compared with placebo. For doxepin 6 mg, an improvement in subjective SOL was found. The safety profile of doxepin for this short-term administration was comparable to placebo, with no evidence of daytime sedation, anticholinergic effects, or memory impairment.

Walsh and colleagues conducted a comparison of zolpidem 10 mg versus trazodone 50 mg versus placebo for two weeks in 306 patients with primary insomnia [35]. After one week, an increase in self-reported TST and a reduction in SOL were significant for both substances versus placebo, but zolpidem produced a greater reduction of SOL than trazodone. After two weeks, the effects on TST were nonsignificant for both substances and the effects on SOL were only maintained in the zolpidem group. The rates of side effects were 75% for trazodone, 76.5% for zolpidem, and 65.4% for placebo. The most frequently reported adverse events were headache and somnolence. Both were slightly more frequent in the trazodone group.

In another study, 55 patients with primary insomnia were randomized to trimipramine at an average dose of 100 mg, lormetazepam 1 mg, or placebo for a treatment period of 28 days [36]. The authors found no significant effects of trimipramine versus placebo on TST, which had been the primary outcome. However, the data show increases in TST by almost 60 minutes in the trimipramine group and 18 minutes in the lormetazepam group, and an almost unaltered TST in the placebo group. Thus, the lack of significance might be due to the small sample size. An effect on sleep efficiency was significant for trimipramine versus placebo, and nonsignificant for lormetazepam versus placebo. The effects diminished after a shift from trimipramine to placebo, but no evidence of rebound insomnia or withdrawal syndrome were reported. No relevant adverse events were found in EEG, vital parameters, physical examination, or laboratory parameters during active treatment.

Side effects

Most antidepressants have far longer half-lives than common BZDs and BZDRAs (see Tables 20.1 and 20.2). For this reason, they are often associated with morning hangover, especially in the first period after treatment onset.

Potential side effects of sedating antidepressants in low dosages have not yet been sufficiently investigated. Common side effects include sedation, anticholinergic effects such as dry mouth, constipation, urinary retention, and glaucoma, antihistaminic effects such as weight gain, orthostatic hypotension, restless legs symptoms, and cardiovascular side effects. In contrast to BZDs and BZDRAs, antidepressants appear not to bear the risk of abuse and dependency.

Antihistaminics

Histamine is an organic nitrogen compound that is known to be involved in local immune responses. As a neurotransmitter, histamine is involved in the maintenance of wakefulness [37], with its H1 receptor subtype being relevant for the regulation of sleep and wakefulness. Diphenhydramine, hydroxyzine, doxylamine, and promethazine are examples of reversible antagonists of histamine at the H1 receptor that are available for the treatment of insomnia.

The efficacy and safety of antihistaminic substances for the treatment of insomnia is not well established. In particular, studies concerning their long-term effects are lacking. Some studies have been conducted on the short-term efficacy and safety of diphenhydramine. Glass et al. compared diphenhydramine (50 mg) with temazepam (15 mg) and placebo in a RCT in elderly patients with insomnia over a period of 14 days [38]. Diphenhydramine was only effective in reducing the number of awakenings, but had no effect on sleep quality, TST, or SOL. The numbers of adverse events were similar in all three groups, but one person in the temazepam group suffered a fall. In another RCT, Morin et al. compared the effects of diphenhydramine (25 mg over 14 days), a valerian–hops combination, and placebo on sleep diary variables and polysomnographically measured sleep in 184 adults with mild insomnia [39]. Diphenhydramine produced significantly greater improvements in sleep efficiency than placebo, but had no significant effect on other sleep variables. No significant adverse events and no rebound insomnia upon discontinuation were observed for both treatments.

In summary, there is some evidence that diphenhydramine produces small to moderate short-term improvements in subjectively reported sleep. However, various side effects have been associated with antihistaminic substances. Impaired psychomotor performance has been reported as a side effect of diphenhydramine. Dizziness, fatigue, tinnitus, decreased appetite, nausea, vomiting, diarrhea, constipation, and weight gain can occur as side effects of antihistaminic substances. Clinical experience suggests a loss of effect over time, indicating that antihistaminic substances are not suitable for the long-term treatment of chronic insomnia.

Antipsychotics

First-generation antipsychotics such as haloperidol are to be distinguished from the so-called atypical or second-generation antipsychotics such as risperidone, quetiapine, olanzapine, and clozapine. The agents of the first generation are assumed to exert their antipsychotic effects by blocking dopamine, mainly at its D2 receptor in the mesolimbic system. However, D2 receptors are not exclusively located in the target regions of the brain, but also exist in other regions such as the basal ganglia. First-generation antipsychotics do not bind selectively to the target receptors. Thus, they are associated with severe side effects such as extrapyramidal dysfunctions (dyskinesia, akathisia, and parkinsonism). Second-generation antipsychotics were developed in order to exert less severe side effects and indeed show a lower incidence of extrapyramidal dysfunction. However, they can produce other side effects, such as massive weight gain. Sedation and sleepiness are also common side effects, which probably result from antagonism of the H1 histaminic receptor. Their sedating effects may suggest the suitability of some antipsychotics for the treatment of insomnia, but to date no controlled studies of antipsychotic agents in patients with primary insomnia have been conducted. Owing to their many side effects, antipsychotics, including the "atypical" agents, are not recommended for the treatment of chronic primary insomnia. Their use as hypnotics should be reserved for patients presenting with severe comorbid psychiatric conditions like schizophrenia and related disorders, who might also benefit from their antipsychotic effects.

Valerian

Valerian is a herbal substance that is extracted from the roots of the plant *Valeriana officinalis*. It is sold as an over-the-counter sleep and anxiolytic medication. Its sedating and anxiolytic effects are assumed to relate to an activity at the GABA receptor. However, the mode of action of valerian is not yet fully understood. A systematic review by Taibi and colleagues identified 29 controlled trials and eight open-label studies on valerian as a sleep aid [40]. The authors concluded that valerian has no side effects but is probably no more effective than placebo for the treatment of insomnia. Many of the reviewed studies were of insufficient methodological quality.

A more recent meta-analysis on the efficacy of valerian for insomnia was conducted by Fernandez-San-Martín and colleagues in 2010. They identified 18 RCTs comparing valerian preparations to placebo [41] and found a mean difference in SOL between valerian and placebo of 0.7 minutes. The relative "risk" of sleep quality improvement (yes/no) with valerian compared with placebo was 1.37. In view of their results, the authors suggested a shift of further research activities to other treatments for insomnia that are more promising than valerian.

Psychological Interventions

Key points

Psychological and behavioral interventions are effective in treating insomnia in the short and long term. The extant literature suggests that the effects of these interventions are more sustainable than those of pharmacological treatment [9]. The improvements in subjective sleep quality, SOL, TST, WASO, and NOA after psychological and behavioral interventions are typically of medium to large effect size. According to a systematic review of the literature published by a task force of the American Academy of Sleep Medicine in 2006, relaxation training, stimulus control therapy, paradoxical intention, sleep restriction, and cognitive–behavioral therapy (CBT) are well-established treatments for patients with chronic primary and comorbid insomnia, including older adults [42]. To date, no complete dismantling studies on the effectiveness of single psychological and behavioral interventions have been conducted

[42]. It remains to be elucidated which techniques are the active components of CBT and whether multicomponent CBT is superior to any single intervention [42]. One example of a treatment manual is the session-by-session guide by Perlis et al. [43].

The following section first summarizes the state of research concerning psychological and behavioral interventions for chronic insomnia. Second, the most relevant interventions are illustrated.

State of research

Effects on insomnia

Five meta-analyses evaluated nonpharmacological interventions for insomnia in adults, two of which exclusively focused on insomnia in older adults. One recent study reviewed the literature on computerized CBT for insomnia.

The first meta-analysis was published by Morin et al. in 1994 and reviewed the literature from 1974 to 1993 [44]. The review included 59 studies ($n = 2012$). Of note, this meta-analysis and most others on psychological and behavioral interventions calculated pre-to-post effect sizes, whereas the meta-analyses on BZDs and BZDRAs cited earlier in the chapter reported between-group effect sizes. Many individual studies compared psychological and behavioral interventions to a waitlist rather than a placebo group, as it is difficult to realize a true placebo group in trials on psychological interventions. Thus, the different kinds of effect sizes for psychological and pharmacological interventions are of limited comparability. Morin et al. reported the following pre versus post effect sizes for nonpharmacological interventions in a total of 2102 patients with primary or comorbid insomnia: 0.88 for SOL, 0.65 for WASO, 0.53 for NOA, and 0.42 for TST. All four effect sizes were significantly greater than zero. Psychological and behavioral interventions contained five hours of therapy time on average. The most effective techniques were stimulus control and sleep restriction, whereas sleep hygiene education alone was not effective. The effects were maintained at follow-up measures (mean follow-up duration six months). Figure 20.1 illustrates the quantitative changes in sleep

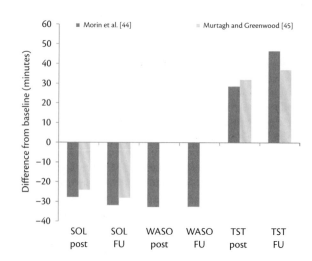

Fig. 20.1 Quantitative improvements in sleep after psychological treatment. SOL, sleep onset latency; WASO, wake time after sleep onset (not reported by Murtagh and Greenwood); TST, total sleep time; post, quantitative change compared with baseline (in minutes) directly after treatment, FU, quantitative change compared with baseline at follow-up. All effects were significantly different from zero.

variables (in minutes) that were found in this meta-analysis and the following one. The figure shows that the improvements were well maintained or even increased at follow-up.

The second meta-analysis was published by Murtagh and Greenwood [45] one year later. The authors reviewed the literature from approximately the same time period, but only included studies on patients with primary insomnia without comorbidities. Sixty-six studies ($n = 1538$) fulfilled the inclusion criteria and were included in the meta-analysis. The reported effect sizes for the pre versus post comparison are similar to those found in the review by Morin et al., with 0.87 for SOL, 0.63 for NOA, and 0.49 for TST (all significant). Similar to the findings of Morin et al., Murtagh and Greenwood found that the sleep improvements after psychological and behavioral interventions were maintained or even augmented during follow-up periods of six months on average.

The first meta-analysis that focused on adults with insomnia at an older age (over 60 years) was conducted by Pallesen and colleagues [46]. Studies that were published between 1966 and 1998, that evaluated a psychological or behavioral treatment for older adults with insomnia, and that investigated quantitative sleep parameters as outcomes were included. The meta-analysis was performed on 13 studies ($n = 388$). Effect sizes directly after treatment were 0.41 for SOL, 0.61 for WASO, 0.25 for NOA, and 0.15 for TST. The effect sizes at follow-up (average duration six months) were 0.61 for SOL, 0.59 for WASO, 0.66 for NOA, and 0.37 for TST (all significant).

Montgomery and Dennis conducted a Cochrane Review on the effects of cognitive–behavioral treatments for sleep problems in the population of patients aged over 60 years [47]. They included only RCTs that met high methodological standards according to a quality checklist. Patients with typical insomnia symptoms (eg, difficulties initiating and maintaining sleep and impaired daytime functioning) as well as patients with delayed or advanced sleep phase syndrome and parasomnias were included. Six RCTs ($n = 224$) met the inclusion criteria. This review found a negligible effect for SOL (−3 minutes) and modest effects for WASO (−22 minutes) and TST (+14.6 minutes). The authors concluded that in elderly patients with sleep problems, cognitive–behavioral interventions are best suited for sleep maintenance problems.

A fifth meta-analysis was published by Irwin et al. in 2006 [48]. Inclusion criteria were RCTs investigating the effects of cognitive–behavioral interventions for primary insomnia with sleep parameters as outcomes. Twenty-three trials were identified. Effect sizes of acute treatment were 0.50 for SOL, 0.69 for WASO, 0.17 (nonsignificant) for TST, 0.74 for sleep efficiency, and 0.79 for subjective sleep quality. The authors analyzed the type of behavioral intervention as a moderating variable and found that combined CBT, relaxation, and behavioral treatment alone did not significantly differ in effect sizes. The interventions were found to be equally effective for middle-aged adults and patients older than 55 years concerning sleep quality, sleep latency, and wakening after sleep onset.

An meta-analysis by Cheng and Dizon evaluated a new trend in psychotherapy: computerized CBT, a low-threshold alternative to face-to-face therapy [49]. The investigated interventions were sleep hygiene education, stimulus control, relaxation, sleep restriction, and cognitive restructuring, delivered through the use of a computer. The authors included six RCTs in their analysis. The effect sizes of computerized CBT for insomnia compared with control groups (waitlist or alternative treatment groups) were 0.41 for sleep quality, 0.40 for sleep efficiency, 0.45 for NOA, and 0.55 for SOL.

The effects on TST (0.22), WASO (0.18), and time in bed (0.25) failed to reach statistical significance.

Adherence

Whereas the efficacy of nonpharmacological interventions for insomnia is undisputed, patients' adherence to the somewhat strenuous recommendations such as restricted bed times is a challenging problem in clinical practice. Matthews et al. reviewed the literature on patients' adherence to CBT for insomnia in a recent systematic review [50]. They included 15 studies published between 1992 and 2012 that investigated short-term adherence to sleep restriction, stimulus control, and sleep hygiene education using measures other than study withdrawal. The authors conclude that despite the relevance of the topic, there is still a dearth of valid research devoted to adherence. Inconsistencies in adherence findings may be due to methodological weaknesses of the included studies, such as small sample sizes, diversity of sample characteristics, and the absence of standardized definitions and measures of adherence. Some of the included studies found a positive relationship between adherence and sleep improvements. The authors suggested that small investments in the improvement of adherence might result in better outcomes. However, the occurrence of side effects, such as sleepiness and fatigue, especially at the beginning of sleep restriction therapy, makes the low adherence of some patients understandable.

Mediators

In a review of potential mechanisms of treatment outcomes of CBT for insomnia, Schwartz and Carney [51] summarized three models of insomnia and derived different theorized mechanisms of action. Behavioral models emphasize that dysfunctional sleep-related behaviors, such as daytime napping or prolonged bedtimes, weaken the homeostatic sleep drive and disrupt a consolidated sleep–wake rhythm. These models thus propose that mechanisms of CBT comprise a reduced time in bed, decreased daytime napping, and a reduced variability of bedtime and rise time. Cognitive models, in contrast, propose that increased worry and rumination, attentional bias toward sleep-related threats, and distorted beliefs about sleep are central to the development and maintenance of chronic insomnia. Based on these models, suggested mechanisms include decreased maladaptive beliefs and attitudes about sleep, increased experience of self-efficacy, and a shift from an external to an internal locus of control about sleep. A third model is the hyperarousal model, which posits that a conditioned cognitive, somatic, and emotional hyperarousal is a central perpetuating factor of insomnia, and thus that effective treatments work through a reduction of this arousal.

The authors found 54 studies that fulfilled their inclusion criteria (RCTs comparing CBT for adults with insomnia versus a control condition, with sleep outcomes as dependent variables). Thirty-nine percent of these (21 studies) included the examination of potential mediating variables. The reviewed studies provided some evidence for each of the three models. The authors concluded that more research is needed to better understand whether CBT works through its theorized mechanisms.

Setting

In their review of the literature published between 1998 and 2004, Morin and colleagues found that psychological treatments were provided over a mean period of 6.5 weeks and included 5.7 sessions on average [42]. Bastien et al. directly compared three different treatment modalities and found no significant differences between group CBT, individual CBT, and telephone consultations in a trial of 45 adults with primary insomnia [52]. In two studies, treatment provided by trained primary care physicians or nurses produced effects that were comparable to those typically found for treatment provided by psychologists [53,54]. CBT is most often conducted in group programs that include psychoeducation, sleep hygiene education, relaxation training, cognitive restructuring, and, as a key component, behavioral interventions such as sleep restriction or stimulus control.

Interventions

Stimulus control

Stimulus control therapy is based on the assumption that in individuals with chronic insomnia, the bed serves as a conditioned stimulus for wakefulness, anxiety, and arousal. Patients often report extended bed times in order to compensate for poor sleep. Thus, compared with healthy sleepers, they spend more time lying in bed awake, worrying about not being able to sleep and consequences of poor sleep. When lying in bed and trying hard to fall asleep without success, patients are assumed to experience a heightened cognitive and somatic arousal and frustration about not being able to sleep. As a consequence of another night with poor sleep, they might decide to spend even more time in bed in order to compensate for their sleep loss. Yet, in fact, they might be too anxious or aroused to fall asleep, they might be "trying too hard," or they might simply not have enough sleep pressure when going to bed early, and thus they consolidate the learning experience that the bed is a cue for wakefulness and arousal instead of relaxation and sleep.

Stimulus control therapy is designed to re-associate the bed with sleep. However, it is also conceivable that the effective mechanism of stimulus control is not, or not exclusively, the re-association of the sleeping environment with deactivation and sleep. It is possible that the technique works, at least in part, by sleep deprivation and a subsequent increased sleep pressure (see the later discussion of sleep restriction therapy).

Stimulus control therapy usually starts with a psychoeducation session. Therapists might start by explaining the two-process model of sleep regulation (cf. [37]). Briefly summarized, sleep and wake behavior is regulated by two processes. The first of these is the circadian rhythm of many biological functions, including body temperature, hormone levels, and a circadian component of sleep propensity. The second process is the homeostatic drive and reduction of sleep pressure. After a long period of wakefulness, sleep pressure grows and leads to faster sleep onset and an increase in slow-wave sleep. The same happens after a night of poor sleep. Thus, there will always be "good nights" following "bad nights," even if patients with insomnia sometimes feel that they do not sleep at all. The model can be used as an introduction to the rationale of stimulus control and sleep restriction therapy.

During stimulus control therapy, patients receive the following instructions:

- Go to bed only when you are sleepy.

- If you are not able to sleep after 20 minutes or wake up at night and cannot return to sleep after 20 minutes, get out of bed, go to another room, and do something relaxing (eg, listening to

soothing music or reading in front of a low-intensity light; go back to bed when feeling drowsy; you can repeat these steps more than once).

- Use the bed only for sleeping (and sex), do not work, watch TV, eat, etc. in the bedroom.

Important, patients should be asked to stand up after *approximately* 20 minutes; they should be instructed not to look at a clock or watch, because this would unnecessarily keep them awake.

Sleep restriction

Similar to stimulus control, sleep restriction therapy is based on the observation that patients with insomnia often report prolonged bed time and daytime napping in order to compensate for poor sleep. This behavior is assumed to produce a destabilization of natural biological sleep–wake rhythms. The rationale for sleep restriction therapy for insomnia is to increase sleep pressure in order to reduce sleep latency and render sleep more restorative. The goal of the therapy is thus not to help patients sleep eight hours per night, but to increase the restorative quality of their sleep. It is assumed that improved sleep continuity can be accomplished by compressing the total time in bed to the actual sleep time and thus increase sleep efficiency. Besides, the individual spends less time awake in bed, which is supposed to dissolve the conditioned connection between the bed as a stimulus and arousal/awakening as a response (see the earlier discussion).

Before starting sleep restriction therapy, patients are required to keep a sleep diary for one to two weeks. The diaries are carefully reviewed together with the therapist, and bed time is restricted to the actual total sleep time (TST). If, for example, TST is an average five hours per night, the time in bed is restricted to five hours per night. However, the total time in bed should not be less than five hours. The patient and the therapist agree on fixed bed times and wake times, which should be followed for seven days a week. Patients are instructed not to nap during the day. Weekly sessions for monitoring and adjustment of sleep behavior are scheduled. Sleep efficiency can be calculated as TST divided by time in bed, multiplied by 100. If sleep efficiency is still below 85% after one week, patients are instructed to decrease time in bed by another 15 minutes. When sleep efficiency is 85% or above, time in bed can be increased in steps of 15–30 minutes per week.

It is important to consider that sleep restriction therapy may produce adverse effects in many patients. In contrast to pharmaceutical approaches, adverse effects of psychotherapy are often neglected by researchers. During sleep restriction therapy, patients may suffer from daytime sleepiness and a reduced level of daytime functioning, especially in the beginning of the sleep restriction treatment [55]. Patients should be instructed only to drive a vehicle and operate machinery if they feel able to stay awake and concentrated. For many patients, the treatment is perceived as aversive, and thus compliance is often insufficient.

Intensive sleep retraining

Intensive sleep retraining (ISR) [56] is a brief conditioning treatment. The rationale is to increase the homeostatic sleep pressure by acute sleep deprivation and realize a series of rapid sleep onsets the following night. This is supposed to dissolve the conditioned insomnia response. In the night before the actual treatment, patients are instructed to restrict their time in bed to five hours. They attend the therapeutic setting (eg, a sleep laboratory) the following night. The treatment is realized during a period of 25 hours, for example from 22:00 to 23:00 the following night. During this period, participants are provided with 50 sleep-onset-opportunities every half-hour. The opportunity for sleep onset is limited to 20 minutes within each trial. If patients fall asleep within this time, they are allowed to sleep for three consecutive minutes and are then awakened. During their wake time, participants undertake relaxing activities such as reading or watching movies. After the intervention period, they receive detailed feedback about their sleep–wake times within each trial.

Potential effective components of ISR are a conditioning effect, a discrimination training of sleep and wake states due to the detailed feedback, and an exposure to sleep deprivation that is highly feared by many individuals with insomnia. In a recent RCT, 79 volunteers with sleep onset insomnia were randomized to IST, stimulus control, a combination of both treatments, or sleep hygiene education as a control condition. All active treatments were superior to the control condition, with few differences between the active treatments. An advantage of ISR appears to be a faster treatment response [56].

Relaxation training

Relaxation training is assumed to work through a reduction in the physiological, cognitive, and emotional hyperarousal that is associated with insomnia. Practitioners may also learn to focus their attention on muscular relaxation and thus interrupt dysfunctional rumination and worry. Sleep improvements have been demonstrated for progressive muscle relaxation (PMR) and other forms of relaxation training such as deep breathing, hypnosis, and autogenic training. PMR has been developed by Edmund Jacobson [57]. The method is based on the conscious tension and subsequent relaxation of different muscle groups. In a second step, the physical relaxation is coupled with an individual signal, such as a word or a mental image, which enables subjects to deliberately recall relaxation.

In addition to the relaxation training itself, patients can also be instructed not to engage in highly activating tasks before bedtime. Patients should be informed that first they will need time to learn the relaxation technique and that therefore sleep improvements are not to be expected from the beginning of the training. At first, relaxation exercises should not be performed directly before bedtime, in order to prevent the experience of failure and subsequent frustration.

Mindfulness

Mindfulness meditation training is another intervention that is sometimes considered a relaxation technique. However, the aim of mindfulness practice is not to achieve a state of relaxation, but to cultivate active awareness of body sensations, thoughts, and feelings in the present moment. Mindfulness is often taught in weekly group meetings over a period of eight weeks. Manualized mindfulness trainings are Mindfulness Based Stress Reduction [58] and Mindfulness Based Cognitive Therapy [59]. Jason Ong and his coworkers developed a mindfulness-based treatment for insomnia that combines intensive mindfulness training with sleep restriction and stimulus control treatment. In an open-label pilot study, the authors found first promising effects that were mainly stable at 12 months follow-up [60,61].

Cognitive interventions

The aims of cognitive therapy for insomnia are restructuring distorted beliefs and attitudes and challenging unrealistic expectations about sleep. Dysfunctional cognitions are critically examined and replaced by more adaptive thoughts. Common distorted beliefs of individuals with insomnia are, for example, the assumption that every person needs eight hours of sleep every night to be healthy and the concern that a night with little sleep inevitably leads to an apparent and dramatic reduction in next-day performance.

Pech and O'Kearney evaluated the efficacy of problem-solving therapy (PST) for primary insomnia [62]. The goal of PST is to reduce engagement in worry in the pre-sleep period and to enhance the feeling of self-efficacy concerning problem solving. The treatment consisted of problem-solving techniques such as setting a fixed time for thinking about problems and noting down possible solutions step by step, action planning, and evaluating solutions. PST was compared with traditional cognitive therapy, as an adjunct to sleep hygiene education, to stimulus control therapy, and to relaxation. Equal effects were found in both groups. However, owing to the design of the study, it cannot be decided whether the behavioral interventions alone were responsible for the treatment effects in both groups. Thus, the results of the study cannot be considered as evidence that PST and/or cognitive therapy are helpful. To date, cognitive interventions alone are not supported by sufficient evidence and thus are not recommended as a standalone treatment for insomnia [42]. The extent to which the cognitive component of CBT plays a role in the efficacy of combined treatments remains to be clarified.

Paradoxical Intention

The rationale of paradoxical intention therapy is to reduce the fear of staying awake and weaken the pressure of having to fall asleep. These are in fact incompatible with falling asleep and often create a vicious circle of fear, pressure to "do it right," and consequent failure to fall asleep in patients with chronic insomnia. In healthy sleepers, in contrast, falling asleep most often happens without any deliberate effort or conscious awareness. The goal of paradoxical intention treatment is to break this vicious circle by instructing patients to stay awake as long as possible after going to bed. Two small RCTs from 1979 and 1986 suggested that paradoxical intention therapy can be equally effective as stimulus control and relaxation training [63,64].

Biofeedback

Different kinds of biofeedback have been suggested for the treatment of insomnia. The most common is electromyography (EMG) biofeedback. Other forms include sensorimotor rhythm (SMR) feedback and theta electroencephalography (EEG) feedback.

EMG biofeedback can be considered a special form of relaxation training that aims at reducing somatic hyperarousal. Patients receive a display of their actual level of tension or relaxation through sensors placed on their skin. While performing relaxation strategies, they can monitor their "success" online and adapt their behavior to the feedback they receive.

The aim of SMR feedback and theta EEG biofeedback is to teach patients to deliberately induce an EEG rhythm that is typically found in human sleep. These interventions are thus designed to actively induce sleep, in contrast to indirectly promoting sleep through the reduction of arousal. Biofeedback meets the American Psychological Association (APA) criteria for "probably efficacious treatments" [65].

Sleep hygiene education

The aim of sleep hygiene education is to eliminate behaviors that are incompatible with healthy sleep. A first step is the thorough examination of the individual sleep behavior: When does the patient go to bed? When does he wake up and when does he get up? What does he do before bedtime? Does he drink alcohol, smoke nicotine, or consume any other stimulants?

According to their individual sleep-related behaviors, patients then receive information and advice. The most important sleep hygiene rules are the following:

- Keep a regular sleep–wake schedule (eg, always go to bed and wake up at approximately the same time, including weekends, and avoid daytime napping).

- Keep to a healthy diet.

- Regularly engage in sporting activities, but avoid sports or other exciting activities before going to bed.

- Reduce the intake of stimulants such as coffee, cola, and black tea to a minimum, and avoid stimulating drinks after noon.

- Avoid nicotine close to bedtime, because nicotine is also a stimulant. Additionally, the sudden withdrawal of nicotine at night may induce awakenings in heavy smokers.

- Avoid alcohol before bedtime. Alcoholic drinks shorten sleep onset latency, but alcohol metabolizes very rapidly and thus produces nightly awakenings as a rebound effect.

- Refrain from amphetamines, cocaine, and other illicit drugs that have sleep-disturbing effects.

- Avoid heavy evening meals.

- Avoid drinking a lot (including non-alcoholic beverages) in the evening.

- Minimize noise and light in the bedroom and avoid a bedroom that is too hot or too cold.

- Do not watch the clock at night, since this often leads to more arousal and more pressure to finally fall asleep, and thus prevents one from doing so.

- Establish a personal bedtime ritual.

Sleep hygiene education is not effective as a standalone treatment for patients with chronic insomnia, but is assumed to be beneficial in nonclinical cases or as an adjunct to other interventions.

Comparative effects of pharmacological and nonpharmacological treatment

The comparative efficacy of pharmacological and nonpharmacological interventions has been evaluated in two systematic reviews. The first was a meta-analysis published by Smith and colleagues in 2002 [66]. The authors included treatment studies on behavior treatments (including stimulus control or sleep restriction) or BZDs and BZDRAs for primary insomnia. Within-subject measures had to be obtained before and after treatment, and patients had to be withdrawn from hypnotic medications before inclusion

in the study. Fourteen behavioral treatment studies ($n = 250$) and eight pharmacological studies ($n = 286$) were included. In this sample, the pre-to-post effect sizes averaged over all included sleep variables (SOL, NOA, WASO, TST, sleep quality) were comparable, at 0.87 for pharmacological and 0.96 for non-pharmacological interventions. Statistical comparisons for the individual variables showed that the weighted effect sizes were comparable for NOA, WASO, TST, and sleep quality. Behavioral interventions were superior to BZDs and BZDRAs concerning SOL (weighted effect sizes were 1.05 versus 0.45).

A systematic review by Mitchell et al. [67] analyzed trials that directly compared CBT for insomnia with any FDA-approved prescription or nonprescription medication in patients with primary insomnia. The levels of evidence were assessed using the GRADE method; i.e, the strength and certainty of evidence was rated as high, moderate, low, or very low for each research question. Five RCTs that met the inclusion criteria were identified. The data were considered too small and too heterogeneous to conduct a meta-analysis. The investigated medications were zolpidem, zopiclone, temazepam, and triazolam. Evidence concerning the short-term comparison of CBT and BZDs/BZDRAs was of very low quality and provided inconsistent results. Long-term comparisons (follow-up periods of 6–24 months) consistently favored CBT, with low to moderate grade of evidence. Quality of life as an outcome was only included in one trial, which found no significant difference between patients treated with CBT versus zopiclone. The study also found no group difference in daytime fatigue as measured by reaction times. The reporting of adverse events was too limited to draw conclusions concerning the comparative safety of the two treatment types.

Conclusion

The current state of research on the treatment of persistent primary and comorbid insomnia in adults is that pharmacological treatment, especially with BZDs or BZDRAs, and non-pharmacological interventions, primarily behavior treatment, are effective for the short-term management. However, both types of interventions bear the risk of adverse effects. Most prominently, BZDs and BZDRAs are associated with the risk of development of tolerance and dependency. Undesired outcomes of psychotherapy are often insufficiently accounted for in clinical trials. Nonpharmacological interventions are superior to medication when long-term effects are considered. Whereas the effects of psychological approaches have been found to remain stable after discontinuation of the treatment for follow-up periods up to two years, insomnia often re-occurs after the discontinuation of medication. Following the present state of evidence, psychological interventions are the first-line treatment for persistent insomnia. Medication is only recommended if psychological treatment alone fails or if patients refuse psychological treatment. If pharmacotherapy is used, it should be limited to a period of up to four weeks.

References

1. Kyle SD, Morgan K, Espie CA. Insomnia and health-related quality of life. Sleep Med Rev 2010;14:69–82.
2. Simon GE, VonKorff M. Prevalence, burden, and treatment of insomnia in primary care. Am J Psychiatry 1997;154:1417–23.
3. Baglioni C, Battagliese G, Feige B, et al. Insomnia as a predictor of depression: a meta-analytic evaluation of longitudinal epidemiological studies. J Affect Disord 2011;135(1–3):10–9.

4. American Academy of Sleep Medicine(AASM). International classification of sleep disorders. 2nd ed. Westchester, IL: AASM, 2005.

5. Schutte-Rodin S, Broch L, Buysse D, et al. Clinical Guideline for the Evaluation and Management of Chronic Insomnia in Adults. J Clin Sleep Med 2008;4:487–504.

6. Morin CM. Definition of acute insomnia: diagnostic and treatment implications. Sleep Med Rev 2012;16:3–4.

7. Riemann D, Nissen C. Substanzinduzierte Schlafstörungen und Schlafmittelmissbrauch. Bundesgesundheitsblatt Gesundheitsforschung Gesundheitsschutz 2011;54:1325–31.

8. Kessler RC, Berglund PA, Coulouvrat C, et al. Insomnia, comorbidity, and risk of injury among insured Americans: results from the America Insomnia Survey. Sleep 2012;35:825–34.

9. Riemann D, Perlis ML. The treatments of chronic insomnia: a review of benzodiazepine receptor agonists and psychological and behavioral therapies. Sleep Med Rev 2009;13:205–14.

10. Walsh JK. Drugs used to treat insomnia in 2002: regulatory-based rather than evidence-based medicine. Sleep 2004;27:1441–2.

11. Mendelson WB. A review of the evidence for the efficacy and safety of trazodone in insomnia. J Clin Psychiatry 2005;66:469–76.

12. Mendelson WB. Hypnotic medications: mechanisms of action and pharmacologic effects. In: Principles and practice of sleep medicine, 4th ed. Philadelphia, PA: Elsevier Saunders, 2005:444–51.

13. National Institute for Clinical Excellence. Guidance on the use of zaleplon, zolpidem and zopiclone for the short-term management of insomnia. Technology Appraisal Guidance 77. 2004; available from http://www.nice.org.uk/TA077guidance.

14. Dündar Y, Dodd S, Strobl J, et al. Comparative efficacy of newer hypnotic drugs for the short-term management of insomnia: a systematic review and meta-analysis. Hum Psychopharmacol. 2004;19(5):305–22.

15. Riemann D, Nissen C. Sleep and psychotropic drugs. In: The Oxford handbook of sleep and sleep disorders, 1st ed. Oxford: Oxford University Press, 2012.

16. Nowell PD, Mazumdar S, Buysse DJ, et al. Benzodiazepines and zolpidem for chronic insomnia: a meta-analysis of treatment efficacy. JAMA 1997; 278:2170–7.

17. Holbrook AM, Crowther R, Lotter A, et al. Meta-analysis of benzodiazepine use in the treatment of insomnia. CMAJ 2000;162:225–33.

18. Glass J, Lanctôt KL, Herrmann N, et al. Sedative hypnotics in older people with insomnia: meta-analysis of risks and benefits. BMJ 2005;331:1169.

19. Kripke DF, Langer RD, Kline LE. Hypnotics' association with mortality or cancer: a matched cohort study. BMJ Open 2012;2(1):e000850.

20. Kripke DF, Garfinkel L, Wingard DL, et al. Mortality associated with sleep duration and insomnia. Arch Gen Psychiatry 2002;59:131–6.

21. Perlis ML, McCall WV, Krystal AD, Walsh JK. Long-term, non-nightly administration of zolpidem in the treatment of patients with primary insomnia. J Clin Psychiatry 2004;65:1128–37.

22. National Institutes of Health. State-of-the-Science Conference statement on manifestations and management of chronic insomnia in adults. NIH Consensus and State-of-the-Science Statements 2005;22(2):1–30.

23. Krystal AD, Walsh JK, Laska E, et al. Sustained efficacy of eszopiclone over 6 months of nightly treatment: results of a randomized, double-blind, placebo-controlled study in adults with chronic insomnia. Sleep 2003;26:793–9.

24. Krystal AD, Erman M, Zammit GK, et al. Long-term efficacy and safety of zolpidem extended-release 12.5 mg, administered 3 to 7 nights per week for 24 weeks, in patients with chronic primary insomnia: a 6-month, randomized, double-blind, placebo-controlled, parallel-group, multicenter study. Sleep 2008;31:79–90.

25. Ancoli-Israel S, Richardson GS, Mangano RM, et al. Long-term use of sedative hypnotics in older patients with insomnia. Sleep Med 2005;6:107–13.

26. Roehrs T, Merlotti L, Zorick F, Roth T. Rebound insomnia in normals and patients with insomnia after abrupt and tapered discontinuation. Psychopharmacology 1992;108:67–71.

27. Korf HW, Schomerus C, Stehle JH. The pineal organ, its hormone melatonin, and the photoneuroendocrine system. Adv Anat Embryol Cell Biol 1998;146:1–100.

28. Buscemi N, Vandermeer B, Hooton N, et al. The efficacy and safety of exogenous melatonin for primary sleep disorders. A meta-analysis. J Gen Intern Med 2005;20:1151–8.

29. Sateia MJ, Kirby-Long P, Taylor JL. Efficacy and clinical safety of ramelteon: an evidence-based review. Sleep Med Rev 2008;12:319–32.

30. Liu J, Wang L-N. Ramelteon in the treatment of chronic insomnia: systematic review and meta-analysis. Int J Clin Pract 2012;66:867–73.

31. Mayer G, Wang-Weigand S, Roth-Schechter B, et al. Efficacy and safety of 6-month nightly ramelteon administration in adults with chronic primary insomnia. Sleep 2009;32:351–60.

32. Buscemi N, Vandermeer B, Friesen C, et al. The efficacy and safety of drug treatments for chronic insomnia in adults: a meta-analysis of RCTs. J Gen Intern Med 2007;22:1335–50.

33. Hajak G, Rodenbeck A, Voderholzer U, et al. Doxepin in the treatment of primary insomnia: a placebo-controlled, double-blind, polysomnographic study. J Clin Psychiatry 2001;62:453–63.

34. Scharf M, Rogowski R, Hull S, et al. Efficacy and safety of doxepin 1 mg, 3 mg, and 6 mg in elderly patients with primary insomnia: a randomized, double-blind, placebo-controlled crossover study. J Clin Psychiatry 2008;69:1557–64.

35. Walsh JK, Erman M, Erwin CW, et al. Subjective hypnotic efficacy of trazodone and zolpidem in DSMIII-R primary insomnia. Hum Psychopharmacol Clin Exp 1998;13:191–8.

36. Riemann D, Voderholzer U, Cohrs S, et al. Trimipramine in primary insomnia: results of a polysomnographic double-blind controlled study. Pharmacopsychiatry 2002;35:165–74.

37. Saper CB, Scammell TE, Lu J. Hypothalamic regulation of sleep and circadian rhythms. Nature 2005;437:1257–63.

38. Glass JR, Sproule BA, Herrmann N, Busto UE. Effects of 2-week treatment with temazepam and diphenhydramine in elderly insomniacs: a randomized, placebo-controlled trial. J Clin Psychopharmacol 2008;28:182–8.

39. Morin CM, Koetter U, Bastien C, et al. Valerian–hops combination and diphenhydramine for treating insomnia: a randomized placebo-controlled clinical trial. Sleep 2005;28:1465–71.

40. Taibi DM, Landis CA, Petry H, Vitiello MV. A systematic review of valerian as a sleep aid: safe but not effective. Sleep Med Rev 2007;11:209–30.

41. Fernández-San-Martín MI, Masa-Font R, Palacios-Soler L, et al. Effectiveness of valerian on insomnia: a meta-analysis of randomized placebo-controlled trials. Sleep Med 2010;11:505–11.

42. Morin CM, Bootzin RR, Buysse DJ, et al. Psychological and behavioral treatment of insomnia: update of the recent evidence (1998–2004). Sleep 2006;29:1398–414.

43. Perlis ML, Jungquist C, Smith MT, Posner D. Cognitive behavioral treatment of insomnia. New York: Springer, 2005.

44. Morin CM, Culbert JP, Schwartz SM. Nonpharmacological interventions for insomnia: a meta-analysis of treatment efficacy. Am J Psychiatry 1994;151:1172–80.

45. Murtagh DR, Greenwood KM. Identifying effective psychological treatments for insomnia: a meta-analysis. J Consult Clin Psychol 1995;63:79–89.

46. Pallesen S, Nordhus IH, Kvale G. Nonpharmacological interventions for insomnia in older adults: a meta-analysis of treatment efficacy. Psychotherapy 1998;35:472–82.

47. Montgomery P, Dennis J. Cognitive behavioural interventions for sleep problems in adults aged 60+. Cochrane Database Syst Rev 2003;(1):CD003161.

48. Irwin MR, Cole JC, Nicassio PM. Comparative meta-analysis of behavioral interventions for insomnia and their efficacy in middle-aged adults and in older adults 55 + years of age. Health Psychol 2006;25:3–14.

49. Cheng SK, Dizon J. Computerised cognitive behavioural therapy for insomnia: a systematic review and meta-analysis. Psychother Psychosom 2012;81:206–16.

50. Matthews EE, Arnedt JT, McCarthy MS, et al. Adherence to cognitive behavioral therapy for insomnia: a systematic review. Sleep Med Rev 2013;17:453–464.

51. Schwartz DR, Carney CE. Mediators of cognitive–behavioral therapy for insomnia: a review of randomized controlled trials and secondary analysis studies. Clin Psychol Rev 2012;32:664–75.

52. Bastien CH, Morin CM, Ouellet M-C, et al. Cognitive–behavioral therapy for insomnia: comparison of individual therapy, group therapy, and telephone consultations. J Consult Clini Psychol 2004;72:653–9.

53. Baillargeon L, Demers M, Ladouceur R. Stimulus-control: nonpharmacologic treatment for insomnia. Can Fam Physician 1998;44:73–9.

54. Espie CA, Inglis SJ, Tessier S, Harvey L. The clinical effectiveness of cognitive behaviour therapy for chronic insomnia: implementation and evaluation of a sleep clinic in general medical practice. Behav Res Ther 2001;39:45–60.

55. Miller CB, Kyle SD, Marshall NS, Espie CA. Ecological momentary assessment of daytime symptoms during sleep restriction therapy for insomnia. J Sleep Res 2013;22:266–72.

56. Harris J, Lack L, Kemp K, et al. A randomized controlled trial of intensive sleep retraining (ISR): a brief conditioning treatment for chronic insomnia. Sleep 2012;35:49–60.

57. Jacobson E. Progressive relaxation, 2nd ed. Oxford: University of Chicago Press, 1938.

58. Kabat-Zinn J. Full catastrophe living: using the wisdom of your body and mind to face stress, pain, and illness, 15th anniversary ed. New York: Delta Trade Paperback/Bantam Dell, 2005.

59. Segal ZV, Williams JMG, Teasdale JD. Mindfulness-based cognitive therapy for depression: a new approach to preventing relapse. New York: Guilford Press, 2002.

60. Ong JC, Shapiro SL, Manber R. Combining mindfulness meditation with cognitive-behavior therapy for insomnia: a treatment-development study. Behav Ther 2008;39:171–82.

61. Ong JC, Shapiro SL, Manber R. Mindfulness meditation and cognitive behavioral therapy for insomnia: a naturalistic 12-month follow-up. Explore (NY) 2009;5:30–6.

62. Pech M, O'Kearney R. A randomized controlled trial of problem-solving therapy compared to cognitive therapy for the treatment of insomnia in adults. Sleep 2013; 36:739–49.

63. Ladouceur R, Gros-Louis Y. Paradoxical intention vs stimulus control in the treatment of severe insomnia. J Behav Ther Exp Psychiatry 1986;17:267–9.

64. Turner RM, Ascher LM. Controlled comparison of progressive relaxation, stimulus control, and paradoxical intention therapies for insomnia. J Consult Clin Psychol 1979;47:500.

65. Morin CM, Hauri PJ, Espie CA, et al. Nonpharmacologic treatment of chronic insomnia. An American Academy of Sleep Medicine review. Sleep 1999;22:1134–56.

66. Smith MT, Perlis ML, Park A, et al. Comparative meta-analysis of pharmacotherapy and behavior therapy for persistent insomnia. Am J Psychiatry 2002;159:5–11.

67. Mitchell MD, Gehrman P, Perlis M, Umscheid CA. Comparative effectiveness of cognitive behavioral therapy for insomnia: a systematic review. BMC Fam Practi 2012;13:40.

SECTION 6

Circadian rhythm disorders

CHAPTER 21

Shift work sleep disorder and jet lag

Vivek Pillai [†] and Christopher L. Drake

Shift work sleep disorder

A considerable proportion of the workforce in the industrialized world engages in shift work, with schedules that are significantly aberrant from the conventional 9-to-5 work day [1]. Prevalence rates of shift work are similar across Europe, South America, Asia, and Africa: 22% in the UK, 25% in Greece and Finland, 24% in the Czech Republic, 15% in Chile, 17.5% in China, and 20% in Senegal [2,3]. In the US, nearly 20% of employed adults are shift workers, and 18–26% begin their shift between 2:00 pm and 6:30 am [4]. Rates of shift work are especially high in service occupations. Almost 50% of protective service (eg, law enforcement and fire safety) and food preparation/service employees, and about a quarter of transportation (eg, train and bus drivers) and healthcare professionals are shift workers [4]. Though a precise, consensus-based classification system for shift work has yet to emerge, the US Bureau of Labor Statistics and the International Classification of Sleep Disorders (ICSD) recognize the following categories: nightshifts, with regular start times between 6:00 pm and 4:00 am; early morning shifts, which start between 4:00 am and 7:00 am; and evening/afternoon shifts, starting between 2:00 pm and 6:00 pm [5]. Finally, 2.7–4.3% of adult workers in the US are involved in rotating shifts, including both rapid shifting (eg, multiples changes in work hours during a week) and slow rotations (eg, three weeks per shift schedule) [6]. However, as most shift workers return to their typical routine of nocturnal sleep during their off-days [7], nearly all shift workers endure rapidly shifting schedules.

Shift work necessitates a sleep–wake schedule that conflicts with the endogenous, physiological regulation of sleep. According to the opponent–process model, sleep and wakefulness result from the interaction between two central nervous system (CNS) processes: a homeostatic sleep drive and a circadian alerting system [8,9]. Homeostatic sleep pressure, marked physiologically by electroencephalographic (EEG) slow-wave activity, accumulates as a function of prior wake time and dissipates with sleep. On the other hand, the suprachiasmatic nucleus (SCN), located in the anterior hypothalamus, confers circadian rhythmicity to the temporal profile of sleep and associated physiological functions, including temperature regulation and cortisol secretion [10,11]. This intrinsic pacemaker actively facilitates wakefulness during the day when endogenous melatonin levels are low, and promotes sleep at night when melatonin levels rise and suppress

CNS arousal [12]. Thus, the circadian alerting signal rises during the day, in effect, opposing the homeostatic sleep pressure that results from wakefulness, until eventually subsiding at night when homeostatic pressure peaks [13]. Desynchrony between these precisely controlled biological rhythms and self-selected sleep–wake schedules can trigger sleep loss and impaired wakefulness.

Shift workers must attempt to sleep during the day when the circadian alerting signal is strong, leading to short, fragmented sleep. The resulting homeostatic sleep debt combines with blunted nighttime circadian arousal to produce excessive sleepiness during the night when the worker must remain awake (Fig. 21.1). However, shift workers, including those working on the same shift, show remarkable diversity in their tolerance to circadian disruption [14,15]. Research suggests that the effects of shift work are moderated by factors such as sleep and circadian physiology, social and familial responsibilities, as well as the frequency and duration of the shift work [16]. These individual differences in the circadian and sleep-related responses elicited by shift work have led to the recognition of shift work sleep disorder (SWD).

Diagnosis and prevalence

Standard diagnostic systems such as the Diagnostic and Statistical Manual of Mental Disorders Fifth Edition (DSM-5) and the ICSD-3 highlight SWD as a specific "type" of circadian rhythm sleep disorder. The cardinal feature of circadian rhythm sleep disorders is sleep disturbance that is the direct result of a mismatch between the endogenous circadian timing of sleep and the patient's desired or, in the case of SWD, required sleep schedule. Specific diagnostic criteria for SWD include insomnia-like symptoms during the sleep period, excessive sleepiness during the wake period, or both. These symptoms must cause clinically significant distress or impairment in one or more areas of functioning. Finally, as we will discuss later in this chapter, it is important to determine whether presenting symptoms are better accounted for by another sleep disorder or general medical condition.

The ubiquity of shift work and the inability of most shift workers to acclimate sufficiently to circadian misalignment would suggest a high prevalence of SWD. However, reliable epidemiological data are presently unavailable owing to a number of diagnostic and methodological challenges. A recent review of the SWD research literature by an American Academy of Sleep Medicine (AASM) taskforce concluded that most prior studies did not apply formal diagnostic criteria in their assessment of this disorder [17]. Further, the distinction between a normal and a pathological response to shift work has yet to be empirically validated. Operationalizations

---

[†] It is with regret that we report the death of Vivek Pillai during the preparation of this edition of the textbook.

(a) **Day worker**

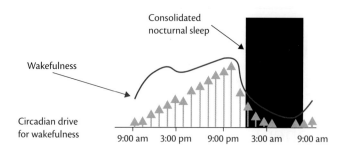

(b) **Night-shift worker**

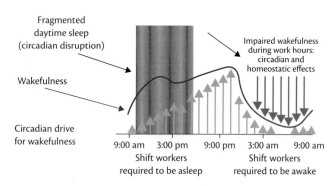

Fig. 21.1 Homeostatic and circadian regulation of sleep. (a) Among day workers, the homeostatic and circadian systems work in tandem to promote wakefulness during the environmental day and sleep during the environmental night. (b) Shift workers attempt to sleep during the day when the circadian alerting signal is strong, leading to short, fragmented sleep. The resulting homeostatic sleep debt combines with blunted nighttime circadian arousal to promote excessive sleepiness during the night when the worker must remain awake.
Adapted from The Journal of Family Practice, 59(1 Suppl), Drake CL, The characterization and pathology of circadian rhythm sleep disorders, pp. S12–7, Copyright (2010), Frontline Medical Communications Inc.

of SWD and "cut-offs" for core symptoms such as excessive sleepiness therefore vary across studies. In a representative community sample of over 2500 conventional day-shift, night-shift, and rotating shift workers, 14–32% of night-shift workers and 8–26% of rotating-shift workers met criteria for SWD based on DSM-IV and a standardized self-report measure of excessive sleepiness [15]. However, this study was unable to establish whether reported sleep symptoms were attributable to shift work. A study of oil rig workers yielded a similar prevalence rate of SWD among shift workers (23%) [18]. In light of the prevalence of shift work in the US, data from these studies suggest that 2–5% of the general population likely meets SWD criteria [5].

Prevalence rates of SWD may also vary as a function of demographic characteristics and individual differences in circadian physiology. The well-documented effects of aging on the homeostatic and circadian sleep systems have prompted the study of age as a risk factor for SWD. Though evidence that tolerance to shift work deteriorates with age is not presently conclusive, studies have shown variously that shift workers over the age of 40 accrue more sleep loss than younger workers [19], older adults (over 50 years old) show less circadian adaptation to shift work [20], reports of sleep disturbance during the sleep period and sleepiness during

the wake period increase with age [17,20,21], and adults over the age of 50 years are less responsive to the circadian phase-delaying effects of bright light (a treatment for SWD, reviewed later in the chapter) [22]. Even fewer data are available on the association between gender and SWD, as most prior research has involved predominantly male samples. Self-report data suggest that female shift workers report more sleep loss, sleepiness, and psychological stress than their male counterparts [23,24]. However, the extent to which these findings reflect gender-related differences in role obligations is not clear.

With respect to circadian physiology, a vulnerability hypothesized to moderate tolerance to shift work is circadian preference or chronotype (morningness versus eveningness), a genetic trait related to the period of the circadian clock and a length polymorphism of the *PER3* clock gene [25–27]. Research shows that the morningness chronotype—these individuals prefer to go to bed early and function optimally during early daytime hours—is associated with reduced tolerance to shift work [27]. Note that as older adults typically espouse morningness [28], this chronotype may also explain some of the age-related vulnerability to SWD. Finally, certain polymorphisms in the coding region of the *PER3* gene may also explain the variance in the cognitive impairments elicited by sleep loss [29], an inevitable consequence of shift work [17].

Morbidity and mortality

A wealth of data supports the link between shift work and various adverse health outcomes, including sleep loss, excessive sleepiness, insomnia, cardiovascular disease, metabolic disturbance, gastrointestinal complaints, cancer, and poor quality of life [16,30]. Increased risk for motor vehicle accidents as a result of excessive sleepiness is another noteworthy and well-documented morbidity in this population. Shift workers, especially those engaged in night and early morning shift work, accrue a significant homeostatic sleep debt due to cumulative sleep loss over successive shifts [31–33]. While sleepiness alone can trigger driving impairments on par with driving under the influence of alcohol [34,35], shift workers often commute to and from work during early morning hours when their circadian alerting signal is at its nadir [10,36]. Not surprisingly, shift work greatly increases the likelihood of on-road accidents [37–39]. Excessive sleepiness during waking hours also raises other safety concerns, such as occupational accidents and injury. The risk of workplace accidents is nearly 60% higher among shift workers than regular day workers, and workplace and motor vehicle accidents attributable to shift work cost the US economy an estimated $71–93 billion per year [40].

However, there have been few attempts to determine whether the morbidity associated with shift work varies as a function of SWD. Drake and colleagues found significantly higher rates of ulcers, sleepiness-related accidents, social and occupational impairments, and depression among shift workers who met criteria for SWD in comparison with both nonsymptomatic shift workers and conventional day workers [15]. Further, in the majority of cases in this study, morbidity indices were significantly higher among shift workers than conventional day workers who reported comparable sleep disturbance. With respect to mental health, a study of radar controllers in the US Air Force revealed a significantly higher risk for anxiety and depression among those with SWD in comparison with nonsymptomatic shift workers [41]. Preliminary data from a recent neuroimaging study also point to significant variations in neurophysiological correlates of attention and memory in individuals with SWD relative to a control group of night shift workers [42].

Clinical evaluation

As with other circadian rhythm disorders, the assessment of SWD involves a careful evaluation of the degree of circadian misalignment, severity and pattern of sleep disturbance, and level of distress or functional impairment. To establish an SWD diagnosis, however, this symptom complex must be attributable to the work–sleep schedule, and, as such, clinicians must be sure to rule out other sleep disorders characterized by excessive sleepiness, including obstructive sleep apnea and narcolepsy. A thorough patient history along with the use of sleep diaries and actigraphy can greatly elucidate the regularity, duration, and timing of sleep and wake cycles. The minimal duration of sleep recording indicated for SWD is 7 days, and it should include sleep and wake episodes during the offending work shift [5]. When feasible, assessing markers of circadian phase such as salivary melatonin or core body temperature (reviewed later in this chapter) can help quantify the degree of circadian desynchrony [43–45]. Finally, in light of the morbidity and mortality associated with core symptoms, such as excessive sleepiness, it is important to assess the severity of these symptoms early in the evaluation process.

Sleepiness

The multiple sleep latency test (MSLT) [46], a measure of sleep latency averaged over consecutive recording intervals roughly two hours apart, is the gold standard for measuring sleepiness. The mean daytime latency on the MSLT for adults in the US is 11.4 minutes, and latencies of 8 minutes or less indicate clinically significant or "pathological" sleepiness [5,47]. However, as these values derive from studies of daytime sleepiness, norms for sleepiness at other phases of the circadian cycle that are more germane to SWD are currently unavailable. In two large ($N = 209$ [48] and $N = 216$ [49]) clinical trials of night workers with an ICSD-3-based diagnosis of SWD, mean nighttime MSLT latencies were approximately 2 minutes. Notably, as one of the inclusion criteria for these studies was a nocturnal MSLT latency of less than 6 minutes, levels of sleepiness in these samples may not reflect the true population average for shift workers. In a smaller sample of 10 night workers with and without SWD, symptomatic workers exhibited a nighttime MSLT latency of 3.6 minutes whereas the asymptomatic group had a 6.8 minute latency [43]. Though this difference was statistically significant, its clinical implications are unknown. Together, these data highlight the need for evidence-based norms to accurately characterize objective sleepiness among shift workers. It is important to note, however, that excessive levels of sleepiness (MSLT < 5 minutes) may still be indicative of a high risk for accident or injury even if consistent with the population norms for the nocturnal phase of the circadian cycle [50].

The high cost of the MSLT precludes routine clinical use among all but narcolepsy patients. On the other hand, self-report measures of sleepiness, such as the Epworth Sleepiness Scale (ESS) [51] or the Karolinska Sleepiness Scale (KSS) [52], can be easily administered and interpreted in most clinical settings. The ESS, for instance, queries respondents about the likelihood of inadvertently falling asleep during routine daily activities, with scores of 10 or greater indicating clinically significant sleepiness. Epidemiological data suggest that roughly 44% of shift workers [15] and 24–33% of conventional day workers [53,54] score in the clinical range on the ESS.

Instruments such as the MSLT and the ESS can also be valuable in distinguishing sleepiness from fatigue, a common presenting problem in SWD [55,56]. While physical or cognitive fatigue may be alleviated by periods of rest or sedentary activity without sleeping, such inactivity will unmask sleepiness. This distinction between fatigue and sleepiness is critical because patients seldom recognize that "dozing off" during quiet periods of relative inactivity is abnormal. If fatigue is suspected, it is important to assess for comorbid major depressive disorder [57]. Finally, the MSLT can differentiate between SWD and narcolepsy, as patients who suffer from the latter exhibit two or more sleep-onset rapid eye movement (REM) periods on the MSLT despite adequate prior sleep [5].

Sleep disturbance

Unlike sleepiness, which is considered a symptom of an underlying sleep or CNS condition, most diagnostic systems now recognize insomnia as a primary disorder [5,58,59]. Describing insomnia as a "symptom" of SWD is hence problematic. A more nuanced approach would be to characterize the insomnia-like sleep symptoms observed in SWD, such as difficulty falling or staying asleep during times of circadian desynchrony, simply as "circadian sleep disturbance." Such a framework allows for the distinction between sleep disturbance that is the direct result of shift-work-related circadian misalignment and those that reflect comorbid insomnia disorder. Indeed, the association between insomnia and SWD may be more complex than current diagnostic systems suggest. Stress-diathesis theories such as the 3Ps model postulate that insomnia disorder results from the interaction between predisposing, precipitating, and perpetuating factors [60]. An environmental trigger or challenge to the sleep system can unmask a premorbid vulnerability to produce sleep disturbance, which is then perpetuated by behavioral or conditioning mechanisms such as poor sleep hygiene. The circadian misalignment imposed by shift work can act as such a precipitant of acute sleep disturbance. Premorbid vulnerabilities and behavioral factors, such as erratic sleep schedules across on- and off-shift days, may determine whether these sleep disturbances evolve into insomnia disorder. Support for this theory comes from studies that find that levels of sleep disturbance following retirement are significantly higher among shift workers than in regular day workers [61,62]. The possibility that shift work represent a trigger for insomnia disorder is intriguing and begs further investigation.

As noted earlier, sleep disturbance in SWD may include difficulty falling asleep, difficulty staying asleep, or nonrestorative sleep. In addition to structured clinical interviews, psychometrically validated instruments, such as the Insomnia Severity Index (ISI) [63] and the Pittsburgh Sleep Quality Index (PSQI) [64], can help quantify the severity of sleep disturbance and waking consequences. An important caveat in the use of these measures in the SWD population, however, is that they do not discriminate between nocturnal and daytime sleep disturbance. Future studies should attempt to adapt and validate these instruments for the assessment of daytime sleep disturbance.

Other comorbidities

Shift work is associated with a wide array of mental and physical health problems. The increased risk for depression, cognitive deficits, cardiovascular disease, and cancer among shift workers stress the importance of regular psychological and physical assessments that are attentive to these comorbidities [30]. Evaluation of alcohol and substance use is also recommended, given that "self-medication" with substances is one of the most commonly reported coping strategies to contend with sleep disturbance in the general population [65,66]. Further, prevalence rates of injurious behaviors such as alcohol use, smoking, and poor diet practices are significantly higher among shift workers than day workers [16,30,67]. A battery of self-report questionnaires, called the Standard Shiftwork Index (SSI) [68], has been used in many studies to quantify these health risks. Recent research on the SSI, however, points to certain psychometric shortcomings in some of the component scales, stressing the need for more validation studies [69,70].

Treatment

As the etiology of SWD is largely unclear, most current treatments are geared toward ameliorating the extent of circadian disruption and managing core symptoms. Step by step, guidelines have emerged in the SWD literature (Box 21.1), and cover all aspects of patient care from circadian adaptation to behavioral and pharmacological interventions for promoting sleep during rest hours and wakefulness during the work shift.

Circadian adaptation: bright light therapy

The SCN, as evidenced by consistent findings across all studied assays of circadian rhythm, has an average period that is slightly longer than the 24 hour day (about 24.2 hours) [10]. However, under normal conditions of diurnal wakefulness and nocturnal sleep, the phase and period of this intrinsic pacemaker are tightly entrained to a 24-hour cycle thanks to environmental cues [71]. Of these environmental zeitgebers, the Earth's light–dark cycle is the most influential. The transmission of photic stimuli via retinohypothalamic and retinogeniculohypothalamic pathways to the SCN regulates the pineal secretion of melatonin [71,72]. The central and peripheral abundance of melatonin receptors, in turn, facilitates photic control of hormone secretion, core body temperature, and rest–wake cycles [72]. As such, carefully timed exposure to photic stimuli of appropriate intensity, wavelength, and duration can "shift" the endogenous circadian clock (see Fig. 21.2) [73]. Among shift workers, such shifts in endogenous rhythms can be adaptive when they realign sleep and wake episodes with the appropriate circadian phase [74]. These principles form the basis of bright light therapy.

As noted earlier, melatonin levels rise in the evening (at about 9 pm)—a phenomenon known as dim light melatonin onset (DLMO)—achieving a peak around mid-darkness and subsequently dropping to low daytime levels shortly before light onset. This temporal profile of melatonin has robust internal consistency per person, and is less sensitive to sleep and posture than other circadian markers such as core body temperature. As such, plasma or salivary melatonin assays can serve as a precise and relatively noninvasive marker of circadian phase. A recent study investigated the melatonin profiles of night workers with SWD and asymptomatic controls during a 25-hour sleep deprivation protocol. Asymptomatic workers showed a significant delay in the timing of DLMO in relation to the SWD group (Fig. 21.3), suggesting that the latter are less adept at shifting their circadian clock to match their sleep–wake schedule. The goal of bright light therapy, therefore, is to reduce misalignment between endogenous and exogenous circadian schedules.

Bright light therapy typically involves short or intermittent exposure to a bright (2000–10 000 lux) light stimulus, scheduled 3–6 hours before the expected nadir of circadian alertness [74]. Though laboratory data support the efficacy of bright light treatment in producing large phase shifts and complete entrainment to shift work [73,75], achieving such effects in the "real world" can prove quite challenging. Therapeutic phase shifting relies on meticulous control over the patient's exposure to environmental light, including bright light exposure at night during the work shift and avoiding sunlight during the day using dark goggles. Further, complete circadian re-entrainment is not only difficult (6–8 hours of bright light exposure at about 10 000 lux), but may be maladaptive as shift workers may revert back to diurnal wakefulness on off-days because of social or familial commitments. As such, recent studies have explored the clinical utility of a stable partial/"compromise" phase delay, such that the nadir of circadian alertness occurs just a few hours after the work shift ends [75,76]. Using intermittent bright light exposure during the night (brief light pulses for 15 minutes each hour for 5 hours) and dark goggles during the day, one simulated night-shift study produced a phase delay of approximately 7.5 hours among its participants, a shift that was associated with better sleep and psychomotor outcomes [76]. In summary, extant evidence supports the efficacy of bright light treatment in conjunction with other behavioral interventions, such as avoiding daylight and careful scheduling of sleep–wake cycles.

Circadian adaptation: other treatments

Studies show that exogenous melatonin administration (0.5–3 mg) can improve circadian adaptation among shift workers, so long as exposure to more potent zeitgebers such as daylight is carefully monitored; poorly timed light exposure can easily counteract any benefits of exogenous melatonin. In a laboratory study of young adults, three days of melatonin administration (3 mg) led to an approximately 1.5-hour shift in circadian phase [77]. Phase-advance effects of 80–90 minutes were reported in another study of young adults who received 1, 2, or 4 mg of the melatonin agonist ramelteon 30 minutes before bedtime for a period of four days [78]. Thus, as a circadian treatment, melatonin may be more suitable for other circadian rhythm disorders, such as jet lag and delayed sleep phase syndrome, where even modest phase shifts can be therapeutic. Note that even low doses (eg, 0.5 mg) of melatonin can produce performance impairments, and therefore cognitively intensive tasks such as operating machinery should be avoided for several hours following administration [79]. The large-scale clinical trials needed to establish the efficacy and safety of melatonin as a chronobiotic for use in SWD have not been undertaken.

Though physical exercise can delay circadian phase, this effect is relatively weak and unlikely to produce therapeutic levels of circadian adjustment. However, the overall health benefits of exercise may help reduce the morbidity associated with SWD, and may therefore be encouraged, especially when scheduled at times when light exposure is desired to shift the circadian clock [80].

Improving sleep

Given that adequate circadian adaptation is challenging for many shift workers, behavioral and pharmacological interventions that directly address sleep disturbance are warranted. Although not all shift workers may experience significant sleep onset difficulties during a daytime sleep episode, circadian misalignment consistently disrupts sleep maintenance during the latter half of the sleep

Box 21.1 Guidelines for the clinical evaluation and treatment of SWD

Assessment

I. Quantify degree of circadian misalignment (sleep diaries and or actigraphy).

II. Assess nature and severity of sleep disturbance both during daytime and nighttime sleep periods.

II. Establish level of sleepiness (ESS); pay special attention to drowsy driving.

III. Determine impact on social and domestic responsibilities.

Management

I. If patient meets criteria for a diagnosis of shift work disorder, cessation of the shift work schedule should be the first option discussed with the patient.

II. Regular physicals with attention to risk for psychological disorders (i.e, depression), gastrointestinal problems, cardiovascular disease, and cancer.

   A. Sleep-related comorbidity: sleep disordered breathing, restless legs syndrome, or other sleep disorder.

   B. Other comorbidity: identify medical or psychiatric disorders that may contribute to insomnia or excessive sleepiness.

III. Determine patient-specific therapeutic approach.

   A. Circadian adaptation:

     1. Consider individual differences (eg, age, phase preference).

     2. Consider compromise phase position (eg, partial phase delay using bright light during first half of night and increased darkness during daytime).

     3. Encourage night workers to adopt a late sleep schedule (bedtime: 3:00–4:00 am) on off-days.

   B. Symptom management:

     1. Insomnia:

       a. Improve sleep hygiene and encourage use of eye masks, ear plugs, and light blocking goggles during daytime sleep.

       b. For sleep maintenance problems, consider an intermediate half-life (5–8 hours) acting hypnotic or melatonin treatment (about 3 mg).

       c. For sleep initiation problems, consider a short-acting hypnotic.

       d. For sleep problems on off-days, consider fixed sleep–wake schedule/anchor sleep.

     2. Excessive sleepiness (i.e, ESS > 10):

       a. Address sleep disturbance if present.

       b. Consider wake-enhancing medication prior to shift (eg, modafinil, armodafinil) or off-label stimulants (eg, amphetamine, methylphenidate).

Box 21.1 Continued

       c. Encourage prophylactic nap prior to work shift.

       d. Recommend use of brief to moderate-length naps (30–60 minutes); consider pre-nap caffeine to reduce sleep inertia.

       e. Consider combined treatment strategies during the work shift (alerting medications, bright light, and naps).

IV. Address additional work, social, and domestic factors.

   A. Social/family/psychological: improve balance between family/social, work, and sleep time; educate patient's family regarding shift workers' need for "protected" sleep times.

   B. Health and safety: promote healthy eating habits (not within 2–4 hours of bedtime), curtail substance use, recommend exercise at appropriate times (not within 2–4 hours of bedtime), stress the risks of working/driving when drowsy or at times of circadian vulnerability.

period [81]. Sleeping regularly for a period of about 4 hours during a particular time of day (eg, 8:00 am to 12:00 noon) on both on- and off-shift days can help anchor circadian rhythms to a particular sleep schedule. Such "anchor" sleep periods combined with another 3- to 4-hour sleep period taken at different times as a function of work schedule can stabilize circadian rhythms and increase sleep duration [82,83]. This strategy may also help accommodate any social or familial obligations the shift worker must keep. Practicing good sleep hygiene can further improve sleep, and involves the following: air-conditioning and blackout shades/curtains to ensure a cool, dark, and quiet sleep environment; use of earplugs and a comfortable night mask; restricting caffeine and alcohol consumption before bedtime; and educating family and flatmates about the importance of the worker's "protected" sleep period [16,80].

Napping prior to the night shift and for brief periods during the night have been shown to improve alertness and performance among shift workers [84,85]. In a study of emergency room physicians and nurses, a 40-minute nap in the middle of a 12-hour night shift improved reaction time, alertness, and fatigue [86]. Notably, alertness during the commute home following the shift was unaffected. Empirical data also support the use of naps in conjunction with other interventions. Laboratory and field studies suggest that the combination of an evening nap and caffeine intake (250–300 mg) 30 minutes before the shift can significantly improve alertness and performance [87]. In a study of professional drivers engaged in shift work, two 20-minute naps followed by 10 minutes of bright light exposure (about 5000 lux) significantly reduced PSG-verified risk of falling asleep during a driving task [85]. Clinicians must, however, advise patients to avoid driving or operating machinery until any post-nap sleep inertia has dissipated, as middle-of-the-night effects of sleep inertia are more severe than those at other times during the circadian cycle [88].

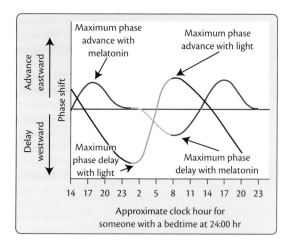

Fig. 21.2 Phase response curves to 1 day of light exposure (green curve) and 3 days of 3–5 mg of melatonin administration (black curve) in a circadian system entrained to local environment time. A phase response curve (PRC) is constructed by plotting the extent of phase shift (hours) in response to a particular stimulus (y-axis) against the circadian phase at which the stimulus occurs (x-axis). Convention dictates that phase delays to later hours be represented as negative numbers, and that phase advances be denoted by positive numbers. As can be seen , the effects of circadian stimuli vary as a function of the time of exposure. Bright light exposure before habitual bedtime and several hours thereafter produces the largest (westward) phase delays, whereas the same stimulus applied just before habitual wake time and several hours thereafter will trigger maximal (eastward) phase advances. At the nadir of core body temperature, which occurs about 2.5 hours before habitual bedtime in young adults (2 hours in older adults), phase delays "cross over" to phase advances. Therefore, bright light exposure too close to this crossover point can cause phase shifts in direction opposite to what is desired. In contrast to light, exogenous melatonin administration in the morning causes a phase delay, but results in a phase advance when given in the morning. On average, the crossover point for exogenous melatonin occurs early in the afternoon.
Adapted from Drake CL, Wright Jr KP, Shift Work, Shift-Work Disorder, and Jet Lag. In: Kryger MH, Roth T, Dement WC, eds, Principles and Practice of Sleep Medicine (Fifth Edition), pp. 784–98, Copyright (2011), with permission from Elsevier.

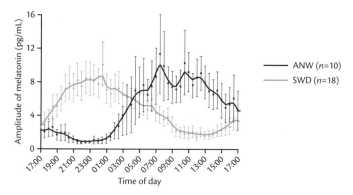

Fig. 21.3 (See colour plate section) Melatonin profiles of night-shift workers with and without SWD. Individuals exhibit remarkable diversity in the degree of circadian adaptation to shift work. A recent study evaluated the dim light salivary melatonin profiles of 10 asymptomatic night workers (ANW) and 18 workers with SWD during a 25-hour sleep deprivation protocol. Though the melatonin profile of the SWD group was similar to that of healthy day workers (20:27 ± 5.0 h), the ANW group exhibited a significantly delayed DLMO (05:00 ± 3.4 h), indicating better circadian adaptation to night work.
Reproduced from Chronobiology International, 29(7), Gumenyuk V, Roth T, Drake CL, Circadian phase, sleepiness, and light exposure assessment in night workers with and without shift work disorder, pp. 928–36, Copyright (2012), with permission from Taylor & Francis.

With respect to pharmacological agents, few well-controlled clinical trials with SWD patients have been carried out. Further, it is difficult to generalize data from clinical trials of hypnotic medications for insomnia to SWD given the added complications of diurnal sleep and nocturnal performance concerns in the latter group. The AASM notes that hypnotic medications, such as triazolam and temazepam, though effective in improving diurnal sleep, have little impact on nocturnal alertness [17,89]. Non-benzodiazepine hypnotics, including zolpidem, can improve subjective sleep quality and achieve modest improvements in nocturnal psychomotor performance, but may trigger side-effects such as "anxious" and "irritable" mood [90]. Exogenous melatonin at doses between 1 and 10 mg and the melatonin-receptor agonists ramelteon and tasimelteon, have shown efficacy in improving daytime sleep in simulation studies, though data from SWD samples are rare [79,91–93]. Common side effects of ramelteon include dizziness, fatigue, and nausea. Melatonin and melatonin agonists may also increase prolactin levels [80].

Improving wakefulness
Though prior studies have investigated the use of stimulants, such as caffeine and amphetamine in samples of shift workers and healthy volunteers, their effects on patients with SWD remain untested. Low doses of amphetamine and repeated low doses of caffeine have

been shown to improve alertness and psychomotor performance over extended periods of wakefulness [94,95]. However, stimulant use can be problematic owing to the tolerance and withdrawal effects associated with caffeine [47] and the high abuse potential of amphetamines and methylphenidate [96]. Empirical support for the wake-promoting effects of commercially available energy drinks is also limited. In a simulated shift work study, two doses of an energy drink (250 mL can; 80 mg caffeine, 1000 mg taurine, and 600 mg glucoronolactone) administered at 1.30 am and 5.30 am improved nocturnal wakefulness, but were associated with shorter sleep durations and poor sleep efficiency during the subsequent sleep episode [97].

Recent clinical trials have examined the suitability of non-amphetamine-based alerting agents for improving SWD-related nocturnal wakefulness. In a sample of SWD patients with excessive nocturnal sleepiness (MSLT < 6 minutes), taking modafinil (200 mg) for a period of 3 months was associated with significant reductions in nocturnal MSLT latencies during the first half of the night (measured at 2:00 am and 4:00 am). Other correlates of alertness, including psychomotor vigilance and driving (self-reported accidents or near-accidents) were also significantly improved in the treatment group, and taking modafinil at the beginning of the night did not impair subsequent daytime sleep. Notably, despite these improvements, levels of nocturnal alertness (mean MSLT 3.77 ± 0.5 minutes) in the treatment group did not reach average daytime values, leaving room for further improvement. In a similar trial, armodafinil (150 mg), an isomer of modafinil with the same half-life (about 15 hours) but a different elimination profile (higher plasma concentrations about 4–6 hours following dosing) [98], significantly improved MSLT-defined nocturnal sleepiness (2.3 ± 1.6 minutes to 5.3 ± 5.0 minutes), as well as performance on neuropsychological measures of memory and attention. Armodafinil was well tolerated and did not impact daytime sleep. The US Food and Drug Administration (FDA) has approved modafinil and armodafinil for improving nocturnal wakefulness in SWD patients;

side effects include headache, nausea, dizziness, and anxiety, with headaches being the most common complaint [48,49].

Occupational adjustments

Though disengaging entirely from shift work is seldom feasible, certain occupational adjustments can be beneficial. First, allowing employees to choose their shift fosters a sense of agency and perceived control among workers, and is associated with health benefits and overall improvements in quality of life [99]. Further, this "self-selection" intervention is not associated with any appreciable increases in institutional costs. That altering the direction of rotation can improve tolerance to shift work is another commonly advocated assertion in the literature [100]. Clockwise or forward transitions in shift work i.e, from day to evening to night, are better suited to the natural tendency of the circadian clock to delay sleep [101]. Such transitions also allow for more time between shifts and are therefore deemed preferable to backward or counterclockwise transitions. However, we are only aware of one study [102] that documented the health benefits of clockwise versus counterclockwise shift rotations. Other studies show that the direction of shift work rotations has no significant impact on the risks associated with SWD [103,104]. Finally, consistent with laboratory studies, some industrial studies suggest that switching from slow to fast rotations, because they require workers to perform at an adverse circadian phase for a shorter period of time, can lead to better outcomes such as fewer sleep disturbances and less fatigue [105–107].

Jet lag

The rapid transmeridian travel afforded by jet planes can significantly derail the synchrony between endogenous circadian functions and environmental time. The slow (1–1.5 hours/day) rate of resynchronization of the circadian clock to environmental zeitgebers lends perspective on the burden exerted by air travel across multiple zones on the sleep system [71,72]. In addition to circadian disruption, the nature of air travel itself can lead to health sequelae. The low cabin pressure inside jet planes can cause gases in the gastrointestinal (GI) system to expand and trigger bloating/discomfort; the relative hypoxia in the cabin atmosphere can exacerbate respiratory conditions; and, finally, many travelers find it difficult to sleep in a plane, thus incurring substantial sleep loss [17,108,109]. The duration and intensity of these consequences of jet travel can vary as a function of the direction (eastward/westward) of travel, the number of time zones crossed, the ability to sleep while traveling, and individual differences in circadian physiology [17]. When clinically significant, the sleep and circadian disturbance elicited by jet travel warrant a diagnosis of jet lag disorder (JLD).

Diagnosis, morbidity, and prevalence

ICSD-3 recognizes JLD as a circadian rhythm disorder that results from rapid air travel across multiple time zones. Core symptoms include daytime sleepiness and nocturnal sleep disturbance in the new time zone, in addition to travel fatigue and general malaise. GI complaints are also common, and may be related to circadian variations in glucose tolerance [110,111]. In terms of duration, jet lag is generally a temporary condition beginning a day or two following arrival in a new time zone, but can last for weeks in some cases depending on the timing and extent of exposure to environmental cues [5]. In a study [112] of elite athletes travelling eastward or westward across six to eight time zones, training performance suffered for 4–7 days following arrival. Furthermore, westward time-zone transitions were associated with a decrease in blood pressure, while eastward travel led to an increase in blood pressure. Other aspects of functioning, including decision making, driving, and general cognitive ability, may also decline owing to circadian misalignment and consequent sleepiness [113]. In a study of pilots flying across seven or eight time zones in either direction, endogenous circadian rhythms were out of phase not only with environmental cues in the destination time zone, but also in relation to each other. Furthermore, following a 2-day layover, pilots operated the return flight during the nadir of circadian alertness and at peak melatonin levels, a finding that highlights the safety risks associated with jet-lag-related circadian disruption. Behavioral and conditioning mechanisms such as poor sleep hygiene and self-medication with recreational substances can further prolong symptoms [5,16,17]. Though the long-term effects of chronic jet travel have not received extensive research consideration, irregularities in menstrual cycles, exacerbation of psychiatric disorders, and cognitive deficits have been reported among frequent long-distance air travelers [113–115].

There are presently no data on the prevalence of JLD, owing most likely to the transient nature of the symptoms and insufficient clarity on the distinction between normal and pathological responses to jet travel; many diagnostic systems, including DSM-V, do not recognize JLD. A few recent studies have examined age and gender as potential moderators of vulnerability to jet lag, though no clear consensus has emerged owing to a lack of standardization in assessment techniques, poor methodology, and contradictory findings [116,117]. Westward travel is typically tolerated better than eastward travel owing to the natural tendency of the circadian clock to delay the onset of sleep [17,118,119]. On the other hand, the period of the SCN in 20–25% of humans is slightly shorter than the 24-hour day [120], potentially making this group more amenable to circadian phase advances and eastward travel. Although the only study thus far on the impact of chronotype on jet lag symptoms did not find an association, the variance in the chronotype variable in this study was quite low: only one of the 85 participants could be classified as an "evening" type [117]. In summary, though a number of potential moderators of jet lag have been proposed based on circadian principles, few have been empirically evaluated with adequate methodological rigor.

Clinical assessment and management

A thorough patient history and physical examination are needed to establish the correspondence between presenting sleep/wake symptoms and jet travel, while ruling out other sleep disorders. Fatigue and other somatic complaints observed in JLD, especially GI or urinary symptoms, may be indicative of an underlying medical condition. Although ICSD-3 does not currently indicate objective laboratory sleep recording for diagnosing JLD [5], research studies have demonstrated PSG-based sleep disruption as a result of jet travel. Beaumont and colleagues measured PSG-based sleep in a sample of 27 healthy volunteers from the US Air Force Reserve Unit for a period of 2 weeks following an eastward flight across seven time zones [121]. In comparison with baseline sleep, participants exhibited significantly delayed sleep onset starting on the fourth night post travel, a disturbance that did not normalize until the ninth night. Increased slow-wave sleep and reduced REM sleep were also observed on the first night in the new time zone, though these changes normalized within three nights.

The ephemeral nature of symptoms and the high costs of recording limit the use of PSG for assessing JLD symptoms in clinical settings. More ambulatory forms of sleep assessment such as actigraphy may serve as an efficient alternative, but have yet to be adequately validated in this population [17]. With respect to self-report, the Columbian Jet Lag Scale is the only empirically validated instrument currently available for the assessment of jet lag symptoms [122]. Respondents endorse the presence and persistence of 14 common jet lag symptoms (eg, "fatigue or tiring easily" and "decreased daytime alertness") on a 5-point Likert-type scale ("not at all" to "extremely"); in a validation study of recent air travelers, overall scores achieved high internal consistency ($\alpha = 0.89$–0.93). Such instruments can be easily administered in clinical settings and can help inform clinicians about the nature and severity of JLD. Finally, when possible, pre-flight assays of a patient's underlying circadian phase, such as DLMO or core body temperature recording, may not only help identify risk for JLD but also inform treatment [123].

There are presently no FDA-approved medications for the management of JLD. Current interventions, derived largely from laboratory studies that simulate travel-related circadian disruption, aim to improve tolerance to jet lag and expedite recovery via three basic mechanisms: improving overall circadian adaptation to the new time zone; promoting sleep during the flight and during the environmental night in the new time zone; and promoting wakefulness during the environmental day in the new time zone.

Circadian adaptation

Entraining endogenous circadian rhythms to the new time zone is the most effective means of alleviating jet lag, especially if the traveler plans to spend a substantial amount of time at the destination [123]. Appropriately timed exogenous melatonin administration can help shift the biological clock during travel. The melatonin phase response curve is well established in humans and is essentially the opposite of that for light (see Fig. 21.2). Melatonin taken after waking in the morning delays circadian phase, whereas afternoon or evening melatonin administration leads to a phase advance [72]. A review of 10 clinical trials of melatonin and JLD concluded that melatonin taken at bedtime at the destination time zone significantly reduced jet lag symptoms, especially for eastward travel and if previous jet travel had triggered JLD symptoms [124]. The review also noted that occasional short-term use was safe and well tolerated, though most reviewed studies were unable to extricate the impact of melatonin on the circadian system from its somnolent effects. Bright light therapy with natural outdoor light or commercial light boxes has also been shown to improve JLD symptoms following both eastward and westward jet travel [125,126]. Finally, though the AASM recommends adjunctive treatment with melatonin and bright light exposure for circadian rhythm disorders [5], the efficacy of such combination treatments has not been investigated in JLD. For eastward travel, melatonin at bedtime in conjunction with early morning bright-light exposure can advance the circadian clock and reduce the burden of JLD symptoms. For westward travel, which is better tolerated as it necessitates a phase delay, bright light exposure in the evening may prove beneficial [118].

Preliminary support has also emerged for interventions aimed at pre-flight circadian adaptation, i.e, shifting the biological clock to suit the new time zone before travel [126,127]. In a laboratory simulation study [126], a sample of 28 healthy young adults received phase-advancement treatment for a period of 3 days: participants shifted their baseline sleep–wake schedule counterclockwise by 1 hour per day and received one of three forms of light exposure for 210 minutes after waking: dim light (<60 lux), intermittent bright light (>3000 lux; 30 minutes on, 30 minutes off), or continuous bright light (>3000 lux). DLMO assessment following treatment revealed that continuous bright light exposure elicited a significantly greater phase advance (2.1 hours) than did dim light exposure (0.6 hours), though the phase advances achieved by intermittent (1.5 hours) and continuous bright light did not significantly differ. Further, scores on the Columbia Jet Lag scale increased significantly during the 3-day phase advancement in the dim light and intermittent bright light groups, but did not change significantly from baseline in the continuous bright light group. Thus, it may be possible for travelers to improve their tolerance to an eastward flight by advancing their sleep–wake schedules and exposing themselves to early morning bright light (going for a walk in the sunshine, or turning up indoor lights). Such a strategy may expedite post-flight environmental entrainment to the desired circadian rhythm and reduce the burden of jet lag [16,17,126].

Promoting sleep

A combination of behavioral adjustments and pharmacological aids can help promote sleep both during the flight as well as upon arrival at the destination. Use of noise-canceling headphones, earplugs, and dark sunglasses can help improve sleep while in flight and at the airport during lengthy layovers. Alcohol use, though commonplace during jet travel, is an ineffective strategy, as the disruptive effects of alcohol on sleep maintenance and architecture are well established [47]. It is generally recommended that travelers begin adapting to the new environmental sleep and wake times immediately after arrival in the new time zone [16]. Melatonin and its agonists, ramelteon and tasimelteon, can be effective in reducing sleep onset latency and improving total sleep duration when taken during the biological day [79,92]. Other medications that have been investigated for improving sleep during and following travel include zolpidem, zopiclone, and benzodiazepines, such as triazolam, temazepam, and midazolam (for a review, see [118]). With few exceptions [128,129], most of these studies involved relatively small samples (N = 6–33), and self-report indices of sleep were the only endpoint in many studies. Moreover, the effects of hypnotic medication on daytime symptoms of jet lag have not been adequately studied. These limitations notwithstanding, results indicate that the use of hypnotic medications to alleviate acute sleep disturbance among travelers is appropriate when carefully weighed against potential side effects [16,17,118]. Clinicians must also remember to discuss the risks of drug interactions with alcohol, because, as mentioned earlier, alcohol use is common during long-distance jet travel [17].

Promoting wakefulness

Staying awake until the appropriate nocturnal bedtime in the new time zone can improve sleep following westward travel. Brief naps (15–20 minutes) during the flight and in the day following arrival can help sustain wakefulness [16,130,131]. However, long naps may lead not only to greater sleep inertia, but also to blunted homeostatic sleep pressure and thus impaired nocturnal sleep [88,132]. Taking caffeine is the most common strategy among travelers for improving wakefulness. In two field studies, slow-release caffeine

(5 mg/day) for 5 days following an eastward flight past seven time zones was associated with quicker circadian entrainment (5 days) than was a placebo (9 days), as evidenced by salivary cortisol assays. Notably, although the caffeine group experienced significantly less daytime sleepiness, PSG-based nocturnal sleep onset latencies and awakenings were higher than those for the placebo group. Thus, there is presently insufficient evidence to recommend caffeine for promoting wakefulness during and post-travel; although caffeine can improve wakefulness, its effects on the subsequent sleep period cannot be discounted.

Conclusion

Shift work has been linked to a variety of negative health outcomes, including GI problems, cardiovascular disease, psychological disorders, and cancer. Though the mechanisms driving the association between shift work and these morbidities are not well understood, the circadian misalignment and chronic sleep disturbance inherent in shift work are important targets for clinical intervention. Educating shift workers about circadian principles and helping them restore the synchrony between endogenous biological rhythms and environmental cues through careful use of bright lights, darkness, and melatonin can prove beneficial. The use of FDA-approved alerting agents can improve wakefulness during work hours and may reduce the risk of workplace accidents and injury. Exercising proper sleep hygiene and the judicious use of hypnotic medications can aid sleep during off-hours.

Rapid transmeridian travel in either direction can disrupt circadian rhythms and trigger nocturnal sleep disturbance, excessive daytimes sleepiness, and functional impairments. Though no FDA-approved medications are presently available for the treatment of JLD, prompt circadian adaptation to the new time zone may be achieved via appropriately timed exposure to bright light and darkness. A combination of behavioral and pharmacological measures can further improve sleep and wakefulness at desired times, and reduce the severity and duration of JLD symptoms.

References

1. Matheson A, O'Brien L, Reid JA. The impact of shift-work on health: a literature review. J Clin Nurs 2014; 23(23–24):3309–20. Sleep 1988;11(1):100–9.
2. Boisard P, Cartron D, Gollac M, Valeyre A. Time and work: duration of work. Dublin: European Foundation for the Improvement of Living and Working Conditions, 2003.
3. Lee S, McCann D, Messenger JC. Working times around the world: trends in working hours, laws and policies in a global comparative perspective. New York: Routledge, 2007.
4. McMenamin TM, Holden RJ, Bahls D. A time to work: recent trends in shift work and flexible schedules. Month Labor Rev 2007;130:3–14.
5. American Academy of Sleep Medicine. International classification of sleep disorders: diagnostic and coding manual, 3rd edn. Darien, IL: American Academy of Sleep Medicine, 2014.
6. US Congress. Biological rhythms—implications for the worker: new developments in neuroscience. Washington, DC: US Government Printing Office, 2005.
7. Lowden A, Kecklund G, Axelsson J, Akerstedt T. Change from an 8-hour shift to a 12-hour shift, attitudes, sleep, sleepiness and performance. Scand J Work Environ Health 1998;24(Suppl 3):69–75.
8. Borbely AA. A two process model of sleep regulation. Human Neurobiol 1982;1(3):195–204.
9. Dijk DJ, Czeisler CA. Contribution of the circadian pacemaker and the sleep homeostat to sleep propensity, sleep structure, electroencephalographic slow waves, and sleep spindle activity in humans. J Neurosci 1995;15(5 Pt 1):3526–38.
10. Czeisler CA, Duffy JF, Shanahan TL, et al. Stability, precision, and near-24-hour period of the human circadian pacemaker. Science (N Y) 1999;284(5423):2177–81.
11. Rosenwasser AM. Neurobiology of the mammalian circadian system: oscillators, pacemakers, and pathways. In: Fluharty SJ, Grill HJ, eds. Progress in psychobiology and physiological psychology: vol. 18. San Diego, CA: Elsevier Academic Press, 2003:1–38.
12. Shanahan TL, Kronauer RE, Duffy JF, Williams GH, Czeisler CA. Melatonin rhythm observed throughout a three-cycle bright-light stimulus designed to reset the human circadian pacemaker. J Biol Rhythm 1999;14(3):237–53.
13. Edgar DM, Dement WC, Fuller CA. Effect of SCN lesions on sleep in squirrel monkeys: evidence for opponent processes in sleep–wake regulation. J Neurosci 1993;13(3):1065–79.
14. Axelsson J, Akerstedt T, Kecklund G, Lowden A. Tolerance to shift work–how does it relate to sleep and wakefulness? Int Arch Occupation Environment Health 2004;77(2):121–9.
15. Drake CL, Roehrs T, Richardson G, Walsh JK, Roth T. Shift work sleep disorder: prevalence and consequences beyond that of symptomatic day workers. Sleep 2004;27(8):1453–62.
16. Drake CL, Wright KP Jr. Shift work, shift-work disorder, and jet lag. In: Kryger MH, Roth T, Dement WC, eds. Principles and practice of sleep medicine, 5th edn. Philadelphia: W.B. Saunders, 2011:784–98.
17. Sack RL, Auckley D, Auger RR, et al. Circadian rhythm sleep disorders: part I, basic principles, shift work and jet lag disorders. An American Academy of Sleep Medicine review. Sleep 2007;30(11):1460–83.
18. Waage S, Moen BE, Pallesen S, et al. Shift work disorder among oil rig workers in the North Sea. Sleep 2009;32(4):558–65.
19. Rosa RR, Harma M, Pulli K, Mulder M, Nasman O. Rescheduling a three shift system at a steel rolling mill: effects of a one hour delay of shift starting times on sleep and alertness in younger and older workers. Occup Environ Med 1996;53(10):677–85.
20. Harma MI, Hakola T, Akerstedt T, Laitinen JT. Age and adjustment to night work. Occup Environ Med 1994;51(8):568–73.
21. Smith L, Mason C. Reducing night shift exposure: a pilot study of rota, night shift and age effects on sleepiness and fatigue. J Human Ergol (Tokyo) 2001;30(1–2):83–7.
22. Duffy JF, Zeitzer JM, Czeisler CA. Decreased sensitivity to phase-delaying effects of moderate intensity light in older subjects. Neurobiol Aging 2007;28(5):799–807.
23. Oginska H, Pokorski J, Oginski A. Gender, ageing, and shiftwork intolerance. Ergonomics 1993;36(1–3):161–8.
24. Shields M. Shift work and health. Health Rep 2002;13(4):11–33.
25. Archer SN, Robilliard DL, Skene DJ, et al. A length polymorphism in the circadian clock gene Per3 is linked to delayed sleep phase syndrome and extreme diurnal preference. Sleep 2003;26(4):413–15.
26. Duffy JF, Rimmer DW, Czeisler CA. Association of intrinsic circadian period with morningness-eveningness, usual wake time, and circadian phase. Behav Neurosci 2001;115(4):895–9.
27. Hilliker NA, Muehlbach MJ, Schweitzer PK, Walsh JK. Sleepiness/alertness on a simulated night shift schedule and morningness-eveningness tendency. Sleep 1992;15(5):430–3.
28. Carrier J, Monk TH, Buysse DJ, Kupfer DJ. Sleep and morningness-eveningness in the "middle" years of life (20–59 y). J Sleep Res 1997;6(4):230–7.
29. Viola AU, Archer SN, James LM, et al. PER3 polymorphism predicts sleep structure and waking performance. Curr Biol 2007;17(7):613–18.
30. Culpepper L. The social and economic burden of shift-work disorder. J Family Pract 2010;59(1 Suppl):S3–11.
31. Folkard S, Lombardi DA, Tucker PT. Shiftwork: safety, sleepiness and sleep. Ind Health 2005;43(1):20–3.

32. Mitler MM, Miller JC, Lipsitz JJ, Walsh JK, Wylie CD. The sleep of long-haul truck drivers. N Engl J Med 1997;337(11):755–61.

33. Pilcher JJ, Lambert BJ, Huffcutt AI. Differential effects of permanent and rotating shifts on self-report sleep length: a meta-analytic review. Sleep 2000;23(2):155–63.

34. Arnedt JT, Wilde GJ, Munt PW, MacLean AW. How do prolonged wakefulness and alcohol compare in the decrements they produce on a simulated driving task? Accid Anal Prev 2001;33(3):337–44.

35. Verster JC, Taillard J, Sagaspe P, Olivier B, Philip P. Prolonged nocturnal driving can be as dangerous as severe alcohol-impaired driving. J Sleep Res 2011;20(4):585–8.

36. Scheer FA, Shea TJ, Hilton MF, Shea SA. An endogenous circadian rhythm in sleep inertia results in greatest cognitive impairment upon awakening during the biological night. J Biol Rhythm 2008;23(4):353–61.

37. Barger LK, Cade BE, Ayas NT, et al. Extended work shifts and the risk of motor vehicle crashes among interns. N Engl J Med 2005;352(2):125–34.

38. Ftouni S, Sletten TL, Howard M, et al. Objective and subjective measures of sleepiness, and their associations with on-road driving events in shift workers. J Sleep Res 2013;22(1):58–69.

39. Smith L, Folkard S, Poole CJ. Increased injuries on night shift. Lancet 1994;344(8930):1137–9.

40. Rajaratnam SM, Howard ME, Grunstein RR. Sleep loss and circadian disruption in shift work: health burden and management. Med J Aust 2013;199(8):S11–15.

41. Puca FM, Perrucci S, Prudenzano MP, et al. Quality of life in shift work syndrome. Funct Neurol 1996;11(5):261–8.

42. Gumenyuk V, Roth T, Korzyukov O, et al. Shift work sleep disorder is associated with an attenuated brain response of sensory memory and an increased brain response to novelty: an ERP study. Sleep 2010;33(5):703–13.

43. Gumenyuk V, Roth T, Drake CL. Circadian phase, sleepiness, and light exposure assessment in night workers with and without shift work disorder. Chronobiol Int 2012;29(7):928–36.

44. Monk TH, Buysse DJ, Billy BD, Fletcher ME, Kennedy KS. Polysomnographic sleep and circadian temperature rhythms as a function of prior shift work exposure in retired seniors. Healthy Aging Clin Care Elder 2013;2013(5):9–19.

45. Wright KP Jr, Drake CL, Lockley SW. Diagnostic tools for circadian rhythm sleep disorders. In: Kushida CA, ed. Handbook of sleep disorders, 2nd ed. London: Informa Healthcare, 2008.

46. Carskadon MA. Evaluation of excessive daytime sleepiness. Neurophysiol Clin 1993;23(1):91–100.

47. Roehrs T, Roth T. Medication and substance abuse. In: Kryger MH, Roth T, Dement WC, eds. Principles and practice of sleep medicine, 5th edn. Philadelphia: W.B. Saunders, 2011:1512–23.

48. Czeisler CA, Walsh JK, Roth T, et al. Modafinil for excessive sleepiness associated with shift-work sleep disorder. N Engl J Med 2005;353(5):476–86.

49. Czeisler CA, Walsh JK, Wesnes KA, Arora S, Roth T. Armodafinil for treatment of excessive sleepiness associated with shift work disorder: a randomized controlled study. Mayo Clin Proc 2009;84(11):958–72.

50. Drake C, Roehrs T, Breslau N, et al. The 10-year risk of verified motor vehicle crashes in relation to physiologic sleepiness. Sleep 2010;33(6):745–52.

51. Johns MW. A new method for measuring daytime sleepiness: the Epworth sleepiness scale. Sleep 1991;14(6):540–5.

52. Kaida K, Takahashi M, Akerstedt T, et al. Validation of the Karolinska sleepiness scale against performance and EEG variables. Clin Neurophysiol 2006;117(7):1574–81.

53. Punjabi NM, Bandeen-Roche K, Young T. Predictors of objective sleep tendency in the general population. Sleep 2003;26(6):678–83.

54. Walsleben JA, Kapur VK, Newman AB, et al. Sleep and reported daytime sleepiness in normal subjects: the Sleep Heart Health Study. Sleep 2004;27(2):293–8.

55. Akerstedt T, Wright KP Jr. Sleep loss and fatigue in shift work and shift work disorder. Sleep Med Clin 2009;4(2):257–71.

56. Shen J, Barbera J, Shapiro CM. Distinguishing sleepiness and fatigue: focus on definition and measurement. Sleep Med Rev 2006;10(1):63–76.

57. Thorpy MJ. Managing the patient with shift-work disorder. J Fam Pract 2010;59(1 Suppl):S24–31.

58. American Psychological Association. Diagnostic and statistical manual of mental disorders: DSM-5™, 5th ed. Arlington, VA: American Psychiatric Publishing, 2013.

59. Harvey AG. Insomnia: symptom or diagnosis? Clin Psychol Rev 2001;21(7):1037–59.

60. Spielman AJ, Glovinsky P. The varied nature of insomnia. In: Hauri PJ, ed. Case studies in insomnia. New York: Plenum Press, 1991.

61. Ingre M, Akerstedt T. Effect of accumulated night work during the working lifetime, on subjective health and sleep in monozygotic twins. J Sleep Res 2004;13(1):45–8.

62. Monk TH, Buysse DJ, Billy BD, et al. Circadian type and bed-timing regularity in 654 retired seniors: correlations with subjective sleep measures. Sleep 2011;34(2):235–9.

63. Morin CM, Belleville G, Belanger L, Ivers H. The Insomnia Severity Index: psychometric indicators to detect insomnia cases and evaluate treatment response. Sleep 2011;34(5):601–8.

64. Buysse DJ, Reynolds CF, Monk TH, Berman SR. The Pittsburgh Sleep Quality Index: a new instrument for psychiatric practice and research. Psychiatry Res 1989;28(2):193–213.

65. Ancoli-Israel S, Roth T. Characteristics of insomnia in the United States: results of the 1991 National Sleep Foundation Survey. I. Sleep 1999;22(Suppl 2):S347–53.

66. Gallup. Sleep in America. Princeton, NJ: Gallup Organization, 1995.

67. Trinkoff AM, Storr CL. Work schedule characteristics and substance use in nurses. Am J Ind Med 1998;34(3):266–71.

68. Barton J, Spelten E, Totterdell P, Smith L, Folkard S, Costa G. The Standard Shiftwork Index: a battery of questionnaires for assessing shiftwork-related problems. Work Stress 1995;9(1):4–30.

69. Smith C, Gibby R, Zickar M, et al. Measurement properties of the Shiftwork Survey and Standard Shiftwork Index. J Hum Ergol 2001;30(1–2):191–6.

70. Tucker P, Knowles SR. Review of studies that have used the Standard Shiftwork Index: evidence for the underlying model of shiftwork and health. Appl Ergon 2008;39(5):550–64.

71. Czeisler CA, Buxton OM. The human circadian timing system and sleep–wake regulations. In: Kryger MH, Roth T, Dement WC, eds. Principles and practice of sleep medicine, 5th edn. Philadelphia: W.B. Saunders, 2011:402–19.

72. Guardiola-Lemaitre B, Quera-Salva MA. Melatonin and the regulation of sleep and circadian rhythms. In: Kryger MH, Roth T, Dement WC, eds. Principles and practice of sleep medicine, 5th ed. Philadelphia: W.B. Saunders, 2011:420–30.

73. Czeisler CA, Allan JS, Strogatz SH, et al. Bright light resets the human circadian pacemaker independent of the timing of the sleep–wake cycle. Science (NY) 1986;233(4764):667–71.

74. Boivin DB, James FO. Light treatment and circadian adaptation to shift work. Ind Health 2005;43(1):34–48.

75. Crowley SJ, Lee C, Tseng CY, Fogg LF, Eastman CI. Complete or partial circadian re-entrainment improves performance, alertness, and mood during night-shift work. Sleep 2004;27(6):1077–87.

76. Smith MR, Eastman CI. Night shift performance is improved by a compromise circadian phase position: study 3. Circadian phase after 7 night shifts with an intervening weekend off. Sleep 2008;31(12):1639–45.

77. Burgess HJ, Revell VL, Eastman CI. A three pulse phase response curve to three milligrams of melatonin in humans. J Physiol 2008;586(2):639–47.

78. Richardson GS, Zee PC, Wang-Weigand S, Rodriguez L, Peng X. Circadian phase-shifting effects of repeated ramelteon administration in healthy adults. J Clin Sleep Med 2008;4(5):456–61.

79. Rajaratnam SM, Polymeropoulos MH, Fisher DM, et al. Melatonin agonist tasimelteon (VEC-162) for transient insomnia after

sleep-time shift: two randomised controlled multicentre trials. Lancet 2009;373(9662):482–91.

80. Wright KP Jr, Bogan RK, Wyatt JK. Shift work and the assessment and management of shift work disorder (SWD). Sleep Med Rev 2013;17(1):41–54.

81. Dawson D, Campbell SS. Timed exposure to bright light improves sleep and alertness during simulated night shifts. Sleep 1991;14(6):511–16.

82. Minors DS, Waterhouse JM. Does "anchor sleep" entrain circadian rhythms? Evidence from constant routine studies. J Physiol 1983;345:451–67.

83. Takeyama H, Kubo T, Itani T. The nighttime nap strategies for improving night shift work in workplace. Ind Health 2005;43(1):24–9.

84. Garbarino S, Mascialino B, Penco MA, et al. Professional shift-work drivers who adopt prophylactic naps can reduce the risk of car accidents during night work. Sleep 2004;27(7):1295–302.

85. Leger D, Philip P, Jarriault P, Metlaine A, Choudat D. Effects of a combination of napping and bright light pulses on shift workers' sleepiness at the wheel: a pilot study. J Sleep Res 2009;18(4):472–9.

86. Smith-Coggins R, Howard SK, Mac DT, et al. Improving alertness and performance in emergency department physicians and nurses: the use of planned naps. Ann Emerg Med 2006;48(5):596–604, e1–3.

87. Schweitzer PK, Randazzo AC, Stone K, Erman M, Walsh JK. Laboratory and field studies of naps and caffeine as practical countermeasures for sleep–wake problems associated with night work. Sleep 2006;29(1):39–50.

88. Wertz AT, Ronda JM, Czeisler CA, Wright KP Jr. Effects of sleep inertia on cognition. JAMA 2006;295(2):163–4.

89. Morgenthaler TI, Lee-Chiong T, Alessi C, et al. Practice parameters for the clinical evaluation and treatment of circadian rhythm sleep disorders. An American Academy of Sleep Medicine report. Sleep 2007;30(11):1445–59.

90. Hart CL, Ward AS, Haney M, Foltin RW. Zolpidem-related effects on performance and mood during simulated night-shift work. Exp Clinl Psychopharmacol 2003;11(4):259–68.

91. Hughes RJ, Badia P. Sleep-promoting and hypothermic effects of daytime melatonin administration in humans. Sleep 1997;20(2):124–31.

92. Markwald RR, Lee-Chiong TL, Burke TM, Snider JA, Wright KP Jr. Effects of the melatonin MT-1/MT-2 agonist ramelteon on daytime body temperature and sleep. Sleep 2010;33(6):825–31.

93. Wyatt JK, Dijk DJ, Ritz-de Cecco A, Ronda JM, Czeisler CA. Sleep-facilitating effect of exogenous melatonin in healthy young men and women is circadian-phase dependent. Sleep 2006;29(5):609–18.

94. Hart CL, Ward AS, Haney M, Nasser J, Foltin RW. Methamphetamine attenuates disruptions in performance and mood during simulated night-shift work. Psychopharmacology 2003;169(1):42–51.

95. Wyatt JK, Cajochen C, Ritz-De Cecco A, Czeisler CA, Dijk DJ. Low-dose repeated caffeine administration for circadian-phase-dependent performance degradation during extended wakefulness. Sleep 2004;27(3):374–81.

96. Wood S, Sage JR, Shuman T, Anagnostaras SG. Psychostimulants and cognition: a continuum of behavioral and cognitive activation. Pharmacol Rev 2014;66(1):193–221.

97. Jay SM, Petrilli RM, Ferguson SA, Dawson D, Lamond N. The suitability of a caffeinated energy drink for night-shift workers. Physiol Behav 2006;87(5):925–31.

98. Darwish M, Kirby M, Hellriegel ET, Robertson P Jr. Armodafinil and modafinil have substantially different pharmacokinetic profiles despite having the same terminal half-lives: analysis of data from three randomized, single-dose, pharmacokinetic studies. Clin Drug Invest 2009;29(9):613–23.

99. Bambra CL, Whitehead MM, Sowden AJ, Akers J, Petticrew MP. Shifting schedules: the health effects of reorganizing shift work. Am J Prev Med 2008;34(5):427–34.

100. Barton J, Folkard S. Advancing versus delaying shift systems. Ergonomics 1993;36(1–3):59–64.

101. Czeisler CA, Moore-Ede MC, Coleman RH. Rotating shift work schedules that disrupt sleep are improved by applying circadian principles. Science (NY) 1982;217(4558):460–3.

102. Orth-Gomer K. Intervention on coronary risk factors by adapting a shift work schedule to biologic rhythmicity. Psychosom Med 1983;45(5):407–15.

103. Cruz C, Boquet A, Detwiler C, Nesthus T. Clockwise and counterclockwise rotating shifts: effects on vigilance and performance. Aviat Space Environ Med 2003;74(6 Pt 1):606–14.

104. Cruz C, Detwiler C, Nesthus T, Boquet A. Clockwise and counterclockwise rotating shifts: effects on sleep duration, timing, and quality. Aviat Space Environ Med 2003;74(6 Pt 1):597–605.

105. Hornberger S, Knauth P. Effects of various types of change in shift schedules: a controlled longitudinal study. Work Stress 1995;9(2–3):124–33.

106. Hornberger S, Knauth P. Follow-up intervention study on effects of a change in shift schedule on shiftworkers in the chemical industry. Int J Ind Ergon 1998;21(3–4):249–57.

107. Ng-A-Tham JEE, Thierry HK. An experimental change of the speed of rotation of the morning and evening shift. Ergonomics 1993;36(1–3):51–7.

108. Nicholson AN. Intercontinental air travel: the cabin atmosphere and circadian realignment. Travel Med Infect Dis 2009;7(2):57–9.

109. Singh B. Sickness pattern among air travellers: review of 735 cases at the Oman airport. Aviat Space Environ Med 2002;73(7):684–7.

110. Rajaratnam SM, Arendt J. Health in a 24-h society. Lancet 2001;358(9286):999–1005.

111. Scheen AJ, Van Cauter E. The roles of time of day and sleep quality in modulating glucose regulation: clinical implications. Horm Res 1998;49(3–4):191–201.

112. Lemmer B, Kern RI, Nold G, Lohrer H. Jet lag in athletes after eastward and westward time-zone transition. Chronobiol Int 2002;19(4):743–64.

113. Cho K. Chronic "jet lag" produces temporal lobe atrophy and spatial cognitive deficits. Nat Neurosci 2001;4(6):567–8.

114. Grajewski B, Nguyen MM, Whelan EA, Cole RJ, Hein MJ. Measuring and identifying large-study metrics for circadian rhythm disruption in female flight attendants. Scand J Work Environ Health 2003;29(5):337–46.

115. Katz G, Knobler HY, Laibel Z, Strauss Z, Durst R. Time zone change and major psychiatric morbidity: the results of a 6-year study in Jerusalem. Compr Psychiatry 2002;43(1):37–40.

116. Moline ML, Pollak CP, Monk TH, et al. Age-related differences in recovery from simulated jet lag. Sleep 1992;15(1):28–40.

117. Waterhouse J, Edwards B, Nevill A, et al. Identifying some determinants of "jet lag" and its symptoms: a study of athletes and other travellers. Br J Sports Med 2002;36(1):54–60.

118. Weingarten JA, Collop NA. Air travel: effects of sleep deprivation and jet lag. Chest 2013;144(4):1394–401.

119. Takahashi M, Nakata A, Arito H. Disturbed sleep–wake patterns during and after short-term international travel among academics attending conferences. Int Arch Occup Environ Health 2002;75(6):435–40.

120. Duffy JF, Wright KP Jr. Entrainment of the human circadian system by light. J Biol Rhythm 2005;20(4):326–38.

121. Beaumont M, Batejat D, Pierard C, et al. Caffeine or melatonin effects on sleep and sleepiness after rapid eastward transmeridian travel. J Appl Physiol 2004;96(1):50–8.

122. Spitzer RL, Terman M, Williams JB, et al. Jet lag: clinical features, validation of a new syndrome-specific scale, and lack of response to melatonin in a randomized, double-blind trial. Am J Psychiatry 1999;156(9):1392–6.

123. Sack RL. The pathophysiology of jet lag. Travel Med Infect Dis 2009;7(2):102–10.

124. Herxheimer A, Petrie KJ. Melatonin for the prevention and treatment of jet lag. Cochrane Database Syst Rev 2002;(2):CD001520.

125. Boulos Z, Macchi MM, Sturchler MP, et al. Light visor treatment for jet lag after westward travel across six time zones. Aviat Space Environ Med 2002;73(10):953–63.

126. Burgess HJ, Crowley SJ, Gazda CJ, Fogg LF, Eastman CI. Preflight adjustment to eastward travel: 3 days of advancing sleep with and without morning bright light. J Biol Rhythm 2003;18(4):318–28.

127. Eastman CI, Gazda CJ, Burgess HJ, Crowley SJ, Fogg LF. Advancing circadian rhythms before eastward flight: a strategy to prevent or reduce jet lag. Sleep 2005;28(1):33–44.

128. Jamieson AO, Zammit GK, Rosenberg RS, Davis JR, Walsh JK. Zolpidem reduces the sleep disturbance of jet lag. Sleep Med 2001;2(5):423–30.

129. Suhner A, Schlagenhauf P, Hofer I, Johnson R, Tschopp A, Steffen R. Effectiveness and tolerability of melatonin and zolpidem for the alleviation of jet lag. Aviat Space Environ Med 2001; 72(7):638–46.

130. Brooks A, Lack L. A brief afternoon nap following nocturnal sleep restriction: which nap duration is most recuperative? Sleep 2006;29(6):831–40.

131. Tietzel AJ, Lack LC. The short-term benefits of brief and long naps following nocturnal sleep restriction. Sleep 2001;24(3):293–300.

132. Spielman AJ, Caruso LS, Glovinsky PB. A behavioral perspective on insomnia treatment. Psychiatric Clin N Am 1987;10(4):541–53.

CHAPTER 22

Advanced, delayed, free-running, and irregular sleep–wake rhythm disorders

Guy Warman and Josephine Arendt

Introduction

Circadian rhythm sleep disorders (CSRDs) should be considered in the differential diagnosis of either hypersomnia or insomnia. While the International Classification of Sleep Disorders, Third Edition (ICSD-3) lists a total of seven types of CRSDs (327.31 delayed sleep phase type; 327.32 advanced sleep phase type; 327.33 irregular sleep–wake type; 327.34 non-entrained type; 327.35 jet-lag type; 327.36 shift work type; 327.37 due to medical condition) [1], here we focus on advanced sleep phase disorder (ASPD), delayed sleep phase disorder (DSPD), free-running (non-24-hour) sleep disorder (FRSD), and irregular sleep–wake rhythm disorder (ISWRD).

As has been outlined in the preceding chapters of this book, human sleep is controlled by the combined actions of the sleep homeostat and the circadian clock in the suprachiasmatic nucleus, which ticks with an inherently inaccurate period (on average approximately 24.2 hours). Although food, exercise, social interaction, and melatonin can adjust (or *entrain*) the clock, light is the most important entraining agent (or *zeitgeber*) for the human clock, and entrains its endogenous period to 24 hours on a daily basis. Circadian photoreception is mediated exclusively by the eye and mainly by the nonvisual pigment "melanopsin" located in a subset of intrinsically photoreceptive ganglion cells (ipRGCs) in the retina.

The human clock is affected by light differently at different times relative to its phase (circadian times). In the biological morning (i.e, the declining phase of the endogenous melatonin profile), light acts to advance the clock to an earlier phase (phase advance), whereas in the evening, light shifts it to a later phase (phase delay). These effects (and those of orally administered melatonin) are best summarized by the "phase response curve" [2,3] (Fig. 22.1). Understanding the differential effects of light and melatonin on the clock at various circadian times is crucial to understanding the theoretical basis of the treatment of CRSDs.

Entrainment of the clock comprises two processes. The first is *period control* (adjustment of the period to 24 hours on a daily basis) and the second is *phase control* (adjustment of the phase of the rhythm to the appropriate time of the daily light–dark cycle). In this chapter, we focus on the CRSDs that result from either a *lack of entrainment* of the human circadian clock (FRSD and ISWRD)

or from a clock that is entrained, but at *a phase that is at odds with societal norms* (ASPD and DSPD).

The primary diagnostic tools for CRSDs are sleep diaries complemented by actigraphs (wrist-worn devices that record overall movement and can be used to objectively determine sleep timing and quality). Measurement of more direct phase markers of the clock such as rhythms in core body temperature and endogenous melatonin production can also be useful (particularly in diagnosing FRSD). Polysomnography (PSG), while not required for the diagnosis of CRSDs, can be beneficial in excluding other primary or secondary insomnias [4].

CRSDs result from one of two different situations. The most common of these is a lack of appropriately timed (or sufficiently strong) environmental light exposure. The second is a consequence of a clock that is unable to entrain with an appropriate

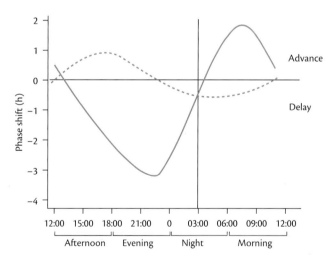

Fig. 22.1 Stylized phase response curves for light (6.7 hours of 10 000 lux) (full line) and melatonin (0.5 mg) (dashed line) in a normally entrained individual. Light late in the biological day (afternoon–evening) (approximately 15:00–00:00) causes a phase delay in the circadian clock, while light in the early biological day (03:00–12:00) causes a phase advance. In contrast, melatonin administered during the late afternoon causes a phase advance and during the biological morning elicits a phase delay.

period and *phase angle*. The two most common environmental situations that cause CRSDs are shift work and rapid transmeridian air travel. From the phase response curve (Fig. 22.1), it can be seen that in most situations the human clock can only shift a maximum of a couple of hours per day. These maximum shifts are described as the "limits of entrainment." Transmeridian travel beyond these limits manifests as "jet lag." On average, without interventions, the circadian clock takes a day to adapt for every time zone crossed. After several days of light exposure in a new time zone, the clock is able to achieve steady state entrainment at an appropriate phase angle (wakening in the morning and sleeping at night). Treatment strategies to expedite entrainment to a new time zone are clearly beneficial if the duration of stay in the new time zone is sufficient [5].

However, for short stopovers, there is little value in attempting to entrain to the new time zone, and the best advice is to try and work and operate (as far as is feasible) during "home" daytime. The rapid changes from diurnal to nocturnal sleep timing experienced in shift work create the same demands on the clock as jet lag, and the advice about whether to try and adapt (or not) is essentially the same (although it is always more difficult to try and entrain to a day at odds with societal norms and the light–dark cycle). Given that an estimated 15–20% of the population in developed countries conduct "shift work," the size of this problem is vast.

The most common cause of CRSDs in people not shift working or conducting transmeridian travel is a lack of exposure to sufficient entraining light (particularly in the morning). Situations in which patients may present with CRSDs as a result of a low morning light exposure include office workers in high latitudes in winter (which in some cases may present as seasonal affective disorder, SAD), residents in rest homes, and patients in dimly lit hospital settings.

In addition to the environmentally driven CRSDs, there are biological causes of CRSDs in people who are exposed to the strong daily light–dark cycles that would normally be expected to entrain their clocks with an appropriate phase angle. The most well characterized of these is blindness, particularly in blind patients who have a lack of conscious light perception. Despite the fact that the primary circadian photoreceptor is nonvisual (as above), conscious perception of light appears to provide an acceptable surrogate to determine whether the circadian light entrainment pathway is intact in blind subjects. CRSDs also occur with psychiatric conditions, particularly with affective disorders. Chronotherapeutic treatments have been shown to be effective in the treatment of SAD, in bipolar, and unipolar depression among others [6].

Advanced sleep phase disorder

Description

ASPD is characterized by disabling sleep times that are too early with respect to societal norms or personal preference. Patients suffering from ASPD will have an early sleep onset (typically between 18:00 and 21:00) and find it very difficult to stay awake past 21:00. They will habitually wake between 02:00 and 05:00 and find it very difficult to sleep past 05:00. The nature of the light exposure that these patients subject themselves to as a consequence of the disease can aggravate, or even maintain their

disorder (i.e, by minimizing evening light exposure and maximizing morning exposure, the circadian clock of ASPD patients is perpetually being phase advanced but not phase delayed; see Fig. 22.1. In addition to an early sleep phase, the phase of endogenous melatonin secretion rhythms and core body temperature are advanced in ASPD sufferers [7].

One of the underlying causes of ASPD is a clock with an inherently short free-running period. This has been demonstrated in the autosomal dominant "familial advanced sleep disorder" (FASPD), which has been shown to be a consequence of a clock with a very short free-running period (23.3 hours) in at least three families studied [8]. FASPD has been associated with a missense mutation in the circadian clock gene *PER2* [9], and extreme morning preference has been associated with a number of polymorphisms, including a length polymorphism, in the *PER3* gene [10], a silent polymorphism in the *PER1* gene [11], and a missense mutation in the *CSNK1D* gene (encoding casein kinase 1δ) (which also predisposes sufferers to migraine) [12]. The pathogenesis of the disease is, however, heterogeneous and there is currently no diagnostic genetic marker for ASPD.

Incidence

The incidence of ASPD is unknown, and it is thought to be underreported as it causes less social/work disruption than some of the other CRSDs. Estimated incidence is, however, rare at less than 1% of the population. Advanced sleep phase appears to increase in frequency with age, and onset is typically in middle age. ASPD is reported in children, however, particularly those with autism spectrum disorders and Smith–Magenis syndrome [13].

Presentation

Prior to ascribing the diagnosis of ASPD, other causes of insomnia and early morning wakening such as major depression, mood disorders, and primary and secondary insomnia should be excluded [14]. Patients with ASPD will present with a chronic history of afternoon or early evening sleepiness and early morning wakening/insomnia. If early sleep onset is not possible owing to social or work commitments, patients will continue to display early morning wakening accompanied by chronic sleep deprivation. If allowed to sleep at their "preferred" sleep times, sleep duration and architecture are normal.

Assessment tools for ASPD

1. Patient sleep diary/sleep log for a minimum of 7 (preferably 14) days. It is important for patients to report their preferred sleep times on "free" (i.e, non-work) days.

2. Objective monitoring of sleep–wake timing using wrist-worn actigraphy (in conjunction with sleep diaries) for a period of at least 7 days [15].

3. ASPD sufferers are likely to score as extreme morning types in morningness–eveningness questionnaires such as the Munich Chronotype Questionnaire [16] and the Horne–Östberg Morningness–Eveningness Questionnaire [17]. However, there are no studies evaluating the sensitivity or specificity of these questionnaires as diagnostic tools, and the AASM recommends that their use be restricted to the confirmation of ASPD rather than diagnosis [4].

Diagnosis

The ICSD-3 diagnostic criteria [1] for ASPD are as follows:

1. An advanced phase of the major sleep episode in relation to the desired sleep time as evidenced by a chronic/recurrent complaint.

2. Symptoms present for at least 3 months.

3. When allowed to select their preferred sleep time, patients have normal sleep duration and quality occurring at a stable (advanced) phase with respect to societal norms.

4. Sleep diaries and objective sleep timing measures (actigraphy) conducted over a minimum of 7 days (preferably 14 days) show stable but advanced sleep timing.

5. The sleep disturbance is not explained by another current sleep, neurological, mental, medical, or substance use disorder.

While not required for diagnosis, investigation of body temperature rhythms or endogenous melatonin onset profiles (dim light melatonin onset) can confirm the advanced phase of the clock in ASPD sufferers. PSG recordings will show "normal" sleep in patients who are sleeping at their preferred phase and may be used to rule out another primary sleep disorder [4].

Management and treatment

Management of ASPD relies on the combination of timed bright evening light exposure and sleep–wake scheduling. Using the principles of the phase response curve (Fig. 22.1), patients' sleep time can potentially be delayed to a desired phase by appropriately timed administration of light (and/or chronobiotics such as melatonin).

Evening light therapy has been reported to be effective in delaying wake time [18] and increasing sleep efficiency in some ASPD sufferers. Two evenings of bright light (4 hours of 2 500 lux) therapy has been reported to phase delay the clock of early waking insomniacs by 2 hours, and subsequently to improve sleep parameters 4 weeks after treatment [19]. Exposure to polychromatic blue-enriched or standard fluorescent white light of approximately 370 $\mu W/cm^2$ 3 hours before bedtime has proven effective in delaying the clock and prolonging the latency to rapid eye movement (REM) sleep in older subjects in the sleep laboratory [20]).

In contrast, a large study of 47 ASPD patients treated with 2–3 hours of "enhanced evening light" (at a relatively modest 265 lux) showed no benefit in altering actigraphically determined sleep phase. Patients in this study did, however, report a subjective benefit of light therapy [21]. The long-term effects of light therapy can dissipate once treatment ceases [22], and patient compliance in maintaining light therapy in the medium to long term can be low.

A second approach to the treatment of ASPD is chronotherapy/ sleep scheduling, which has been shown to be effective in the treatment of ASPD in one case report in which a gradual advance of bedtime by 3 hours every 2 days has successfully resulted in a desired sleep phase at a 5-month follow-up [23].

The administration of low-dose oral melatonin has been reported to be efficacious in delaying the clock when administered after the body temperature nadir (in the early subjective morning) (Fig. 22.1). Thus, theoretically at least, it could be useful in delaying the clock of ASPD sufferers. There are, however, no systematic reports of its use for the treatment of ASPD [14] and the mild sleep-promoting effects of melatonin may negate its usefulness in the morning.

Recommended treatment for ASPD comprises evening bright (up to 10 000 lux) light therapy accompanied by minimization of morning light exposure. Sleep scheduling (where practicable) may also be used in conjunction with bright light therapy.

Delayed sleep phase disorder

Description

DSPD, first described in 1981 [24], is characterized by stable sleep times that are too late with respect to societal norms or personal preference. Patients suffering from DSPD will have a late sleep onset (typically between 02:00 and 06:00) and wake typically between 10:00 and 13:00. DSPD patients present with sleep onset insomnia and have extreme sleep inertia when trying to conform to work or social schedules [14] owing to a delay in their "wake maintenance zone." They will describe undisturbed sleep when sleeping at their (late) preferred sleep phase on free days and holidays. As with ASPD, the nature of the light exposure these patients receive (little phase-advancing morning light and increased phase-delaying evening light exposure) may aggravate or maintain their disorder.

While the etiology of DSPD is unknown, possible causes include a circadian clock with a longer than average endogenous period [25,26], a hypersensitivity to evening (phase-delaying) light exposure that results in more profound delays than advances in "normal" light exposure settings [27], and an abnormal phase relationship between the circadian clock and the sleep homeostatic process regulating sleep and wakefulness.

There are reported cases of familial DSPD [28], and a number of polymorphisms in circadian clock genes appear to correlate with extreme evening-type behavior (including polymorphisms in *PER3* [10,29–31], *CLOCK* [32], *ARNTL2* (33), and *PER1* [11]). As with ASPD, however, none of these polymorphisms provide a diagnostic tool for DSPD.

A delay in the major sleep episode is usually accompanied by a delayed phase of circadian phase markers (such as melatonin and core temperature) in DSPD patients, although recent evidence suggests there may be two subtypes of DSPD patients: those with shifted circadian phase markers and those with shifted sleep but "normally" phased markers of the clock.

Incidence

DSPD is by far the most common of the CRSDs, representing over 80% of CRSD diagnoses, but the prevalence of DSPD in the general population is largely unknown, with estimates between 0.17% and 9% in the community and primary healthcare setting [34–36]. The condition is more common in adolescence (7–16%) and is reported in approximately 10% of patients presenting to sleep clinics with insomnia [1]. Onset is common in adolescence, with the incidence of generally "late chronotypes" peaking in males at 21 years and females at 17 years [16].

Presentation

DSPD can present at any age, but most commonly manifests in adolescence (90% of DSPD patients report the onset of their symptoms in adolescence [37]). Onset in childhood also occurs, particularly in familial cases. The incidence of DSPD is much less common at older ages. Patients present with disabling sleep onset insomnia, great difficulty waking, and an inability to adapt to a "normal" phase even after several days or weeks. Chronic sleep deprivation is common (as evidenced by reduced total sleep time), as is associated morning sleepiness. When allowed to sleep at their preferred phase, sleep quality and duration are normal. DSPD sufferers will score as evening types on chronotyping questionnaires and will report being most alert in the evening. Their inability to rise in the morning can lead to issues maintaining work or academic careers, and in children and adolescents DSPD is frequently accompanied by truancy and academic failure. DSPD may be associated with psychopathologies such as a mood disorders (major depression/bipolar), severe obsessive/compulsive disorder, autism spectrum disorder, and attention deficit hyperactivity disorder (ADHD) [1].

Assessment tools for DSPD

1. Patient sleep diary/sleep log for a minimum of 7 (preferably 14) days. It is important for patients to report their preferred sleep times on "free" (i.e, non-work) days.

2. Objective monitoring of sleep–wake timing using wrist-worn actigraphy (in conjunction with sleep diaries) for a period of at least 7 days (preferably 14 days) [15].

3. DSPD sufferers typically score as evening types in morningness–eveningness questionnaires such as the Munich Chronotype Questionnaire [16] and the Horne–Östberg Morningness–eveningness Questionnaire [17]. The Basic Language Morningness Scale (BALM) is also useful in screening for DSPD [38].

As with ASPD, the measurement of circadian phase markers such as core temperature and melatonin profiles (either analysis of dim light melatonin onsets in salivary or plasma samples or the rhythm of 6-sulphatoxymelatonin in urine) can be used to confirm the delayed phase of the clock. PSG will confirm both normal sleep architecture and duration when patients are sleeping at their preferred phase.

Diagnosis

The ICSD-3 diagnostic criteria [1] for DSPD are as follows:

1. A significant delay in the phase of the major sleep episode in relation to the desired sleep/wake time.

2. Symptoms present for at least 3 months.

3. When allowed to choose their preferred sleep phase, patients show improved duration and quality of sleep and maintain a delayed (but 24-hour) sleep pattern.

4. Sleep logs/actigraphy for a minimum of 7 (preferably 14) days show a delay in the timing of the habitual sleep period.

5. The sleep disturbance is not explained by another current sleep, neurological, mental, medical, or substance use disorder.

DSPD must be distinguished from primary and secondary chronic insomnia (in which sleep initiation and maintenance are not improved when patients are able to sleep at their preferred phase). Excessive daytime sleepiness may be caused by other sleep disorders (eg, insomnias or breathing disorders). DSPD must also be distinguished from "normal" delayed sleep phase (particularly in adolescents), which does not impair functioning or work or school schedules.

Management and treatment

As with ASPD, the theory underlying the treatment of DSPD is based on the phase response curve (Fig. 22.1). By maximizing morning (phase-advancing) light exposure and minimizing phase-delaying evening light exposure, the patient's phase can be adjusted.

There is good evidence to support the use of morning bright light therapy in the treatment of DSPD. A number of case reports and placebo-controlled trials have shown the efficacy of bright light therapy administered in the morning (prior to or on waking) for 1–2 weeks in phase-advancing sleep timing and circadian rhythms in DSPD sufferers [25,39]. Morning light therapy has even proven to be effective when administered through closed eyelids [40]. The level of light necessary to advance sleep timing and the clock depends on the wavelength used. As circadian photoreception is mediated by a blue-light sensitive opsin, blue light is more effective than other wavelengths in shifting the clock [41]. However, compliance with light therapy can be problematic, particularly with long-term therapy.

Oral melatonin administered during the phase advance portion of the melatonin phase response curve (in the subjective evening) (Fig. 22.1) is known to elicit phase advances of the human circadian clock [3,42], and afternoon and evening melatonin administration (0.3–5 mg up to 8 hours prior to sleep onset for 4 weeks) has been used to phase advance the clock in DSPD sufferers [43,44]. Low doses of melatonin (0.3–0.5 mg) prove to be as effective as high doses (3–5 mg) [44], and early timing is more effective than later [44]. Melatonin also has mild sleep-promoting effects that can be useful when administered in the subjective evening/bedtime. While compliance with melatonin treatment is better than that of light therapy, relapse of symptoms can occur when treatment is discontinued [45]. There are few data on the very long-term effects of melatonin treatment in adults, but there is little evidence for any adverse effects to date [46].

As the phase-advancing effects of morning light therapy and evening melatonin treatment are additive [47], their use together is effective in the treatment of DSPD [48–50].

Cognitive–behavioral therapy (CBT) and chronotherapy/sleep scheduling together with bright light therapy have also been used to treat DSPD in adults [51] and adolescents [52]. Adolescents with DSPD receiving six 1-hour weekly sessions of CBT together with an advance in daily wake time of 30 minutes, and 30–120 minutes of morning light therapy until their target waking time of 06:00, showed improved sleep and reduced daytime impairments, with effects persisting at 6 months [52]. Phase-advancing chronotherapy/sleep scheduling can be particularly difficult for DSPD sufferers, and an effective alternative [25] is phase-delaying chronotherapy (progressively delaying sleep time by 3 hours every 2 days until the desired sleep time is achieved). This is, however, disruptive in patients trying to maintain a regular work and social life.

Recommended treatment for DSPD comprises daily morning bright (up to 10 000 lux) light therapy (either before or on waking) accompanied by minimization of evening light exposure (after 21:00) and afternoon/evening melatonin administration. Sleep scheduling/chronotherapy (where practicable) and CBT may be used in conjunction with these approaches.

Free-running (non-entrained type/non-24-hour) sleep disorder

Description

FRSD results when the circadian clock is not properly entrained to the 24-hour day and thus "free-runs" with its endogenous period (on average longer than 24 hours). The etiology of FRSD is unknown, but it is assumed to result either from an inability of light (or other non-photic zeitgebers) to entrain the clock, or from a clock with such an extreme free-running period that it is out of the range of entrainment of a 24-hour day. Subjectively, sufferers will often report sleep that drifts later each day. Objectively, however, they may not show sleep–wake patterns that "free-run," as their work or societal demands may not allow their sleep to follow their circadian drive. The result can be either a clearly drifting sleep pattern or a pattern of alternating periods of "good" nocturnal sleep interspersed with periods of very short nocturnal sleep episodes and daytime naps (when the circadian clock has drifted out of phase with the 24-hour day and is promoting sleep during the day and wakefulness at night) [53] (Fig. 22.2). In the latter case, it is only when a marker that faithfully represents the phase of the circadian clock (such as melatonin or core body temperature) is measured that the "free-running" pattern is revealed.

Incidence

Estimates of the prevalence of CRSDs in blind or visually impaired populations vary, with some studies suggesting that up to 70% of blind subjects suffer from a CRSD [54–58]. The severity and magnitude of CRSDs in the blind appears to correlate with the degree of light perception of patients. As light is the primary zeitgeber that entrains the human circadian clock, FRSD is most common in the blind, and particularly people with no or little conscious light perception. Subjective estimates of the prevalence of FRSD in the community range from 17% to 50% in blind individuals with no conscious light perception (NLP) or reduced light perception (RLP) and from 4% to 8% in blind individuals with light perception (LP) [58,59]. The objectively determined incidence of FRSD (via the measurement of 6-sulphatoxymelatonin rhythms in urine) is 39% in NLP and 10% LP [60]. Almost all bilaterally enucleated patients show free-running rhythms [61].

From these numbers, it is clear that FRSD does not affect all people who have no conscious perception of light. Entrainment in these individuals may be explained by (a) intact circadian photoreception (from melanopsin-containing retinal ganglion cells in an intact inner retina), (b) entrainment by non-photic cues (such as social interaction, meals, or exercise), or (c) a free-running period that is so close to 24 hours as to be indistinguishable from an entrained rhythm. Although extremely rare, free-running sleep patterns have been reported in sighted individuals in low light environments in the laboratory, at high latitudes [62,63], in patients following chronotherapy for DSPD, as a result of traumatic brain injury [1], and in recovery from offshore night-shift work [64].

Presentation

FRSD can be differentiated from DSPD (in which some patients with severe DSPD display delays in sleep onset over several days) by measuring circadian phase markers (eg, melatonin and/or

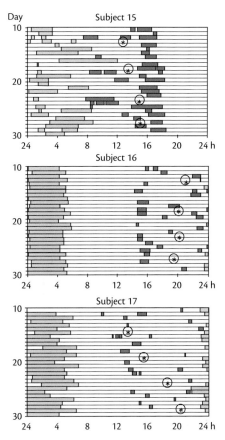

Fig. 22.2 Three blind subjects (no perception of light) showing abnormal sleep and melatonin rhythms. Subjectively recorded sleep is shown by the gray bars, and naps (classified as such by the subjects) are shown by the black bars. Melatonin was assessed as 6-sulphatoxymelatonin (aMT6s) in sequential urine collections for 48 h weekly, and the asterisks indicate the calculated peak times (acrophase) of the aMT6s rhythms. Note the abnormal timing of aMT6s, which normally peaks between 24:00 and 06:00, and the association of naps with daytime melatonin production. Subject 17 is clearly "free-running" (i.e, showing endogenous periodicity), with a steady daily delay of the aMT6s rhythm. Nearly all blind subjects with no eyes have shown this phenomenon. Subject 16 is synchronized to 24 hours, but with an abnormal phase position. Cortisol and core body temperature rhythms show abnormalities similar to those of melatonin. These and other observations in the blind underline the importance of light for synchronizing rhythms and the association of daytime endogenous melatonin production with poor night time sleep and daytime naps.

core body temperature) to determine whether their clock is truly "free-running."

Patients with FRSD frequently report "drifting sleep patterns" and present with alternating periods of insomnia and excessive daytime sleepiness and hypersomnia. Given that the average free-running period in humans is longer than 24 hours [65], when drifting sleep is reported, it is usually described as drifting a little later each day. When sufferers' circadian phase is aligned with the external environment, they may be asymptomatic. As their clock drifts, patients describe increasing sleep latency, sleep onset insomnia, and excessive daytime sleepiness. Depression and mood disorders can occur as comorbidities. Approximately 25% of sighted individuals with FRSD have related psychiatric diagnoses [1].

Onset of FRSD can occur at the onset of blindness or any time thereafter. In congenitally blind infants, it can be apparent early. FRSD has been reported in children with intellectual disabilities and blindness, particularly those with optic nerve hypoplasia. It has also been described in children with Rett syndrome [66], Angelman syndrome [67], and autism spectrum disorders. Drifting sleep can be more readily apparent in children than adults, but is frequently described by parents or caregivers as "waking too early/late" or "sleeping at abnormal times" [1].

Assessment tools for FRSD

1. Patient sleep diary/sleep log for a minimum of 14 days (preferably longer). It is important for patients to report their preferred sleep times on "free" (i.e, non-work/non-school) days.

2. Objective monitoring of sleep–wake timing using wrist-worn actigraphs (in conjunction with sleep diaries) for a period of at least 14 days.

3. Measurement of circadian phase markers (such as dim light melatonin onset (DLMO) from serially collected saliva or blood samples over the course of an evening, or urinary 6-sulpha-toxymelatonin analysis for a minimum of 24 and preferably 48 hours) repeated at weekly intervals on ideally four occasions to confirm "free-running" status.

Diagnosis

The ICSD-3 diagnostic criteria [1] for FRSD are as follows:

1. A history of alternating periods of asymptomatic periods and insomnia and/or excessive daytime sleepiness.

2. Symptoms persisting over the course of at least 3 months.

3. Daily sleep logs (and actigraphy) for a minimum of 14 days (preferably longer in blind patients) demonstrate a pattern that typically delays each day with a period (usually) of longer than 24 hours.

4. The sleep disorder is not better explained by another current sleep, neurological, mental, medical, or substance use disorder.

As illustrated in Fig. 22.2, patients with FRSD may or may not display drifting sleep–wake patterns when analyzed by sleep diary or actigraphy. Thus, measurement of direct phase markers of the clock such as melatonin [68] or core body temperature [69] may be necessary in order to diagnose FRSD.

Management and treatment

Given that the overwhelming majority of patients with FRSD are blind and are not able to entrain to photic cues, it is necessary to use non-photic entraining agents (zeitgeber) to entrain the circadian clock of these patients to a 24-hour period.

Melatonin has been shown to be particularly effective in entraining the clock of blind "free-runners" [70–72] (see Fig. 22.3). A single melatonin treatment (5 mg fast-release) at the correct phase can advance the clock by up to 1.5 hours (Fig. 22.1) [73]. Given that the endogenous period of the clock in blind free-runners is (on average) 24.5 hours, entrainment with melatonin is entirely feasible [74]. Recent studies suggest that lower "physiological" doses (between 0.3 and 0.5 mg) may be more effective in achieving entrainment than higher "pharmacological" doses, but with great individual variability. There is little evidence so far for an advantage of slow-release formulations over fast-release. In general, the lowest

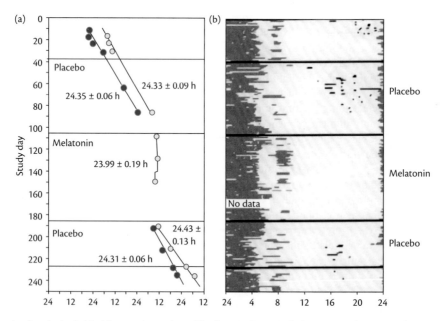

Fig. 22.3 Entrainment of the circadian clock of a blind free-running patient with a free-running period of approximately 24.3–24.4 hours using daily melatonin. (a) Days 0–100: urinary analysis of 6-sulphatoxymelatonin (filled circles) and cortisol (open circles) rhythms shows a free-running clock with a period of 24.3 hours when the patient is treated with placebo. Days 105–180: the rhythm is entrained to 24 hours by the daily administration of 0.5 mg oral melatonin (at 21:00). Days 185–250: the patient free-runs again when melatonin administration is ceased and placebo is resumed. (b) The corresponding subjective sleep diary data shows cyclic appearance of daytime naps and reduction in nighttime sleep duration in patient on placebo, which are not apparent during melatonin treatment [70].

Adapted from Journal of Biological Rhythms, 18(5), Hack LM, Lockley SW, Arendt J, Skene DJ, The Effects of Low-Dose 0.5-mg Melatonin on the Free-Running Circadian Rhythms of Blind Subjects, pp. 420–9, Copyright (2003), with permission from SAGE Publications.

effective dose should be used. Successful entrainment is accompanied by a consolidation of the nocturnal sleep episode, a decrease in daytime somnolence, and an improvement in mood.

Increasing the structure of other non-photic cues (eg, meal timing, social interaction, and exercise) may also be helpful in entraining the clock of FRSD sufferers [75], although evidence in support of this is somewhat limited.

In sighted individuals or blind individuals with light perception who have intact circadian photo-entrainment pathways, light may be used to entrain the clock. In this case, morning (phase-advancing) light (Fig. 22.1) is effective in eliciting the required phase change required to entrain the clock to 24 hours.

Recommended treatment for FRSD in blind patients lacking circadian photo-entrainment comprises daily evening melatonin administration (between 0.3 and 5 mg), starting if possible during a period of good sleep, accompanied by increased structure of non-photic cues (meals, social interaction, etc.). In blind patients with light perception and in sighted individuals, morning bright light therapy can be used (with or without evening melatonin and increased structure of non-photic cues).

Irregular sleep–wake rhythm disorder

Description

ISWRD is characterized by a lack of consolidation of the sleep–wake cycle [76]. Total sleep time is essentially normal for age in ISWRD patients, but sleep is fragmented across 24 hours and there is no major nocturnal sleep episode present. This disorder is common in people with Alzheimer's and other dementias [77]. The etiology is unclear, but possible causes include changes in the hypothalamus as a result of neurological disease, a reduction in the light input to the suprachiasmatic nucleus as a result of vision or optic tract disorders, and/or a decreased strength of daily light–dark cycles and lack of activity associated with institutionalization in a rest-home environment.

Incidence

The incidence of ISWRD is unknown, but it is commonly associated with brain injury or mental retardation in children and with dementia in older adults [14]. Age *per se* is not a risk factor for ISWRD but comorbidities in older adults such as Alzheimer's disease and neurological dysfunction are, particularly for those patients with evening agitation and sun-downing [77–79]. The risk factors for ISWRD are Alzheimer's, Parkinson's, and Huntington's diseases in adults and developmental disorders in children [1]. ISWRD has been reported in children with Angelman syndrome, William syndrome, autism spectrum disorders, and Smith–Magenis syndrome [13,67].

Presentation

Patients with ISWRD will present with sleep maintenance insomnia/nocturnal restlessness and daytime sleepiness with frequent daytime naps (depending on the time of day). Sleep occurs in three or more short (<4 hour) intervals across 24 hours [79]. Total sleep time across the 24 hours is, however, normal and the longest sleep period is often between 02:00 and 06:00. The fragmented nature of the sleep in demented patients with ISWRD can make home or family care particularly demanding, and it is cited as a driver of institutionalization of these patients.

Assessment tools for ISWRD

1. Patient sleep diary/sleep log for a minimum of 14 days (preferably longer) [80].

2. Objective monitoring of sleep–wake timing using wrist-worn actigraphy (in conjunction with sleep diaries) for a period of at least 14 days [80]. However, compliance with wearing wrist actigraphs can be low in dementia patients.

3. Measurement of dim light melatonin onset rhythms in saliva or plasma, or 6-sulphatoxymelatonin in urine, may show decreased amplitude in ISWRD patients.

Diagnosis

The ICSD-3 diagnostic criteria [1] for ISWRD are as follows:

1. The patient or caregiver reports a chronic or recurrent pattern of irregular sleep–wake episodes over 24 hours characterized by insomnia, excessive daytime sleepiness (napping), or both.

2. Symptoms are present for at least 3 months.

3. Sleep diaries and actigraphy (where possible) over 7–14 days demonstrate no major sleep period and multiple irregular sleep bouts (at least three per 24 hours).

4. The sleep disturbance is not explained by another current sleep, neurological, mental, medical, or substance use disorder.

PSG is not required for diagnosis, but may be used to exclude an alternative diagnosis and when conducted over 24 hours will show the loss of a consolidated sleep episode and normal total sleep time.

Management and treatment

Increasing the amplitude of the daily light–dark signal by bright light treatment is the most effective therapeutic intervention (particularly in institutional settings) for ISWRD sufferers [4,81]. A number of studies have shown an improvement in rest–activity rhythms and sleep (including consolidated nocturnal sleep, reduced nocturnal agitation and napping, and improvement of daytime alertness) in rest-home patients as a result of bright light exposure (1 500–8 000 lux for around 2 hours) (reviewed in [4,14]). Light treatment has also been proven effective in treating ISWRD in some children with mental retardation who have not been responsive to CBT or hypnotics [82].

There is little evidence for the efficacy of melatonin in the treatment of ISWRD. Neither fast-release nor controlled-release melatonin appear to convincingly improve actigraphically determined sleep parameters in ISWRD patients [4,14,76]. Controlled-release melatonin may, however, prove useful in improving sleep maintenance in some patient populations, and the use of combined morning light and evening melatonin (2.5 mg) therapy has been shown to improve sleep duration and reduce sleep latency in Alzheimer's patients [83]. There is also some weak evidence that melatonin may be beneficial in treating ISWRD in children with psychomotor retardation [84].

There have been several reports of the successful use of melatonin in treating sleep problems in children with neurodevelopmental disorders (including a large UK-based randomized controlled trial: the MENDS trial) [85].

In these studies, escalating doses of melatonin (0.5–to 12—mg before bedtime) resulted in an increase in sleep duration and a shortening of sleep latency (by up to 45 minutes). Although it is unclear whether the underlying sleep problems are circadian in nature, these findings are noteworthy as melatonin is prescribed for these children in the UK.

Structured physical and social activity, the improvement of sleep hygiene (by reducing nighttime light exposure and noise and controlling bedroom temperature), and informing patients and caregivers on sleep changes in dementia have all been shown to be beneficial for the treatment of ISWRD, particularly in conjunction with light therapy [86,87].

Recommended treatment for ISWRD is an increase in the strength of the daily light–dark cycle (primarily by means of morning/daytime light therapy). Scheduled exercise and social activity together with improved sleep hygiene are also effective, particularly in conjunction with light therapy. There is limited evidence that melatonin (in conjunction with light therapy) may be effective in treating ISWRD.

References

1. American Academy of Sleep Medicine. International classification of sleep disorders, 3rd ed. Darien, IL: American Academy of Sleep Medicine.
2. Khalsa SBS, Jewett ME, Cajochen C, Czeisler CA. A phase response curve to single bright light pulses in human subjects. J Physiol 2003;549(3):945–52.
3. Lewy AJ, Ahmed S, Jackson JM, Sack RL. Melatonin shifts human circadian rhythms according to a phase-response curve. Chronobiol Int 1992;9(5):380–92.
4. Morgenthaler TI, Lee-Chiong T, Alessi C, et al. Practice parameters for the clinical evaluation and treatment of circadian rhythm sleep disorders. An American Academy of Sleep Medicine report. Sleep 2007;30(11):1445–59.
5. Arendt J. Managing jet lag: some of the problems and possible new solutions. Sleep Med Rev 2009;13(4):249–56.
6. Wirz-Justice A, Benedetti FF, Terman M. Chronotherapeutics for affective disorders: a clinician's manual for light and wake therapy. Basel: Karger, 2009.
7. Reid KJ, Chang AM, Dubocovich ML, et al. Familial advanced sleep phase syndrome. Arch Neurol 2001;58(7):1089–94.
8. Jones CR, Campbell SS, Zone SE, et al. Familial advanced sleep-phase syndrome: a short-period circadian rhythm variant in humans. Nat Med 1999;5(9):1062–5.
9. Toh KL. An hPer2 phosphorylation site mutation in familial advanced sleep phase syndrome. Science 2001;291(5506):1040–3.
10. Archer SN, Robilliard DL, Skene DJ, et al. A length polymorphism in the circadian clock gene Per3 is linked to delayed sleep phase syndrome and extreme diurnal preference. Sleep 2003;26(4):413–15.
11. Carpen JD, Schantz M, Smits M, Skene DJ, Archer SN. A silent polymorphism in the PER1 gene associates with extreme diurnal preference in humans. J Hum Genet 2006;51(12):1122–5.
12. Brennan KC, Bates EA, Shapiro RE, et al. Casein kinase I mutations in familial migraine and advanced sleep phase. Sci Transl Med 2013;5(183):183ra56–6.
13. Novakova M, Nevšímalová S, Příhodová I, SlAdek M, Sumova A. Alteration of the circadian clock in children with Smith–Magenis syndrome. J Clin Endocrinol Metab 2012;97(2):E312–18.
14. Sack RL, Auckley D, Auger RR, et al. Circadian rhythm sleep disorders: part II, advanced sleep phase disorder, delayed sleep phase disorder, free-running disorder, and irregular sleep–wake rhythm. An American Academy of Sleep Medicine review. Sleep 2007;30(11):1484–501.
15. Van Someren EJW. Actigraphic monitoring of sleep and circadian rhythms. In: Montagna P, Chokroverty S, eds. Handbook of clinical neurology, vol 98. Sleep disorders. Amsterdam: Elsevier B.V., 2011:55–63.
16. Roenneberg T, Kuehnle T, Pramstaller PP, et al. A marker for the end of adolescence. Curr Biol 2004;14(24):R1038–9.
17. Horne JG, Ostberg O. A self-assessment questionnaire to determine morningness–eveningness in human circadian rhythms. Int J Chronobiol 1976;4:97–110.
18. Lack L, Wright J. The effect of evening bright light in delaying the circadian rhythms and lengthening the sleep of early morning awakening insomniacs. Sleep 1993;16(5):436–43.
19. Lack L, Wright J, Kemp K, Gibbon S. The treatment of early-morning awakening insomnia with 2 evenings of bright light. Sleep 2005;28(5):616–23.
20. Munch M, Scheuermaier KD, Zhang R, et al. Effects on subjective and objective alertness and sleep in response to evening light exposure in older subjects. Behav Brain Res 2011;224(2):272–8.
21. Palmer CR, Kripke DF, Savage HC, et al. Efficacy of enhanced evening light for advanced sleep phase syndrome. Behav Sleep Med 2002;1(4):213–26.
22. Suhner AG, Murphy PJ, Campbell SS. Failure of timed bright light exposure to alleviate age-related sleep maintenance insomnia. J Am Geriatr Soc 2002;50(4):617–23.
23. Moldofsky H, Musisi S, Phililipson EA. Treatment of a case of advanced sleep phase syndrome by phase advance chronotherapy. Sleep 1986;9:61–5.
24. Weitzman ED, Czeisler CA, Coleman RM, et al. Delayed sleep phase syndrome. A chronobiological disorder with sleep-onset insomnia. Arch Gen Psychiatry 1981;38(7):737–46.
25. Czeisler CA, Richardson GS, Coleman RM, et al. Chronotherapy: resetting the circadian clocks of patients with delayed sleep phase insomnia. Sleep 1981;4(1):1–21.
26. Micic G, de Bruyn A, Lovato N, et al. The endogenous circadian temperature period length (tau) in delayed sleep phase disorder compared to good sleepers. J Sleep Res 2013;22(6):617–24.
27. Aoki H, Ozeki Y, Yamada N. Hypersensitivity of melatonin suppression in response to light in patients with delayed sleep phase syndrome. Chronobiol Int 2001;18:263–71.
28. Ancoli-Israel S, Schnierow B, Kelsoe J, Fink R. A pedigree of one family with delayed sleep phase syndrome. Chronobiol Int 2001;18(5):831–40.
29. Ebisawa T, Uchiyama M, Kajimura N, et al. Association of structural polymorphisms in the human period3 gene with delayed sleep phase syndrome. EMBO Rep 2001;2(4):342–6.
30. Archer SN, Carpen JD, Gibson M, et al. Polymorphism in the PER3 promoter associates with diurnal preference and delayed sleep phase disorder. Sleep 2010;33(5):695.
31. Hida A, Kitamura S, Katayose Y, et al. Screening of Clock gene polymorphisms demonstrates association of a PER3 polymorphism with morningness–eveningness preference and circadian rhythm sleep disorder. Sci Rep 2014;4:6309.
32. Mishima K, Tozawa T, Satoh K, Saitoh H, Mishima Y. The 3111T/C polymorphism of hClock is associated with evening preference and delayed sleep timing in a Japanese population sample. Am J Med Genet 2005;133B(1):101–4.
33. Parsons MJ, Lester KJ, Barclay NL, et al. Polymorphisms in the circadian expressed genes PER3 and ARNTL2 are associated with diurnal preference and GNβ3 with sleep measures. J Sleep Res 2014;23(5):595–604.
34. Arroll B, Fernando A, Falloon K, et al. Prevalence of causes of insomnia in primary care: a cross-sectional study. Br J Gen Pract 2012;62(595):e99–103.
35. Schrader H, Bovim G, Sand T. The prevalence of delayed and advanced sleep phase syndromes. J Sleep Res 1993;2(1):51–5.

36. Paine SJ, Gander PH, Travier N. The epidemiology of morningness/eveningness: influence of age, gender, ethnicity, and socioeconomic factors in adults (30–49 years). J Biol Rhythm 2006;21(1):68–76.

37. Dagan Y, Eisenstein M. Circadian rhythm sleep disorders: toward a more precise definition and diagnosis. Chronobiol Int 1999;16(2):213–22.

38. Rhee MK, Lee H-J, Rex KM, Kripke DF. Evaluation of two circadian rhythm questionnaires for screening for the delayed sleep phase disorder. Psychiatry Invest 2012;9(3):236.

39. Rosenthal NE, Joseph-Vanderpool JR, Levendosky AA, et al. Phase-shifting effects of bright morning light as treatment for delayed sleep phase syndrome. Sleep 1990;13(4):354–61.

40. Cole RJ, Smith JS, Alcal YC, Elliott JA, Kripke DF. Bright-light mask treatment of delayed sleep phase syndrome. J Biol Rhythm 2002;17(1):89–101.

41. Warman VL, Dijk DJ, Warman GR, Arendt J, Skene DJ. Phase advancing human circadian rhythms with short wavelength light. Neurosci Lett 2003;342(1–2):37–40.

42. Arendt J, Bojkowski C, Folkard S, et al. Some effects of melatonin and the control of its secretion in humans. Ciba Foundation Symp 1985;117:266–83.

43. Dahlitz M, Alvarez B, Vignau J, et al. Delayed sleep phase syndrome response to melatonin. Lancet 1991;337(8750):1121–4.

44. Mundey K, Benloucif S, Harsanyi K, Dubocovich ML, Zee PC. Phase-dependent treatment of delayed sleep phase syndrome with melatonin. Sleep 2005;28(10):1271–8.

45. Dagan Y, Yovel I, Hallis D, Eisenstein M, Raichik I. Evaluating the role of melatonin in the long-term treatment of delayed sleep phase syndrome (DSPS). Chronobiol Int 1998;15(2):181–90.

46. Arendt J, Skene DJ. Special considerations for the treatment of circadian rhythm sleep disorders. In: Kushida CA, ed. Handbook of sleep disorders, 2nd ed. London: Informa Healthcare, 2008:207–22.

47. Revell VL, Burgess HJ, Gazda CJ, et al. Advancing human circadian rhythms with afternoon melatonin and morning intermittent bright light. J Clin Endocrinol Metab 2006;91(1):54–9.

48. Samaranayake CB, Fernando A, Warman G. Outcome of combined melatonin and bright light treatments for delayed sleep phase disorder. Aust N Z J Psychiatry 2010;44(7):676.

49. Saxvig IW, Wilhelmsen-Langeland A, Pallesen S, et al. A randomized controlled trial with bright light and melatonin for delayed sleep phase disorder: effects on subjective and objective sleep. Chronobiol Int 2014;31(1):72–86.

50. Wilhelmsen-Langeland A, Saxvig IW, Pallesen S, et al. A randomized controlled trial with bright light and melatonin for the treatment of delayed sleep phase disorder: effects on subjective and objective sleepiness and cognitive function. J Biol Rhythm 2013;28 (5):306–21.

51. Sharkey KM, Carskadon MA, Figueiro MG, Zhu Y, Rea MS. Effects of an advanced sleep schedule and morning short wavelength light exposure on circadian phase in young adults with late sleep schedules. Sleep Med 2011;12(7):685–92.

52. Gradisar M, Dohnt H, Gardner G, et al. A randomized controlled trial of cognitive-behavior therapy plus bright light therapy for adolescent delayed sleep phase disorder. Sleep 2011;34(12):1671–80.

53. Lockley S, Tabandeh H, Skene D, et al. Day-time naps and melatonin in blind people. Lancet 1995;346(8988):1491.

54. Lockley SW, Arendt J, Skene DJ. Visual impairment and circadian rhythm disorders. Dialog Clin Neurosci 2006;9(3):301–14.

55. Lockley SW, Skene DJ, Tabandeh H, et al. Relationship between napping and melatonin in the blind. J Biol Rhythm 1997;12(1):16–25.

56. Tabandeh H, Lockley SW, Buttery R, et al. Disturbance of sleep in blindness. Am J Ophthalmol 1998;126(5):707–12.

57. Leger D, Guilleminault C, Defrance R, Domont A, Paillard M. Prevalence of sleep/wake disorders in persons with blindness. Clin Sci 1999;97(2):193–9.

58. Warman GR, Pawley MDM, Bolton C, et al. Circadian-related sleep disorders and sleep medication use in the New Zealand blind population: an observational prevalence survey. PLoS ONE 2011;6(7):e22073.

59. Leger D, Guilleminault C, Defrance R, Domont A, Paillard M. Blindness and sleep patterns. Lancet 1996;348(9030):830–1.

60. Flynn-Evans EE, Tabandeh H, Skene DJ, Lockley SW. Circadian rhythm disorders and melatonin production in 127 blind women with and without light perception. J Biol Rhythm 2014;29(3):215–24.

61. Lockley SWS, Skene DJD, Arendt JJ, et al. Relationship between melatonin rhythms and visual loss in the blind. J Clin Endocrinol Metab 1997;82(11):3763–70.

62. Kennaway DJ, Van Dorp CF. Free-running rhythms of melatonin, cortisol, electrolytes, and sleep in humans in Antarctica. Am J Physiol 1991;260(6 Pt 2):R1137–44.

63. Arendt J. Biological rhythms during residence in polar regions. Chronobiol Int 2012;29(4):379–94.

64. Gibbs M, Hampton S, Morgan L, Arendt J. Predicting circadian response to abrupt phase shift: 6-sulphatoxymelatonin rhythms in rotating shift workers offshore. J Biol Rhythm 2007;22(4):368–70.

65. Duffy JF, Wright KP Jr. Entrainment of the human circadian system by light. J Biol Rhythm 2005;20(4):326–38.

66. Young D, Nagarajan L, de Klerk N, et al. Sleep problems in Rett syndrome. Brain Dev 2007;29(10):609–16.

67. Takaesu Y, Komada Y, Inoue Y. Melatonin profile and its relation to circadian rhythm sleep disorders in Angelman syndrome patients. Sleep Med 2012;13(9):1164–70.

68. Sack RL, Lewy AJ, Blood ML, Keith LD, Nakagawa H. Circadian rhythm abnormalities in totally blind people: incidence and clinical significance. J Clin Endocrinol Metab 1992;75(1):127–34.

69. Klein T, Martens H, Dijk DJ, et al. Circadian sleep regulation in the absence of light perception: chronic non-24-hour circadian rhythm sleep disorder in a blind man with a regular 24-hour sleep–wake schedule. Sleep 1993;16(4):333–43.

70. Hack LM, Lockley SW, Arendt J, Skene DJ. The effects of low-dose 0.5-mg melatonin on the free-running circadian rhythms of blind subjects. J Biol Rhythm 2003;18(5):420–9.

71. Lockley SW, Skene DJ, James K, Thapan K, JJ W, Arendt J. Melatonin administration can entrain the free-running circadian system of blind subjects. J Endocrinol 2000;164(1):R1–6.

72. Sack RL, Brandes RW, Kendall AR, Lewy AJ. Entrainment of free-running circadian rhythms by melatonin in blind people. N Engl J Med 2000;343(15):1070–7.

73. Deacon S, Arendt J. Melatonin-induced temperature suppression and its acute phase-shifting effects correlate in a dose-dependent manner in humans. Brain Res 1995;688(1):77–85.

74. Arendt J, Skene DJ. Melatonin as a chronobiotic. Sleep Med Rev 2005;9(1):25–39.

75. Weber AL, Cary MS, Connor N, Keyes P. Human non-24-hour sleep–wake cycles in an everyday environment. Sleep 1980;2(3):347–54.

76. Zee PC, Vitiello MV. Circadian rhythm sleep disorder: irregular sleep wake rhythm. Clin Sleep Med 2009;4(2):213–18.

77. Van Someren EJ, Hagebeuk EE, Lijzenga C, et al. Circadian rest–activity rhythm disturbances in Alzheimer's disease. Biol Psychiatry 1996;40(4):259–70.

78. Martin JL, Webber AP, Alam T, et al. Daytime sleeping, sleep disturbance, and circadian rhythms in the nursing home. Am J Geriatr Psychiatry 2006;14(2):121–9.

79. Zee PC, Attarian H, Videnovic A. Circadian rhythm abnormalities. Continuum (Minneap Minn) 2013;19(1 Sleep Disorders):132–47.

80. Van Someren EJW. Improving actigraphic sleep estimates in insomnia and dementia: how many nights? J Sleep Res 2007;16(3):269–75.

81. Van Someren EJ, Swaab DF, Colenda CC, et al. Bright light therapy: improved sensitivity to its effects on rest–activity rhythms in Alzheimer patients by application of nonparametric methods. Chronobiol Int 1999;16(4):505–18.

82. Guilleminault C, McCann CC, Quera-Salva M, Cetel M. Light therapy as treatment of dyschronosis in brain impaired children. Eur J Pediatr 1993;152(9):754–9.

83. Riemersma-Van Der Lek RF, Swaab DF, Twisk J, et al. Effect of bright light and melatonin on cognitive and noncognitive function in elderly residents of group care facilities: a randomized controlled trial. JAMA 2008;299(22):2642–55.

84. Pillar G, Shahar E, Peled N, et al. Melatonin improves sleep–wake patterns in psychomotor retarded children. Pediatr Neurol 2000;23(3):225–8.

85. Gringras P, Gamble C, Jones AP, et al. Melatonin for sleep problems in children with neurodevelopmental disorders: randomised double masked placebo controlled trial. BMJ 2012;345:e6664–4.

86. McCurry SM, Gibbons LE, Logsdon RG, Vitiello MV, Teri L. Nighttime insomnia treatment and education for Alzheimer's disease: a randomized, controlled trial. J Am Geriatr Soc 2005;53(5):793–802.

87. Schnelle JF, Cruise PA, Alessi CA, et al. Sleep hygiene in physically dependent nursing home residents: behavioral and environmental intervention implications. Sleep 1998;21(5):515–23.

Sleep neurology

CHAPTER 23

Sleep-related movement disorders

Alessandro Gradassi and Federica Provini

Introduction

Sleep-related movement disorders are conditions characterized by simple and usually stereotyped movements. They disturb sleep's physiological occurrence and must entail (by definition) either daytime sleepiness or fatigue as consequence of their presence, owing to the continuous interruptions of the sleep cycle [1]. The category also includes other sleep-related monophasic movement disorders, such as sleep-related leg cramps [1].

Some movements, such as bruxism, might occur during both wakefulness and sleep, but a clear worsening of the symptoms during sleep is necessary in order to include the condition among sleep-related movement disorders [1]. Like other movements, such as sleep starts (hypnic jerks), sleep-related movement disorders might occasionally be present in healthy individuals. Setting a dividing line between normal and pathological is very difficult in such cases.

Once it has been determined that the patient suffers from a sleep-related movement disorder, the patient's age and the part of the body involved provide an idea about which movement disorder might be affecting them. In some cases, following these clues, it is possible to make a clinical diagnosis, while in some others, the use of all-night polysomnography with synchronized video recording (video-polysomnography, VPSG) is necessary to describe properly the neurophysiological features of the phenomenon, the time and the stage of occurrence during the night, and the patient's level of consciousness in order to reach a correct diagnosis.

Sleep-related movement disorders must be distinguished from parasomnias, such as sleepwalking or REM sleep behavior disorder (RBD), which normally show complex muscular patterns and complex behaviors that may appear purposeful, although they may be unconscious too.

This chapter describes the conditions classified as sleep-related movement disorders, excluding restless legs syndrome (RLS), which is dealt with in Chapter 24 of this volume.

Periodic limb movement disorder

Periodic limb movement disorder (PLMD) is characterized by periodic episodes of repetitive, highly stereotyped limb movements that occur during sleep (PLMS: see the next paragraph) and by clinical sleep disturbance that cannot be accounted for by another primary sleep disorder [1].

Periodic limb movements (PLM) are involuntary muscular contractions that occur periodically about every 20–30 s and involve the limbs, most often the lower ones. They usually consist of a toe extension with foot dorsiflexion and despite occurring mostly while asleep (periodic limb movements during sleep, PLMS), they also take place while awake (periodic limb movements of wakefulness, PLMW). PLMS were first clinically reported by Symonds in 1953, who described a patient, among five patients with different diseases, with jerks during relaxed wakefulness and sleep, and coined the term "nocturnal myoclonus" [2]. Some years later, Lugaresi and Coccagna first recorded and defined PLMS polysomnographically using the term "nocturnal myoclonus" in Symonds' honor [3]. Subsequently, Coleman suggested the term "periodic movements in sleep" [4], which was then substituted by "periodic limb movements in sleep," to emphasize the observation that arms may be involved as well.

Epidemiology

The prevalence of PLMS varies between 2% and 15% in the general population [5–7]. The simultaneous presence of PLMS and sleep complaints (periodic limb movement disorder) [1] had a prevalence of 3.9% in a large epidemiological study [8]. PLMS are less common in children [9–11] and their prevalence increases with age; this includes patients not affected by sleep disturbances [12–17]. The prevalence of PLMS reaches 80% in patients with other medical and neurological diseases, the first among which is RLS, where PLMS prevalence can reach about 95% [18,19] of RLS patients. An elevated prevalence of PLMS can be found among patients with other sleep disorders such as narcolepsy [20] and in elderly patients with hypersomnia [12]. PLMS may be seen in obstructive sleep apnea (OSAS), and in cases of severe OSAS, PLMS may become more noticeable during the continuous positive airway pressure (CPAP) treatment [21,22]. There may be an increased prevalence of PLMS in patients with RBD. In a study of 40 RBD patients, 70% exhibited PLMS, which were also seen during REM sleep [23]. Several studies have documented PLMS in patients with various non-sleep-related disorders (eg, essential hypertension, migraine, and end-stage renal disease), but the significance of the reported data remains undetermined [6].

Clinical aspects and polysomnographic features

PLM represent a heterogeneous motor phenomenon. In their simplest and most common form, they consist of periodic extensions of the big toe and/or the foot. When the phenomenon becomes more intense and diffuse, there may be knee and hip flexion. Sometimes,

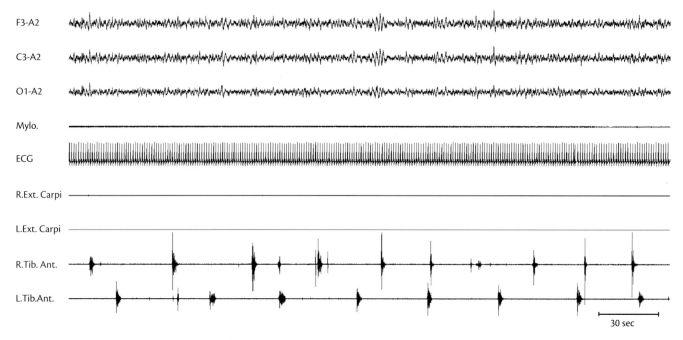

Fig. 23.1 Periodic limb movements during sleep (PLMS). Polygraph recording of PLMS during stage 2 NREM sleep. EMG bursts on the tibialis anterior muscles occur with a characteristic periodicity showing different patterns of muscular contraction. Mylo.: mylohyoideus; Ext.: extensor; Tib. Ant.: tibialis anterior; R.: right; L.: left.

the forearm may also flex at the elbow. PLM may begin with one or repeated myoclonic jerks, followed, after a short pause, by a tonic contraction, or it may consist of a single prolonged tonic contraction (Fig. 23.1). PLM may affect only one or both legs; more often, both extremities are involved, but usually not symmetrically or simultaneously. Sometimes the phenomenon alternates in each leg (Figs. 23.1 and 23.2). According to standard criteria, PLMS must occur in series of four or more consecutive movements, split by an inter-movement interval of at least 5 seconds and a maximum of 90 seconds (from onset to onset) [24,25]. The duration of each PLMS may last between 0.5 and 10 s. PLMS are polygraphically scored only when the amplitude of the EMG activation exceeds 8 μV; the activation ends when the EMG amplitude falls below 2 μV.

The number of PLMS per hour of sleep constitutes the PLMS Index (PLMSI). A PLMSI greater than 5 was formerly considered pathological, but more recently, many authors, taking account of age-related effects and night-to-night variations, have accepted a PLMSI greater than 15 as pathological in adults [1,26]. Because of

the evident limitations of the PLMI for the description and evaluation of PLMS, especially with regard to their presence in different neurological and medical conditions and to the response to treatment, new parameters have been described. The Periodicity Index (PI), a sophisticated, automatic method developed to describe the time structure of limb movement activity [27,28]. The PI value ranges from 0 to 1, where 0 indicates a total absence of periodicity, and 1 complete periodicity [29]. PI is higher in RLS patients and lower in patients with RBD, probably reflecting differences in the mechanisms involved in the generation of these different conditions. PLMS can also be described in terms of the time distribution of limb movement throughout the night, which, in general, is not uniform, and is also linked to the co-presence of other disturbances [30]. PLMS, alone or associated with RLS, mostly manifest themselves after falling asleep, in the first half of the night, and then decrease dramatically toward the morning [31–33]. In addition, sleep stages are known to modulate PLMS frequency and periodicity, at least in patients with RLS, occurring mainly during stages 1

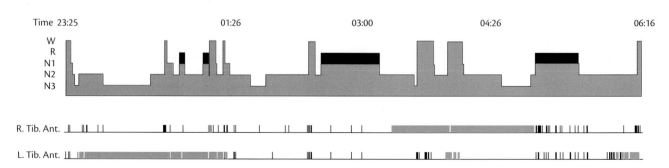

Fig. 23.2 PLMS. Evolution throughout the night (upper trace) of severe nocturnal myoclonus (lower traces) in a 62-year-old man. The jerks are present during relaxed wakefulness before sleep onset and in infra-sleep wakefulness. PLMS persist during all sleep stages, affecting in particular the left leg (L. Tib. Ant.: left tibialis anterior) in the first part of the night and then the right leg (R. Tib. Ant.: right tibialis anterior) in the last part of the night.

and 2 of NREM sleep and decreasing with deepening sleep stage [34,35]. Even in subjects with only PLMS, the limb movements show a circadian rhythm, peaking at sleep onset, preceding the evening rise in melatonin secretion [36].

PLMS may be associated with EEG arousals or microarousals [35], or with pure autonomic activation alone, in the absence of an EEG arousal as defined by the ASDA criteria [37]. Spectral EEG and heart rate analyses have revealed a wide variety of complex and stereotyped variations in cortical activity and heart rate associated with PLMS. These include increases in heart rate and in alpha, theta, and delta power in the EEG [38–40]. The concomitant cerebral and autonomic responses before and during PLMS suggest that these do not trigger cardiac and EEG activation but are part of the entire arousal response, which recruits several neural networks from the brainstem up to the cortical level [41,42].

Clinical relevance

It is still debated whether isolated PLMS have a clinical meaning or not, and whether PLMS alone, without the complaint of non-restorative sleep or associated daytime symptoms, in the absence of other sleep disorders, may be an independent cause of sleep disturbances [6]. Subjects with PLMS may or may not be aware of the movements, and the complaints might be referred by the bed partner only. Moreover, it is common experience that PLMS could be only an incidental finding during a VPSG recording, not being responsible for any clinical sleep–wake consequence. On the other hand, the hypothesis of a direct pathological role of PLMS disruption is weakened by the observation that pramipexole can suppress PLMS without affecting arousals [43]. No correlation has been found among PLMSI, arousals, and sleep structure in patients with insomnia/hypersomnia [44,45], and in many cases, despite treatment of PLMS, no improvement in daytime sleepiness was noted. Some authors support the view that PLMS may cause insomnia, but only when correlated with a corresponding EEG arousal, and the lack of an arousal indicates that these may be a normal sleep characteristic [46]. Owing to autonomic activation associated with PLMS, especially in patients with RLS but also in controls, resulting in increases in heart rate and blood pressure, an intimate relationship among RLS/PLMS on the one hand and hypertension, heart disease, stroke, and increasing mortality in patients with renal failure on the other has been described, but the causality is far from established [47–54].

Pathophysiology

The exact pathophysiology of PLMS is still unknown. A cortical origin seems unlikely, in the absence of a cortical prepotential in EEG–EMG back-averaging, and the absence of a Bereitschaftspotential before PLMS indicates that PLMS are not voluntarily generated [55]. Studies with functional magnetic resonance imaging (fMRI) indicate activation of the brainstem but not the cerebral cortex during PLMS [56]. The fact that PLMS almost never involve the face suggests that the generator of PLMS is below the level of the facial nucleus in the brainstem. The existence of PLMS in patients with a complete spinal cord lesion, such as during spinal anesthesia or as a result of spinal transection, indicates that the generator may be in the spinal cord [57,58]. The peripheral nervous system theory has not been abandoned yet, mainly because of the presence of small-fiber neuropathy in some RLS patients often coexisting with PLMS, but it is still an unresolved question whether the peripheral

dysfunction triggers PLMS or is simply coincidental. Moreover, direct repetitive electrical stimulation [59] of the peroneal nerve during sleep triggers a tonic contraction similar to what was previously called nocturnal myoclonus, and modifies the rhythm of the spontaneously occurring phenomenon, suggesting that PLMS are in some way triggered by a sensory input [59]. Studies aimed at finding the muscle recruitment patterns in PLMS have shown that leg muscles are most frequently involved, with no hierarchical order and no caudal or rostral propagation typical of propriospinal myoclonus, suggesting the engagement of different, independent, and sometimes unsynchronized generators. Taken together, all these data suggest that the spinal cord hyperexcitability is induced by supraspinal factors, changing with sleep phases acting as trigger for PLMS [60,61].

A pathogenetic role for the dopaminergic system is certainly plausible, but still controversial. The results of neuroimaging studies, improvement of symptoms with dopaminergic drugs, and the coexistence of PLMS with conditions such as RLS and Parkinson's disease where a dopaminergic dysfunction has been postulated would support such a theory [6].

Recently PLMS, together with RLS, has been demonstrated to have a genetic risk factor based on a significant genomewide association study with a common variant of *BTBD9* on chromosome 6p21.2 for PLMS in patients with or without RLS, but no such association has been found in RLS patients without PLMS [62].

Differential diagnosis

PLMS have to be differentiated from other sleep motor manifestations that might mimic leg movements, since the legs are mainly involved in almost every sleep-related movement disorder. The characteristics of the muscular contraction, its distribution, and its periodic pattern make recognition of PLMS on polygraphic recordings quite simple. In some cases, VPSG study could be mandatory to allow a correct diagnosis to be made. *Sleep starts* are physiological, consisting of sudden jerks of trunk and extremities occurring on falling asleep or during light sleep [1]. *Propriospinal myoclonus* is a type of spinal myoclonus characterized by rhythmic or arrhythmic spontaneous contraction of the axial muscles, usually spreading to limb muscles [63]. Propriospinal myoclonus may arise at sleep onset and disappear during sleep [64]. Excessive *fragmentary myoclonus* is characterized by short and nonperiodic muscle potentials (10–100 ms), that often do not end with any distal movement but when intensified may disrupt sleep [65]. Further differential diagnosis must include *nocturnal leg cramps* (see the next section) and *alternating leg muscle activation (ALMA)*, in which a single contraction of one leg alternates with a similar contraction of the other leg, occurring in all sleep stages at a frequency of 0.5–3 Hz, each lasting for 0.1–0.5 s in sequences of at least four ALMAs [1].

Treatment

Before describing the management of PLMS, it is necessary to reiterate that PLMS that do not disturb the patient's sleep and therefore do not represent any clinical issue are not to be treated [66]. PLMS are treated only when the patient reports sleep complaints and when other sleep disorders, likely to be responsible for them, have been ruled out. It should be noted that several medications (eg, selective serotonin reuptake inhibitors (SSRIs), tricyclic antidepressants, and neuroleptics) have also been reported to worsen PLMS, so a drug history must be taken before any treatment [6,67–69].

There is insufficient evidence to comment on the role of pharmacological therapies in isolated PLMD, because most trials have been open studies including small patient groups. Many of the studies in RLS patients involving dopaminergic medications (eg, pramipexole, ropinirole, and rotigotine) demonstrated statistically significant decreases in PLMS. In addition, gabapentin (300–2400 mg/daily), pregabalin (150–600 mg/daily), and valproate (125–600 mg/daily) have also been shown to decrease PLM indices in subjects with RLS. Oxycodone decreases both the number of PLMS and arousals [66,67]; lamotrigine (100 mg/daily), melatonin (3 mg, 30 min before bedtime), and bupropion have shown a positive effect, reducing PLMS and sleep fragmentation [6,66,67].

Nocturnal leg cramps

Nocturnal leg cramps are sudden and painful contractions of the calf muscles, sometimes also accompanied by contractions of the intrinsic muscles of the feet. They occur during sleep or while at rest, are usually unilateral, and last from a few seconds up to as many as 10 minutes [70–72]. When they occur during sleep, the patient wakes up suddenly owing to the painful sensation felt in the leg. Massage, movement, or heat usually relieves the pain, but a residual tenderness can persist for up to half an hour. Cramps can occur at any age, but tend to be more common in middle-aged and older people. Between 20% and 25% of adults have experienced leg cramps, especially those over 80 years [71,72]. Leg cramps can be either idiopathic or secondary to systemic or focal pathological conditions [73]. They are most commonly noted in otherwise healthy individuals after excessive physical exercise. Some authors have hypothesized that the lack of repetitive leg squatting to stretch the leg tendons and muscles, typical of our "civilized" lifestyle, results in the occurrence of these cramps [74,75].

Leg cramps may be triggered by peripheral vascular diseases, prolonged standing, and varicose veins. The high prevalence of cramps among patients with neurological disorders, such as parkinsonism and peripheral neuropathy, suggests a possible association with nerve dysfunction or damage [76]. Leg cramps may arise in pregnancy and some medical conditions, including electrolyte disturbances such as uremia, diabetes, thyroid diseases, hypomagnesemia, hypocalcemia, hyperphosphatemia, hypokalemia, and hyponatremia. The cramps in these conditions may occur predominantly or exclusively during sleep. Also, certain drugs may trigger leg cramps, eg, β-agonists, calcium antagonists, potassium-sparing diuretics, thiazide-like and loop diuretics, steroids, lithium, and statins [77]. About 60% of patients with cirrhosis of liver also complain of leg cramps [78]. There has also been a report of familial nocturnal leg cramping with an autosomal dominant inheritance [79].

Polysomnographic recordings are useful to clarify the nature of leg cramps, which may occur during any sleep stage, and to determine whether each cramp is associated with an awakening. According to the American Academy of Sleep Medicine [1], the diagnostic criteria for sleep-related leg cramps are as follows: (A) a painful sensation in the leg or foot is associated with sudden muscle hardness or tightness, indicating strong muscle contraction; (B) the painful muscle contractions in the legs or feet occur during the sleep period, although they may arise from either wakefulness or sleep; (C) the pain is relieved by forceful stretching of the affected muscles, releasing the contraction.

Muscle strain, dystonias, ischemic or neuropathic claudication, and nerve root disease might mimic leg cramps. Myopathic and neuropathic conditions are usually characterized by muscle cramps, generally during the day and not just at nighttime and not exclusively involving the legs. It is important not to confound nocturnal leg cramps with other motor disturbances that may occur during sleep, such as PLMS and RLS, sleep starts, painful legs and moving toes syndrome persisting during sleep, and excessive fragmentary myoclonus. However, the clinical features of nocturnal leg cramps are distinctive, and polysomnography is rarely necessary. No treatment has been proven to be both safe and effective against leg cramps. Quinine sulfate (200–325 mg) before bedtime has shown a modest benefit, but the clinician must be aware of the serious risk of its hepatic, blood, and renal toxicity [80]. The evidence of benefit from other therapies is insufficient or conflicting. Magnesium citrate, potassium, gabapentin, and botulinum toxin may also be effective, as may multivitamin supplementation with vitamins E and C, especially in patients with cramps during hemodialysis. Sodium supplementation also improves the symptoms, but there is a potential risk of hypertension. Gastrocnemius stretching and deep tissue massages have long been suggested as therapies against leg cramps, but a systematic review has found limited evidence for the use of nonpharmacological treatment for leg muscle cramps [81].

Sleep bruxism

Sleep bruxism (SB) is characterized by grinding or clenching teeth during sleep [1]. It is produced by either phasic or tonic muscle activity in jaw-closing muscles associated with tooth-grinding sounds [82–84]. Series of phasic muscle contractions, termed rhythmic masticatory muscle activity (RMMA), are present in about 60% of people at a frequency of about two times per hour of sleep without tooth grinding [85]. The exaggerated occurrence of RMMA is characteristic of patients with SB (Fig. 23.3).

In contrast to normal subjects, sleep bruxers have more episodes of RMMA, more bursts per episode, and bursts of larger amplitude and shorter duration [85]. Most people brux at some period during their lives, but most are unaware of their behavior. Bruxism does not usually interrupt the patient's sleep, but it can be a problem for the bed partner owing to the noise caused. These factors have led to discrepancies in the reported prevalence of bruxism, namely around 8% in the healthy adult population, with a linear decrease with age [86]. The incidence of bruxism is thought to be highest between the second and fifth decades of life, without a gender dominance. Many childhood bruxers stop doing so by their teens, although self-reported bruxism appears to increase between adolescence and young adulthood [87]. The repetitive nocturnal clenching may be associated with muscle and joint pain, temporal headache, tooth damage, and hypersensitivity of the teeth to cold liquids or air.

Bruxism, whether occurring during wakefulness or sleep, is classified into primary, secondary, or iatrogenic [84]. SB is classified as secondary sleep bruxism if associated with medical, psychiatric, or neurological disorders, including sleep disorders associated either with drug administration or with withdrawal from a number of medications (antidopaminergic drugs, SSRIs, and calcium antagonists) and recreational substances (alcohol, caffeine, cigarettes, cocaine, and amphetamine) (Table 23.1). Anxiety and vulnerability

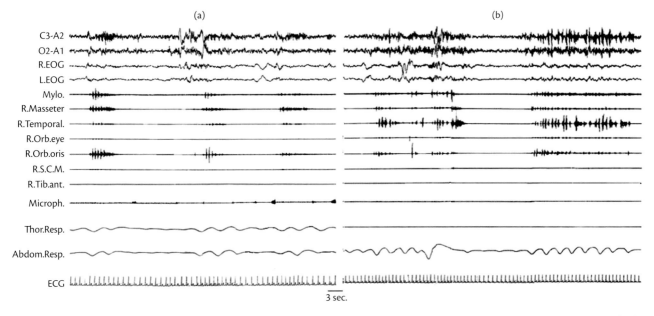

Fig. 23.3 Rhythmic masticatory muscle activity. Polysomnographic excerpts (a and b) showing clusters of myoclonic jerks and tonic activity involving the orofacial, masticatory and cervical muscles during REM sleep. EOG: electro-oculogram; Mylo: mylohyoideus; Temporal.: temporalis; Orb.: orbicularis; S.C.M.:sternocleidomastoideus; Tib. Ant.: tibialis anterior; Microph.: microphone; Thor.: thoracic; Abdom.: abdominal; Resp.: respirogram; R.: right; L.: left.

to psychosomatic disorders are common findings among patients with bruxism, although the contribution of these factors has not yet been fully established [84]. The real nature of the pathophysiology of bruxism is still debated, but two main theories have been proposed: a peripheral one, based on the assumption that malocclusion triggers masticatory activity, and a central theory, supporting a loss of cortical or basal ganglial inhibition of brainstem motor generators as the main cause of bruxism [82]. The relationship between SB and chronic use of medications with antidopaminergic properties suggests that the CNS dopaminergic system plays a role. Additionally, genetic factors appear to play an important role in the generation of bruxism in both children and adults.

The diagnosis of SB aims to demonstrate the presence of tooth grinding, since this is the pathognomonic feature of sleep bruxism. The patient interview investigates the patient's awareness of jaw clenching, the presence of pain in the jaw muscles, temporomandibular dysfunction, tooth damage or fracture, the possible presence of headache on waking up in the morning, or excessive daytime sleepiness. Clinical examination includes examination of the head and neck muscles to identify the presence of contingent masseter hypertrophy as an indicator of a clenching habit, rule out temporomandibular disorders, and estimate the jaw opening and lateral mobility, and examination of the oral mucosa to search for tooth grooving or ridging on the side of the tongue and on the cheeks, suggesting a concomitant oral habit. Video-polygraphic monitoring in bruxism demonstrates increased masseter and temporalis muscle activity during sleep, along with grinding sounds, especially during stages 1 and 2 of NREM sleep. Sleep bruxism is established in the presence of tooth grinding noise, associated with at least three EMG events, or with a burst lasting 0.5 s or more, or with one contraction lasting 2 s or more. The confirmed episodes are classified by patterns into phasic events (three or more bursts), tonic-sustained events (one episode lasting more than 2 s), or mixed events (showing both patterns). The cut-off of four

EMG episodes per hour of sleep (Brux Index) allows a good distinction between patients with minor episodes of bruxism and complaints about pain and headaches and patients with a current history of tooth grinding [84,88]. RMMA is often associated with sleep microarousals and a shift in sympatho-vagal balance toward increased sympathetic activity starting some minutes preceding SB onset, in particular in subjects with moderate to severe SB [89]. The association between respiratory sleep disturbances and bruxism is hard to establish, because of a lack of studies and the absence of standard apnea–hypopnea diagnostic criteria in patients with bruxism. It is widely known that sleep apneas evoke arousals, which may facilitate bruxism. The reported prevalence of bruxism–apnea concomitance varies between 30% and 50%. Sleep bruxism might be misdiagnosed as different pathologies of various kinds. It is very important to distinguish clenching (while awake) from sleep bruxism (while asleep), since these conditions probably have different pathophysiologies and etiologies. Typically, diurnal bruxism is silent, whereas nocturnal bruxism may be annoying.

Sleep-related faciomandibular myoclonus (SFMM) consists of sudden and brief contractions (lasting less than 0.25 s) originating from the masseter and temporalis muscles, and spreading to the orbicularis oris, oculi, and eventually to the sternocleidomastoideus muscles. This myoclonus may be familial, never shows any kind of tonic or phasic activity, and is mostly present during NREM sleep, decreasing in REM sleep. Despite the presence of tooth tapping sounds, SFMM is characterized by occasional bleeding of the posterolateral sides of the tongue and an absence of masseter hypertrophy [90].

Since no specific cure exists, the main goal in the management of SB lies in the prevention or reduction of complaints related to damages to orofacial structures [84]. Of high importance is the treatment of possibly comorbid sleep disorders, and an improvement in sleep bruxism will improve sleep quality. Psychological therapies aiming to decrease the psycho-emotional factors underlying sleep bruxism may

Table 23.1 Effect of drugs on sleep bruxism (SB)-related oromotor activity

Drug	Dosage	Effect	Time of use	Side effects
Diazepam	5–10 mg/night	↓ SB-related oromotor activity	Short periods: 1–2 nights	
Methocarbamol	1–2 g/night	↓ SB-related oromotor activity		
Clonazepam	1 mg/night	↓ SB-related EMG activity by 30% in SB patients with other sleep disorders	Short-term use	Dizziness, somnolence and dependence–addiction
L-dopa	Two doses of 100 mg/night	↓ SB activity by 30%		
Clonidine	0.3 mg/night	↓ SB by 60%		Severe morning hypotension
Botulin toxin type A		↓ Jaw muscle EMG activity during sleep in SB patients		Further studies are needed to evaluate benefit/risk
Propranolol	Two doses of 60 mg/night	↓ SB activity or not effective		
Bromocriptine	7.5 mg	Not effective		
Amitriptyline	25 mg/night	Failed to control SB		
Selective serotonin-reuptake inhibitor (SSRI) antidepressants		↑ the risk of SB		

Source data from Kato T, Blanchet PJ, Huynh NT, Montplaisir JY, Lavigne GJ, Sleep bruxism and other disorders with orofacial activity during sleep. In: Chokroverty S, Allen RP, Walters AS, Montagna P, [eds], Sleep and Movement Disorders, pp. 555–72, Copyright (2013), Oxford University Press.

be useful [84]. Pharmacological therapy should be used only during periods of high emotional stress, which normally leads to exacerbation of sleep bruxism symptoms. Botulinum toxin A, benzodiazepines and other muscle relaxants, anticonvulsants, β-blockers, dopaminergic drugs, antidepressants, and clonidine are among the available drugs used as part of an interdisciplinary approach (Table 23.1) [84].

Orthopedic devices have not shown any medium- to long-term benefit in reducing muscular contraction while asleep. Thus, although they may be used to deal with and prevent tooth damage or painful muscular symptoms, they are not appropriate for long-term use.

Rhythmic movement disorder

Rhythmic movement disorder (RMD) is characterized by repetitive and stereotyped movements occurring immediately after sleep onset and during light sleep, although they may appear in any sleep stage. It is also called jactatio capitis or corporis nocturna, headbanging, or headrolling, but the term RMD is a better description, since many body areas are involved in the movement activity, such as axial muscles, head, neck, and trunk, and sometimes legs as well [1]. RMD is usually common among normal children, as a sleep-facilitating tool [91,92], with a prevalence up to 66% at the age of 9 months and decreasing to 8% in 4-year-old children. The symptoms of many of these patients do not cease as they grow, but may persist into adulthood, although not involving any psychopathology [92,93]. A late onset of RMD (in adolescence or adulthood) is relatively rare and has been associated with RLS or arousal on resumption of breathing after apneic or hypopnic episodes [94–96]. In some cases, RMD may persist during wakefulness, particularly in autistic or mentally retarded individuals.

During a common RMD episode, normally one of the following movements occurs: while supine, the head (headrolling type) or the whole body (bodyrolling type) is moved laterally; while prone, the whole body rocks on the hands and knees (bodyrocking type). The phenomenon usually lasts a few to several minutes, repeating at a frequency of 0.5–2 per second [1,97] (Fig. 23.4).

Serious injuries from RMD are rare, but bone and skull injuries have been reported in association with headbanging.

The specific causes and physiological mechanisms underlying RMD remain uncertain. The absence of organic causes, in the majority of cases, has led to behavioral and psychological theories. A recent hypothesis proposes that RMD is linked to arousal fluctuations and mediated via central motor pattern generators of the brainstem. Rare cases of familial occurrence have been reported, but genetic studies had never been performed [98].

RMD must be distinguished from other types of sleep-related motor manifestations. Sleep bruxism, thumb sucking, tics, dyskinesias, and nocturnal seizures must be ruled out through an accurate clinical description of the episodes and a VPSG recording.

Rhythmic foot movement (RFM, or *hypnagogic foot tremor*) is characterized by asynchronous oscillations of the whole foot or toes in both legs at about 0.3–4 Hz occurring during pre-sleep wakefulness and light sleep; it may be considered a new kind of RMD arising in adults, sometimes associated with insomnia, OSAS, PLMS, and RLS.

The treatment of RMD is first of all based on reassuring the patient that the condition will resolve in most cases, but devices protecting the head might be necessary to ensure safe sleep, particularly for children with learning disabilities. Usually, RMD does not affect sleep quality. Pharmacological therapy should be considered only in patients with self-inflicted injuries and poor sleep quality: benzodiazepines (clonazepam 1 mg/nightly or oxazepam 10–20 mg/nightly), dopamine agonists, citalopram, and tricyclic antidepressants have shown a beneficial effect on disturbances, but with variable success [97].

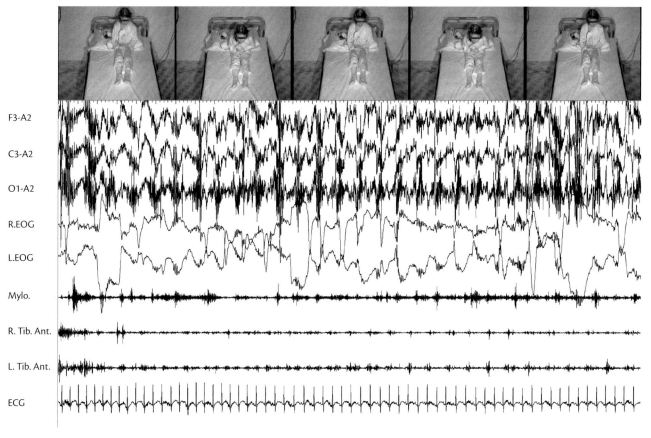

Fig. 23.4 Rhythmic movement disorders. Polysomnographic excerpt of rhythmic forward and backward movements of the trunk and head arising during wakefulness before sleep onset. Note the high-amplitude 1 Hz movement artifact on EEG leads reflecting rhythmic body movements. Upper panel: video-clips synchronous with polysomnographic recording. EOG: electro-oculogram; Mylo.: mylohyoideus; Tib. Ant.: tibialis anterior; R.: right; L.: left (due to the courtesy of Prof. Giuseppe Plazzi).

Conclusions

Sleep-related abnormal movements or excessive normal movements are disorders that can disrupt the quality of sleep, resulting in discomfort, sometimes injuries, and daytime symptoms. The severity of these abnormal movements at nighttime varies, but a precise diagnosis is always necessary because treatment and management of movement disorders occurring during sleep depend on the underlying problem. Diagnosis of a *sleep movement disorder* involves taking a detailed patient history, a review of medications used, and physical examination. Most movement disorders can be simply diagnosed from a patient's or bed partner's description of the symptoms. Sleep studies, monitoring EEG, and recording of multiple muscle activity along with video documentation are required in doubtful cases to identify the type of abnormality, its severity, and its response to therapy.

References

1. American Academy of Sleep Medicine. International classification of sleep disorders, 3rd ed. Diagnostic and coding manual. Darien, IL: American Academy of Sleep Medicine, 2014.
2. Symonds CP. Nocturnal myoclonus. J Neurol Neurosurg Psychiatry 1953;16:166–71.
3. Lugaresi E, Tassinari CA, Coccagna G, Ambrosetto C. Particularités cliniques et polygraphiques du syndrome d'impatience des membres inferieurs. Rev Neurol (Paris) 1965;113:545–55.
4. Coleman RM. Periodic movements in sleep (nocturnal myoclonus) and restless legs syndrome. In Guilleminault C, ed. Sleep and waking disorders: indications and techniques. Menlo Park, CA: Addison-Wesley, 1982:265–95.
5. Bixler EO, Kales A, Vela-Bueno A, et al. Nocturnal myoclonus and nocturnal myoclonic activity in the normal population. Res Commun Chem Pathol Pharmacol 1982;36:129–40.
6. Hornyak M, Feige B, Riemann D, Voderholzer U. Periodic leg movements in sleep and periodic limb movement disorder: prevalence, clinical significance and treatment. Sleep Med Rev 2006;10:169–77.
7. Scofield H, Roth T, Drake C. Periodic limb movements during sleep: population prevalence, clinical correlates, and racial differences. Sleep 2008;31:1221–7.
8. Ohayon MM, Roth T. Prevalence of restless legs syndrome and periodic limb movement disorder in the general population. J Psychosom Res 2002;53:547–54.
9. Kirk VG, Bohn S. Periodic limb movements in children: prevalence in a referred population. Sleep 2004;27:313–15.
10. Picchietti MA, Picchietti DL, England SJ, et al. Children show individual night-to-night variability of periodic limb movements in sleep. Sleep 2009;32:530–5.
11. O'Brien LM, Holbrook CR, Faye Jones V, Gozal D. Ethnic difference in periodic limb movements in children. Sleep Med 2007;8:240–6.
12. Coleman RM, Pollak CP, Weitzman ED. Periodic movements in sleep (nocturnal myoclonus): relation to sleep disorders. Ann Neurol 1980;8:416–21.
13. Ancoli-Israel S, Kripke DF, Klauber MR, et al. Periodic limb movements in sleep in community-dwelling elderly. Sleep 1991;14:496–500.

14. Youngstedt SD, Kripke DF, Klauber MR, et al. Periodic leg movements during sleep and sleep disturbances in elders. J Gerontol A Biol Sci Med Sci 1998;53:M391–4.

15. Carrier J, Frenette S, Montplaisir J, et al. Effects of periodic leg movements during sleep in middle-aged subjects without sleep complaints. Mov Disord 2005;20:1127–32.

16. Pennestri MH, Whittom S, Adam B, et al. PLMS and PLMW in healthy subjects as a function of age: prevalence and interval distribution. Sleep 2006; 29:1183–7.

17. Ferri R, Manconi M, Lanuzza B, et al. Age-related changes in periodic leg movements during sleep in patients with restless legs syndrome. Sleep Med 2008;9:790–8.

18. Montplaisir J, Boucher S, Poirier G, et al. Clinical, polysomnographic, and genetic characteristics of restless legs syndrome: a study of 133 patients diagnosed with new standard criteria. Mov Disord 1997;12:61–5.

19. Rye DB, Trotti LM. Restless legs syndrome and periodic leg movements of sleep. Neurol Clin 2012;30:1137–66.

20. Pizza F, Tartarotti S, Poryazova R, et al. Sleep-disordered breathing and periodic limb movements in narcolepsy with cataplexy: a systematic analysis of 35 consecutive patients. Eur Neurol 2013;70:22–6.

21. Baran AS, Richert AC, Douglass AB, et al. Change in periodic limb movement index during treatment of obstructive sleep apnea with continuous positive airway pressure. Sleep 2003;26:717–20.

22. Hedli LC, Christos P, Krieger AC. Unmasking of periodic limb movements with the resolution of obstructive sleep apnea during continuous positive airway pressure application. J Clin Neurophysiol 2012;29:339–44.

23. Fantini ML, Michaud M, Gosselin N, et al. Periodic leg movements in REM sleep behavior disorder and related autonomic and EEG activation. Neurology 2002;59:1889–94.

24. American Sleep Disorders Association. Recording and scoring leg movements. The Atlas Task Force. Sleep 1993;16:748–59.

25. Zucconi M, Ferri R, Allen R, et al. The official World Association of Sleep Medicine (WASM) standards for recording and scoring periodic leg movements in sleep (PLMS) and wakefulness (PLMW) developed in collaboration with a task force from the International Restless Legs Syndrome Study Group (IRLSSG). Sleep Med 2006;7:175–83.

26. Hornyak M, Kopasz M, Feige B, et al. Variability of periodic leg movements in various sleep disorders: implications for clinical and pathophysiologic studies. Sleep 2005;28:331–5.

27. Ferri R, Zucconi M, Manconi M, et al. New approaches to the study of periodic leg movements during sleep in restless legs syndrome. Sleep 2006;29:759–69.

28. Ferri R, Fulda S, Manconi M, et al. Night-to-night variability of periodic leg movements during sleep in restless legs syndrome and periodic limb movement disorder: comparison between the periodicity index and the PLMS index. Sleep Med 2013;14:293–6.

29. Ferri R. The time structure of leg movement activity during sleep: the theory behind the practice. Sleep Med 2012;13:433–41.

30. Ferri R, Manconi M, Plazzi G, et al. Leg movements during wakefulness in restless legs syndrome: time structure and relationships with periodic leg movements during sleep. Sleep Med 2012;13:529–35.

31. Culpepper WJ, Badia P, Shaffer JI. Time-of-night patterns in PLMS activity. Sleep 1992;15:306–11.

32. Hening WA, Walters AS, Wagner M, et al. Circadian rhythm of motor restlessness and sensory symptoms in the idiopathic restless legs syndrome. Sleep 1999;22:901–12.

33. Trenkwalder C, Hening WA, Walters AS, et al. Circadian rhythm of periodic limb movements and sensory symptoms of restless legs syndrome. Mov Disord 1999;14:102–10.

34. Pollmächer T, Schulz H. Periodic leg movements (PLM): their relationship to sleep stages. Sleep 1993;16:572–7.

35. Sforza E, Jouny C, Ibanez V. Time course of arousal response during periodic leg movements in patients with periodic leg movements and restless legs syndrome. Clin Neurophysiol 2003;114:1116–24.

36. Duffy JF, Lowe AS, Silva EJ, Winkelman JW. Periodic limb movements in sleep exhibit a circadian rhythm that is maximal in the late evening/early night. Sleep Med 2011;12:83–8.

37. Atlas Task Force of the American Sleep Disorders Association; Guilleminault C, Chairman. EEG arousals: scoring rules and examples. Sleep 1992;15:173–84.

38. Ferrillo F, Beelke M, Canovaro P, et al. Changes in cerebral and autonomic activity heralding periodic limb movements in sleep. Sleep Med 2004;5:407–12.

39. Ferri R, Zucconi M, Rundo F, et al. Heart rate and spectral EEG changes accompanying periodic and non-periodic leg movements during sleep. Clin Neurophysiol 2007;118:438–48.

40. Guggisberg AG, Hess CW, Mathis J. The significance of the sympathetic nervous system in the pathophysiology of periodic leg movements in sleep. Sleep 2007;30:755–66.

41. Lugaresi E, Coccagna G, Mantovani M, Lebrun R. Some periodic phenomena arising during drowsiness and sleep in man. Electroencephalogr Clin Neurophysiol 1972;32:701–5.

42. Parrino L, Boselli M, Buccino GP, et al. The cyclic alternating pattern plays a gate-control on periodic limb movements during non-rapid eye movement sleep. J Clin Neurophysiol 1996;13:314–23.

43. Manconi M, Ferri R, Zucconi M, et al. Dissociation of periodic leg movements from arousals in restless legs syndrome. Ann Neurol 2012;71:834–44.

44. Mendelson WB. Are periodic leg movements associated with clinical sleep disturbance? Sleep 1996;19:219–23.

45. Karadeniz D, Ondze B, Besset A, Billiard M. Are periodic leg movements during sleep (PLMS) responsible for sleep disruption in insomnia patients? Eur J Neurol 2000;7:331–6.

46. Gooneratne NS, Bellamy SL, Pack F, et al. Case-control study of subjective and objective differences in sleep patterns in older adults with insomnia symptoms. J Sleep Res 2011;20:434–44.

47. Walters AS, Rye DB. Review of the relationship of restless legs syndrome and periodic limb movements in sleep to hypertension, heart disease, and stroke. Sleep 2009;32:589–97.

48. Siddiqui F, Strus J, Ming X, Lee IA, et al. Rise of blood pressure with periodic limb movements in sleep and wakefulness. Clin Neurophysiol 2007;118:1923–30.

49. Coelho FM, Georgsson H, Narayansingh M, et al. Higher prevalence of periodic limb movements of sleep in patients with history of stroke. J Clin Sleep Med 2010;6:428–30.

50. Cuellar NG. The effects of periodic limb movements in sleep (PLMS) on cardiovascular disease. Heart Lung 2013;42:353–60.

51. Winkelman JW, Shahar E, Sharief I, Gottlieb DJ. Association of restless legs syndrome and cardiovascular disease in the Sleep Heart Health Study. Neurology 2008;70:35–42.

52. Winkelman JW, Finn L, Young T. Prevalence and correlates of restless legs syndrome symptoms in the Wisconsin Sleep Cohort. Sleep Med 2006;7:545–52.

53. Koo BB, Blackwell T, Ancoli-Israel S, et al; Osteoporotic Fractures in Men (MrOS) Study Group. Association of incident cardiovascular disease with periodic limb movements during sleep in older men: outcomes of sleep disorders in older men (MrOS) study. Circulation 2011;124:1223–31.

54. Portaluppi F, Cortelli P, Calandra-Buonaura G, et al. Do restless legs syndrome (RLS) and periodic limb movements of sleep (PLMS) play a role in nocturnal hypertension and increased cardiovascular risk of renally impaired patients? Chronobiol Int 2009;26:1206–21.

55. Trenkwalder C, Bucher SF, Oertel WH, et al. Bereitschaftspotential in idiopathic and symptomatic restless legs syndrome. Electroencephalogr Clin Neurophysiol 1993;89:95–103.

56. Bucher SF, Seelos KC, Oertel WH, et al. Cerebral generators involved in the pathogenesis of the restless legs syndrome. Ann Neurol 1997;41:639–45.

57. Watanabe S, Ono A, Naito H. Periodic leg movements during either epidural or spinal anesthesia in an elderly man without sleep-related (nocturnal) myoclonus. Sleep 1990;13:262–6.

58. de Mello MT, Lauro FA, Silva AC, Tufik S. Incidence of periodic leg movements and of the restless legs syndrome during sleep following acute physical activity in spinal cord injury subjects. Spinal Cord 1996;34:294–6.

59. Lugaresi E, Cirignotta F, Coccagna G, Montagna P. Nocturnal myoclonus and restless legs syndrome. Adv Neurol 1986;43:295–307.

60. Provini F, Vetrugno R, Meletti S, et al. Motor pattern of periodic limb movements during sleep. Neurology 2001;57:300–4.

61. de Weerd AW, Rijsman RM, Brinkley A. Activity patterns of leg muscles in periodic limb movement disorder. J Neurol Neurosurg Psychiatry 2004;75:317–19.

62. Stefansson H, Rye DB, Hicks A, et al. A genetic risk factor for periodic limb movements in sleep. N Engl J Med 2007;357:639–47.

63. Chokroverty S, Walters A, Zimmerman T, Picone M. Propriospinal myoclonus: a neurophysiologic analysis. Neurology 1992;42:1591–5.

64. Montagna P, Provini F, Plazzi G, et al. Propriospinal myoclonus upon relaxation and drowsiness: a cause of severe insomnia. Mov Disord 1997;12:66–72.

65. Vetrugno R, Plazzi G, Provini F, et al. Excessive fragmentary hypnic myoclonus: clinical and neurophysiological findings. Sleep Med 2002;3:73–6.

66. Provini F, Vetrugno R, Ferri R, Montagna P. Periodic limb movements in sleep. In: Hening W, Allen RP, Chokroverty S, Earley CJ, eds. Restless legs syndrome. Philadelphia: Saunders Elsevier, 2009;119–33.

67. Aurora RN, Kristo DA, Bista SR, et al. The treatment of restless legs syndrome and periodic limb movement disorder in adults-an update for 2012: practice parameters with an evidence-based systematic review and meta-analyses: an American Academy of Sleep Medicine Clinical Practice Guideline. Sleep 2012;35:1039–62.

68. Yang C, White DP, Winkelman JW. Antidepressant and periodic leg movements of sleep. Biol Psychiatry 2005;58:510–14.

69. Hoque R, Chesson AL Jr. Pharmacologically induced/exacerbated restless legs syndrome, periodic limb movements of sleep, and REM behavior disorder/REM sleep without atonia: literature review, qualitative scoring, and comparative analysis. J Clin Sleep Med 2010;6:79–83.

70. Leung AK, Wong BE, Chan PY, Cho HY. Nocturnal leg cramps in children: incidence and clinical characteristics. J Natl Med Assoc 1999;91:329–32.

71. Abdulla AJ, Jones PW, Pearce VR. Leg cramps in the elderly: prevalence, drug and disease associations. Int J Clin Pract 1999;53:494–6.

72. Haskell SG, Fiebach NH. Clinical epidemiology of nocturnal leg cramps in male veterans. Am J Med Sci 1997;313:210–14.

73. Kanaan N, Sawaya R. Nocturnal leg cramps. Clinically mysterious and painful—but manageable. Geriatrics 2001;56:34–42.

74. Sontag SJ, Wanner JN. The cause of leg cramps and knee pains: an hypothesis and effective treatment. Med Hypotheses 1988;25:35–41.

75. Weiner IH, Weiner HL. Nocturnal leg muscle cramps. JAMA1980;244:2332–3.

76. Allen RE, Kirby KA. Nocturnal leg cramps. Am Fam Physician 2012;86:350–5.

77. Garrison SR, Dormuth CR, Morrow RL, et al. Nocturnal leg cramps and prescription use that precedes them: a sequence symmetry analysis. Arch Intern Med 2012;172:120–6.

78. Baskol M, Ozbakir O, Coskun R, et al. The role of serum zinc and other factors on the prevalence of muscle cramps in non-alcoholic cirrhotic patients. J Clin Gastroenterol 2004;38:524–29.

79. Jacobsen JH, Rosenberg RS, Huttenlocher PR, Spire JP. Familial nocturnal cramping. Sleep 1986;9:54–60.

80. Leroy F, Bridoux F, Abou-Ayache R, et al. Quinine-induced renal bilateral cortical necrosis. Nephrol Ther 2008;4:181–6.

81. Blyton F, Chuter V, Walter KE, Burns J. Non-drug therapies for lower limb muscle cramps. Cochrane Database Syst Rev 2012;(1):CD008496.

82. Lavigne GJ, Khoury S, Abe S, et al. Bruxism physiology and pathology: an overview for clinicians. J Oral Rehabil 2008;35:476–94.

83. Carra MC, Rompre PH, Kato T, et al. Sleep bruxism and sleep arousal: an experimental challenge to assess the role of cyclic alternating pattern. J Oral Rehabil 2011;38:635–42.

84. Kato T, Blanchet PJ, Huynh NT, et al. Sleep bruxism and other disorders with orofacial activity during sleep. In: Chokroverty S, Allen RP, Walters AS, Montagna P, eds. Sleep and movement disorders. New York:Oxford University Press, 2013:555–72.

85. Lavigne GJ, Rompre PH, Poirier G, et al. Rhythmic masticatory muscle activity during sleep in humans. J Dent Res. 2001;80:443–8.

86. Ohayon MM, Li KK, Guilleminault C. Risk factors for sleep bruxism in the general population. Chest 2001;119:53–61.

87. Strausz T, Ahlberg J, Lobbezoo F, et al. Awareness of tooth grinding and clenching from adolescence to young adulthood: a nine-year follow-up. J Oral Rehabil 2010;37:497–500.

88. Dutra KM, Pereira FJ, Rompre PH, et al. Oro-facial activities in sleep bruxism patients and in normal subjects: a controlled polygraphic and audio-video study. J Oral Rehabil 2009;36:86–92.

89. Huynh N, Kato T, Rompré PH, et al. Sleep bruxism is associated to micro-arousals and an increase in cardiac sympathetic activity. J Sleep Res 2006;15:339–46.

90. Vetrugno R, Provini F, Plazzi G, et al. Familial nocturnal facio-mandibular myoclonus mimicking sleep bruxism. Neurology 2002;58:644–7.

91. Dyken ME, Rodnitzky RL. Periodic, aperiodic, and rhythmic motor disorders of sleep. Neurology 1992;42:68–74.

92. Mayer G, Wilde-Frenz J, Kurella B. Sleep related rhythmic movement disorder revisited. J Sleep Res 2007;16:110–16.

93. Stepanova I, Nevsimalova S, Hanusova J. Rhythmic movement disorder in sleep persisting into childhood and adulthood. Sleep 2005;28:851–7.

94. Lombardi C, Provini F, Vetrugno R, et al. Pelvic movements as rhythmic motor manifestation associated with restless legs syndrome. Mov Disord 2003;18:110–13.

95. Vitello N, Bayard S, Lopez R, et al. Rhythmic movement disorder associated with restless legs syndrome. Sleep Med 2012;13:1324–5.

96. Gharagozlou P, Seyffert M, Santos R, Chokroverty S. Rhythmic movement disorder associated with respiratory arousals and improved by CPAP titration in a patient with restless legs syndrome and sleep apnea. Sleep Med 2009;10:501–3.

97. Montagna P. Sleep-related non epileptic motor disorders. J Neurol 2004;251:781–94.

98. Bonakis A, Kritikou I, Vagiakis E, et al. A familial case of sleep rhythmic movement disorder persistent into adulthood; approach to pathophysiology. Mov Disord 2011;26:1770–2.

CHAPTER 24

Restless legs syndrome/ Willis–Ekbom disease

Luigi Ferini-Strambi and Sara Marelli

Epidemiological aspects

Restless legs syndrome (RLS), recently renamed Willis–Ekbom disease (WED), is a common neurological disorder characterized by uncomfortable and unpleasant sensations in the legs, with an urge to move. The most common adult RLS/WED descriptors are "restless," "uncomfortable," "twitchy," "need to stretch," "urge to move," and "legs want to move on their own." About one-third of patients express their RLS/WED sensations as painful, and, it has been reported that these patients had more severe RLS/WED symptoms [1].

The clinical spectrum of RLS/WED is broad, ranging from individuals suffering from the disease only during short periods in their lives up to those severely affected, with daily symptoms. Considering all the clinical factors, it is the age of onset that appears to be the unique characteristic item qualifying as an endophenotype [2]. Two different phenotypes of RLS/WED have been reported: (1) early-onset primary or idiopathic RLS/WED, the most frequent form, with a peak onset around 20–40 years of age, frequent familial history, slow disease progression, and low cerebrospinal fluid (CSF) ferritin level [2,3]; (2) Late-onset RLS/WED with a peak onset after 40 years of age, less frequent RLS/WED familial history, rapid disease progression, and frequent association with other diseases, including renal failure, anemia, neuropathy, myelopathy, multiple sclerosis, and diabetes [2–4].

RLS/WED prevalence in the general population has been estimated to be approximately 5% [5], but studies conducted in Asian countries thus far indicate a lower prevalence. In most studies, prevalence increases with age up to 60–70 years, except in Asian populations where an age-related increase has not been found [6]. In adults over age 40, RLS/WED occurs about twice as often in women than men, but there is no gender preference in children [7] or young adults [6]. In an epidemiological survey conducted in the USA and five European countries [6], RLS/WED symptoms of any frequency were reported by 7.2% of the general population, while symptoms occurring at least twice a week and described as moderately or severely distressing were reported by 2.7%. The authors defined these latter subjects as those who probably require treatment for their RLS/WED.

Some studies have evaluated ethnic differences in prevalence. A population-based study conducted among 1,754 Hispanics of Mexican descent (HMD) and 1,913 non-Hispanic whites (NHW) 18 years of age or older [8] showed that the prevalence was significantly lower in HMD than in NHW, and significantly greater in high-acculturation HMD.

Another study evaluated the prevalence among African American (AA) and non-African American (NAA) racial groups [9]. RLS/WED prevalence in the NAA population was approximately three times higher than in the AA group.

A study [10] that evaluated the incidence and correlates of RLS/WED in a US population-based sample (535 participants aged 40 years or more) found an incidence of RLS/WED of 1.7% per year. Use of estrogen and history of obstructive lung disease were associated with a significantly higher incidence of RLS/WED. RLS/WED, in turn, was associated with insomnia and increased sleepiness.

Two other population-based cohort prospective studies have evaluated RLS/WED incidence in Germany: the cumulative incidence was 9.1% and 7.0%, respectively, and the persistence of RLS/WED symptoms from baseline to follow-up was 47.4% in one study (mean follow-up 2.2 years) and 41.5% in the second (mean follow-up 5.2 years) [11]. Another prospective Japanese study reported that RLS/WED may not be persistent in more than 50% of the affected population: the frequency of RLS/WED symptoms, but not the severity, may predict the persistence of the disorder [12].

Diagnostic criteria and clinical aspects

In 1995, the international RLS/WED Study Group (IRLSSG) established four essential criteria for the diagnosis of RLS/WED that have provided reliable diagnostic standards for clinical practice. In 2012, the IRLSSG revised the criteria by introducing a fifth criterion in order to improve the issues of differential diagnosis, stating that the symptoms are not due to another medical or behavioral condition.

No biological assay is available to make a diagnosis of RLS/WED. Clinical diagnosis is based on clinician interaction with the patient. Concerning the first criterion, several patients will not be able to separate symptomatically or temporally the two components: an urge to move the legs and dysesthesias. RLS/WED may also involve the arms, as well as other body parts in the severe forms of the disease [13]. Arm involvement is reported in up to 50% of cases [14], but usually the legs are affected earlier and more severely than the arms.

RLS/WED typically involves symptoms in both legs, but not always at the same time or symmetrically [14].

Concerning the criterion that the urge to move the legs and the accompanying unpleasant sensations are partially or totally relieved by movement, it must be noted that patients with very severe RLS/WED may report minimal or no relief of symptoms even after a prolonged period of activity such as walking or bending.

RLS/WED symptoms in the afternoon are not uncommon, particularly in the case of long periods of inactivity [15]; however the symptoms are most pronounced during the evening and night. The circadian variation in symptoms occurs independently of activity, sleep deprivation, or sleep–wake state [16–18]. Those patients affected by very severe RLS/WED may have symptoms persisting throughout the day and night without any clear circadian variation.

Myalgia, venous stasis, leg edema, arthritis, leg cramps, positional discomfort, and habitual foot tapping are the mimicking conditions that must be excluded in the diagnosis of RLS/WED. It has been reported that adding differential diagnosis to the diagnostic criteria in diagnostic questionnaires or scales produces a greatly improved agreement with clinical expert diagnosis exceeding 90% [19,20].

Patients with RLS/WED can, however, have one of these other conditions in addition to RLS/WED: the comorbidity of RLS/WED and peripheral neuropathy is a typical example [21].

In the 2012 IRLSSG Consensus Diagnostic Criteria, specifiers for clinical course and clinical significance have been added in order to more completely characterize RLS/WED.

Clinical course is generally considered an important aspect among these patients. Some patients have sporadic episodes of symptoms, while others have them regularly. The latter, seen most frequently in clinical practice, are more likely to seek treatment. The REST general population survey found that of all those reporting RLS/WED symptoms during the previous year, 57.5% had symptoms occurring twice a week or more; the majority (66%) also reported the symptoms as moderate to severely disturbing [6]. As already mentioned, it is this latter group of RLS/WED sufferers who are often considered to be in need of treatment.

The 2012 IRLSSG Revised Criteria include the following specifiers for clinical course of RLS/WED:

A. Chronic-persistent RLS/WED: symptoms when not treated would occur on average at least twice weekly for the past year.

B. Intermittent RLS/WED: symptoms when not treated would occur on average less than twice weekly for the past year, with at least five lifetime events.

Concerning the "clinical significance" of RLS/WED, it is known that the symptoms of RLS/WED may cause significant distress or impairment in social, occupational, and educational contexts owing to their impact on sleep, energy/vitality, daily activities, behavior, cognition, or mood.

No consensus has been reached in defining "clinical significance" in terms of the specific frequency and duration of RLS/WED. However, using classical health-related quality of life (HRQoL) measures, physical and mental health scores have been reported to be lower in severe cases, and impairments are strongly associated with RLS/WED severity [22,23]. This finding has been confirmed in a population-based study [24] that also showed that the impairment in activities of daily function was mediated by poor sleep quality and depressive symptoms.

The 2012 IRLSSG Consensus Diagnostic Criteria also reported some patterns that can support a diagnosis, particularly when there is some lack of diagnostic certainty.

RLS/WED has one identified sign, namely, periodic leg movements (PLM). PLM can occur in sleep (PLMS) or wakefulness (PLMW). A PLMS index (number of PLMS per hour of sleep) above five per hour is considered pathological: this index may be observed in almost 80% of RLS/WED patients.

It is well known that PLMS is a sensitive but not specific motor sign of RLS/WED. However, it has been reported that the PLMS index shows high night-to-night variability, requiring multiple nights for its reliable estimation. This is not the case for the degree of periodicity of leg movements, quantified by the periodicity index [25]. Moreover, some other studies have documented a bimodal distribution of the inter-movement intervals for PLM that divide into short (<10 seconds) and long (10–90 seconds) inter-movement intervals [26], with the second interval range being representative of the typical periodic activity. The PLMW of RLS/WED patients during the sleep period have mostly short inter-movement intervals (<10 seconds), while the PLMS have mostly long inter-movement intervals (10–90 seconds) [27].

Concerning the distribution of PLMS, patients with RLS/WED show a prevalence of movements in the first two hours of sleep and a progressive decrease throughout the night, in contrast to other disorders with PLMS, such as narcolepsy and REM sleep behavior disorder (RBD) (Fig. 24.1).

PLMS occur with significant transient changes in EEG, heart rate, and blood pressure [28], which have been suggested to reflect an increased risk of cardiovascular disease observed with RLS/WED in some but not all studies [28].

RLS/WED has been observed to occur commonly in families, indicating significant genetic or shared environmental factors for the syndrome. Some authors found that 20% of consecutive RLS/WED patients in two clinical settings reported RLS/WED among

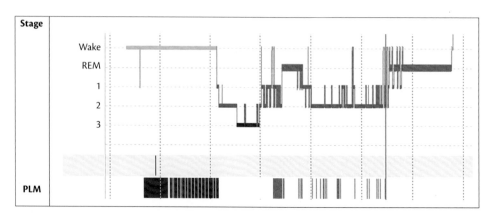

Fig. 24.1 Hypnogram of a patient with RLS/WED.

their first-degree relatives [29]. Moreover, twin studies have shown high concordance for RLS/WED [30,31]. Thus, the presence of RLS/WED among first-degree relatives is supportive of the diagnosis.

Sleep disturbance is a common and distressing aspect of RLS/WED [6,32]. Epidemiological data indicate that about 75% of RLS/WED patients are likely to seek treatment for sleep disturbance characterized by a long sleep latency or nocturnal awakenings. Most patients report difficulty falling asleep, but some patients fall asleep rapidly and wake up shortly after with unpleasant leg sensations that force them to get up and walk around. Individuals with moderate to severe RLS/WED have chronic sleep loss with total sleep times of 4.5–6 hours a night [6,32,33], and the sleep disturbance correlates with RLS/WED severity [34,35]. However, individuals with moderate to severe RLS/WED usually do not report a level of daytime sleepiness that would be expected for the degree of sleep loss [36,37]. They can suffer other consequences of sleep deprivation such as fatigue, reduced concentration, and depression, but do not usually nap. In RLS/WED cases where there is excessive sleepiness, a possible comorbid sleep apnea should be suspected.

The recently released International Classification of Sleep Disorders, Third Edition (ICSD-3) [38] diagnostic criteria for RLS/WED include five essential criteria of the IRLSSG, in addition to a clinical significance criterion that is similarly worded to the IRLSSG diagnostic specifier for clinical significance. For the ICSD-3 diagnosis of RLS/WED, this clinical significance criterion "must be met."

ICSD-3 also include a part dedicated to the "associated features." It has been underlined that sleep onset and maintenance complaints in RLS/WED are notably higher than in controls, with odds ratios (OR) between 1.7 and 3.5. Daytime fatigue and daytime sleepiness are also common complaints; however, the sleepiness is not as severe as expected for the degree of sleep disruption, implying hyperarousal in RLS/WED. Moreover, some patients with RLS/WED may choose to work at night, thereby shifting quiet activities and their sleep schedule away from the circadian peak of their RLS/WED symptoms.

ICSD-3 considers that PLM, a family history of RLS/WED, and response to dopaminergic therapy are supportive of the diagnosis.

In the Diagnostic and Statistical Manual of Mental Disorders, Fifth edition (DSM-5) [39], RLS/WED is elevated to a separate diagnostic entity, in contrast to the previous edition, based on the public health relevance of the condition, scientific progress made by RLS/WED researchers, and the need to provide a definition of a clinically significant condition that is frequently encountered in daily psychiatric practice.

In comparison with other diagnostic criteria, DSM-5 requires frequency (at least three times per week) and duration (at least three months) of symptoms. While the imposition of arbitrary cutoffs to restrict RLS/WED diagnosis to a more frequently occurring and longer-duration condition might lead to improved diagnostic specificity and reliability in primary care or psychiatric practice, this would also minimize the potential clinical significance of the intermittent subtype or recent-onset RLS/WED.

Moreover, in comparison with the 2012 IRLSSG Revised Criteria, which define a full spectrum of RLS/WED, the DSM-5 criteria define a narrower clinical spectrum of RLS/WED by requiring the RLS/WED symptoms to be "accompanied by significant distress or impairment in social, occupational, education, academic, behavioral, or other important areas of functioning."

Furthermore, in the "diagnostic marker" section, polysomnographic findings like an increased latency to sleep and higher arousal index have been introduced. Thus, there has been an unfortunate confusion in the RLS/WED diagnostic criteria created by three different professional physician organizations.

Physiopathology

The physiopathology of RLS/WED is not fully established. Genetics, central nervous system dopamine dysregulation, and brain iron deficiency seem to be the primary involved factors, but some data support the hypothesis that peripheral phenomena also contribute to the pathophysiology of RLS/WED. One study has demonstrated peripheral hypoxia in the legs of patients with RLS/WED [40]. According to the authors, peripheral hypoxia could be a primary trigger of RLS, irritating peripheral afferent nerves, or it could be a secondary phenomenon resulting from deficiencies in iron metabolism, often associated with RLS/WED.

There is clear evidence for a genetic contribution to RLS/WED, considering that more than 50% of idiopathic cases report a positive family history [41]. Moreover, in most pedigrees, RLS/WED segregates in an autosomal dominant fashion, with over 90% penetrance rate [42].

However, several linkage studies of familial RLS/WED have identified mostly marginal associations over a wide range of chromosomes. It must be stressed that no specific gene associated with RLS/WED has been identified in these studies. In contrast, genome-wide association studies (GWAS) have identified common susceptibility alleles of modest (OR 1.2–1.7) risk at six genomic loci on chromosomes 2p, 6p, 15q, and 16q [43–45].

The increased risk of RLS/WED occurs at loci for genomic regions of *MEIS1*, *BTBD9*, *PTPRD*, *MAP2K/SKOR1*, and *TOX3/BC034767* and at an intergenic region on chromosome 2 (rs6747972). It is known that a *MEIS1* risk variant influences iron metabolism [46] and that *BTBD9* regulates brain dopamine levels and controls iron homeostasis through the iron regulatory protein-2 [47]. These findings clearly suggest that dopaminergic neurotransmission and iron dysregulation can contribute to the pathogenesis of RLS.

The strong positive effects of L-DOPA and dopamine agonists on RLS/WED and PLMS clearly support the role of the dopaminergic system in the physiopathology of these conditions. Moreover, dopamine antagonists generally exacerbate RLS/WED symptoms.

The few post-mortem studies that have been performed have shown no histopathological abnormalities in RLS/WED brains, including the major dopaminergic areas [48,49].

In general, standard MRI studies have shown no morphological abnormalities in RLS/WED. An MRI study with a voxel-based morphometric analysis showed significant regional decreases in gray matter volume in the left hippocampal gyrus, both parietal lobes, medial frontal areas, and cerebellum of RLS/WED patients [50].

Also, white matter may be decreased in multiple subcortical areas in close proximity to the primary and associated motor and somatosensory areas of RLS/WED patients [51]. Notably, the reported abnormal loss of myelination is consistent with that found in iron-deprived animals [52].

Concerning brain functional studies on the dopaminergic system, SPECT and PET studies showed inconsistent alterations in basal ganglia postsynaptic and presynaptic D2/3 receptor binding, with reports of increases, decreases, and no change [53].

However, some recent intriguing findings in RLS/WED patients suggest an overly activated dopaminergic system. PET studies in the striatum of patients with RLS/WED have reported a decrease in dopamine transport, which might be expected to increase synaptic dopamine concentrations [54]. A more recent PET study showed that patients with RLS/WED had lower dopamine-2 receptor binding potentials in the putamen and caudate, but not the ventral striatum [55]. A neuropathological study showed in RLS/WED brain tissue a significant decrease in D2 receptors in the putamen that correlated with RLS severity, without any changes in D1 receptor or dopamine transport. Brain RLS/WED tissues showed significant increases in tyrosine hydroxylase in the substantia nigra, but not in the putamen [56]. The decreases in dopamine transport and the D2 receptors are consistent with increased striatal dopamine.

Moreover, CSF studies on dopamine metabolites are inconsistent in RLS/WED, but one study showed a significant increase in 3-o-methyldopa and homovanillic acid, which suggests a possible increase in dopaminergic activity in severe RLS/WED patients [57].

It has been hypothesized that the increased presynaptic dopamine state occurs with a balanced decreased postsynaptic response [58]. This balance may not suffice at certain times in the daily variation of dopamine. In the evening, dopaminergic activity drops below a critical threshold, which triggers the RLS/WED symptoms. Administering l-DOPA or a dopamine agonist in the evening would be expected to restore the pre- and postsynaptic balance, thereby reducing symptoms.

Of note, increased extracellular dopamine and decreased dopamine transporter (DAT) and D1 and D2 receptors in the striatum have also been found in both animal and cell models of iron insufficiency [53, 59].

Neuropathological, biological, and neuroimaging studies support the role of iron in the physiopathology of RLS/WED. Conditions associated with secondary RLS/WED, such as end-stage renal disease and pregnancy, are characterized by inadequate iron. Moreover, iron supplements have been used in several studies to successfully improve symptoms of both idiopathic and secondary RLS/WED.

A neuropathological study showed a marked decrease in iron and H-ferritin (the heavy-chain subunit of ferritin) staining in the substantia nigra, a mild decrease in transferrin receptor staining on neuromelanin-containing cells, and morphological differences in the cells staining for L-ferritin (the light-chain subunit of ferritin) in idiopathic RLS/WED brains compared with control brains [48]. Another study demonstrated a decreased concentrations of iron transport proteins (DMT1 and ferroportin) in the substantia nigra of RLS/WED patients [60].

MRI and ultrasound studies of regional brain iron content in RLS/WED patients compared with controls have consistently shown reduced brain iron, particularly in the substantia nigra [61,62].

A study performed using voxel-based MRI relaxometry showed that the reduction in brain iron in RLS/WED patients seems to extend beyond the substantia nigra to other brain regions, including the cerebellum and subcortical white matter [63]. Another MRI study with more sensitive methods for measuring iron (a phase-imaging technique) found that the brain iron deficiency in RLS/WED includes other areas beside the substantia nigra and the striatum, in particular the thalamus [64].

This raises the question whether RLS/WED is related to a regional or a global brain iron deficiency. The mechanisms underlying the decreased iron concentration in RLS/WED brains remains unclear. However, some authors hypothesized that the source of the brain iron deficit is at the blood–brain interface [65]. They analyzed the expression of iron management proteins in the epithelial cells of the choroid plexus and the brain microvasculature in post-mortem tissues of individuals with RLS/WED. The presence of an iron regulatory protein was demonstrated in the brain microvasculature, and the activity of this protein was decreased in RLS/WED with the consequence of insufficient iron storage in endothelial cells.

The role of iron in dopaminergic transmission in the CNS is noteworthy. A possible link between the iron and dopamine might be represented by the additional function of iron as a cofactor of tyrosine hydroxylase, which is the rate-limiting enzyme for dopamine synthesis. An iron-deficient diet can induce RLS/WED-like sensory and motor symptoms in rodents [66]. Furthermore, iron deficiency is associated with increased extracellular dopamine, decreased DAT, and decreased D2 and D1 receptors in the striatum of rats similar to the findings in RLS/WED.

Treatment

In the management of RLS/WED, it is important to inform the patient of the need to maintain good sleep hygiene to prevent the development of the insomnia that is frequently observed. Indeed, some patients go to bed later at night and remain active during hours when their symptoms make sleep difficult, and some severe RLS/WED patients may even change their working schedule for that purpose. Moreover, dysfunctional thinking about sleep is a central aspect in the perpetuation of primary insomnia and a target symptom of cognitive behavioral therapy (CBT) for insomnia. A proof-of-concept study on CBT tailored to RLS/WED (eight group 90 minute sessions on a weekly basis) showed favorable results in both medicated and unmedicated RLS/WED patients [67].

Patients should avoid alcohol, caffeine, and heavy meals in the evening, since these may aggravate RLS/WED symptoms. Improvement in RLS/WED symptoms has been anecdotally reported when the mind has been kept alert by performing tasks requiring a large amount of concentration.

There have been few studies on nonpharmacological treatments for RLS/WED. A 12-week randomized controlled trial evaluated the effectiveness of an exercise program: participants were randomized to either exercise (a conditioning program of aerobic and lower-body resistance training three days per week) or control groups. At the end of the 12 weeks, a significant improvement in RLS/WED symptoms was observed in the exercise group compared with controls [68]. In another study, a six-month exercise training regime was as effective as six-month low-dosage dopamine agonist treatment in reducing RLS/WED symptoms in uremic patients [69].

It has been also reported that pneumatic compression devices [70], acupuncture [71], and near-infrared light treatment [72] may reduce symptoms of RLS/WED, but further well-designed, large-scale clinical trials are needed.

According to the pathophysiological concept of spinal cord hyperexcitability in idiopathic RLS/WED, a pilot study evaluated the effect of transcutaneous spinal direct current stimulation in patients compared with controls [73]: one session of cathodal, anodal, and sham stimulation of the thoracic spinal cord for 15 minutes during their symptomatic phase in the evening produced a reduction in RLS/WED symptoms.

On the other hand, five sessions of transcranial direct current stimulation with electrodes on the sensorimotor areas showed no significant effect in subjects with drug-naive RLS/WED [74].

It should be noted that some common classes of drugs can exacerbate RLS/WED. Dopaminergic antagonistic antiemetics or antipsychotics may worsen RLS/WED [75–77], as may antidepressants [75,78].

Pharmacological treatment of RLS has undergone considerable changes over the last few years. Several classes of medication have demonstrated efficacy, including dopaminergic agents, the $\alpha_2\delta$ ligands, and opioids. According to published practice recommendations [79,80] pharmacological therapy should be limited to those patients who suffer from clinically relevant RLS/WED symptoms, including intermittent RLS/WED with impaired sleep quality or quality of life.

Levodopa was the drug most frequently studied in earlier small RLS/WED trials. The immediate response to levodopa without a long titration period is really appreciated by the patient, and a positive response to this drug with the first dosage strongly supports the diagnosis of RLS/WED [81]. However, a possible side effect of levodopa is morning rebound, as well as augmentation. Augmentation [82] refers to the worsening of RLS/WED symptom severity from pretreatment levels following an initial therapeutic benefit for most days of the week, associated with an earlier onset of symptoms by at least two to four hours. A shorter latency to symptom onset with immobility, and involvement of previously unaffected limbs, can also be observed. Prevalence rates of augmentation in open-label trials range from 18.6% to 72% [83–85].

In recent years, three non-ergoline derivative agonists, pramipexole, ropinirole, and transdermal rotigotine patches, have been extensively studied for RLS/WED treatment (Table 24.1). Overall, the dopamine agonists have been found to be effective in short- and longer-duration placebo-controlled studies for the treatment of RLS/WED and PLMS [86]. Trials of dopamine agonists have tried to determine the lowest effective dose, and currently one-sixth to one-eighth of the maximum dose used to treat Parkinson disease is recommended for treatment of RLS/WED [87].

Another class of drugs that has demonstrated efficacy for RLS/WED and PLMS are the $\alpha_2\delta$ ligands, including gabapentin, gabapentin enacarbil, and pregabalin [88] (Table 24.1). A double-blind study has shown a greater reduction in RLS/WED symptoms with 300 mg/day pregabalin than with pramipexole at a dose of either 0.25 or 0.5 mg, over periods of 12 and 52 weeks. Augmentation rates were significantly lower with pregabalin than with 0.5 mg of pramipexole [89]. Another randomized, double-blinded, crossover trial [90] demonstrated improvements in objective and subjective measures of sleep maintenance and sleep architecture with pregabalin (300 mg/day) compared with placebo and pramipexole (0.5 mg/day). In particular, the effects of pregabalin on PLM-arousal index were comparable to those of pramipexole.

The therapeutic effects of opioids in RLS/WED have been examined in several open-label and controlled clinical trials [79]. A 12-week placebo-controlled study evaluated a fixed-dose-combination drug, oxycodone–naloxone, administered twice a day in RLS/WED patients who had failed previous treatments owing to lack of benefit or side effects [91]. Two hundred and seventy-six patients were randomized to either placebo or oxycodone 5 mg–naloxone 2.5 mg twice a day and titrated up to either benefit or a maximum dose of oxycodone 40 mg–naloxone 20 mg twice a day. All patients then entered a 40-week open-label extension. Oxycodone–naloxone was superior to placebo, and, in the extension period, provided continued benefit for a median of 281 days at a mean dose of oxycodone 18.1 mg and naloxone 9.1 mg. Side effects from active treatment included fatigue, constipation, nausea, somnolence, and headache. Augmentation was not observed [91].

Table 24.1 Drugs most frequently used in RLS/WED

Drug	Time to maximum blood level (h)	Elimination half-life (h)	Initial daily dose (mg)	Usual dose range
Dopaminergic agonists				
Pramipexole	2	8–12 (increase with decreasing glomerular filtration rate and age)	0.125	0.125–1.000 mg daily approximately 1–3 h before bedtime
Ropinirole	1–1.5	6	0.25(–0.5)	0.50–4.00 mg daily approximately 1–3 h before bedtime
Rotigotine (transdermal patch)	Stable plasma levels over 24 h	Stable plasma levels over 24 h (elimination half-life biphasic: 3 and 6)	1	1–3 mg daily
α₂δ ligands				
Gabapentin	2	5–7	300	300–1200 mg daily; may be in split dosing with an afternoon and bedtime dose
Gabapentin enacarbil	7–9	Relatively stable plasma levels over 18–24 h (elimination half-life: 6)	600	600–1800 mg daily about 1 h before bedtime
Pregabalin	1.5	6	25	Up to 300 mg
Opioids				
Oxycodone–naloxone prolonged-release	—	5	5 mg oxycodone–2.5 mg naloxone twice daily	10 mg oxycodone–5 mg naloxone to 20 mg oxycodone–10 mg naloxone twice daily

Current treatment guidelines based on long-term studies recommend that chronic/persistent RLS/WED should be treated with either a non-ergot dopamine agonist or an $\alpha_2\delta$ calcium channel ligand [92,93]. Patients should be advised that these drugs are symptomatic therapies that cannot cure the condition and might not completely or permanently relieve the symptoms. Moreover, some different aspects must be evaluated in the choice of agent, including the severity of RLS/WED symptoms, cognitive status of the patient, comorbid conditions, and licensing of drugs in a given country. The clinician should consider the most common long-term side effects specific to each class of drug.

Since $\alpha_2\delta$ ligands can alleviate chronic pain and may be helpful in treating anxiety and insomnia, the presence of any of these comorbidities may favor their use. However, these ligands can cause depression and weight gain, and therefore a dopamine agonist is a more appropriate choice in the presence of these conditions. On the other hand, dopamine agonists may occasionally cause impulse control disorders (ICDs), such as compulsive gambling or binge eating. All patients should be warned about the possibility of ICDs prior to starting a dopamine agonist, and these compounds are relatively contraindicated in those with a history of ICDs.

Another important aspect that can influence the choice of the treatment is the duration of RLS/WED symptoms. For RLS/WED present through much of the day and night, the use of long-acting agents, such as rotigotine patches or gabapentin enacarbil, should be considered. In refractory RLS/WED, combination therapy with drugs of different classes or oral prolonged-release oxycodone–naloxone should be considered. An open-label study involving refractory RLS/WED patients showed generally favorable results with 1 g of high-molecular-weight intravenous iron dextran [94]. Several trials with different iron formulations have been conducted, but no formulation has proved to be reliably effective in all patients [87]. Not all patients with iron deficiency benefit from iron supplementation; however, it has been suggested that patients with RLS/WED who have low serum ferritin concentration (<75 ng/mL), either with or without anemia, should be treated with iron formulations before starting dopaminergic therapy [95]. It is notable that very low ferritin (≤20 ng/mL) seems to increase the risk of augmentation [96].

Nevertheless, since the severity and frequency of symptoms vary widely among RLS/WED patients, individualized treatment approaches should be considered. Moreover, further studies are needed to identify the long-term treatment needs of patients with RLS/WED, which is often a chronic condition.

References

1. Cho YW, Song ML, Earley CJ, Allen RP. Prevalence and clinical characteristics of patients with restless legs syndrome with painful symptoms. Sleep Med 2015;16:775–78.
2. Winkelmann J, Wetter TC, Collado-Seidel V, et al. Clinical characteristics and frequency of the hereditary restless legs syndrome in a population of 300 patients. Sleep 2000;23:597–602.
3. Whittom S, Dauvilliers Y, Pennestri MH, et al. Age-at-onset in restless legs syndrome: a clinical and polysomnographic study. Sleep Med 2007;9:54–9.
4. Allen RP, Picchietti D, Hening WA, et al; Restless Legs Syndrome Diagnosis and Epidemiology Workshop at the National Institutes of Health; International Restless Legs Syndrome Study Group. Restless legs syndrome: diagnostic criteria, special considerations, and epidemiology. A report from the Restless Legs Syndrome Diagnosis and Epidemiology Workshop at the National Institutes of Health. Sleep Med 2003;4:101–19.
5. Garcia-Borreguero D, Egatz R, Winkelmann J, Berger K. Epidemiology of restless legs syndrome: the current status. Sleep Med Rev 2006;10:153–67.
6. Allen RP, Walters AS, Montplaisir J, et al. Restless legs syndrome prevalence and impact: REST general population study. Arch Intern Med 2005;165:1286–92.
7. Picchietti D, Allen RP, Walters AS, et al. Restless legs syndrome: prevalence and impact in children and adolescents—the Peds REST study. Pediatrics 2007;120:253–66.
8. Sawanyawisuth K, Palinkas LA, Ancoli-Israel S, et al. Ethnic differences in the prevalence and predictors of restless legs syndrome between Hispanics of Mexican descent and non-Hispanic whites in San Diego County: a population-based study. J Clin Sleep Med 2013;9:47–53.
9. Alkhazna A, Saeed A, Rashidzada W, Romaker AM. Racial differences in the prevalence of restless legs syndrome in a primary care setting. Hosp Pract (1995) 2014;42:131–37.
10. Budhiraja P, Budhiraja R, Goodwin JL, et al. Incidence of restless legs syndrome and its correlates. J Clin Sleep Med 2012;8:119–24.
11. Szentkiralyi A, Fendrich K, Hoffmann W, et al. Incidence of restless legs syndrome in two population-based cohort studies in Germany. Sleep Med 2011;12:815–20.
12. Kagimura T, Nomura T, Kusumi M, et al. Prospective survey on the natural course of restless legs syndrome over two years in a closed cohort. Sleep Med 2011;12:821–26.
13. Buchfuhrer MJ. Restless legs syndrome (RLS) with expansion of symptoms to the face. Sleep Med 2008;9:188–90.
14. Karroum EG, Leu-Semenescu S, Arnulf I. Topography of the sensations in primary restless legs syndrome. J Neurol Sci 2012;320:26–31.
15. Tzonova D, Larrosa O, Calvo E, et al. Breakthrough symptoms during the daytime in patients with restless legs syndrome (Willis–Ekbom disease). Sleep Med 2012;13:151–5.
16. Hening WA, Walters AS, Wagner M, et al. Circadian rhythm of motor restlessness and sensory symptoms in the idiopathic restless legs syndrome. Sleep 1999;22:901–12.
17. Trenkwalder C, Hening WA, Walters AS, et al. Circadian rhythm of periodic limb movements and sensory symptoms of restless legs syndrome. Mov Disord 1999;14:102–10.
18. Michaud M, Dumont M, Selmaoui B, et al. Circadian rhythm of restless legs syndrome: relationship with biological markers. Ann Neurol 2004;55:372–80.
19. Popat RA, Van Den Eeden SK, Tanner CM, et al. Reliability and validity of two self-administered questionnaires for screening restless legs syndrome in population-based studies. Sleep Med 2010;11:154–60.
20. Benes H, Kohnen R. Validation of an algorithm for the diagnosis of restless legs syndrome: the restless legs syndrome-diagnostic index (RLS-DI). Sleep Med 2009;10:515–23.
21. Ferini-Strambi L. RLS-like symptoms: differential diagnosis by history and clinical assessment. Sleep Med 2007;8 Suppl 2:S3–6.
22. Kushida C, Martin M, Nikam P, et al. Burden of restless legs syndrome on health-related quality of life. Qual Life Res 2007;16:617–24.
23. McCrink L, Allen RP, Wolowacz S, et al. Predictors of health-related quality of life in sufferers with restless legs syndrome: a multi-national study. Sleep Med 2007;8:73–83.
24. Hanewinckel R, Maksimovic A, Verlinden VJ, et al. The impact of restless legs syndrome on physical functioning in a community-dwelling population of middle-aged and elderly people. Sleep Med 2015;16:399–405.
25. Ferri R, Fulda S, Manconi M, et al. Night-to-night variability of periodic leg movements during sleep in restless legs syndrome and periodic limb movement disorder: comparison between the periodicity index and the PLMS index. Sleep Med 2013;14:293–96.
26. Ferri R, Zucconi M, Manconi M, et al. Different periodicity and time structure of leg movements during sleep in narcolepsy/cataplexy and restless legs syndrome. Sleep 2006;29:1587–94.

27. Ferri R, Manconi M, Plazzi G, et al. Leg movements during wakefulness in restless legs syndrome: time structure and relationships with periodic leg movements during sleep. Sleep Med 2012;13:529–35.
28. Ferini-Strambi L, Walters AS, Sica D. The relationship among restless legs syndrome (Willis–Ekbom disease), hypertension, cardiovascular disease, and cerebrovascular disease. J Neurol 2014;261:1051–68.
29. Allen RP, La Buda MC, Becker P, Earley CJ. Family history study of the restless legs syndrome. Sleep Med 2002;3 Suppl:S3–7.
30. Ondo WG, Vuong KD, Wang Q. Restless legs syndrome in monozygotic twins: clinical correlates. Neurology 2000;55:1404–6.
31. Xiong L, Jang K, Montplaisir J, et al. Canadian restless legs syndrome twin study. Neurology 2007;68:1631–33.
32. Allen RP, Stillman P, Myers AJ. Physician-diagnosed restless legs syndrome in a large sample of primary medical care patients in western Europe: prevalence and characteristics. Sleep Med 2010;11:31–7.
33. Saletu B, Gruber G, Saletu M, et al. Sleep laboratory studies in restless legs syndrome patients as compared with normals and acute effects of ropinirole. 1. Findings on objective and subjective sleep and awakening quality. Neuropsychobiology 2000;41:181–89.
34. Winkelman JW, Finn L, Young T. Prevalence and correlates of restless legs syndrome symptoms in the Wisconsin Sleep Cohort. Sleep Med. 2006;7:545–52.
35. Winkelman JW, Redline S, Baldwin CM, et al. Polysomnographic and health-related quality of life correlates of restless legs syndrome in the Sleep Heart Health Study. Sleep 2009;32:772–8.
36. Gamaldo C, Benbrook AR, Allen RP, et al. Evaluating daytime alertness in individuals with restless legs syndrome (RLS) compared to sleep restricted controls. Sleep Med 2009;10:134–8.
37. Allen RP, Barker PB, Horska A, Earley CJ. Thalamic glutamate/glutamine in restless legs syndrome: increased and related to disturbed sleep. Neurology 2013;80:2028–34.
38. American Academy of Sleep Medicine. International classification of sleep disorders, 3rd ed. Darien, IL: American Academy of Sleep Medicine, 2014.
39. American Psychiatric Association. Diagnostic and statistical manual of mental disorders, 5th ed. Arlington, VA: American Psychiatric Association, 2013.
40. Salminen AV, Rimpilä V, Polo O. Peripheral hypoxia in restless legs syndrome (Willis–Ekbom disease). Neurology 2014;82:1856–61.
41. Allen RP, Picchietti DL, Garcia-Borreguero D, et al; International Restless Legs Syndrome Study Group. Restless legs syndrome/Willis–Ekbom disease diagnostic criteria: updated International Restless Legs Syndrome Study Group (IRLSSG) consensus criteria—history, rationale, description, and significance. Sleep Med 2014;15:860–73.
42. Winkelmann J, Muller-Myhsok B, Wittchen HU, et al. Complex segregation analysis of restless legs syndrome provides evidence for an autosomal dominant mode of inheritance in early age at onset families. Ann Neurol 2002;52:297–302.
43. Winkelmann J, Schormair B, Lichtner P, et al. Genome-wide association study of restless legs syndrome identifies common variants in three genomic regions. Nat Genet 2007;39:1000–1006.
44. Stefansson H, Rye DB, Hicks A, et al. A genetic risk factor for periodic limb movements in sleep. N Engl J Med 2007;357:639–47.
45. Winkelmann J, Czamara D, Schormair B, et al. Genome-wide association study identifies novel restless legs syndrome susceptibility loci on 2p14 and 16q12.1. PLoS Genet 2011;7:e1002171. Erratum: PLoS Genet 2011;7(8).
46. Catoire H, Dion PA, Xiong L, et al. Restless legs syndrome-associated MEIS1 risk variant influences iron homeostasis. Ann Neurol 2011;70:170–75.
47. DeAndrade MP, Johnson RL Jr, Unger EL, et al. Motor restlessness, sleep disturbances, thermal sensory alterations and elevated serum iron levels in Btbd9 mutant mice. Hum Mol Genet 2012;21:3984–92.
48. Connor JR, Boyer PJ, Menzies SL, et al. Neuropathological examination suggests impaired brain iron acquisition in restless legs syndrome. Neurology 2003;61:304–9.
49. Earley CJ, Allen RP, Connor JR, et al. The dopaminergic neurons of the A11 system in RLS autopsy brains appear normal. Sleep Med 2009;10:1155–57.
50. Chang Y, Chang HW, Song H, et al. Gray matter alteration in patients with restless legs syndrome: a voxel-based morphometry study. Clin Imaging 2015;39:20–5.
51. Unrath A, Muller HP, Ludolph AC, et al. Cerebral white matter alterations in idiopathic restless legs syndrome, as measured by diffusion tensor imaging. Mov Disord 2008;23:1250–5.
52. Connor JR, Ponnuru P, Lee BY, et al. Postmortem and imaging based analyses reveal CNS decreased myelination in restless legs syndrome. Sleep Med 2011;12:614–19.
53. Dauvilliers Y, Winkelmann J. Restless legs syndrome: update on pathogenesis. Curr Opin Pulm Med. 2013;19:594–600.
54. Earley CJ, Kuwabara H, Wong DF, et al. The dopamine transporter is decreased in the striatum of subjects with restless legs syndrome. Sleep 2011;34:341–7.
55. Earley CJ, Kuwabara H, Wong DF, et al. Increased synaptic dopamine in the putamen in restless legs syndrome. Sleep 2013;36:51–7.
56. Connor JR, Wang XS, Allen RP, et al. Altered dopaminergic profile in the putamen and substantia nigra in restless leg syndrome. Brain 2009;132:2403–12.
57. Allen RP, Connor JR, Hyland K, Earley CJ. Abnormally increased CSF 3-ortho-methyldopa (3-OMD) in untreated restless legs syndrome (RLS) patients indicates more severe disease and possibly abnormally increased dopamine synthesis. Sleep Med 2009;10:123–8.
58. Earley CJ, Connor J, García-Borreguero D, et al. Altered brain iron homeostasis and dopaminergic function in restless legs syndrome (Willis–Ekbom disease). Sleep Med 2014;15:1288–301.
59. Hyacinthe C, De Deurwaerdere P, Thiollier T, et al. Blood withdrawal affects iron store dynamics in primates with consequences on monoaminergic system function. Neuroscience 2015;290:621–35.
60. Connor JR, Wang XS, Patton SM, et al. Decreased transferrin receptor expression by neuromelanin cells in restless legs syndrome. Neurology 2004;62:1563–7.
61. Allen RP, Barker PB, Wehrl F, et al. MRI measurement of brain iron in patients with restless legs syndrome. Neurology 2001;56:263–5.
62. Godau J, Schweitzer KJ, Liepelt I, et al. Substantia nigra hypoechogenicity: definition and findings in restless legs syndrome. Mov Disord 2007;22:187–92.
63. Lee BJ, Farace E, Wang J. In vivo measurement of iron deficiency in RLS with voxel-based MRI relaxometry. Neurology 2007;68:A356 [abst].
64. Rizzo G, Manners D, Testa C, et al. Low brain iron content in idiopathic restless legs syndrome patients detected by phase imaging. Mov Disord 2013;28:1886–90.
65. Connor JR, Ponnuru P, Wang XS, et al. Profile of altered brain iron acquisition in restless legs syndrome. Brain 2011;134:959–68.
66. Dowling P, Klinker F, Amaya F, et al. Iron-deficiency sensitizes mice to acute pain stimuli and formalin-induced nociception. J Nutr 2009;139:2087–92.
67. Hornyak M, Grossmann C, Kohnen R, et al. Cognitive behavioral group therapy to improve patients' strategies for coping with restless legs syndrome: a proof-of-concept trial. J Neurol Neurosurg Psychiatry 2008;79:823–5.
68. Aukerman MM, Aukerman D, Bayard M, et al. Exercise and restless legs syndrome: a randomized controlled trial. J Am Board Fam Med 2006;19:487–93.
69. Giannaki CD, Sakkas GK, Karatzaferi C, et al. Effect of exercise training and dopamine agonists in patients with uremic restless legs syndrome: a six-month randomized, partially double-blind, placebo-controlled comparative study. BMC Nephrol 2013;14:194.
70. Lettieri CJ, Eliasson AH. Pneumatic compression devices are an effective therapy for restless legs syndrome: a prospective, randomized, double-blinded, sham-controlled trial. Chest 2009;135:74–80.
71. Pan W, Wang M, Li M, et al. Actigraph evaluation of acupuncture for treating restless legs syndrome. Evid Based Complement Alternat Med 2015;2015:343201.

72. Mitchell UH, Johnson AW, Myrer B. Comparison of two infrared devices in their effectiveness in reducing symptoms associated with RLS. Physiother Theory Pract 2011;27:352–9.

73. Heide AC, Winkler T, Helms HJ, et al. Effects of transcutaneous spinal direct current stimulation in idiopathic restless legs patients. Brain Stimul 2014;7:636–42.

74. Koo YS, Kim SM, Lee C, et al. Transcranial direct current stimulation on primary sensorimotor area has no effect in patients with drug-naïve restless legs syndrome: a proof-of-concept clinical trial. Sleep Med 2015;16:280–7.

75. Bliwise DL, Zhang RH, Kutner NG. Medications associated with restless legs syndrome: a case-control study in the US Renal Data System (USRDS). Sleep Med 2014;15:1241–5.

76. Zhao M, Geng T, Qiao L, et al. Olanzapine-induced restless legs syndrome. J Clin Neurosci 2014;21:1622–5.

77. Rittmannsberger H, Werl R. Restless legs syndrome induced by quetiapine: report of seven cases and review of the literature. Int J Neuropsychopharmacol 2013;16:1427–31.

78. Hoque R, Chesson AL. Pharmacologically induced/exacerbated restless legs syndrome, periodic limb movements of sleep, and REM behavior disorder/REM sleep without atonia: literature review, qualitative scoring, and comparative analysis. J Clin Sleep Med 2010;6:79–83.

79. Oertel WH, Trenkwalder C, Zucconi M, et al. State of the art in restless legs syndrome: practice recommendations for treating restless legs syndrome. Mov Disord 2007;22 Suppl 18:S466–75.

80. Garcia-Borreguero D, Stillman P, Benes H, et al. Algorithms for the diagnosis and treatment of restless legs syndrome in primary care. BMC Neurol 2011;27;11–28.

81. Stiasny-Kolster K, Kohnen R, Moller JC, Oertel W. Validation of "L-dopa test" for diagnosis of restless legs syndrome. Mov Disord 2006;21:1333–9.

82. Garcia-Borreguero D, Allen RP, Kohnen R, et al; International Restless Legs Syndrome Study Group. Diagnostic standards for dopaminergic augmentation of restless legs syndrome: report from World Association of Sleep Medicine–International Restless Legs Syndrome Study Group consensus conference at the Max Planck Institute. Sleep Med 2007;8:520–30.

83. Vignatelli L, Billiard M, Clarenbach P, et al.; EFNS Task Force. EFNS guidelines on management of restless legs syndrome and periodic limb movement disorder in sleep. Eur J Neurol 2006;13:1049–65.

84. Collado-Seidel V, Kazenwadel J, Wetter TC, et al. A controlled study of additional sr-L-dopa in L-dopa-responsive restless legs syndrome with late-night symptoms. Neurology 1999;52:285–90.

85. Garcia-Borreguero D, Kohnen R, Hogl B, et al. Validation of the Augmentation Severity Rating Scale (ASRS): a multicentric, prospective study with levo-dopa in RLS. Sleep Med 2007;8:455–63.

86. Ferini-Strambi L, Marelli S. Pharmacotherapy for restless legs syndrome. Expert Opin Pharmacother 2014;15:1127–38.

87. Trenkwalder C, Winkelmann J, Inoue Y, Paulus W. Restless legs syndrome—current therapies and management of augmentation. Nat Rev Neurol 2015;11:434–45.

88. Garcia-Borreguero D, Larrosa O, de la Llave Y, et al. Treatment of restless legs syndrome with gabapentin. Neurology 2002;59:1573–9.

89. Allen RP, Chen C, Garcia-Borreguero D, et al. Comparison of pregabalin with pramipexole for restless legs syndrome. N Engl J Med 2014;370:621–31.

90. Garcia-Borreguero D, Patrick J, DuBrava S, et al. Pregabalin versus pramipexole: effects on sleep disturbance in restless legs syndrome. Sleep 2014;37:635–43.

91. Trenkwalder C, Benes H, Grote L, et al.; RELOXYN Study Group. Prolonged release oxycodone–naloxone for treatment of severe restless legs syndrome after failure of previous treatment: a double-blind, randomised, placebo-controlled trial with an open-label extension. Lancet Neurol 2013;12:1141–50.

92. Silber MH, Becker PM, Earley C, et al.; Medical Advisory Board of the Willis–Ekbom Disease Foundation. Willis–Ekbom Disease Foundation revised consensus statement on the management of restless legs syndrome. Mayo Clin Proc 2013;88:977–86.

93. Garcia-Borreguero, D, Kohnen R, Silber MH, et al. The long-term treatment of restless legs syndrome/Willis–Ekbom disease: evidence-based guidelines and clinical consensus best practice guidance: a report from the International Restless Legs Syndrome Study Group. Sleep Med 2013;14:675–84.

94. Ondo WG. Intravenous iron dextran for severe refractory restless legs syndrome. Sleep Med 2010;11:494–6.

95. Earley CJ. The importance of oral iron therapy in restless legs syndrome. Sleep Med 2009;10:945–6.

96. Trenkwalder C, Högl B, Benes H, Kohnen R. Augmentation in restless legs syndrome is associated with low ferritin. Sleep Med 2008;9:572–4.

CHAPTER 25

An overview of sleep dysfunction in Parkinson disease

Elisaveta Sokolov and K. Ray Chaudhuri

Introduction

Disturbances in nocturnal sleep and their consequences during waking in Parkinson disease (PD) were recognized by James Parkinson himself in 1817. Parkinson described sleep problems in his case series as follows: "His attendants observed, that of late the trembling would sometimes begin in his sleep, and increase until it awakened him: when he always was in a state of agitation and alarm" [1]. Sleep disturbance in PD is complex, with a prevalence of up to 98%, and has been shown to be a key determinant of quality of life (QoL) These sleep disturbances are heterogeneous, ranging from insomnia to drug-induced sleep disorders, and now can be assessed by simple validated bedside tools such as the Parkinson's Disease Sleep Scale (PDSS) [2,3]. Also, sleep, contrary to previous perceptions, can be disordered not just in advanced PD, but also in the pre-motor as well as the untreated states [4,5].

Epidemiology

Nocturnal sleep disturbances of varying severity affect virtually all people with PD [6]. Assessment of the epidemiology of sleep disorder in PD and prevalence figures are variable, based on whether the concept includes sleep dysfunction as a whole (holistic) or addresses individual aspects of sleep dysfunction in PD such as insomnias, parasomnias (mostly REM sleep behavior disorder, RBD), excessive daytime sleepiness (EDS), sleep apnea, or drug-induced sleep disorders (Tables 25.1 and 25.2).

Controlled studies

The validation study of the non-motor symptoms (NMS) questionnaire (NMSQuest) compared 123 PD patients with 96 age-matched controls and reported that sleep-related complaints such as insomnia (41%), intense/vivid dreams (31%), acting out during dreams (33%), restless legs (37%), and daytime sleepiness (28%) are significantly more prevalent in PD [7]. In another community-based study, Tandberg et al. [8] reported that 60% of patients with PD (144 of 239) had a range of sleep problems, compared with 33% of healthy controls (33 of 100) with similar age and sex distribution. A multicenter assessment of NMS and their impact on quality of life in PD was carried out, demonstrating that in over 1000 PD patients studied, sleep disturbances (64%) were the second most reported symptom after psychiatric symptoms (67%). The prevalence of sleep disturbance in untreated subjects was approximately 40%, which increased to approximately 82% in more advanced disease [9].

In two recent studies, untreated and early PD patients were compared with healthy controls with respect to NMS, including sleep. Mollenhauer et al. [10] studied 159 untreated PD cases with 110 age-matched controls and reported a significantly worse PDSS score: 15.3 (mean 8.55, range 0–41.00) for PD versus 10.2 (6.34, 0–44.50) for healthy controls; $p < 0.001$. In another study, Khoo et al. [5] studied 159 patients with early PD and 99 healthy controls and reported a significantly greater number of NMS compared with controls: 8.4 versus 2.8. In particular daytime somnolence, dream re-enactment, vivid dreams, restless legs and night-time pain were significantly worse in PD compared to controls. These studies confirm observations from an older study by Dhawan et al. [11], who used PDSS and polysomnography (PSG) in untreated, advanced PD, and healthy controls (Table 25.2).

Sleep as a determinant of QoL and NMS

It has been shown that NMS, including sleep disturbance, are more intrusive for PD patients than their motor symptoms. In an observational study, Hely and colleagues [12] evaluated PD patients followed for a period of 15–18 years after being recruited to a bromocriptine versus levodopa trial: 33% of the original cohort were assessed at 15 years. The majority had significant NMS, including sleep disorders that they regarded as more bothersome than their motor symptoms or levodopa-induced dyskinesias. A study by Politis et al. [13] surveyed early and late PD patients, who were asked to rate their most bothersome symptoms. In both groups, sleep dysfunction was self-rated as one of the most bothersome symptoms by patients. A recent study by Kurtis et al. [14] investigated 388 PD patients in a cross-sectional, multicenter study and reported that fatigue, depression, and urinary, cardiovascular, and thermoregulatory dysfunctions were significant contributors to the SCOPA sleep scale nighttime (SCOPA-NS) score (variance 23%), while cognitive impairment, urinary, cardiovascular, and pupillomotor disorders influenced the SCOPA-daytime score less (variance 14%) . However, fragmentation of sleep occurred much more frequently in PD patients and the impact on their QoL was considered greater. In addition, a community-based study involving 239 PD patients reported that 60% experienced sleep disturbance, compared with 33% of healthy controls with the same demographics [15]. The NMSQuest study in 2006 [7] has enabled delineation of NMS in PD. By using the validated NMSQuest, it was found that symptoms such as nocturia (67%) are common in controls, whereas other sleep-related complaints, such as insomnia (41%),

Table 25.1 Epidemiological studies of sleep studies with healthy controls

Authors [reference]	Year	Study type	Methodology	Numbers	Overall results
Dhawan et al. [11]	2006	Comparative study	PDSS and PSG	DNPD: 25 APD: 34 HC: 131	DNPD: 105.72 ± 21.5 APD: 86.95 ± 20.78 Nocturia, nighttime cramps, dystonia, tremor, and daytime somnolence related to nocturnal disabilities in DNPD
Chaudhuri et al. [7]	2006	NMSQuest	Questionnaire	PD: 123 HC: 96	Nocturia (67%) was common in controls. Insomnia (41%), vivid dreams (31%), acting out during dreams (33%), restless legs (37%), and daytime sleepiness (28%) were more prevalent in PD
Tandberg et al. [15]	1999	Community	Clinical	PD: 239 HC: 100	15.5% of patients experienced EDS compared with only 1% of controls
Van Hilten et al. [72]	1994	Holistic	Clinical		Compared with controls, patients with PD had a raised nocturnal activity level and raised duration of movement, indicative of a more disturbed sleep. Fragmentation of sleep was more frequent in PD patients, and impact on QoL was considered greater than in controls

QoL: quality of life; PSG: polysomnography; EDS: excessive daytime sleepiness; DNPD: drug-naive PD; APD: advanced PD; HC: healthy controls.

Table 25.2 Published sleep studies reporting varying outcomes

Authors [reference]	Year	Type of sleep dysfunction	Type of study	Outcomes
Wetter et al. [73]	2000	PLM	Clinical and PSG	Sleep disruption and increased motor activity during REM and NREM sleep were a frequent finding in PD. 50% showed REM sleep features
Chaudhuri et al. [3]	2002	Holistic	PDSS validation	The mean difference between controls and patients with early/moderate PD was 18%. Mean difference between controls and patients with advanced PD was 35%. PDSS discriminated well between sleep problems of patients with advanced PD and those of patients with early PD
Fabbrini et al [85].	2002	EDS	Clinical and PSG	EDS was significantly higher in treated PD than untreated PD or controls
Stiasny-Kolster et al. [43]	2005	RBD and olfactory dysfunction	Clinical and Imaging	97% of the RBD patients had a pathologically increased olfactory threshold. RBD patients had profound impairments of olfactory function
Hely et al. [12]	2005	Holistic	Questionnaire	The majority had significant NMS, including sleep disorders that they regarded as more bothersome than their motor symptoms or levodopa-induced dyskinesias
Gjerstaad et al. [23]	2006	EDS	Questionnaire	8-year prevalence of 54.2%. EDS was a persistent feature in the majority of patients. EDS was related to age, gender, and use of dopamine agonists
Barone et al. [9]	2009	Holistic	Questionnaire	Sleep disturbances were present in 64% of cohort. Sleep disturbance in untreated subjects was 40%, Sleep disturbance in advanced disease was 82%
Dusek et al. [66]	2010	Daytime REM	Clinical	RPR demonstrated an improvement in sleep scale scores compared with RIR. 43% reported disappearance of sleep attacks on RPR
Bliwise et al. [30]	2013	Daytime REM	MWT	Sizeable proportion of PD patients demonstrated REM sleep and daytime sleep tendency during daytime nap testing. These data confirmed similarities in REM intrusions between PD and narcolepsy

PSG: polysomnography; PDSS: Parkinson's Disease Sleep Scale; EDS: excessive daytime sleepiness; REM: rapid eye movement; RPR: ropinirole prolonged-release; RIR: ropinirole immediate-release; MWT: maintenance of wakefulness testing.

intense/vivid dreams (31%), acting out during dreams (33%), restless legs (37%), and daytime sleepiness (28%), are more prevalent in PD. This was observed in 123 PD patients and 96 age-matched controls in an international multicenter setting (Table 25.1). The overall prevalence figures vary because of the non-homogenous methodology of ascertainment and range from 25% to 98%.

Classification of sleep problems and their impact in PD

Sleep disturbances in PD can be categorized as follows: insomnia, parasomnias, EDS, motor symptom-related sleep disturbances, and sleep disordered breathing (Table 25.3). There are some unifying features in terms of sleep architecture in PD patients, including reduced total sleep time, multiple sleep arousals, sleep efficiency, and fragmentation of sleep [16–18]. We suggest a sleep classification as described in the following subsections.

Excessive daytime sleepiness

This can be defined as the desire and the necessity to sleep during the daytime to such a degree that it interferes with normal function. EDS may be experienced by patients as feeling sleepy or feeling fatigued; however, it is different from fatigue. This phenomenon may be so severe that activities such as driving have to be discontinued [19]. The somnolence can be generalized, or present as sudden onset of sleep or as secondary narcolepsy without cataplexy, the last of these in particular being precipitated by dopamine agonists such as pramipexole and ropinirole, possibly through a D_3 receptor-mediated action [20]. Tests such as the Multiple Sleep Latency test can be carried out in order to delineate and subtype EDS in PD [21].

Generalized somnolence

EDS is an important aspect of sleep-related morbidity in PD and may be caused by underlying dopaminergic denervation or may be due to poor nocturnal sleep. It is prevalent in up to 50% of those with a PD diagnosis, it has been related to age and gender, and it is thought to be a progressive problem [21–23]. The pathophysiology of EDS is unclear. and both disease-related and drug-related factors play a part. Rye et al. [24] and others have argued the case for sleep dysfunction in PD being a manifestation of the dopamine-denervated state, an argument supported by MPTP studies in monkey models. The role of drugs and somnolence in PD is discussed later in this chapter. Fatigue could be a confounder of sleep and EDS in PD. One study by Valko and colleagues [22] demonstrated that fatigued patients were almost twice as likely to suffer from EDS than non-fatigued patients (60% versus 31%). Of these patients, 50% were taking a combination of levodopa and a dopamine agonist, 38% were just taking levodopa, and 10% were just receiving a dopamine agonist. Dopaminergic treatment had a greater effect on EDS than on fatigue. In addition, EDS was more common and severe with prolonged disease course, but the same pattern was not observed when it came to fatigue. The pathophysiology may involve a denervation of the wakefulness flip–flop switch and may also be exacerbated by dopaminergic therapies [25,26].

Sudden onset of sleepiness

In the 1990s, it was reported that some patients with PD may fall asleep suddenly while driving when taking dopamine agonists [27]. This became known as sudden onset of sleep and is now recognized

Table 25.3 Classification of sleep problems in PD

Category	Subtype
Insomnia	Sleep onset
	Sleep maintenance
	Mixed
Parasomnias	*Mainly during non-REM sleep (NREM parasomnias)*
	Commonly observed:
	Confusional arousals
	Sleep terrors
	Nightmares
	Sleep-talking
	Rare:
	Catathrenia
	During REM sleep (REM parasomnias)
	RBD
	REM loss of atonia
EDS	Generalized somnolence
	Episodes of sudden onset of sleep
	Secondary narcolepsy without cataplexy
	Postprandial hypotension
RLS type symptoms	Typical RLS
	Akathisia
	RLS-L (recently reported)
	PLM
Sleep disordered breathing	OSA
Drug-induced	EDS
	SooS
	Insomnia
	Night-eating and impulse control disorder
Nocturia	

REM: rapid eye movement; RBD: REM behavior disorder; EDS: excessive daytime sleepiness; RLS: restless legs syndrome; RLS-L: restless legs syndrome-like; PLM: periodic limb movements; SooS: sudden onset of sleepiness.

as a complication of dopamine agonist therapies as well as a subtype of PD being particularly prone to sleep attacks. The events can occur without any pre-warning (similar to narcolepsy), though in some patients sleepiness typically occurs prior to attacks [26,28].

Narcolepsy without cataplexy

Narcolepsy is a chronic, disabling condition that is recognized by a tetrad of symptoms comprising EDS, cataplexy, sleep paralysis, and hypnagogic hallucinations. Approximately 25% of narcoleptics do not have cataplexy. Of these, the majority have normal levels of hypocretin in their cerebrospinal fluid (CSF), unlike those presenting with narcolepsy with cataplexy (Figs. 25.1 and 25.2).

Narcolepsy without cataplexy can be caused by a partial loss of hypocretin cells [29]. Hypocretin-1 and -2 (also called orexin A and B) are neuropeptides produced from prepro-hypocretin. Hypocretin-containing cells are found within the lateral hypothalamus, with widespread projections to the whole neuraxis. It has been demonstrated that with advancing motor PD, there is a

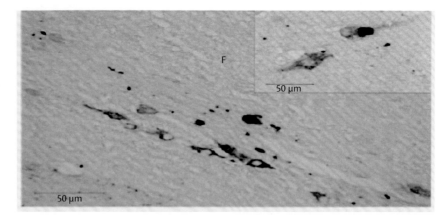

Fig. 25.1 (See colour plate section) Example of hypocretin neurons (DAB staining: dark) that contain a Lewy body (alpha-synuclein, AP-body) in PD patients. Several hypocretin neurons that do not show this colocalization are also present. "F" indicates the fornix.
Reproduced from Brain, 130(6), Hegeman I, van Pelt J, van Duinen S, Jan Lammers G and Swaab DF, Fronczek R, Overeem S, Lee S, Hypocretin (orexin) loss in Parkinson's disease, pp. 1577–1585, Copyright (2007), with permission from Oxford University Press.

progressive loss of hypocretin neurons. Many PD patients have daytime sleep attacks that present similarly to narcoleptic sleep attacks, and those may be increased with the use of dopaminergic agonists, but can also arise independently of these drugs [26]. A recent study by Bliwise et al. [30] showed that a large proportion of PD patients studied demonstrated REM sleep and daytime sleep tendency during daytime nap testing. The authors concluded that there were similarities in REM intrusions between narcolepsy and PD, and a parallel neurodegeneration of hypocretin deficiency was suggested. The loss of hypocretin neurons may be a cause of the narcolepsy-type symptoms of PD, and it has been postulated, but not confirmed, that symptoms may be improved by therapies to reverse the hypocretin deficiency [31]. CSF has been studied in terms of hypocretin level; however, analysis of hypocretins in these PD patients has been inconclusive. Some studies have reported particularly low levels from ventricular CSF sampling, and others have reported normal values. A recent PET imaging study utilizing the serotonin receptor-active ligand DASB suggest that there may be serotonergic dysfunction in the raphe area of the brain underpinning EDS in PD [25] (Table 25.4).

Dopamine agonists, sleep attacks, and somnolence

Korner et al. found that in their cohort of 6620 PD patients, 42.9% had sudden onset of sleepiness (SooS), and 10% of these arose without warning. Notably, the risk of SooS was significantly increased with monotherapy using non-ergot derivatives compared with ergot derivatives or the combination of non-ergot derivatives with L-DOPA in patients younger than 70 years. These findings were independent of duration of drug intake [31]. Dopamine agonists

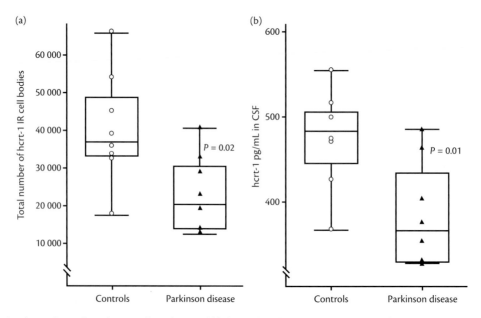

Fig. 25.2 Boxplots showing the median, 25th–75th percentiles and range of (a) the number of hypocretin neurons and (b) the hypocretin-1 (hcrt-1) concentration in post-mortem ventricular cerebrospinal fluid in PD patients and controls. Open circles represent controls and filled triangles represent PD patients.
Reproduced from Brain, 130(6), Hegeman I, van Pelt J, van Duinen S, Jan Lammers G and Swaab DF, Fronczek R, Overeem S, Lee S, Hypocretin (orexin) loss in Parkinson's disease, pp. 1577–1585, Copyright (2007), with permission from Oxford University Press.

Table 25.4 Studies reporting orexin/hypocretin measurements in PD

Authors [reference]	Year	Type of study	Outcomes
Thannickal et al. [29]	2009	Post-mortem human brain/immunohistochemistry	PD characterized by massive hypocretin cell loss, with greater loss with disease progression and severity
Fronczek et al. [74]	2007	Post-mortem/immunoassay	Significant decrease between PD patients and controls in the number of hypocretin neurons (40% lower in prefrontal cortex and 25% lower in CSF)
Compta et al. [75]	2009	Clinical CSF studies	CSF hypocretin-1 levels were unrelated to either Epworth sleepiness scale. Excessive daytime sleepiness was more frequent in
			PD patients with dementia than PD patients without dementia, but lumbar CSF hypocretin-1 levels were normal and unrelated to severity of sleepiness or the cognitive status
Weinecke et al. [76]	2012	Clinical	Progressive loss of hypocretin cells over the course of PD
Bridoux et al. [77]	2013	Clinical (ventriculography during DBS)	High levels of hypocretin-1 in PD may be associated with loss of REM muscle atonia

CSF: cerebrospinal fluid; REM: rapid eye movement; DBS: deep brain stimulation.

are known to have a variable effect on sleep. They impact sleep architecture, causing EDS or SooS in susceptible patients. Onset insomnia and maintenance insomnia may be an effect. During NREM sleep, night-eating syndromes have been reported, possibly as part of impulse control disorder, as well as hallucinations and night terrors [32].

REM sleep behavior disorder

This is a parasomnia that involves abnormal behavior during the sleep phase with rapid eye movements. It was first described in 1986 by Schenk et al. [33]. RBD is characterized by loss of skeletal muscle atonia with prominent motor activity and dreaming [34]. There is a loss of motor inhibition that triggers various behaviors during sleep, ranging from limb twitches to more complex movements such as kicking, boxing, and other purposeful movements. This is often associated with frightening dreams or nightmares [35] during which the patient will shout out or act out their thoughts [36–39]. The REM Sleep Behavior Disorder Screening Questionnaire (RBD-SQ), and REM-Sleep-Behavior Disorder Severity Scale (RBD-SS) are available for bedside screening [40,41]. Diagnosis of definite RBD requires PSG and is usually made using the criteria established by Schenck and colleagues and the International Classification of Sleep Disorders, Second Edition (ICSD-2) [42].

RBD in pre-motor PD

RBD is a strong predictor of development of synucleinopathy [43], and studies suggest that it could be a robust pre-motor marker of PD, with up to 82% of older men diagnosed with RBD going on to develop parkinsonism or dementia [44]. The sublaterodorsal nucleus (SLD) inhibits locomotor generators and spinal interneurons throughout REM sleep. It is therefore possible that muscle atonia may be due to degeneration of these nuclei [45]. The pathological basis of RBD is unknown; however, the key structures potentially implicated in RBD pathology include the locus coeruleus, lateral pontine tegmentum, pedunculopontine nucleus, ventrolateral preoptic (VLPO) nucleus, and SLD. Psychosis can be experienced by

at least 50–60% of patients with advanced PD, and an association between vivid dreams and PD psychosis has been shown in some cases [46–48]. Arnulf et al. [49] found that REM periods during wakefulness were present in patients with PD and psychosis. A prospective two-year study showed that patients with RBD and hallucinations tended to be older, with a greater extent of loss of executive function than those who did not experience hallucinations [50].

Daytime REM intrusion

The interruption of REM sleep into the daytime is a feature of narcolepsy. The importance of these interruptions is, however, yet to be determined. Some PD patients demonstrated REM sleep and daytime sleepiness during daily nap assessments. This verifies similarities between REM interruptions in narcolepsy and PD. This could implicate a similar hypocretin deficiency in both conditions [30].

Sleep disordered breathing

Sleep disordered breathing is increasingly recognized in PD. Obstructive sleep apnea (OSA) is thought to be prevalent in 50% of PD patients [51], resulting in daytime tiredness or sleepiness. Upper airway dysfunction in PD may promote OSA, leading yo symptoms such as daytime fatigue and somnolence, as well as loud and/or irregular snoring accompanied by intermittent gasping. However, unlike non-PD subjects with OSA, PD patients do not have a large body habitus or a thick neck circumference. OSA may coexist with restless legs syndrome (RLS), RBD, or periodic limb movements (PLM). However, some studies have found the link between OSA and PD to be tenuous [52]. Formal PSG will identify sleep apnea in the majority of patients [53].

Nocturia

Nocturia is a common cause of sleep disruption in PD and was shown to affect 43% of patients in one study [54], with an estimated prevalence of 30–80% [10,55–57]. Studies using bedside scales such as the Non-Motor Symptoms Scale (NMSS) and the

Table 25.5 Animal models of PD demonstrating sleep disturbance

Authors [reference]	Study title	Animal model	Symptoms studied
Jenner et al. [78]	Animal models of Parkinson's disease: a source of novel treatments and clues to the cause of the disease	6-OHDA-lesioned rodents.	Sleep/wakefulness, circadian rhythms, RBD
Chesselet et al. [79]	Progressive mouse model of parkinson's disease: the Thy1-aSyn (Line 61) mice	Alpha-synuclein over-expressor (ASO = Thy1-aSYN) mice	Circadian rhythm, insomnia
Jenner et al. [78]	Animal models of Parkinson's disease: a source of novel treatments and clues to the cause of the disease	MPTP-treated primates	Sleep–wake cycle. REM sleep/RBD
Taylor et al. [69]	Non-motor symptoms of Parkinson's disease revealed in an animal model with reduced monoamine storage capacity	VMAT2-deficient mice	Altered sleep latency

6-OHDA: 6-hydroxydopamine; MPTP: 1-methyl-4-phenyl-1,2,3,6-tetrahydropyridine; VMAT2: vesicular monoamine transporter 2; REM: rapid eye movement; RBD: REM sleep behavior disorder.

PDSS have consistently identified nocturia as one of the most prevalent symptoms in PD, becoming more intrusive to sleep as the disease advances [58]. More than 50% of PD patients have severe bladder symptoms, commonly symptoms of overactive bladder [59]. Furthermore, in patients with comparable levels of nocturia, poorer sleep as defined on PSG is regarded as more bothersome [60]. In terms of causation, one theory is that the micturition reflex is normally inhibited by the basal ganglia. Degeneration then occurs, leading to a loss of this D_1-mediated inhibition and subsequent detrusor overactivity [56]. Uchiyama et al. [61] found that the effects of apomorphine on bladder function in rats are both time- and dose-dependent. At low doses, it decreased voiding frequency and increased micturition volume (which reflected an increase in bladder capacity). At medium and high doses of apomorphine, there was an initial increase and then a subsequent decrease in frequency and an initial decrease and a subsequent increase in volume. The pharmacodynamics of dopamine receptor agonists on nocturia and urgency are clearly more complicated than anticipated. This fresh perspective may be useful in understanding the often conflicting data on the effects of dopamine receptor agonists on NMS in PD. Rotigotine, for instance, has been shown to be effective for nocturia in open-label studies, while the RECOVER study (randomized and placebo-controlled) failed to confirm this observation [62].

Insomnias

The ICSD describes insomnia as "difficulty in initiating and/or maintaining sleep." Broadly insomnia is of two types: sleep initiation insomnia (SII) and sleep maintenance insomnia (SMI). The latter is reported to be one of the five most bothersome symptoms of advanced PD [20]. Patients with PD have problems with sleep fragmentation and early awakening compared with controls, whereas sleep initiation problems are equally frequent among patients and healthy elderly people [13]. SMI may be due to frequent waking at night as a result of nocturnal akinesia and off periods [63].

Sleep disturbance secondary to anti-parkinsonian medications

Dopaminergic therapy can affect the sleep–wake cycle and in high dose induces wakefulness and disrupts typical sleep patterns by reducing slow-wave and REM sleep. Dopaminergic medications in low doses increases sleep duration at night and induce somnolence. Several studies, such as the RECOVER study suggest that sustained overnight dopaminergic stimulation can reduce nocturnal akinesia, RLS, and PLM and thereby improve sleep quality and quantity [62]. Drugs, including amantadine, selegiline, and anticholinergics aggravate sleep initiation and may induce insomnia, while selective serotonin reuptake inhibitors (SSRIs) may need to be avoided in the evening as they promote wakefulness [64]. Insomnia may also be caused by giving inhibitors of monoamine oxidase B (MAO-B) inhibitors such as selegiline late at night; in the case of selegiline, this is likely due to it having an amphetamine metabolite [65]. Evidence suggests that dopamine agonists such as short-acting ropinirole and pramipexole may potentiate SooS, with levodopa doing so to a lesser extent [66].

Pathophysiology

Animal models

Studies in both cats and rats have demonstrated important structures involved in the condition [67]. It has been suggested that degeneration of brainstem nuclei such as the locus coeruleus, pedunculopontine nucleus, and sublaterodorsal nucleus may be important in the pathophysiology of RBD. These nuclei have been shown to be closely interconnected, either activating or inhibiting one another. Muscle atonia and enactment during REM sleep may be due to disturbances in the sublaterodorsal nucleus, which has inhibitory effects on locomotor generators and spinal interneurons [68]. Thus, animal studies have shown a close relationship between dopamine and sleep (Table 25.5). Degeneration of central sleep regulatory neurons and related thalamocortical pathways is implicated in the sleep disturbance evident in PD [69–70]. This essentially arises as an indirect effect of dopaminergic cell depletion in the brainstem. The ventral tegmental area and the pars compacta of the substantia nigra both display connections to areas related to sleep regulation. Stimulation of D_1-like receptors is wake-related, whereas stimulation of D_2-like receptors is biphasic. Stimulation occurs at low doses, and sleep-inducing effects precipitate at higher doses. In addition, D_3 agonists promote sleep [71].

Table 25.6 Validated scales for the assessment of sleep in PD

Reference	Scale
[80]	Parkinson's Disease Sleep Scale (PDSS) Versions 1 and 2
[81]	Pittsburgh Sleep Quality Index (PSQI)
[82]	Scales for Outcomes in Parkinson's Disease (SCOPA) Sleep Scale
[83]	Epworth Sleepiness Scale (ESS)
[84]	Inappropriate Sleep Composite Score (ISCS)
[84]	Stanford Sleepiness Scale (SSS)

Diagnostic tools for sleep disorders in PD

Clinical tools

The systematic use of a sleep questionnaire is recommended in order to accurately recognize these NMS in PD, and the Movement Disorders Society (MDS) task force has reviewed and recommended a number of PD validated scales for use in the clinic and at the bedside. Table 25.6 illustrates scales fulfilling the criteria outlined by the MDS that are recommended for use. In addition to assessment of the PD patient using one of these scales, measurement of sleep and wake is indicated in patients with potential sleep apnea or parasomnias. For a brief screen in the clinic, the patient-completed NMSQuest, which has a sleep domain, can be used.

Treatment

The nature of sleep disturbance in PD is multifactorial and, as such, treatment has to be tailored to individual cases and etiology. The evidence base in most cases remains poor and recently both the American Academy of Neurology (AAN) and the MDS have issued guidance on evidence-based management of NMS of PD that includes sleep disorders. Recommended treatments from these guidelines are shown in Table 25.7.

Conclusions

Overall, sleep dysfunction is a key NMS of PD and a major determinant of QoL of patients as well as caregivers. Sleep dysfunction in PD is multifactorial and complex and can be present from the pre-motor to the palliative stage. It is essential that sleep dysfunction be correctly identified and treated by healthcare professionals. Exciting new developments suggest that aspects of sleep problems could function as possible clinical biomarkers for PD and also subtypes of PD. Several validated clinical sleep scales for bedside use are available and serve to refine accurate management of aspects of sleep dysfunction in PD and subsequent improvement in patients' QoL.

Acknowledgements

This chapter presents independent research funded by the National Institute for Health Research (NIHR) Mental Health Biomedical Research Centre and Dementia Unit at South London and Maudsley NHS Foundation Trust and King's College London.

Table 25.7 Treatment of sleep disturbance in PD

Insomnia-related symptoms: fragmented sleep with problems in sleep onset and maintenance	Pharmacological strategies	Short-acting benzodiazepines Non-benzodiazepine hypnotics: zopiclone Tricyclic antidepressants: amitriptyline
	Nonpharmacological measures	Avoid alcohol at night, caffeine, tobacco Daytime exercise and exposure to sunshine Relaxation and cognitive therapies
Motor symptoms: fidgeting, cramps, posturing, tremor, akinesia	Pharmacological strategies	Trial of sustained dopaminergic stimulation (nighttime dosing of): levodopa + COMT inhibitor; long-acting dopamine agonists (rotigotine patch therapy has level 1 evidence to support nighttime use) Nocturnal apomorphine infusion (only in specialized centers)
	Nonpharmacological measures	Use of satin bed sheets and bed straps to help movement in bed
RBD	Pharmacological strategies	Clonazepam Melatonin Pramipexole + clonazepam Donepezil, levodopa (have been tried)
Urinary symptoms: nocturia	Pharmacological strategies	Low-dose amitriptyline Consider transdermal rotigotine patch. If detrusor instability: oxybutynin, tolterodine If morning hypotension: desmopressin nasal spray; do not use evening diuretics, antihypertensives, or vasodilators
	Nonpharmacological strategies	Decrease evening fluid intake Empty bladder prior to bed Catheters/bedside commode If associated with postural hypotension, head-up tilt of bed
Sleep apnea		NIV, CPAP, MRS, soft palate implants
EDS		Modafinil, caffeine tablets
RLS/PLM		Dopamine agonist, gabapentin

COMT: catechol O-methyltransferase; RBD: REM sleep behavior disorder; CPAP: continuous positive airway pressure; NIV: noninvasive ventilation; MRS: mandibular responding splint; EDS: excessive daytime sleepiness; RLS: restless legs syndrome; PLM: periodic limb movements.

References

1. Parkinson J. An essay on the shaking palsy 1817. J Neuropsychiatry Clin Neurosci 2002;14:223–36; discussion 222.

2. Lees AJ, Blackburn NA, Campbell VL. The night time problems of Parkinson's disease. Clin Neuropharmacol;1988;11:512.

3. Chaudhuri KR, Pal S, DiMarco A, et al. The Parkinson's disease sleep scale: a new instrument for assessing sleep and nocturnal disability in Parkinson's disease. J Neurol Neurosurg Psychiatry 2002;73:629–35.

4. Karlsen KH, Larsen JP, Tandberg E, Maeland JG. Influence of clinical and demographic variables on quality of life in patients with Parkinson's disease. J Neurol Neurosurg Psychiatry 1999;66:431–5.

5. Khoo, TK, Yarnall AJ, Duncan GW, et al. The spectrum of nonmotor symptoms in early Parkinson disease. Neurology 2013;80(3):276–81.

6. Chaudhuri KR, Healy DG, Schapira AH. Non-motor symptoms of Parkinson's disease: diagnosis and management. Lancet Neurol 2006;5:235–45.

7. Chaudhuri KR, Martinez-Martin P, Schapira AH, et al. International multicenter pilot study of the first comprehensive self-completed nonmotor symptoms questionnaire for Parkinson's disease: the NMSQuest study. Mov Disord 2006;21:916–23.

8. Tandberg E, Larsen J, Karlsen K. A community based study of sleep disorders in patients with Parkinson's disease. Mov Disord 1998;13:895–9.

9. Barone P, Antonini A, Colosimo C, et al. The PRIAMO study: a multicenter assessment of nonmotor symptoms and their impact on quality of life in Parkinson's disease. Mov Disord 2009;24:1641–9.

10. Mollenhauer B, Trautmann E, Sixel-Döring F, et al. Nonmotor and diagnostic findings in subjects with de novo Parkinson disease of the DeNoPa cohort. Neurology 2013;81(14):1226–34.

11. Dhawan V, Dhoat S, Williams et al. The range and nature of sleep dysfunction in untreated Parkinson's disease (PD). A comparative controlled clinical study using the Parkinson's disease sleep scale and selective polysomnography. J Neurol Sci 2006;248:158–62.

12. Hely MA, Morris JG, Reid WG, Trafficante R. Sydney Multicenter Study of Parkinson's disease: non-L-dopa-responsive problems dominate at 15 years. Mov Disord 2005; 20:190–9.

13. Politis M, Molloy S, Bain P, Chaudhuri KR, Piccini P. Parkinson's disease symptoms: the patient's perspective. Mov Disord 2010;25:1646–51.

14. Kurtis M, Rodriguez-Blazquez C, Martinez-Martin P. Relationship between sleep disorders and other non-motor symptoms in Parkinson's disease. Parkinsonism Relat Disord 2013;19:1152–5.

15. Tandberg E, Larsen JP, Karlsen K. Excessive daytime sleepiness and sleep benefit in Parkinson's disease: a community-based study. Mov Disord 1999;14:922–7.

16. Adler CH, Thorpy MJ. Sleep issues in Parkinson's disease. Neurology 2005;64:S12–20.

17. Arnulf I, Konofal E, Merino-Andreu M, et al. Parkinson's disease and sleepiness: an integral part of PD. Neurology 2002;58:1019–24.

18. Rye DB, Jankovic J. Emerging views of dopamine in modulating sleep/wake state from an unlikely source: PD. Neurology 2002;58:341–6.

19. Meindorfner C, Körner Y, Möller JC, et al. Driving in Parkinson's disease: mobility, accidents, and sudden onset of sleep at the wheel. Mov Disord 2005;20(7):832–42.

20. Chaudhuri KR. Nocturnal symptom complex in PD and its management. Neurology 2003;61:S17–23.

21. Arnulf I. Excessive daytime sleepiness in Parkinsonism. Sleep Med Rev 2005;9:185–200.

22. Valko PO, Waldvogel D, Weller M, et al. Fatigue and excessive daytime sleepiness in idiopathic Parkinson's disease differently correlate with motor symptoms, depression and dopaminergic treatment. Eur J Neurol 2010;17(12):1428–36.

23. Gjerstaad MD, Alves G, Wentzel-Larsen T, Aarsland D, Larsen JP. Excessive daytime sleepiness in Parkinson disease. Neurology 2006;67(5):853–8.

24. Rye D. Seeing beyond one's nose: sleep disruption and excessive sleepiness accompany motor disability in the MPTP treated primate. Exp Neurol 2010;222(2):179–80.

25. Pavese N, Metta V, Simpson BS, et al. Sleep regulatory centres dysfunction in Parkinson's disease patients with excessive daytime sleepiness. An in vivo PET study. Parkinsonism Relat Disord 2012;18(2):S24–5.

26. Saper CB, Chou TC, Scammell TE. The sleep switch: hypothalamic control of sleep and wakefulness. Trends Neurosci 2001;24:726–31.

27. Frucht S, Rogers JD, Greene PE, Gordon MF, Fahn S. Falling asleep at the wheel: motor vehicle mishaps in persons taking Pramipexole and Ropinirole. Neurology 1999;52:1908–10.

28. Körner Y, Meindorfner C, Möller JC, et al. Predictors of sudden onset of sleep in Parkinson's disease. Mov Disord 2004;19:1298–305.

29. Thannickal TC, Nienhuis R, Siegel JM. Localized loss of hypocretin (orexin) cells in narcolepsy without cataplexy. Sleep S 2009;32(8):993–8.

30. Bliwise DL, Trotti LM, Juncos JJ, et al. Daytime REM sleep in Parkinson's disease. Parkinsonism Relat Disord 2013;19(1):101–3.

31. Nishino S, Ripley B, Overseem S, et al. Hypocretin (orexin) deficiency in human narcolepsy. Lancet 2000;355:39–40.

32. Neto M, Pereira M, Sobreira E, et al. Sleep-related eating disorder in two patients with early-onset Parkinson's disease. Eur Neurol 2011;66:106–9.

33. Schenck CH, Bundlie SR, Ettinger MG, Mahowald MW. Chronic behavioral disorders of human REM sleep: a new category of parasomnia. Sleep 1986;9:293–308.

34. Olsen EJ, Boeve BF, Silber MH. Rapid eye movement sleep behaviour disorder; demographic, clinical and laboratory findings in 93 cases. Brain 2000;123(Pt 2):331–9.

35. Schenck CH, Mahowald MW. REM sleep behavior disorder: clinical, developmental, and neuroscience perspectives 16 years after its formal identification in SLEEP. Sleep 2002;25:120–38.

36. Schenck CH, Bundlie SR, Mahowald MW. Delayed emergence of a parkinsonian disorder in 38% of 29 older men initially diagnosed with idiopathic rapid eye movement sleep behaviour disorder. Neurology 1996; 46:388–93.

37. Olson EJ, Boeve BF, Silber MH. Rapid eye movement sleep behaviour disorder: demographic, clinical and laboratory findings in 93 cases. Brain 2000;123:331–9.

38. Fantini ML, Ferini-Strambi L, Montplaisir J. Idiopathic REM sleep behaviour disorder: toward a better nosologic definition. Neurology 2005;64:780–6.

39. Comella CL, Nardine TM, Diederich NJ, Stebbins GT. Sleep-related violence, injury, and REM sleep behavior disorder in Parkinson's disease. Neurology 1998;51:526–9.

40. Stiasny-Kolster K, Mayer G, Schafer S, et al. The REM sleep behavior disorder screening questionnaire—a new diagnostic instrument. Mov Disord 2007;22:2386–93.

41. Martinez-Martin P, Visser M, Rodriguez-Blazquez C, et al. SCOPA-sleep and PDSS: two scales for assessment of sleep disorder in Parkinson's disease. Mov Disord 2008;23(12):1681–8.

42. American Academy of Sleep Medicine. REM sleep behavior disorder. The international classification of sleep disorders diagnostic and coding manual, 2nd ed. Westchester, IL: American Academy of Sleep Medicine, 2005:148–52.

43. Stiasny-Kolster K, Doerr Y, Möller JC, et al. Combination of "idiopathic" REM sleep behaviour disorder and olfactory dysfunction as possible indicator for alpha-synucleinopathy demonstrated by dopamine transporter FP-CIT-SPECT. Brain 2005;128:126–37.

44. Schenck CH, Boeve BF, Mahowald MW. Delayed emergence of a parkinsonian disorder or dementia in 81% of older males initially diagnosed with idiopathic REM sleep behavior disorder (RBD): 16 year update on a previously reported series. Sleep Med 2013;14:744–8.

45. Bradley F, Boeve MD, Silber MH, et al. Association of REM sleep behavior disorder and neurodegenerative disease may reflect an underlying synucleinopathy. Mov Disord 2001;16(4):622–30.

46. Thanvi BR, Lo TCN, Harsh DP. Psychosis in Parkinson's disease. Postgrad Med J 2005;81:644–6.

47. Goetz CG. Scales to evaluate psychosis in Parkinson's disease. Parkinsonism Relat Disord 2009;15(Suppl 3):S38–41.

48. Ravina B, Marder K, Fernandez HH, et al. Diagnostic criteria for psychosis in Parkinson's disease; report of an NINDS, NIMH work group. Mov Disord 2007;22(8):1061–8.

49. Arnulf I, Bonnet AM, Damier P, et al. Hallucinations, REM sleep, and Parkinson's disease; a medical hypothesis. Neurology 2000;55(5):281–8.

50. Sinforiani E, Pacchetti C, Zangaglia R, et al. REM behaviour disorder, hallucinations and cognitive impairment in Parkinson's disease; a two year follow-up. Mov Disord 2008;23(10):1441–5.

51. Diederich NJ, Vaillant M, Leischen M, et al. Sleep apnea syndrome in Parkinson's disease. A case-control study in 49 patients. Mov Disord 2005;20:1413–18.

52. Leu S, Oudiette D, Roze E, et al. Is obstructive sleep apnoea a problem in Parkinson's disease? Sleep Med 2010;11:247–52.

53. Uemura Y, Nomura T, Inoue Y, et al. Validation of the Parkinson's disease sleep scale in Japanese patients: a comparison study using the Pittsburgh Sleep Quality Index, the Epworth sleepiness scale and polysomnography. J Neurol Sci 2009;287:36–40.

54. Stocchi F, Barbato L, Nordera G, Berardelli A, Ruggieri S. Sleep disorders in Parkinson's disease. Adv Neurol 2001;86:289–93.

55. Grandas F, Iranzo A. Nocturnal problems occurring in Parkinson's disease. Neurology 2004;63:S8–11.

56. Blackett H, Walker R, Wood B. Urinary dysfunction in Parkinson's disease: a review. Parkinsonism Relat Disord 2009;15:81–7.

57. Oerlemans W, de Weerd AW. The prevalence of sleep disorders in patients with Parkinson's disease. Sleep Med 2003;3:147–9.

58. Garcia-Borreguero D, Larrosa O, Bravo M. Parkinson's disease and sleep. Sleep Med Rev 2003;7:115–29.

59. Winge K, Nielsen KK. Bladder dysfunction in advanced Parkinson's disease. Neurourol Urodyn 2012;31(8):1279–83.

60. Vaughan CP, Juncos JL, Trotti LM, Johnson TM 2nd, Bliwise DL. Nocturia and overnight polysomnography in Parkinson disease. Neurourol Urodyn 2013;32(8):1080–5.

61. Uchiyama T, Sakakibara R, Yoshiyama M, et al. Biphasic effect of apomorphine, an anti-parkinsonian drug, on bladder function in rats. Neuroscience 2009;162(4):1333–8.

62. Trenkwalder C, Kies B, Rudsinska M, et al. Rotigotine effects on early morning motor function and sleep in Parkinson's disease: a double-blind, randomised, placebo-controlled study (RECOVER). Mov Disord 2011;26(1):90–9.

63. Nico J, Mcintyre D. Sleep disorders in Parkinson's disease: many causes, few therapeutic options. J Neurol Sci 2012;314(1–2):12–19.

64. Heinonnen EH, Myllyla V. Safety of Selegeline (deprenyl) in the treatment of Parkinson's disease. Drug Saf 1998;19:11–22.

65. Lyons KE, Friedman JH, Hermanowicz N, et al. Orally disintegrating Selegeline in Parkinson's patients with dopamine agonist-related adverse effects. Clin Neuropharmacol 2010;33: 5–10.

66. Dusek P, Busková J, Růzicka E, et al. Effects of ropinirole prolonged-release on sleep disturbances and daytime sleepiness in Parkinson disease. Clin Neuropharmacol 2010;33(4):186–90.

67. Duty S, Jenner P. Animal models of Parkinson's disease: a source of novel treatments and clues to the cause of the disease. Br J Pharmacol 2011;164:1357–91.

68. Shouse MN, Siegel JM. Pontine regulation of REM sleep components in cats: integrity of the pedunculopontine tegmentum (PPT) is important for phasic events but unnecessary for atonia during REM sleep. Brain Res 1992;571:50–63.

69. Taylor TN, Caudle WM, Shepherd K, et al. Non-motor symptoms of Parkinson's disease revealed in an animal model with reduced monoamine storage capacity. J Neurosci 2009;29(25):8103.

70. Boeve BF, Silber MH, Saper CB, et al. Pathophysiology of REM sleep behaviour disorder and relevance to neurodegenerative disease. Brain 2007;130:2770–88.

71. Monti J, Monti D. The involvement of dopamine in the modulation of sleep and waking. Sleep Med Rev 2007;11:113–33.

72. van Hilten B, et al. Arch Neurol 1994;51(9):922–8.

73. Wetter TC, Collado-Seidel V, Pollmächer T, Yassouridis A, Trenkwalder C. Sleep and periodic leg movement patterns in drug-free patients with Parkinson's disease and multiple system atrophy. 2000;23(3):361–7.

74. Fronczek R, Overeem S, Hegeman I, Lammers G, et al. Hypocretin (orexin) loss in Parkinson's disease. Brain 2007;1577–85.

75. Compta Y, Santamaria J, Ratti L, Tolosa E, et al. Cerebrospinal hypocretin, daytime sleepiness and sleep architecture in Parkinson's disease dementia. Brain 2009;3308–17.

76. Wienecke M, Werth E, Poryazova R, Bauman-Vogel H, et al. Progressive dopamine and hypocretin deficiencies in Parkinson's disease: is there an impact on sleep and wakefulness? Journal of Sleep Research 2012;21(6):710–17.

77. Bridoux A, Moutereau S, Covali-Noroc A, Margarit L, Palfi S, et al. Ventricular orexin-A (hypocretin-1) levels correlate with rapid-eye-movement sleep without atonia in Parkinson's disease. Nat Sci Sleep 2013;5:87–91.

78. Jenner, et al. Animal models of Parkinson's disease: a source of novel treatments and clues to the cause of the disease. Br J Pharmacol 2011;164(4):1357–91. doi: 10.1111/j.1476-5381.2011.01426.x.

79. Chesselet, et al . Progressive mouse model of Parkinson's disease: the Thy1-aSyn (Line 61) mice. Neurotherapeutics 2012;9(2):297–314.

80. Parkinson's Disease Sleep Scale (PDSS). The Parkinson's disease sleep scale: a new instrument for assessing sleep and nocturnal disability in Parkinson's disease. J Neurol Neurosurg Psychiatry 2002;73:629–35. doi:10.1136/jnnp.73.6.629.

81. Buysse DJ, Reynolds CF, Monk TH, et al. The Pittsburgh Sleep Quality Index: a new instrument for psychiatric practice and research. Psychiatry Res 1989;28:193–213.

82. Scales for Outcomes in Parkinson's Disease (SCOPA). A short scale for the assessment of motor impairments and disabilities in Parkinson's disease: the SPES/SCOPA. J Neurol Neurosurg Psychiatry 2004;75:388–95. doi:10.1136/jnnp.2003.017509.

83. The Parkinson's disease sleep scale: a new instrument for assessing sleep and nocturnal disability in Parkinson's disease. J Neurol Neurosurg Psychiatry 2002;73:629–35. doi:10.1136/jnnp.73.6.629.

84. Goetz, et al. Scales to assess sleep impairment in Parkinson's disease: Critique and recommendations. Movement disorders 2010;25(1615):2704–16.

85. Fabbrini G, Barbanti P, Aurilia C, et al. Excessive daytime sleepiness in de novo and treated Parkinson's disease. Mov Disord. 2002;17(5):1026–30.

CHAPTER 26

Sleep disorders in neurodegenerative diseases other than Parkinson disease and multiple system atrophy

Raffaele Manni and Michele Terzaghi

Introduction

The twenty-first century will witness an unprecedented increase in the aging of the population [1]. Between 2000 and 2050, the proportion of the world's population aged over 60 years will double, rising from about 11% to about 22%. Since there is a strong link between aging and the likelihood of developing neurodegenerative diseases, the number of people suffering from these conditions is expected to rise. Thus, the assessment and management of neurodegenerative diseases is set to play an increasingly prominent role in clinical practice in the coming decades.

Patients affected by neurodegenerative diseases frequently report sleep–wake disturbances of various kinds [2–4]. There is growing evidence that sleep alterations are associated with a higher incidence of cognitive and neuropsychiatric problems, leading to a reduced quality of life [5–7]. Furthermore, sleep alterations result in an increased caregiver burden [8,9] and can ultimately be a factor leading to the institutionalization of affected patients [10,11].

Yet, in spite of these considerations, there are no large-scale systematic studies of sleep in neurodegenerative diseases other than Alzheimer disease (AD) and other dementias.

Changes in sleep patterns, in particular greater nocturnal sleep fragmentation and the development of a tendency to nap during the day, are part of the normal aging process [12–14]. In this setting, neurodegeneration, in affected patients, causes further disruption of sleep patterns [15]. Accumulating evidence indicates that sleep disturbances in neurodegenerative diseases should not be considered merely ancillary symptoms, but rather that their presence is directly related to the neurodegenerative process. Although the mechanisms underlying sleep alterations in neurodegenerative conditions are still to be fully clarified, it is possible that they can be attributed both to direct structural alterations to the networks orchestrating sleep generation and to a variety of indirect mechanisms acting against them [16].

The neuronal degeneration leading to the central nervous system-related manifestations typically characterizing neurodegenerative diseases affects multiple neurotransmitter pathways [17]. The resulting dysfunctions are likely to impact on the three main systems involved in sleep regulation: the homeostatic system, which determines sleep, including its duration and structure; the circadian system, which regulates sleep propensity in relation to the time of day/night; and the ultradian system, which regulates NREM/REM alternation.

Age-related changes in sleep

Age-related changes in homeostatic as well as circadian processes may account for the sleep fragmentation, difficulty in falling asleep, and decreased slow-wave sleep (SWS) typically observed in the elderly [12–14,18]. Objective sleep changes occurring in this population include a lower density of phasic events (i.e, a decrease in K-complexes and sleep spindles), more frequent stage shifts, lower sleep efficiency, and lower percentages of SWS and REM sleep [18,19]. Sleep efficiency, in particular, continues to decrease with increasing age (Table 26.1).

The modifications in sleep architecture and schedule that are induced by alterations in the circadian modulation of sleep occurring with advancing age potentially contribute to a variety of age-related disorders [13,14]. Moreover, the prevalence of sleep disorders such as sleep-related breathing disorder (SRBDs), restless legs syndrome (RLS), and periodic limb movements (PLM) in sleep increases with age [18].

In neurodegenerative disorders, however, the prominence of sleep alterations is much greater than that which can be attributed to aging per se [4]. Furthermore, comorbid conditions (cardiovascular, metabolic, osteomuscular, respiratory, gastrointestinal, nycturia, etc.) or the effects of the medications for these comorbidities further contribute to the sleep disruption [19–23].

Alzheimer disease

Sleep disturbances in AD patients frequently occur in association with behavioral and psychiatric symptoms of dementia [24–26]; for this reason, they tend to be overlooked, especially in the early stages of the disease.

However, recent studies report sleep disorders among the core non-cognitive symptoms in mild cognitive impairment (MCI) [27],

Table 26.1 PSG findings in normal aging and neurodegenerative diseases

Sleep macrostructure	Aging	Alzheimer disease	Dementia with Lewy bodies	Progressive supranuclear palsy	Huntingtondisease
Reduced sleep efficiency	x	x	x	x	x
Long sleep latency			x		x
Long REM sleep latency			x		
Lower percentages of SWS	x	x	x		x
Lower percentages of REM sleep	x	x	x	x	x
Diminished total sleep time				x	x
Increased arousal index			x		
Lower density of phasic events	x				
Increased frequency of stage shifts	x				

x: present.

and, globally, 45–50% of patients with AD report sleep complaints such as early morning or recurrent nocturnal awakenings and daytime sleepiness [28–31]. Sleep disruption in AD patients is reportedly the main reason for their institutionalization [12,32].

Polysomnographic (PSG) studies in patients with AD (Table 26.1) indicate that their sleep is characterized by longer and more frequent awakenings, decreased SWS and REM sleep, and more daytime napping [30,33–35]. Sleep disordered breathing (SDB), in the form of sleep apnea, may be present with a prevalence ranging from 33% to 53% of patients with probable AD. The prevalence of obstructive sleep apnea (OSA) increases with aging, but it seems that patients with AD are at an even higher risk, with 40–70% of patients experiencing five or more apneas/hypopneas per hour of sleep [36–38].

No studies have specifically assessed the prevalence of PLM in dementia, and it should be noted that the effective role of PLM in sleep fragmentation needs to be clarified: a higher PLM index was found to be associated with longer sleep latency, but assessment of the effective correlates of PLM is difficult, as it has been reported that PLM (in sleep) may occur in subjects without any sleep complaints and are more frequent with aging [39,40]. RLS is reported in up to 24% of demented subjects [41].

Abnormal nocturnal behaviors during sleep are significantly more frequent and appear earlier in dementia with Lewy bodies (DLB) than in AD [42]. Furthermore, as far as REM parasomnias are concerned, it should be remembered that a substantial burden of coexisting Lewy body pathology was found to be present in a majority of patients affected by REM sleep behavior disorder (RBD) plus dementia submitted to post-mortem analysis [43]. Thus, clinicians should be aware that careful differential diagnosis is always warranted in the presence of suspected or video-PSG-documented RBD in demented subjects. This should focus, in particular, on any features indicative or reminiscent of parkinsonism.

The presence of agitation in the later hours of the day is reported in only a minority of nursing home residents with dementia, and is a less frequent occurrence in AD than in DLB subjects. This agitation, together with other time-of-day-related behavioral abnormalities, constitutes a phenomenon known as sundowning [44]. Occurring in subjects with dementia, sundowning is a set of symptoms (including sleep–wake disruption) that can build up into a delirious state; these symptoms peak in the evening and can continue into the night.

Actigraphic investigations have revealed disruption of circadian rhythms in about half of AD patients [45]. Neuropathological studies have indicated that deterioration of the suprachiasmatic nucleus (SCN) in the hypothalamus can be documented in AD patients, as can alterations in the 24-hour melatonin secretion profile [46,47]. Furthermore, retinal abnormalities have been documented in AD patients, potentially affecting the transmission of light stimuli to the SCN [48]. The SCN is considered to be the main biological clock regulating circadian rhythms.

The neurodegeneration per se, however, is likely to be only a part of the overall determinants of sleep disorders in AD. A role of genetic susceptibility as well as environmental factors, namely, sleep hygiene and light exposure within the 24-hour cycle, can be postulated [49]. A greater deterioration of sleep parameters in apolipoprotein E (*APOE*) ε4-negative AD patients has been reported [50], although this finding awaits further confirmation, and particular forms of the monoamine A oxidase (*MAOA*) polymorphism may influence the occurrence of sleep disturbances [51]. Some variables—such as poor sleep hygiene, unfavorable environmental conditions, and medications—seem to be responsible for the sleep architecture alterations and for the predisposition to sundowning in AD patients. Disrupted sleep cycles and nighttime wakefulness may underlie this phenomenon. In particular, dysregulation of circadian mechanisms has been suggested to play a role in the pathophysiology of delirium, and various possible relationships have been hypothesized. Indeed, a vicious cycle involving delirium and circadian integrity has been conjectured: it is suggested that the cognitive and psychiatric disturbances of delirium affect circadian integrity by interfering with external cues entraining the circadian rhythms (zeitgebers); circadian alterations, in turn, impairing wakefulness, result in a worsening of the delirium [52]. Several papers in the literature have explored the role of interventions of various kinds (light exposure, melatonin administration, educational interventions, etc.) intended to stabilize rest–activity rhythms and prevent sundowning [13,14,53]. In extreme cases, the circadian sleep rhythms are disrupted to such a degree that the subject displays a complete day–night reversal of sleep patterns, with the main sleep period occurring during daytime.

The question of whether sleep disorders contribute to the cognitive deterioration processes occurring in neurodegenerative diseases is debated in the literature. However, there is preliminary evidence suggesting that disordered sleep may worsen cognitive deterioration (memory and executive functioning) in the MCI stage of these diseases [49,54]. Furthermore, negative effects of sleep disorders on cognitive functions have been reported in patients with dementia as well as in non-demented elderly subjects [55,56]. On the basis of this evidence, treating sleep disorders and preserving good sleep quality for as long as possible may be hypothesized to delay cognitive and functional decline.

The decrease in REM sleep documented in AD has been found to correlate with dementia severity [30,31,57–59]. Dementia severity has also been suggested to correlate with the severity of RBD, while an association between *APOE4* genotype, sleep apnea, and cognitive impairment has been hypothesized [49,50]. There is a growing interest in the potential interaction between sleep apnea and AD [23,38,60]. Several studies have reported the occurrence of delirium associated with OSA and central sleep apnea (CSA), and its resolution with continuous positive airway pressure (CPAP) treatment [61–67]. A prospective study systematically using validated screening tools for delirium and OSA showed OSA to be a predictive risk factor for the occurrence of delirium in elderly surgical subjects [68].

A possible association of RLS with cognitive impairment has been reported in the literature [69,70]. Sleep reduction/fragmentation due to RLS might worsen cognitive symptoms or even accelerate neurocognitive degeneration.

Clinical/instrumental assessment of sleep disorders

Sleep disturbances should be evaluated in AD patients in the early stages of the disease. In MCI and dementia, studies based on subjective reports of sleep often mingle the direct experiences of bed partners with the reports of caregivers/nurses, who might over- or underestimate the frequency and severity of the sleep disorders. In AD patients, the diagnosis of sleep disturbances should be based primarily on a detailed and targeted medical history, and corroborated whenever possible by data collected using questionnaires [71]. Unfortunately, the questionnaires and scales used to investigate sleep in the general population have not been formally validated in individuals with cognitive decline. Nevertheless, evidence-based recommendations for the assessment of sleep disorders in older people can be applied to individuals with MCI or dementia within the same age range. The use of a rapidly and easily administered sleep questionnaire able to identify sleep patterns potentially associated with clinical and functional disease variables in AD appears to be suitable for the early identification and longitudinal monitoring of AD subjects [72]. A scale investigating sleep fragmentation was recently constructed and found to correlate significantly with variables considered indexes of cognitive and functional deterioration in AD: Mini Mental State Examination (MMSE), Activities of Daily Living (ADL), and Clinical Dementia Rating (CDR) scores [73].

Actigraphy, shown to be an appropriate and reliable method in clinical practice, is an interesting support tool for the study of sleep in AD [74]. It allows long-term evaluation (over periods ranging from days to several weeks) of sleep–wake cycles in a patient-friendly environment (the patient's own home). The patient is therefore free to follow his or her habitual sleep–wake schedule throughout the 24-hour cycle. Actigraphy is useful in patients with AD both for initial evaluations of sleep patterns and for assessing the effects of interventions. In patients with dementia, the degree of correlation with PSG findings has been reported to be fairly good [45]. However, even though actigraphy has been shown to be a suitable method for the assessment of sleep patterns in the elderly, video-PSG continues to be the gold standard under certain circumstances. Although video-PSG can introduce an important bias in the evaluation of sleep structure (due to the well-known first-night effect), it offers the possibility of evaluating polygraphic and video traces in a synchronized way, which is essential when investigating sleep movement disorders, parasomnias, and SDB. Furthermore, ambulatory video-PSG will increasingly allow patients to be recorded outside the sleep laboratory, for instance in the ward or at home. Furthermore, 24-hour ambulatory PSG recordings allow the evaluation of nighttime sleep as well as daytime functioning, including napping and daytime somnolence.

Dementia with Lewy bodies

DLB, the second most common cause of dementia in the elderly [75], is frequently associated with changes in sleep patterns [76,77]. Questionnaire-based surveys indicate that patients with DLB have a wide range of sleep disorders, including impaired sleep quality or reduced sleep efficiency, vivid dreams and confusion on awakening, and abnormal motor control during sleep in the form of probable RLS and probable PLM during sleep [76,77]. PSG data show that a high percentage of DLB subjects display a mixture of different sleep pathologies ranging from unstable and fragmented sleep to SDB and various motor-behavioral abnormalities. Objective PSG data (Table 26.1) show that DLB patients have poor sleep continuity, long sleep latency, long REM sleep latency, reduced REM sleep, and a significant number of arousals not accounted for by a movement or breathing disorder [78,79]. The observation that sleep comorbidities do not seem to fully explain the sleep instability in DLB [78] highlights the possibility that a complex pathophysiology, potentially linked to neurodegenerative changes, underlies the sleep fragmentation in these patients. DLB subjects who show a more severe cognitive impairment and an early onset of visual hallucinations are more likely to display the simultaneous presence of distinctive elements of wakefulness, NREM sleep, and REM sleep in the absence of identifiable conventional sleep stages (dissociated sleep), which represents an extreme form of disorganization of sleep architecture [79].

RBD is the most prominent sleep disorder in DLB, reported in 50–80% of patients. Indeed, the presence of RBD supports a diagnosis of DLB, potentially heralding its onset by years [80], and the inclusion of RBD in the DLB diagnostic criteria was found to improve the classification accuracy in autopsy-confirmed DLB cases [81]. Numerous cases of RBD have been reported in association with clinically diagnosed DLB.

Furthermore, nocturnal motor-behavioral episodes in DLB are more complex than generally assumed, since they include not only RBD, but also confusional arousals with or without hallucinations and other arousal-related episodes during NREM or REM sleep and reported as RBD-like at clinical interview [67,82]. Nocturnal sleep enactment behaviors have been found to occur even more frequently in patients with DLB than in those with Parkinson disease (PD); these episodes consisted of isolated RBD in about one-third of the cases, whereas in the majority they took the form of abnormal arousal-related motor-behavioral episodes.

Clinicians evaluating patients with DLB should be aware of the complex disordered sleep patterns these individuals may present and thus of the possibility of misleading symptoms, and the risk of overlooking sleep comorbidities. Accordingly, they should consider performing PSG sleep investigations; nocturnal video-PSG, overcoming the limits of questionnaire-based investigations and yielding an objective analysis of sleep patterns, should allow them to make a correct diagnosis and achieve optimal treatment of disrupted sleep in DLB. In particular, video-PSG should be used to examine disruptive sleep behaviors suggesting dream enactment, since RBD is only one of the possible causes of these behaviors.

The question of whether and how sleep disorders may contribute to cognitive decline in DLB is a complex one. Literature data [42] show that altered sleep patterns are not associated with a more pronounced cognitive decline in DLB, as measured by MMSE, or with substantial deficits in specific cognitive domains.

Limited evidence indicates that DLB subjects reporting a sleep-related disturbance as the presenting symptom, particularly those whose onset symptom was RBD, obtain higher MMSE scores and perform better on tests of logic and executive functions than those with other symptoms at onset [67]. Starting from these data, and assuming that the evolution of clinical features reflects the topography of the degeneration over time, it can be suggested that different patterns of neurodegeneration could occur in DLB [83–85], reflecting different neuronal susceptibility to degeneration. This pattern of progression may explain the presence of less severe cognitive impairment and slower progression of dementia in those with RBD as the presenting symptom. In this context, it is possible to hypothesize a "bottom-up" (ascending) and patchy progression of neurodegeneration [83,84], wherein more resilient neuronal groups in networks implicated in cognition are affected later than those responsible for the critical expression of RBD. The presence of a sleep disturbance (eg, RBD) as the prodromal symptom of DLB was found to indicate a different disease phenotype, characterized by earlier appearance of parkinsonism, visual hallucinations, and delayed emergence of dementia [86], supporting the "bottom-up" hypothesis of progression of neurodegeneration from the brainstem to the cortex.

A "top-down" (descending) progression [83,84,87] from the neocortex/limbic system to the brainstem networks may explain the occurrence early in the disease course of cognitive impairment that is not associated with RBD, which would not appear until a later stage of neurodegeneration. Neuropathological studies are needed to determine whether neuronal loss and Lewy body-related neurodegeneration in the brainstem nuclei and corticolimbic areas are different in subjects with RBD as opposed to those without RBD.

Respiratory patterns during sleep in DLB subjects have been poorly investigated; only two papers have reported PSG-based findings [78,79]. The Mayo Clinic group reported retrospective data on 78 patients diagnosed with possible or probable DLB, submitted to video-PSG to evaluate the presence of suspected comorbid sleep disorders. On video-PSG, 60% of the sample had evidence of SDB (respiratory disorder index RDI > 5); 36% of the patients had an RDI ≥ 10. The mean RDI was 11.9±15.8. No data were presented about the distribution according to SDB severity. Our group, conducting a study on this topic, evaluated 29 consecutive subjects diagnosed with probable DLB according to agreed consensus criteria for DLB [67]. Video-PSG revealed SDB in 34.8% subjects, mainly consisting of OSA, which was mild (AHI values between 5 and 15) in 8.6%, moderate (AHI between 16 and 30) in 17.4%, and severe (AHI >30) in 8.6% of the subjects. The frequency of sleep apnea in our patient series (mean age 75.4 ± 5.1 years) was in line with that reported in the literature in elderly patients (30.5% of >65-year-olds having an AHI of 5 or higher, versus 33.3% of 70-year-olds and 39.5% of 80-year-olds) [88,89] and in PD patients unselected for sleep complaints [90]. Moderate to severe sleep apnea (AHI > 15) was found in 26.1% of DLB subjects.

Progressive supranuclear palsy

Progressive supranuclear palsy (PSP) is a neurodegenerative disease characterized by gaze dysfunction, extrapyramidal symptoms, and cognitive dysfunction. Sleep disturbances are present in most cases of PSP [34,91]. Sleep studies (Table 26.1) in patients with PSP showed increased awakenings, diminished total sleep time, and reduced REM sleep. Marked insomnia, characterized by increased sleep latency and increased awakenings, was the most common complaint [34]. Insomnia severity was related to overall disease severity, the number of awakenings increasing with greater motor impairment, and total sleep time declining with progressing dementia. Insomnia has been found to be worse in PSP than in AD or PD. Nocturnal motor-behavioral events, in the form of RBD, have been reported to occur in PSP [92]. REM sleep without atonia (RSWA) is found in up to 27% of patients with PSP [93]. Standardized sleep questionnaires have identified possible RLS in more than half of PSP patients, and the condition has also been associated with significantly increased PLM in sleep [94].

Corticobasal degeneration

The most common sleep disorder in corticobasal degeneration is insomnia, although PLM and RBD can also be present [94]. It has been shown that focal dystonia, and "alien limb" phenomenon, can potentially persist unchanged throughout wakefulness, NREM sleep (all stages), and even REM sleep. In an anecdotal case report, the occurrence of dystonia was not found to be triggered by EEG arousal, which instead tended to follow the dystonic manifestations, and indeed appeared to be evoked by them [95].

Huntington disease

In Huntington disease (HD), as in PD, there is a growing awareness that, alongside the motor symptoms, sleep and circadian abnormalities are important non-motor features of the disease. Although the long-term impact of sleep disruption in HD is unknown, sleep alterations are deemed to contribute to the progressive evolution of the condition [96]. Sleep disturbances in HD are likely to be underdiagnosed, because of underreporting by patients, who might lack the insight necessary to provide information about their sleep pattern in relation to their psychiatric features [97]. Nevertheless, up to 90% of patients may complain of sleep problems, which have a moderate to severe impact on their overall health [98]. HD patients report insomnia and have a tendency to experience increased daytime somnolence [98,99]. The few PSG studies (Table 26.1) available show multiple sleep pattern alterations: reductions of REM sleep and of SWS, increased sleep latency, impaired sleep continuity, reduced sleep efficiency, reduced total sleep time, and increased wakefulness after sleep onset [96].

Genetic neurodegenerative disorders—spinocerebellar ataxias

Patients affected by other neurodegenerative disorders of genetic origin may present several sleep disturbances. The spinocerebellar ataxias (SCAs) are a large group of heterogeneous disorders in which sleep disorders can be frequent. Different SCA subtypes are characterized by different patterns of sleep disturbances [100].

SCA1, SCA2, SCA3, SCA4, and SCA6 patients can exhibit RLS and PLM in sleep; the highest prevalence of RLS is found in SCA3 [101,102].

SCA2 is characterized by good subjective sleep quality, paralleled by reduced REM sleep, reduced REM density, the presence of RSWA and PLM. REM sleep alterations and PLM are related to SCA2 severity; in particular, REM alterations are related to increases in ataxia scores, whereas RSWA is related to the number of cytosine–adenine–guanine repeats. More advanced SCA2 can be associated with disappearance of REM sleep and an increase of SWS [103].

SCA3 is characterized by impaired sleep efficiency and decreased REM sleep. Subjects with SCA3 may also complain of RLS, PLM, vocal cord paralysis and RBD [104–106].

SCA6 is characterized by only minor sleep abnormalities in the form of RLS and PLM [107].

Status dissociatus

In subjects with the most advanced and severe neurodegenerative diseases, as well as in patients affected by some prion diseases like fatal familial insomnia, an extreme form of sleep alteration can occur [108]. The term status dissociatus refers to the simultaneous coexistence of three different states of being: wakefulness, NREM sleep, and REM sleep. When the clear-cut distinctions between these states are lacking, they may inappropriately overlap, leading to an intermediate state of being that is characterized by a wide range of clinical phenomena [109]. In particular, patients affected by status dissociatus show subcontinuous behavioral manifestations of vivid dreams and oneirism, persisting throughout the 24-hour sleep–wake cycle.

Key points for the treatment of disrupted sleep in neurodegenerative disorders

In view of the multiple and complex mechanisms potentially underlying disrupted sleep in neurodegenerative disorders, evaluation of sleep patterns should include a comprehensive workup, a full assessment of sleep hygiene, and a careful evaluation of primary and other sleep comorbidities (eg, SDB, movement disorders during sleep, parasomnias, and comorbid medical, psychiatric, or iatrogenic conditions). Table 26.2 outlines principles of treatment.

Inappropriate sleep habits and environmental conditions (especially inadequate exposure to natural light) should be corrected whenever found. Once a correct diagnosis has been established, sleep comorbidities should be properly treated. In particular, associated medical and psychiatric conditions should be specifically treated, as these conditions can contribute to disturbed sleep patterns.

The efficacy of nonpharmacological interventions to improve sleep continuity is supported by a growing body of evidence. Re-establishing correct sleep hygiene can improve sleep continuity,

Table 26.2 Principles of treatment

Global approach	Screening for sleep comorbidities—medical or psychiatric illness—undesired side effects
Insomnia	Nonpharmacological interventions: Sleep hygiene—cognitive–behavioral therapy—daytime bright light exposure—sleep restriction
	Pharmacological interventions: Z-drugs—short-life benzodiazepines—melatonin—trazodone—neuroleptics (quetiapine)—antidepressants
REM sleep behavior disorder	Clonazepam—melatonin—melatoninergic agents—quetiapine
Confusional spells/ hallucinations	ACh inhibitors—second-generation neuroleptics (quetiapine)
Excessive daytime sleepiness	Modafinil—caffeine—activating antidepressants
Restless legs syndrome/ periodic limb movement disorder	Dopaminergic agonists—clonazepam—gabapentin—pregabalin—opioids

particularly in institutionalized subjects [13,14,52]. It is important to be aware that many drugs, such as diuretics, beta-blockers, bronchodilators, corticosteroids, cardiovascular drugs, and H_2 blockers, can cause or exacerbate insomnia. Alcohol and caffeine should be consumed in minimal quantities, especially during the evening and just before going to sleep.

The sleep environment should be favorable to sleep onset and maintenance; at night, noise and ambient light should be reduced to a minimum. External interventions (by caregivers or nurses) potentially triggering arousal from sleep should also be kept to a minimum.

Reinforcement of the distinction between night and day may strengthen the circadian rhythm, and external cues entraining circadian rhythms should also be reinforced by avoiding or limiting daytime napping, maintaining regular meal times, eating a light meal in the evening, doing regular physical activity, and ensuring regular exposure to bright light in the morning [53,110–112].

The pharmacological management of disrupted sleep in subjects with neurodegenerative disorders, and particularly in those at risk of experiencing delirium, usually culminates in the use of atypical antipsychotics. It should be remembered that sedative drugs should be chosen paying careful consideration to their side effects, their interactions with other drugs, and the risk of excessive sedation, which could worsen neuropsychological deficits.

Every drug treatment should be started and conducted at the minimum effective doses, and reduction or suspension of treatment considered whenever possible.

References

1. United Nations, Department of Economic and Social Affairs, Population Division. World population ageing 2013. ST/ESA/SER. A/348.
2. Gagnon JF, Petit D, Latreille V, Montplaisir J. Neurobiology of sleep disturbances in neurodegenerative disorders. Curr Pharm Des 2008;14:3430–45.

3. Raggi, R. Ferri. Sleep disorders in neurodegenerative diseases. Eur J Neurol 2010,17:1326–38.

4. Auger RR, Boeve BF. Sleep disorders in neurodegenerative diseases other than Parkinson's disease. Handb Clin Neurol 2011;99:1011–50.

5. Vendette M, Gagnon JF, Decary A, et al. REM sleep behavior disorder predicts cognitive impairment in Parkinson disease without dementia. Neurology 2007;69:1843–9.

6. Forsaa EB, Larsen JP, Wentzel-Larsen T, et al. Predictors and course of health-related quality of life in Parkinson's disease. Mov Disord 2008;23:1420–7.

7. Naismith SL, Hickie IB, Lewis SJ. The role of mild depression in sleep disturbance and quality of life in Parkinson's Disease. J Neuropsych Clin Neurosci 2010;22:384–9.

8. Gallagher-Thompson D, Brooks JO III, Bliwise D, et al. The relations among caregiver stress, "sundowning" symptoms, and cognitive decline in Alzheimer's disease. J Am Geriatr Soc 1992;40:807–10.

9. Happe S, Berger K. The association between caregiver burden and sleep disturbances in partners of patients with Parkinson's disease. Age Ageing 2002;31:349–54.

10. Pollak CP, Perlick D, Linsner JP, et al. Sleep problems in the community elderly as predictors of death and nursing home placement. J Community Health 1990;15:123–35.

11. Pollak CP, Perlick D. Sleep problems and institutionalization of the elderly. J Geriatr Psychiatry Neurol 1991;4:204–10.

12. Van Someren EJ. Circadian and sleep disturbances in the elderly. Exp Gerontol 2000;35:1229–37.

13. Espiritu JR. Aging-related sleep changes. Clin Geriatr Med. 2008;24:1–14.

14. Gibson EM, Williams WP 3rd, Kriegsfeld LJ. Aging in the circadian system: considerations for health, disease prevention and longevity. Exp Gerontol 2009;44:51–6.

15. Bliwise DL. Review: sleep in normal aging and dementia. Sleep 1993;16:40–81.

16. Zhong G, Naismith SL, Rogers NL, Lewis SJ. Sleep–wake disturbances in common neurodegenerative diseases: a closer look at selected aspects of the neural circuitry. J Neurol Sci. 2011;307:9–14.

17. Slats D, Claassen JA, Verbeek MM, Overeem S. Reciprocal interactions between sleep, circadian rhythms and Alzheimer's disease: focus on the role of hypocretin and melatonin. Ageing Res Rev 2013;12:188–200.

18. Cooke JR, Ancoli-Israel S. Normal and abnormal sleep in the elderly. Handb Clin Neurol 2011;98:653–65.

19. Van Cauter E, Leproult R, Plat L. Age-related changes in slow wave sleep and REM sleep and relationship with growth hormone and cortisol levels in healthy men. JAMA 2000;284:861–8.

20. Ohayon MM, Carskadon MA, Guilleminault C, Vitiello MV. Meta-analysis of quantitative sleep parameters from childhood to old age in healthy individuals: developing normative sleep values across the human lifespan. Sleep 2004;27:1255–73.

21. Cole C, Richards K. Sleep disruption in older adults. Harmful and by no means inevitable, it should be assessed for and treated. Am J Nurs 2007;107:40–9.

22. Cuellar NG, Rogers AE, Hisghman V, Volpe SL. Assessment and treatment of sleep disorders in the older adult. Geriatr Nurs 2007;28:254–64.

23. Ancoli-Israel S, Palmer BW, Cooke JR, et al. Cognitive effects of treating obstructive sleep apnea in Alzheimer's disease: a randomized controlled study. J Am Geriatr Soc 2008;56:2076–81.

24. Vitiello MV, Prinz PN. Alzheimer's disease. Sleep and sleep/wake patterns. Clin Geriatr Med 1989;5:289–99.

25. Pat-Horenczyk R, Klauber MR, Shochat T, Ancoli-Israel S. Hourly profiles of sleep and wakefulness in severely versus mild-moderately demented nursing home patients. Aging Clin Exp Res 1998;10:308–15.

26. Moran M, Lynch CA, Walsh C, et al. Sleep disturbance in mild to moderate Alzheimer's disease. Sleep Med 2005; 6:347–52.

27. Naismith SL, Rogers NL, Hickie IB, et al. Sleep well, think well: sleep–wake disturbance in mild cognitive impairment. J Geriatr Psychiatry Neurol 2010;23:123–30.

28. Benca RM, Obermeyer WH, Thisted RA, Gillin JC. Sleep and psychiatric disorders. A meta-analysis. Arch Gen Psychiatry 1992;49:651–68.

29. McCurry SM, Logsdon RG, Teri L, et al. Characteristics of sleep disturbance in community-dwelling Alzheimer's disease patients. J Geriatr Psychiatry Neurol 1999;12:53–59.

30. Vitiello MV, Borson S. Sleep disturbances in patients with Alzheimer's disease: epidemiology, pathophysiology and treatment. CNS Drugs 2001;15:777–96.

31. Bliwise DL. Sleep disorders in Alzheimer's disease and other dementias. Clin Cornerstone 2004;6:S16–28.

32. Bianchetti A, Scuratti A, Zanetti O, et al. Predictors of mortality and institutionalization in Alzheimer disease patients 1 year after discharge from an Alzheimer dementia unit. Dementia 1995;6:108–12.

33. Petit D, Gagnon GF, Fantini ML, et al. Sleep and quantitative EEG in neurodegenerative disorders. J Psychosom Res 2004;56:487–96.

34. Bhatt MH, Podder N, Chokroverty S. Sleep and neurodegenerative diseases. Semin Neurol 2005;25:39–51.

35. Gagnon JF, Petit D, Fantini ML, et al. REM sleep behavior disorder and REM sleep without atonia in probable Alzheimer disease. Sleep 2006;29:1321–25.

36. Reynolds CF 3rd, Kupfer DJ, Taska LS, et al. Sleep apnea in Alzheimer's dementia: correlation with mental deterioration. J Clin Psychiatry 1985;46:257–61.

37. Hoch CC, Reynolds CF 3rd, Kupfer DJ, et al. Sleep-disordered breathing in normal and pathologic aging. J Clin Psychiatry 1986;47:499–503.

38. Ancoli-Israel S, Klauber MR, Butters N, et al. Dementia in institutionalized elderly: relation to sleep apnea. J Am Geriatr Soc 1991;39:258–63.

39. Ancoli-Israel S, Kripke D, Klauber MR, et al. Periodic limb movements in sleep in community dwelling elderly. Sleep 1991;14:496–500.

40. Mendelson WB. Are periodic leg movements associated with sleep disturbance? Sleep 1996;19:219–23

41. Guarnieri B, Adorni F, Musicco M, et al. Prevalence of sleep disturbances in mild cognitive impairment and dementing disorders: a multicenter Italian clinical cross-sectional study on 431 patients. Dement Geriatr Cogn Disord 2012;33:50–8.

42. Bliwise DL, Mercaldo ND, Avidan AY, et al. Sleep disturbance in dementia with Lewy bodies and Alzheimer's disease: a multicenter analysis. Dement Geriatr Cogn Disord 2011;31:239–46.

43. Schenck CH, Mahowald MW, Anderson ML, et al. Lewy body variant of Alzheimer's disease (AD) identified by postmortem ubiquitin staining in a previously reported case of AD associated with REM sleep behavior disorder. Biol Psychiatry 1997;42:527–8.

44. Bliwise DL. What is sundowning? J Am Geriatr Soc 1994;42:1009–11.

45. Ancoli-Israel S, Clopton P, Klauber MR, et al. Use of wrist activity for monitoring sleep/wake in demented nursing-home patients. Sleep 1997;20:24–7.

46. Cardinali DP, Brusco LI, Liberczuk C, Furio AM. The use of melatonin in Alzheimer's disease. Neuro Endocrinol Lett 2002;23:20–3.

47. Wu Y-H, Swaab DF. Disturbance and strategies for reactivation of the circadian rhythm system in aging and Alzheimer's disease. Sleep Med 2007;8:623–36.

48. Volicer L, Harper DG, Manning BC, et al. Sundowning and circadian rhythms in Alzheimer's disease. Am J Psychiatry 2001;158:704–11.

49. Peter-Derex L, Yammine P, Bastuji H, Croisile B. Sleep and Alzheimer's disease. Sleep Med Rev 2015;19:29–38.

50. Yesavage JA, Friedman L, Kraemer H, et al. Sleep/wake disruption in Alzheimer's disease: APOE status and longitudinal course. J Geriatr Psychiatry Neurol 2004;17:20–24.

51. Craig D, Hart DJ, Passmore AP. Genetically increased risk of sleep disruption in Alzheimer's disease. Sleep 2006;29:1003–7.

52. Fitzgerald JM, Adamis D, Trzepacz PT, et al. Delirium: a disturbance of circadian integrity? Med Hypotheses 2013;81:568–76

53. Ancoli-Israel S, Martin JL, Kripke DF, et al. Effect of light treatment on sleep and circadian rhythms in demented nursing home patients. J Am Geriatr Soc 2002;50:282–9.

54. Rauchs G, Harand C, Bertran F, et al. Sleep and episodic memory: a review of the literature in young healthy subjects and potential links

between sleep changes and memory impairment observed during aging and Alzheimer's disease. Rev Neurol (Paris) 2010;166: 873–81.

55. Schlosser Covell GE, Dhawan PS, Lee Iannotti JK, et al. Disrupted daytime activity and altered sleep–wake patterns may predict transition to mild cognitive impairment or dementia: a critically appraised topic. Neurologist 2012;18:426–9.

56. Lim AS, Kowgier M, Yu L, et al. Sleep fragmentation and the risk of incident Alzheimer's disease and cognitive decline in older persons. Sleep 2013;36:1027–32.

57. Hatfield CF, Herbert J, van Someren EJ, et al. Disrupted daily activity/rest cycles in relation to daily cortisol rhythms of home-dwelling patients with early Alzheimer's dementia. Brain 2004;127:1061–74.

58. Harper DG, Volicer L, Stopa EG, et al. Disturbance of endogenous circadian rhythm in aging and Alzheimer disease. Am J Geriatr Psychiatry 2005;13:359–68

59. Vecchierini MF. Sleep disturbances in Alzheimer's disease and other dementias. Psychol Neuropsychiatr Vieil 2010;8:15–23.

60. Chong MS, Ayalon L, Marler M, et al. Continuous positive airway pressure reduces subjective daytime sleepiness in patients with mild to moderate Alzheimer's disease with sleep disordered breathing. J Am Geriatr Soc 2006;54:777–81.

61. Munoz X, Marti S, Sumalla J, et al. Acute delirium as a manifestation of obstructive sleep apnea syndrome. Am J Respir Crit Care Med 1998;158:1306–7.

62. Becker K, Poon C, Zeidler M, Wang T. An unusual cause of delirium. J Clin Sleep Med 2010;6:290–1.

63. Lee JW. Recurrent delirium associated with obstructive sleep apnea. Gen Hosp Psychiatry 1998;20:120–2.

64. Sandberg O, Franklin KA, Bucht G, Gustafson Y. Sleep apnea, delirium, depressed mood, cognition, and ADL ability after stroke. J Am Geriatr Soc 2001;49:391–7.

65. Lombardi C, Rocchi R, Montagna P, et al. Obstructive sleep apnea syndrome: a cause of acute delirium. J Clin Sleep Med 2009;5:569–70.

66. Whitney JF, Gannon DE. Obstructive sleep apnea presenting as acute delirium. Am J Emerg Med 1996;14:270–1.

67. Terzaghi M, Sartori I, Rustioni V, Manni R. Sleep disorders and acute nocturnal delirium in the elderly: a comorbidity not to be overlooked. Eur J Intern Med 2014;25:350–5.

68. Flink BJ, Rivelli SK, Cox EA, et al. Obstructive sleep apnea and incidence of postoperative delirium after elective knee replacement in the nondemented elderly. Anesthesiology 2012;116:788–96.

69. Pearson VE, Allen RP, Dean T, et al. Cognitive deficits associated with restless legs syndrome (RLS). Sleep Med 2006;7:25–30.

70. Gamaldo C, Benbrook AR, Allen RP, et al. Evaluating daytime alertness in individuals with restless legs syndrome (RLS) compared to sleep restricted controls. Sleep Med 2009;10:134–8.

71. Guarnieri B, Musicco M, Caffarra P, et al. Recommendations of the Sleep Study Group of the Italian Dementia Research Association (SINDem) on clinical assessment and management of sleep disorders in individuals with mild cognitive impairment and dementia: a clinical review. Neurol Sci 2014;35:1329–48.

72. Manni R, Sinforiani E, Terzaghi M, et al. Sleep Continuity Scale in Alzheimer's Disease (SCADS): application in daily clinical practice in an Italian center for dementia. Neurol Sci 2015;36:469–71.

73. Manni R, Sinforiani E, Zucchella C, et al. Sleep continuity scale in Alzheimer's disease: validation and relationship with cognitive and functional deterioration. Neurol Sci 2013;34:701–5.

74. Camargos EF, Louzada FM, Nóbrega OT. Wrist actigraphy for measuring sleep in intervention studies with Alzheimer's disease patients: application, usefulness, and challenges. Sleep Med Rev2013;17:475–88.

75. McKeith I, Mintzer J, Aarsland D, et al.; International Psychogeriatric Association Expert Meeting on DLB. Dementia with Lewy bodies. Lancet Neurol 2004;3:19–28.

76. Rongve A, Boeve BF, Aarsland A. Frequency and correlates of caregiver-reported sleep disturbances in a sample of persons with early dementia. J Am Geriatr Soc 2010;58:480–6.

77. Grace JB, Walker MP, McKeith IG. A comparison of sleep profiles in patients with dementia with Lewy bodies and Alzheimer's disease. Int J Geriatr Psychiatry 2000;15:1028–33.

78. Pao WC, Boeve BF, Ferman TJ, et al. Polysomnographic findings in dementia with Lewy bodies. Neurologist 2013;19:1–6.

79. Terzaghi M, Arnaldi D, Rizzetti MC, et al. Analysis of video-polysomnographic sleep findings in dementia with Lewy bodies. Mov Disord 2013;28:1416–23.

80. Claassen DO, Josephs KA, Ahlskog JE, et al. REM sleep behavior disorder preceding other aspects of synucleinopathies by up to half a century. Neurology 2010;75:494–9.

81. Ferman TJ, Boeve BF, Smith GE, et al. Inclusion of RBD improves the diagnostic classification of dementia with Lewy bodies. Neurology 2011;77:875–82.

82. Manni R, Terzaghi M, Repetto A, et al. Complex paroxysmal nocturnal behaviors in Parkinson's disease. Mov Disord 2010;25:985–90.

83. Molano J, Boeve B, Ferman T, et al. Mild cognitive impairment associated with limbic and neocortical Lewy body disease: a clinicopathological study. Brain 2010;133:540–56.

84. Frigerio R, Fujishiro H, Ahn TB, et al. Incidental Lewy body disease: do some cases represent a preclinical stage of dementia with Lewy bodies? Neurobiol Aging 2011;32:857–63.

85. Uchikado H, Lin WL, DeLucia MW, Dickson DW. Alzheimer disease with amygdala Lewy bodies: a distinct form of alpha-synucleinopathy. J Neuropathol Exp Neurol 2006;65:685–97.

86. Dugger BN, Boeve BF, Murray ME, et al. Rapid eye movement sleep behaviour disorder and subtypes in autopsy-confirmed dementia with Lewy bodies. Mov Disord 2012;27:72–8.

87. Beach TG, Adler CH, Lue L, et al.; Arizona Parkinson's Disease Consortium. Unified staging system for Lewy body disorders: correlation with nigrostriatal degeneration, cognitive impairment and motor dysfunction. Acta Neuropathol 2009;117:613–34.

88. Bixler EO, Vgontzas AN, Ten Have T, et al. Effects of age on sleep apnea in men: I. Prevalence and severity. Am J Respir Crit Care Med 1998;157:144–8.

89. Hoch CC, Reynolds CF 3rd, Monk TH, et al. Comparison of sleep-disordered breathing among healthy elderly in the seventh, eighth, and ninth decades of life. Sleep 1990;13:502–11.

90. Cochen De Cock V, Abouda M, Leu S, et al. Is obstructive sleep apnea a problem in Parkinson's disease? Sleep Med 2010;11:247–52.

91. Aldrich MS, Foster NL, White RF, et al. Sleep abnormalities in progressive supranuclear palsy. Ann Neurol 1989;25:577–81.

92. Pareja JA, Caminero AB, Masa JF, Dobato JL. A first case of progressive supranuclear palsy and preclinical REM sleep behavior disorder presenting as inhibition of speech during wakefulness and somniloquy with phasic muscle twitching during REM sleep. Neurologia 1996;11:304–6.

93. Arnulf I, Merino-Andreu N, Bloch F, et al. REM sleep behavior disorder and REM sleep without atonia in progressive supranuclear palsy. Sleep 2005;28:349–54.

94. Abbott SM, Videnovic A. Sleep disorders in atypical parkinsonism. Mov Disord Clin Pract (Hoboken) 2014;1:89–96.

95. Terzaghi M, Sartori I, Rustioni V, Manni R. Paroxysmal dystonia persisting during sleep in asymmetric parkinsonism: disinhibition of a central pattern generator? Eur J Neurol 2008;15:e78–9.

96. Morton JA. Circadian and sleep disorder in Huntington's disease. Exp Neurol 2013;243:34–44.

97. Goodman AO, Rogers L, Pilsworth S, et al. Asymptomatic sleep abnormalities are a common early feature in patients with Huntington's disease. Curr Neurol Neurosci Rep 2011;11:211–17.

98. Goodman AO, Morton AJ, Barker RA. Identifying sleep disturbances in Huntington's disease using a simple disease-focused questionnaire. PLoS Curr 2010;15:2.

99. Videnovic A, Leurgans S, Fan W, et al. Daytime somnolence and nocturnal sleep disturbances in Huntington disease. Parkinsonism Relat Disord 2009;15:471–4.

100. Pedroso JL, Braga-Neto P, Felicio AC, et al. Sleep disorders in cerebellar ataxias. Arq Neuropsiquiatr 2011;69:253–7.

101. Schols L, Haan J, Riess O, et al. Sleep disturbance in spinocerebellar ataxias: is the SCA3 mutation a cause of restless legs syndrome? Neurology 1998;51:1603–7.

102. Abele M, Burk K, Laccone F, et al. Restless legs syndrome in spinocerebellar ataxia types 1, 2, and 3. J Neurol 2001;248:311–14.

103. Velázquez-Pérez L, Voss U, Rodríguez-Labrada R, et al. Sleep disorders in spinocerebellar ataxia type 2 patients. Neurodegener Dis 2011;8:447–54.

104. Pedroso JL, França MC, Braga-Neto P, et al. Nonmotor and extracerebellar features in Machado–Joseph disease: a review. Mov Disord 2013;28:1200–8.

105. Iranzo A, Munoz E, Santamaria J, et al. REM sleep behavior disorder and vocal cord paralysis in Machado–Joseph disease. Mov Disord 2003;18:1179–83.

106. Syed BH, Rye DB, Singh G. REM sleep behavior disorder and SCA-3 (Machado–Joseph disease). Neurology 2003;60:148.

107. Boesch SM, Frauscher B, Brandauer E, et al. Restless legs syndrome and motor activity during sleep in spinocerebellar ataxia type 6. Sleep Med 2006;7:529–32.

108. Provini F. Agrypnia excitata. Curr Neurol Neurosci Rep 2013;13:341

109. Mahowald MW, Schenck CH. Insights from studying human sleep disorders. Nature 2005;437:1279–85.

110. Yang J, Choi W, Ko YH, et al. Bright light therapy as an adjunctive treatment with risperidone in patients with delirium: a randomized, open, parallel group study. Gen Hosp Psychiatry 2012;34:546–51.

111. Friedman L, Spira AP, Hernandez B, et al. Brief morning light treatment for sleep/wake disturbances in older memory-impaired individuals and their caregivers. Sleep Med 2012;13:546–9.

112. Mishima K, Okawa M, Hishikawa Y, et al. Morning bright light therapy for sleep and behavior disorders in elderly patients with dementia. Acta Psychiatr Scand 1994;89:1–7.

CHAPTER 27

Sleep and stroke

Mark Eric Dyken, Kyoung Bin Im,
George B. Richerson, and Deborah C. Lin-Dyken

Stroke and sleep: background

Stroke and sleep disorders are both common individually. Stroke is the second major cause of death and the leading cause of long-term disability worldwide. It is responsible for half of all acute neurological hospital admissions in the USA, with a prevalence of 6.5 million among adults aged 20 years and older and a yearly incidence of 795 000 [1–2]. The National Sleep Foundation's "Sleep in America" poll from 2002 reported that 93% of people with fair or poor health had sleep problems (55% complaining that sleepiness interfered with daily activities) [3]. Given the large numbers of patients with stroke, treating concomitant sleep problems can improve quality of life, potentially reducing morbidity and mortality in many cases. Major sleep disorders are defined in the International Classification of Sleep Disorders, Third Edition (ICSD-3) under sleep-related breathing disorders (SRBDs), insomnia, hypersomnias of central origin, circadian rhythm sleep disorders, parasomnias, and sleep-related movement disorders [4].

Stroke and SRBDs

In 2006, SRBDs, including obstructive sleep apnea (OSA, a problem with a prevalence up to 24% in men and 9% in women in the general adult population), were first considered "less well-documented or potentially modifiable risk factors" for stroke, suggesting a potential cause-and-effect relationship between OSA and stroke [5,6].

An association

In 1962, reports suggested that sleep apnea could be caused by central nervous system (CNS) injury [7]. Automatic respiration (i.e, that which occurs in the absence of any conscious effort, such as during sleep) is generated by a network of interconnected neurons within the medulla and pons, including the ventrolateral portion of the nucleus of the solitary tract (corresponding approximately to the dorsal respiratory group (DRG), which is not defined anatomically, but as a region containing neurons that fire bursts in phase with respiratory output), the Bötzinger complex, pre-Bötzinger complex, nucleus ambiguus, nucleus para-ambigualis, and nucleus retroambigualis (together forming a column corresponding approximately to the ventral respiratory group (VRG), also defined functionally, not anatomically) (Figs. 27.1 and 27.2) [8,9]. Neurons in the medulla that generate the respiratory output are stimulated by peripheral chemoreceptors that detect a decrease in blood PO_2 and/or an increase in blood

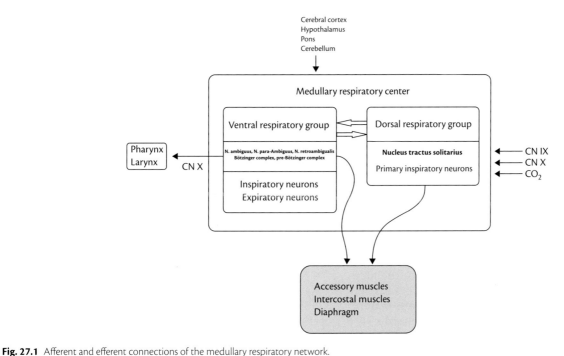

Fig. 27.1 Afferent and efferent connections of the medullary respiratory network.

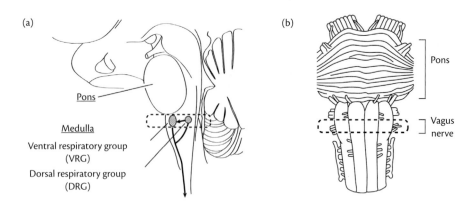

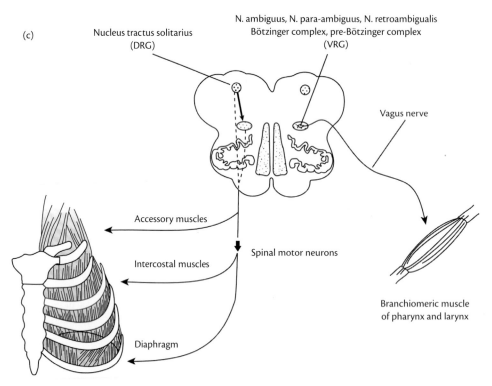

Fig. 27.2 Neuroanatomy of the medullary respiratory network: the brainstem showing in a parasagittal section (a) the location of the dorsal and ventral respiratory groups (DRG and VRG) and their projection to the spinal cord; in a basal brain view (b) the vagus nerve rootlets exiting the lateral surface of the medulla, and in a transverse section of the medulla (c) projections from the DRG to VRG, and the output from both groups to respiratory muscles.
Reproduced from Dyken et al, Stroke in Sleep. In: Chokroverty S, Sahota P, [eds], Acute and Emergent Events in Sleep Disorders, Copyright (2011), with permission from Oxford University Press.

PCO_2, as well as central respiratory chemoreceptors (CRCs) that respond to an increase in PCO_2, but not to hypoxia. Neurons in the raphe nuclei, the retrotrapezoid nucleus, the locus coeruleus, and the nucleus of the solitary tract all have been proposed to be CRCs [10–11], but the relative importance of each group is unknown. Of these candidates, there is greatest support for Phox2b-expressing neurons of the retrotrapezoid nucleus [12] and for serotonin neurons of the raphe nuclei [13], both in the medulla. Central sleep apnea (CSA) has been reported following stroke of the nucleus of the solitary tract, and OSA has been observed after stroke of the nucleus ambiguus, with dysfunctional vagal motor innervation to the larynx and pharynx [14]. Case reports suggest that diffuse CNS injury can also affect these areas, causing apnea [10,15].

Snoring

In 1989, Palomake et al. studied 167 men with stroke (36% during sleep) [16]. Snoring, using stepwise multiple logistic regression analysis, was the only potential risk factor significantly related to stroke in sleep [16]. In 1991, Palomake found that the odds ratio (OR) of snoring as a risk factor for ischemic stroke increased when obesity and sleepiness (classical OSA signs and symptoms) were also present [17].

PSG studies
Case reports

In 1982, Chaudhary et al. reported a man with right lateral medullary stroke, an apnea index (average number of apneas/hour of sleep) of 18, and an oxygen saturation (SaO_2) low of 60% [18].

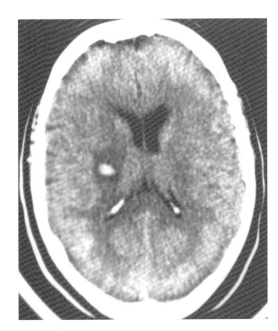

Fig. 27.3 This brain CT without contrast was performed in a 34-year-old man who awoke with stroke, after which he was diagnosed with obstructive sleep apnea. This study reveals a hemorrhage, with a surrounding area, greater than 1 cm in diameter, of low density, consistent with edema, involving the putamen and posterior limb of the right internal capsule.

Reproduced from Dyken ME, Cerebrovascular disease and sleep apnea. In: Bradley DT, Floras JS, [eds], Sleep Apnea: Implications in Cardiovascular and Cerebrovascular Disease (Lung Biology in Health and Disease), pp. 285–306, Copyright (2000), with permission from Informa Healthcare.

Hypothetically, nucleus ambiguus injury caused this OSA; nevertheless, pre-stroke weight gain, snoring, and sleepiness suggested that OSA was present prior to stroke. In 1985, Tikare et al. diagnosed OSA in a patient with recent stroke (brain computerized tomography (CT) showed paraventricular low attenuation), and suggested that OSA-induced hypoxia and cardiac arrhythmia caused the stroke [19]. In 1991, Dyken et al. diagnosed OSA in a sleepy, sonorous, obese 34-year-old man, after he awoke with left hemiparesis (brain CT suggested a hypertensive hemorrhagic stroke: Fig. 27.3) [20,21]. Hemodynamic studies reporting elevated blood pressures following sleep-related respiratory obstructions supported the hypothesis that OSA precipitated this hypertensive bleed [22,23].

Case-controlled studies

In 1992, Dyken et al. published preliminary data of a 4-year follow-up study of 24 consecutively encountered inpatients admitted for stroke, along with 27 healthy gender- and age-matched controls [24,25]. OSA was diagnosed in 71% of strokes: 10 of 13 males (77%) and 7 of 11 females (64%). However, it was diagnosed in only 3 of 13 males without stroke (23%) ($p = 0.169$) and in only 2 of 14 females without stroke (14%) ($p = 0.0168$).

A risk factor

Transient ischemic attacks

Reports of patients with transient ischemic attacks (TIAs, or "ministrokes," that is to say, focal neurological deficits resolving within 24 hours) during sleep, subsequently diagnosed with OSA and whose treatment for OSA was followed by long-term resolution of TIA, suggest a cause-and-effect relationship between OSA and stroke, as 15% of strokes are preceded by TIAs (90-day risk up to 17.3%) [3,26–27].

Cohort studies

Table 27.1 shows the results of incidence studies for OSA and stroke risk.

Population-based studies

In 2001, Shahar et al. studied the cross-sectional association between SRBDs and self-reported cardiovascular disease in 6424 subjects using home polysomnography (PSG) [28]. The relative odds of prevalent stroke (upper versus lower AHI quartile) was 1.58 (95% confidence interval, CI, 1.02–22.46).

In 2005, Arzt et al., utilizing logistic regression (using 12 years of data from a stratified random sample), performed a cross-sectional analysis of 1475 subjects (30–60 years) [29]. A baseline AHI ≥ 20 independently increased the OR for stroke (3.83; 95% CI 1.17–12.56; $p = 0.03$) compared with a reference group with an AHI < 5, after adjusting for sex, age, body mass index (BMI: weight in kilograms/square of height in meters), alcohol, smoking, diabetes, and hypertension.

A longitudinal analysis of 1189 individuals tested whether SRBD was associated with increased incident stroke at 4-year intervals. A baseline AHI ≥ 20 had significantly higher OR for incident stroke compared with the reference group (4.48; 95% CI 1.31–15.33; $p = 0.02$), when controlling for sex and age.

Clinic-based studies

In 2005, Yaggi et al. examined an observational cohort of 1022 subjects with suspected SRBD and compared the risk of developing stroke, TIA, or death from any cause in 697 subjects with OSA (AHI ≥ 5) with the risk in individuals with an AHI < 5 [30]. Many with SRBD were treated (diet, upper-airway surgery, and positive airway pressure (PAP) therapies).

Over 3.3–3.4 years, the OSA group had 22 incident strokes and/or TIAs and 50 deaths (the comparison group had 2 strokes and/or TIAs and 14 deaths). OSA was associated with significant risk for composite stroke, TIA, or death (hazard ratio (HR) 1.97; 95% CI 1.12–3.48; $p = 0.01$), after adjusting for sex, age, race, smoking, BMI, diabetes, hyperlipidemia, atrial fibrillation, and hypertension. Trend analysis found that increased OSA severity was associated with increased risk of stroke, TIA, or death from any cause ($p = 0.005$).

In 2006, Munoz et al. studied a non-institutionalized, elderly population (range 70–100 years, median 77.28), drawn from a random one-stage cluster sampling stratified by sex, age, and census area [31]. After adjusting for sex, a baseline AHI ≥ 30 was a risk factor for incident ischemic stroke or TIA (HR 2.52; 95% CI 1.04–6.1; $p = 0.04$).

In 2008, Valham et al. studied a population (≤70 years), with angina and coronary artery disease (verified by angiography and left ventriculography) [32]. Initial PSGs (without electroencephalography (EEG), using a pressure sensitive bed to monitor respiration) of 392 randomly selected subjects showed sleep apnea (AHI ≥ 5) in 54%. A 10-year follow-up, during which 9 apneics received OSA therapy, showed that 47 subjects (12%) suffered strokes. Sleep apnea was associated with an increased stroke risk; HR of 2.89 (95% CI 1.37–6.09, $p = 0.005$), independent of treatment, previous stroke or TIA, sex, age, BMI, smoking, diabetes, hypertension, left-ventricular function, hypertension, and atrial fibrillation. Compared with individuals without apnea, subjects with an AHI > 5 but < 15, and subjects with an AHI > 15, respectively, had 2.44 (59% CI 1.08–5.52, $p = 0.011$) and 3.56 (95% CI 1.56–8.16, $p = 0.011$) times increased risk of stroke, independent of confounders.

Table 27.1 OSA and stroke risk: incidence studies

Incidence studies	Subjects studied	Population size	AHI used to define SDB group	SDB prevalence	AHI used to define comparison group	Mean follow-up period (years)	Group outcome: total number of subjects in a given group with outcome	Risk estimate of SDB as risk factor for outcome (95% CI)
Authors/year								
Arzt et al. 2005	Population-based General adult 30–60 years	† 1475 †† 1189	≥20	7% (N = 99)	<5	Three intervals of 4 years	Stroke SDB = 4 Comparison = 9	*OR = 4.48 (1.31–15.33; p = 0.02)
Yaggi et al. 2005	Clinic-based Referred for suspected SDB ≥50 years	1022	≥5	68% (N = 697)	<5	3.4 SDB 3.3 CG	Stroke, TIA, or death SDB = 72 Comparison = 16	**HR = 1.97 (1.12–3.48; p = 0.01)
Munoz et al. 2006	Clinic-based: Random sample, non-institutional elderly 70–100 years	394	≥30	25% (N = 98)	<30	4.5	TIA or ischemic stroke SDB = 9 Comparison = 11	***HR = 2.52 (1.04–6.1; p = 0.04)
Valham et al. 2008	Clinic based Symptomatic angina and CAD	392	≥5	54%	<5	10.0	Stroke SDB = 38 Comparison = 9	****HR = 2.89 (1.37–6.09; p = 0.005)
Redline et al. 2010	Community-based ≥40 years	5,422	>15	Male 44% (N = 1095) Female 24% (N = 720)	<4.1	8.7	Ischemic stroke Male SDB = 54 Female SDB = 37	Male: *****HR = 2.86 (1.1–7.4) Female: ****** A 2% increase in HR (0–5) after threshold OAHI of 25

AHI, apnea/hypopnea index = the average number of apneas and hypopneas per hour of sleep; SDB, sleep-disordered breathing; CG, comparison group; CI, confidence interval; P, probability; OR, odds ratio; HR, hazard ratio; CAD, coronary artery disease; OAHI, obstructive apnea hypopnea index.

† Original population providing original cross-sectional prevalence data.

†† Population used for longitudinal analysis of incident stroke.

* In a model adjusted for age and sex.

** In a model adjusted for age, sex, race, smoking, BMI, diabetes mellitus, hyperlipidemia, atrial fibrillation and hypertension.

*** In a model adjusted for sex.

**** In a model adjusted for age, BMI, left ventricular function, diabetes, sex, intervention, hypertension, atrial fibrillation, previous stroke or TIA.

***** In a model for male subjects comparing the risk for ischemic stroke and the OAHI in the top quartile (quartile IV; OAHI > 19) to the lowest quartile (quartile I; OAHI < 4.1) of the overall population studied.

****** In a model using non-linear, covariate adjusted associations between OAHI and the female sex.

Adapted from Chest, 136(6), Dyken MD, Im KB, Obstructive sleep apnea and stroke, pp. 1668–1677, Copyright (2009), with permission from American College of Chest Physicians.

In 2010, Redline et al. followed 5422 subjects, without stroke for a median of 8.7 years, during which 193 ischemic strokes occurred [33]. Men with an obstructive AHI (OAHI) > 19.1 (the top quartile) had an adjusted HR for stroke of 2.86 (95% CI 1.1–7.4), compared with men with an OAHI < 4.1 (quartile I). Stroke risk did not associate with OAHI quartile or oxygen desaturation in women. Nevertheless, using nonlinear covariate-adjusted associations with the OSA exposures and interactions with gender, there was a 2% increase (95% CI 0–5) in stroke HR with each unit increment in OAHI above a threshold of 25.

Treatment versus no treatment

Morbidity and mortality

In 1996, a 4-year follow-up by Dyken et al. of a 1992 prevalence study of OSA and stroke showed that all stroke subjects who died had OSA ($n = 5$; one used continuous positive airway pressure (CPAP), dying from urosepsis) [27,28]. Only one male control, an individual without OSA, died (prostatic carcinoma). Respectively, stroke subjects dead versus alive at 4 years had original diagnostic mean AHIs of 41.3 and 22.1, suggesting that the diagnosis and severity of OSA in stroke was associated with worse long-term mortality.

A 1990, prospective, treatment versus non-treatment study by Partinen et al. suggested a cause-and-effect relationship between OSA and stroke [34,35]. Seven years after treating 198 OSA subjects with weight loss ($n = 127$) or tracheostomy ($n = 71$), 5.2% of the weight loss group had stroke (17.3% died, 11% from vascular etiologies), whereas only 1.2% with tracheostomy suffered stroke (2.8% died).

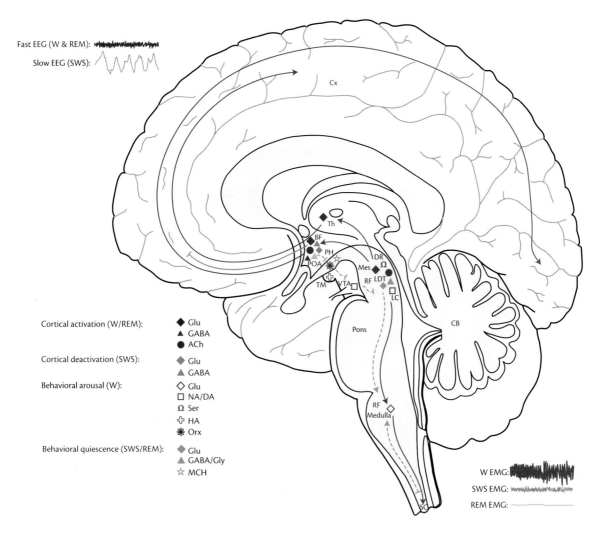

Fast EEG (W & REM):

Slow EEG (SWS):

Cortical activation (W/REM):
◆ Glu
▲ GABA
● ACh

Cortical deactivation (SWS):
◆ Glu
▲ GABA

Behavioral arousal (W):
◇ Glu
□ NA/DA
Ω Ser
✛ HA
✳ Orx

Behavioral quiescence (SWS/REM):
◆ Glu
▲ GABA/Gly
☆ MCH

W EMG:

SWS EMG:

REM EMG:

Fig. 4.1 Sleep–wake state substrates. Sagittal schematic view of the human brain depicting neurons with their chemical neurotransmitters and pathways by which they influence cortical activity or behavior across the sleep-wake cycle. Neurons that are active during waking (red symbols) include cells with ascending projections toward the cortex, which stimulate cortical activation, and cells with descending projections toward the spinal cord, which stimulate behavioral arousal with postural muscle tone. Those with predominantly ascending projections discharge in association with fast, gamma EEG activity and cease firing with slow, delta activity to be active during both W and REM sleep (W/REM or W/PS, filled red symbols); they include neurons that release glutamate (Glu, diamonds), GABA (triangles) or acetylcholine (ACh, circles) (W/PS-max active, Fig. 4.2). Those with more diffuse or descending projections discharge in association with behavioral arousal and EMG activity and cease firing with muscle atonia to be active during W and silent during REM (W, empty red symbols); they include neurons that release glutamate (Glu, diamonds), noradrenaline (NA, square), serotonin (Ser, omega), histamine (HA, cross) or orexin (Orx, asterisk) (W-max active, Figs. 4.4 and 4.7). Neurons that are active during sleep (blue or aqua symbols) include cells with ascending projections toward the cortex, which dampen fast cortical activity, and those with descending projections toward the hypothalamus, brainstem or spinal cord, which diminish behavioral arousal and muscle tone. Those sleep-active neurons with ascending projections to the cortex or local relay neurons discharge in association with slow EEG activity during SWS (SWS, blue triangle; SWS-max active, Fig. 4.3). They include GABAergic neurons that can inhibit other W/REM cortical or subcortical neurons. Those sleep-active neurons with descending projections to the spinal cord or local relay neurons discharge in association with decreasing muscle tone and EMG (SWS/REM, aqua diamonds and triangles; PS-max active see Figs. 4.5 and 4.6). They include GABAergic neurons in the basal forebrain, preoptic area, hypothalamus and brainstem that can inhibit other W neurons, including Glu, MA or Orx neurons. They also include MCH neurons (aqua star, PS-max active, Fig. 4.7), which have more diffuse projections but can exert an inhibitory influence upon other neurons of the arousal systems including the MA, HA and Orx neurons. SWS/REM GABAergic neurons, which can also contain glycine (GABA/Gly), in the ventral medullary RF can inhibit motor neurons in the brainstem and spinal cord, particularly during REM sleep. BF, basal forebrain; CB, cerebellum; Cx, cortex; DR, dorsal raphe; LC, locus coeruleus nucleus; LDT, laterodorsal tegmental nucleus; Mes, mesencephalon; PH, posterior hypothalamus; POA, preoptic area; RF, reticular formation; SC, spinal cord; Th, thalamus; TM, tuberomammillary nucleus; VTA, ventral tegmental area.

Adapted from Jones BE, "Neurobiology of waking and sleeping" from Vinken PJ and Bruyn GW (eds), Handbook of clinical neurology, pp. 131–49, Copyright (2011), with permission from Elsevier.

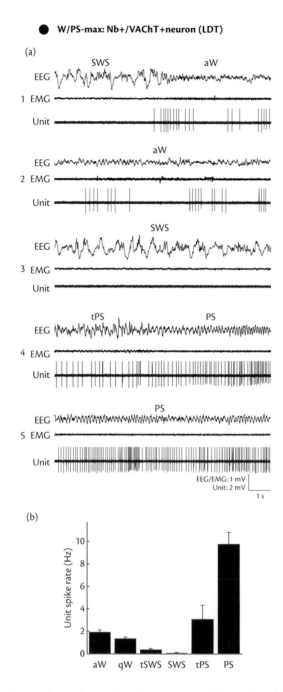

Fig. 4.2 Discharge of cholinergic W/ PS-max active unit across sleep–wake states in rat. Data from a recorded, Neurobiotin (Nb)-labeled cell (#CBS28U03) that was identified as immunopositive for vesicular ACh transporter (VAChT) and located in the LDT. (a) Polygraphic records from 10 s epochs or periods of the unit together with EEG (from retrosplenial cortex) and EMG activity during a transition from SWS to aW (1), aW (2), SWS (3), a transition from tPS to PS (4), and PS (5). (b) Bar graph showing mean spike rate of the unit across sleep–wake stages. Note that during W (2), the unit discharged tonically at a slow rate (1.91 Hz) with prominence of fast EEG activity, ceased firing during SWS (3) (0.06 Hz) in association with slow EEG activity (~1– 4 Hz), and discharged maximally and tonically to reach its highest rates during PS (5) (9.70 Hz) in association with prominent rhythmic theta (~6– 8 Hz) along with fast EEG activity. It changed its rate of discharge prior to cortical activation in the transition from SWS to aW (1) and prior to PS during tPS (4) as EEG activity progresses to theta. The unit discharge was significantly positively correlated with EEG gamma ($r = 0.37$) along with theta activity ($r = 0.93$). aW: active wake; qW: quiet wake; tSWS: transition to slow-wave sleep; SWS: slow-wave sleep; tPS: transition to paradoxical sleep; PS: paradoxical sleep.

Reproduced from J Neurosci, 34(13), Boucetta S, Cisse Y, Mainville L, Morales M, Jones BE, Discharge Profiles across the Sleep–Waking Cycle of Identified Cholinergic, GABAergic, and Glutamatergic Neurons in the Pontomesencephalic Tegmentum of the Rat, pp. 4708– 27, Copyright (2014), with permission from Society for Neuroscience.

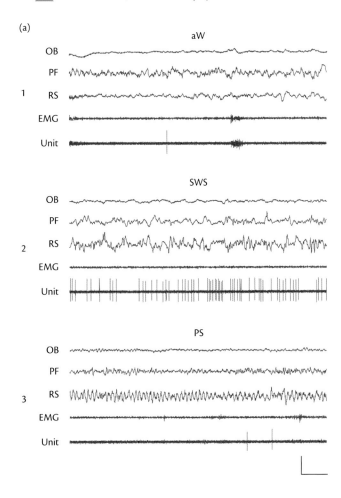

SWS-max: Nb+/GAD+ neuron (BF)

(a)

aW

OB
PF
RS
EMG
Unit

1

SWS

OB
PF
RS
EMG
Unit

2

PS

OB
PF
RS
EMG
Unit

3

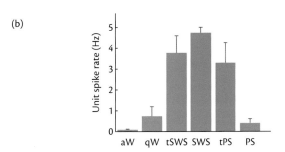

(b)

Fig. 4.3 Discharge of GABAergic SWS-max active unit across sleep–wake states in rat. Data from a recorded, Nb-labeled cell (c120u04) that was identified as immunopositive for glutamic acid decarboxylase (GAD) and located in the BF. (a) Polygraphic records from 10 s epochs of the unit spiking together with EEG and EMG activity during aW (1), SWS (2), and PS (3). (b) Bar graph showing mean spike rate of the unit across sleep–wake stages. Note that the unit was virtually silent during aW (0.1 Hz), increased slightly during qW, then increased substantially with tSWS to reach the highest rates during SWS (4.74 Hz), decrease slightly during tPS, and decrease substantially during PS (0.4 Hz). Across sleep– wake stages, the unit's discharge rate was significantly, positively correlated with delta EEG amplitude ($r = 0.60$). Calibrations: horizontal, 1 s; vertical, 1 mV (EEG, EMG), 2 mV (unit). OB: olfactory bulb; PF: prefrontal cortex; RS: retrosplenial cortex.

Reproduced from J Neurosci., 29(38), Hassani OK, Lee MG, Henny P, Jones BE, Discharge profiles of identified GABAergic in comparison to cholinergic and putative glutamatergic basal forebrain neurons across the sleep–wake cycle, pp. 11828– 40, Copyright (2009), with permission from Society for Neuroscience.

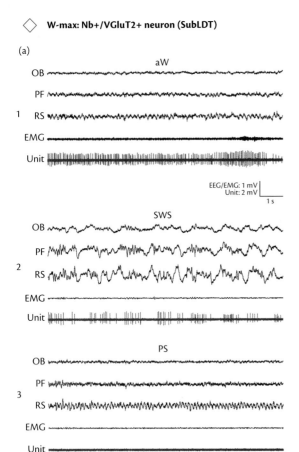

◇ **W-max: Nb+/VGluT2+ neuron (SubLDT)**

(a)

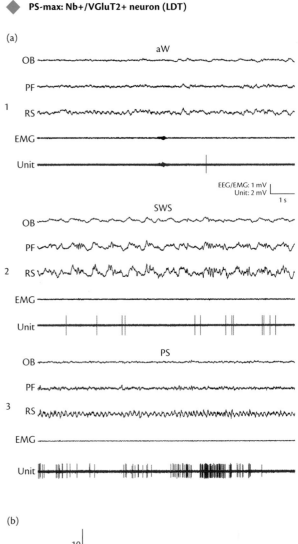

◆ **PS-max: Nb+/VGluT2+ neuron (LDT)**

(a)

(b)

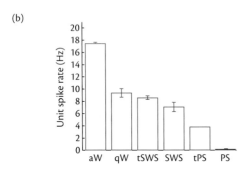

Fig. 4.4 Discharge of glutamatergic W-max active unit across sleep–wake states in rat. Data from a recorded, Nb-labeled cell (#CBS47U02) that was identified by in situ hybridization as expressing the vesicular Glu transporter (VGluT2) and was located in the SubLDT. (a, b) Note that this VGluT2+ cell discharged maximally and tonically during aW (1) (17.40 Hz) with fast EEG activity and high neck muscle tone, decreased its firing during SWS (2) (6.83 Hz) in association with slow EEG activity and low muscle tone, and ceased firing during PS (3) (0.78 Hz) in association with theta EEG activity and muscle atonia. The unit discharge was positively correlated with EMG activity ($r = 0.69$).

(b)

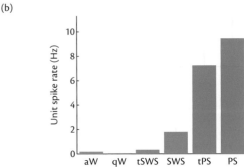

Fig. 4.5 Discharge of glutamatergic PS-max active unit across sleep–wake states in rat. Data from a recorded, Nb-labeled cell (#CBS46U02) that that was identified by in situ hybridization as expressing VGluT2 and was located in the LDT. (a, b) Note that this VGluT2+ cell discharged at its lowest rates during aW (1) (0.13 Hz) with fast EEG activity and high neck muscle tone, increased its firing during SWS (2) (1.77 Hz) in association with slow EEG activity and low muscle tone, and discharged maximally to reach its highest rate during PS (3) (9.42 Hz) in association with theta EEG activity and muscle atonia. It increased its rate most markedly immediately preceding PS during tPS.

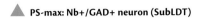

PS-max: Nb+/GAD+ neuron (SubLDT)

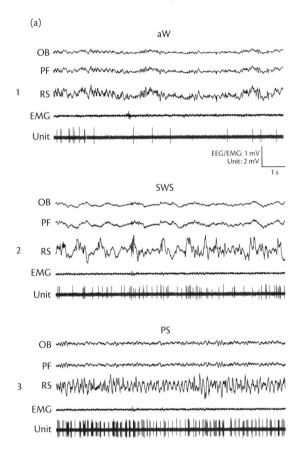

(a)

aW

OB

PF

1   RS

EMG

Unit

EEG/EMG: 1 mV
Unit: 2 mV
1 s

SWS

OB

PF

2   RS

EMG

Unit

PS

OB

PF

3   RS

EMG

Unit

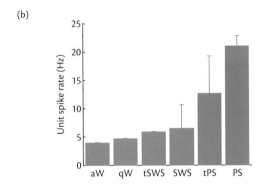

(b)

Fig. 4.6 Discharge of GABAergic PS-max active unit across sleep–wake states in rat. Data from recorded, Nb-labeled cell (#CBS28U04) that was immunopositive for GAD and located in the SubLDT. (a, b) Note that this GAD+ cell discharged at relatively low rates during aW (1) (3.90 Hz) with fast EEG activity and high EMG amplitude, increased firing during SWS (2) (6.05 Hz) in association with slow delta EEG activity and low muscle EMG, and discharged maximally during PS (3) (20.98 Hz) with theta and fast EEG activity accompanied by muscle atonia. It increased its discharge most markedly immediately preceding PS during tPS. The unit discharge was positively correlated with EEG theta activity ($r = 0.53$) and negatively correlated with EMG amplitude ($r = -0.45$).

Reproduced from J Neurosci, 34(13), Boucetta S, Cisse Y, Mainville L, Morales M, Jones BE, Discharge Profiles across the Sleep- Waking Cycle of Identified Cholinergic, GABAergic, and Glutamatergic Neurons in the Pontomesencephalic Tegmentum of the Rat, pp. 4708–27, Copyright (2014), with permission from Society for Neuroscience.

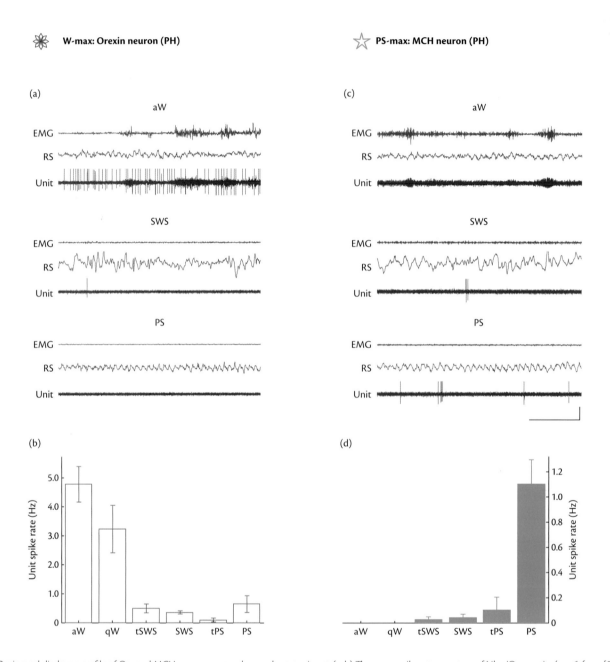

Fig. 4.7 Reciprocal discharge profile of Orx and MCH neurons across sleep–wake states in rat. (a, b) The mean spike rate per stage of Nb+/Orx+ units (*n* = 6; from [53]) varies in a reciprocal manner to that of Nb+/MCH+ units (c, d). The reciprocal firing profiles were not correlated with EEG gamma or delta activity, but were correlated in an inverse manner with EMG amplitude, positively for the wake-active Orx neurons and negatively for the MCH sleep-active neurons.

Reproduced from Proc Natl Acad Sci U S A, 106(7), Hassani OK, Lee MG, Jones BE, Melanin-concentrating hormone neurons discharge in a reciprocal manner to orexin neurons across the sleep–wake cycle, pp. 2418–22, Copyright (2009), with permission from National Academy of Sciences.

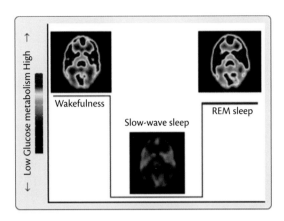

Fig. 11.1 Schematic representation of the variations in global cerebral glucose metabolism in resting wakefulness, slow-wave sleep, and REM sleep. The images represent the cerebral glucose metabolism measured in a single subject during three different sessions with [18F]fluorodeoxyglucose positron emission tomography (FDG- PET). Functional images are displayed at the same brain level and using the same color scale. Similar rates of brain glucose metabolism are measured during wakefulness and REM sleep. Brain glucose metabolism is significantly decreased during slow-wave sleep relative to both wakefulness and REM sleep.

Adapted from Brain Res, 513(1), Maquet P, Dive D, Salmon E, et al, Cerebral glucose utilization during sleep– wake cycle in man determined by positron emission tomography and [^{18}F]2-fluoro-2-deoxy-D-glucose method, pp. 136– 43, Copyright (1990) with permission from Elsevier.

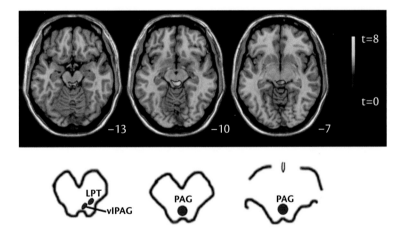

Fig. 11.2 Statistical parametric mapping (t) axial maximum intensity projection maps rendered onto a stereotactically normalized MRI scan, showing areas of significant decreases of fractional anisotropy values (color code, yellow to orange) in a cohort of patients with idiopathic REM sleep behavior disorder versus healthy control subjects. The number at the bottom right corner of each MRI scan corresponds to the z-coordinate in Talairach space. The schematic drawings below the scans correspond to the MRI and visualize proposed nuclei involved in REM sleep control (modified from Boeve et al. [94]). The REM-off region is represented by the ventrolateral part of the periaqueductal gray matter (vlPAG)/ periaqueductal gray matter (PAG) and the lateral pontine tegmentum (LPT).

Reproduced from Annals of Neurology, 69(2), Scherfler C, Frauscher B, Schocke M, Iranzo A, Gschliesser V, Seppi K, Santamaria J, Tolosa E, Hogl B, Poewe W, White and gray matter abnormalities in idiopathic rapid eye movement sleep behavior disorder: a diffusion- tensor imaging and voxel- based morphometry study, pp. 400–407, Copyright (2011), with permission from John Wiley and Sons.

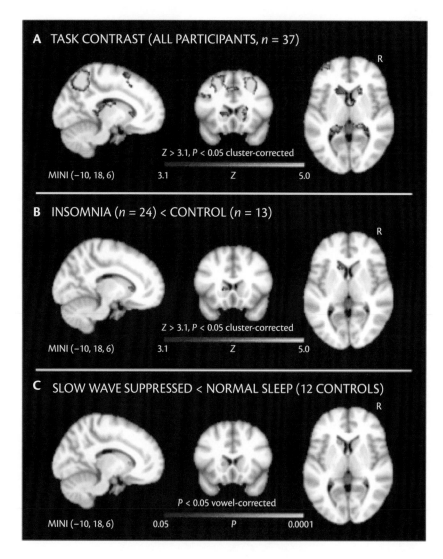

Fig. 11.3 Reduced caudate recruitment in insomnia and after slow-wave sleep fragmentation. (A) The head of the left caudate shows increased BOLD signal during executive functioning relative to baseline trials across all participants. (B) Patients with insomnia show an attenuated task-elicited BOLD response in the head of the left caudate nucleus when compared to controls (Z_{max} = 4.31 at MNI coordinates (−12, 18, 2); cluster size = 43 voxels = 344 mm³). (C) Controls show an attenuated task-elicited BOLD response in the head of the left caudate nucleus after a night of slow-wave sleep suppression relative to a night of normal sleep (Z_{max} = 3.32 at MNI coordinates (−12, 18, 4); 36 of 43 voxels in the region of interest = 84%). Significant clusters (A and B) or voxels (C) are shown in a gradient from red to yellow overlaid on the most informative orthogonal slices from the averaged MNI152 brain, displayed according to neurological convention (left = left). MNI coordinates for the orthogonal slices, statistical thresholds, and a color bar indicating Z-value or significance level are shown at the bottom.

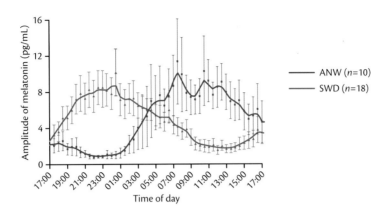

Fig. 21.3 Melatonin profiles of night-shift workers with and without SWD. Individuals exhibit remarkable diversity in the degree of circadian adaptation to shift work. A recent study evaluated the dim light salivary melatonin profiles of 10 asymptomatic night workers (ANW) and 18 workers with SWD during a 25-hour sleep deprivation protocol. Though the melatonin profile of the SWD group was similar to that of healthy day workers (20:27 ± 5.0 h), the ANW group exhibited a significantly delayed DLMO (05:00 ± 3.4 h), indicating better circadian adaptation to night work.

Reproduced from Chronobiology International, 29(7), Gumenyuk V, Roth T, Drake CL, Circadian phase, sleepiness, and light exposure assessment in night workers with and without shift work disorder, pp. 928–36, Copyright (2012), with permission from Taylor & Francis.

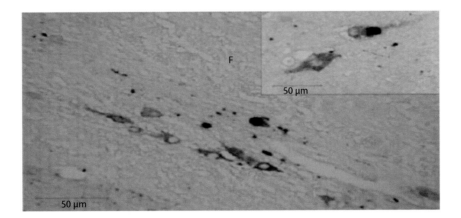

Fig. 25.1 Example of hypocretin neurons (DAB staining: dark) that contain a Lewy body (alpha-synuclein, AP-body) in PD patients. Several hypocretin neurons that do not show this colocalization are also present. "F" indicates the fornix.

Reproduced from Brain, 130(6), Hegeman I, van Pelt J, van Duinen S, Jan Lammers G and Swaab DF, Fronczek R, Overeem S, Lee S, Hypocretin (orexin) loss in Parkinson's disease, pp. 1577–1585, Copyright (2007), with permission from Oxford University Press.

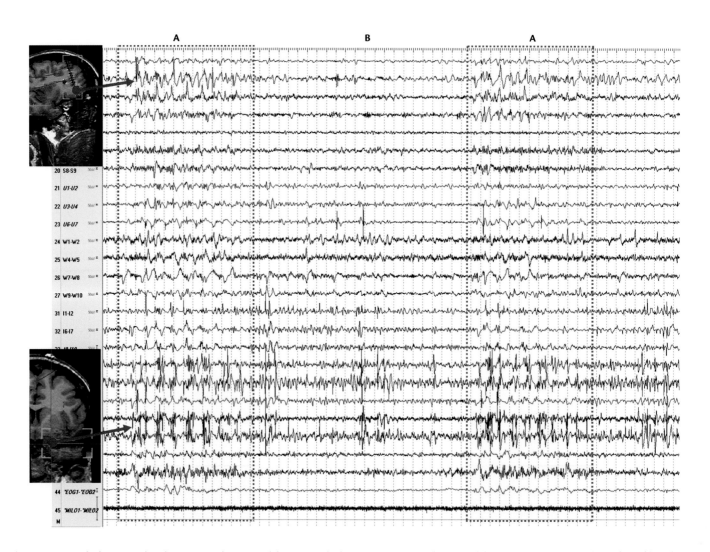

Fig. 28.4 Intracerebral EEG recording during NREM sleep in an adult patient with pharmacoresistant mesial temporal lobe epilepsy. During the A phase of CAP (dotted boxes) IEDs in the mesial temporal lobe (lower MRI image) are more numerous and spread to the orbital region (upper MRI image). During the B phase of CAP, IEDs are reduced and circumscribed to the temporal lobe.

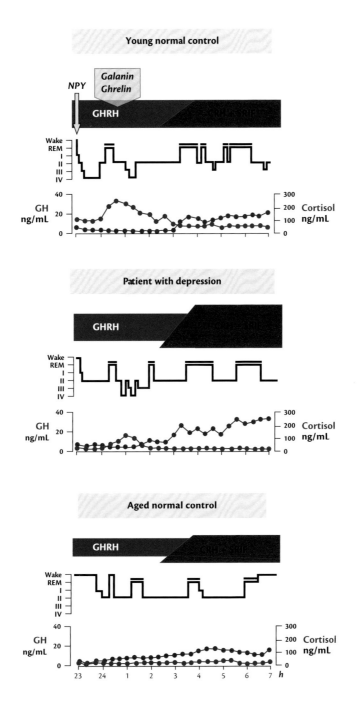

Fig. 44.2 Model of peptidergic sleep regulation. A reciprocal interaction between the neuropeptides growth hormone-releasing hormone (GHRH) and corticotropin-releasing hormone (CRH) appears likely, at least in male subjects. GHRH is thought to preponderate during the first half of the night, whereas CRH (and SRIF, somatostatin) dominate during the second half of the night. Neuropeptide Y (NPY) influences the time of sleep onset. Ghrelin and galanin are cofactors to GHRH. The balance between GHRH and CRH is changed during aging (reduced GHRH activity) and during depression (CRH overactivity). Therefore, similar sleep–endocrine changes are found during aging and in patients with depression.

Reproduced from Der Nervenarzt, 66, Steiger A, Schlafendokrinologie, pp. 15–27, Copyright (1995), with permission from Springer.

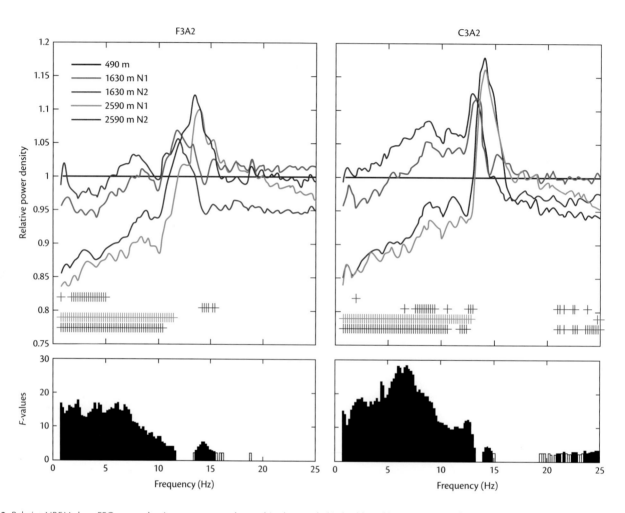

Fig. 54.3 Relative NREM sleep EEG power density spectra at moderate altitude recorded in healthy subjects. Upper panels: Spectra at altitude (1630 and 2590 m, N1 (first night) and N2 (second night)) are plotted relative to baseline sleep (490 m; line at 1). Significant differences ($p < 0.05$) between baseline and altitude are indicated by "+" ($n = 44$). Frequency resolution: 0.2 Hz. Lower panels: F-values of the frequency bins with significant p- values for factor Condition (490 m N1, 1630 m N1, 1630 m N2, 2590 m N1 and 2590 m N2) of mixed model ANOVA with factors Condition and Order. F3A2: frontal derivation; C3A2: central derivation.

CPAP

In 2005, Martinez-Garcia et al. showed that of 51 patients with recent stroke and minimum AHI of 20, only 15 (29.4%) tolerated CPAP after 1 month [36]. Those not tolerating CPAP had a fivefold (OR 5.09) increase in the probability of suffering a new vascular event.

In 2006, Palombini et al. showed that only 22% of 32 patients with recent stroke tolerated CPAP for 8 weeks owing to difficulties from facial weakness, motor impairment, and discomfort [37]. Brown et al. found that patients with stroke took longer putting on and taking off ($p < 0.01$) traditional CPAP headgear compared with one-piece systems [38]. Palombini et al. stated, "Better education and support of patients and families, and special training session in rehabilitation services, will be needed to improve compliance" [42]. Disler et al. showed that, with better "support," patients with moderately severe motor and cognitive functional independence measurement scores tolerated CPAP [39].

Positional therapy

Positional OSA (worse supine, from gravitational effect) is common in acute stroke [40]. In 2008, Dziewas et al. diagnosed OSA in 78% of 55 subjects within 72 hours of stroke (65% positional) [45]. After 6 months, only 49% had OSA (33% positional). The authors stated that "positional sleep apnea is a predominant feature in acute stroke and its incidence decreases significantly during the following months. These findings may have implications for sleep apnea treatment in patients with acute stroke." They suggested that serial PSG studies may permit modifying, reducing, and eventually withdrawing OSA treatment.

Medications

Brunner evaluated mirtazapine as an alternative treatment in elderly stroke patients with sleep apnea in an open trial [41]. Ten subjects, all of whom refused CPAP, underwent PSG before and after a course of mirtazapine. Four individuals showed worsening of apnea, and although six had significantly reduced apnea, some experts hypothesize that this improvement may be related to the natural progression of the disorder over time after stroke, as suggested by Dziewas et al. [45].

Other therapeutic considerations

The evaluation and treatment in acute stroke must be tailored, because critical illness in an intensive care setting may require portable PSG with end-tidal CO_2 monitoring, complemented with arterial blood gases when hypoventilation, CO_2 retention, and underlying lung or neuromuscular compromise are suspected. Although positional therapy should be considered, even simple head-of-bed elevation may be contraindicated because of perfusion pressure issues; as such, the utilization of positional devices preventing supine sleep might be preferable. Various PAP therapies (including CPAP, bilevel PAP (BPAP), and noninvasive positive pressure ventilatory units such as auto-adjusting BPAP, which includes adaptive servo-ventilation for CSA, and volume-assured pressure support for severe hypoventilation) may need to be presented in a supportive educational manner with close follow-up for adherence. Initially, severe cases may require intubation and tracheostomy.

Pediatric stroke and OSA

There is a relative paucity of information about the relationship between stroke and sleep apnea in the pediatric population. The majority of reports involve sickle cell disease (SCD), an inherited hemoglobinopathy where hypoxemia leads to red blood cell thickening, resulting in painful vaso-occlusion. In 1988, a case report described a 6.5-year-old with SCD and multiple ischemic strokes, in whom PSG diagnosed severe OSA from adenotonsillar enlargement [42]. The authors suggested that apnea-associated hypoxemia contributed to these strokes. A 1989 study reported that 13 of 21 children with OSA and SCD had resolution of symptoms and improvement in hypoventilation after tonsillectomy/adenoidectomy (T&A) [43]. A French group reported that two boys, ages 5 and 6 years, with SCD and snoring, had elevated middle cerebral artery blood flow velocities (≥ 200 cm/s), as determined by transcranial Doppler (TCD), that normalized (<170 cm/se) after T&A [44].

A retrospective study evaluated children ≤17 years with SCD, who underwent T&A, matched to patients without T&A [45]. T&A was associated with a significantly reduced rate of hospital visits in subjects with OSA and cerebrovascular ischemia (stroke and TIAs). PSG was used in a cross-sectional study to assess the prevalence of SDB in children with SCD [46]. Sixty-four subjects, aged 2–14 years, were evaluated with the Pediatric Sleep Questionnaire, and PSG was performed in those with snoring. The prevalence of SDB was 23.7%, but no association was found between elevated TCD velocity and SDB. Finally, a review article, not limited to SCD, concluded that there is strong evidence for an association between SDB and cardiovascular morbidity in children and that treatment of SDB results in improvements in blood pressure, cardiovascular control, and inflammation and endothelial function [47].

Potential mechanisms for OSA-induced stroke

Metabolic syndrome

The odds of having the metabolic syndrome is increased up to ninefold in individuals with OSA (53% of newly diagnosed apneics) [48–49]. A cross-sectional case–control study found the metabolic syndrome more often in apneics than controls (men 49.5% versus 22.0%, $p < 0.01$; women 32.0% versus 6.7%, $p < 0.01$) [50].

OSA is independently associated with obesity, hypertension, and insulin resistance/diabetes (stroke risk factors of the metabolic syndrome) [3,51–52]. Elevation of the BMI by one standard deviation increases the OR for SRBD (AHI ≥ 5) by 4.17 [7]. A prospective population-based study showed that after 4 years, the OR for developing hypertension of subjects with AHI between 5.0 and 14.9, and those with AHI ≥ 15.0 was respectively two versus three times greater compared with non-apneics [53]. A community-based cross-sectional study of 69 non-diabetics showed that those individuals with mild and moderately severe OSA had reduced insulin sensitivity when compared with non-apneics (AHI < 5), independent of sex, race, age, and body fat percentage [54].

Autonomic activity

Microneurography (a direct measure of efferent sympathetic neural activity, SNA), supports the hypothesis that OSA-induced hypertensive events, from elevated SNA (secondary to reflex effects of hypoxia, hypercapnia, and decreased input from thoracic stretch receptors), can cause stroke (Figs. 27.4 and 27.5) [24]. In 1995, Somers et al. studied 10 subjects with OSA and found that SNA increased by 246% during the last 10 s of apnea, with a mean blood pressure increase from 92 mmHg waking to 127 mmHg in rapid eye movement (REM, stage R) sleep [55]. Persistently elevated waking sympathetic tone in apneics suggested that OSA might induce chronic changes predisposing to stroke.

Autonomic effects could contribute to cardiac arrhythmias in up to 48% of apneics [56–57]. In 1992, Somers et al. showed that

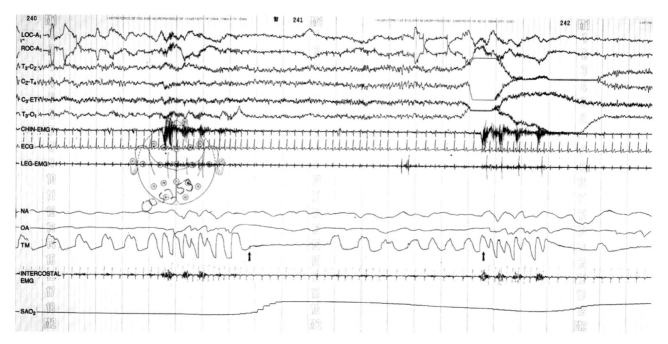

Fig. 27.4 A PSG tracing (paper speed 10 mm/s) has been reduced to correspond to the temporally related microneurographic tracing shown in Fig. 27.5 (paper speed 5 mm/s). Arrows indicate a prolonged mixed apnea of approximately 26 s duration occurring during REM sleep, associated with severe oxygen desaturation. LOC: left outer canthus; ROC: right outer canthus; T: temporal; C: central; ET: ears tied; O: occipital; EMG: electromyogram; N: nasal airflow; OA: oral airflow; TM: thoracic movement.

Adapted from Dyken ME, Cerebrovascular disease and sleep apnea. In: Bradley DT, Floras JS, [eds], Sleep Apnea: Implications in Cardiovascular and Cerebrovascular Disease (Lung Biology in Health and Disease), pp. 285–306, Copyright (2000), with permission from Informa Healthcare.

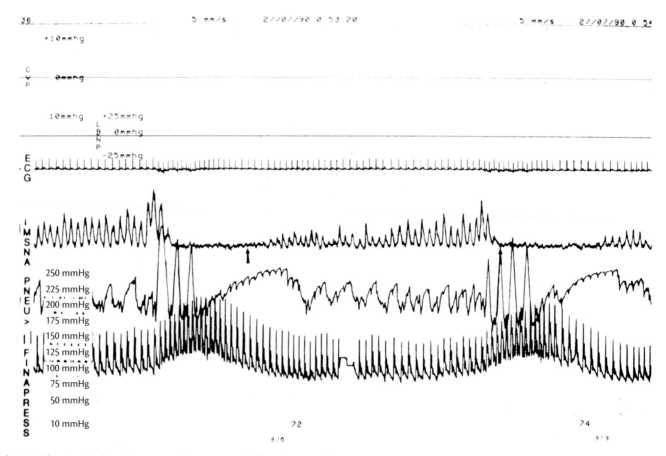

Fig. 27.5 The arrows in this microneurographic tracing recorded from the peroneal nerve indicate a gradual elevation of efferent nerve activity during a mixed apnea. The activity peak is immediately followed by cessation of the apnea, with a subsequent marked elevation of arterial blood pressure to 215/130 mmHg from a baseline of 135/80 mmHg. MSNA: muscle sympathetic nerve activity; PNEU: chest excursion; FINAPRESS; fingertip blood pressure.

Adapted from Dyken ME, Cerebrovascular disease and sleep apnea. In: Bradley DT, Floras JS, [eds], Sleep Apnea: Implications in Cardiovascular and Cerebrovascular Disease (Lung Biology in Health and Disease), pp. 285–306, Copyright (2000), with permission from Informa Healthcare.

obstructive apneas (inspiration against a closed glottis with hypoxemia) could cause excessive parasympathetic response with episodic sinus arrest and dramatic blood pressure reductions (180/100 mmHg prior to obstructions, to systolic pressures < 50 mmHg during obstructions) [58].

Cardiogenic

The diagnosis of atrial fibrillation also carries with it a 49% risk for OSA, and CPAP non-compliance is associated with greater recurrence after cardioversion [59,60]. Atrial fibrillation might contribute to stroke in some patients with OSA, as it is a strong risk factor for stroke [3].

A patent foramen ovale (PFO) is a well-known stroke risk factor found in approximately 30% of patients with ischemic stroke [61]. OSA is associated with increased right heart pressure, and during obstructive events a PFO can result in right-to-left shunting. Beelke et al. observed right-to-left shunting in 9 of 10 subjects with PFO and OSA [62]. The number of microembolic signals during apneas positively correlated with the number during waking Valsalva maneuvers. In one patient, Pinet and Orehek showed resolution of apnea-associated shunting after 1 week of CPAP [63].

Circadian rhythms

Dyken et al. hypothesized that if stroke has an equal probability of occurring at anytime during a 24-hour time period, 33% of all strokes should occur during an 8-hour period of sleep [28]. Nevertheless, stroke tends to occur during early morning, and their prospective prevalence study showed that a higher than expected percentage of subjects with OSA had strokes during sleep (54%; $p = 0.0304$) [28,64].

REM sleep

Prolonged REM sleep occurs in early morning (coinciding with greatest stroke risk). Normal REM sleep physiological phenomena negatively affect OSA: hypotonia (worsens obstructions), elevated SNA and blood pressure (reaching waking levels with surges during muscle twitches of phasic REM), and increased cerebral blood flow (apneas increase intracranial pressure and reduce cerebral perfusion pressure) [65–66].

Early morning is associated with low fibrinolytic activity and high levels of catecholamines, blood viscosity, and platelet aggregability, when REM SNA activation might potentiate platelet aggregation and plaque development [67]. Effects of OSA on this otherwise normal hematological milieu might include further elevations in catecholamines and platelet activation, increasing thrombus and embolus formation and stroke risk [76–68].

Elevated platelet activation proteins, soluble CD40 ligand (sCD40L) and soluble P-selectin (sP-selectin), have been linked to silent brain infarctions (SBIs) [69]. Using magnetic resonance imaging (MRI) Minoguchi et al. showed SBIs in 25% of patients with moderate to severe OSA but in only 6.7% of controls, with higher serum levels of sCD40L and sP-selectin that reduced significantly after CPAP [79].

Arousal

Definition

PSG arousal from non-REM (NREM) sleep is defined as an abrupt shift of EEG including alpha, theta, and/or frequencies > 16 Hz (not including sleep spindles) lasting ≥ 3 s, with ≥ 10 s of stable sleep preceding the change [70]. An arousal from REM sleep also requires an increase in submental electromyographic (EMG) activity, lasting ≥ 1 s [80].

Studies suggest that obstructions induce arousals from NREM sleep after inspiratory effort reaches a variable arousal threshold [71]. One study hypothesized that impaired arousal led to prolonged apneas, EEG flattening, and generalized tonic spasms, "cerebral anoxic attacks" [72]. Dyken et al. described cases involving critically ill patients with OSA, where elevated arousal thresholds led to prolonged obstructions, resulting in diffuse cerebral hypoxemic EEG patterns, clinical encephalopathy, and death (Figs. 27.6–27.8) [11,73].

White et al. showed that sleep deprivation can increase the arousal threshold to hypoxia and hypercapnia [74]. As sleep deprivation is common in acutely ill patients, they "speculate—as to the clinical significance of these findings as they apply to the patient with a precarious respiratory status." OSA, a "precarious respiratory status," can also increase the arousal threshold, possibly as a result of sleep fragmentation and hypoxemia.

Mechanisms of arousal during OSA

An apnea often resolves with an arousal or "micro-arousal" (of which the patient is usually not aware) [75]. This protective reflex allows obstruction relief, with an increase in tidal volume and respiratory frequency, and without the arousal the apnea might not terminate. During apnea, several stimuli induce arousal, including hypercapnia, hypoxia, and increased airway resistance/respiratory effort.

Increasing partial pressure of carbon dioxide (PCO_2) in arterial blood is a powerful stimulus for arousal. Healthy sleeping humans exposed to 8% CO_2 in ambient air will usually awaken within 60 s [76]. As described above, an increase in blood PCO_2 is detected by serotonin neurons in the medulla that stimulate breathing. Serotonin neurons in the midbrain also respond to an increase in blood PCO_2 and they cause arousal from sleep. Both groups of serotonin neurons are found in close association with large branches of the basilar artery [77,78]. They sense variations in arterial CO_2, responding indirectly to brain pH changes by increasing their excitatory drive to other neurons (possibly thalamic, cortical, and parabrachial) that mediate arousal [16,79]. Transgenic mice with selective deletion of the transcription factor Lmxlb in serotonin neuron precursors fail to develop virtually all brain serotonin neurons [80]. These mice do not awaken from sleep in response to an increase in ambient CO_2 to as high as 10% [81].

Hypoxic air alone can induce arousal without hypercapnia [82]. Arterial PO_2 reductions are sensed by peripheral arterial chemoreceptors in the carotid and aortic bodies. Central mechanisms, although not clear, do not involve serotonergic neurons, but may include raphe and solitary tract nuclei [91,83]. Although upper airway obstruction can induce arousal by increasing work of breathing, prolonged apneas imply that the concomitant development of hypoxia and hypercapnia is critical in the arousal phenomena associated with OSA [84].

Stroke and insomnia

Insomnia—"repeated difficulty with sleep initiation, duration, consolidation, or quality that occurs despite adequate time and opportunity for sleep and results in some form of daytime impairment"—resulting from stroke is formally referred to as "insomnia due to medical condition" [6]. Stroke patients have a high incidence of insomnia [85]. In a study of 277 subjects, 18.7% had insomnia acutely and 56.7% developed insomnia within 3–4 months of stroke [86].

Contributing factors include initial shock, adjustments to physical and cognitive limitations, post-stroke depression, and

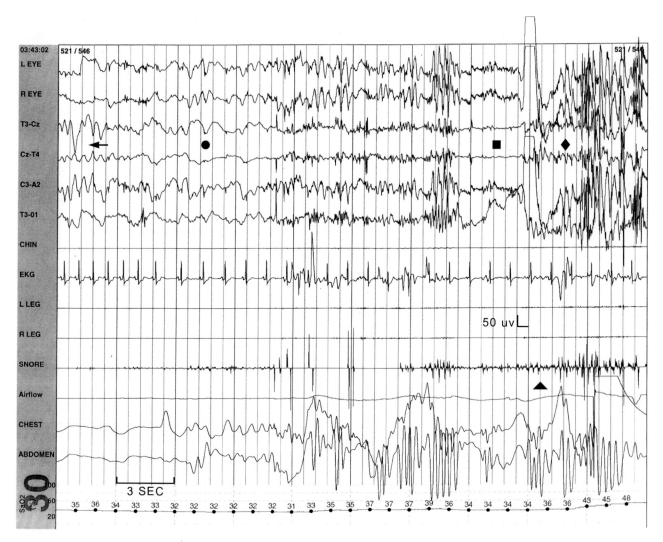

Fig. 27.6 This patient suffered a prolonged obstructive apnea, which eventually resulted in a sudden EEG change from a classic REM sawtooth pattern (arrows) to a poorly organized, diffuse delta slow-wave pattern (black circle), followed by a general flattening of all activity (black square) that led to attempts to arouse the patient (as evidenced by diffuse movement artifact: black diamond). Nevertheless, persistent obstruction (black triangle) necessitated emergency rescue breathing maneuvers. Persistent EEG flattening followed by slowing and eventual recovery of normal waking patterns was appreciated in subsequent epochs. L: left; R: right; T: temporal; C: central; O: occipital; CHIN: mentalis EMG; L LEG: left anterior tibialis EMG; R LEG: right anterior tibialis EMG; SNORE: snoring microphone; ABDOMEN: abdominal effort; SaO_2: oxygen saturation.

Adapted from Neurology, 62(3), Dyken ME, Yamada T, Glenn CL, et al, Obstructive sleep apnea associated with cerebral hypoxemia and death, pp. 491–93, Copyright (2004), with permission from Wolters Kluwer Health, Inc.

medication effects. Damage to the CNS "sleep switch" (nuclei in the preoptic area of the hypothalamus) can also contribute to insomnia (Fig. 27.9) [87,88]. A study of 336 elderly stroke patients showed insomnia to be most prevalent with hemorrhage and with lesions in the brainstem, frontal lobe, and basal ganglion [95].

The sleep switch uses γ-aminobutyric acid (GABA) in reciprocal inhibitory relays with variable waking centers of the reticular activating system (Fig. 27.9) [97,98]. Benzodiazepine receptor agonists include those with nonselective affinity for the GABA receptor complex (eszopiclone) and others with selective affinity for the $GABA_A$ receptor (zolpidem and zaleplon) [89,90]. Although various benzodiazepine and non-benzodiazepine hypnotics and antidepressants have been used to treat insomnia in stroke, many have CNS depressant effects that could exacerbate OSA [91,92]. Reducing dopaminergic stimulation

may improve insomnia in stroke, and a recent sham-controlled randomized trial in patients hospitalized with acute stroke experiencing insomnia for ≥ three days found acupuncture to be therapeutic [93,94]. Cognitive–behavioral therapy (CBT) has been supported in the treatment of insomnia in geriatric populations; however no study has focused specifically on post-stroke patients [103,95].

Stroke and hypersomnia

Hypersomnia due to a medical condition is diagnosed when stroke directly causes sleepiness [6]. The ascending reticular activating system promotes wakefulness through monoaminergic and cholinergic neurotransmitter systems (Fig. 27.10) [98]. Stroke affecting the hypothalamus (the orexin/hypocretin-containing lateral

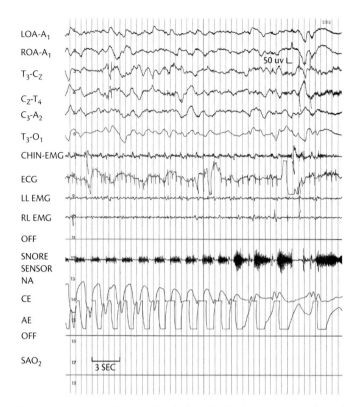

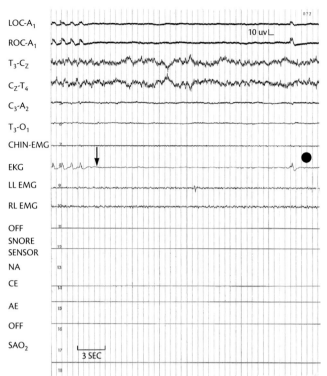

Fig. 27.7 An 80-year -old man with multiple medical problems, who was admitted with exacerbation of pulmonary and cardiac disease under a do-not-resuscitate/do-not-intubate status (for whom signed consent had been given for PSG as part of an IRB-approved study) had a 30 s obstruction that was associated with an SaO_2 low of 12%. At that time, the EEG showed progressive development of a disorganized slow-wave pattern over a 2.5-minute period, followed by electrocerebral silence (using a recording sensitivity of 1.0 µV/mm). A1: left ear reference; A2: right ear reference; T: temporal; C: central; O: occipital; LL: left leg; RL: right leg; NA: nasal airflow; CE: chest effort; AD: abdominal effort; SaO_2: oxygen saturation.
Reproduced from Dyken et al, Stroke in Sleep. In: Chokroverty S, Sahota P, [eds], Acute and Emergent Events in Sleep Disorders, Copyright (2011), with permission from Oxford University Press.

Fig. 27.8 After the patient in Fig. 27.7 (upon whom no heroic therapeutic interventions were allowed) had a final series of apneic events, no discernible EEG activity was captured while utilizing a recording sensitivity or 1.0 µV/mm. A prolonged period of asystole (see arrow) was followed by cardiac arrest, at which time the patient was declared dead (black circle). LOC: left outer canthus; A1: left ear reference; A2: right ear reference; T: temporal; C: central; O: occipital; LL: left leg; RL: right leg; NA: nasal airflow; CE: chest effort; AD: abdominal effort; SaO_2: oxygen saturation.
Adapted from Neurology, 62(3), Dyken ME, Yamada T, Glenn CL, et al, Obstructive sleep apnea associated with cerebral hypoxemia and death, pp. 491–93, Copyright (2004), with permission from Wolters Kluwer Health, Inc.

nucleus and the histaminergic tuberomammillary nucleus), the brainstem (the noradrenergic locus coeruleus and the "REM sleep-on" cholinergic cells of the pedunculopontine/laterodorsal nuclear complex), and cholinergic and GABAergic cells in the basal forebrain could result in hypersomnolence.

Hypersomnia can follow lesions of pontine tegmental reticular formation and the paramedian nuclei of the thalamus. In a prospective observational study of 100 consecutively hospitalized patients, the prevalence of CNS hypersomnia in acute ischemic stroke patients was estimated as 22% [96].

Hypersomnia can be a side effect of a medical regimen. A 52-year-old woman with an ischemic infarction in the upper brainstem tegmentum from subarachnoid hemorrhage developed sleep attacks and cataplectic-like events on valproic acid and diphenylhydantoin seizure prophylaxis [97]. Her sleep symptoms resolved immediately after discontinuing anticonvulsants. Neurotransmitters associated with CNS waking centers rationalize pharmacological treatments that include modafinil, methylphenidate, levodopa and antidepressants with stimulant effects [98]. Modafinil may be useful in hypersomnolence associated with anticonvulsant treatment of post-stroke seizures [99].

Reductions in hypersomnolence have been reported following bilateral mesodiencephalic paramedian infarction using 200 mg of modafinil, and during stroke rehabilitation using methylphenidate (5–30 mg/day) and levodopa (100 mg/day) [100–101]. Bromocriptine 20–40 mg/day may improve hypersomnolence, apathy, and behaviors counterproductive to good sleep [102].

Stroke and circadian rhythm sleep disorders

A circadian rhythm disorder (CRSD) is a persistent or recurrent pattern of sleep disturbance due to alterations of the circadian timekeeping system or misalignment between the endogenous circadian rhythm and exogenous factors that affect the timing or duration of sleep and lead to insomnia or excessive daytime sleepiness and impairment of functioning [6]. Multi-infarct dementia, the second leading dementia type in the USA, may cause greater circadian sleep disruption than Alzheimer disease [103,104].

Circadian rhythms are maintained by the suprachiasmatic nucleus of the anterior hypothalamus, and lesions result in asynchrony of circadian rhythms of sleep and wakefulness, possibly

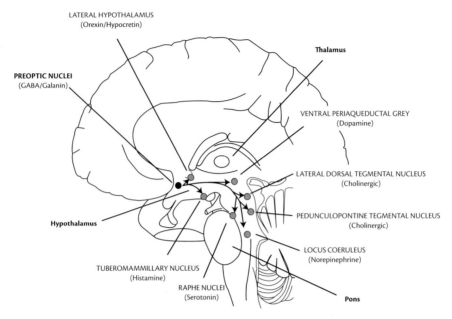

Fig. 27.9 Basic sleep onset systems. Diagrammatic representation of the brainstem in the parasagittal plane showing the proposed structures and mechanism involved in sleep onset. Excited nuclei in the preoptic nuclei of the hypothalamus (the ventrolateral and median preoptic nuclei) use inhibitory neurotransmitters (GABA and galanin) in reciprocal inhibitory relays with waking centers, and in direct thalamic projections. In addition, gradual inhibition of REM-off cells that function in part through cholinergic cells of the pedunculopontine tegmental nucleus and lateral dorsal tegmental nucleus complex leads to disinhibition of GABAergic reticular thalamic nuclei that assist in the generation of NREM sleep through intrathalamic connections to limbic forebrain structures that include the orbitofrontal cortex. Sleep is also facilitated by the solitary tract nucleus, utilizing unknown neurotransmitters, through direct connections with the hypothalamus, amygdala, and other forebrain structures. Serotonergic neurons in the midline (raphe) of the medulla, pons, and mesencephalon of the brainstem help modulate sleep. The black circle and lines indicate inhibitory nuclei and tracts during sleep onset; green circles indicate wakefulness nuclei.

Reproduced from Chest, 141(2), Dyken et al, Sleep-Related Problems in Neurologic Diseases, pp. 528–544, Copyright (2012), with permission from American College of Chest Physicians.

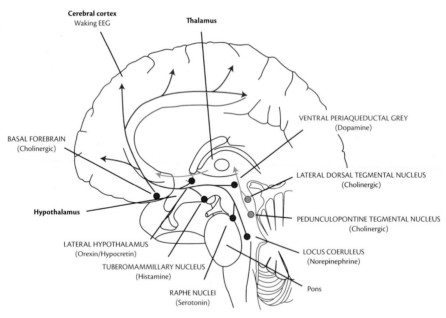

Fig. 27.10 Basic wake systems. This diagrammatic representation of the brain/brainstem in the parasagittal plane shows the very basic structures and mechanism hypothesized to be involved in the generation of wakefulness in humans. There are two ascending independent waking pathways that travel through the pontomesencephalic junction that eventually lead to diffuse cortical projections: (1) the neuronal tracts and nuclear areas in dark green define a ventral system through the hypothalamus (involving hypothalamic nuclei in the tuberomammillary nucleus and the lateral hypothalamus, LH), which relays to cholinergic basal forebrain (BF) cells and the cerebral cortex; and (2) the neuronal tracts and nuclear areas in light green define a dorsal thalamic route that leads to stimulation of thalamic relay, nonspecific midline and intralaminar nuclei (while inhibiting the reticular nucleus of the thalamus). The orexin/hypocretin neurons in the LH reinforce the waking activity of all these nuclei and directly innervate the BF (the nucleus basalis, diagonal band of Broca, and medial septal nuclei), and the cerebral cortex. In the BF, there are cholinergic cells that excite cortical pyramidal neurons and GABAergic cells that inhibit cortical inhibitory neurons (thus disinhibiting the cortex). Both groups are active during wakefulness and REM sleep, but relatively inactive (or at least less active) during NREM sleep.

Reproduced from Chest, 141(2), Dyken et al, Sleep-Related Problems in Neurologic Diseases, pp. 528–544, Copyright (2012), with permission from American College of Chest Physicians.

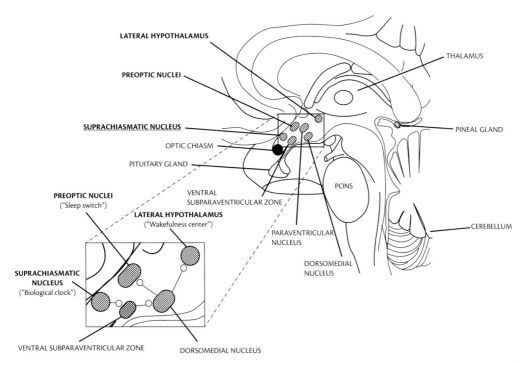

Fig. 27.11 Diagrammatic representation of the brainstem in the parasagittal plane showing the close proximity of the suprachiasmatic nucleus (the "biological clock") to the waking and sleep centers of the hypothalamus. The major neuronal pathway mediating the SCN-generated circadian rhythm of sleep and wakefulness is through a projection to the ventral subparaventricular zone (vSPZ), followed by second-order projection from the vSPZ to the dorsomedial nucleus (DMN). The DMN sends primarily GABA projections to the preoptic nuclei (the "sleep switch") and glutamatergic projections to the lateral hypothalamus (the "wakefulness center"). Open circle: facilitatory.

Reproduced from Chest, 141(2), Dyken et al, Sleep-Related Problems in Neurologic Diseases, pp. 528–544, Copyright (2012), with permission from American College of Chest Physicians.

related to damage to vasopressin- and neurotensin-containing neurons (Fig. 27.11) [98,105]. Stroke affecting these mechanisms can disrupt the sleep–wake cycle, classically evidenced as "sundowning"—nocturnal exacerbation of delirium (agitation and confusion), often associated with daytime sleepiness [6].

When addressing dementia, sundowning, and stroke, OSA should always be considered. A randomized double-blind placebo-controlled trial utilizing CPAP in 52 men and women with dementia showed significantly improved neuropsychological scores after 3 weeks [106]. Medical problems such as renal and hepatic disease, systemic infection, hypovolemia, acid–base and electrolyte imbalances, and hypovitaminosis should also be corrected. Restricting naps, and incorporating cognitive–behavioral strategies emphasizing good sleep hygiene (comfortable, quiet, dark sleep environment), can reduce nighttime behavioral disturbances [107].

Light is a powerful zeitgeber (external cue synchronizing the sleep–wake cycle). Sundowning tends to be worse when daytime illumination is low. Exposure to bright light may help optimize the sleep–wake cycle (the best time has not been defined). Increasing activities with outdoor sunlight exposure is valuable. A 14-week intervention trial showed benefits of daytime physical activity when combined with improved nighttime sleep hygiene practices [108].

Anecdotes report successful sundowning treatment with propranolol, trazodone, and clonidine, but general avoidance of narcotics, sedative–hypnotics, H_2 receptor blockers, anti-parkinsonian medications, and anticholinergics is recommended, as all have been associated with delirium [109]. A majority of 30 stroke patients with sleep rhythm disorders had "good results" with melatonin; nevertheless, studies suggest that melatonin may promote vasoconstriction [110,111].

Psychoactive medications (thioridazine 25–50 mg or haloperidol 1–2 mg at bedtime) have been used for sundowning, but often cause orthostasis and extrapyramidal side effects, while benzodiazepines often exacerbate agitation. Agonists such as zolpidem and zaleplon that preferentially bind to $GABA_A$ sleep-promoting receptors in the frontal cortex may be more effective, with fewer side effects than traditional hypnotics [112].

A multicenter double-blind placebo-controlled trial of atypical antipsychotics (olanzapine, quetiapine, and risperidone), involving 421 subjects with dementia psychosis, aggression, or agitation, found no significant difference between drug and placebo in outcomes measured by the Clinical Global Impression of Change, but there was a significant increase in adverse events with every antipsychotic compared with placebo [113]. In addition, risperidone may increase cerebrovascular disease risk in older patients [114].

Stroke and parasomnia

REM sleep behavior disorder (RBD) generally occurs in older men, with violent behaviors from REM sleep, followed by arousals where the patient describes dreams paralleling observed behaviors (isomorphism), with up to 77.1% reporting dream-related injuries [6]. Normally, REM sleep is associated with relative paralysis preventing dream enactment. This is due to activated pontine "REM sleep-on" cells that project caudally to stimulate medullary centers in the brainstem that subsequently inhibit alpha motor neurons in the spinal cord (Fig. 27.12) [98].

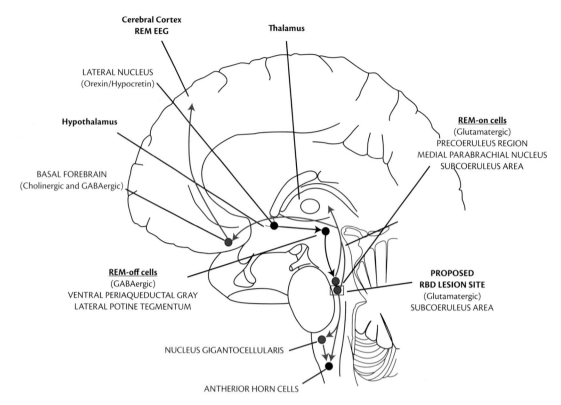

Fig. 27.12 This parasagittal section of the brain and brainstem shows the suspected pathology explaining RBD, based upon the recently proposed "flip-flop" model of sleep state transitions by Saper et al. [115]. In normal REM sleep, glutamatergic REM-on cells in what would be considered the subcoeruleus area (SCA) in cats and the sublaterodorsal nucleus (SLD) in rats (an area presently not well defined in humans), directly and indirectly (through the nucleus gigantocellularis, one of the ventromedial groups of reticular nuclei in the medulla oblongata) cause hyperpolarization of anterior horn cells in the spinal cord, resulting in atonia. From animal studies, it has been hypothesized that in RBD, degeneration of the SCA disrupts descending tracts that would normally lead to atonia/paresis, thus allowing violent behaviors during REM (dreaming/paralyzed) sleep. Black circles and lines nuclei and neuronal tracts normally inhibited during REM sleep; green circles and lines indicate nuclei and neuronal tracts normally activated during REM sleep; the rectangle indicates the proposed lesion site in RBD.
Reproduced from Chest, 141(2), Dyken et al, Sleep-Related Problems in Neurologic Diseases, pp. 528–544, Copyright (2012), with permission from American College of Chest Physicians.

Atonia of REM sleep is dependent upon two brainstem systems: a motor-inhibitory system (activated in REM sleep) and a motor-excitatory system (inhibited in REM sleep) [115,116]. Experiments suggest that the motor-inhibitory system uses midbrain atonic regions to control caudal brainstem areas. A stroke affecting these atonic regions anywhere from the mesencephalon to their point of colocalization with the excitatory motor system (the subcoeruleus area) could lead to RBD (reported with stroke affecting the pontine tegmentum bilaterally and in unilateral right paramedian pontine tegmental infarction) [116,117].

Clonazepam successfully treats up to 90% of idiopathic RBD, and its recommended use in RBD with neurodegenerative disorders such as Parkinson disease has been without significant tolerance or abuse [6,118]. Although significant improvements are usually noticed within a week using 0.5–1.0 mg, it could precipitate sundowning or exacerbate OSA. Taking clonazepam 2 hours prior to sleep may also address insomnia, restless legs syndrome, and/or periodic limb movements in sleep, and reduce the risk of morning hangover effects.

Clonazepam's benefits in RBD may be from a "serotonergic effect." Lesions in the raphe nucleus (which is the source of brain serotonin) increases REM sleep phasic motor activity [119]. The serotonin effect is suspected to be inhibition of a specific excitatory motor system for RBD (rather than a general excitation of inhibitory motor systems), as REM without atonia (a classic PSG finding in RBD) tends to persist after successful clonazepam treatment. Therapy also includes providing a safe sleeping environment (mattress on the floor, etc.) [119].

Stroke and sleep-related movement disorders

Restless legs syndrome (RLS), defined by the acronym "URGE"— Urge to move (usually legs), worse Resting, relieved by Going (moving limbs), and most disturbing in the Evening—can lead to problems with insomnia, sleepiness, concentration, memory, motivation, anxiety, and depression [6]. PSG-defined periodic limb movements during sleep (PLMS) are found in up to 90% of RLS patients. If they cause insomnia and sleepiness, periodic limb movement disorder (PLMD) is diagnosed.

Walters and Rye suggest that sympathetic hyperactivity associated with RLS/PLMS may lead to hypertension, heart disease, and stroke [120]. Case reports document RLS/PLMS with basal ganglia infarctions involving the lenticulostriatum [121]. Sechi et al. hypothesized that a "lesion in this area (nuclear complex or fiber systems) may exert both an ascending disinhibition on sensorimotor cortex, and a disinhibition of descending inhibitory pathways, resulting in a facilitation of RLS and PLM." This

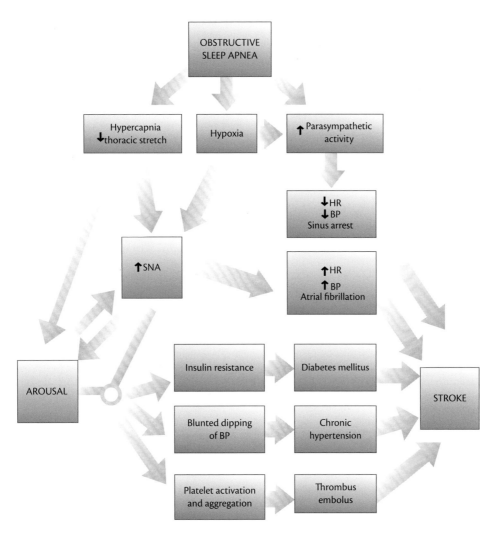

Fig. 27.13 This over-simplistic diagram highlights some of the major suspected factors linking OSA, arousal, and stroke. OSA can lead to autonomic instability. Inspiration against a closed airway with hypoxemia can increase parasympathetic activity, potentially leading to bradycardia, sinus arrest, and hypotensive events. Increased sympathetic neural activity (SNA) from the reflex effects of hypoxia, hypercapnia, and decreased input from thoracic stretch receptors can lead to tachycardia, blood pressure surges, and potentially to arrhythmias such as atrial fibrillation. While an acute arousal can be protective in preventing untoward effects of a single prolonged apnea, chronic concomitant SNA elevations have been hypothesized to help explain the known associations with a variety of stroke risk factors, including the development of thrombus/emboli, diabetes mellitus, and chronic hypertension.

Reproduced from Dyken ME, Richerson GB, Im KB, Sleep apnea, stroke risk factors, and the arousal response. In: Culebras A, [ed], Sleep, Stroke, and Cardiovascular Disease, Copyright (2013), with permission from Cambridge University Press.

is consistent with evidence relating RLS/PLMS to dopamine deficiency/dysfunction. The ventral striatum receives its major dopaminergic innervation via mesolimbic pathways from mesencephalic A10 cells of the ventral tegmentum. Correction of the deficiency/dysfunction may explain successful treatment of post-stroke RLS/PLMS with dopamine agonists [122]. Levodopa is associated with augmentation (chronic therapy worsening RLS), whereas agonists specific for the D_2 family of dopamine receptors may reduce augmentation [123].

Conclusions

There is a strong relationship between stroke and sleep problems, as stroke can precipitate, and may be caused by, some specific sleep disorders. OSA is the most frequent and dangerous sleep disorder associated with stroke. Although no scientifically proven cause-and-effect relationships exists between OSA and stroke, the known pathophysiology of untreated OSA mandates therapeutic intervention whenever reasonably possible (Fig. 27.13). Symptoms of OSA often suggest other primary sleep disorders. If OSA is ruled out, good sleep hygiene practices through the implementation of cognitive–behavioral techniques should be considered, as stroke patients may be prone to the adverse effects of many medications otherwise routinely used to treat sleep-related problems.

References

1. Murray CJ, Lopez AD. Mortality by cause for eight regions of the world: Global Burden of Disease Study. Lancet 1997;349:1269–76.
2. American Heart Association. Heart Disease and Stroke Statistics, 2009 Update At-A-Glance. Available at: http://www.americanheart.org/downloadable/heart/1240250946756LS-1982%20Heart%20and%20Stroke%20Update.042009.pdf

3. National Sleep Foundation "Sleep in America" Poll. National Sleep Foundation Web site. http://www.sleepfoundation.org/sites/default/files/2002SleepinAmericaPoll.pdf

4. American Academy of Sleep Medicine. International classification of sleep disorders, 3rd ed. Diagnostic and coding manual. Darien, IL: American Academy of Sleep Medicine, 2014.

5. Young T, Palta M, Dempsey J, et al. The occurrence of sleep-disordered breathing among middle-aged adults. N Engl J Med 1993;328:1230–5.

6. Goldstein LB, Adams R, Alberts MJ, et al. Primary prevention of ischemic stroke: a guideline from the American Heart Association/American Stroke Association Stroke Council. Stroke 2006;37:1583–633.

7. Severinghaus JW, Mitchell RA. Ondine's curse-failure of respiratory center automaticity while awake [abstract]. Clin Res 1962;10:122.

8. Hugelin A. Forebrain and midbrain influence on respiration. In: Fishman AP, Cherniak NS, Widdecombe JG, Geige SR, eds. Handbook of physiology. Section 3. The respiratory system, vol 2. Control of breathing, part 1. Bethesda, MD: American Physiological Society 1986;69–91.

9. Dyken ME, Afifi AK, Im KB. Stroke in sleep. In: Chokroverty S, Sahota P, eds. Acute and emergent events in sleep disorders. New York: Oxford University Press, 2011:328–48.

10. Mulkey DK, Stornetta RL, Weston MC, et al. Respiratory control by ventral surface chemoreceptor neurons in rats. Nat Neurosci 2004;7(12):1360–9.

11. Dean JB, Bayliss DA, Erickson JT, et al. Depolarization and stimulation of neurons in nucleus tractus solitarii by carbon dioxide does not require chemical synaptic input. Neuroscience 1990;36(1):207–16.

12. Guyenet PG, Bayliss DA, Mulkey DK, et al. The retrotrapezoid nucleus and central chemoreception. Adv Exp Med Biol 2008;605:327–32.

13. Richerson GB. Serotonergin neurons as carbon dioxide sensors that maintain pH homeostasis. Nat Rev Neurosci 2004;5:449–61.

14. Dyken ME, Im KB. Obstructive sleep apnea and stroke. Chest 2009;136(6):1668–77.

15. Dyken ME, Yamada T, Berger HA. Transient obstructive sleep apnea and asystole in association with presumed viral encephalopathy. Neurology 2003;60(10):1692–4.

16. Palomake H, Partinen M, Juvela S, et al. Snoring as a risk factor for sleep-related brain infarction. Stroke 1989;10:1311–15.

17. Palomake H. Snoring and the risk of ischemic brain infarction. Stroke 1991;22:1021–5.

18. Chaudhary BA, Elguindi AS, King DW. Obstructive sleep apnea after lateral medullary syndrome. South Med J 1982;75:65–7.

19. Tikare SK, Chaudhary BA, Bandisode MS. Hypertension and stroke in a young man with obstructive sleep apnea syndrome. Postgrad Med 1985;78:59–66.

20. Dyken ME, Somers VK, Yamada T. Hemorrhagic stroke; part of the natural history of severe obstructive sleep apnea? [abstract]. Sleep Res 1991;20:371.

21. Dyken ME. Cerebrovascular disease and sleep apnea. In: Bradley DT, Floras JS, eds. Sleep disorders and cardiovascular and cerebrovascular disease. New York: Marcel Dekker 2000:285–306.

22. Tilkian AG, Guilleminault C, Schroeder JS, et al. Hemodynamics in sleep-induced apnea: studies during wakefulness and sleep. Ann Intern Med 1976;85:714–19.

23. Dyken ME, Somers VK, Yamada T. Stroke, sleep apnea and autonomic instability. In: Togawa K, Katayama S, Hishikawa Y, eds. Sleep apnea and rhonchopathy. Basel: Karger, 1993:166–8.

24. Dyken ME, Somers VK, Yamada T, et al. Investigating the relationship between sleep apnea and stroke [abstract]. Sleep Res 1992;21:30.

25. Dyken ME, Somers VK, Yamada T, et al. Investigating the relationship between stroke and obstructive sleep apnea. Stroke 1996;27:401–7.

26. Ovbiagele B, Kidwell CS, Saver JL. Epidemiological impact in the United States of a tissue-based definition of transient ischemic attack. Stroke 2003;34:919–24.

27. Pressman MR, Schetman WR, Figueroa WG, et al. Transient ischemic attacks and minor stroke during sleep. Stroke 1995;26:2361–5.

28. Shahar E, Whitney CW, Redline S, et al. Sleep-disordered breathing and cardiovascular disease. Cross-sectional results of the Sleep Heart Health Study. Am J Resp Crit Care Med 2001;163:19–25.

29. Arzt M, Young T, Finn L, et al. Association of sleep-disordered breathing and the occurrence of stroke. Am J Resp Crit Care Med 2005;172:1147–51.

30. Yaggi KH, Concato J, Kernan WN, et al. Obstructive sleep apnea as a risk factor for stroke and death. N Engl J Med 2005;19:2034–41.

31. Munoz R, Duran-Cantolla J, Martinez-Vila E, et al. Severe sleep apnea and risk of ischemic stroke in the elderly. Stroke 2006;37:2317–21.

32. Valham F, Mooe T, Rabben T, et al. Increased risk of stroke in patients with coronary artery disease and sleep apnea: a 10-year follow-up. Circulation 2008;118:955–60.

33. Redline S, Yenokyan G, Gottlieb DJ, et al. Obstructive sleep apnea–hypopnea and incident stroke; the Sleep Heart Health Study. Am J Respir Crit Care Med 2010;182:269–77.

34. Partinen M, Jamieson A, Guilleminault C. Long-term outcome for obstructive sleep apnea syndrome patients: mortality. Chest 1988;94:1200–4.

35. Partinen M, Guilleminault C. Daytime sleepiness and vascular morbidity at seven-year follow-up in obstructive sleep apnea patients. Chest 1990;97:27–32.

36. Martinez-Garcia MA, Galiano-Blancart R, Roman-Sanches P, et al. Continuous positive airway pressure treatment in sleep apnea prevents new vascular events after ischemic stroke. Chest 2005;4:2123–9.

37. Palombini L, Guilleminault C. Stroke and treatment with nasal CPAP. Eur J Neurol 2006;13:198–200.

38. Brown DL, Concannon M, Kare AB, et al. Comparison of two headgear systems for sleep apnea treatment of stroke patients. Cerebrovasc Dis 2009;27:183–6.

39. Disler P, Hansford A, Skelton J, et al. Diagnosis and treatment of obstructive sleep apnea in a stroke rehabilitation unit: a feasibility study. Am J Phys Med Rehabil 2002;81:622–5.

40. Dziewas R, Hopmann B, Humpert M, et al. Positional sleep apnea in patients with ischemic stroke. Neurol Res 2008;30:645–8.

41. Brunner H. Success and failure of mirtazapine as alternative treatment in elderly stroke patients with sleep apnea—a preliminary open trial. Sleep Breath 2008;12(3):281–5.

42. Robertson PL, Aldrich MS, Hanash SM, Goldstein GW. Stroke associated with obstructive sleep apnea in a child with sickle cell anemia. Ann Neurol 1988;23(6):614–16.

43. Maddern BR, Reed HT, Ohene-Frempong K, Beckerman RC. Obstructive sleep apnea syndrome in sickle cell disease. Ann Otol Rhinol Laryngol 1989;98(3):174–8.

44. Bader-Meunier B, Francois M, Verlhac S, et al. Increased cerebral blood flow velocity in children with sickle cell disease: adenotonsillectomy or transfusion regimens? Pediatrics 2007;120(1):235.

45. Tripathi A, Jerrell JM, Stallworth JR. Cost-effectiveness of adenotonsillectomy in reducing obstructive sleep apnea, cerebrovascular ischemia, vaso-occlusive pain, and ACS episodes in pediatric sickle cell disease. Ann Hematol 2011;90:145–50.

46. Goldstein NA, Keller R, Rey K, et al. Sleep-disordered breathing and transcranial Dopplers in sickle cell disease. Arch Otolaryngol Head Neck Surg 2001;137(12):1263–8.

47. Vlahandonis A, Walter LM, Horne RSC. Does treatment of SDB in children improve cardiovascular outcome? Sleep Med Rev 2013;17:75–85.

48. Coughlin SR, Mawdsley L, Mugarza JA, et al. Obstructive sleep apnoea is independently associated with an increased prevalence of metabolic syndrome. Eur Heart J 2004;25:735–41.

49. Ambrosetti M, Lucioni AM, Conti S, et al. Metabolic syndrome in obstructive sleep apnea and related cardiovascular risk. J Cardiovasc Med 2006;7:826–9.

50. Sasanabe R, Banno K, Otake K, et al. Metabolic syndrome in Japanese patients with obstructive sleep apnea syndrome. Hypertens Res 2006;29:315–22.

51. Roger VL, Go AS, Lloyd-Jones D, et al. Heart disease and stroke statistics—2012 update: a report from the American Heart Association.

Available from: http://circ.ahajournals.org/content/early/2011/12/15/CIR.0b013e31823ac046

52. Tishler PV, Larkin EK, Schluchter MD, Redline S. Incidence of sleep-disordered breathing in an urban adult population. JAMA 2003;289:2230–7.

53. Peppard PE, Young T, Palta M, et al. Prospective study of the association between sleep-disordered breathing and hypertension. N Engl J Med 2000;342:1378–84.

54. Aurora RN, Polak J, Punjabi NM, et al. Obstructive sleep apnea is associated with insulin resistance independent of visceral fat. Am J Respir Crit Care Med 2011;183:A6075.

55. Somers VK, Dyken ME, Clary MP, et al. Sympathetic neural mechanisms in obstructive sleep apnea. J Clin Invest 1995;96:1897–904.

56. Guilleminault C, Connolly SJ, Winkle RA. Cardiac arrhythmia and conduction disturbances during sleep in 400 patients with sleep apnea syndrome. Am J Cardiol 1983;52:490–4.

57. Wolk R, Somers VK. Obesity-related cardiovascular disease: implications of obstructive sleep apnea. Diabetes Obes Metab 2006;8:250–60.

58. Somers VK, Dyken ME, Mark AL, et al. Parasympathetic hyperresponsiveness and bradyarrhythmias during apnea in hypertension. Clin Auton Res 1992;2:171–6.

59. Gami AS, Pressman G, Caples SM, et al. Association of atrial fibrillation and obstructive sleep apnea. Circulation 2004;110:364–7.

60. Kanagala R, Murali NS, Friedman PA, et al. Obstructive sleep apnea and the recurrence of atrial fibrillation. Circulation 2003;107:2589–94.

61. Gupta V, Yesilbursa D, Huang WY, et al. Patent foramen ovale in a large population of ischemic stroke patients: diagnosis, age distribution, gender, and race. Echocardiography. 2008;25(2):217–27.

62. Beelke M, Angeli S, Del Sette M, et al. Prevalence of patent foramen ovale in subjects with obstructive sleep apnea: a transcranial Doppler ultrasound study. Sleep Med 2003;4(3):219–23.

63. Pinet C, Orehek J. CPAP suppression of awake right-to-left shunting through patent foramen ovale in a patient with obstructive sleep apnoea. Thorax 2005;60(10):880–1.

64. Marsh E, Biller J, Adams H, et al. Circadian variation in onset of acute ischemic stroke. Arch Neurol 1990;47:1178–80.

65. Somers VK, Dyken ME, Mark AL, et al. Sympathetic nerve activity during sleep in normal humans. N Engl J Med 1993;328:303–7.

66. Jennum P, Borgesen SE. Intracranial pressure and obstructive sleep apnea. Chest 1989;95:279–83.

67. Tofler GH, Brezinski D, Schafer AI, et al. Concurrent morning increase in platelet aggregability and the risk of myocardial infarction and sudden cardiac death. N Engl J Med 1987;316:1514–18.

68. Geiser T, Buck F, Meyer BJ, et al. In vivo platelet activation is increased during sleep in patients with obstructive sleep apnea syndrome. Respiration 2002;69:229–34.

69. Minoguchi K, Yokoe T, Tazaki T, et al. Silent brain infarction and platelet activation in obstructive sleep apnea. Am J Resp Crit Care Med 2007;175:612–17.

70. Berry RB, Brooks R, Gamaldo CE, et al. for the American Academy of Sleep Medicine. The AASM manual for the scoring of sleep and associated events: rules, terminology and technical specifications, version 2.0. Darien, IL: American Academy of Sleep Medicine, 2012.

71. Berry RB, Kouchi KG, Der DE, et al. Sleep apnea impairs the arousal response to airway occlusion. Chest 1996;109:1490–6.

72. Cirignotta F, Zucconi M, Mondini S, et al. Cerebral anoxic attacks in sleep apnea syndrome. Sleep 1989;12:400–4.

73. Dyken ME, Yamada T, Glenn CL, et al. Obstructive sleep apnea associated with cerebral hypoxemia and death. Neurology 2004;62:491–3.

74. White DP, Douglas NJ, Pickett CK, et al. Sleep deprivation and the control of ventilation. Am Rev Respir Dis 1983;198:984–6.

75. Martin SE, Engleman HM, Kingshott RN, et al. Microarousals in patients with sleep apnoea/hypopnoea syndrome. J Sleep Res 1997;6:276–80.

76. Berthon-Jones M, Sullivan CE. Ventilation and arousal responses to hypercapnia in normal sleeping humans. J Appl Physiol 1984; 57:59–67.

77. Severson CA, Wang W, Pieribone VA, et al. Midbrain serotonergic neurons are central pH chemoreceptors. Nat Neurosci 2003;6(11):1139–40.

78. Bradley SR, Pieribone VA, Wang W, et al. Chemosensitive serotonergic neurons are closely associated with large medullary arteries. Nat Neurosci 2002;5(5):401–2.

79. Steriade M, McCormick DA, Sejnowski TJ. Thalamocortical oscillations in the sleeping and aroused brain. Science 1993;262(5134):679–85.

80. Zhao ZQ, Scott M, Chiechio S, et al. Lmx1b is required for maintenance of central serotonergic neurons and mice lacking central serotonergic system exhibit normal locomotor activity. J Neurosci 2006;26(49):12781–8.

81. Buchanan GF, Richerson GB. Central serotonin neurons are required for arousal to CO_2. Proc Natl Acad Sci 2010;107:16354–9.

82. Berthon-Jones M, Sullivan CE. Ventilatory and arousal responses to hypoxia in sleeping humans. Am Rev Respir Dis 1982;125:632–9.

83. Darnall RA, Schneider RW, Tobia CM, et al. Arousal from sleep in response to intermittent hypoxia in infant rodents is modulated by medullary raphe GABAergic mechanisms. Am J Physiol Regul Integr Comp Physiol 2012;302:R551–60.

84. Issa FG, Sullivan CE. Arousal and breathing responses to airway occlusion in healthy sleeping adults. J Appl Physiol 1983;55:1113–19.

85. Li HC, Chen XG, Tian X. Analysis on somnipathy related factors in elderly patients with stroke and comparative study on the efficacy of treatment by traditional Chinese medicine and by estazolam. Zhongguo Zhong Xi Yi Jie He Za Zhi 2009;29(3):204–7.

86. Leppävuoria A, Pohjasvaarab T, Vatajaa R, et al. Insomnia in ischemic stroke patients. Cerebrovasc Dis 2002;14:90–7.

87. Saper CB, Chou TC, Scammel TE. The sleep switch: hypothalamic control of sleep and wakefulness. Trends Neurosci 2001;24:726–31.

88. Dyken ME, Afifi AK, Lin-Dyken DC. Sleep-related problems in neuro-logic diseases. Chest 2012;141:528–44.

89. Kim CR, Chun MH, Han EY. Effect of hypnotics on sleep patterns and functional recovery of patients with subacute stroke. Am J Phys Med Rehabil 2010;89(4):315–22.

90. Im KB, Strader S, Dyken ME. Management of sleep disorders in stroke. Curr Treatm Opin Neurol 2010;12(5):379–95.

91. Li Pi Shan RS, Ashworth NL. Comparison of lorazepam and zopiclone for insomnia in patients with stroke and brain injury: a randomized, crossover, double-blinded trial. Am J Phys Med Rehabil 2004;83(6):421–7.

92. Palomaki H, Berg A, Meririnne E, et al. Complaints of poststroke insomnia and its treatment with mianserin. Cerebrovasc Dis 2003;15(1–2):56–62.

93. Jennum P, Santamaria J. Members of the Task Force. Report of an ENFS task force on management of sleep disorders in neurologic disease (degenerative neurologic disorders and stroke. Eur J Neurol 2007;14(11):1189–200.

94. Lee SY, Baek YH, Park SU, et al. Intradermal acupuncture on shen-men and nei-kuan acupoints improves insomnia in stroke patients by reducing the sympathetic nervous activity: a randomized clinical trial. Am J Chin Med 2009;37(6):1013–21.

95. Ancoli-Israel S, Ayalon L. Diagnosis and treatment of sleep disorders in older adults. Am J Geriat Psychiat 2006;14(2):95–103.

96. Bassetti C, Valko P. Poststroke hypersomnia. Sleep Med Clinics 2006;1:139–55.

97. Matsuda Y, Neshige R, Endo C, et al. A case of upper brainstem infarction developing symptomatic narcolepsy after the administration of anti-convulsant drugs. Rinsho Shinkeigaku 1991;31(7):750–3.

98. Hermann DM, Bassetti CL. Sleep-related breathing and sleep–wake disturbances in ischemic stroke. Neurology 2009;73(16):1313–22.

99. Smith BW. Modafinil for treatment of cognitive side effects of antiepileptic drugs in a patient with seizures and stroke. Epilepsy Behav 2003;4(3):352–3.

100. Bassetti CL. Sleep and stroke. In: Kryger MH, Roth T, Dement WC, eds. Principles and practice of sleep medicine, 4th ed. Philadelphia: Elsevier Saunder, 2005:811–30.

101. Scheidtmann K, Fries W, Muller F, Koenig E. Effect of levodopa in combination with physiotherapy on functional recovery after stroke: a prospective, randomized, double-blind study. Lancet 2001;358:787–90.

102. Catsman-Berrevoets CE, Harskamp F. Compulsive pre-sleep behaviour and apathy due to bilateral thalamic stroke. Neurology 1988;38:647–9.

103. Plassman BL, Langa KM, Fisher GG, et al. Prevalence of dementia in the United States: the aging, demographics, and memory study. Neuroepidemiology 2007;29:133–5.

104. Meguro K, Ueda M, Kobayashi I, et al. Sleep disturbance in elderly patients with cognitive impairment, decreased daily activity and periventricular white matter lesions. Sleep 1995;18:109–14.

105. Goncharuk VD, Van Heerikhuize J, Dai JP, et al. Neuropeptide changes in the suprachiasmatic nucleus in primary hypertension indicate functional impairment of the biological clock. J Comp Neurol 2001;431:320–30.

106. Ancoli-Israel S, Palmer BW, Cooke JR, et al. Cognitive effects of treating obstructive sleep apnea in Alzheimer's disease: a randomized controlled study. J Am Geriatr Soc 2008;56:2076–81.

107. McCurry SM, Logsdon RG, Vitiello MV, Teri L. Treatment of sleep and nighttime disturbances in Alzheimer's disease: a behavior management approach. Sleep Med 2004;5(4):373–7.

108. Alessi C, Yoon EJ, Schnelle JF, et al. A randomized trial of a combined physical activity and environmental intervention in nursing home residents: do sleep and agitation improve? J Am Geriatr Soc 1999;47:784–91.

109. Little JT, Satlin A, Sunderland T, Volicer L. Sundown syndrome in severely demented patients with probable Alzheimer's disease. J Geriatr Psychiatry Neurol 1995;8:103–6.

110. Domzal TM, Kaca-Orynska M, Zaleski P. Melatonin in sleep rhythm disorders after cerebral stroke. Pol Merkur Lekarski 2000;8(48):411–12.

111. Krause DN, Barrios VE, Duckles SP. Melatonin receptors mediate potentiation of contractile responses to adrenergic nerve stimulation in rat caudal artery. Eur J Pharmacol 1995;276:207–13.

112. Shaw SH, Curson H, Coquelin JP. A double-blind, comparative study of zolpidem and placebo in the treatment of insomnia in elderly psychiatric in-patients. J Int Med Res 1992;20:150–61.

113. Schneider LS, Tariot PN, Dagerman KS, et al. Effectiveness of atypical antipsychotic drugs in patients with Alzheimer's disease. N Engl J Med 2006;355(15):1525–38.

114. Wooltorton E. Risperidone (Risperdal): increased rate of cerebrovascular events in dementia trials. CMAJ 2002;167(11):1269–70.

115. Saper CB, Fuller PM, Pedersen NP, et al. Sleep state switching. Neuron 2010;68(6):1023–42.

116. Lai YY, Siegel JM. Muscle tone suppression and stepping produced by stimulation of midbrain and rostral pontine reticular formation. J Neurosci 1990;10:2727–34.

117. Tachibana N. Historical overview of REM sleep behavior disorder in relation to its pathophysiology. Brain Nerve 2009;61(5):558–68.

118. Xi Z, Luning W. REM sleep behavior disorder in a patient with pontine stroke. Sleep Med 2009;10(1):143–6.

119. Mahowald MW, Schenck CH. REM sleep parasomnias. In: Kryger MH, Roth T, Dement WC, eds. Principles and practice of sleep medicine, 4th ed. Philadelphia: Elsevier Saunders, 2005:897–916.

120. Walters AS, Rye DB. Review of the relationship of restless legs syndrome and periodic limb movements in sleep to hypertension, heart disease, and stroke. Sleep 2009;32(5):589–97.

121. Sechi G, Agnetti V, Galistu P, et al. Restless legs syndrome and periodic limb movements after ischemic stroke in the right lenticulostriate region. Parkinsonism Relat Disord 2008;14(2):157–60.

122. Unrath A, Kassubek J. Symptomatic restless leg syndrome after lacunar stroke: a lesion study. Mov Disord 2006;21(11):2027–8.

123. Littner MR, Kushida C, Anderson WM, et al. Practice parameters for the dopaminergic treatment of RLS and PLMD. Sleep 2004;27:557–9.

CHAPTER 28

Sleep and epilepsy

Lino Nobili, Paola Proserpio,
Steve Gibbs, and Giuseppe Plazzi

Introduction

The relationship between sleep and epilepsy has intrigued research-ers and thinkers since antiquity. Descriptions of episodes of epi-leptic seizures occurring during sleep can be found in the extant writings of both Aristotle and Hippocrates. Yet, a precise account of seizure occurrence in relation to the sleep–wake cycle was revealed only at the end of the nineteenth century when pioneer studies derived from clinical observations revealed that seizure occurrence did not follow a random distribution over the 24 hours but rather clustered at certain times of the day [1–3]. Following these pivotal observations, further advances in the field were brought about by the development and wider use of the EEG. In 1947, in a landmark paper [4], Gibbs and Gibbs reported that sleep could activate epi-leptiform discharges on the EEG.

In recent years, the combination of clinical and EEG observa-tions along with advanced brain imaging and signal analysis meth-ods has confirmed and helped to further understand the complex and reciprocal interactions between sleep and epilepsy.

In this chapter, an overview of the relationships between sleep and epilepsy will be presented, focusing on the strong link between the physiology of the sleep state and the pathological mechanisms of epileptic seizures.

Interrelationship between sleep and epilepsy: physiological mechanisms

Neuronal synchronization and interactions between neurons and neuronal populations are the basic features of brain function. Alterations of synchronization and neuronal hyperexcitability are also central factors in epilepsy that may transform an interictal state to an ictal one [5]. Factors enhancing synchronization are condu-cive to active ictal precipitation in susceptible individuals. These factors include nonspecific influences, such as sleep and sleep deprivation.

Sleep consists of repetitive cycles where NREM and REM sleep alternate with a periodicity of about 90–100 minutes. These two neurophysiological conditions (NREM and REM) generally exert opposite effects on interictal and ictal epileptic activity (EA). Indeed, many studies show that NREM sleep can enhance visuali-zation of interictal epileptiform discharges (IEDs) on the scalp EEG in both partial and generalized seizures, while REM sleep reduces the production and spread of EA (Fig. 28.1) [6–9].

Indeed, during NREM sleep, the discharges may spread ipsilat-erally and contralaterally from the primary focus, whereas during REM sleep, the discharges seem to focalize maximally (Fig. 28.2), especially in temporal lobe epilepsy [8].

From a physiological point of view, NREM sleep seems to act as a proconvulsant because this state is characterized by diffuse cortical synchronization mediated by the thalamocortical input, which can favor an already hyperexcitable cortex to generate seizures. On the other hand, during the transition to REM sleep, inputs from activat-ing cholinergic pontine REM-on cells lead to a relative depolariza-tion of the thalamocortical cells, thus blocking the thalamocortical oscillations in both the spindle and the delta range and giving rise to a low-amplitude desynchronized EEG pattern (slow α and θ frequencies) [10]. Such a desynchronized state reduces the spread of EA, thereby reducing its visibility on the scalp EEG, as well as reducing seizure occurrence. This also explains the attenuation of bilaterally synchronous epileptiform discharges during REM sleep. The descending brainstem pathways responsible for lower motor neuron inhibition during REM sleep also appear to protect against generalized motor seizures during REM sleep [11]. As for gener-alized epilepsy, REM sleep has been considered the most potent antiepileptic state in the sleep–wake cycle. Notably, Cohen et al. found a lowered convulsive threshold during REM deprivation in cats [12]. REM deprivation may thus exacerbate epilepsy.

Furthermore, Busek et al. found a negative correlation between the occurrence of rapid eye movements during REM sleep and EA on the scalp [13], suggesting that the desynchronizing effect of this stage of sleep seems to be accentuated during phasic REM sleep events, probably as a consequence of a further cholinergic activity increase caused by phasic disinhibition of cholinergic neurons of the pontomesencephalic tegmentum.

Different clinical studies have revealed that in the majority of focal and generalized epilepsies, during NREM sleep, interictal EAs are more likely to occur and propagate to other brain regions. However there are considerable controversies surrounding the issue of whether light NREM or deep NREM sleep exerts a stronger facilitating effect on spiking. Data from the literature suggest that this may depend on the type of epilepsy syndrome being studied. Indeed, it has been observed that in a range of focal childhood epi-leptic syndromes characterized by a marked activation of interictal spikes during NREM sleep (benign rolandic epilepsy, Landau–Kleffner syndrome, and electrical status epilepticus during sleep), interictal EA seems to be modulated mainly by spindle oscillatory

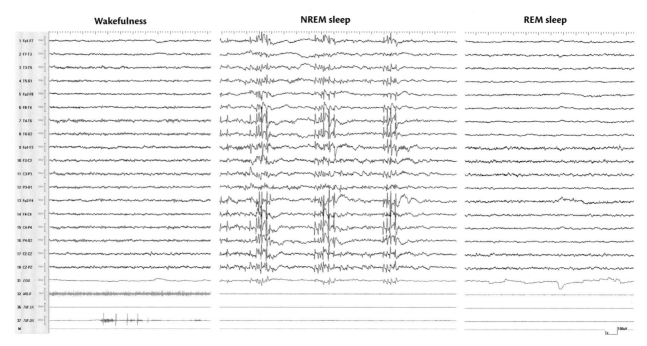

Fig. 28.1 Scalp EEG during the sleep–wake cycle in an epileptic child. In this example, no clear epileptiform discharges are visualized during wakefulness and REM sleep. On the contrary, NREM sleep is a known enhancer of interictal epileptiform discharges (IEDs) on scalp EEGs. Bursts of IEDs are visible (and more diffuse) during NREM sleep. EEG recorded according to the 10–20 international nomenclature. EOG, electro-oculogram; MILO, chin electromyography; TIB SX, left tibialis electromyography; TIB DX, right tibialis electromyography.

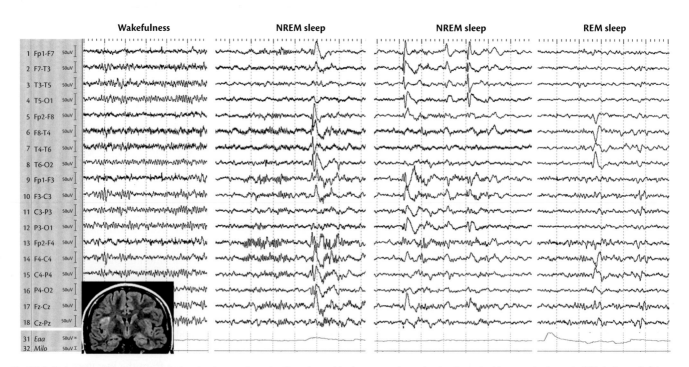

Fig. 28.2 Scalp video-EEG monitoring during the sleep–wake cycle of a patient with pharmacoresistant focal epilepsy. In this example, the scalp EEG during wakefulness is within normal limits. During NREM sleep, IEDs are clearly evident, but appear asynchronously in the right and the left frontotemporal regions (and are therefore nonlocalizing). During REM sleep, the IEDs are more circumscribed and located in the right temporal region, localizing to the known MRI lesion. The inset at lower left is a brain MRI coronal section showing a hypersignal in the right fronto-operculo-insular region compatible with a focal cortical dysplasia. EEG recorded according to the 10–20 international nomenclature. Eog, electro-oculography; Milo, chin electromyography.

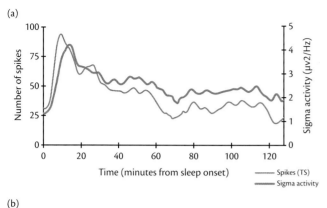

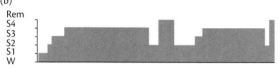

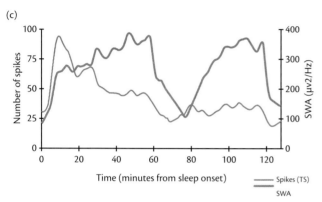

Fig. 28.3 Spectral analysis of the scalp EEG signal during the first two sleep cycles of the night in a patient with Landau–Kleffner syndrome. (a) Temporal series of the number of spikes/min plotted against sigma activity (SA, bold line). On scalp EEG, interictal spikes follow the SA distribution from sleep onset, suggesting modulation of the interictal spikes by the spindle oscillatory mechanisms. (b) Representative hypnogram during the first two sleep cycles of the night. (c) Temporal series of spikes/min plotted against slow-wave activity (SWA, bold line). Note the discrepancy in the distribution of spikes in relation to SWA compared with the SA in (a).

Adapted from Epilepsia, 41, Nobili L, Baglietto MG, Beelke M, De Carli F, De Negri E, Tortorelli S, Ferrillo F, Spindles-inducing mechanism modulates sleep activation of interictal epileptiform discharges in the Landau-Kleffner syndrome, pp. 201–206, Copyright (2000), with permission from John Wiley and Sons.

mechanisms (mostly evident in the N2 stage of sleep; Fig. 28.3) [14–16]; conversely, in adult focal epilepsies, interictal EA is generally modulated by ultraslow arousal fluctuations (expressed by the so-called cyclic alternating pattern, CAP; Fig. 28.4) and follow the intra-night dynamics of EEG delta activity (Fig. 28.5) [17].

It is frequently stated that it is the increase in neuronal synchronization by the thalamocortical system that favors seizure occurrence during NREM sleep. However, clinical studies clearly show that sleep-related seizures occurring during NREM sleep occur predominantly in stage N2 (61–68%) and not during N3 or slow-wave sleep, where the maximum level of synchronization is achieved (9–14%) [18]. Independently of NREM sleep stage, electroclinical studies have shown that seizures occur mostly during transitional unstable states, when the EEG shows fluctuating levels

of synchronization as expressed by the CAP [19,20] . Intracerebral recordings of this phenomenon show that during these intervals of the sleep–wake cycle, brain activity is in a transitional unbalanced state, showing important fluctuations in the level of synchronization, both spatially and temporally, with the possible coexistence of sleep-like and wake-like electrophysiological activity [21,22]. These features seem to constitute the electrophysiological substrate favoring the occurrence of seizures during sleep [23].

Video-EEG studies have shown that the distribution of focal-onset seizures throughout the sleep–wake cycle is influenced mainly by the location of the epileptogenic zone: frontal lobe seizures are more likely to occur during sleep, whereas patients affected by temporal lobe epilepsy or with a posterior epilepsy (originating from the occipital or parietal lobes) have a reduced probability of sleep-related seizures [18]. On the other hand, temporal lobe seizures tend to generalize more frequently during sleep.

Specific histopathology has also been linked to sleep-related seizures, more precisely to sleep-related hypermotor seizures. Case series of patients with pharmacoresistant seizures have associated a common epileptogenic lesion, namely, type II focal cortical dysplasia (FCD) or Taylor type, with a significant increase in sleep-related seizures—much more so than for other histopathological substrates, regardless of its location inside the brain [24].

Since many MRI-negative cases of pharmacoresistant patients with sleep-related seizures submitted to surgical intervention are associated with type II FCD after histopathological analysis, it has been suggested that the propensity of some type II FCDs to manifest during sleep might be partly related to their size [25]. Indeed, a small type II FCD might not be able to recruit sufficient non-dysplastic cortex for seizure propagation during wakefulness owing to a low critical mass of neurons, and therefore hijacks the sleep oscillatory mechanisms during the night in order to manifest itself [25,26].

Clinical features

Sleep has a well-documented and strong association with syndromic and nonsyndromic epilepsies (Table 28.1). The current ILAE classification highlights the fact that specific epileptic syndromes have a particular tendency for seizures to present exclusively or predominantly during sleep or upon wakening. Here we discuss their electroclinical features.

Grand mal seizures on awakening

Awakening epilepsy [27] is an age-related syndrome of idiopathic generalized epilepsy characterized by generalized tonic–clonic seizures (GTCS) occurring predominantly on awakening (independently of the time of day). The EEG is characterized by frequent generalized spike waves, rare focal abnormalities, and increased photosensitivity. The common denominator among external influences precipitating seizures is lack of sleep. With regard to sleep habit, patients with awakening epilepsy can roughly be described as late sleepers and late risers, which may predispose them to a chronic sleep deficit. Polygraphic studies have shown the presence of a disturbance in sleep stability in these patients.

Juvenile myoclonic epilepsy

Juvenile myoclonic epilepsy (JME) is a prototype of idiopathic generalized epilepsy, commonly presenting with myoclonic jerks

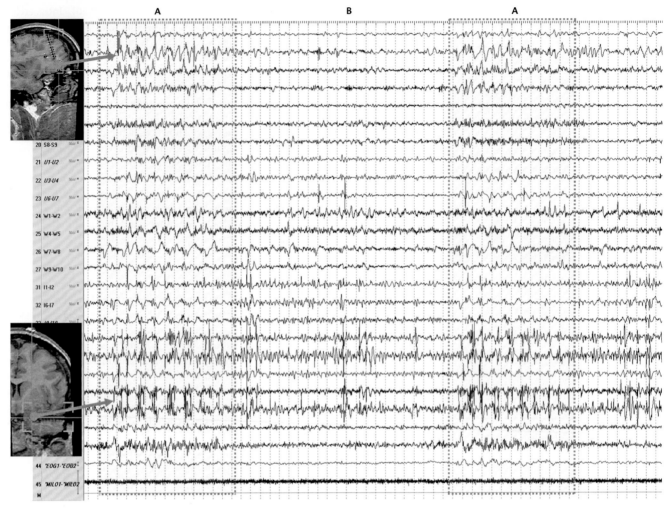

Fig. 28.4 (See colour plate section) Intracerebral EEG recording during NREM sleep in an adult patient with pharmacoresistant mesial temporal lobe epilepsy. During the A phase of CAP (dotted boxes) IEDs in the mesial temporal lobe (lower MRI image) are more numerous and spread to the orbital region (upper MRI image). During the B phase of CAP, IEDs are reduced and circumscribed to the temporal lobe.

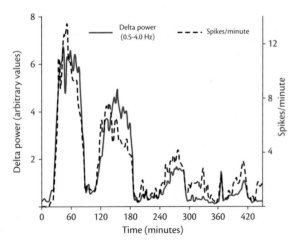

Fig. 28.5 Spectral analysis of the scalp EEG signal during the whole night in a patient with temporal lobe epilepsy. IEDs (dotted line) follow the temporal distribution of delta power (full line) and its known decay during the night.

during adolescence, and is characterized by a strong genetic predisposition [28]. Generalized tonic–clonic seizures can occur independently or precede the myoclonus. Seizures tend to occur in the early morning hours shortly after awakening, with a second peak of occurrence in some patients in the early evening. Myoclonic seizures can be subtle and overlooked for many years as simple clumsiness. These patients also have daytime absence seizures with staring spells, which can mimic daytime sleep attacks. Patients may be exceedingly sensitive to sleep deprivation and alcohol consumption. Using transcranial magnetic stimulation, it has been shown that cortical excitability is increased early in the morning in patients with idiopathic generalized epilepsy, particularly in JME, but not in subjects with focal epilepsy or controls without epilepsy [29]. This finding may explain the increased seizure susceptibility in these patients at this time of the day. Interictal discharges in these patients are prominent at sleep onset and on awakening. During NREM sleep, EA is facilitated by arousal fluctuations [30], and conversely it may promote sleep instability which will foster further EA, and conceivably seizures.

Table 28.1 Sleep-related epilepsies

Generalized epilepsies and syndromes
Grand mal seizures on awakening
Juvenile myoclonic epilepsy
Lennox–Gastaut syndrome
West syndrome
Focal epileptic syndromes
Benign epilepsy with centrotemporal spikes
Childhood epilepsy with occipital paroxysms
Nocturnal frontal lobe epilepsy*
Undetermined (focal or generalized) epileptic syndromes
Epileptic encephalopathy with continuous spikes and slow waves during slow sleep (CSWS/ESES)
Landau–Kleffner syndrome

* Sleep-related complex motor attacks can also have an extrafrontal origin.

Lennox–Gastaut syndrome

In Lennox–Gastaut syndrome, the clinical features consist of multiple primary generalized seizure types, including prominent nocturnal tonic, astatic/atonic, atypical absence, myoclonic, and generalized tonic–clonic seizures with accompanying psychomotor and cognitive maldevelopment [31]. Tonic seizures, typically activated by sleep, are much more frequent during NREM sleep than during wakefulness, and are never seen during REM sleep. They may only be characterized by subtle and frequently undetected brief apneas, but are often very frequent, being associated with characteristic paroxysmal fast activity on EEG; such sleep-related tonic seizures are seen in over 90% of patients with Lennox–Gastaut syndrome. EEG typically demonstrates slow spike-and-wave complexes at 1.5–2.5 Hz, multifocal epileptiform abnormalities, and generalized background slowing [32]. In sleep, the spike-and-wave discharges characteristically increase in NREM sleep and may be intermixed with trains of fast spikes of 10–25 Hz lasting 2–10 seconds (so-called grand mal discharges) as interictal abnormalities [33].

West syndrome (infantile spasms)

In West syndrome, spasms consist of brisk myoclonic-like muscle contractions, in flexion or extension, that usually start between 3 and 7 months of age [34]. They are usually repeated in clusters and are usually observed in relation to arousal from sleep or before going to sleep. The characteristic high-amplitude "hypsarrhythmic" interictal EEG pattern is seen most prominently in NREM sleep, particularly at onset, which therefore constitutes the best period in which to perform a diagnostic EEG [35]. Less than 3% of spasms occur during sleep [34]. However, clusters of subclinical ictal EEG discharges not associated with motor spasms may occur during REM sleep and may become associated with clinical spasms if the patient awakens from REM sleep during the cluster [36]. Response to treatment is variable, and a majority of patients continue to have seizures at follow-up, sometimes evolving into Lennox–Gastaut syndrome, and with a poor developmental outcome.

Benign epilepsy with centrotemporal spikes

Benign epilepsy with centrotemporal spikes is the most common partial epilepsy syndrome in the pediatric age group, with an onset between ages 3 and 13 years and with remission in adolescence [37]. The clinical seizures are characterized by focal clonic facial seizures, often preceded by perioral numbness. In many cases, patients have generalized tonic–clonic seizures that appear to be a secondary generalization. On occasion, there is speech arrest. Consciousness is preserved. The seizures are mostly nocturnal, with 55–59% of patients having seizures exclusively during sleep. The EEG shows centrotemporal or rolandic spikes or sharp waves with the typical morphology of a triphasic sharp wave of high amplitude localized to the centrotemporal region but sometimes spreading to the contralateral hemisphere. The activation of interictal epileptic discharges (IEDs) by NREM sleep is a well-known feature of benign epilepsy of childhood with rolandic spikes [38]. The discharge rate is increased during drowsiness and light sleep when compared with the waking record, with no change in spike morphology. Despite the increased frequency of seizures and interictal EA during sleep, the sleep architecture is not affected and no sleep disruption is seen in these children [39]. The response to medication is excellent and the epilepsy prognosis is universally benign. However, mild neuropsychological deficits may be seen when interictal EA during sleep is high [40].

Childhood epilepsy with occipital paroxysms

Panayiotopoulos syndrome is an interesting benign epilepsy syndrome seen in children aged 2–6 years and is approximately half as common as rolandic epilepsy [41] Autonomic seizures and autonomic status epilepticus are the main clinical manifestations. Seizures are characterized by autonomic instability (thermoregulatory alterations, tachycardia, hyperpnea, high blood pressure, and pallor), frequently accompanied by nausea and emesis. Seizures mostly start in sleep, with the child waking up or found confused or unconscious [42]. The same child may have seizures both during sleep and during wake. Impairment of consciousness is typically followed by prolonged periods of eye deviation, which can last from minutes to hours in the case of status epilepticus. Interictal EEG shows a predominance of interictal multifocal spikes with a preference for occipital paroxysms (more than 50%). Electrographic seizures also seem to emanate from the occipital region during these events. Sleep typically accentuates the spike abnormalities. Panayiotopoulos syndrome has a very benign course, with complete spontaneous remission within a few years. The majority of patients do not require any antiepileptic treatment, which is best reserved for more severe and distressing cases [42,43].

Epileptic encephalopathy with continuous spikes and waves during slow sleep

Epileptic encephalopathy with continuous spikes and waves during slow sleep (CSWS), formerly known as electrical status epilepticus during sleep (ESES), is a disease of childhood characterized by a triad of epilepsy, cognitive or behavioral impairment, and continuous spike-and-wave EEG discharges during slow-wave sleep [44]. All-night PSG study is necessary for diagnosis. In this syndrome, it is the dramatic decline of the neuropsychological state that is the most disturbing and problematic clinical feature. The regression of skills is usually of insidious onset and progressive.

Most diagnosed patients have a prior history of epilepsy. The characteristic EEG finding consists of 2.0–2.5 Hz generalized spike-and-wave discharges seen during at least 85% of NREM sleep and greatly reduced during REM sleep. Occasional bursts of spike-and-wave discharges or focal frontal spikes are seen during REM sleep. There are a few bursts of generalized spike-and-wave discharges seen in the EEG during wakefulness. These EEG discharges disrupt the stages of NREM sleep. In particular, the vertex sharp waves, K complexes, and spindles are usually difficult to recognize. However, a normal cyclic pattern of REM–NREM persists. Generally, no sleep disturbances are observed, but some children have difficulty awakening in the morning [45].

CSWS is now considered an epileptic encephalopathy of childhood. The EEG findings of continuous epileptic discharges generally disappear within three years of appearance. Focal abnormalities in the EEG may persist, however. It is not clear whether CSWS is a focal epilepsy or a generalized epilepsy with heterogeneous presentation, and hence it is classified under the category of undetermined epileptic syndromes. Seizures show a benign course and respond well to antiepileptic medications, with disappearance of seizures by the mid-teens. The psychological impairment, however, persists.

Landau–Kleffner syndrome

Landau–Kleffner syndrome (LKS) is an acquired disorder with epileptic aphasia in which children, usually 3–8 years of age, who have developed age-appropriate speech experience language regression with verbal auditory agnosia, abnormal epileptiform activity, behavioral disturbances, and sometimes overt seizures [46]. There are several similarities between ESES and LKS. In both conditions, a normal EEG background during wakefulness, with generalized spike-wave discharges or focal epileptiform activity, can be found. However, in ESES, discharges during sleep are generalized, while in LKS, spike waves tend to be more localized in the temporal derivations. Compared with ESES, patients with LKS also have fewer seizures, as well as more focal cognitive impairment and less psychological impairment. Consequently, overall prognosis is usually better in LKS [47].

Nocturnal frontal lobe epilepsy

Nocturnal frontal lobe epilepsy (NFLE) is a syndrome of heterogeneous etiology, with genetic, lesional, and cryptogenic forms having been described [48–50]. NFLE is usually considered a benign clinical epileptic syndrome because seizures occur almost exclusively during sleep, and in the majority of patients pharmacological treatment is effective; however, severe and drug-resistant forms, occasionally associated with mental retardation, have been described [51]. Although heterogeneous, NFLE is a syndrome that has been extensively studied and characterized during recent decades.

In the 1990s, the occurrence of sleep-related motor attacks in numerous individuals belonging to the same family was observed, and the definition of autosomal dominant nocturnal frontal lobe epilepsy (ADNFLE) was introduced for the first time [52]. The genetic origin of the disease was confirmed by a linkage study in Australian kindred. More specifically, a locus was identified at chromosome 20q13.2–q13.3, and two different mutations were detected in the gene (CHRNA4) encoding the α_4 subunit of the neuronal nicotinic acetylcholine receptor (nAChR) [53]. Three de novo or inherited CHRNA4 mutations, occasionally associated with mild to moderate mental retardation, were later reported. ADNFLE was quickly recognized as a genetically heterogeneous disorder, since most of the described families did not show mutations in CHRNA4, and new loci and genes were reported in the following years. In particular, another linkage site was later reported at chromosome 15q24, and mutations were found in CHRNB2, the gene encoding for the B2 subunit of the ACh neural receptor and localized on chromosome 1. Another linkage locus at chromosome 8p12.3–8q12.3 and a missense mutation in the gene CHRNA2 encoding the neural ACh receptor A2 subunit have been reported in familial seizures characterized by complex ictal behavior resembling epileptic nocturnal wanderings, as well as mutations in the corticotropin-releasing hormone gene (for a review, see [54]).

The findings of genetic alterations of the cholinergic system may give some insight into the relationships among genes, epileptogenesis, and arousal-regulating processes. Indeed, the nAChR are extensively distributed in the brain and contribute to the regulation of sleep and arousal oscillations, at both the cortical and subcortical levels. Experimental studies have shown that a mutation of the nicotinic receptors may facilitate the occurrence of an unbalanced excitation/inhibition circuitry within GABAergic reticular thalamic neurons, thus generating seizures through the synchronizing effect of spontaneous oscillations in thalamocortical connections [55]. Conversely, other experimental investigations have shown a physiological involvement of nAChR in the regulation of NREM and REM stability, notably in the regulation of transient events such as microarousals [56]. Thus, it seems that a genetic alteration observed in NFLE might facilitate both the epileptogenesis and the occurrence of arousal instability. With these assumptions, the high prevalence of parasomnias in the personal and family histories of individuals with NFLE [57] might rely on a common alteration of the arousal-regulating system. However, ADNFLE is related not only to mutations in the cholinergic system. Since 2005, other genes, not belonging to the nACh receptor subunit family, have been identified (the corticotropin-releasing hormone gene, a gene encoding the sodium-activated potassium channel subunit 1, and the DEPDC5 gene) [51,58,59].

From a clinical point of view, given the high intra-familial variability and overlapping features of the clinical manifestations, ADNFLE patients do not show a clear distinction from sporadic NFLE cases, except for certain ADNFLE mutations frequently associated with specific additional neurological or psychiatric symptoms. In the great majority of NFLE patients, seizures begin before the age of 20 years, with a peak during childhood, although onset during adulthood has been also reported. Seizure frequency is usually high, and patients generally experience many seizures a night, although the frequency may diminish during adulthood. Of note, occasional seizures during wakefulness can occur. Subjective seizure manifestations, uncommon during the night, have been reported by patients during these diurnal events; however, frontal auras generally have poor localizing and lateralizing values [48,49,54].

NFLE patients may show different sleep-related motor events of increasing complexity and duration, even during a single night. These include (1) short-lasting (2–4 seconds) stereotyped movements involving the limbs, the axial musculature, and/or the head [60,61]; (2) paroxysmal arousals (PAs), characterized by sudden and brief arousals (5–10 seconds in duration) sometimes accompanied by stereotyped movements, vocalization, frightened expression, and fear [62]; (3) major attacks, lasting 20–30 seconds, characterized by asymmetric tonic or dystonic posturing, or complex movements such as pelvic thrusting, pedaling, choreoathetoid, and ballistic movements of the limbs [49]; (4) epileptic nocturnal wandering, consisting of ictal deambulatory behaviors often associated with a frightened expression and fear [63]. The increasing complexity of NFLE ictal motor behaviors, from minor to major events, reflects different durations and propagations of the discharge within the frontal lobe [62]. Owing to the recurrence of nocturnal motor events, some NFLE patients may complain of nonrestorative sleep and of daytime sleepiness.

Studies with intracerebral electrodes (stereo-EEG) conducted in drug-resistant patients with NFLE have shown that seizure onset in patients with asymmetric tonic or dystonic posturing is generally localized in the posterior portion of the frontal cingulated gyrus and in the posterior mesial frontal cortex with a primary involvement of the supplementary motor area [64]. In patients with seizures characterized by hyperkinetic automatisms and complex motor behaviors, the region of seizure onset may involve the dorsolateral and anterior frontal regions (frontopolar and frontal anteromesial regions). Seizures characterized by the association of fear and nocturnal wandering seem to involve a cerebral network including the anterior cingulate, orbitopolar, and temporal regions. Some of these clinical manifestations have been interpreted as a release of inhibition (provoked by the seizure) of innate behavioral automatisms and survival behaviors, programmed in cortical and subcortical central pattern generators [65].

Often, interictal and ictal scalp EEG features of NFLE patients are uninformative, owing to the inaccessibility of much of the frontal lobes to surface electrodes and to the presence of movement artifacts related to seizures [49,64]. Moreover, the reduced contribution of scalp EEG is accompanied by a low incidence of significant MRI findings, even in symptomatic cases.

In recent years, it has been shown that sleep-related complex motor attacks, similar to those occurring in NFLE patients, may also originate from the temporal lobe [66,67], the insular–opercular region [68], and the posterior cerebral regions [69] rendering the term NFLE somewhat misleading. To address this issue and the fact that seizures are not "nocturnal" per se but rather facilitated by NREM sleep, a recent consensus conference has proposed that NFLE be renamed "sleep-related hypermotor epilepsy" (SHE), a term deemed to better represent this heterogeneous syndrome [70].

To identify an extrafrontal onset in NFLE patients, a careful analysis of aura features may be particularly useful in the differential diagnosis of NFLE. Indeed, these patients may report subjective manifestations that could suggest an origin of seizure outside the frontal lobe, such as epigastric and acoustic sensations, and/or déjà vu in temporal lobe onset; laryngeal and throat sensations, dysarthria, hypersalivation, and diffuse or bilateral cutaneous paresthesias of unpleasant or electrical character in opercular and/or insular onset; and visual hallucinations in occipital seizures.

As stated earlier, studies conducted in patients with drug-resistant epilepsy have shown that type II focal cortical dysplasia (type II FCD; Taylor-type cortical dysplasia) is the most frequent etiological substrate of NFLE. Regardless of its anatomical localization, frontal or extrafrontal, type II FCD increases the risk of sleep-related epilepsy, in particular type IIb [24,71]. During wakefulness, type IIb FCD shows a peculiar pattern of interictal activity that is characterized by the occurrence of rhythmic and subcontinuous spike and polyspike waves with a frequency usually between 1 and 3 Hz, alternating with short bursts of fast discharges interrupted by suppression of activity. These bursts of fast discharges are relatively rare and sporadic during wakefulness, but become numerous during slow-wave sleep, when they tend to recur pseudoperiodically and often spread over surrounding nonlesional areas and develop into a seizure.

With regard to the pharmacological treatment of NFLE, the first-choice drug is carbamazepine, which can be administered before sleep, resulting in satisfactory seizure control in this population. Other drugs have shown efficacy in the treatment of NFLE, but usually as a second choice: topiramate, oxcarbazepine (OXC), and levetiracetam (LEV). It has been shown that surgery can also provide excellent results in drug-resistant NFLE patients, with 76% of cases being completely seizure-free [64].

Many of the differences between NFLE and non-epileptic sleep-related events have now been clarified, and a number of clinical features have been categorized to help physicians in the differential diagnosis (Table 28.2). However, considering the similarities and the possible coexistence of parasomnias in people with NFLE, the diagnostic process may be complicated, especially if it is based only on anamnestic investigations. Efforts to obtain a systematic assessment of the diagnostic reliability of clinical history have led to two instruments: the Frontal Lobe Epilepsy and Parasomnias Scale (FLEPS) [72] and the Structured Interview for NFLE [73]. Despite their clinical usefulness, these tools are limited by contradictory diagnostic accuracy.

Sleep V-PSG is unanimously considered the "gold-standard" diagnostic test, but it is expensive, with limited availability, and does not always capture the event in a single-night recording. Moreover, even when the nocturnal episode has been recorded, the diagnosis can remain doubtful because ictal scalp EEG often fails to disclose epileptiform abnormalities or because the episode captured is a minor motor event for which the diagnosis is not reliable, even among experts. To make video analysis of nocturnal paroxysmal events more reliable, a diagnostic algorithm focusing on the semiological features of the arousal parasomnias and NFLE has been proposed [74]. Despite the limits of V-PSG, the possibility of analyzing a video of the nocturnal attack remains an important diagnostic tool, making home video recording a useful adjunct when episodes are infrequent, even if the onset of the episode is missed [75].

Comorbidities: epilepsy and sleep disorders

Patients suffering from nocturnal epilepsy, and from epilepsy in general, can have sleep disorders [76]. These can manifest independently from the epileptic events, but can also negatively influence the epilepsy itself; conversely, the expression of sleep disorders can be negatively influenced by the epileptic condition in a bidirectional influenced system [77]. The possible occurrence of comorbidities also brings about the problem of differential diagnosis, as previously discussed, because of the potential difficulty in distinguishing referred non-epileptic nocturnal events from epileptic attacks, which in the majority of cases need individualized therapeutic approaches.

Parasomnias

Parasomnias and epileptic seizures may occur in a subject either simultaneously or at different times in his or her life, the clinical

Table 28.2 Clinical features useful in the differential diagnosis between nocturnal frontal lobe epilepsy (NFLE) and NREM parasomnia

	NFLE	NREM parasomnia
Age at onset	Any age (usually before the age of 20 years)	3–8 years
Family history of parasomnias	Possible	Frequently present
Time of occurrence during the night	Any time	Usually during the first third
Sleep-stage onset of episodes	NREM sleep (usually N2)	NREM sleep (usually N3)
Frequency during one night	Several episodes/night	Usually one episode/night
Frequency in a month	Almost every night	Sporadic
Duration	Seconds–3 minutes	1-10 minutes
Evolution	Stable, increased frequency, rare remission	Tend to disappear
Triggering factors	Rare	Frequent (sleep deprivation, febrile illness)
Stereotypic motor pattern	Yes	No
Consciousness if awakened	Usually preserved	Usually impaired
Recall of the episode on awakening	Variable	No

pattern of this comorbidity varying according to the patient's age and epileptic syndrome [57,76,78].

NREM arousal parasomnias have been reported to be common in sporadic as well as in familial forms of NFLE. A systematic investigation of the presence of NREM arousal parasomnias in the personal and family histories of subjects with NFLE found this comorbidity to be present in up to 34% and 39%, respectively [57].

As previously stated in the discussion of NFLE, it can be hypothesized that these two disorders, even if etiologically different, could share a common, possibly genetically determined, pathophysiological substrate involving a defective arousal system favoring the occurrence of both disorders [79]. Although not yet identified, the cholinergic system and related pathways could represent a model unifying the pathogenesis of both disorders. It has been further speculated that the clinical manifestations of NFLE and NREM arousal parasomnias may arise from the activation of innate motor behaviors underlain by central pattern generators, via different processes in which arousal is a triggering mechanism [65].

Lastly, REM parasomnias, in particular REM sleep behavior disorder (RBD), may coexist with SRE and can lead to diagnostic difficulties or misdiagnosis as well, especially in elderly people, where RBD is more frequent [80].

Obstructive sleep apnea

Obstructive sleep apnea (OSA) is a very common sleep disorder and is likely to be diagnosed in an epileptic patient, given the high prevalence of the two diseases in the general population. Although unrelated to the epileptic process, possible pathophysiological interactions can explain, to a certain extent, the coexistence of the two pathologies in a non-negligible portion of epileptic patients.

OSA has been seen in up to 10.2% of an unselected group of patients with epilepsy with no other sleep or cerebral disorder [81]. In patients with refractory epilepsy, OSA might be even more frequent, and has been reported in one-third of patients investigated for epilepsy surgery. OSA has also been seen in up to 20% of children with epilepsy undergoing polysomnography because of complaints about sleep disturbance [82]. Predisposing factors for OSA in epileptic subjects are male gender, obesity, nocturnal seizures, and a later age of seizure onset. In general, OSA in epileptic patients is reported to be mild or moderate. OSA can be facilitated by weight gain (a well-known risk factor for OSA), as a consequence of reduced physical activity and of antiepileptic drug (AED) therapy, for example with valproate (VPA) or carbamazepine (CBZ). Women taking VPA show a significantly increased risk of polycystic ovarian syndrome, which in turn is associated with obesity and so indirectly can lead to sleep apneas. Some AEDs, such as phenobarbital (PB), benzodiazepines (BDZs), and possibly phenytoin (PHT), can cause upper airway tone reduction, thus facilitating sleep apneas. Nonpharmacological treatment of epilepsy with vagus nerve stimulation has also been shown to worsen OSA. On the other hand, remission of OSA as well as of seizures has been seen anecdotally in a patient following frontal lobe resection [83].

Conversely, OSA can negatively influence epilepsy, because sleep fragmentation induced by snoring and apneas produces sleep instability (a high CAP index), thus promoting seizure occurrence. An improvement in seizure control after treatment of OSA with continuous positive airway pressure (CPAP) has been described along with a parallel improvement in sleep architecture [84]. Therefore, identifying and treating a coexisting breathing disorder in an epileptic patient allows better management of the epileptic disease and can direct the neurologist toward a more appropriate pharmacological choice among the available AEDs.

Excessive daytime sleepiness

Epileptic patients frequently complain of excessive daytime sleepiness (EDS). This is found in about 30–50% of people with epilepsy [85] and may result from clinical seizures, particularly nocturnal seizures and ictal or interictal EEG epileptiform discharges; comorbid conditions; and effects of antiepileptic medication. The AEDs most commonly associated with EDS are PHT, BDZs, and gabapentin (GBP). Frequently used AEDs that are less sedating are CBZ, VPA, topiramate (TPM), and lamotrigine (LTG).

Independently of drug therapy, it has been shown that sleep architecture is abnormal in many epileptic patients, and this can lead to EDS. Some studies have described an increased number of arousals, awakenings and stage shifts, and reduced total sleep time, slow-wave sleep, REM sleep, and sleep efficiency. These alterations are seen even in the absence of nocturnal seizures in both generalized and focal epilepsies. Subjective sleepiness is also frequently reported in patients with refractory seizures undergoing investigations for epilepsy surgery, with improvement after surgery [86]. Other contributing factors for EDS in epileptic patients are coexistence of OSA, restless legs syndrome. or inadequate sleep hygiene, which should all be sought out during patient consultation and follow-up [87,88].

Therapeutic approach and pharmacological implications

When a sleep disorder and epilepsy coexist, the best strategy is to use a single drug to treat the two pathologies. CBZ taken at night for NFLE can sometimes be efficacious in the treatment of NREM and REM parasomnias, for which the mainstay treatment is usually clonazepam (CNZ). On the other hand, the chronic use of CNZ and other sedative AEDs, such as PB, should be avoided in NFLE patients because, by increasing light NREM sleep and arousals, they can exacerbate seizures. If an epileptic patient presents with symptoms of restless legs syndrome, then an AED such as CNZ (but also CBZ, OXC, GBP, or VPA) can be effective in the treatment of both disorders [89]. Finally, some patients with epilepsy may complain of insomnia related to sleep fragmentation and repeated arousals as a result of nocturnal seizures and interictal EEG epileptiform discharges, AED side effects, depression, anxiety, or withdrawal or tapering of AEDs. Indeed, some AEDs are known to cause insomnia. Sadler reported a 6.4% incidence of dose-dependent lamotrigine-related insomnia [90]. In contrast, Foldvary et al. failed to observe any effect of lamotrigine on sleep efficiency, sleep latency, or total sleep time in a PSG study of seven subjects with epilepsy [91]. The other AED that has been found to have stimulant-like effects in patients with epilepsy is felbamate; however, because of serious toxicity, this has largely been withdrawn from the market and is rarely used nowadays to treat epilepsy.

AEDs have variable effects on nocturnal sleep and daytime vigilance (for reviews, see [85,87,92]. The effects of AEDs on sleep can be divided into general effects consisting of reduction of REM and slow-wave sleep, reduction of sleep latency, and increased percentage of NREM stages 1 and 2, and specific effects depending on the individual AED (Table 28.3).

Studies suggest that the short- and long-term effects of CBZ on sleep differ. CBZ in acute administration leads to a reduction in REM sleep, with REM fragmentation and increased sleep stage shifts, as well as an increase in daytime somnolence. These effects are not observed during chronic CBZ use, where sleep consolidation with reduced awakenings and increased slow-wave sleep and sleep efficiency have been observed. Whether these effects vary significantly between different populations is still unknown.

VPA in general has minimal effects on sleep architecture in patients with epilepsy. At higher doses, it can cause an increase in slow-wave sleep and a decrease in REM sleep. However, different VPA-related effects have been described: difficulty initiating sleep, daytime sleepiness, and an increase in stage 1 and a decrease in stage 2 sleep. Furthermore, an absence of sleep structure modification and even a stabilizing effect have also been described.

The acute administration of PB usually shortens sleep latency, increases stage 2 sleep, reduces REM sleep, and decreases arousals, but the chronic use of PB can increase sleep fragmentation.

Primidone (PRM) in chronic use produces shortened sleep latency and a reduction in REM density, but not REM percentage.

PHT in acute administration causes reduced sleep latency, a reduction in stage 1 and 2 sleep, and an increase in slow-wave sleep but also of arousals, with no change in REM sleep and no relationship with serum drug levels. The long-term effects consist mostly of a reversal of the observed short-term effects, together with an increase in NREM sleep stages 1 and 2 and a decrease in slow-wave sleep. REM sleep remains unaltered.

The BZD group of drugs is generally used for status epilepticus (eg, lorazepam, diazepam, and midazolam), but sometimes clonazepam and clobazam are used in some drug-resistant seizures and certain types of seizures (eg, myoclonic seizures and Lennox–Gastaut syndrome). These drugs generally cause decreased sleep efficiency, sleep onset latency, stage 1 NREM, slow-wave sleep, and arousals.

Ethosuximide can reduce slow-wave sleep and increase stage 1 and REM sleep, as well as increasing the tendency to wake after sleep onset (WASO).

Several newer AEDs have come onto the market to treat patients with seizure disorders; most of these have been approved as add-on therapy, but some are now being used as primary AEDs. These drugs have not been studied extensively to determine their effects on sleep architecture.

Vigabatrin does not seem to affect sleep structure. GBP increases REM sleep and slow-wave sleep, reducing stage 1 and arousals and awakenings, contributing to sleep consolidation, and allowing, above all if taken only at night, a improvement in daytime alertness. It seems to act on sleep through a serotonergic mechanism. Lamotrigine has minimal effects on sleep in general. It may cause increased REM sleep and decreased slow-wave sleep [92]. TPM does not seem to modify sleep architecture. Tiagabine can increase slow-wave sleep and sleep efficiency. LEV in healthy volunteers increases total sleep time, sleep efficiency and stage 2 and slow-wave sleep, while reducing stage shifts and WASO, without affecting daytime vigilance [93]. Hypersomnia after LEV treatment in epileptic patients has been described [94,95]. Studies of the effects of OXC and zonisamide on human sleep are lacking.

Finally, it should also be mentioned that conflicting reports have been published on the effects of melatonin on seizure control. Definitive data supporting its recommendation in the absence of a circadian sleep disorder are still lacking. Vagus nerve stimulation

Table 28.3 Effects of antiepileptic drugs (AEDs) on sleep architecture

AED	Sleep efficiency	Sleep latency	N1	N2	N3	REM
Carbamazepine	I	D	–	–	I	D
Valproate	–	–	?	D	I	D
Phenobarbital	D	D	I	I	–	D
Primidone	?	D	?	?	I	D
Phenytoin	D	D	I	I	D	–
Benzodiazepines	D	D	D	I	D	?
Ethosuximide	D	I	I	–	D	I
Vigabatrin	?	–	?	?	?	?
Gabapentin	I	D	D	–	I	I
Lamotrigine	–	–	–	–	D	I
Tiagabine	I	–	–	–	I	–
Topiramate	–	–	–	–	–	–
Levetiracetam	I	–	–	I	I	–
Oxcarbazepine	?	?	?	?	?	?

I, increase; D, decrease; -, no change; ?, unknown.

(VNS) therapy, frequently used for refractory epilepsy, can affect respiration during sleep, worsening preexisting OSA and interfering with effective CPAP titration [87]. On the other hand, chronic VNS can improve alertness and reduce REM sleep in patients with refractory epilepsy.

Sleep and sudden unexpected death in epilepsy

Sudden unexpected death in epilepsy (SUDEP) is the most distressing potential outcome of epilepsy. This possibility has been under-recognized by the medical community in the past, but has been increasingly studied in recent years. In epileptic patients, especially in those with pharmacoresistant epilepsy, the risk of SUDEP is 24–40 times higher compared with the general population [96]. It is considered to be the result of a peri-ictal concurrence of a number of predisposing and precipitating factors, such as early-onset epilepsy, male gender, learning disability, generalized tonic–clonic seizures, high seizure frequency, AED polypharmacy, subtherapeutic AED levels, and long duration of epilepsy [97,98]. Nevertheless, SUDEP remains predominantly a sleep-related phenomenon. Indeed, a retrospective study of autopsy-confirmed SUDEP has identified at least 58% of cases as occurring during sleep. Patients with sleep-related SUDEP were also more likely to have a history of nocturnal seizures than those with non-sleep-related SUDEP [99]. Therefore, sleep-related seizures seem to be an independent risk factor for SUDEP. Autonomic factors such as cardiac or respiratory dysfunctions, or both, have been implicated in SUDEP; however, conclusive evidence on their role is still lacking, and the way in which they might be related to one another or to an epileptic seizure, eventually leading to sudden death, has not yet been elucidated [97,100]. Although much remains to be explained about the pathophysiology and prevention of SUDEP, informing patients about SUDEP is strongly recommended, since it can optimize epilepsy self-management and engage the patient as a partner in their own care [101]. No data on the effectiveness of any particular clinical strategy are presently available; however, reducing the occurrence of tonic–clonic seizures, exercising caution in changing AEDs, and improving postictal surveillance are likely to be beneficial [98].

References

1. Echeverria MC. De l'épilepsie nocturne. Ann Med Psychol Paris 1879;5:177.
2. Gowers WR. Course of epilepsy. In: Gowers WR, ed. Epilepsy and other chronic convulsive diseases: their causes, symptoms and treatment. London: William Wood, 1885:157–64.
3. Fere L. Les Épilepsies et les Épileptiques. Paris: Alcan, 1890.
4. Gibbs EL, Gibbs FA. Diagnostic and localizing value of electroencephalographic studies in sleep. Res Publ Assoc Res Nerv Ment Dis 1947;26:366.
5. Engel J Jr, Dichter MA, Schwartzkroin A. Basic mechanisms of human epilepsy. In: Engel Jr J, Pedley TA, eds. Epilepsy: a comprehensive textbook, 2nd ed. Philadelphia: Lippincott Williams & Wilkins, 2008:495.
6. Montplaisir J, Laverdiere M, Saint-Hilaire JM, Rouleau I. Nocturnal sleep recording in partial epilepsy: a study with depth electrodes. J Clin Neurophysiol 1987;4:383.
7. Malow BA, Lin X, Kushwaha R, Aldrich MS. Interictal spiking increases with sleep depth in temporal lobe epilepsy. Epilepsia 1998;39:1309.
8. Sammaritano M, Gigli JL, Gotman J. Interictal spiking during wakefulness and sleep and the localization of foci in temporal lobe epilepsy. Neurology 1991;23:4.
9. Ferrillo F, Beelke M, Nobili L. Sleep EEG synchronization mechanisms and activation of interictal epileptic spikes. Clin Neurophysiol 2000;111 Suppl 2:S65–73.
10. Shouse MN, Martins da Silva A, Sammaritano M. Circadian rhythm, sleep and epilepsy. J Clin Neurophysiol 1996;13:32.
11. Shouse MN, Siegel JM, Wu MF, et al. Mechanisms of seizure suppression during rapid-eye-movement (REM) sleep in cats. Brain Res 1989;505:271–82.
12. Cohen HB, Thomas J, Dement WC. Sleep stages, REM deprivation and electroconvulsive threshold in the cat. Brain Res 1970;19:317.
13. Busek P, Buskova J, Nevsimalova S. Interictal epileptiform discharges and phasic phenomena of REM sleep. Epileptic Disord 2010;12:217–21.
14. Nobili L, Baglietto MG, Beelke M, et al. Modulation of sleep interictal epileptiform discharges in partial epilepsy of childhood. Clin Neurophysiol 1999;110:839–45.
15. Nobili L, Baglietto MG, Beelke M, et al. Spindles-inducing mechanism modulates sleep activation of interictal epileptiform discharges in the Landau–Kleffner syndrome. Epilepsia 2000;41:201–6.
16. Beelke M, Nobili L, Baglietto MG, et al. Relationship of sigma activity to sleep interictal epileptic discharges: a study in children affected by benign epilepsy with occipital paroxysms. Epilepsy Res 2000;40:179–86.
17. Ferrillo F, Beelke M, De Carli F, et al. Sleep-EEG modulation of interictal epileptiform discharges in adult partial epilepsy: a spectral analysis study. Clin Neurophysiol 2000;111:916–23.
18. Herman ST, Walczak TS, Bazil CW. Distribution of partial seizures during the sleep/wake cycle: differences by seizure onset. Neurology 2001;56:1453.
19. Ferri R, Rundo F, Bruni O, et al. Dynamics of the EEG slow-wave synchronization during sleep. Clin Neurophysiol 2005;116:2783–95.
20. Parrino L, Halasz P, Tassinari CA, Terzano MG. CAP, epilepsy and motor events during sleep: the unifying role of arousal. Sleep Med Rev 2006;10:267–85.
21. Nir Y, Staba RJ, Andrillon T, et al. Regional slow waves and spindles in human sleep. Neuron 2011;70:153–69.
22. Nobili L, Ferrara M, Moroni F, et al. Dissociated wake-like and sleep-like electro-cortical activity during sleep. Neuroimage 2011;58:612–19.
23. Gibbs SA, Proserpio P, Terzaghi M, et al. Sleep-related epileptic behaviors and non-REM-related parasomnias: insights from stereo-EEG. Sleep Med Rev 2016;25:4–20.
24. Nobili L, Cardinale F, Magliola U, et al. Taylor's focal cortical dysplasia increases the risk of sleep-related epilepsy. Epilepsia 2009;50:2599–604.
25. Chassoux F, Landré E, Mellerio C, et al. Type II focal cortical dysplasia: electroclinical phenotype and surgical outcome related to imaging. Epilepsia 2012;53:349–58.
26. Beenhakker MP, Huguenard JR. Neurons that fire together also conspire together: is normal sleep circuitry hijacked to generate epilepsy? Neuron 2009;62:612–32.
27. Janz D. Epilepsy with grand mal on awakening and the sleep–waking cycle. Clin Neurophysiol 2000;111:S103.
28. Janz D. Epilepsy with impulsive petit mal (juvenile myoclonic epilepsy). Acta Neurol Scand 1985;72:449.
29. Badawy RA, Curatolo JM, Newton M, et al. Sleep deprivation increases cortical excitability in epilepsy: syndrome-specific effects. Neurology 2006;67:1018–22.
30. Gigli GL, Calia E, Marciani MG, et al. Sleep microstructure and EEG epileptiform activity in patients with juvenile myoclonic epilepsy. Epilepsia 1992;33:799–804.
31. Gastaut H, Roger J, Soulayrol R, et al. Childhood epileptic encephalopathy with diffuse slow spike-waves (otherwise known as "petit mal variant") or Lennox syndrome. Epilepsia 1966;7:139–79.
32. Markand ON. Lennox–Gastaut syndrome (childhood epileptic encephalopathy). J Clin Neurophysiol 2003;20:426–41.
33. Erba G, Moschen R, Ferber R. Sleep-related changes in EEG discharge activity and seizure risk in patients with Lennox–Gastaut syndrome. Sleep Res 1981;10:247.

34. Kellaway P, Hrachovy RA, Frost JD, Zion T. Precise characterization and quantification of infantile spasms. Ann Neurol 1979;6:214–18.

35. Hrachovy RA, Frost JD. Infantile epileptic encephalopathy with hypsarrhythmia (infantile spasms/West syndrome). J Clin Neurophysiol 2003;20:408–25.

36. Hrachovy RA, Frost JD, Kellaway P. Hypsarrhythmia: variations on the theme. Epilepsia 1984;25:317–25.

37. Beaumanoir A, Ballis T, Varfis G, Ansari K. Benign epilepsy of childhood with Rolandic spikes. A clinical, electroencephalographic, and telencephalographic study. Epilepsia 1974;15:301–15.

38. Dalla Bernardina B, Pajno-Ferrara F, Beghini G. Proceedings: rolandic spike activation during sleep in children with and without epilepsy. Electroencephalogr Clin Neurophysiol 1975;39:537.

39. Clemens B, Majoros E. Sleep studies in benign epilepsy of childhood with rolandic spikes. II. Analysis of discharge frequency and its relation to sleep dynamics. Epilepsia 1987;28:24–27.

40. Baglietto MG, Battaglia FM, Nobili L, et al. Neuropsychological disorders related to interictal epileptic discharges during sleep in benign epilepsy of childhood with centrotemporal or rolandic spikes. Dev Med Child Neurol 2001;43:407–12.

41. Caraballo R, Cersósimo R, Fejerman N. Panayiotopoulos syndrome: a prospective study of 192 patients. Epilepsia 2007;48:1054–61.

42. Panayiotopoulos CP, Michael M, Sanders S, et al. Benign childhood focal epilepsies: assessment of established and newly recognized syndromes. Brain 2008;131:2264–86.

43. Ferrie C, Caraballo R, Covanis A, et al. Panayiotopoulos syndrome: a consensus view. Dev Med Child Neurol 2006;48:236–40.

44. Tassinari CA, Michelucci R, Forti A, et al. The electrical status epilepticus syndrome. In: Degen R, Dreyfuss SE, eds. Benign localized and generalized epilepsies of early childhood. Amsterdam: Elsevier, 1992:111.

45. Tassinari CA, Cantalupo G, Rios-Pohl L, et al. Encephalopathy with status epilepticus during slow sleep: "the Penelope syndrome." Epilepsia 2009;50 Suppl 7:4–8.

46. Landau WN, Kleffner FR. Syndrome of acquired aphasia with convulsive disorder in children. Neurology 1957;50:1772.

47. McVicar KA, Shinnar S. Landau–Kleffner syndrome, electrical status epilepticus in slow wave sleep, and language regression in children. Ment Retard Dev Disabil Res Rev 2004;10:144–9.

48. Oldani A, Zucconi M, Asselta R, et al. Autosomal dominant nocturnal frontal lobe epilepsy. A video-polysomnographic and genetic appraisal of 40 patients and delineation of the epileptic syndrome. Brain 1998;121 Pt 2:205–23.

49. Provini F, Plazzi G, Tinuper P, et al. Nocturnal frontal lobe epilepsy. A clinical and polygraphic overview of 100 consecutive cases. Brain 1999;122 Pt 6:1017–31.

50. Moroni F, Nobili L, Curcio G, et al. Sleep in the human hippocampus: a stereo-EEG study. PLoS One 2007;2:e867.

51. Heron SE, Smith KR, Bahlo M, et al. Missense mutations in the sodium-gated potassium channel gene KCNT1 cause severe autosomal dominant nocturnal frontal lobe epilepsy. Nat Genet 2012;44:1188–90.

52. Scheffer IE, Bhatia KP, Lopes-Cendes I, et al. (1994) Autosomal dominant frontal epilepsy misdiagnosed as sleep disorder. Lancet 1994;343:515–17.

53. Steinlein OK, Magnusson A, Stoodt J, et al. An insertion mutation of the CHRNA4 gene in a family with autosomal dominant nocturnal frontal lobe epilepsy. Hum Mol Genet 1997;6:943–47.

54. Nobili L, Proserpio P, Combi R, et al. Nocturnal frontal lobe epilepsy. Curr Neurol Neurosci Rep 2014;14:424.

55. Klaassen A, Glykys J, Maguire J, et al. Seizures and enhanced cortical GABAergic inhibition in two mouse models of human autosomal dominant nocturnal frontal lobe epilepsy. Proc Natl Acad Sci U S A 2006;103:19152–57.

56. Xu J, Cohen BN, Zhu Y, et al. Altered activity–rest patterns in mice with a human autosomal-dominant nocturnal frontal lobe epilepsy mutation in the beta2 nicotinic receptor. Mol Psychiatry 2011;16:1048–61.

57. Bisulli F, Vignatelli L, Naldi I, et al. Increased frequency of arousal parasomnias in families with nocturnal frontal lobe epilepsy: a common mechanism? Epilepsia 2010;51:1852–60.

58. Combi R, Dalpra L, Ferini-Strambi L, Tenchini ML. Frontal lobe epilepsy and mutations of the corticotropin-releasing hormone gene. Ann Neurol 2005;58:899.

59. Picard F, Makrythanasis, P, Navarro V, et al. DEPDC5 mutations in families presenting as autosomal dominant nocturnal frontal lobe epilepsy. Neurology 2014;82:2101–6.

60. Terzaghi M, Sartori I, Mai R, et al. Sleep-related minor motor events in nocturnal frontal lobe epilepsy. Epilepsia 2007;48:335–41.

61. Halasz P, Kelemen A, Szucs A. The role of NREM sleep micro-arousals in absence epilepsy and in nocturnal frontal lobe epilepsy. Epilepsy Res 2013;107:9–19.

62. Nobili L, Francione S, Mai R, et al. Nocturnal frontal lobe epilepsy: intracerebral recordings of paroxysmal motor attacks with increasing complexity. Sleep 2003;26:883–6.

63. Plazzi G, Tinuper P, Montagna P, et al. Epileptic nocturnal wanderings. Sleep 1995;18:749–56.

64. Nobili L, Francione S, Mai R, et al. Surgical treatment of drug-resistant nocturnal frontal lobe epilepsy. Brain 2007;130:561–73.

65. Tassinari CA, Rubboli G, Gardella E, et al. Central pattern generators for a common semiology in fronto-limbic seizures and in parasomnias. A neuroethologic approach. Neurol Sci 2005;26 Suppl 3:s225–32.

66. Nobili L, Cossu M, Mai R, et al. Sleep-related hyperkinetic seizures of temporal lobe origin. Neurology 2004;62:482–5.

67. Vaugier L, Aubert S, McGonigal A, et al. Neural networks underlying hyperkinetic seizures of "temporal lobe" origin. Epilepsy Res 2009;86:200–8.

68. Proserpio P, Cossu M, Francione S, et al. Insular–opercular seizures manifesting with sleep-related paroxysmal motor behaviors: a stereo-EEG study. Epilepsia 2011;52:1781–91.

69. Proserpio P, Cossu M, Francione S, et al. Epileptic motor behaviors during sleep: anatomo-electro-clinical features. Sleep Med 2011;12 Suppl 2:S33–8.

70. Tinuper P, Bisulli F, Cross JH, Hersdorffer D et al. Definition and diagnostic criteria of sleep-related hypermotor epilepsy. Neurology 2016; 86(19):1834-42.

71. Tassi L, Garbelli R, Colombo N, et al. Electroclinical, MRI and surgical outcomes in 100 epileptic patients with type II FCD. Epileptic Disord 2012;14:257–66.

72. Derry CP, Davey M, Johns M, et al. Distinguishing sleep disorders from seizures: diagnosing bumps in the night. Arch Neurol 2006;63:705–9.

73. Bisulli F, Vignatelli L, Naldi I, et al. Diagnostic accuracy of a structured interview for nocturnal frontal lobe epilepsy (SINFLE): a proposal for developing diagnostic criteria. Sleep Med 2012;13:81–7.

74. Derry CP, Harvey AS, Walker MC, et al. NREM arousal parasomnias and their distinction from nocturnal frontal lobe epilepsy: a video EEG analysis. Sleep 2009;32:1637–44.

75. Nobili L. Can homemade video recording become more than a screening tool? Sleep 2009;32:1544–5.

76. Manni R, Terzaghi M. Comorbidity between epilepsy and sleep disorders. Epilepsy Res 2010;90:171–7.

77. Gibbs SA, Proserpio P, Lo Russo G, et al. [Anatomo-electro-clinical features of nocturnal epileptic motor behaviors and non-REM parasomnias: data from intracerebral recordings]. Prat Neurol—FMC 2014;5:121–8.

78. Tinuper P, Provini F, Bisulli F, et al. Movement disorders in sleep: guidelines for differentiating epileptic from non-epileptic motor phenomena arising from sleep. Sleep Med Rev 2007;11:255–67.

79. Bisulli F, Vignatelli L, Provini F, et al. Parasomnias and nocturnal frontal lobe epilepsy (NFLE): lights and shadows—controversial points in the differential diagnosis. Sleep Med 2011;12 Suppl 2:S27–32.

80. Manni R, Terzaghi M, Zambrelli E. REM sleep behaviour disorder in elderly subjects with epilepsy: frequency and clinical aspects of the comorbidity. Epilepsy Res 2007;77:128–33.

81. Manni R, Terzaghi M, Arbasino C, et al. Obstructive sleep apnea in a clinical series of adult epilepsy patients: frequency and features of the comorbidity. Epilepsia 2003;44:836–40.

82. Kaleyias J, Cruz M, Goraya JS, et al. Spectrum of polysomnographic abnormalities in children with epilepsy. Pediatr Neurol 2008;39:170–6.

83. Foldvary-Schaefer N, Stephenson L, Bingaman W. Resolution of obstructive sleep apnea with epilepsy surgery? Expanding the relationship between sleep and epilepsy. Epilepsia 2008;49:1457–9.

84. Devinsky O, Ehrenberg B, Barthlen GM, et al. Epilepsy and sleep apnea syndrome. Neurology 1994;44:2060–4.

85. Foldvary-Schaefer N. Sleep complaints and epilepsy: the role of seizures, antiepileptic drugs and sleep disorders. J Clin Neurophysiol 2002;19:514–21.

86. Zanzmera P, Shukla G, Gupta A, et al. Effect of successful epilepsy surgery on subjective and objective sleep parameters—a prospective study. Sleep Med 2013;14:333–8.

87. Foldvary-Schaefer N, Grigg-Damberger M. Sleep and epilepsy: what we know, don't know and need to know. J Clin Neurophysiol 2006;23:4.

88. Derry CP, Duncan S. Sleep and epilepsy. Epilepsy Behav 2013;26:394–404.

89. Trenkwalder C, Hening WA, Montagna P, et al. Treatment of restless legs syndrome: an evidence-based review and implications for clinical practice. Mov Disord 2008;23:2267–302.

90. Sadler M. Lamotrigine associated with insomnia. Epilepsia 1999;40:322–5.

91. Foldvary N, Perry M, Lee J, et al. The effects of lamotrigine on sleep in patients with epilepsy. Epilepsia 2001;42:1569–73.

92. Placidi F, Diomedi M, Scalise A, et al. Effect of anticonvulsants on nocturnal sleep in epilepsy. Neurology 2000;54:S25–32.

93. Cicolin A, Magliola U, Giordano A, et al. Effects of levetiracetam on nocturnal sleep and daytime vigilance in healthy volunteers. Epilepsia 2006;47:82–85.

94. Khatami R, Siegel AM, Bassetti CL. Hypersomnia in an epilepsy patient treated with levetiracetam. Epilepsia 2005;46:588–9.

95. Zhou J-Y, Tang X-D, Huang L-L, et al. The acute effects of levetiracetam on nocturnal sleep and daytime sleepiness in patients with partial epilepsy. J Clin Neurosci 2012;19:956–60.

96. Mohanraj R, Norrie J, Stephen LJ, et al. Mortality in adults with newly diagnosed and chronic epilepsy: a retrospective comparative study. Lancet Neurol 2006;5:481–7.

97. Nobili L, Proserpio P, Rubboli G, et al. Sudden unexpected death in epilepsy (SUDEP) and sleep. Sleep Med Rev 2011;15:237–46.

98. Shorvon S, Tomson T. Sudden unexpected death in epilepsy. Lancet 2011;378:2028–38.

99. Lamberts RJ, Thijs RD, Laffan A, et al. Sudden unexpected death in epilepsy: people with nocturnal seizures may be at highest risk. Epilepsia 2012;53:253–7.

100. Massey CA, Sowers LP, Dlouhy BJ, Richerson GB. Mechanisms of sudden unexpected death in epilepsy: the pathway to prevention. Nat Rev Neurol 2014;10:271–82.

101. Donner E, Buchhalter J. Commentary: It's time to talk about SUDEP. Epilepsia 2014;55:1501–3.

CHAPTER 29

Autonomic dysfunction and sleep disorders

Giovanna Calandra-Buonaura and Pietro Cortelli

Introduction

There is a close relationship between the autonomic nervous system (ANS) and sleep, which are interdependent on each other by virtue of their common controls, neurobiological substrates, and functions. Sleep induces profound changes in the activity of the ANS, and disorders of the ANS adversely affect vital functions during sleep. As a consequence of this intimate interconnection between the ANS and sleep, several neurological and general medical disorders present both autonomic dysfunctions and sleep disturbances. This chapter focuses on the description of autonomic dysfunctions associated with sleep disorders [1]. This association may result from a common pathogenetic mechanism that affects both the autonomic and sleep functions, as in fatal familial insomnia, or from a prevalent expression of a primary disorder of autonomic regulation during sleep, as in congenital central hypoventilation syndrome. Alternatively, the autonomic dysfunction may be mainly caused by the sleep disorder, as observed in obstructive sleep apnea syndrome (OSAS), or the causal mechanism resulting in an association between autonomic dysfunction and a sleep disorder has not yet been defined with certainty, as in narcolepsy with cataplexy and REM sleep behavior disorder. Autonomic dysfunction may results in an overactivity or a failure of ANS functions. In both cases, it has been demonstrated that the autonomic disorder, particularly when this involves cardiovascular or respiratory control, not only impairs the patient's quality of life, but also has a significant negative impact on the prognosis of the associated sleep disorder and may represent a risk factor for the development of other chronic diseases or for life-threatening events. Therefore, prompt recognition of autonomic disturbances is of crucial importance to achieve the correct diagnosis, choose the most proper therapeutic approach, and treat the risk factors that could severely influence prognosis.

The autonomic nervous system

The ANS regulates visceral functions (circulation, respiration, thermoregulation, neuroendocrine secretion, and gastrointestinal and genitourinary functions) and integrated processes that control vital functions in response to internal and external demands with the final aim to maintain the homeostasis [2]. The ANS comprises the central autonomic network (CAN), which includes several interconnected areas distributed throughout the central nervous system (CNS) (insular cortex, anterior cingulate cortex, amygdala, hypothalamus, periaqueductal gray, parabrachial nucleus, nucleus of the solitary tract, ventrolateral reticular formation, and raphe nuclei)

that receive and integrate humoral, viscerosensory, and environmental inputs to generate specific autonomic, endocrine, and somatomotor responses, and two efferent pathways, the sympathetic and parasympathetic nervous system. Each efferent pathway is composed of a two-neuron system consisting of preganglionic neurons located in the brainstem and spinal cord connected with ganglionic neurons, which in turn make synapses with the target organ. The preganglionic neurons of both systems act through the neurotransmitter acetylcholine (Ach), which is also released by the postganglionic neurons of the parasympathetic nervous system. Norepinephrine (noradrenaline) (NE) is the primary postganglionic sympathetic neurotransmitter in all organs (except the sweat glands) receiving Ach. The sympathetic action is also amplified by the neurohormone epinephrine (adrenaline) (EPI), released by the adrenal medulla. Other neurochemical transmitters involved in ANS control include adenosine triphosphate, nitric oxide, and vasoactive intestinal polypeptide. The effects of each system in the regulation of visceral functions are listed in Table 29.1.

As dysfunction of the autonomic control of the cardiovascular system is frequently associated with sleep disorders leading to harmful consequences, it is important to bear in mind the main mechanism by which blood pressure (BP) is regulated in humans. BP is determined by cardiac output and total peripheral resistance. Cardiac output depends on venous return to the heart, cardiac contractility, and heart rate (HR). The moment-to-moment control of the arterial BP is exerted through a complex integration between cardiovascular reflexes and central autonomic influences. The baroreceptor reflex, or baroreflex, is the most important mechanism involved in this physiological task. The arterial baroreceptors are mechanoreceptors mainly located in the carotid sinuses and aortic arch, innervated by the glossopharyngeal and vagus nerves, respectively, which respond to changes in carotid or aortic stretch elicited by rise or fall in arterial BP. Activation of the baroreceptors in response to an increase in BP elicits a decrease in sympathetic activity and an increase in parasympathetic control of the heart, which cause a decrease in total peripheral resistance and HR and a subsequent reduction of venous return and cardiac output. Opposite consequences, tachycardia and vasoconstriction, are evoked by a decrease in arterial BP. The baroreflex also inhibits the release of vasopressin by magnocellular neurons of the supraoptic and paraventricular nuclei of the hypothalamus; vasopressin is involved in the long-term modification of BP. Primary baroreceptor afferents provide excitatory input to the nucleus of the solitary tract. This nucleus through its connections with the ventrolateral medulla,

Table 29.1 Main effects of the sympathetic and parasympathetic branches of the autonomic nervous system on visceral functions

Organ	Sympathetic branch	Parasympathetic branch
Pupil	Dilation	Constriction
Blood Vessel (arterioles)	Constriction	None
Lungs	Bronchodilation	Bronchodilation
Heart	Increase rate	Decrease rate
	Increase myocardial contractility	Decrease myocardial contractility
Gastrointestinal tract	Decrease motility	Increase motility
Kidney	Decrease output	None
Bladder	Relax detrusor	Relax sphincter
	Contract sphincter	Contract detrusor
Penis	Ejaculation	Erection
Sweat glands	Secretion	Palmar sweating
Piloerection	Increase	none
Lacrimal gland	Slight secretion	Secretion
Parotid gland	Slight secretion	Secretion
Submandibular gland	Slight secretion	Secretion

is responsible for the sympatho-inhibitory effect described above and, with a direct input to vagal preganglionic neurons in the nucleus ambiguus, elicit increased parasympathetic modulation of the heart. The activity of the baroreflex is continuously modulated in relation to prevailing behavioral and physiological conditions, by reciprocal connections of the CAN with the hypothalamus, contributing to both short- and long-term control of BP, including the circadian changes in BP between daytime activities and night-time sleep [3,4]. Finally, the arterial chemoreceptors, which are located within the carotid bodies and the aortic arch and primarily monitor blood oxygen variations, participate in the regulation of cardiovascular parameters. Their stimulation induced by hypoxia may lead to sympathetically mediated vasoconstriction with subsequent increase in BP and vagally mediated decrease in HR. This respiratory–cardiovascular interaction may be involved in the pathophysiology of harmful cardiovascular consequences of sleep disordered breathing, such as sympathetic overactivity and hypertension in OSAS [5–7].

Modulation of autonomic control during sleep

The sleep–wake cycle may be viewed as a rhythmic alternation between two contrasting systems, the arousal and anti-arousal system, which act as a kind of flip–flop switch allowing the transition from wake to sleep states and vice versa, with stability in any one of these states of vigilance allowed by the action of neurotransmitters, such as the orexin system [8].

The anti-arousal system, which promotes sleep, originates from the ventrolateral preoptic hypothalamic nucleus and inhibits the dorsal and ventral arousal systems at the level of their nuclei. The

neuronal populations that participate in the transition from wake to sleep and in the subsequent development of different sleep stages are localized nearby several areas of the CAN and also act through the same neurotransmitter. As a consequence the modulation of the ANS on vital functions changes according to behavioral state (wakefulness, NREM sleep, and REM sleep). A sympathetic prevalence is observed during wakefulness, while the parasympathetic tone is dominant during most of the sleep period, with variations during different sleep stages. Sympathetic activity is lower during NREM sleep compared with wakefulness and parasympathetic activity prevails, while during REM sleep, sympathetic activity is enhanced to levels comparable to those during wakefulness [9]. As a consequence, during NREM sleep, progressive decreases in arterial BP and HR, which become more pronounced from stage 1 to stage 3 NREM, are observed. Healthy normotensive persons show a BP decline during sleep of 10–20% compared with mean daytime values, a phenomenon generally referred to as "dipping" [10]. Similarly, sympathetic nerve activity, recorded in skeletal muscle and skin nerves, is decreased by more than half from wakefulness to deep NREM sleep [11]. The baroreflex function is differently modulated by central influences during the different sleep phases; in particular, during NREM sleep, the baroreflex maintains a slow HR despite a decrease in BP.

REM sleep is characterized by consistent variations in cardiovascular parameters and also in baroreflex activity. During tonic REM sleep, a marked bradycardia and decreased peripheral resistance are observed, resulting in a BP decrease below the levels reached in NREM sleep. This BP decrease is interrupted during bursts of rapid eye movements and muscle twitches by large transient increases in BP and HR, which are consequences of phasic inhibition of parasympathetic and phasic increase of sympathetic activity.

Changes in ventilation also occur during sleep, as breathing control is different during wake, NREM, and REM sleep. In the transition from wakefulness to sleep, a progressive inactivation of voluntary control of ventilation occurs, and during NREM sleep, ventilation is only automatically driven by chemical feedback related to arterial CO_2 and O_2 levels. Sleep onset is characterized by oscillations in breathing amplitude and sporadic central apneas, while during steady NREM sleep, breathing becomes progressively regular. In this stage, a reduction in minute ventilation is observed due to a decrease in tidal volume and respiratory frequency. REM sleep is characterized by breathing variability, which seems to be of central origin and is characterized by sudden changes in breathing amplitude and frequency concurrently with REM bursts.

During the entire sleep period, oscillations of EEG activity, systemic arterial BP, HR, and ventilation occur periodically, every 20–30 seconds [12,13] or transiently as part of the physiological response to an arousing stimulus [14].

Finally, body temperature decreases during NREM sleep, together with decreases in metabolic activity, glucose consumption, and cerebral blood flow. The regulation of body temperature is controlled by the ANS, which uses many sources of information to generate specific thermoregulatory responses (eg, sweating, shivering, and skin vasomotor adjustments). These mechanisms are still active during NREM sleep, whereas they are mostly suspended during REM sleep, characterized by an abolition of the thermoregulatory responses to environmental heating and cooling [15]. However, sleep and temperature are more widely interrelated, and thermoregulation also plays important role in initiating sleep, whose onset typically occurs on the declining portion of the circadian body temperature curve, when body heat loss is maximal [16].

Assessment of autonomic functions

Autonomic disorders may result from an overactivity or a failure of ANS functions and may present with a wide variety of symptoms and signs (Table 29.2). Their diagnosis may be arduous because of the overlap with other conditions and because mild symptoms might be concealed for years because of compensatory mechanisms. For these reasons, a carefully taken history and a detailed examination, including the detection of BP response to upright posture, are necessary when an autonomic dysfunction is suspected. The majority of ANS functions cannot be directly evaluated; therefore, the assessment of ANS integrity frequently relies on indirect methods, which measure the reflex responses of the target organs to physiological and pathological stimuli. Laboratory investigations are performed with the aims of detecting the presence of the autonomic dysfunction and its severity, determining whether the dysfunction is due to an impairment of the ANS or is secondary to other causes like drugs, assessing which branch of the ANS is mostly impaired, and locating the site of the lesion [17].

For example, the cardiovascular reflex tests (head-up tilt test (HUTT), Valsalva maneuver, handgrip, deep breathing and cold face) assess HR and BP changes in response to specific maneuvers and allow to reveal dysfunctions of the autonomic control of the cardiovascular system and to separately examin the integrity of the parasympathetic and sympathetic branches and the baroreceptor reflex. These tests are easy to perform, reproducible, sensitive, and specific, and are therefore suitable as first-line methods for both diagnosis and longitudinal evaluations. Blood samples can also be collected during the tests to quantify catecholamine levels, which provide measures of adrenal medullary and sympathetic neural activity. When an impairment of the physiological circadian variation of the autonomic parameters is suspected or the autonomic disturbances are manifested mainly during sleep, 24-hour or nocturnal polygraphic recordings may be performed to evaluate these parameters (eg, BP, HR, respiratory rate, oxygen saturation (SaO_2), temperature, and sudomotor activity) in relation to different physiological states (wakefulness, NREM sleep, and REM sleep) or degree of alertness (eg, autonomic arousal response). Several indirect techniques have also been applied to estimate baroreflex function. In particular, the slope of the HR changes in response to BP changes evoked by these methods is commonly referred to as baroreflex sensitivity (BRS, measured in ms/mmHg) [18]. BRS has a prognostic value in cardiovascular diseases like myocardial infarction and heart failure, and is impaired in pathological conditions, including sleep disorders like OSAS [4]. Spectral analysis of HR variability (HRV) calculated from the interval between two consecutive R-waves of QRS complexes (RR interval) in the ECG trace is also used to estimate sympathetic or parasympathetic modulation in autonomic cardiac control. The power spectrum of HRV comprises high-frequency components (HF: 0.15–0.4 Hz), reflecting parasympathetic outflow and breathing activity, low-frequency components (LF: 0.04–0.15 Hz), mediated mainly by sympathetic activity, and very low-frequency components (VLF: 0–0.04 Hz) whose physiological correlates are not fully understood. Even if the interpretation of the LF component as a pure marker of sympathetic activity

Table 29.2 Main clinical manifestations of autonomic dysfunction

Pupil	Abnormal miosis
	Abnormal mydriasis
Cardiovascular	Orthostatic hypotension
	Supine hypertension
	Paroxysmal hypertension
	Bradycardia
	Tachycardia
Urinary	Frequency
	Nocturia
	Urgency
	Incomplete bladder emptying
	Incontinence
Sexual	Erectile failure
	Priapism
	Retrograde ejaculation
	Ejaculatory failure
Sudomotor	Hypohidrosis
	Anhidrosis
	Hyperhidrosis
	Heat intolerance
	Hyperpyrexia

is still debated, the LF/HF ratio is widely used as a reliable indicator of sympathetic and parasympathetic outflow balance [19]. Finally, pharmacological probes (eg, growth hormone release in response to arginine or clonidine) [17] or imaging studies with radioactive tracers may distinguish the central or postganglionic site of the autonomic lesion. For example, cardiac 123-meta-iodo-benzylguanidine (MIBG) scintigraphy is used to assess cardiac sympathetic innervation which is impaired in postganglionic autonomic disorders [20]. As these tests are not available in all centers and are more invasive and expensive, they should be performed only as a second-line approach to better define an autonomic dysfunction that has not yet been ascertained.

Fatal familial insomnia

Fatal familial insomnia (FFI) is a rare prion disease whose clinical hallmark is agrypnia excitata syndrome, which is characterized by a progressive and untreatable sleep loss associated with motor and autonomic sympathetic overactivation persisting night and day and with a peculiar oneiric behavior (oneiric stupor) [21,22]. Somatomotor abnormalities also occur with variable latency and degree during the disease course [21,23]. The disease arises at a mean age of 50–51 years and is uniformly fatal, leading to death after either a short (<12 months) or a long (12–72 months) course following onset of insomnia. FFI is transmitted as an autosomal dominant trait and is linked to a missense mutation at codon 178 (D178N) of the prion protein gene located on chromosome 20 co-segregating with methionine at codon 129, the site of a common methionine–valine polymorphism [24,25]. Methionine-homozygous patients at codon 129 have on average shorter disease duration and a clinical phenotype slightly different to that of heterozygotes, who usually display fewer sleep and autonomic disturbances at onset but earlier and more severe motor abnormalities [26]. A sporadic form of fatal insomnia has also been described, sharing clinical and neuropathological features with FFI but lacking the D178N mutation [27]. From a clinical point of view, at disease onset, patients usually complain of progressive inability to initiate and maintain sleep. They also appear taciturn and apathetic and may look drowsy owing to sleep deprivation. An early progressive impairment of attention and vigilance is observed, whereas intellectual function remains substantially intact until the advanced stages of the disease. Autonomic signs accompany insomnia, such as a tendency to perspire, salivate, and lacrimate, tachycardia, hypertension, urgency, impotence, and slight evening pyrexia. Fluctuating diplopia is also a common early manifestation. Worsening of sleep and autonomic disturbance are associated with episodes of oneiric stupor, a peculiar hallucinatory behavior during which patients lose contact with the environment and display motor gestures mimicking daily life activities that they link to the content of a dream. These episodes initially last only a few seconds, but with disease progression patients become more confused, alternating between wakefulness and oneiric confusional states. Patients then develop disturbances of gait, spontaneous and evoked myoclonus, dysarthria, dysphagia, and pyramidal signs (hyper-reflexia and Babinski's sign), and finally progress into incomprehensible speech, inability to stand and walk, recurrent spasms, and occasional convulsive seizures. Death occurs from sudden cardiorespiratory failure or ensuing infections [21]. Longitudinal 24-hour polysomnographic studies document a progressive wake–sleep cycle derangement characterized by a drastic reduction in total sleep time, with loss of physiological sleep structures (sleep spindles, K-complexes, and delta waves). The dominant EEG pattern is characterized by stage 1 NREM sleep interspersed with short episodes of REM sleep with or without atonia, which can arise directly from wake [28]. Motor activity is markedly increased, with loss of physiological circadian motor rhythmicity [29]. Heart and breathing rate, BP, and core body temperature are higher in FFI patients compared with controls in 24-hour polysomnographic recordings. The circadian rhythms of HR and BP show a dominant 24-hour rhythm, with a progressive reduction in amplitude and a shift in phase. An early loss of the physiological nocturnal fall in BP with maintenance of nocturnal bradycardia, which is due mainly to parasympathetic activation, is also observed [30]. The rhythmic components of HR and BP, despite reductions in amplitude, persist even after the total disappearance of sleep, and only in the pre-terminal stage of FFI all the 24-hour variations are abolished. Further serial 24-hour monitoring of hormonal and catecholamine levels reveals a persistently increased plasma concentration of cortisol, which is known to modulate the vascular response to catecholamines and to act centrally to increase sympathetic activity, in contrast to a normal adrenocorticotropin level in the early stage of the disease. This pattern is followed by the appearance of a pathological nocturnal peak of cortisol and adrenocorticotropin, and then by a norepinephrine and epinephrine elevation. In contrast, melatonin secretion is reduced and it lacks the physiological nocturnal peak (Fig. 29.1).

All these data point toward an imbalanced autonomic control in FFI characterized by normal parasympathetic activity and a higher background and stimulated sympathetic activity. Sympathetic overactivity in these patients is also supported by the following observations: (1) an elevated norepinephrine plasma level at rest, increasing further under orthostatic stress; (2) an exaggerated BP increase in response to physiological stimuli (HUTT, Valsalva maneuver, or isometric handgrip); (3) absent BP rise after

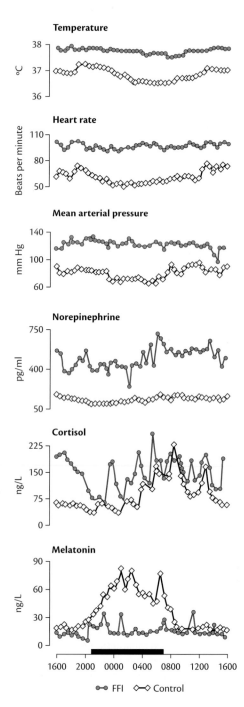

Fig. 29.1 The 24-hour circadian rhythms of body core temperature, heart rate, mean arterial pressure, norepinephrine, cortisol, and melatonin in a FFI 129 Met/Val patient compared with a normal sex- and age-matched control. The dark bar represents the dark period.

norepinephrine infusion due to down regulation of adrenoceptors; (4) abnormal HR increase after atropine infusion; (5) diminished depressor and sedative effects of clonidine, which usually inhibits central sympathetic activity; (6) increased mean level of resting awake muscle sympathetic nerve activity measured by microneurography [23,31,32]. Both sleep and autonomic disturbances in FFI are thought to be related to damage to the medial thalamus, which is severely affected in the disease. Neuropathological studies disclosed severe neuronal loss and reactive astrogliosis in the thalamus, especially the anterior ventral and mediodorsal nuclei, and PET studies showed a severe thalamic hypometabolism at the onset of insomnia and dysautonomia [23]. These nuclei belong to the circuits that connect the limbic prefrontal cortex to the hypothalamus and brainstem. In particular, the mediodorsal nucleus is deeply interconnected with several areas involved in autonomic control (anterior cingulate, insula, amygdala, and hypothalamus). The interruption of these circuits, disconnecting the limbic cortical areas that control instinctive behavior and the structures responsible for sleep and autonomic control, results in sleep loss associated with a persistent generalized activation syndrome [21,28].

Congenital central alveolar hypoventilation syndrome

The term "congenital central alveolar hypoventilation syndrome" (CCHS) defines a syndrome characterized by failure of automatic central control of breathing, resulting in hypoventilation during sleep and to a lesser degree during wakefulness, usually presenting in the newborn period. The diagnosis is made in the absence of other causes of hypoventilation, such as primary lung, cardiac, or neuromuscular diseases, other sleep or neurological disorders, brainstem lesions, or medication use. In the International Classification of Sleep Disorders (ICSD-3), CCHS is included under the category "Sleep-related hyperventilation disorders" [1]; however, this condition, despite long being considered a unique disorder of respiratory control, has recently been more correctly recognized as a disorder of autonomic regulation, owing to the coexistence of autonomic dysfunctions in other systems. Central hypoventilation is therefore the most severe manifestation of a generalized ANS dysfunction [33–36]. CCHS is also associated with neural crest tumors (neuroblastoma, ganglioneuroblastoma, and ganglioneuroma) and with Hirschsprung disease (congenital absence of ganglion cells in the myenteric plexus causing bowel obstruction) [35,37].

A genetic basis of the disease has been recognized with the discovery of mutations of the paired-like homeobox gene 2B (PHOX2B) on chromosome 4p12 [38,39], which encodes a transcription factor that plays a role in the regulation of neural crest cell migration and embryologic development of the ANS. Nearly 90% of CCHS patients are heterozygous for PHOX2B mutations causing expansion of the 20-residue polyalanine region of this transcription factor (polyalanine repeat mutations, PARMs), adding 4–13 copies and producing genotypes 20/24 to 20/33. The remaining 10% are heterozygous for nonpolyalanine repeat mutations (NPARMs), including missense, nonsense, and frameshift mutations of the PHOX2B gene. Most mutations occur de novo in CCHS, but 5–10% are inherited from a mosaic typically unaffected parents. The inheritance of the PHOX2B mutation from CCHS cases and from mosaic parents is autosomal dominant. A PHOX2B mutation is required

for the diagnosis of CCHS, and different mutations aid in predicting different phenotypes, including severity of the ventilatory control disorder and the autonomic dysfunction, risk of associated disorders, and adverse consequences like sudden cardiac death [35]. The disease usually manifests in the newborn period in otherwise healthy infants who do not breathe spontaneously or breathe only shallowly or erratically or experience episodes of hypoventilation or apnea, frequently requiring mechanical ventilation immediately after birth. Occasionally, patients may present in the first few months of life with acute life-threatening events (cyanosis, respiratory arrest, or hypoxic neurologic damage) or in childhood with signs of end-organ damage from chronic hypoxemia and hypercarbia (cor pulmonale, seizures, or developmental delay). Later-onset presentation has also been described and may be related to variable penetration of the PHOX2B mutations, to the possibility that environmental cofactors are needed to elicit the phenotype, or as a consequence of a delayed diagnosis due to unrecognized mild disease manifestations at an early age [35].

During sleep, the pattern of breathing in CCHS patients is characterized by hypoventilation with decreased tidal volume and respiratory rate, which is more severe during NREM than REM sleep. Central apnea may also occur, particularly at sleep onset [40,41]. Ventilation is generally adequate during wakefulness, but more severely affected children hypoventilate also during wakefulness.

Previous studies showed that children with CCHS lack ventilatory responsiveness to hypercapnia and hypoxemia, suggesting an abnormality of both central and peripheral chemoreceptor function. However it has also been demonstrated that during sleep, the arousal response to hypercapnia is not impaired in CCHS patients. This suggests as an alternative hypothesis that chemoreceptors are functionally intact, while the abnormality in CCHS may be located in areas of the brain involved in integration of chemoreceptor afferent pathways for ventilation [42,43].

A diffuse autonomic modulation impairment of both the sympathetic and parasympathetic branches of the ANS is observed in CCHS and includes abnormalities of pupillary response to light, esophageal dysmotility, swallowing dysfunction, decreased basal body temperature, poor heat tolerance and sporadic profuse sweating, elevated HR and reduced HR variability at rest, blunted BP response to actively standing, reduced BRS, reduced respiratory sinus arrhythmia, and abrupt asystole [34,44,45]. This diffuse autonomic modulation impairment supports the hypothesis of significant functional alterations of brain areas involved in autonomic control. Macey and co-workers [46] used functional magnetic resonance imaging (fMRI) techniques to examine signal responses in the brains of CCHS patients compared with controls while performing a voluntary Valsalva maneuver, which elicits a sequence of sympathetic and parasympathetic actions. Increased signals emerged in control over CCHS patients in the cingulate, right parietal cortex, cerebellar cortex, fastigial nucleus, and basal ganglia, whereas anterior cerebellar cortical sites and deep nuclei, dorsal midbrain, and dorsal pons showed increased signals in the patient group. The dorsal and ventral medulla showed delayed responses in CCHS patients. The authors suggested that the delayed responses in medullary sensory and output regions and the aberrant reactions in cerebellar and pontine sensorimotor coordination areas may be implicated in the rapid cardiorespiratory integration deficits in CCHS.

A further fMRI study, assessing neural response patterns to Valsalva maneuver in 9 CCHS patients and 25 controls, demonstrated abnormal responses in limbic areas such as the amygdala and hippocampus, and muted responses across other multiple brain areas, in particular in the insulae and ventral cerebellum in patients compared with controls [47].

Patients with CCHS require lifetime mechanically assisted ventilation during sleep to ensure adequate ventilation and oxygenation, and to prevent acute and long-term consequences. Some patients (from 6% to 33%) require ventilatory support during both wakefulness and sleep. Positive-pressure ventilators via tracheostomy, bilevel positive airway pressure, negative-pressure ventilators, and diaphragm pacing can all be used in these patients. The mortality rate varies from 8% to 38% among studies and has been reduced with modern techniques for home ventilation [35,43].

Obstructive sleep apnea syndrome

Obstructive sleep apnea syndrome (OSAS) is characterized by repetitive episodes of complete (apnea) or partial (hypopnea) upper airway obstruction occurring during sleep, which usually result in blood oxygen desaturation and often terminate by brief arousal [1]. The apneic episodes are associated with peculiar fluctuations in HR characterized by an HR decrease at onset of apnea, followed by abrupt tachycardia on resumption of breathing generally accompanied by an arousal [48]. In addition, hyperactivity of the sympathetic nervous system, recorded through muscle sympathetic nerve activity, has been documented in relation to these respiratory events [5–7] and confirmed also by spectral analysis of HRV, which demonstrated increased LF and LF/HF ratio during sleep apnea episodes [49].

Chemoreflex stimulation induce by repeated hypoxia is the main mechanism implicated in enhanced sympathetic activity during sleep apnea [7]. However, a depression of spontaneous BRS, which has been demonstrated in severe OSAS patients, may also contribute to a further increase in sympathetic activity [50].

OSAS is associated with an impaired autonomic control of cardiovascular parameters and an enhanced sympathetic tone not only during sleep but also during wakefulness. Cortelli and co-workers [51] demonstrated that normotensive OSAS patients have higher HR and norepinephrine plasma levels at rest during wakefulness and a higher BP response to HUTT compared with controls, suggesting sympathetic overactivity.

Analysis of the circadian rhythm of HRV confirmed an enhanced sympathetic modulation from morning to noon (lower mean HF value and higher mean LF/HF ratio) in OSAS patients compared with controls [52]. Finally, elevated levels of plasma and urinary catecholamines have been demonstrated in these patients while awake [53]. The main consequence of the described alterations of autonomic control of the cardiovascular system in OSAS patients is an increased risk of developing cardiovascular and cerebrovascular diseases (hypertension, myocardial infarction, arrhythmias, heart failure, and stroke). There are now several epidemiological studies supporting a direct contribution of sleep apnea to hypertension, and many hypotheses have been advanced to explain the causal relationship between the two conditions [53,54]. However, the sympathetic overactivity demonstrated in OSAS patients during both wakefulness and sleep seems to have the prominent role in the etiology of OSAS-related hypertension [53].

In OSAS patients, still normotensive during the day, a reduced BRS and a hyperactive chemoreflex function were demonstrated in the awake state. This peculiar combination of reduced baroreflex and hyperactive chemoreflex function suggested that a central remodeling of autonomic cardiovascular control may precede the development of daytime hypertension [4,51]. It has been hypothesized that sympathetic activation, which occurs as an acute effect of OSAS, when repeated over a long period of time in predisposed subjects, may change the afferent regulation of the barosensitive neurons located in the nucleus of the solitary tract. This could attenuate their inhibitory effect on the sympatho-excitatory neurons, which could in turn be responsible for the sustained chronic peripheral sympathetic overactivation and its cardiovascular consequence [4].

The alteration of cardiac autonomic modulation and risk of developing cardiovascular diseases, in particular hypertension, have also been correlated with presence of excessive daytime sleepiness in OSAS patients. In fact, patients with both OSAS and excessive daytime sleepiness, when compared with patients without, had significantly lower BRS and significantly higher LF/HF ratio during the different stages of sleep [55]. In addition the association between sleep disordered breathing and hypertension is stronger in patients who report daytime sleepiness than in those who do not [56]. Lombardi and co-workers hypothesized that the common mechanism causing excessive daytime sleepiness and cardiac autonomic dysfunction may lie in the occurrence of apnea-related autonomic arousals from sleep, resulting in further sympathetic overactivation [55].

Finally, findings from cross-sectional studies suggest a high prevalence of cardiac arrhythmias in patients with OSAS and a high prevalence of OSAS in those with cardiac arrhythmias. Bradycardia, sinus pauses, second-degree heart block, atrial fibrillation, ventricular repolarization disturbances, ventricular premature complexes, and ventricular tachycardia have been associated with OSAS. Further, OSAS-related arrhythmogenesis has also been implicated in sudden cardiac death [57–60].

Several mechanisms have been involved in the genesis of dysrhythmias in OSAS, including (1) intermittent hypoxia associated with both ANS activation and increased oxidative stress, which could in turn lead to cardiac cellular damage and alteration in myocardial excitability; (2) recurrent arousals from sleep, causing further sympathetic activation; (3) increased negative intrathoracic pressure, which may mechanically stretch the myocardial walls and thus promote acute changes in myocardial excitability as well as structural remodeling of the myocardium [59].

Treatment of OSAS with continuous positive-airway pressure has been demonstrated to significantly improve cardiovascular autonomic modulation, reducing sympathetic overactivity and the risk of development of cardiovascular diseases like hypertension. Preliminary evidence from uncontrolled interventional studies suggests also that treatment of OSAS may prevent cardiac arrhythmias. However randomized studies are still needed to address this important issue [53,54,59].

Narcolepsy with cataplexy

Narcolepsy with cataplexy (NC) is a sleep disorder characterized by excessive daytime sleepiness and cataplexy (sudden loss of bilateral muscle tone provoked by emotions) and usually associated with sleep paralysis, hypnagogic hallucinations, and nocturnal sleep disruption [1]. Loss of orexin neurons of the lateral and posterior hypothalamus has been demonstrated in NC. These neurons are connected with cerebral areas involved in central autonomic control (prefrontal cortex, hypothalamus, limbic structures, and brainstem autonomic nuclei). Orexins, also known as hypocretin 1 and 2, are neuropeptides implicated in several physiological functions (arousal, energy homeostasis, feeding, thermoregulation, and neuroendocrine and cardiovascular control), which are mediated by changes in the ANS [61]. Autonomic dysfunctions in NC patients have been observed [62], including abnormal pupillometry function [63–65], erectile dysfunction [66], impaired autonomic control of the cardiovascular system during sleep [67,68], and wakefulness [69]. Furthermore, increased body mass index and increased risk of type 2 diabetes have been frequently reported in NC patients. Although association could reflect a disturbance in food intake and energy metabolism related to orexin deficiency, both the pathophysiological mechanism and the relationship between orexin deficit and metabolic syndrome remain unclear [70–73]. Particular interest has recently been directed at dysfunctions of the autonomic control of the cardiovascular system in NC patients owing to their possible contribution to an increased cardiovascular risk in this population. The effect of orexins on the cardiovascular system is controversial. The initial animal studies indicated that the orexin system triggered sympathetic activation, as intracerebroventricular or brain tissue microinjections of orexin in rats caused increases in HR, BP, and body temperature. Further orexin-knockout or orexin-neuron-depleted mice showed an attenuated sympatho-excitatory response to stress. However, opposite results were found in these models of orexin-deficient mice during sleep, as they demonstrated a blunted decrease in BP on passing from wakefulness to NREM sleep and an enhanced increase in BP on passing from NREM to REM sleep compared with controls. Similarly, recent studies suggested that orexin deficit in humans is not unequivocally associated with reduced sympathetic tone but may be associated with sympathetic cardiovascular activation, parasympathetic withdrawal, or both. Grimaldi and colleagues [67] demonstrated in drug-free NC patients compared with controls significantly higher systolic BP values during nighttime REM sleep and a blunted decrease in nocturnal BP (non-dipping pattern) (Fig. 29.2). These data were confirmed by a further study, which found a high percentage of NC patients showing a non-dipper profile [68], suggesting an increase in sympathetic modulation during sleep. However, an attenuated HR response to leg movements [74] and arousal [75] during sleep pointing toward a decrease sympathetic tone was also observed.

Three studies carried out spectral analyses of HRV in NC patients and obtained different results. Fronczek and colleagues found a higher power in all frequency bands in the supine awake condition, associated with a similar LF/HF ratio, and hypothesized a reduced sympathetic tone in NC patients [76]. In contrast, an increase LF/HF ratio (increased sympathetic modulation) during wakefulness preceding sleep [69] and an enhanced sympathetic activity at rest [77] were observed in NC patients compared with controls.

In conclusion, impaired autonomic control of the cardiovascular system in NC patients has been observed, and despite the fact that the direction of the cardiovascular autonomic changes is not unequivocally ascertained, the clinical importance of these findings, particularly if it is confirmed that an overactivity of the sympathetic branch exists in NC, may be relevant due to a possible increased cardiovascular risk in this population.

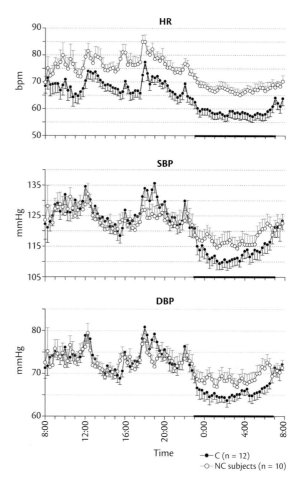

Fig. 29.2 Mean ± standard error (SE) values of heart rate (HR), systolic blood pressure (SBP), and diastolic blood pressure (DBP) during 24 hours in control subjects (C) and patients with narcolepsy with cataplexy (NC). The dark bar represents the dark period. SE has been reported in one direction for clarity.

REM sleep behavior disorder

REM sleep behavior disorder (RBD) is a sleep parasomnia characterized by dream-enacting behaviors, often violent and injurious, occurring during REM sleep and associated with loss of the physiological REM muscle atonia [1]. This condition may be either idiopathic (iRBD) or associated with another neurologic disorder [78]. RBD has been frequently observed in the α-synucleinopathies, neurodegenerative disorders characterized by the presence of intracellular inclusions containing α-synuclein, namely, Parkinson disease (PD), Lewy body dementia (LBD), and multiple system atrophy (MSA), which can also present dysfunctions of the ANS. The onset of RBD can precede, by years, the onset of these diseases [79–82]. For this reason, several studies have tried to disclose signs predictive of the future development of a neurodegenerative disease in patients with iRBD by means of clinical, neuropsychological, electrophysiological, and neuroradiological modalities. Impairment of autonomic functions, in particular a dysfunction in the autonomic control of the cardiovascular system, has been observed in iRBD. Mahowald and Schenck first reported a lack of HR increase in association with the vigorous behaviors during REM sleep shown by these patients [83]. Three subsequent studies demonstrated a blunted HR response associated with sleep-related movements in iRBD patients compared with controls and subjects with restless legs syndrome [84–86]. In addition, the physiological parasympathetic withdrawal and sympathetic prevalence observed during REM sleep compared with NREM sleep is lacking in iRBD patients [87]. As autonomic cardiac dysfunction and in particular a sympathetic failure is also common in patients with α-synucleinopathies, several studies have investigated whether the presence of this dysfunction in iRBD predicts the subsequent development of neurodegenerative diseases.

Frauscher and colleagues [88] evaluated 15 patients with iRBD and an equal number of patients with PD and healthy controls using cardiovascular autonomic function testing and the Composite Autonomic Scoring Scale [89], a validated, self-completed questionnaire on autonomic symptoms, and demonstrated the presence of an autonomic dysfunction in patients with iRBD of an intermediate degree between controls and PD patients. The authors suggested that iRBD could be an early manifestation of α-synucleinopathies and that iRBD patients with autonomic dysfunctions might be at particular risk for developing one of these diseases. However, previous studies led to different conclusions. A retrospective study showed an impairment of cardiac autonomic control in patients initially diagnosed with iRBD compared with controls; however, no difference was detected among RBD patients who subsequently did or did not develop a neurodegenerative disease [90]. Similarly, it was observed that autonomic dysfunction was no worse in patients with both PD and RBD than in patients with iRBD, suggesting that RBD predicts autonomic dysfunction better than the presence of PD [91,92]. Consistent with these clinical studies, Miyamoto and colleagues [93], by means of cardiac MIBG scintigraphy, which assesses cardiac sympathetic innervations, showed a similar loss of sympathetic terminals in patients with iRBD and PD, while Kashihara and co-authors [94] demonstrated that MIBG uptake is more markedly reduced in iRBD compared with PD patients. These studies suggested that autonomic dysfunction is integrally related to the pathogenesis of RBD rather than a preclinical sign of a specific neurodegenerative disease. The importance of finding early markers of neurodegenerative disease indicates that systematic prospective autonomic investigations are required in iRBD patients to better clarify the association between autonomic dysfunction and RBD and their predictive role in the early diagnosis of neurodegenerative diseases.

Conclusions

Over the past several years, many experimental and human studies have shown that autonomic disorders may influence the physiology of sleep, and conversely sleep disorders may affect ANS functions. Sleep and the ANS are interdependent by virtue of their common controls, neurobiological substrates, and functions.

Indeed, taking into account ANS and sleep with bidirectional interactions, it is possible to understand the complexity of many sleep disorders and their impact on health and to open new insights into the regulation of sleep and the integrative function of ANS.

References

1. American Academy of Sleep Medicine (AASM), The international classification of sleep disorders, 3rd edition: diagnostic and coding manual. Darien, IL: American Academy of Sleep Medicine, 2014.
2. Benarroch EE, ed. Central autonomic network: functional organization and clinical correlations. Armonk, NY: Futura, 1997.
3. Benarroch EE. The arterial baroreflex: functional organization and involvement in neurologic disease. Neurology 2008;71:1733–8.
4. Cortelli P, Lombardi C, Montagna P, Parati G. Baroreflex modulation during sleep and in obstructive sleep apnea syndrome. Auton Neurosci 2012;169:7–11.
5. Hedner J, Ejnell H, Sellgren J, et al. Is high and fluctuating muscle nerve sympathetic activity in the sleep apnoea syndrome of pathogenetic importance for the development of hypertension? J Hypertens 1988; Suppl 6:S529–31.
6. Watanabe T, Mano T, Iwase S, et al. Enhanced muscle sympathetic nerve activity during sleep apnea in the elderly. J Auton Nerv Syst 1992;37:223–6.
7. Somers VK, Dyken ME, Clary MP, Abboud FM. Sympathetic neural mechanisms in obstructive sleep apnea. J Clin Invest 1995;96:1897–904.
8. Saper CB, Scammell TE, Lu J. Hypothalamic regulation of sleep and circadian rhythms. Nature 2005; 437:1257–63.
9. Mancia G. Autonomic modulation of the cardiovascular system during sleep. N Engl J Med 1993;328:347–9.
10. Smolensky MH, Hermida RC, Castriotta RJ, Portaluppi F. Role of sleep–wake cycle on blood pressure circadian rhythms and hypertension. Sleep Med 2007; 8:668–80.
11. Somers VK, Dyken ME, Mark AL, Abboud FM. Sympathetic-nerve activity during sleep in normal subjects. N Engl J Med 1993;328:303–7.
12. Lugaresi E, Coccagna G, Mantovani M, Lebrun R. Some periodic phenomena arising during drowsiness and sleep in man. Electroencephalogr Clin Neurophysiol 1972;32:701–5.
13. Terzano M, Mancia D, Salati M, et al. The cyclic alternating pattern as a physiologic component of normal NREM sleep. Sleep 1985;8:137–45.
14. Sforza E, Jouny C, Ibanez V. Cardiac activation during arousal in humans: further evidence for hierarchy in the arousal response. Clin Neurophysiol 2000; 111: 1611–9.
15. Parmeggiani PL. Interaction between sleep and thermoregulation: an aspect of the control of behavioral states. Sleep 1987;10:426–35.
16. Krauchi K. The thermophysiological cascade leading to sleep initiation in relation to phase of entrainment. Sleep Med Revs 2007;11:439–51.
17. Mathias CJ. Autonomic diseases: clinical features and laboratory evaluation. J Neurol Neurosurg Psychiatry 2003;74 Suppl 3:iii31–41.
18. Parati G, Di Rienzo M, Mancia G. How to measure baroreflex sensitivity: from the cardiovascular laboratory to daily life. J Hypertens 2000; 18, 7–19.
19. Task Force of the European Society of Cardiology and the North American Society of Pacing and Electrophysiology. Heart rate variability: standards of measurement, physiological interpretation, and clinical use. Circulation 1996;93:1043–65.
20. Yamashina S, Yamazaki J. Neuronal imaging using SPECT. Eur J Nucl Med Mol Imaging 2007; 34:939–50
21. Montagna P, Gambetti P, Cortelli P, Lugaresi E. Familial and sporadic fatal insomnia. Lancet Neurol 2003; 2:167–76.
22. Guaraldi P, Calandra-Buonaura G, Terlizzi R, et al. Oneiric stupor: the peculiar behavior of agrypnia excitata. Sleep Med 2011;12 Suppl 2:S64–7.
23. Cortelli P, Parchi P, Contin M, et al. Cardiovascular dysautonomia in fatal familial insomnia. Clin Auton Res 1991;1:15–21.
24. Medori R, Tritschler HJ, LeBlanc A, et al. Fatal familial insomnia, a prion disease with a mutation at codon 178 of the prion protein gene. N Engl J Med 1992 13;326:444–9.
25. Goldfarb LG, Petersen RB, Tabaton M, et al. Fatal familial insomnia and familial Creutzfeldt–Jakob disease: disease phenotype determined by a DNA polymorphism. Science 1992;258:806–8.
26. Montagna P, Cortelli P, Avoni P, et al. Clinical features of fatal familial insomnia: phenotypic variability in relation to a polymorphism at codon 129 of the prion protein gene. Brain Pathol 1998;8:515–20.
27. Parchi P, Petersen RB, Chen SG, et al. Molecular pathology of fatal familial insomnia. Brain Pathol 1998;8:539–48.
28. Lugaresi E, Provini F, Cortelli P. Agrypnia excitata. Sleep Med 2011;12 Suppl 2:S3–10.

29. Plazzi G, Schutz Y, Cortelli P, et al. Motor overactivity and loss of motor circadian rhythm in fatal familial insomnia: an actigraphic study. Sleep 1997;20:739–42.

30. Portaluppi F, Cortelli P, Avoni P, et al. Diurnal blood pressure variation and hormonal correlates in fatal familial insomnia. Hypertension 1994;23:569–76.

31. Benarroch EE, Stotz-Potter EH. Dysautonomia in fatal familial insomnia as an indicator of the potential role of the thalamus in autonomic control. Brain Pathol 1998;8:527–30.

32. Donadio V, Montagna P, Pennisi M, et al. Agrypnia excitata: a microneurographic study of muscle sympathetic nerve activity. Clin Neurophysiol 2009;120:1139–42.

33. Mellins RB, Balfour HH Jr, Turino GM, Winters RW. Failure of automatic control of ventilation (Ondine's curse). Report of an infant born with this syndrome and review of the literature. Medicine (Baltimore) 1970;49:487–504.

34. Weese-Mayer DE, Silvestri JM, Huffman AD, et al. Case/control family study of autonomic nervous system dysfunction in idiopathic congenital central hypoventilation syndrome. Am J Med Genet 2001;100:237–45.

35. Weese-Mayer DE, Berry-Kravis EM, Ceccherini I, et al.; ATS Congenital Central Hypoventilation Syndrome Subcommittee. An official ATS clinical policy statement. Congenital central hypoventilation syndrome: genetic basis, diagnosis, and management. Am J Respir Crit Care Med 2010;181:626–44.

36. Rand CM, Patwari PP, Carroll MS, Weese-Mayer DE. Congenital central hypoventilation syndrome and sudden infant death syndrome: disorders of autonomic regulation. Semin Pediatr Neurol 2013;20:44–55.

37. Haddad GG, Mazza NM, Defendini R, et al. Congenital failure of automatic control of ventilation, gastrointestinal motility and heart rate. Medicine (Baltimore) 1978; 57:517–26.

38. Amiel J, Laudier B, Attié-Bitach T, et al. Polyalanine expansion and frameshift mutations of the paired-like homeobox gene *PHOX2B* in congenital central hypoventilation syndrome. Nat Genet 2003;33:459–61.

39. Weese-Mayer DE, Berry-Kravis EM, Zhou L, et al. Idiopathic congenital central hypoventilation syndrome: analysis of genes pertinent to early autonomic nervous system embryologic development and identification of mutations in *PHOX2B*. Am J Med Genet A 2003;123:267–78.

40. Commare MC, Francois B, Estournet B, Barois A. Ondine's curse: a discussion of five cases. Neuropediatrics 1993;24:313–18.

41. Huang J, Colrain IM, Panitch HB, et al. Effect of sleep stage on breathing in with central hypoventilation. J Appl Physiol 2008;105:44–53.

42. Marcus CL, Bautista DB, Amihyia A, Ward SL, Keens TG. Hypercapneic arousal responses in children with congenital central hypoventilation syndrome. Pediatrics 1991;88:993–8.

43. Healy F, Marcus CL. Congenital central hypoventilation syndrome in children. Paediatr Respir Rev 2011;12:253–63.

44. Trang H, Girard A, Laude D, Elghozi JL. Short-term blood pressure and heart rate variability in congenital central hypoventilation syndrome (Ondine's curse). Clin Sci (Lond) 2005;108:225–30.

45. Patwari PP, Stewart TM, Rand CM, et al. Pupillometry in congenital central hypoventilation syndrome (CCHS): quantitative evidence of autonomic nervous system dysregulation. Pediatr Res 2012;71:280–5.

46. Macey KE, Macey PM, Woo MA, et al. fMRI signal changes in response to forced expiratory loading in congenital central hypoventilation syndrome. J Appl Physiol 2004;97:1897–907.

47. Ogren JA, Macey PM, Kumar R, et al. Central autonomic regulation in congenital central hypoventilation syndrome. Neuroscience 2010;167:1249–56.

48. Guilleminault C, Connolly S, Winkle R, et al. Cyclical variation of the heart rate in sleep apnea syndrome. Mechanisms, and usefulness of 24 h electrocardiography as a screening technique. Lancet 1984;1:126–31.

49. Vanninen E, Tuunainen A, Kansanen M, et al. Cardiac sympathovagal balance during sleep apnea episodes. Clin Physiol 1996;16:209–16.

50. Parati G, Di Rienzo M, Bonsignore MR, et al. Autonomic cardiac regulation in obstructive sleep apnea syndrome: evidence from spontaneous baroreflex analysis during sleep. J Hypertens 1997;15:1621–6.

51. Cortelli P, Parchi P, Sforza E, et al. Cardiovascular autonomic dysfunction in normotensive awake subjects with obstructive sleep apnoea syndrome. Clin Auton Res 1994;4:57–62.

52. Noda A, Yasuma F, Okada T, Yokota M. Circadian rhythm of autonomic activity in patients with obstructive sleep apnea syndrome. Clin Cardiol 1998;21:271–6.

53. Fletcher EC. Sympathetic over activity in the etiology of hypertension of obstructive sleep apnea. Sleep 2003;26:15–19.

54. Bradley TD, Floras JS. Obstructive sleep apnoea and its cardiovascular consequences. Lancet 2009;373:82–93.

55. Lombardi C, Parati G, Cortelli P, et al. Daytime sleepiness and neural cardiac modulation in sleep-related breathing disorders. J Sleep Res 2008;147:231–4.

56. Kapur VK, Resnick HE, Gottlieb DJ; Sleep Heart Health Study Group. Sleep disordered breathing and hypertension: does self-reported sleepiness modify the association? Sleep 2008;31:1127–32.

57. Gami AS, Howard DE, Olson EJ, Somers VK. Day–night pattern of sudden death in obstructive sleep apnea. N Engl J Med 2005;352:1206–14.

58. Leung RS. Sleep-disordered breathing: autonomic mechanisms and arrhythmias. Prog Cardiovasc Dis 2009;51:324–38.

59. Rossi VA, Stradling JR, Kohler M. Effects of obstructive sleep apnoea on heart rhythm. Eur Respir J 2013;41:1439–51.

60. Gami AS, Olson EJ, Shen WK, et al. Obstructive sleep apnea and the risk of sudden cardiac death: a longitudinal study of 10,701 adults. J Am Coll Cardiol 2013;62:610–6.

61. Grimaldi D, Silvani A, Benarroch EE, Cortelli P. Orexin/hypocretin system and autonomic control: new insights and clinical correlations. Neurology 2014;82:271–8.

62. Plazzi G, Moghadam KK, Maggi LS, et al. Autonomic disturbances in narcolepsy. Sleep Med Rev 2011;15:187–96.

63. Yoss RE, Moyer NJ, Ogle KN. The pupillogram and narcolepsy. A method to measure decreased levels of wakefulness. Neurology 1969;19:921–8.

64. Norman ME, Dyer JA. Ophthalmic manifestations of narcolepsy. Am J Ophthalmol 1987;103:81–6.

65. O'Neill WD, Oroujeh AM, Keegan AP, Merritt SL. Neurological pupillary noise in narcolepsy. J Sleep Res 1996;5:265e71.

66. Karacan I. Erectile dysfunction in narcoleptic patients. Sleep 1986;9:227–31.

67. Grimaldi D, Calandra-Buonaura G, Provini F, et al. Abnormal sleep-cardiovascular system interaction in narcolepsy with cataplexy: effects of hypocretin deficiency in humans. Sleep 2012;35:519–28.

68. Dauvilliers Y, Jaussent I, Krams B, et al. Non-dipping blood pressure profile in narcolepsy with cataplexy. PLoS One 2012;7(6):e38977

69. Ferini-Strambi L, Spera A, Oldani A, et al. Autonomic function in narcolepsy: power spectrum analysis of heart rate variability. J Neurol 1997;244:252–5.

70. Schuld A, Hebebrand J, Geller F, Pollmächer T. Increased body-mass index in patients with narcolepsy. Lancet 2000; 355:1274–5.

71. Honda Y, Doi Y, Ninomiya R, Ninomiya C. Increased frequency of non-insulin-dependent diabetes mellitus among narcoleptic patients. Sleep 1986;9:254–9.

72. Heier MS, Jansson TS, Gautvik KM. Cerebrospinal fluid hypocretin 1 deficiency, overweight, and metabolic dysregulation in patients with narcolepsy. J Clin Sleep Med 2011;7:653–8.

73. Poli F, Plazzi G, Di Dalmazi G, et al. Body mass index independent metabolic alterations in narcolepsy with cataplexy. Sleep 2009;32:1491–7.

74. Dauvilliers Y, Pennestri MH, Whittom S, et al. Autonomic response to periodic leg movements during sleep in narcolepsy–cataplexy. Sleep 2011;34:219–23.

75. Sorensen GL, Knudsen S, Petersen ER, et al. Attenuated heart rate response is associated with hypocretin deficiency in patients with narcolepsy. Sleep 2013;36:91–8.

76. Fronczek R, Overeem S, Reijntjes R, et al. Increased heart rate variability but normal resting metabolic rate in hypocretin/orexin-deficient human narcolepsy. J Clin Sleep Med 2008;4:248–54.

77. Grimaldi D, Pierangeli G, Barletta G, et al. Spectral analysis of heart rate variability reveals an enhanced sympathetic activity in narcolepsy with cataplexy. Clin Neurophysiol 2010;121:1142–7.

78. Boeve BF. REM sleep behavior disorder: updated review of the core features, the REM sleep behavior disorder–neurodegenerative disease association, evolving concepts, controversies, and future directions. Ann N Y Acad Sci 2010;1184:15–54.

79. Schenck CH1, Boeve BF, Mahowald MW. Delayed emergence of a parkinsonian disorder or dementia in 81% of older men initially diagnosed with idiopathic rapid eye movement sleep behavior disorder: a 16-year update on a previously reported series. Sleep Med 2013;14:744–8.

80. Boeve BF, Silber MH, Ferman TJ, Lin SC, et al. Clinicopathologic correlations in 172 cases of rapid eye movement sleep behavior disorder with or without a coexisting neurologic disorder. Sleep Med 2013;14:754–62.

81. Iranzo A, Tolosa E, Gelpi E, et al. Neurodegenerative disease status and post-mortem pathology in idiopathic rapid-eye-movement sleep behaviour disorder: an observational cohort study. Lancet Neurol 2013;12:443–53.

82. Iranzo A, Fernández-Arcos A, Tolosa E, et al. Neurodegenerative disorder risk in idiopathic REM sleep behavior disorder: study in 174 patients. PLoS One 2014;9(2):e89741.

83. Mahowald MW, Schenck CH. REM sleep behavior disorder. In: Kryger MH, Roth T, Dement WC, eds. Principle and practice of sleep medicine, 2nd ed. Philadelphia, PA: WB Saunders, 1994:574–88.

84. Ferini-Strambi L, Oldani A, Zucconi M, Smirne S. Cardiac autonomic activity during wakefulness and sleep in REM sleep behavior disorder. Sleep 1996;19:367–9.

85. Fantini ML, Michaud M, Gosselin N, et al. Periodic leg movements in REM sleep behavior disorder and related autonomic and EEG activation. J Neurol 2002;59:1889–94.

86. Sorensen GL, Kempfner J, Zoetmulder M, et al. Attenuated heart rate response in REM sleep behavior disorder and Parkinson's disease. Mov Disord 2012;27:888–94.

87. Lanfranchi PA, Fradette L, Gagnon JF, et al. Cardiac autonomic regulation during sleep in idiopathic REM sleep behavior disorder. Sleep 2007;30:1019–25.

88. Frauscher B, Nomura T, Duerr S, et al. Investigation of autonomic function in idiopathic REM sleep behavior disorder. J Neurol 2012;259:1056–61.

89. Suarez GA, Opfer-Gehrking TL, Offord KP, et al. The autonomic symptom profile: a new instrument to assess autonomic symptoms. Neurology 1999;52:523–8.

90. Postuma RB, Lanfranchi PA, Blais H, et al. Cardiac autonomic dysfunction in idiopathic REM sleep behavior disorder. Mov Disord 2010;25:2304–10.

91. Postuma RB, Gagnon JF, Vendette M, Montplaisir JY. Markers of neurodegeneration in idiopathic rapid eye movement sleep behaviour disorder and Parkinson's disease. Brain 2009;132:3298–307.

92. Postuma RB, Montplaisir J, Lanfranchi P, et al. Cardiac autonomic denervation in Parkinson's disease is linked to REM sleep behavior disorder. Mov Disord 2011;26:1529–33.

93. Miyamoto T, Miyamoto M, Inoue Y, et al. Reduced cardiac ^{123}I-MIBG scintigraphy in idiopathic REM sleep behavior disorder. Neurology 2006;67:2236–8.

94. Kashihara K, Imamura T, Shinya T. Cardiac ^{123}I-MIBG uptake is reduced more markedly in patients with REM sleep behavior disorder than in those with early stage Parkinson's disease. Parkinsonism Relat Disord 2010;16:252–5.

CHAPTER 30

Neuromuscular disorders and sleep

Katerina Sajgalikova, Erik K. St. Louis, and Peter Gay

Introduction

This chapter examines the range of sleep disturbances seen in patients with neuromuscular disorders, particularly emphasizing sleep-related breathing disorders, which may be a presenting manifestation of neuromuscular disorders, and which significantly contribute to morbidity and mortality in this patient population. It provides an overview of physiological and pathological alterations in neuromuscular breathing mechanisms and control during sleep. The symptoms and forms of sleep disordered breathing (SDB) seen in specific neuromuscular disorders such as amyotrophic lateral sclerosis (ALS), myopathies, and disorders of neuromuscular junction transmission are reviewed. The chapter concludes with a discussion of management strategies for neuromuscular disorder patients with SDB, which is common in such patients, requiring generalists, neurologists, and sleep physicians to work together toward prompt diagnosis and optimal treatment approaches.

Neuromuscular contributions to sleep-related breathing

Patients afflicted by neuromuscular disorders may develop respiratory muscle weakness causing impairment of pulmonary gas exchange, which may in turn lead to sleep-related breathing disorders. SDB often manifests earlier than daytime respiratory symptoms and may be the presenting manifestation in patients with neuromuscular disorders. Hence, unrecognized and untreated SDB may result in chronic or acute respiratory failure, which is the most common cause of morbidity and mortality in up to 80% of patients with neuromuscular diseases [1].

Pulmonary function abnormalities in neuromuscular patients most often include reduced vital capacity (VC), which is particularly useful for following disease progression, treatment response, or evaluation in the acute setting, since VC measurement assesses both inspiration and expiration. Inspiratory muscle weakness demonstrates restrictive physiology with decreased VC, total lung capacity (TLC), functional residual capacity (FRC), and normal FEV1/FVC (forced vital capacity) ratio. Residual volume (RV) progressively increases as expiratory muscle weakness progresses [2] (Fig. 30.1). VC generally remains normal (or minimally reduced) until respiratory muscle strength pressures are under 50% of predicted values [3]. As respiratory muscle weakness progresses, VC falls in a curvilinear fashion [3]. Diaphragmatic paralysis may result in marked orthopnea due to markedly decreased supine VC. Maximum expiratory and inspiratory flow–volume curves show a decline in inspiratory flow, and reduced peak expiratory flow at higher volumes, correlating with the reduction in FVC, with blunting of the expiratory curve contour and abrupt expiratory flow cessation immediately prior to reaching RV. Maximum voluntary ventilation is also proportionately reduced to lost respiratory muscle function [4]. Diffusing capacity is usually normal in neuromuscular patients unless an additional parenchymal or infiltrative pulmonary process is also present.

During sleep, particularly rapid eye movement (REM) sleep, upper airway resistance increases, while chemosensitivity and skeletal muscle tone decrease, with the exception of the diaphragm and extraocular muscles, resulting in suppressed ventilation. Breathing is more rapid, superficial, and irregular and sleep is fragmented; total sleep time is shorter, accompanied by frequent breathing-related arousals [5,6]. While these changes in ventilation are not prominent in healthy patients, these alterations are accentuated in patients with respiratory muscle weakness and may lead to hypercapnic respiratory insufficiency and failure. Hypercapnia becomes particularly likely when respiratory muscle strength is less than 30% of normal and when vital capacity is less than 55% of the predicted value [4]. Significant hypercapnia is therefore usually a late manifestation of respiratory muscle failure. Patients suffering from neuromuscular disorders may present with impairment at the levels of the upper motor neuron (in the case of amyotrophic lateral sclerosis, ALS), lower motor neuron, neuromuscular junction, or muscle, including weakness of respiratory muscles that may result in SDB. Nocturnal symptoms of SDB include shorter total sleep time, sleep fragmentation due to frequent respiratory-related arousals, intermittent snoring or suppressed breathing, insomnia, and oxyhemoglobin desaturation, which in turn may lead to daytime symptoms of impaired functioning and quality of life in patients with neuromuscular diseases. Daytime symptoms resulting from sleep fragmentation include fatigue and tiredness, sleepiness, morning headaches, and waking with breathlessness. However, patients with neuromuscular disorders may have isolated SDB with relative preservation of daytime respiratory function. SDB is more likely to occur in patients with rib-cage and spinal deformities, obesity, and craniofacial abnormalities. Secondary restrictive lung disease due to atelectasis, recurrent pneumonia, and pulmonary fibrosis may occur in addition to respiratory muscle weakness. Pneumonia occurs following repeated aspiration and retention of secretions

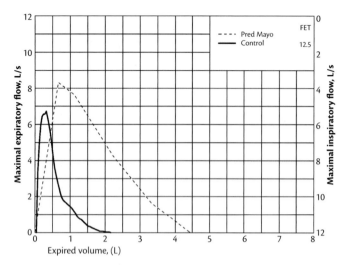

Fig. 30.1 Impaired flow–volume curve in neuromuscular disease. This was obtained during pulmonary function tests in a 58-year-old man with bilateral isolated phrenic neuropathies resulting in hypercapnic respiratory failure. Note the severe limitation of expiratory flow and the reduction in expired volume.

due to a weak cough reflex. With chronic hypoventilation, hypoxemia and hypercapnia develop, which may be complicated by subsequent heart failure and autonomic dysfunction.

The respiratory muscles include the diaphragm, intercostal, and abdominal muscles, in addition to accessory respiratory muscles of the sternocleidomastoid and neck strap muscles. Upper airway patency depends on adequate muscle tone and strength of the tongue, pharyngeal wall, hypopharynx, and larynx. The diaphragm is the most important muscle for inspiration during wakefulness or sleep, and the severity of hypoventilation parallels the degree of diaphragmatic weakness. According to the severity of respiratory muscle weakness, REM sleep may further reduce respiratory muscle function, which can lead to life-threatening hypoxia and hypercapnia.

The most common forms of SDB in neuromuscular diseases are nocturnal hypoventilation, obstructive sleep apnea (OSA), and central sleep apnea (CSA). Alveolar hypoventilation in patients with neuromuscular diseases typically appears during REM sleep. Respiration during REM sleep depends on metabolic control, while voluntary control diminishes. Chemosensitivity may, however, accustom to the changes in blood gases, potentially leading to longer periods of hypoxia during REM sleep. Prolonged hypoventilation stimulates bicarbonate retention and additional decrease in respiratory drive, leading to more marked REM sleep hypoventilation. As a neuromuscular disease advances, hypoventilation may also be observed in non-REM (NREM) sleep and during the daytime [7]. Hence, daytime respiratory function most often occurs later in the course of advancing neuromuscular weakness and accordingly has markedly greater prognostic value for imminent respiratory demise than earlier-presenting nighttime signs. In patients with neuromuscular disorders, sleep is fragmented by frequent arousals, which may disturb sleep, with arousal serving as a protective mechanism to blunt deleterious changes in blood gases [8].

Nocturnal hypoventilation is defined as an increase in $PaCO_2$ greater than 45 mmHg, or disproportionately increased relative to

levels while awake (according to the International Classification of Sleep Disorders, ICSD). Sleep-related hypoxemia is defined as oxyhemoglobin saturation less than 90% not related to discrete obstructive or central apneas or hypopneas for 5 or more consecutive minutes. Sleep-related hypoventilation in adults increases $PaCO_2$ by 10 mmHg or more compared with waking levels. Features indicating sleep-related hypoventilation such as abdominal paradox in the supine position, daytime hypercapnia with $PaCO_2 > 45$ mmHg, impairment of pulmonary function tests (FVC < 50%, maximal inspiratory pressure < 40 cmH_2O), awake oxyhemoglobin saturation < 91%, or SpO_2 saturation < 88% for 5 minutes or more on nocturnal pulse oximetry suggest that a polysomnography (PSG) study should be performed, and that ventilatory support should be introduced. Evidence to guide when supportive noninvasive positive pressure ventilation (NIV) should be initiated remains weak given the absence of randomized controlled trial evidence; however, expert consensus has established guideline thresholds for the initiation of NIV in patients having chronic respiratory insufficiency associated with restrictive thoracic disorders, with the Centers for Medicare and Medicaid generally following these recommended thresholds for coverage determination, as shown in Table 30.1 [9,10].

Sleep-related breathing in specific neuromuscular disorders

Amyotrophic lateral sclerosis

ALS, also called motor neuron disease or Lou Gehrig's disease, is a degenerative disorder based on progressive premature death of upper and lower motor neurons in the motor cortex of the brain, brainstem, and spinal cord. ALS is characterized by progressive muscle weakness and atrophy, fasciculations, hyperreflexia, spasticity, dysarthria, dysphagia, and dyspnea. The major cause of morbidity and mortality in ALS is progressive respiratory muscle weakness and ultimately respiratory failure. The sporadic form of the disease is most common, with the average age of onset being in the sixth and seventh decades. Familial ALS comprises only 5–10% of cases, and onset may be at a younger age. Weakness in ALS often begins focally in a specific muscle group or body region. Three types of disease onset in ALS can be distinguished: limb (60%), bulbar (30%), and respiratory (2%).

Sleep in ALS patients is disturbed by dyspnea and hypoxemia. Patients often experience frequent nocturnal awakenings, and sleep quality is unrefreshing, often with daytime sleepiness and morning headaches. The main cause of hypoxemia is REM sleep hypoventilation, which is most often induced by phrenic nerve dysfunction and resultant diaphragmatic weakness. Pulmonary function tests are prognostically valuable in monitoring the progression and survival of ALS patients [11,12]. Significant respiratory insufficiency during sleep should be treated with NIV, initially for in-home care with bilevel positive airway pressure (BPAP). Bulbar symptoms and frontotemporal dementia may partially account for intolerance of NIV [9]. When considering initiation of NIV, the measurements of nocturnal gas exchange, muscle strength, and symptomatic complaints must be taken into consideration. FVC < 50%, possibly even earlier to achieve better survival, maximal inspiratory pressure (MIP) < −60 cmH_2O, supine vital capacity nasal inspiratory pressure (SNIP) < 40 cmH_2O, oxygen saturation of 88% or less for

Table 30.1 Recommended guidelines for initiation of noninvasive positive pressure ventilatory devices in chronic respiratory insufficiency associated with restrictive thoracic disorders

Consensus Guidelines (1999) [9]	1. Symptoms of hypoventilation (one or more needed): Daytime sleepiness Fatigue Morning headache 2. Physiological criteria (one or more needed): $PaCO_2 \geq 45$ mmHg Oxyhemoglobin saturation < 88% for ≥ 5 minutes MIP < −60 cm FVC < 50% predicted
CMS Criteria [10]: all Consensus Guidelines criteria above, plus:	1. Requires both Consensus Guideline Categories above 2. COPD does not contribute significantly 3. Both $PaCO_2$ and nocturnal oximetry are on patient's usual FiO_2

at least 5 consecutive minutes, and $PaCO_2 > 45$ mmHg are suggested thresholds for NIV initiation [9,13–15]. NIV improves nocturnal breathing and often improves sleep quality, energy, speech clarity, quality of life, and survival time. NIV increases oxygenation, but has no significant effect on objective sleep efficiency or arousal index [16]. Oronasal masks are often poorly tolerated by ALS patients with severe sialorrhea and jaw closure weakness. Excessive salivation can be reduced by tricyclic antidepressants or a scopolamine patch, or ultrasound-guided submandibular injection of botulinum toxin [9]. Diaphragmatic pacing stimulation to induce phrenic nerve function may delay chronic mechanical ventilation up to 24 months [17]. ALS patients ultimately face the decision concerning whether to choose life-prolonging long-term mechanical ventilation by tracheostomy, which is postponed to the late stages of the disease to reduce consequences of immobility and limited communication. Dyspnea in terminal stages can be palliated with morphine.

Duchenne muscular dystrophy

Duchenne muscular dystrophy (DMD) is a hereditary X-linked muscle disease in the gene encoding the synthesis or expression of the protein dystrophin. Afflicted boys are born without initial disability, but clinical manifestations develop later between 3 and 5 years of age with progressive muscular weakness involving respiratory muscles, ultimately causing respiratory failure, the most common cause of death in DMD by the third decade of life. In the first decade, SDB, including OSA, occurs with the gradual progression of muscle weakness to relative atonia, affecting particularly the upper airway dilator muscles and deforming the rib cage. As DMD advances in the second decade, patients suffer from alveolar hypoventilation mainly during REM sleep, marked by hypercapnia and oxyhemoglobin desaturation despite normal waking respiratory function. Therefore, the severity of SDB must be evaluated by PSG and CO_2 evaluation, since daytime pulmonary function tests may not reveal the full impact of functional impact and resultant hypoxia and hypercapnia during sleep [18,19]. The contribution of

PSG to identifying SDB in DMD patients increases when $PaCO_2$ exceeds 45 mmHg and the patient develops apparent daytime symptoms such as excessive sleepiness, morning headaches, and fatigue caused by sleep fragmentation and REM sleep deprivation.

In patients suffering from sleep-related hypoventilation and daytime symptoms, NIV should be considered. This can improve the patient's quality of life by decreasing daytime sleepiness, as well as improving oxygenation and increasing survival. Significant nocturnal and later daytime respiratory insufficiency and ineffective coughing occur as muscular weakness progresses, leading to complications such as aspiration pneumonia and atelectasis, and patients may need to receive 24-hour ventilatory support. Tracheostomy is indicated in patients with recurrent respiratory infections when direct airway suctioning is necessary, and in DMD patients with severely compromised chest wall compliance [18,19].

Since nocturnal hypoxemia is caused by hypoventilation, oxygen should not be utilized alone without ventilatory support, since patients with chronic hypercapnia are dependent upon hypoxemic breathing drive, and oxygen alone could result in a further blunted breathing drive with resultant severe hypercapnia and respiratory failure.

Scoliosis is associated with increased arousals and decreased sleep efficiency and REM sleep time. DMD patients with scoliosis are usually treated with steroids, which can decelerate the progression of scoliosis and delay spinal corrective surgery. Correction of scoliosis does not improve vital capacity or ameliorate sleep disturbances or diurnal consequences, although corrective surgery plays a significant role in improving DMD patients' quality of life and nursing care [18].

Myotonic dystrophy

Myotonic dystrophy (dystrophia myotonica, DM) is an autosomal dominant multisystem disease. Two subtypes of this disorder have been identified, according to the chromosomal location and type of intron defect. Both are caused by untranslated repeat expansions of RNA, forming a pathological change of a chloride channel protein. Myotonic dystrophy subtype 1 (Steinert disease, DM1) is the result of a CTG trinucleotide repeat expansion (ranging from 50 to thousands of repeats), resulting in mutation in the gene for myotonin protein kinase (*DMPK*) [19,20]. The greater the number of repeats, the more severe is the manifestation of the disease [21], leading to the phenomenon of genetic anticipation, with progressively more severe phenotypes in successive generations given a progressively lengthened number of repeats. DM1 is characterized by a variety of different severity of phenotypes, which vary according to temporal onset through the lifespan, including congenital-type DM1. A defect in the zinc finger protein 9 (*ZNF9*) gene characterizes myotonic dystrophy type 2 (DM2, also previously known as proximal myotonic myopathy, or PROM). In most patients, symptoms of DM2 typically appear during the third decade. DM2 is usually a milder disease than DM1, but may involve a different spectrum of sleep disturbances, including prominent restless legs syndrome (RLS) [22]. DM affects skeletal and cardiac muscles, respiratory, endocrine and central nervous systems, the gastrointestinal tract, and lens, and is associated with a variety of sleep disorders. Interestingly, DM also impacts the central nervous system; in the brain, DM appears to predominantly involve the white matter, especially in the callosal body and the limbic system [20].

Sleep disorders are very common in both DM subtypes and, compared with other neuromuscular diseases, show great variability.

Sleep disturbances in DM may include SDB, central hypersomnia resembling narcolepsy or idiopathic hypersomnia, prominent fatigue, insomnia, RLS, and periodic limb movement disorder [20–26]. SDB is the most common sleep manifestation in DM1, with a spectrum of disordered breathing including OSA or CSA and sleep-related hypoventilation. In some patients with congenital DM1, mixed obstructive and central apneas develop. Owing to severe diaphragmatic, intercostal, upper airway, and tongue muscle weakness, patients may demonstrate significant alveolar hypoventilation with hypoxemia and hypercapnia, especially during REM sleep. Patients with DM tend to have a high BMI, so the degree of nocturnal desaturation is greater than in other neuromuscular patients with similar degrees of muscle weakness. SDB in DM may lead to early respiratory failure, and pulmonary function tests and arterial blood gases while awake often may underestimate the degree of sleep-related respiratory function compromise. CSA may be due to direct involvement of the brainstem and diencephalon by DM pathology [24]. PSG shows different patterns of SDB, including obstructive, central, or mixed apneas and hypopneas, respiratory-effort-related arousals, shallow and periodic breathing, and non-apneic sustained sleep-related hypoxemia due to hypoventilation. Other PSG features seen frequently in DM include frequent spontaneous arousals (which may be associated with muscle pain and stiffness, especially in DM2), decreased sleep efficiency, and frequent periodic leg movements of sleep with movement arousals. SDB and excessive daytime sleepiness (EDS) can be the presenting symptoms heralding a DM diagnosis [23–26].

EDS is present in DM1 patients and has also been described, although less frequently, in the DM2 subtype [26,27]. Sleepiness in DM may be attributed to sleep disturbances caused by respiratory muscle weakness or sleep apnea, but also results from dysfunction of sleep–wakefulness control. Hypersomnia often persists after SDB has been effectively treated by continuous positive airway pressure (CPAP) as a result of central hypersomnia caused by DM brain pathology [24,25]. The central hypersomnia disorder of DM is thought to result from a decrease in serotonergic raphe and superior central nucleus neurons, reduction of medullary reticular catecholaminergic neurons, as well as dysfunction of hypothalamic hypocretinergic function proven by reduced cerebrospinal fluid hypocretin levels [28].

Early PSG to evaluate for SDB may help prevent early respiratory failure. Positive PSG results inform the implementation of either CPAP or NIV with BPAP during sleep. In patients with EDS resulting from OSA, CPAP is preferred. In those presenting with daytime hypercapnia or sustained non-apneic hypoxemia due to sleep-related hypoventilation, BPAP is necessary to provide NIV. If the sleep study is normal, or symptoms of EDS remain in spite of otherwise effective therapy for SDB, then evaluation for central hypersomnia and stimulant medications (eg, modafinil, methylphenidate, or dexamphetamine) can be considered.

Neuromuscular junction disorders

Neuromuscular junction disorders include myasthenia gravis, Lambert-Eaton myasthenic syndrome, congenital myasthenic syndrome, and botulism.

Myasthenia gravis

Myasthenia gravis (MG) is an autoimmune disorder. IgG antibodies against the postsynaptic acetylcholine receptor are found in the plasma of most patients with MG. Antibodies cause receptor degeneration or blockade resulting in reduction of functional postsynaptic acetylcholine receptors (AChR). Even though the proper amount of acetylcholine is released from the presynaptic neuron, there is decreased muscle contraction, given compromise of the postsynaptic AChR function by anti-AChR antibodies. IgG-positive MG is associated with thymoma or thymic hyperplasia. The autoimmune process in MG is thought to be initiated by reaction of thymic B cells with thymic cells that have similar antigenic characteristics to skeletal muscle cells. Muscle-specific tyrosine kinase antibodies (MuSK) are found in the blood of a subset of patients with MG.

MG is characterized by fatigable muscle weakness due to reduced muscle contraction. The majority of MG patients present with abnormalities of eye movements or eye opening, with diplopia and ptosis. Other manifestations are limb muscle weakness, dysarthria, and dysphagia. MG symptoms typically worsen as the day progresses, especially following repeated activity, and are classically worse in the evening hours and better in the morning. With progressive disease, particularly during subacute periods of worsening known as myasthenic crisis, respiratory muscle weakness is present. Myasthenic or iatrogenic cholinergic crisis (the latter resulting from excessive doses of pyridostigmine) may lead to pronounced SDB, respiratory insufficiency, and eventual respiratory failure.

Respiratory and sleep disturbances can be detected by subjective symptoms such as morning headache, fatigue, nocturnal breathlessness, daytime somnolence, and cognitive dysfunction, or by objective testing demonstrating oxygen desaturation or hypercapnia.

SDB is especially prominent during REM sleep given the dependence of effective ventilation on diaphragmatic function during REM, making patients with diaphragmatic weakness particularly vulnerable to severe desaturations. SDB in MG may involve obstructive, central, or mixed sleep apnea. CSA has been associated with the presence of AChR-antibodies in cerebrospinal fluid. OSA in MG patients occurs mainly as a result of oropharyngeal weakness, and OSA frequency may be up to 15–20% higher in MG than in the normal population, although evidence has been conflicting and further studies are needed [29,30]. Daytime pulmonary function tests are usually normal when MG is in clinical remission, or if there are no risk factors for respiratory compromise such as older age or obesity, steroid-induced myopathy of the oropharyngeal muscles, or decreased TLC [31,32].

MG treatment only rarely induces complete remission. Treatments for MG include cholinesterase inhibitors, thymectomy in anti-AChR antibody-positive cases, corticosteroids, immunosuppressive drugs, and plasmapheresis or IVIG during myasthenic crisis. Most MG symptoms respond at least transiently to symptomatic therapy with slow-release cholinesterase inhibitors such as pyridostigmine. Thymectomy is helpful in reducing disease severity and frequently induces remission in anti-AcChR antibody-positive MG cases, and has been reported to reduce the frequency of sleep apnea episodes, nocturnal hypoxia, and weakness of the oropharyngeal muscles [7,33]. Corticosteroids can induce weight gain that may in turn increase OSA severity, and steroid therapy often induces severe and brittle insomnia [32]. SDB can be symptomatically treated by introduction of nasal CPAP or NIV. Nocturnal hypoventilation and sleep apnea may be severe and occasionally require assisted ventilation.

Lambert–Eaton myasthenic syndrome, botulism, and congenital myasthenic syndrome

SDB has also been described in Lambert–Eaton myasthenic syndrome (LEMS), botulism, and congenital myasthenic syndrome (CMS), and although it is thought to be less frequent than in MG [7], it may be underdiagnosed [34]. Significant muscle weakness can lead to severe respiratory impairment that may require assisted ventilation. Regular screening of muscle strength is indicated; clinical examination of the bulbar muscles, as well as cervical flexion and extension, can help identify segmental weakness that may assist in portending diaphragmatic weakness and the need for NIV or mechanical ventilation.

Other myopathies

Other less common myopathies that may manifest sleep disorders are facioscapulohumeral muscular dystrophy (FSHD), congenital muscular dystrophies (CMDs), metabolic, mitochondrial, and inflammatory myopathies, and limb-girdle muscular dystrophy (LGMD).

Facioscapulohumeral muscular dystrophy

FSHD is the third most common hereditary muscular dystrophy. Most cases of FSHD are inherited in an autosomal dominant fashion, while the remainder is due to sporadic mutations. FSHD is a slowly progressive myopathy resulting from chromosomal deletion of 4q35. The onset of FSHD is usually in the second decade, but it may also manifest in early childhood. The greater the chromosomal impairment or mutation, the more severe are the manifestations of FSHD. FSHD is characterized by craniocaudal spreading of muscle weakness, usually sparing respiratory muscles.

Poor sleep quality results particularly from reduced nocturnal mobility correlating with weakness severity. Body movement is essential to obviate peripheral nerve compressions and subsequent pain and paresthesias [35]. OSA is a frequent cause of sleep disturbance in FSHD patients owing to pharyngeal muscle weakness. Kyphoscoliosis resulting from asymmetrical FSHD involvement of the trunk and scapular muscles may also induce sleep-related hypoventilation. PSG shows longer sleep latency, frequent spontaneous arousals, reduced overall sleep time, and shortened REM sleep time [36–37].

Congenital muscular dystrophies

CMDs are a genetically heterogeneous group of autosomal recessive, slowly progressive muscle disorders. Clinical manifestations depend on mutations in specific genes encoding proteins such as laminin. Muscle weakness is obvious at birth or during the first months of life. Examples of CMDs are laminin-α_2-deficient CMD, Ullrich CMD, and muscle–eye–brain disease. Sleep is disrupted by CSA due to a central ventilatory control disorder, or by OSA resulting from upper airway muscle weakness [38]. Mixed apnea/hypopnea may also occur. Accessory respiratory and intercostal muscle atonia during REM sleep may cause nocturnal oxyhemoglobin desaturation and hypercapnia, fragmented sleep with frequent arousals, and reduced REM and total sleep times [38]. Clinical examination and diurnal respiratory function tests are in most cases normal, but it is important to identify SDB in asymptomatic CMD patients early enough to prevent respiratory failure. PSG is therefore an important part of screening, and, if needed, ventilatory support should be introduced.

Limb-girdle muscular dystrophy

LGMD is a rare autosomal dominant muscle disorder with clinical similarities to Duchenne and Becker muscular dystrophies. The age of onset ranges from the first to third decades of life. Earlier disease onset correlates with more severe symptoms and more rapid progression. As LGMD progresses, respiratory muscle function decreases, resulting in sleep disruption. Sleep abnormalities are similar to those in DMD. SDB appears owing to both CSA on account of failure of respiratory control and OSA due to upper airway muscular weakness [39]. LGMD patients with SDB should be adequately treated with nocturnal NIV or, if needed, by tracheostomy and mechanical ventilation.

Metabolic myopathies

Metabolic myopathies are rare hereditary disorders characterized by impairment of biochemical metabolism of muscle tissue, with defects in a wide variety of proteins. The most important metabolic myopathy that significantly affects respiratory muscle function and results in SDB is acid maltase deficiency (AMD), also known as Pompe disease. AMD is a glycogen storage disorder resulting in muscle tissue function failure. AMD may manifest in both childhood and adulthood forms and, given slow progression, survival time is long. The most frequent cause of death is respiratory muscle failure. Diaphragmatic insufficiency is frequent and may manifest earlier than other muscle group weakness in AMD [40]. The failure of diaphragmatic muscle function is most pronounced during REM sleep, resulting in SDB characterized by profound and long-duration periods of sleep-related hypoventilation, apneas, substantial oxyhemoglobin desaturation, and hypercapnia. SDB and sleep-related hypoventilation may be predicted by diurnal pulmonary function tests [9,39]. In order to improve quality of life and prevent early respiratory failure, NIV should be administered [40].

Mitochondrial myopathies

Mitochondrial myopathies are characterized by respiratory chain impairment, and are also known as oxidative phosphorylation disorders. These disorders result in reduced energy metabolism affecting the most energy-demanding tissues, the muscles and brain, earliest and primarily. Therefore, these disorders are also called mitochondrial encephalomyopathies. Prominent fatigue is typical, and respiratory compromise has been reported [41].

Inflammatory myopathies

Inflammatory myopathies, including dermatomyositis (DM), polymyositis (PM), and sporadic inclusion-body myositis (sIBM), are rare systemic connective tissue diseases that may lead to mobility impairment and loss of muscle tone. Weakness of respiratory muscles, particularly the oropharyngeal muscles, may result in OSA and respiratory compromise [42].

Isolated phrenic neuropathy

Isolated phrenic neuropathy (IPN) is a rare cause of acute or subacute unexplained dyspnea and orthopnea, and can lead to hypercapnic respiratory failure when bilateral involvement of the phrenic nerves occurs (Fig. 30.1). Acute diaphragmatic palsy can develop in association with a variety of disorders, such as Parsonage–Turner syndrome, immune brachial plexus neuropathy, diabetic polyneuropathy, Guillain–Barré syndrome, motor neuron disease, large artery vasculitis, and von Recklinghausen disease. Unilateral phrenic neuropathy is most often asymptomatic, and is a relatively frequent incidentally detected finding as hemidiaphragmatic elevation on chest radiography. Bilateral IPN (BIPN) usually has an acute, painless onset, without an antecedent trigger. To distinguish diaphragmatic weakness from other causes of dyspnea such as pulmonary embolism or cardiac failure, the examiner should lay the patient supine, which results in worsened dyspnea, and often accessory muscle (sternocleidomastoid and neck strap muscles) use and abdominal paradox may be seen. There may be an up to 50% decrease in vital capacity when transferring between the upright and supine positions when upright and supine pulmonary functions are formally measured [7]. Chest X-rays show bilateral diaphragmatic elevation, electrophysiological testing demonstrates reduced or absent phrenic nerve conductions and active diaphragmatic denervation, and diaphragmatic ultrasound and fluoroscopy show reduced diaphragmatic movement [44].

Patients with bilateral or severe unilateral IPN are at significant risk of SDB. Severe nocturnal hypoventilation and desaturation during REM sleep can occur. Unlike many other neuromuscular disorders, SDB often occurs independently of BMI. Patients suffer from fragmented sleep and consequently from fatigue, morning headaches, and hypersomnia. To evaluate disordered sleep, PSG is indicated. The phrenic nerve may take years to regenerate, and in some cases may never fully recover. During this time, patients require NIV to improve quality of life and prevent respiratory failure, and NIV often reduces sleeping problems and the ability to rest in a recumbent position [43,44]. Diaphragmatic plication can also be considered for patients who suffer permanent diaphragmatic paralysis.

Spinal cord disorders

Spinal cord disorders manifesting sleep impairment are primarily spinal cord injuries, postpoliomyelitis syndrome (PPS), and spinal muscular atrophy (SMA).

Spinal cord injury

The severity and manifestations of sleep disorders in patients with spinal cord injury depends on the location of the lesion. If spinal cord injury extends to the brainstem and alters reticular formation (RF) function, altered sleep–wake regulation may occur, so the more rostral the spinal cord damage, the poorer the sleep quality may be. Concomitant closed head injury often accompanies spinal cord injury, which may also impact sleep–wake regulation, cause central posttraumatic hypersomnia, and impact melatonin secretion. Melatonin plays important roles in circadian rhythms and sleep promotion. Consequences of low plasma melatonin concentration include shortened total sleep duration, repeated arousals, long wakefulness periods, and shortened REM latency and decreased REM percentage [45]. Defective melatonin secretion can be treated with replacement by 2–6 mg of exogenous melatonin dosed before bedtime. Insomnia and daytime sleepiness resulting from head injuries can be treated with prescribed hypnotics and modafinil or other psychostimulant medications [45,46]. Pain, spasms, immobilization, supine position, and bladder distension each may influence sleep as well, so optimal treatment of these complications is also important to optimize sleep in this patient population.

The most common type of SDB in patients with spinal cord injury is OSA. Sleep-related hypoventilation may occur, given reduced activity of intercostal and respiratory accessory muscles, especially during REM sleep, and the ventilatory function of the diaphragm may be altered during NREM sleep. CSA may appear after high cervical spinal cord injury, especially when the injury also extends to brainstem respiratory centers. Other possible causes of CSA are syringomyelia and syringobulbia. A recent study found that the mode of administration of intrathecal baclofen also impacted the severity of SDB, with bolus administration leading to more frequent and severe respiratory events (especially central apneas) than continuous infusion [47]. Treatment of SDB and central hypoventilation syndrome includes both symptomatic measures such as avoiding the supine position and respiratory suppressant drugs, as well as the use of NIV, tracheostomy, and diaphragmatic pacing [17,48].

Postpoliomyelitis syndrome

PPS occurs in approximately 25% of patients with a remote history of acute poliomyelitis caused by poliovirus. The onset of PPS ranges from two to five decades after the primary disease. In the acute poliomyelitis infection, poliovirus destroys spinal cord anterior horn motor neurons, thus denervating skeletal muscles acutely. However, chronically during recovery, reinnervation of muscle fibers occurs by axonal sprouting from surviving motor neurons. PPS usually occurs in patients who had the paralytic form of poliomyelitis, and mainly affects previously involved muscles, although it may also affect muscles that appeared to have been spared during the earlier acute attack of poliovirus. PPS is thought to develop owing to normal loss of motor neurons consequent to aging, and possibly also to overuse of the affected muscles. In PPS, the process of ongoing chronic denervation due to motor neuron loss related to aging exceeds the capacity for reinnervation of the muscle by healthy motor neurons. In patients who previously had the bulbar form of poliomyelitis, PPS patients may develop impaired respiration and swallowing. Capacity for recovery depends on the ability of the surviving motor neurons to successfully reinnerrvate the affected muscles.

Sleep disorders in PPS are usually due to underlying impaired respiratory function in patients experiencing worsening of ventilatory function, mostly affecting patients whose respiratory muscles were involved during their primary illness with acute poliomyelitis. PSG demonstrates nocturnal hypoventilation, hypopneas, apneas, hypoxemia, delayed REM sleep latency and reduced REM time, recurrent arousals, and sleep fragmentation [49]. Morning headaches, EDS, or frank respiratory insufficiency may appear. Most apneas are obstructive or mixed. Musculoskeletal deformities such as kyphoscoliosis may induce restrictive ventilatory impairment associated with respiratory accessory muscle weakness [7]. Therapeutic options for respiratory disorders in PSS are introduction of NIV and, rarely, tracheostomy with mechanical ventilation.

Spinal muscular atrophy

SMA describes a heterogeneous group of hereditary autosomal recessive disorders characterized by deterioration of spinal cord anterior horn motor neurons and, in some cases, nuclei of caudal cranial nerves ranging from the trigeminal to hypoglossal nerves. In SMA, four subtypes may occur, according to age of onset. Patients may have intercostal and diaphragmatic muscle weakness and different degrees of bulbar symptoms, leading to respiratory dysfunction and SDB. Also, chest wall deformities and scoliosis may worsen the extent of SDB, which can eventually lead to respiratory failure, especially in childhood-onset forms I and II. SDB is characterized by OSA, hypercapnia, and oxyhemoglobin desaturation during REM sleep. Sleep is disrupted by frequent arousals and sweating, morning headaches and nausea, daytime sleepiness, and school performance difficulties in children and adolescents [50]. NIV can improve subjective and objective symptoms of SDB.

Diagnostic assessment and approach to the patient with neuromuscular disease and sleep-related breathing disorders

Patients with chronic neuromuscular disease should be routinely assessed for sleep complaints. The presence of symptoms is the primary consideration to initiate evaluation for OSA, CSA, or hypoventilation. However, some patients may have SDB without any evident symptoms. Therefore, evaluation by a sleep specialist and screening for SDB should be considered, with at least an initial unattended in-home study such as portable overnight oximetry. No single test is completely accurate for detecting the presence of nocturnal desaturation or respiratory failure. Therefore, several different means of evaluation should be used in concert to assess for possible SDB and hypoventilation, beginning with a thorough clinical history and examination. Patients should be carefully questioned about past and present sleep history, including whether they have a history of loud disruptive snoring, whether snoring varies by sleep position, whether snort or gasp arousal or witnessed pauses in breathing have been noted, and whether symptoms of morning predominant headache, dry mouth, or sore throat are regularly present. Inquiring about restless legs symptoms (an uncomfortable urge to move the legs, with rest onset and worsening, relief by movement or getting up to walk, and evening predominance of symptoms) is also important, especially in patients with myotonic dystrophy. Taking a thorough family history and drug, alcohol, and medication use history is also important. Psychiatric history may also play an important role in further diagnostic assessment.

Pulmonary function tests (PFT) help to evaluate the likelihood of sleep-related hypoventilation, evaluate the ventilatory control system, and exclude intrinsic bronchopulmonary disease, and may have prognostic value [11]. PFT include vital capacity, forced expiratory volume, total lung volume, minimal residual volume, and gas distribution and transfer measurements [7–9] Vital capacity (VC) is a global respiratory function test using both inspiratory and expiratory muscles. VC can be measured in both upright and supine positions. VC in the supine position sensitively differentiates the origin of respiratory impairment. If VC values fall within the normal range, then respiratory muscle weakness is probably not responsible for ventilation problems. PFT findings consistent with diaphragmatic weakness and probable nocturnal hypoventilation include a fall in FVC values between the sitting to supine positions of 15–20%, or when sitting FVC is less than 80%. FVC less than 50%, along with recurrent respiratory tract infections, is typical of patients with neuromuscular disease with nocturnal hypoventilation disorders. Owing to fluctuation of muscle weakness in myasthenia gravis, assessment of FVC must be done carefully. Sleep hypoventilation is very likely to be seen when FVC is less than 50% of predicted value, or if a greater than 20% decrement is seen between the upright and supine positions. In this case, a PSG should be performed, and NIV should be considered.

Supine vital capacity nasal inspiratory pressure (SNIP) is able to measure the function of inspiratory muscle strength, predominantly the diaphragm. SNIP > 70 cmH_2O (in an adult male) and SNIP > 60 cmH_2O (in an adult female) exclude the presence of clinically significant respiratory muscle weakness. SNIP has been shown to be a very good predictor of nighttime desaturation and respiratory failure in ALS [15]. NIV should be considered when SNIP decreases to less than 40 cmH_2O [51,52].

Mouth pressures (maximum inspiratory and expiratory pressures, MIP and MEP, also known as bugle pressures) characterize global inspiratory and expiratory muscle strength. Inspiratory muscle strength includes assessment of the diaphragm, respiratory accessory, and intercostal muscles, while expiratory muscle strength encompasses expiratory muscles through evaluation of cough strength. Mouth pressures should be measured at the time of diagnosis and follow-up to aid identification of deterioration, and may also be used in acute situations to decide whether mechanical ventilation is needed. In patients with facial muscle weakness, the mouth pressure is inaccurate because of insufficient mouth sealing.

Arterial blood gas (ABG) values remain in the normal range during wakefulness until the underlying neuromuscular disorder becomes chronic and involves signs of respiratory failure, or in cases of acute respiratory insufficiency. Abnormal ABG values correlate with significant weakness of respiratory muscles. Respiratory failure in neuromuscular patients is characterized by a chronic, compensated respiratory acidosis, with findings on ABG of elevated $PaCO_2$ and bicarbonate, accompanied by normal or slightly reduced pH. Nocturnal hypoventilation is diagnosed by nighttime oxyhemoglobin desaturation (SpO_2 < 88%) for five or more consecutive minutes, together with a morning ABG demonstrating daytime hypercapnia ($PaCO_2$ > 45 mmHg) with raised pH and bicarbonate values [5,7]. Findings consistent with nocturnal hypoventilation can support an indication for NIV initiation.

Portable overnight oximetry is useful to screen for sustained oxyhemoglobin desaturation associated with nocturnal hypoventilation and for frequent oscillatory desaturation events associated with OSA or CSA. When patients develop diaphragm dysfunction, they may show characteristic oximetry patterns heralding impending progressive respiratory muscle dysfunction as shown in Fig. 30.2. As diaphragmatic failure becomes more advanced, the oximetry findings become more profound and show the characteristic clustered periodic deep episodic desaturations dependent on REM stage sleep. Again, this is because of the superimposed influence of normal REM sleep stage muscle atonia upon preexisting diaphragmatic weakness that further compromises respiratory function, given that the diaphragm is the sole muscle supporting respiratory function in the REM sleep state. Overnight oximetry is recommended when relevant symptoms suggestive of SDB are observed, including daytime sleepiness, loud disruptive snoring, morning headaches, and repeated arousals and restlessness during sleep.

Portable screening devices are not very sensitive and are able to detect only moderate to severe OSA; therefore, if typical symptoms of SDB are present, PSG should still be considered to detect mild OSA or the upper airway resistance syndrome.

In-lab PSG is the most sensitive assessment of sleep in patients with neuromuscular disorders, and provides polygraphic data concerning respiratory function, movement, and sleep architecture. PSG is indicated in patients with symptoms of SDB, unexplained cor pulmonale, inspiratory VC < 50% of predicted value, and

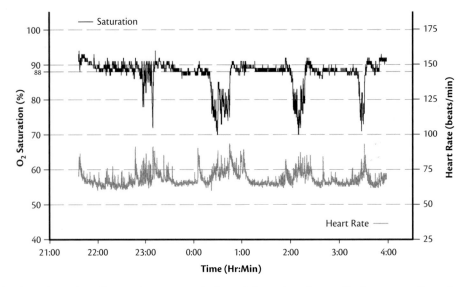

Fig. 30.2 Portable overnight oximetry in a patient with progressive neuromuscular disease. Oximetry shows features of both recurrent oscillatory desaturation typical of obstructive sleep disordered breathing, in addition to sustained hypoxemia representing hypoventilation from diaphragmatic weakness. Note the periodic worsening of sustained hypoxemia, especially in the first third of the night, which was verified during polysomnography to correspond to periods of worsened hypoxemia during REM sleep stage.

reduced peak inspiratory pressure < 2.5 kPa. The absence of REM sleep appears to correlate with a poor prognosis in neuromuscular disorders, and suggests impending respiratory failure. Other typical findings include reduced total sleep time, an increased numbers of arousals, sleep fragmentation and disorganization, obstructive, central and mixed sleep apneas, oxyhemoglobin desaturation, or delayed initial sleep latency and prolonged wake after sleep onset time consistent with initial and sleep-maintenance insomnia. Addition of transcutaneous or end-tidal CO_2 monitoring can be very helpful to more directly assess hypoventilation, and can help guide NIV treatment [7,53].

Management of sleep-related breathing disorders in neuromuscular diseases

Timely recognition and treatment of sleep disorders in patients with neuromuscular disorders can significantly improve quality of life. SDB is often the first indicator of impaired respiratory functions in neuromuscular patients, and can be detected earlier than other ventilatory problems that may ultimately lead to respiratory failure, the chief cause of morbidity and mortality in these patients.

Chronic management considerations

The aims of long-term treatment are to prolong survival and improve quality of life. General options applicable to all neuromuscular patients include lifestyle changes (loss of weight if obese), sufficient nutrition, proper sleep hygiene with regular sleep schedule, and avoidance of caffeine, alcohol, or sedative drugs that may disturb sleep or suppress breathing. If possible, exercise and rehabilitation of respiratory muscles should also be introduced.

Positive airway pressure and noninvasive positive pressure ventilation

Noninvasive positive pressure ventilation (NIV) is the preferred initial treatment for SDB, as well as daytime ventilatory support when necessary. There are two types of delivery: continuous positive airway pressure (CPAP) and bilevel positive airway pressure (BPAP).

The latter is often better tolerated by neuromuscular patients and is more effective for nocturnal ventilation. CPAP should be initiated only in neuromuscular patients with normal nocturnal ventilation, since it may increase the burden on weak respiratory muscles. NIV can be applied via mouthpiece, nasal mask, nasal pillows, or a full face mask interface.

Since SDB and respiratory impairment are first detected during REM sleep, patients usually need initial ventilatory support only during nighttime, allowing them to breathe on their own during the day. When daytime hypercapnia evolves, nocturnal ventilation should be introduced. The level of nocturnal ventilation must be determined in the sleep laboratory or at the hospital bedside with careful monitoring [54]. Contraindications for NIV include bulbar involvement, swallowing impairment, inability to clear secretions, and lack of patient cooperation with inability to tolerate a mask interface.

NIV ventilatory support may prevent decline in lung function and improve sleep quality, quality of life, and survival [11,55,56]. Initiation of NIV is recommended when patients become symptomatic with EDS, loud disruptive snoring, orthopnea, and morning headaches, or when they reach an FVC < 50% of predicted value, SNIP < 40 cmH_2O, $PaCO_2$ > 45 mmHg, or oxyhemoglobin saturation < 88% [9,51,52]. In stable chronic hypoventilation syndromes, NIV should be initiated with inspiratory and expiratory PAP (IPAP and EPAP) set at 8 cmH_2O and 4 cmH_2O, respectively, with titration as necessary to adequately support hypoxemia toward the maximum IPAP and EPAP of 30 cmH_2O and 20 cmH_2O, respectively. Use of NIV is dependent on patient compliance, interface fit and seal (avoiding air leakage), and tolerability of NIV, as well as severity of scoliosis [51]. The earlier the initiation and patient's successful adoption of NIV, the better the tolerance that may be achieved [55]. NIV becomes ineffective when ability to clear secretions decreases or the primary disease progresses, especially when bulbar symptoms become more severe.

Invasive mechanical ventilation

Tracheostomy is usually considered when NIV becomes ineffective, when severity of bulbar impairment progresses or scoliosis undergoes marked deterioration, for increasing patient safety when unable to clear secretions, for avoiding cognitive impairment, and for prolonging survival [53–54,56]. The benefits of mechanical ventilation are complete control of gas volumes, ability to administer higher ventilatory pressures, permitting direct airway suctioning of secretions, and treatment of acute respiratory failure. However, many complications can occur such as hemorrhage, tracheal necrosis or stenosis, tracheoesophageal fistulae, bacterial colonization, increased secretions and risk of aspiration, and swallowing problems. Tracheostomy impairs communication, so is usually considered by patients as the last resort for treatment of SDB and respiratory impairment and should be carefully discussed with them. Another major secondary result is that the performance of a tracheostomy commonly results in other major life-altering decisions, such as displacement to a skilled nursing facility and separation from family members.

Oxygen therapy

Oxygen therapy may improve hypoxemia, but at the risk of masking underlying hypoventilation or atelectasis. Oxygen therapy may lead to deterioration in central respiratory drive by blunting the hypoxic drive to breathe in the context of chronic hypercapnia, and may lead to acute respiratory failure. Therefore, oxygen may be dangerous to use alone, and should be delivered as a supplementary adjunct to NIV or assisted cough therapy. Specific indications for oxygen administration may include infection with pneumonia. Monitoring of $PaCO_2$ should be considered during oxygen treatment to ensure there is no evolving hypercapnia.

Diaphragm pacing stimulation

Diaphragm pacing stimulation (DPS) may replace long-term mechanical ventilation in patients with failure of brainstem respiratory control centers or malfunction of upper motor neurons subserving the diaphragm. DPS provides direct electrical phrenic nerve stimulation to drive diaphragmatic movement. Possible candidates for DPS include patients with spinal cord injury above the C3 level and those with ALS. DPS may delay institution of tracheostomy and mechanical ventilation by up to 24 months [17,48]. Prior to DPS, laparoscopic diaphragm mapping is required to identify the best contractible motor point and to evaluate for diaphragmatic atrophy [17,48,57]. Before weaning patients from ventilatory support, the diaphragm's fast fatigable anaerobic-type muscle fibers must be conditioned during daily 15–30 minute sessions to enable conversion to slow-conducting aerobic oxidative fibers [17,48,57].

Acute, urgent, and emergent management considerations

Respiratory failure can manifest as an acute situation emerging from an otherwise healthy and stable-appearing state in Guillain–Barré syndrome or high-level spinal cord injury, or during acute respiratory decompensation in chronic neuromuscular disorders such as myasthenia gravis, ALS, or DMD.

For acutely deteriorating unstable neuromuscular patients, invasive mechanical ventilation should be initiated in an intensive care unit to avoid respiratory arrest. Endotracheal intubation with positive pressure ventilation is the preferred initial approach. Prior to invasive ventilation, comorbidities, quality of life after extubation, and respect for the patient's wishes must be considered. Rapid progression of muscle weakness, bulbar symptoms, VC < 20 mL/kg,

MIP > −30 cmH$_2$O, or MEP < 40 cmH$_2$O are predictors of impending respiratory failure and an indication for invasive ventilation in Guillain–Barré syndrome, and similar values are generally favored in neurocritical care settings for other acutely deteriorating neuromuscular patients in the consideration of intubation and mechanical ventilation [58]. Tracheostomy does not have to be considered immediately, nor is it necessarily a permanent solution when the patient is expected to recover from an acute bout of neuromuscular weakness, but should be considered after 7–10 days of mechanical ventilation through an endotracheal tube to prevent tracheal erosion or superinfection [59].

NIV is used acutely during some episodes of ventilatory insufficiency ($PaCO_2 \geq 45$ mmHg, pH ≤ 7.35) and to treat respiratory failure when invasive ventilation is considered inappropriate, or when avoiding endotracheal intubation is desirable. NIV should be initiated when patients with chronic neuromuscular respiratory insufficiency develop daytime symptoms of sleepiness, fatigue, or morning headache, or when hypercapnia is found, and acutely during respiratory infection to prevent respiratory failure, in palliative care settings, and as supportive ventilation in stabilized patients after tracheostomy is no longer needed. Oxygen therapy should be reserved for acute infections, such as pneumonia, to improve hypoxemia, and should be accompanied by other ventilatory support and not used alone, to avoid blunting hypoxemic breathing drive.

Conclusions

SDB is common in patients with neuromuscular disorders, and is a significant contributor to morbidity and mortality in this patient population. SDB often manifests earlier than daytime respiratory symptoms and may be the presenting manifestation of a neuromuscular disorder. The most common forms of SDB in patients with neuromuscular disorders are nocturnal hypoventilation, OSA, and CSA. During REM sleep in particular, altered upper airway resistance and chemosensitivity impair sleep-related breathing, and effective respiration depends upon diaphragmatic effort due to generalized muscle atonia, so that REM-related hypopneas, apneas, and hypoventilation are common early in the course of neuromuscular bellows failure. Typical early symptoms of SDB in neuromuscular patients include daytime symptoms resulting from sleep fragmentation, such as fatigue and tiredness, sleepiness, morning headaches, and orthopnea. PSG should be considered early in the course of neuromuscular disorders when clinical features of sleep-related hypoventilation such as supine abdominal paradox, daytime hypercapnia with $PaCO_2 > 45$ mmHg, or impaired pulmonary function tests (FVC < 50%, MEP < 40 cmH$_2$O) are seen, as NIV is likely necessary. Timely application of NIV reduces morbidity and may delay mortality in patients with a variety of neuromuscular problems, including ALS, the myotonic dystrophies and other myopathies, myasthenia gravis, isolated phrenic neuropathies, or spinal cord injury. Oxygen therapy alone should be avoided in neuromuscular patients, since it may further blunt the hypoxic drive to breathe in the setting of chronic hypercapnia. In most cases, NIV satisfactorily ameliorates hypoxemia and improves related symptoms of SDB. A team approach involving generalists, neurologists, and sleep physicians is necessary to promptly diagnose and effectively treat SDB problems in neuromuscular patients.

Acknowledgements

The work described here was supported in part by the European Regional Development Fund—Project FNUSA-ICRC (No. CZ.1.05/1.1.00/02.0123), European Social Fund and the State Budget of the Czech Republic, and the National Center for Research Resources and the National Center for Advancing Translational Sciences, National Institutes of Health, through Grant Number 1 UL1 RR024150-01. The content of this chapter is solely the responsibility of the authors and does not necessarily represent the official views of the NIH.

References

1. Wagner MH, Berry RB. Disturbed sleep in a patient with Duchenne muscular dystrophy. J Clin Sleep Med 2008;4(2):173–5.
2. Kreitzer SM, Saunders NA, Tyler HR, Ingram RH. Respiratory muscle function in amyotrophic lateral sclerosis. Am Rev Respir Dis 1978;117(3):437–47.
3. De Troyer A, Borenstein S, Cordier R. Analysis of lung volume restriction in patients with respiratory muscle weakness. Thorax 1980;35(8):603–10.
4. Braun NM, Arora NS, Rochester DF. Respiratory muscle and pulmonary function in polymyositis and other proximal myopathies. Thorax 1983;38(8):616–23.
5. Misuri G, Lanini B, Gigliotti F, et al. Mechanism of CO_2 retention in patients with neuromuscular disease. Chest 2000;117(2):447–53.
6. Brack T, Jubran A, Tobin MJ. Dyspnea and decreased variability of breathing in patients with restrictive lung disease. Am J Respir Crit Care Med 2002;165(9):1260–4.
7. Desai H, Mador MJ. Sleep in patients with respiratory muscle weakness. Sleep Med Clin 2008;3(4):541–50.
8. Perrin C, Unterborn JN, Ambrosio CD, Hill NS. Pulmonary complications of chronic neuromuscular diseases and their management. Muscle Nerve 2004; 29(1):5–27.
9. Clinical indications for noninvasive positive pressure ventilation in chronic respiratory failure due to restrictive lung disease, COPD, and nocturnal hypoventilation—a consensus conference report. Chest 1999;116:521–34.
10. US Department of Health and Human Services. Centers for Medicare & Medicaid Services, "PAP devices for the treatment of OSA"(L11528, L11528, L11518, L171), revision effective date 10/1/2011. Washington, DC: US Department of Health and Human Services.
11. Gay PC, Westbrook PR, Daube JR, et al. Effects of alterations in pulmonary function and sleep variables on survival in patients with amyotrophic lateral sclerosis. Mayo Clin Proc 1991;66(7):686–94.
12. David WS, Bundlie SR, Mahdavi Z. Polysomnographic studies in amyotrophic lateral sclerosis. J Neurol Sci 1997;152(Suppl):S29–35.
13. Atkeson AD, RoyChoudhury A, Harrington-Moroney G, et al. Patient-ventilator asynchrony with nocturnal noninvasive ventilation in ALS. Neurology 2011;77(6):549–55.
14. Carratù P, Spicuzza L, Cassano A, et al. Early treatment with noninvasive positive pressure ventilation prolongs survival in amyotrophic lateral sclerosis patients with nocturnal respiratory insufficiency. Orphanet J Rare Dis 2009;4:10.
15. Benditt JO, Boitano LJ. Pulmonary issues in patients with chronic neuromuscular disease. Am J Respir Crit Care Med 2013;187(10):1046–55.
16. Katzberg HD, Selegiman A, Guion L, et al. Effects of noninvasive ventilation on sleep outcomes in amyotrophic lateral sclerosis. J Clin Sleep Med 2013;9(4):345–51.
17. Onders RP, Elmo M, Khansarinia S, et al. Complete worldwide operative experience in laparoscopic diaphragm pacing: results and differences in spinal cord injured patients and amyotrophic lateral sclerosis patients. Surg Endosc 2009;23(7):1433–40.
18. Polat M, Sakinci O, Ersoy B, Sezer RG, Yilmaz H. Assessment of sleep-related breathing disorders in patients with duchenne muscular dystrophy. J Clin Med Res 2012;4(5):332–7.
19. Prendergast P, Magalhaes S, Campbell C. Congenital myotonic dystrophy in a national registry. Paediatr Child Health 2010;15(8):514–18.
20. Minnerop M, Weber B, Schoene-Bake J-C, et al. The brain in myotonic dystrophy 1 and 2: evidence for a predominant white matter disease. Brain 2011;134(Pt 12):3530–46.
21. Savić Pavićević D, Miladinović J, Brkušanin M, et al. Molecular genetics and genetic testing in myotonic dystrophy type 1. Biomed Res Int 2013;2013:391821.
22. Lam EM, Shepard PW, St Louis EK, et al. Restless legs syndrome and daytime sleepiness are prominent in myotonic dystrophy type 2. Neurology 2013;81(2):157–64.
23. Tieleman AA, Knoop H, van de Logt A-E, et al. Poor sleep quality and fatigue but no excessive daytime sleepiness in myotonic dystrophy type 2. J Neurol Neurosurg Psychiatry 2010;81(9):963–7.
24. Romigi A, Albanese M, Liguori C, et al. Sleep–wake cycle and daytime sleepiness in the myotonic dystrophies, critical care medicine: principles of diagnosis and management in the adult. J Neurodegener Dis 2013;201:483–7.
25. Van der Meché FG, Bogaard JM, van der Sluys JC, et al. Daytime sleep in myotonic dystrophy is not caused by sleep apnoea. J Neurol Neurosurg Psychiatry 1994;57(5):626–8.
26. Yu H, Laberge L, Jaussent I, et al. Daytime sleepiness and REM sleep characteristics in myotonic dystrophy: a case-control study. Sleep 2011;34(2):165–70.
27. Shepard P, Lam EM, St Louis EK, Dominik J. Sleep disturbances in myotonic dystrophy type 2. Eur Neurol 2012;68(6):377–80.
28. Martínez-Rodríguez JE, Lin L, Iranzo A, et al. Decreased hypocretin-1 (Orexin-A) levels in the cerebrospinal fluid of patients with myotonic dystrophy and excessive daytime sleepiness. Sleep 2003;26(3):287–90.
29. Fernandes Oliveira E, Nacif SR, Alves Pereira N, et al. Sleep disorders in patients with myasthenia gravis: a systematic review. J Phys Ther Sci 2015;27(6):2013–18.
30. Nicolle MW, Rask S, Koopman WJ, et al. Sleep apnea in patients with myasthenia gravis. Neurology 2006;67(1):140–2.
31. Quera-Salva MA, Guilleminault C, Chevret S, et al. Breathing disorders during sleep in myasthenia gravis. Ann Neurol 1992;31(1):86–92.
32. Martínez De Lapiscina EH, Aguirre MEE, Blanco TA, Pascual IJ. Myasthenia gravis: sleep quality, quality of life, and disease severity. Muscle Nerve 2012;46(2):174–80.
33. Amino A, Shiozawa Z, Nagasaka T, et al. Sleep apnoea in well-controlled myasthenia gravis and the effect of thymectomy. J Neurol 1998;245(2):77–80.
34. Culebras A. Disorders and neurologic diseases, 2nd ed. Boca Raton: CRC Press, 2007.
35. Della Marca G, Frusciante R, Vollono C, et al. Sleep quality in facioscapulohumeral muscular dystrophy. J Neurol Sci 2007;263(1–2):49–53.
36. Della Marca G, Frusciante R, Dittoni S, et al. Decreased nocturnal movements in patients with facioscapulohumeral muscular dystrophy. J Clin Sleep Med 2010;6(3):276–80.
37. Della Marca G, Frusciante R, Dittoni S, et al. Sleep disordered breathing in facioscapulohumeral muscular dystrophy. J Neurol Sci 2009;285(1–2):54–8.
38. Pinard J-M, Azabou E, Essid N, et al. Sleep-disordered breathing in children with congenital muscular dystrophies. Eur J Paediatr Neurol 2012;16(6):619–24.
39. Grigg-Damberger MM, Wagner LK, Brown LK. Sleep hypoventilation in patients with neuromuscular diseases. Sleep Med Clin 2012;7:667–87.
40. Mellies U, Ragette R, Schwake C, et al. Sleep-disordered breathing and respiratory failure in acid maltase deficiency. Neurology 2001;57(7):1290–5.
41. Sharp LJ, Haller RG. Metabolic and mitochondrial myopathies. Neurol Clin 2014;32(3):777–99.

42. Selva-O'Callaghan A, Sampol G, Romero O, et al. Obstructive sleep apnea in patients with inflammatory myopathies. Muscle Nerve 2009;39(2):144–9.

43. Jinnur P, Kumar N, Vassallo R, St Louis EK. A 54-year-old man with acute onset orthopnea and sleep-related hypoxia. J Clin Sleep Med 2014;10(5):595–8.

44. McCool FD, Tzelepis GE. Dysfunction of the diaphragm. N Engl J Med 2012;366(10):932–42.

45. Giannoccaro MP, Moghadam KK, Pizza F, et al. Sleep disorders in patients with spinal cord injury. Sleep Med Rev 2013;17(6):399–409.

46. Biering-Sørensen F, Jennum P, Laub M. Sleep disordered breathing following spinal cord injury. Respir Physiol Neurobiol 2009;169(2):165–70.

47. Bensmail D, Marquer A, Roche N, et al. Pilot study assessing the impact of intrathecal baclofen administration mode on sleep-related respiratory parameters. Arch Phys Med Rehabil 2012;93(1):96–9.

48. Posluszny JA, Onders R, Kerwin AJ, et al. Multicenter review of diaphragm pacing in spinal cord injury: successful not only in weaning from ventilators but also in bridging to independent respiration. J Trauma Acute Care Surg 2014;76(2):303–9; discussion 309–10.

49. Hsu AA, Staats BA. "Postpolio" sequelae and sleep-related disordered breathing. Mayo Clin Proc 1998;73(3):216–24.

50. Mellies U, Dohna-Schwake C, Stehling F, Voit T. Sleep disordered breathing in spinal muscular atrophy. Neuromuscul Disord 2004;14(12):797–803.

51. Bourke SC, Bulloc RE, Williams TL, Shaw PJ, Gibson CJ. Noninvasive ventilation in ALS: indications and effects on quality of life. Neurology 2003;61:171–7.

52. Ritsma BR, Berger MJ, Charland DA, et al. NIPPV: prevalence, approach and barriers to use at Canadian ALS centres. Can J Neurol Sci 2010;37(1):54–60.

53. Wolfe LF, Joyce NC, McDonald CM, Benditt JO, Finder J. Management of pulmonary complications in neuromuscular disease. Phys Med Rehabil Clin N Am 2012;23(4):829–53.

54. Finder JD, Birnkrant D, Carl J, et al. Respiratory care of the patient with Duchenne muscular dystrophy: ATS consensus statement. Am J Respir Crit Care Med 2004;170(4):456–65.

55. Lo Coco D, Marchese S, Pesco MC, et al. Noninvasive positive-pressure ventilation in ALS: predictors of tolerance and survival. Neurology 2006;67(5):761–5.

56. Radunovic A, Annane D, Rafiq MK, Mustfa N. Mechanical ventilation for amyotrophic lateral sclerosis/motor neuron disease. Cochrane Database Syst Rev 2013;3:CD004427.

57. Onders RP, Dimarco AF, Ignagni AR, Aiyar H MJ. Mapping the phrenic nerve motor point: the key to a successful laparoscopic diaphragm pacing system in the first human series. Surgery 2004;4(136):819–26.

58. Lawn ND, Fletcher DD, Henderson RD, Wolter TD, Wijdicks EF. Anticipating mechanical ventilation in Guillain-Barré syndrome. Arch Neurol 2001;58(6):893–8. Available from: http://www.ncbi.nlm.nih.gov/pubmed/11405803

59. Durbin CG Jr. Indications for and timing of tracheostomy. Respir Care 2005;50(4):483–7.

CHAPTER 31

Sleep in other neurological disorders—headache

Pradeep Sahota and Niranjan N. Singh

Introduction

Headache and sleep disorder are among the most commonly reported problems in clinical practice and often coexist in the same patient. The two are related in several ways, though the relationship is very complex and still not very well understood [1–8].

In 1873, Living published the very first observation on the relationship between sleep and headache [1]. However, he did not offer any explanation. In 1929, Hans Berger recorded the first EEG and demonstrated the difference in electrical activity between awake and sleep [9], with subsequent development of polysomnography (PSG). In 1945, Bing described headaches on awakening [2]. In 1970, Dexter and Weitzman described a relationship between headache and sleep stages [6]. Relationship between chronic paroxysmal hemicrania and REM sleep was described in 1978. A relationship between dreams and headache has been also reported [10]. In 1990, Sahota and Dexter published a review describing the spectrum of this relationship between headache and sleep [11].

PSG has become more widely available in the last 30 years, and there is now increased access to trained physicians who treat sleep disorders, headaches or both with better understanding of the relationship between sleep and headache. We will review the spectrum of this relationship between these two entities and then focus on treatment of headaches related to sleep.

Epidemiology

Headache may be intrinsically related to sleep (migraine with and without aura, cluster headaches, hypnic headaches, and paroxysmal hemicrania). It can also cause chronic sleep disturbance (chronic migraine, chronic tension-type headache, and medication-overuse headache) or may be the manifestation of a sleep disorder (eg, sleep apnea-related headache). Headache and sleep disorder may be a common manifestation of systemic illness like infection, anemia, hypoxia, or any metabolic disturbance.

According to a population-based study from the United States, the 1-year prevalence of migraine in the general population is 11.7% (17.1% for females and 5.6% for males) [12]. Cluster headache is relatively rare, with a prevalence of 0.1–0.3%, and more common in males [13]. Headaches on awakening or nocturnal headaches were reported in 17% of patients attending a headache clinic [14]. According to Rasmussen, 24% of migraineurs and 12% of tension-type headache patients have headaches during sleep or upon awakening [15].

Snoring and headache have also been examined in various studies. According to a Swedish study, morning headaches were present in 18% of snorers versus 5% of controls [16]. Headache frequency in sleep apnea varies from 15% to 50% and occurs more frequently than in insomniacs [16]. Hence, headaches in sleep or related to sleep are common (see Boxes 31.1 and 31.2).

Relationship between headache and sleep

This relationship can be divided into two aspects:

1. Headache may affect sleep.
2. Sleep may affect headache.

Headache may affect sleep

Headache may or may not be associated with sleep disruption. Kayed et al. reported 17/18 attacks of paroxysmal hemicrania during REM sleep [17]. Headaches disrupted the sleep architecture, leading to decreased total sleep time, diminished REM sleep, and an eightfold increase in awakenings during REM sleep.

Wolff reported that "in two-thirds of the patients with cluster headache, the headache always began during sleep and the pain is so severe that the patient frequently jumps out of the bed before he is fully awake" [18]. Dexter and Weitzman reported four patients with cluster headache, when they noticed significant decrease in total REM sleep along with increases in stage III and IV sleep [6].

There is also experimental data to suggest a common anatomical and physiological substrate for headache and sleep. Recent advancement in functional imaging and biochemistry suggest a potential central generator regulating both headaches and sleep [19–21].

Sleep may affect headache

Headache may occur during sleep, after sleep, and in relation to different stages of sleep [2,6–8,11,14]. Headache may be triggered by sleep dysregulation. Lack of sleep and excessive sleep are both considered among the most common triggers for migraine headache [22].

According to a large migraine and sleep study in over 1283 migraineurs, sleep disturbance and oversleeping were recognized as headache triggers in 50% and 37% patients, respectively, while 85% of patients reported sleep as a deactivator. More than two-thirds of these patients reported early morning headaches. Less than 6 hours

Box 31.1 Extent of relationship between sleep and headache (sleep and headache are known to be related in several ways)

Sleep-related headaches (during and after sleep)

- Migraine with and without aura
- Paroxysmal hemicrania (PH)
- Cluster headache (CH)
- Hypnic headache (HH)

Sleep-phase-related headaches

With stage N3 and REM sleep

- Migraine with and without aura

With REM sleep

- Episodic cluster headache
- Migraine with and without aura
- Paroxysmal hemicrania
- Hypnic headache

Length of sleep and headaches (excessive deep sleep, lack of sleep, and sleep disruption)

- Migraine with and without aura
- Tension-type headache (TTH)

Sleep relieves headaches

- Migraine with and without aura

Sleep disorders and headaches

- Obstructive sleep apnea syndrome (OSAS) and headaches
- Somnambulism and headaches
- Other parasomnias and headaches

Effect of headaches on sleep (minimal to significant sleep disruption)

- Migraine with and without aura
- Cluster headache
- Hypnic headache

Dreams and Headaches

- Migraine with and without aura

Adapted from Headache, 30(2), Sahota PK, Dexter JD, Sleep and headache syndromes: a clinical review, pp. 80–4, Copyright (1990), with permission from John Wiley and Sons.

Box 31.2 Interrelationship between headache and sleep

- Headache is a symptom of a primary sleep disturbance
- Sleep disturbance is a symptom of a primary headache disorder
- Sleep disturbance and headache are symptoms of an unrelated medical disorder
- Sleep disturbance and headache are both manifestations of a similar underlying pathogenesis

Source data from Headache, 5(10), Paiva T, Batista A, Martins P, Martins A, The relationship between headaches and sleep disturbances, pp. 590–6, Copyright (1995), John Wiley and Sons.

headaches were common in patients with sleep disorder: 34% versus 7% in controls. Twenty-five percent of patients reported morning headache versus 3% of controls [24].

A variety of sleep disorders were associated with headache, including obstructive sleep apnea (OSA) syndrome (OSAS), insomnia, restless legs syndrome (RLS), hypersomnia, and parasomnias [24]. Compared with insomniacs, morning headaches are more common in OSA: 74% versus 40% in controls [25].

Sleep–headache relationship: anatomical and physiological basis

While the relationship between headache and sleep is complex and is still not well understood, there are some common neural substrates. Sleep and trigeminal pain processing share several common pathways with respect to neurotransmission and function of distinct brain areas. The central structure involving both headache and sleep include the hypothalamus (especially orexinergic neurons) and periaqueductal gray areas (PAG) [26].

The transition from wake to sleep and vice versa is thought to be mediated via a flip-flop switch [27]. The anatomical basis of this flip-flop mechanism is an interconnection between the arousal-generating centers and sleep-regulatory centers in the brain. The arousal-associated network consists of the orexinergic perifornical hypothalamus, tuberomammillary nucleus, locus coeruleus, and dorsal median raphe, which are inhibited by the sleep-regulatory ventrolateral preoptic nucleus of the hypothalamus via γ-aminobutyric acid (GABA) and galanin. A circadian mechanism also exists to regulate sleep in a 24-hour cycle. The ventrolateral portion of the periaqueductal gray matter (vlPAG) is a region that regulates both sleep and pain. Stimulation of this region may lead to REM sleep and antinociception [28]. Involvement of the hypothalamus ia also suggested by clinical aspects of headache—such as the autonomic activation, yawning, and sleepiness associated with migraine [29].

Neurophysiological and positron emission tomography (PET) imaging studies have shown hypothalamic activation in cluster headache and brainstem activation in migraine headaches [30]. There is evidence that dysfunctional hypothalamic activity contributes to both altered sleep–wake function and headache via orexinergic neurons, which are exclusively localized in the perifornical hypothalamus and synthesize two neuropeptides (orexins A and B) that bind to receptors found throughout the neuraxis, including the brainstem [31].

sleep was noticed in 38% of patients [22]. In another study of 289 headaches, the prevalence of insomnia was reported to be 60% [23]. Goder et al. reviewed association between sleep and headache in 432 patients who underwent PSG and 30 controls without any sleep problem and reported that combined nocturnal and early morning

Melatonin also has an important role to play in sleep and headache. It is synthesized from serotonin by the pineal gland. The control of melatonin secretion involves the suprachiasmatic nucleus, which integrates light-independent activity of the retinal hypothalamic pathway. Cluster headache shows a decrease in peak and median melatonin secretion [32].

The brainstem and hypothalamic nuclei are hypothesized to regulate both sleep and headache. The hypothalamus has a role in descending control of pain perception, with connections to the periaqueductal gray, the locus coeruleus, and the median raphe nuclei. The hypothalamus and interconnected brainstem areas likely represent the neural sites responsible for the chronobiological features of some headaches, in particular the sleep-related attacks typical of trigeminal autonomic cephalalgia (TAC), migraines, and hypnic headaches [33].

Functional imaging studies using $H_2^{15}O$-PET and functional magnetic resonance imaging (fMRI) have shown activation of the hypothalamus during cluster headache, short-lasting unilateral neuralgiform headache with conjunctival injection and tearing (SUNCT syndrome), and hemicrania continua [34,35]. PET scans have already demonstrated brainstem activation in spontaneous migraine attacks [36].

The locus coeruleus and dorsal raphe nuclei are repositories of norepinephrine (noradrenaline) and serotonin (5-hydoxytryptamine, 5-HT). The serotonergic system has an inherent rhythm, under the control of the suprachiasmatic nucleus. The role of 5-HT in migraine is well established. Intravenous 5-HT can abort migraine attacks, by supplementing the depletion that induces migraine attacks [37]. This has led to the development of serotonin receptor agonists (triptans), which are the mainstay of treatment of acute migraines. Serotonin depletion is also observed during REM sleep, which may account for a relationship between REM and migraine. The trigeminovascular system is involved in migraine headache.

There is overwhelming evidence that cluster headaches and hypnic headaches are chronobiological disorders with a strong association with sleep and hypothalamus. Cluster headache shows a remarkable periodicity (circannual and circadian), suggesting a linkage to the circadian rhythm. In cluster headache, pain is located peri-orbitally in the trigeminal nerve distribution, with ipsilateral parasympathetic (rhinorrhea and lacrimation) and sympathetic (Horner syndrome) manifestations and with periodicity and clustering (hypothalamic dysfunction and suprachiasmatic nuclei). The regulatory role of the suprachiasmatic nucleus on the sleep–wake cycle and circadian rhythm provides strong evidence of an inherent relationship between sleep and headache.

Differential diagnosis of headache during sleep

Headache in relationship to sleep has a wide differential diagnosis. Important differential considerations include sleep apnea-related headache, hypnic headache, cluster headache, exploding head syndrome, episodic and chronic migraine headaches, and tension-type headaches. A diagnosis of these primary headache disorders is based on the recurring pattern of the headache with normal interval examination. Secondary causes of the headache should be excluded by a careful history, examination, and appropriate diagnostic testing including neuroimaging and other tests as required.

Simple questionnaires can provide key information. The headache and sleep diaries are important tools which can help to characterize the headache and its relationship to sleep. In the following sections, we will give a brief overview of sleep-related headaches, followed by a discussion of their management.

Sleep-related headaches and their management

Cluster headache

Cluster headache is a trigeminal autonomic cephalalgia that presents as episodes of severe excruciating unilateral retro-orbital pain with profound autonomic features of Horner syndrome including miosis, anhydrosis, ptosis, rhinorrhea, lacrimation, nasal congestion, and redness of eye. A single episode may last 15–180 minutes. The episodes may happen in a cluster of one to nine attacks in one day, clustered over months, or throughout the year [38].

Russell found a preponderance of attacks beginning during sleep, with the majority of daytime attacks happening when the patient was physically relaxed [39]. Cluster headache has been reported to occur during REM sleep [6,40]. Dexter and Weitzman recorded nine cluster headache episodes in three patients, of which seven episodes occurred during REM sleep within 9 minutes of REM onset [6].

The majority of the headaches occur between 9 pm and 10 am [41]. It has also been reported in several studies that patients with cluster headache have a high incidence of OSA [40,41] There is an 8- to 24-fold increase in the incidence of OSA in cluster headache [41].

Nocturnal hypoxia related to OSA could be a trigger for cluster headache [42].

Hypothalamic involvement has also been implicated, as there is a correlation between improvement of headache and sleep architecture with deep brain stimulation [43].

Hypnic headache

Raskin in 1988 described six elderly patients with headaches occurring exclusively during sleep. [44]. This is a rare headache syndrome, with only 174 cases reported in the literature by 2011 and with a prevalence of less than 0.1% in the headache clinic [45].

Hypnic headache is also called alarm clock headache. It is characterized by dull headache occurring exclusively during waking up from sleep at a constant time, usually between 1 am and 3 am, and lasting for an hour, with an average frequency of one per week to six per night. It is more common in elderly females. It is distinct from cluster headache, being less severe, with a lack of unilateralism and an absence of cranial autonomic symptoms [44,46,47]. A meta-analysis of data pulled from 71 published cases of hypnic headache revealed a duration of 67 ± 44 minutes with a frequency of 1.2 ± 0.9 per 24 hours [46].

The relationship between hypnic headache and sleep stages is complex and controversial. In the initial description, Raskin hypothesized that hypnic headache is related to REM sleep [44]. There have been anecdotal reports of association between hypnic headache, OSA, and REM sleep [47]. Recently, this hypothesis was challenged by Holle et al., who reported that 73% of hypnic headache attacks occur during non-REM (NREM) sleep [48].

Migraine

The relationship between migraine and sleep is very complex. Sleep is a known deactivator for a migraine, but patients can wake up with a migraine attack as well. Migraine can emerge during nocturnal sleep, or following a brief period of nap, or in relation to a change in sleep duration (either over- or under-sleeping). Patients with migraine without aura have much higher prevalence of sleep abnormalities [49]. Various sleep abnormalities, including insomnia, parasomnia, RLS, narcolepsy, excessive daytime sleepiness (EDS), and feeling sleepy when waking up, have been found to be associated with episodic and chronic migraine. The exact pathophysiology remains unclear. In the following subsections, important sleep disturbances with migraine will be described.

Migraine with and without aura is an episodic throbbing headache of moderate to severe intensity lasting between 4 and 72 hours. It can be unilateral or bilateral in location. The headache may be preceded by a visual or other somatosensory aura. The patient becomes sensitive to light, sound, movement, and smell in various combinations. Approximately 15–20% of patients may experience reversible focal neurological deficits lasting less than 60 minutes, the most common being visual symptoms.

As early as 1970, Dexter and Weitzman studied three migraine patients and reported eight arousals. Six of these were during REM sleep, within 3–9 minutes [6]. Another study by Dexter revealed a consistent relationship between morning headache and arousals during nights with larger amounts of stage III and IV and REM sleep [7]. In a recent, larger study of over 3 years, involving 1698 migraine patients (3582 migraine attacks), the chance of waking up with a migraine attack per hour was more than twice between 4 am and 9 am (254 attacks/hour) compared with any other hour (115 attacks/hour). This trend associates the later parts (REM predominant) of the sleep cycle with the occurrence of migraine [50]. However, these data were not confirmed by Goder et al., who found no association between sleep stages and migraine headache [24]. Migraine is associated with a variety of known sleep disorders, some of which will be described here.

Migraine and restless legs syndrome

The frequency of RLS in migraine patients in the pediatric age group is significantly higher than in adults (22% versus 5%) [51]. A strong association between migraine and RLS is reported in women [52]. Rhode et al., in a case–control study of patients with migraine, found a significant higher lifetime prevalence of RLS than the control group [53]. Similar correlation has been reported by d'Onofrio et al. [54] and by Chen et al. [55]. The underlying pathophysiology has been linked to the dysfunction of dopaminergic metabolism in migraine [53,56].

Migraine and narcolepsy

The association between migraine and narcolepsy is controversial. Dahmen et al. reported a two- to fourfold increase in migraine prevalence in patients with narcolepsy [57, 8]. On the contrary, in a multicenter case–control study of 96 patients with narcolepsy, there was no significant association with migraine [59]. The patients with narcolepsy showed nonspecific headache due to sleep disturbance, not fulfilling the diagnostic criteria for migraine.

Migraine and insomnia

In a survey by Lateef et al., adults with migraine reported more frequent difficulty in initiating sleep, difficulty with staying asleep, early morning awakening, and daytime fatigue when compared with the individual without headache [60].

In population-based study from Hong Kong, in Chinese women with different headache diagnoses, early waking up was noted in 29% of patients, difficulty in staying asleep in 28%, and difficulty in falling asleep in 24.4% [61].

In another population-based study from Sweden, difficulty in initiating sleep, a high degree of sleepiness when waking up, and daytime sleepiness were more common in patients with migraine than in those without [62]. Insomnia was not common in patients with migraine in this study.

Migraine and excessive daytime sleepiness

A high prevalence of EDS has been reported in patients with migraine. Peres et al. reported EDS in migraine patients with an Epworth Sleepiness Scale (ESS) score of more than 10 in 37% [63]. EDS was more frequent in migraineurs than in controls [64].

In a recent population-based study from Sweden addressing the relationship between headache and sleep, among 297 participants (77 headache-free subjects, 135 diagnosed with tension-type headache, 51 with migraine, and 34 with other headaches, including hangover headache, caffeine withdrawal headache, headache attributed to systemic viral infection, medication-overuse headache, and possible migraine with tension-type headache), ESS over 10 was more common in those with migraine than in those without [62].

Migraine and other sleep disturbances

An increased prevalence of parasomnias, including bruxism, sleep-talking and sleepwalking, and night terrors, has been reported in children with migraine [65].

Chronic migraine and sleep

The relationship between chronic migraine and sleep is different from that between episodic migraine and sleep. Patients with chronic migraine present with headache of more than 15 days in a month, each episode lasting more than 4 hours for at least 3 months. These headaches arise from episodic migraine. There is often a component of medication-overuse headache defined as use of pain medications more than 15 days in a month or triptans more than 10 days in a month on a regular basis. There are often associated psychiatric comorbidities including insomnia. The Nord-Trondelag Health Study revealed that subjects with chronic migraine had a 17 times higher risk of severe sleep disturbance [62] than those without chronic migraine.

Sleep apnea headache

According to the International Classification of Sleep Disorders, Third Edition (ICSD-3), sleep apnea headache is classified as a secondary headache attributed to disorders of homeostasis. A typical sleep apnea-related headache is a bilateral pressing quality pain occurring more than 15 days in a month—without nausea, photophobia, phonophobia, or vomiting, the headache improves within 30 minutes of waking up, with complete resolution within 72 hours of effective treatment of sleep apnea. Prevalence of sleep apnea headaches is variable. According to Aldrich et al., the frequency of morning headaches was 18% in patients with OSA versus 21–38% in patients with other sleep disorders [66]. Morning headaches have been reported in habitual snorers as well as in their bed partners [67].

In a recent population based cross-sectional study from Norway, sleep apnea headache was reported in 11.8% of patients with OSA versus 4.6% of participants without sleep apnea. The prevalence of headache was also related to the severity of sleep apnea, with higher prevalence in severe sleep apnea with apnea–hypopnea index AHI > 30 [68]. Similarly, in a Turkish study, morning headache was reported in 33.6% of patients with OSA with AHI > 5. These headaches resolved with effective treatment of sleep apnea using positive pressure [69]. In a large telephone survey of 18 980 participants from Europe, the prevalence of chronic morning headache was found to be 7.6%. The headache was more common in patients with depression, insomnia, and sleep-related breathing disorders [70].

It is still unclear whether hypoxia or degree of oxygen desaturation is the underlying pathophysiology for morning headache.

Exploding head syndrome

First described by Armstrong-Jones in 1920, this is unique and a rare syndrome of sudden loud painless explosive sound in the head without any actual headache. The condition may be frightening, awakening the patient from sleep [71].

In a polysomnographic evaluation of nine patients with exploding head syndrome, the episode occurred during nocturnal awakening when the subject was relaxed but temporarily awake. In ICSD-3, exploding head syndrome is listed among the parasomnias [72].

Tension-type headache

Various sleep abnormalities, including insufficient sleep and oversleeping, have been associated with tension-type headache (TTH). In a study by Karly et al., 12.9% of the patients with TTH reported oversleeping as a precipitating factor [73]. Insufficient sleep has been noted as an aggravating factor for TTH [74,75].

Results from the third Nord–Trøndelag Health Survey indicated that subjects with chronic headache were 17 times more likely to have severe sleep disturbances, with the association being somewhat stronger for chronic migraine than for chronic TTH [62].

In a recent study using actigraphy and computerized ecological momentary assessment, a longer total sleep time along with poor sleep quality was associated with TTH [76]. In a cross-sectional study from Norway, sleep apnea did not have any association with TTH in the general population [77].

Paroxysmal hemicranias

Attacks with characteristics of pain and associated symptoms and signs similar to those of cluster headache have been described in paroxysmal hemicranias, but they are shorter-lasting, more frequent than in cluster headache, occur more commonly in women than men, and respond very well to indomethacin. Each attack consists of severe unilateral, hemicranial headache with ipsilateral cranial autonomic features (miosis, ptosis, lacrimation, and rhinorrhea) lasting from 2 to 45 minutes, and occurs more frequently within a 24-hour period.

Paroxysmal hemicrania has been called "REM-locked" headache. Kayed et al. reported 17 out of 18 attacks during REM sleep [17]. The headaches also disrupted the sleep architecture, leading to decreased total sleep time and REM sleep.

Management of headaches and sleep

Primary headache syndromes such as migraine and cluster headaches occurring during the night must be differentiated from acute severe secondary headache seen in patient with brain tumors, intracranial hemorrhage, and meningitis. Headaches on awakening or early morning headaches can be observed in patients with sleep apnea, depression, anxiety, chronic TTH, substance abuse, and medication-overuse headache. Red flags in the history and examination include first and worst headache, progressive worsening of headache, intractable vomiting, fever, signs of encephalopathy, stiff neck, and weakness, and these necessitate careful workup, including a neurological consultation along with neuroimaging and lumbar puncture, depending upon the headache characteristics. A careful sleep history along with a sleep diary should be obtained in the context of 24-hour sleep–wake cycle. A combined sleep–wake and headache diary is most helpful in delineating the occurrence of headache in relationship to sleep. The Berlin Sleep Questionnaire has a positive predictive value of 89% for sleep apnea [28]. An insomnia calendar is helpful for the patient with significant insomnia and headache, inquiring about bedroom environment, sleep schedule, daytime naps, whether caffeine and medication promote insomnia, and whether nicotine leads to emotional and cognitive arousals [28].

PSG may be required for better assessment of sleep factors, including sleep apnea, parasomnia, and other sleep disorders.

Treatment of different headache syndromes

Migraine with and without aura, chronic migraine, and medication-overuse headache

The treatment of headache can divided into pharmacological and nonpharmacological options.

Nonpharmacological management

There should be an individualized approach, depending upon the patient's comorbid conditions. The following are some general guidelines:

1. Maintenance of the biorhythms with regular sleep schedule, regular meals, aerobic exercises, and avoiding triggers.

2. Diet has an important role in the management of migraine headaches, with avoidance of high carbohydrate food and caffeine being very important.

3. Patients with medication overuse will require detoxification, limiting pain medication to fewer than 10 days in a month. Naproxen has been shown to be effective during the weaning period [78].

4. Smoking cessation and maintaining an appropriate weight are very important.

5. Appropriate screening for sleep disorders in patients with a headache, including detailed history and PSG if needed, cannot be overemphasized.

6. Patients with insomnia or poor sleep hygiene should be encouraged to undergo behavioral sleep modification. Referral for more intensive behavioral insomnia treatment may be needed.

7. A five-component intervention used by Calhoun and Ford may be useful [79]:

   I. Schedule a consistent bedtime that allows 8 hours in bed.

   II. Avoid watching TV, reading, and listening to music in bed.

   III. Use visualization techniques to shorten the time to sleep onset.

IV. Supper should be at least 4 hours before bedtime and only limited amounts of fluids should be taken within 2 hours of bedtime.

V. Discontinue daytime naps.

8. Psychiatric comorbidities should be identified and treated as well.

Pharmacological treatment

Acute treatment is needed to abort a single severe attack of migraine headache. The appropriate medications can be used at home, in the emergency room or urgent care center, or in an inpatient setting. They consist of analgesics and migraine-specific therapies (triptans and ergotamines).

Triptans and nonsteroidal anti-inflammatory drugs (NSAIDs) are considered the first-line treatment for an acute attack of migraine headache. Antiemetics (including ondansetron and promethazine), neuroleptics (including chlorpromazine and prochlorperazine), ketorolac, magnesium, divalproex sodium, and a steroid (methylprednisolone oral or IV) have been used to abort a short or protracted course of headache in office, home and inpatient settings.

Triptans

Triptans are selective serotonin 5-HT_{1B} and 5-HT_{1D} receptor agonists [80]. Three postulated mechanisms of action of these medications are the following: intracranial vasoconstriction (1B), peripheral neuronal inhibition (1D) and presynaptic dorsal horn stimulation (1D).

Efficacy has been reported in multiple randomized trials [81]. Current evidence suggests nearly equivalent efficacy among oral triptans except frovatriptan, which is less efficacious but has a longer half-life [82]. The choice of agent may often be determined by insurance coverage and patient preference.

Ergots

Ergots are less specific than triptans in their serotonin receptor agonism, which possibly explains their more robust side effects [83]. Dihydroergotamine (DHE) is currently the only widely available ergot alkaloid. Available preparations include a nasal spray and injections. The nasal spray is used as one puff of 0.5 mg in each nostril, repeated after 15 minutes, with 2 mg maximum daily dose. Injectable DHE is 0.5–1 mg repeated after 1 hour, with a 3 mg maximum daily dose. It is usually administered in the emergency department and inpatient setting, but can be self-administered [84]. Repetitive intravenous administration of DHE over several days (according to the Raskin and other protocols) is helpful in managing chronic migraine and status migrainosus.

Preventive treatment

There are several medications used as preventive treatment for high-frequency migraine, chronic migraine, and medication-overuse headache. Possible mechanism of action include stabilization of the reactive nervous system, enhancement of the anti-nociceptive pathway, inhibition of central and peripheral sensitization, and inhibition of cortical spreading depression [80,85–87]. Preventive treatment is used to reduce the frequency, duration, and intensity of headache, along with improved responsiveness to acute therapy. It has also been shown that preventive treatment slows progression to chronic migraine.

Methysergide was the first preventive medication used in the 1960s. Since then, no specific medication has been developed for the preventive treatment of migraine. There are several classes of medications used in preventive therapy, including antiepileptics (eg, topiramate and divalproex soldium), antidepressants (eg, amitriptyline), beta-blockers (eg, propranolol), calcium channel blockers (eg, verapamil), and botulinum toxin. A detailed discussion of these agents is beyond the scope of this chapter. Patients with three or more episodes per month may be candidates for preventive treatment. Generally, these medications should be started at a small dose and slowly titrated to the maximum recommended and tolerated dose. An adequate trial of 2–3 months is reasonable. Comorbid conditions, insurance coverage, drug interactions, and side effects should be considered when making a choice.

Migraine in women

Women present with unique issues in the management of migraine headaches. There are several unique features that may impact headaches and their treatment. Menarche, pregnancy, pre-menopause, menopause, and late-life migraine are different phases in women's life related to changes in hormones.

Menstrual migraine and menstrual-related migraine are unique conditions related to fluctuations in estrogen level [88]. Standard abortive and preventative treatment can be applied, with a special precaution of contraception failure and teratogenic effects. Folic acid 0.4–0.8 mg is recommended for every woman on migraine-preventive treatment. Women with a history of migraine and a history of thrombosis, ischemic heart disease, stroke, or smoking should not be offered combined oral contraceptives [88]. Women with migraines should not smoke if using oral contraceptives. Triptans are designated category C for use during pregnancy, but approved during breastfeeding.

Pregnancy may lead to improvement in more than 55% of patients with migraine, mostly in the second half of pregnancy.

Improvement in migraine has been noted in one-third of women after spontaneous menopause, but worsening is reported in more than two-thirds after surgical menopause. High-dose hormone replacement treatment has been shown to increase the risk for stroke.

Finally, a history of physical and sexual abuse in women with chronic migraine is common and needs to be addressed at the time of treatment.

Emerging treatments

In late 2009, antagonists to calcitonin gene-related peptide (CGRP), known as gepants, became a new hope for the treatment of acute migraine [89]. The absence of vasoconstrictive effects with gepants can be considered an advantage over triptans. Gepants are in different phases of development.

Oral lasmiditan, a 5-HT_{1F} receptor agonist that is centrally acting and highly selective, without the vasoconstrictive effects of triptans and DHE, has shown to be effective in a small placebo-controlled trial. [90].

Interventional treatments

There have been several open label non-randomized studies using neuromodulation: the ONSTIM (Occipital Nerve Stimulation for the Treatment of Chronic Migraine Headache) study, the PRISM (Precision Implantable Stimulator for Migraine) study, and a St Jude's study involving around 1200 patients with chronic migraine. Results have shown some promise, but several questions (including that of cost) need to be answered before any further recommendations can be made [91].

Occipital nerve stimulation (ONS) is a surgical procedure for refractory headache, including chronic migraine. A 60% improvement was seen in 17 patients with chronic daily headache after ONS, including two patients with chronic migraine [92]. Lead migration and infections were common problems after ONS replacement in area studies. Peripheral procedures such as occipital nerve blocks or trigger point injections are promising rescue treatments for migraine and may be effective in medication-overuse and chronic migraine. Tobin and Flitman reported a 56% improvement in medication-overuse patients [92]. In a single blinded randomized controlled trial with chronic migraine patients, occipital nerve block with triamcinolone combined with lidocaine was not superior to lidocaine alone [93].

Cluster headaches

The medical management of cluster headache includes both acute therapy aimed at aborting individual attacks and prophylactic therapy aimed at preventing recurrent attacks and clustering [94]. Agents used for acute therapy include inhalation of oxygen and sumatriptan. Transitional prophylaxis involves a short course of steroid (prednisone). The mainstay of prophylaxis is verapamil, but methysergide (which entails a risk of retroperitoneal fibrosis but may be used in refractory cases after proper patient education and explanation of risks), lithium, and divalproex sodium can also be used. Some patients may benefit from topiramate and melatonin [95].

Acute treatment
High flow oxygen, 100% at 12–15 L/min for 15–20 minutes has been shown to be very effective [96]. Injectable sumatriptan 6 mg is the only US-approved treatment for cluster headache. Nasal sprays of sumatriptan 20 mg and zolmitriptan 5 mg are also effective [97,98].

The choice of agent may often be determined by insurance coverage and patient preference (see Tables 31.1 and 31.2]).

Prophylactic treatment
For the prophylactic treatment of cluster headache, verapamil and lithium remains the mainstay of treatment, bridging with a short course of steroid (prednisone) [99,100].

Nonpharmacological treatment
Diet and lifestyle modification
Cluster headache is a chronobiological disorder, with attacks occurring during REM sleep. Alcohol is a known trigger and should be avoided during the cluster period. The prevalence of sleep apnea is very high in patients with cluster headache, and therefore maintenance of ideal weight and treatment of sleep apnea are highly recommended.

Table 31.1 Summary of practical clinical pharmacology of the medication used in acute headache management

Drug	Indications	Dose (maximum dose/day)	Drug interactions and contraindications	Typical adverse effects	Cost-effectiveness
Almotriptan: tablets	Migraine	6.25–12.5 mg (25 mg)	Contain sulfur; Dose reduction with CYP3A4 inhibitors	Dizziness, chest pressure, nausea, abnormal taste, paresthesias, vasospasm	Expensive
Eletriptan: tablets	Migraine	20-40 mg (80 mg)	Dose reduction with CYP3A4 inhibitors	Dizziness, chest pressure, nausea, abnormal taste, paresthesias, vasospasm	Expensive
Rizatriptan: tablets	Migraine and cluster headache	5-10 mg (30 mg, 15 mg if propranolol)	Dose reduction with propranolol; Do not use within 2 weeks of monoamine oxidase inhibitor (MAOI)	Dizziness, chest pressure, nausea, abnormal taste, paresthesias, vasospasm	Expensive
Sumatriptan: tablets, nasal spray, and injection; Combination with naproxen (85/500 mg)	Migraine and cluster headache	25–100 mg tablet (200 mg); 5–20 mg spray (40 mg); 4–6 mg injection (12 mg)	Do not use within 2 weeks of MAOI	Dizziness, chest pressure, nausea, abnormal taste, paresthesias, vasospasm	Moderate
Zolmitriptan: tablets and nasal spray	Migraine and cluster headache	2.5–5 mg (10 mg)	Do not use within 2 weeks of MAOI		Expensive
Frovatriptan: tablets	Migraine	2.5 mg (7.5 mg)			Expensive
Naratriptan: tablets	Migraine	1–2.5 mg (5 mg)			Expensive
Dihydroergotamine: tablets, injection, and nasal spray	Migraine and cluster headache	1–3 mg (3 mg)	Do not combine with triptans	Dizziness, chest pressure, nausea, vomiting, abdominal pain, vasospasm	Inexpensive

Table 31.2 Preventive treatment for migraine, cluster headache, and hypnic headache

Drug	Indications	Usual daily dose	Drug interactions and contraindications	Typical adverse effects	Cost-effectiveness
Propranolol: tablets	Migraine	80–240 mg	Contraindicated in asthma Major interaction with thioridazine and calcium channel blockers	Dizziness, bronchospasm, Bradycardia	Inexpensive
Verapamil: tablets	Migraine and cluster headache	180–480 mg	Major interactions with lomitapide and clozapine	Dizziness, Bradycardia, constipation	Inexpensive
Amitriptyline: tablets	Migraine	25–150 mg	Major interaction with MAOIs	Dizziness dry mouth and dry, constipation	Inexpensive
Topiramate	Migraine and cluster headache	25–150 mg	Major interaction with metformin	Dizziness weight loss, renal stones, anomia and paresthesias	Inexpensive
Divalproex sodium	Migraine and cluster headache	250–1500 mg	Do not use in hepatic failure	Weight gain, hair loss, tremor	Inexpensive
Indomethacin	Hypnic headache and migraine headache	75–150 mg	Renal failure	Dizziness, abdominal pain	Inexpensive
Lithium	Cluster headache and hypnic headache	300–600 mg	Major interaction with several medications. Monitor lithium level	Tremor, ataxia, dizziness, multisystem adverse effects	Inexpensive
Caffeine	Hypnic headache	40–60 mg at bedtime	None	Dizziness, insomnia	Inexpensive
Botulinum toxin	Chronic migraine	155 units IM every 3 months	None	Weakness, headache	Expensive

Interventional procedures

Posterior hypothalamic neurostimulation may be considered in medically refractory cases of cluster headache. There is now enough experience with this approach to suggest that about two-thirds of patients benefit [101]. ONS is an alternative approach [102]. Recently, sphenopalatine ganglion stimulation has been proposed

Hypnic headache

Treatment of an acute attack of hypnic headache is limited because of the short duration of headaches. Triptans, oxygen, and NSAIDs are ineffective. Because of the rarity of this condition, most recommendations are based on case reports. A cup of coffee or caffeine 40–60 mg at bedtime can be used as a prophylactic treatment. Sustained-release indomethacin 75 mg at bedtime or lithium 300–600 mg daily can be used as a second-line treatment [103].

There are case reports of successful treatment with topiramate 25–100 mg at bedtime and oxeterone 60–120 mg at bedtime

Diet and lifestyle modification are important in the management of hypnic headaches.

There is a high association of OSA in patients with hypnic headache, and this should be carefully screened and treated.

Maintaining sleep hygiene, appropriate weight, and diet and smoking cessation cannot be overemphasized.

Sleep apnea-related headaches

Sleep apnea may present as an independent generator of headache or associated with cluster or hypnic headaches. OSA requires treatment according to the published guidelines using continuous positive airway pressure (CPAP), oral appliances, surgical intervention, or conservative treatment [104]. The headache is expected to improve with treatment of sleep apnea. Avoiding sedation with hypnotics or opiates until effective treatment of sleep apnea has been established is very important. Treatment of headache that persists despite standard treatment of sleep apnea requires evaluation before a symptomatic treatment can be provided on long-term basis. A reevaluation is required in 2–3 months to monitor the effectiveness of treatment.

Based on case series and uncontrolled studies, improvement in headache is expected in one-third to one-half of patients after effective treatment of sleep apnea [104].

Tension-type headaches

The diagnostic problem encountered most often is discriminating between TTH and mild migraines. Significant comorbidities, including anxiety, depression, and insomnia, should be identified and treated.

Triggers frequently reported with TTH include stress, irregular meals, high intake of coffee and other caffeine-containing drinks, dehydration, sleep disorders (including too much or too little sleep), reduced or inappropriate physical exercise, psychological problems, and hormonal swings in females during the menstrual cycle [105].

Nonpharmacological management

This should be considered for all patients. Physical therapy is the most frequently used nonpharmacological treatment of TTH and includes improvement of posture, relaxation, exercise programs, hot and cold packs, ultrasound, and electrical stimulation [106].

Psychological treatment, including electromyographic (EMG) biofeedback and relaxation training, reduces muscle tension and autonomic arousal that can precipitate headaches. Cognitive-behavioral therapy or stress management aim to teach patients to identify thoughts and beliefs that may be stressful [106].

Pharmacological treatment

Simple analgesics, including aspirin, 500–1000 mg and acetaminophen (paracetamol) 1000 mg, are effective for acute treatment. NSAIDs, including ibuprofen, naproxen, and ketoprofen, are more effective than acetaminophen and aspirin. Triptans, muscle relaxants, and opiates have no role in the treatment of TTH.

Prophylactic pharmacotherapy for chronic TTH includes amitriptyline 10–75 mg/day and mirtazapine 15–30 mg/day.

Treatment of other rare headaches

Paroxysmal hemicrania

This is an indomethacin-responsive headache. A standard dose of 25–50 mg of indomethacin three times a day is recommended, which can be used both as a diagnostic test and as treatment [107]. In patients intolerant to indomethacin, COX-2 inhibitors, topiramate, subcutaneous sumatriptan, and occipital nerve block have been tried, with successful results according to case reports.

Exploding head syndrome

So far, there have been no trials for therapies for this syndrome, although there is a report of three patients responding to clomipramine [107,108]. Reassurance that the condition is benign is very helpful.

Summary

Headache and sleep disorders are among the most common problems encountered in clinical practice. The relationship is complex and not fully understood. Management requires careful history, examination, and appropriate diagnostic tools, including a sleep and headache diary and PSG, when needed. Pharmacological treatment includes acute and preventive treatment and consideration of nonpharmacological treatment options, including diet, behavioral, and lifestyle modification along with management of sleep problems such as sleep apnea.

References

1. Living E. On megrim, sick headache and some allied disorder. London: Churchill, 1873.
2. Bing R. Lehrbuch der nerver krankhesten. Basel: B Schwabe, 1945.
3. Gans M. Part II. Treating migraine by "sleep rationing." J Nerv Ment Dis 1951;113:405–29.
4. Levitan H. Dreams which culminate in migraine headaches. Psychother Psychosom 1984;41:161–6.
5. American Academy of Sleep Medicine. International classification of sleep disorders, 2nd ed. Diagnostic and coding manual. Westchester, IL: American Academy of Sleep Medicine, 2005.
6. Dexter JD, Weitzman ED. The relationship of nocturnal headaches to sleep headaches to sleep stage patterns. Neurology 1970;20:413–519.
7. Dexter JD. The relationship between stages III + IV + REM sleep and arousals with migraine. Headache 1979;19(7):364–9.
8. Kayed K, Sjaastad O. Nocturnal and early morning headaches. Ann Clin Res 1985;17:243–6.
9. Berger H. Über das Elektroenkephalogramm des Menschen. J Psychol Neurol 1930;40:160–79.
10. Levitan H. Dreams which culminate in migraine headaches. Psychother Psychosom 1984;41(4):161–6.
11. Sahota PK, Dexter JD. Sleep and headache syndromes: a clinical review. Headache 1990;30(2):80–4.
12. Stovner LJ, Hagen K, Jensen R, et al. The global burden of headache: a documentation of headache prevalence and disability worldwide. Cephalalgia 2007;27:193–210.
13. Sjaastad O, Bakketeig LS. Cluster headache prevalence. Vaga study of headache epidemiology. Cephalalgia 2003;23:528–33.
14. Paiva T, Batista A, Martins P, Martins A. The relationship between headaches and sleep disturbances. Headache 1995;35:590–6.
15. Rasmussen BK. Migraine and tension-type headache in a general population: precipitating factors, female hormones, sleep pattern and relation to lifestyle. Pain 1993;53(1):65–72.
16. Alberti A, Mazzotta G, Gallinella E, Sarchielli P. Headache characteristics in obstructive sleep apnea syndrome and insomnia. Acta Neurol Scand 2005;111(5):309–16.
17. Kayed K, Godtlibsen OB, Sjaastad O. Chronic paroxysmal hemicranias IV: "REM sleep locked" nocturnal headache attacks. Sleep 1978;1(1):91–5.
18. Wolff HG. Headache and other head pain, 2nd ed. Oxford: Oxford University Press, 1963:455.
19. Lance JW, Lambert GA, Goadsby PJ, Duckworth JW. Brainstem influences on the cephalic circulation: experimental data from cat and money of relevance to the mechanism if migraine. Headache 1983;23(6):258–65.
20. Raskin NH, Hosouchi Y, Lamb S. Headache may arise from perturbation of brain. Headache 19087;27(8):416–20.
21. Bruyn GW. The biochemistry of migraine. Headache 1980;20(5):235–46.
22. Kelman L, Rains CJ. Headache and sleep: examination of sleep patterns and complains in large clinical sample of migraineurs. Headache 2005;45:904–10.
23. Maizels M, Burchette R. Somatic symptoms in headache patients; the influence of headache diagnosis, frequency and comorbidity. Headache 2004;44:983–93.
24. Goder R, Fritzer G, Kapsokalvyas A, et al. 19 Polysomnographic findings in nights preceeding a migraine attack. Cephalalgia 2001;21:31–7.
25. Alberti A. Headache and sleep. Sleep Med Rev 2006;10:431–7.
26. Evers S. Sleep and headache: the biological basis. Headache 2010;50(7):1246–51.
27. Lu J, Sherman D, Devor M, Saper CB. A putative flip-flop switch for control of REM sleep. Nature 2006;441:589–94.
28. Brennan KC, Charles A. Sleep and headaches. Semin Neurol 2009;29(4):406–18.
29. Rains JC, Poceta JS. Sleep-related headaches. Neurol Clin 2012;30(4):1285–98.
30. Aurora SK, Barrodale PM, Tipton RL, et al. Brainstem dysfunction in chronic migraine as evidenced by neurophysiological and positron emission tomography studies. Headache 2007;47(7):996–1003.
31. Holland P, Goadsby PJ. The hypothalamic orexinergic system: pain and primary headaches. Headache 2007;47(6):951–62.
32. Leone M, Lucini V, D'Amico D, et al. Twenty-four hour melatonin and cortisol plasma levels in relation to timing of cluster headache. Cephalalgia 1995;15:224–9.
33. Montagna P. Hypothalamus, sleep and headaches. Neurol Sci 2006;27(Suppl 2):S138.
34. May A, Bahra A, Buhel C, Frackowiak RS, Goadsby PJ. Hypothalamic activation in cluster headache attacks. Lancet 1998;352:275–8.
35. Sprenger T, Boecker H, Toelle TR, et al. Specific hypothalamic activation during a spontaneous cluster headache attack. Neurology 2004;3:62–3.
36. Weiller C, May A, Limmroth V, et al. Brain stem activation during a spontaneous cluster headache attack. Neurology 2004;3:62–3.
37. Dodick DW, Eross EJ, Parish JM, Silber M. Clinical, anatomical, and physiologic relationship between sleep and headache. Headache 2003;43(3):282–92.

38. Headache Classification Subcommittee of the International Headache Society. The International Classification of Headache Disorders: 2nd edition. Cephalalgia 2004;24(Suppl 1):9–160.

39. Russell D. Cluster headache: severity and temporal profiles of attacks and patient activity prior to and during attacks. Cephalalgia 1981;1(4):209–16.

40. Kudrow L, McGinty DJ, Phillips ER, Stevenson M. Sleep apnea in cluster headache. Cephalalgia 1984;4(1):33–8.

41. Nobre ME, Leal AJ, Filho PM. Investigation into sleep disturbance of patients suffering from cluster headache. Cephalalgia 2005;25(7):488–92.

42. Graff-Radford SB, Teruel A. Cluster headache and obstructive sleep apnea: are they related disorders? Curr Pain Headache Rep 2009;13(2):160–3.

43. Vetrugno R, Pierangeli G, Leone M, et al. Effect on sleep of posterior hypothalamus stimulation in cluster headache. Headache 2007;47(7):1085–90

44. Raskin NH. The hypnic headache syndrome. Headache 1988;28(8):534–6.

45. Rains JC, Poceta JS. Sleep-related headaches. Neurol Clin 2012;30(4):1285–98.

46. Evers S, Goadsby PJ. Hypnic headaches, clinical features, pathophysiology and treatment. Neurology 2003;60:905–9.

47. Pinessi L, Rainero I, Cicolin A, et al. Hypnic headache syndrome: association with REM sleep. Cephalalgia 2003;23:150–4.

48. Holle D, Wessendorf TE, Zaremba S, et al. Serial polysomnography in hypnic headache. Cephalalgia 2011;31(3):286–90.

49. Karthik N, Kulkarni GB, Taly AB, Rao S, Sinha S. Sleep disturbances in "migraine without aura"—a questionnaire based study. J Neurol Sci 2012;321(1–2):73–6.

50. Russell D. Cluster headache: severity and temporal profiles of attacks and patient activity prior to and during attacks. Cephalalgia 1981;1(4):209–16.

51. Seidel S, Bock A, Schlegel W, et al. Increased RLS prevalence in children and adolescents with migraine: a case-control study. Cephalalgia 2012;32(9):693–9.

52. Schurks M, Winter AC, Berger K, Buring JE, Kurth T. Migraine and restless legs syndrome in women. Cephalalgia 2012;32(5):382–9.

53. Rhode AM, Hosing VG, Happe S, Comorbidity of migraine and restless legs syndrome—a case-control study. Cephalalgia 2007;27(11):1255–60.

54. d'Onofrio F, Bussone G, Cologno D, et al. Restless legs syndrome and primary headaches: a clinical study. Neurol Sci 2008;29(Suppl 1):S169–72.

55. Chen PK, Fuh JL, Chen SP, Wang SJ. Association between restless legs syndrome and migraine. J Neurol Neurosurg Psychiatry 2010;81(5):524–8.

56. Cannon PR, Larner AJ. Migraine and restless legs syndrome: is there an association? J Headache Pain 2011;12(4):405–9.

57. Dahmen N, Kasten M, Wieczorek S, et al. Increased frequency of migraine in narcoleptic patients: a confirmatory study. Cephalalgia 2003;23(1):14–19.

58. Dahmen N, Querings K, Grun B, Bierbrauer J. Increased frequency of migraine in narcoleptic patients. Neurology 1999;52(6):1291–3.

59. DMKG Study Group. Migraine and idiopathic narcolepsy—a case-control study. Cephalalgia 2003;23(8):786–9.

60. Lateef T, Swanson S, Cui L, et al. Headaches and sleep problems among adults in the United States: findings from the National Comorbidity Survey-Replication study. Cephalalgia 2011;31(6):648–53.

61. Yeung WF, Chung KF, Wong CY. Relationship between insomnia and headache in community-based middle-aged Hong Kong Chinese women. J Headache Pain 2010;11(3):187–95.

62. Zwart JA, Dyb G, Hagen K, et al. Depression and anxiety disorders associated with headache frequency. The Nord–Trøndelag Health Study. Eur J Neurol 2003;10(2):147–52.

63. Peres MF, Stiles MA, Siow HC, Silberstein SD. Excessive daytime sleepiness in migraine patients. J Neurol Neurosurg Psychiatry 2005;76(10):1467–8.

64. Barbanti P, Fabbrini G, Aurilia C, Vanacore N, Cruccu G. A case-control study on excessive daytime sleepiness in episodic migraine. Cephalalgia 2007;27(10):1115–19.

65. Cevoli S, Giannini G, Favoni V, Pierangeli G, Cortelli P. Migraine and sleep disorders. Neurol Sci 2012;33(Suppl 1):S43–6.

66. Aldrich MS, Chauncey JB. Are morning headaches part of obstructive sleep apnea syndrome? Arch Internal Med 1990;150(6):1265–7.

67. Seidel S, Frantal S, Oberhofer P, et al. Morning headaches in snorers and their bed partners: a prospective diary study. Cephalalgia 2012;32(12):888–95.

68. Kristiansen HA, Kvaerner KJ, Akre H, et al. Sleep apnoea headache in the general population. Cephalalgia 2012;32(6):451–8.

69. Goksan B, Gunduz A, Karadeniz D, et al. Morning headache in sleep apnoea: clinical and polysomnographic evaluation and response to nasal continuous positive airway pressure. Cephalalgia 2009;29(6):635–41.

70. Ohayon MM. Prevalence and risk factors of morning headaches in the general population. Arch Internal Med 2004;164(1):97–102.

71. Armstrong-Jones R. "Snapping of the brain." Lancet 1920; 196(5066):720.

72. American Academy of Sleep Medicine. International Classification of Sleep Disorders, 3rd ed. Diagnostic and coding manual. Darien, IL: American Academy of Sleep Medicine, 2014.

73. Karli N, Zarifoglu M, Calisir N, Akgoz S. Comparison of pre-headache phases and trigger factors of migraine and episodic tension-type headache: do they share similar clinical pathophysiology? Cephalalgia 2005;25(6):444–51.

74. Koseoglu E, Nacar M, Taslaslioglu A, Cetinkaya F. Epidemiological and clinical characteristics of migraine and tension type headache in 1146 females in Kayseri, Turkey. Cephalalgia 2003;23(5):381–8.

75. Spierings EL, Ranke AH, Honkoop PC. Precipitating and aggravating factors of migraine versus tension-type headache. Headache 2001;41(6):554–8.

76. Kikuchi H, Yoshiuchi K, Yamamoto Y, Komaki G, Akabayashi A. Does sleep aggravate tension-type headache? An investigation using computerized ecological momentary assessment and actigraphy. Biopsychosoc Med 2011;5:10.

77. Kristiansen HA, Kvaerner KJ, Akre H, Overland B, Russell MB. Tension-type headache and sleep apnea in the general population. J Headache Pain 2011;12(1):63–9.

78. Tepper SJ. Medication-overuse headache. Continuum (Minneap Minn) 2012;18(4):807–22.

79. Calhoun AH, Ford S. Behavioral sleep modification may revert transformed migraine to episodic migraine. Headache 2007;47(8):1178–83.

80. Rizzoli PB. Acute and preventive treatment of migraine. Continuum (Minneap Minn) 2012: 18(4):764–82.

81. Ferrari MD, Goadsby PJ, Roon KI, Lipton RB. Triptans (serotonin, 5-HT1B/1D agonists) in migraine: detailed results and methods of a meta-analysis of 53 trials. Cephalalgia 2002; 22(8):633–58.

82. Loder E. Triptan therapy in migraine. N Engl J Med 2010;363(1):63–70.

83. Saper JR, Silberstein S. Pharmacology of dihydroergotamine and evidence for efficacy and safety in migraine. Headache 2006; 46(4):S171–81.

84. Klapper JA, Stanton J. Clinical experience with patient administered subcutaneous dihydroergotamine mesylate in refractory headaches. Headache 1992;32(1):21–3.

85. Ramadan NM. Current trends in migraine prophylaxis. Headache 2007;47(Suppl 1):S52–7.

86. Solomon S. Major therapeutic advances in the past 25 years. Headache 2007; 47(Suppl 1):S20–22.

87. Evans RW, Rizzoli P, Loder E, Bana D. Beta-blockers for migraine. Headache 2008; 48(3):455–60.

88. Brandes LS, Green M. Migraine in women. Continuum (Minneap Minn) 2012;18(4):835–52.

89. Ho TW, Ferrari MD, Dodick DW, et al. Efficacy and tolerability of MK-0974 (telcagepant), a new oral antagonist of calcitonin gene-related

peptide receptor, compared with zolmitriptan for acute migraine: a randomized, placebo-controlled, parallel-treatment trial. Lancet 2008;372(9656):2115–23.

90. Färkkilä M, Diener HC, Géraud G, et al. Efficacy and tolerability of lasmiditan, an oral 5-HT(1F) receptor agonist, for the acute treatment of migraine: a phase 2 randomized, placebo-controlled, parallel-group, dose-ranging study. Lancet Neurol 2012;11(5):405–13.

91. Silberstein SD, Dodick D, Saper, J, et al. Safety and efficacy of peripheral nerve stimulation of the occipital nerves for the management of chronic migraine: results from a randomized, prospective, multicenter double-blinded, controlled study. Cephalalgia 2014;0(0):1–15.

92. Tobin J, Flitman S. Occipital nerve blocks: when and what to inject? Headache 2009; 49:1521–33.

93. Ashkenazi A, Matro R, Shaw JW, et al. Greater occipital nerve block using local anaesthetics alone or with triamcinolone for transformed migraine: a randomised comparative study. J Neurol Neurosurg Psychiatry 2008;79:415–17.

94. Dodick DW, Capobianco DJ. Treatment and management of cluster headache. Curr Pain Headache Rep 2001;5(1):83–91.

95. Nesbitt AD, Goadsby PJ. Cluster headache. BMJ 2012;344:e2407.

96. Cohen AS, Burns B, Goadsby PJ. High-flow oxygen for treatment of cluster headache: a randomized trial. JAMA 2009;302(22):2451–7.

97. Cittadini E, May A, Straube A, et al. Effectiveness of intranasal zolmitriptan in acute cluster headache: a randomized, placebo-controlled, double-blind crossover study. Arch Neurol 2006;63(11):1537–42.

98. van Vliet JA, Bahra A, Martin V, et al. Intranasal sumatriptan in cluster headache: randomized placebo-controlled double-blind study. Neurology 2003;60(4):630–3.

99. Bussone G, Leone M, Peccarisi C, et al. Double blind comparison of lithium and verapamil in cluster headache prophylaxis. Headache 1990;30(7):411–17.

100. Goadsby PJ. Trigeminal autonomic cephalalgias. Continuum (Minneap Minn) 2012;18(4):883–95.

101. Leone M, Proietti Cecchini A, et al. Lessons from 8 years' experience of hypothalamic stimulation in cluster headache. Cephalalgia 2008;28(7):787–97.

102. Burns B, Watkins L, Goadsby PJ. Treatment of medically intractable cluster headache by occipital nerve stimulation: long-term follow-up of eight patients. Lancet 2007;369(9567):1099–106.

103. Lanteri-Minet M, Donnet A. Hypnic headache. Curr Pain Headache Rep 2010;14(4):309–15.

104. Kiely JL, Murphy M, McNicholas WT. Subjective efficacy of nasal CPAP therapy in obstructive sleep apnoea syndrome: a prospective controlled study. Eur Respir J 1999;13(5):1086–90.

105. Kaniecki RG. Tension-type headache. Continuum (Minneap Minn) 2012;18(4):823–34.

106. Fumal A, Schoenen J. Tension-type headache: current research and clinical management. Lancet Neurol 2008;7(1):70–83.

107. Cohen AS, Kaube H. Rare nocturnal headaches. Curr Opin Neurol 2004;17(3):295–9.

108. Sachs C, Svanborg E. The exploding head syndrome: polysomnographic recordings and therapeutic suggestions. Sleep 1991;14(3):263–6.

CHAPTER 32

Sleep after traumatic brain injury

Christian R. Baumann

In the last ten years or so, it has become increasingly obvious that sleep–wake disorders (SWDs) after traumatic brain injury (TBI) are frequent and chronic conditions. TBI, which is defined as an "an alteration in brain function, or other evidence of brain pathology, caused by an external force," is a frequent condition, with an incidence of up to 600 per 100 000 [1,2]. Given the observation that more than half of TBI patients suffer from SWDs, a yearly incidence of about 300 patients with post-traumatic SWDs must be assumed [3].

This brief chapter is intended to offer a short clinical introduction to the variety of SWDs that may emerge after TBI.

Post-traumatic pleiosomnia

After TBI, patients sleep significantly more than carefully matched controls [4]. To avoid confusion with the term hypersomnia (which is used for both increased sleep need and increased sleepiness), we coined the term pleiosomnia for increased sleep need of 2 hours or more per 24 hours compared with pre-TBI conditions [5]. Six months after trauma, pleiosomnia is present in about 20–25% of TBI patients [3]. Excessive daytime sleepiness (EDS) is not present in all pleiosomnia patients, but increased slow-wave sleep (SWS) appears to be common in this condition [5]. The severity of TBI, as assessed by the presence of intracranial hemorrhage, is a predictor for the development of post-traumatic pleiosomnia [4].

Post-traumatic excessive daytime sleepiness

A variety of studies applying questionnaires or sleep laboratory tests, including the multiple sleep latency test (MSLT), identified EDS as a prevalent complication after head trauma, occurring in up to 50–60% of TBI patients [3,4,6–10]. On comparing subjective with objective measures of sleepiness in the same population, there is growing evidence that TBI patients often underestimate the presence and severity of EDS [3,4]. In a proportion of TBI patients, EDS is linked to underlying sleep–wake comorbidities such as obstructive sleep apnea (OSA) syndrome and periodic limb movements during sleep (PLMS), but in many patients, no other causes of sleepiness than the trauma itself could be identified [3,6,9]. In contrast to pleiosomnia, severity of TBI is not associated with the development of EDS.

Post-traumatic insomnia

Most studies report a prevalence of insomnia of about 30–70% in TBI patients, but some other studies, including our own, have delivered markedly lower frequencies [3,11]. The most likely explanation for this very large range is the heterogeneity of the methods used to assess insomnia, the different definitions of insomnia, and the heterogeneous intervals between TBI and insomnia assessments. For instance, an early study showed that insomnia symptoms might prevail shortly after TBI, but then fade and unmask enhanced sleep pressure [12]. On the other hand, and in contrast to findings regarding sleepiness, there is some evidence that TBI might overestimate insomnia symptoms, when comparing objective with subjective assessments [13].

Post-traumatic sleep-related breathing disorders

Extensive evaluations of pre-TBI sleep–wake behavior, including detailed interviews with bed partners, suggest that OSA emerges in a large proportion of TBI survivors as a de novo post-traumatic feature [14]. The prevalence of OSA after TBI ranges from 11% to36% [15]. After all, it is still unclear whether or not the prevalence of OSA is higher in the TBI than in the general population, and whether de novo sleep-related breathing disorders persist or constitute a transient phenomenon.

Post-traumatic sleep-related movement disorders

Evidence on post-traumatic sleep-related movement disorders is scarce. In our own controlled prospective study, we did not find increased periodic limb movement indices after TBI [4]. Some of our colleagues identified 6 of 87 TBI patients with PLMS [9]. The entity of post-traumatic restless legs syndrome probably does not exist.

Post-traumatic circadian rhythm sleep–wake disorders

Again, there is not much evidence on circadian malfunctioning after TBI. Some authors used actigraphy studies, saliva melatonin measurements, and body temperature assessments in 42 TBI subjects with insomnia complaints and found circadian rhythm disorders in 36% [16]. This well-designed study suggests that circadian rhythm SWDs may be frequent after TBI, and that they can be easily misdiagnosed as insomnia. Others confirmed the existence of post-traumatic circadian rhythm disorders such as delayed sleep–wake phase disorder or non-24-hour sleep–wake rhythm disorder [17,18].

Pathophysiology of post-traumatic sleep–wake disorders

There are many independent factors that potentially cause or contribute to SWDs after TBI, including psychiatric sequelae (depression, anxiety, post-traumatic stress disorder), medication (sedatives, analgesics, anticonvulsants, etc.), pain, neuroendocrine disturbances, psychosocial problems, and genetic background. There is some evidence that trauma-induced brain damage might contribute. First, a significant loss of a variety of sleep–wake regulating neuronal systems, particularly histaminergic neurons in the tuberomammillary nucleus, has been found in patients who died from fatal TBI [19]. Thus, a reduction of wake drive might contribute to pleiosomnia and EDS. Furthermore, a case–control study revealed that evening melatonin production is significantly lower in TBI patients, suggesting that impaired melatonin synthesis might contribute to circadian rhythm SWDs [20].

Diagnosis of post-traumatic sleep–wake disorders

Sleep–wake questionnaires that have been developed for other populations of patients can also be used in the TBI population, but the clinician has to keep in mind that none of these instruments have been validated in TBI patients [21]. Even more, there is increasing evidence that TBI patients suffer from some misperception of their SWDs [3,4,5,13]. Therefore, objective sleep laboratory tests should be performed in any patient with the slightest doubt about the insight into his or her own sleep–wake behavior.

Treatment of post-traumatic sleep–wake disorders

Contributing factors or comorbidities should be identified and treated, if possible. For TBI patients with insomnia, cognitive–behavioral therapy should be considered [22,23]. Stimulants such as modafinil can be tried to treat EDS after TBI [24,25]. There is no report or even any suggestion about the treatment of post-traumatic pleiosomnia.

References

1. Menon DK, Schwab K, Wright DW, Maas AI. Position statement: definition of traumatic brain injury. Arch Phys Med Rehabil 2010;91(11):1637–40.
2. Langlois Orman JA, Kraus JF, et al. Epidemiology. In: Silver JM, McAllister TW, Yudofsky MD, eds. Textbook of traumatic brain injury. Arlington, VA: American Psychiatric Publishing, 2011:3–22.
3. Baumann CR, Werth E, Stocker R, et al. Sleep–wake disturbances 6 months after traumatic brain injury: a prospective study. Brain 2007;130:1873–83.
4. Imbach LL, Valko PO, Li T, et al. Increased sleep need and daytime sleepiness 6 months after traumatic brain injury: a prospective controlled clinical trial. Brain 2015;138:726–35.
5. Sommerauer M, Valko PO, Werth E, Baumann CR. Excessive sleep need following traumatic brain injury: a case-control study of 36 patients. J Sleep Res 2013;22:634–9.
6. Masel BE, Scheibel RS, Kimbark T, Kuna ST. Excessive daytime sleepiness in adults with brain injuries. Arch Phys Med Rehabil 2001;82:1526–32.
7. Guilleminault C, Faull KF, Miles L, van den Hoed J. Posttraumatic excessive daytime sleepiness: a review of 20 patients. Neurology 1983;33:1584–9.
8. Watson NF, Dikmen S, Machamer J, et al. Hypersomnia following traumatic brain injury. J Clin Sleep Med 2007;3:363–8.
9. Castriotta RJ, Wilde MC, Lai JM, et al. Prevalence and consequences of sleep disorders in traumatic brain injury. J Clin Sleep Med 2007;3:349–56.
10. Castriotta RJ, Murthy JN. Sleep disorders in patients with traumatic brain injury: a review. CNS Drugs 2011;25:175–85.
11. Zeitzer JM, Friedman L, O'Hara R. Insomnia in the context of traumatic brain injury. J Rehabil Res Dev 2009;46:827–36.
12. Cohen M, Oksenberg A, Snir D, et al. Temporally related changes of sleep complaints in traumatic brain injured patients. J Neurol Neurosurg Psychiatry 1992;55:313–15.
13. Ouellet MC, Morin CM. Subjective and objective measures of insomnia in the context of traumatic brain injury: a preliminary study. Sleep Med 2006;7:486–97.
14. Guilleminault C, Yuen KM, Gulevich MG, et al. Hypersomnia after head-neck trauma: a medicolegal dilemma. Neurology 2000;54:653–9.
15. Valko PO, Baumann CR. Sleep disorders after traumatic brain injury. In: Kryger ME, Roth T, Dement WC, eds. Principles and practice of sleep medicine, 6th ed. Philadelphia: Elsevier, 2016:959–68.
16. Ayalon L, Borodkin K, Dishon L, et al. Circadian rhythm sleep disorders following mild traumatic brain injury. Neurology 2007;68:1136–40.
17. Quinto C, Gellido C, Chokroverty S, Masdeu J. Posttraumatic delayed sleep phase syndrome. Neurology 2000;54:250–2.
18. Boivin DB, James FO, Santo JB, et al. Non-24-hour sleep-wake syndrome following a car accident. Neurology 2003;60:1841–3.
19. Valko PO, Gavrilov YV, Yamamoto M, et al. Damage to histaminergic tuberomammillary neurons and other hypothalamic neurons with traumatic brain injury. Ann Neurol 2015;77:177–82.
20. Shekleton JA, Parcell DL, Redman JR, et al. Sleep disturbance and melatonin levels following traumatic brain injury. Neurology 2010;74:1732–8.
21. Mollayeva T, Kendzerska T, Colantonio A. Self-report instruments for assessing sleep dysfunction in an adult traumatic brain injury population: a systematic review. Sleep Med Rev 2013;17:411–23.
22. Ouellet MC, Morin CM. Cognitive behavioral therapy for insomnia associated with traumatic brain injury: a single-case study. Arch Phys Med Rehabil 2004;85:1298–302.
23. Ouellet MC, Morin CM. Efficacy of cognitive-behavioral therapy for insomnia associated with traumatic brain injury: a single-case experimental design. Arch Phys Med Rehabil 2007;88:1581–92.
24. Jha A, Weintraub A, Allshouse A, et al. A randomized trial of modafinil for the treatment of fatigue and excessive daytime sleepiness in individuals with chronic traumatic brain injury. J Head Trauma Rehabil 2008;23:52–63.
25. Kaiser PR, Valko PO, Werth E, et al. Modafinil ameliorates excessive daytime sleepiness after traumatic brain injury. Neurology 2010;75:1780–5.

CHAPTER 33

Sleep disorders in multiple sclerosis

Luigi Ferini-Strambi and Sara Marelli

Introduction

Multiple sclerosis (MS) is an inflammatory condition of the central nervous system (CNS) presumably induced by an environmental trigger(s) in a genetically susceptible subject. Sleep disorders are common, although clinically under-recognized, in MS patients. Approximately half of all patients with MS report sleep-related problems [1–3]. It is clear that some physical and psychological factors, such as pain, anxiety and mood disorders, sleep disordered breathing, nocturia, and nocturnal spasticity-related discomfort, may all contribute to sleep disturbances. Moreover, it is also well known that disease-modifying and symptomatic therapies commonly used in MS can also affect sleep, by causing either insomnia or hypersomnia [4]. The list of these therapies includes interferon beta, methylprednisolone, baclofen, tizanidine, gabapentin, pregabalin, and oxybutynin. A recent study showed dynamic changes of sleep architecture in mice with experimental autoimmune encephalomyelitis (EAE), a model of multiple sclerosis [5]. The changes of sleep patterns were mainly reflected by altered sleep stage distribution and increased sleep fragmentation; the extent of sleep fragmentation correlated with the severity of disease. This is the first study of sleep profile in EAE mice demarcating specific changes related to the autoimmune disorder without confounding factors such as psychosocial impact and treatment effects. Since several immunological factors in serum (including tumor necrosis factor α and other cytokines) have been implicated in the development of sleep disorders and since MS is shown to have immune abnormalities, it is reasonable to think that MS and sleep disorders share a similar background [6].

Common sleep disorders in patients with MS include insomnia, sleep apnea, restless legs syndrome (RLS), narcolepsy, and rapid eye movement (REM) sleep behavior disorder (RBD). In a cross-sectional epidemiological survey, Patel and colleagues [7] evaluated middle-aged women ($n = 60 028$) who reported a habitual sleep duration of 7 hours or more. MS (odds ratio (OR) 3.7, 95% confidence interval (CI) 3.0–4.5) was the factor most strongly associated with prolonged sleep. It has been reported that sleep disturbance in MS is a predictive factor and contributor to fatigue [8], supporting the hypothesis that recurrent arousals from sleep (sleep fragmentation) lead to excessive CNS activation with subsequent excessive fatigue [8–10]. More than 80% of MS patients complain of fatigue and approximately one out of four considers fatigue as the most burdensome symptom of the illness [11]. On the other hand, fatigue is a major reason for early retirement in MS [12].

It has recently been reported that treatment of the underlying sleep disorder led to an improvement of MS-related fatigue [13]. Thus, an increased clinical awareness of sleep-related problems is warranted in the MS population because they are extremely common and have the potential to negatively impact overall health and quality of life.

Insomnia in multiple sclerosis

Insomnia is a widespread complaint, estimated to affect at least 10% of the adult population, but only 6% fulfill the criteria of the Diagnostic and Statistical Manual, Fourth Edition, Text Revision (DSM-IV-TR) [14]. Causes of insomnia common in the MS population include pain associated with muscle spasms, periodic limb movements (PLM), RLS, nocturia, medication effect, and psychiatric illness such as depression. Chronic insomnia can also predispose an individual to the development of major depression [15]. In patients with MS, sleep difficulties have been shown to be associated with the yearly exacerbation rate and with disease severity [16]. Table 33.1 lists studies investigating insomnia in MS.

Only the study of Tachibana et al. [1] reported a prevalence of insomnia similar to that of the general population. However, none of the studies investigating insomnia in MS have used standardized diagnostic criteria, except for a cross-sectional study by Veauthier et al. [17], which reported insomnia in 25% of MS samples using the criteria of the International Classification of Sleep Disorders, Second Edition (ICSD-2) [18]. The multifactorial etiology of insomnia in MS patients must be considered before any decision is made on therapeutic strategy.

Pain

Pain is a common finding, but often under-recognized, in MS patients. It is estimated to affect 29–86% of MS patients in various stages of the disease and severely influences rehabilitation and quality of life [22]. The pain experienced by MS patients is generally caused by nervous system damage during the course of the disease and can usually be characterized as central neuropathic pain (less frequently as peripheral or nociceptive pain). In a large study that examined 364 MS patients [23], 57.5% reported pain during the course of their disease (21% nociceptive, 2% peripheral neuropathic, and 1% related to spasticity); 27.5% had central pain. It has been reported that chronic pain in MS is not significantly related to age, disease duration, or disease course, but is correlated with aspects of health-related quality of life [24]. Pain has the potential

Table 33.1 Insomnia in MS patients

Authors	Study site	Number of subjects	Mean age (years)	Findings
Tachibana et al., 1994 [1]	UK	28	Range 22–67	Three patients had non-organic insomnia
Stanton et al., 2006 [19]	UK	60	41 (median)	Sleep diaries for 1 week: 42% of patients had an incapability of initiating sleep (>30 min) at least two nights per week. 53% of patients had disrupted sleep at least two nights per week. Nocturia was the most common cause of disrupted nights (72.5%)
Bamer et al., 2008 [20]	Washington, USA	1063	50.9	Using the Medical Outcomes Study Sleep Scale [21], moderate or severe sleep problems in 33.1%
Veauthier et al., 2011 [17]	Germany	66	43.2	25% of patients had insomnia according to ICSD-2 criteria
Pokryszko-Dragan et al., 2013 [8]	Poland	100	42	Sleep complaints in 49% of patients (non-validated sleep questionnaire)

to disrupt sleep, with consequent daytime somnolence, worsening fatigue, and a lower pain threshold [25]. Indeed, the presence of chronic pain can be associated with a vicious cycle pattern. A day with intense pain can be followed by a night of poor sleep quality, and a night of poor sleep can increase pain the next day. Treatment options include medications such as gabapentin and pregabalin, which have been shown to improve nocturnal pain and promote restorative sleep [26,27]. Other medication options include carbamazepine and pharmacotherapy directed at treating muscle spasticity (baclofen, dantrolene, tizanidine, botulinum toxin, and diazepam). Cannabis-based medicine may also be effective in reducing pain and sleep disturbance in MS patients with central neuropathic pain [28,29].

Nocturia

Urinary bladder dysfunction is a common problem for MS patients. The severity of symptoms often correlates with the degree of spinal cord involvement and hence the patient's general level of disability [30]. Nocturia or urinary incontinence affects 70–80% of patients with MS [31]. Spasticity or involuntary contraction of the bladder causing nocturia and incontinence can lead to frequent awakenings and sleep fragmentation [32].

Awareness and treatment of this sometimes under-recognized cause of sleep disruption may lead to significant improvements in the quality of life in patients with MS. Treatment options for nocturnal bladder spasticity include fluid restriction, intermittent catheterization, anticholinergic agents such as propantheline or oxybutynin, and the hormone desmopressin [33]. Botulinum neurotoxin-A injection represents a significant advance in the management of voiding dysfunction among MS patients failing first-line therapy. It significantly improves patients' urodynamic parameters and quality of life, with efficacy sustained by repeated injections with minimal risk of adverse events [34].

Depression

The association between MS and depression has been well established. A survey of 115 071 adults living in Canada confirmed an elevated 12-month prevalence of depression in patients with MS,

relative to both healthy individuals and those with other long-term medical illnesses [35].

In particular, patients with MS aged 18–45 years had a one in four chance of developing depression over the course of 1 year. Further epidemiological data from a community sample of 1374 patients with MS revealed a 41.8% prevalence of depression, and the authors noted the importance of disease severity as a robust correlate [36].

McGuigan and Hutchinson [37] performed a study to assess the point prevalence of previously unrecognized symptoms of depression in a community-based population with MS. They found that one in four patients had unrecognized and therefore untreated symptoms of depression. These data are consistent with the findings of another study [38] that evaluated 260 MS patients and found 25.8% of patients with major depressive disorder: among these depressed patients, 65.6% received no antidepressant medication and 4.7% received sub-threshold doses. Depression in patients with MS has a complex and multifactorial pathogenesis: adverse psychosocial impact of a chronic, usually progressive, disabling illness, atrophy of frontal and temporal regions, a lack of family support, and possible depressogenic effects of drugs such as corticosteroids and interferon [39].

Depression has the potential to cause insomnia, leading to excessive daytime sleepiness (EDS) and worsening fatigue. Early recognition and treatment can prevent psychiatric sequelae and improve sleep and the overall quality of life [40]. Treatment options for patients with depression and MS include psychotherapy and medications such as the selective serotonin reuptake inhibitors (SSRIs), tricyclic antidepressants, and non-tricyclic antidepressants. However, it should be considered that several studies have found that antidepressant use is associated with increased PLM in sleep (PLMS), a possible cause of sleep fragmentation [41,42].

Nocturnal movement disorders

The incidence of RLS and PLMS is higher in patients with MS than in the general population [43,44]. In the general population, conservative estimates report RLS affecting between 5% and 15% [45] and PLMS affecting 5% between the age of 30 and 50 years [46]. A recent meta-analysis that reviewed 24 studies found that the RLS prevalence ranged from 12.12% to 57.50% among patients with MS and from 2.56% to 18.33% among people without MS: pooled analysis further indicated that the odds of RLS among patients with MS were fourfold higher compared with people without MS [47].

A study estimated the prevalence of RLS in 82 MS patients, and compared the neurological damage between patients with and without RLS using conventional and diffusion tensor (DT) MRI [48]. Thirty patients were affected by RLS. Patients affected by RLS showed a higher disability according to the Expanded Disability Status Scale (EDSS) score than patients without RLS. No difference between the two groups was found in whole-brain, cerebellar, and brainstem T_2 lesion loads or in T_2 lesion loads of the two cerebral and cerebellar hemispheres when considered separately. Among the MRI metrics analyzed, cervical cord fractional anisotropy was significantly reduced in patients with RLS compared with MS patients without RLS, suggesting that cervical cord damage represents a significant risk factor for RLS among MS patients.

Other studies have also reported a relation between cord involvement caused by different pathologies (eg, intramedullary lesions, schwannoma, and MS) and RLS and/or PLMS [49–53]. A possible explanation is that cord damage may interrupt descending or ascending pathways, resulting in brain–spinal disconnection, which in turn leads to the appearance of RLS. The hypothesis that impairment of a descending cerebrospinal inhibitory pathway could lead to a higher spinal motor excitability in RLS patients is indeed supported by several clinical and neurophysiological data [54,55]. A possible target of the spinal lesion could be represented by the dopaminergic descending neurons projecting from the A11 hypothalamic area to D_3 receptors located in the dorsal and intermediolateralis spinal nuclei [56]. Several findings support the notion that this nervous pathway is central in RLS genesis: the A11 area receives a diffuse innervation from the suprachiasmatic nucleus, which is the main physiological drive for the circadian rhythm; artificial lesions of A11, as well as systemic administration of selective D_3 antagonists, increase locomotor activity in rats; knockout mice for D_3 receptors exhibit hyperactivity; and D_3 agonists indeed represent the first-choice drugs in RLS [56,57]. Moreover, the hypothesis that the spinal lesion related to RLS is a consequence of ascending pathway damage cannot be excluded. The RLS may indeed be the result of a central somatosensory processing dysfunction due to an abnormal peripheral afferent input [58].

Treatment options for RLS and PLMS are similar and include dopaminergic agents (levodopa/carbidopa, pramipexole, ropinirole, and rotigotine), anticonvulsants (gabapentin, pregabalin, and clonazepam), and opioids [59]. These compounds should be also considered for the treatment of RLS and PLMS in MS patients.

Medication

Immunomodulatory therapy for the treatment of MS has been associated with hypersomnolence, increasing fatigue, depression, and insomnia. In patients with relapsing MS, 5% of those treated with interferon-β1a three times a week in one series had hypersomnolence, as compared with 1% of controls [32]. In another study [60], 3–17% of patients treated with interferon-β1b for 1 month had insomnia and described fatigue as a common (33%) side effect. Corticosteroids are widely believed to disrupt sleep. The most consistent effect of corticosteroids on polysomnographic (PSG) data in normal subjects is a marked decrease in REM sleep [61]. Approximately 50% of patients treated with prednisone for optic neuritis reported sleep disturbance, compared with 20% on placebo [62]. Preliminary data [63] also demonstrated that treatment of MS patients with methylprednisolone causes sleep electroencephalogram (EEG) changes typically seen in patients with depression (reduced REM sleep latency, decreased REM sleep density, and decreased slow-wave sleep). Earlier data suggesting that treatment with interferon-β therapy predisposes patients to depression has been questioned. However, Mohr et al. [38] suggested that, considering the uncertainty of a link between interferon and depression, a well as the complete remission of psychiatric complications after interferon discontinuation, physicians should closely monitor the psychiatric status of patients. To date, disrupted sleep, depression, and increased fatigue have not been described with the use of glatiramer acetate [64], mitoxantrone [65], or immunoglobulins [66]. Insomnia has been reported in MS patients treated with laquinimod [67], while there are no specific data on natalizumab and fingolimod.

Sleep disordered breathing

The medullary reticular formation is responsible for controlling automatic breathing during sleep. In MS patients, demyelinating lesions in this area could affect nocturnal respiratory effort, leading to sleep disordered breathing and even nocturnal death (Ondine's curse) [68]. CNS and brainstem-related nocturnal respiratory abnormalities such as paroxysmal hyperventilation, hypoventilation, respiratory muscle weakness, and respiratory arrest have all been described [68,69], and these should be considered in MS patients in the evaluation of symptoms of daytime somnolence, increased fatigue, and nonrestorative sleep.

Concerning the prevalence of obstructive sleep apnea (OSA) in MS patients, the estimates based on PSG studies vary widely (0–58%, Table 33.2). Differences in PSG acquisition and scoring methods may in part explain variability in study results. Of note,

Table 33.2 OSA in MS patients

Authors	Study site	Number of subjects	Mean age (years)	Prevalence of OSA (%)
Ferini-Strambi et al., 1994 [73]	Italy	25	39.9	12
Kaynak et al., 2006 [74]	Turkey	37	37	0
Veauthier et al., 2011 [75]	Germany	66	43.2	9.1
Neau et al., 2012 [76]	France	205	40 (for 25 subjects selected for PSG)	0 (from 205 patients selected to undergo PSG)
Kaminska et al., 2012 [71]	Canada	62	47.3	58

a recent cross-sectional study suggests that progressive MS sub-types and increased level of disability are risk factors for OSA in MS [70].

Kaminska et al. [71] found that OSA (apnea–hypopnea index ≥ 15) was frequent in MS (36 of 62 patients) and was associated with fatigue but not sleepiness, independent of MS-related disability. A recent study showed that CPAP therapy in some MS patients with OSA was associated with a significant reduction in Fatigue Severity Scale scores [72]. Future work on large samples of MS patients is needed to understand the real impact of CPAP therapy on quality of life in this patient group.

Narcolepsy

Narcoleptic symptoms have long been recognized in patients with MS. Studies published in the first half of the twentieth century report cases of MS associated with sleep attacks termed "narcolepsy" [77,78]. Symptoms of narcolepsy may appear before or after other symptoms of MS [79,80].

There is a coincidence of genetic susceptibility between narcolepsy and MS [81]. Studies involving Caucasian Americans, Japanese, Afro-Brazilians, and African Americans show a strong association (>90%) between narcolepsy with cataplexy and certain human leukocyte antigens: *HLA-DR2, -DQB1*0602, -DQA1*0102,* and *-DQw1* [82].

The susceptibility to MS is coded by genes within or close to the *HLA-DR–DQ* subregion. Indeed, in the MS population, an increased prevalence (50-70%) of *HLA-DR2, -DQB1, -DQA1, -A3, -DQw1,* and *-B7* has also been found [83]. The finding that both narcolepsy and MS are strongly linked to similar HLA expression, a hallmark of most autoimmune diseases, suggests that similar autoimmune factors may play a role in the development of both diseases and may be partially responsible for similar symptoms of fatigue and somnolence. Hypocretin-1 and -2 (orexin-A and -B) are neuropeptides released by lateral hypothalamic neurons that are involved in wake promotion and sleep regulation [82]. These neurons are reduced in patients with idiopathic narcolepsy. Most sporadic, *HLA-DQB1*0602*-positive, narcoleptic patients with cataplexy have undetectable levels of hypocretin-1 in the cerebrospinal fluid (CSF). This evidence, taken in the context of a strong narcolepsy HLA association, suggests the possibility of an autoimmune disorder directed against hypocretin-containing cells in the lateral hypothalamus, although no direct cause-and-effect relationship has been established. Hypothalamic MS plaques have been shown to cause hypersomnia and narcoleptic symptoms in the context of low CSF hypocretin-1 levels [84]. Additionally, abnormally low levels of hypocretin-1 in MS patients with hypothalamic plaques have been found. Therefore, it is possible for CNS inflammation and demyelination, in this area, to cause somnolence by altering CSF hypocretin-1 levels [85]. One study evaluated lesions on magnetic resonance imaging (MRI), CSF hypocretin-1 levels, and serum anti-aquaporin 4 (AQP4) antibody titer in seven MS patients with narcolepsy [86]. Bilateral and symmetrical hypothalamic lesions associated with marked or moderate hypocretin deficiency were found in all seven cases. Four of these patients met the ICSD-2 narcolepsy criteria. Three patients, including two with narcolepsy, were seropositive for anti-AQP4 antibody and diagnosed to have neuromyelitis optica-related disorder.

Modafinil is a CNS activating and wake-promoting agent, and is pharmacologically distinct from other CNS stimulants. Preclinical studies [87] have demonstrated that modafinil can selectively activate lateral hypothalamic neurons that produce wake-promoting hypocretin-1. It is well known that modafinil significantly improves EDS associated with narcolepsy [88], and a preliminary study [89] showed that it effectively manages fatigue associated with MS. However, a recent meta-analysis [90] showed that existing trials of modafinil for fatigue and EDS associated with MS provided inconsistent results. Thus, modafinil is not yet sufficient to be recommended for EDS and fatigue in MS until solid data are available.

REM sleep behavior disorder

RBD is a parasomnia characterized by complex motor behaviors, such as kicking, punching, and dream enactment, which occur during REM sleep. RBD may be idiopathic or associated with various neurological conditions such as brainstem neoplasm, MS affecting the brainstem, olivopontocerebellar atrophy, diffuse Lewy body disease, Parkinson disease, Alzheimer dementia, progressive supranuclear palsy, or Shy–Drager syndrome and pure autonomic failure [91,92]. RBD has been described as an initial presenting symptom in a 25-year-old woman with MS, and subsequently resolved after treatment with adrenocorticotropic hormone [93]. However, in that study, no MRI images documenting the described pontine and bilateral periventricular cerebral lesions were presented. More recently, another RBD case in a 51-year-old woman with MS has been reported [94], and the RBD onset was attributed to the large MS plaque in the dorsal brainstem: MRI showed a large confluent area of increased T_2 signal in the dorsal pons lesion similar to that provoked in animal models (eg, cats, with bilateral peri-locus coeruleus lesions inducing REM sleep without atonia accompanied by motor behaviors). A study showed that the estimated prevalence of RBD in MS was 1.4% [95].

Clonazepam is first-line therapy for RBD. However, if RBD occurs in association with an acute brainstem inflammatory lesion, high doses of methylprednisolone should be tried first [4].

In relation to the reported association between MS and depression, the literature over the last three decades has provided evidence for tricyclic antidepressants causing REM sleep without muscle atonia and inducing RBD in healthy subjects as well as in patients with neuropsychiatric disorders [96,97]. There are similar reports of RBD symptoms being triggered by SSRIs, and a systematic PSG study of patients taking serotonergic antidepressants, such as fluoxetine, paroxetine, citalopram, sertraline, and venlafaxine, found an increase in REM sleep electromyographic (EMG) tonic activity compared with control subjects [97,98]. MS patients taking such medications may be at an increased risk for developing RBD, particularly with increasing age.

In conclusion, the association between MS and sleep disorders is common. Though often unrecognized, sleep disorders in MS are seen at higher frequency than in the general population, and they may contribute to pain, fatigue, and depression—symptoms commonly observed in MS patients. An increased clinical awareness and appropriate treatment of sleep disorders in MS population may significantly improve the overall quality of life in these patients. As has recently been suggested [13], it would be desirable to create more sensitive and specific questionnaires for sleep disorders in the MS population to screen patients who may require further sleep medical investigations. Extended controlled trials treating sleep disorders in MS patients with fatigue will determine whether the treatments provide symptomatic relief and improve quality of life. Moreover, given how MS and sleep disruption both generate pro-inflammatory cytokines, it would be interesting to evaluate the effects of treatment for the sleep disorders in MS patients on cytokines.

References

1. Tachibana N, et al. Sleep problems in multiple sclerosis. Eur Neurol 1994;34:320–3.
2. Figved N, et al. Neuropsychiatric symptoms in patients with multiple sclerosis. Acta Psychiatr Scand 2005;112:463–8.
3. Merlino G, et al. Prevalence of "poor sleep" among patients with multiple sclerosis: an independent predictor of mental and physical status. Sleep Med 2009;10:26–34.
4. Brass SD, et al. Sleep disorders in patients with multiple sclerosis. Sleep Med Rev 2010;14(2):121–9.
5. He J, et al. Increased sleep fragmentation in experimental autoimmune encephalomyelitis. Brain Behav Immun 2014;38:53–8.
6. Barun B. Pathophysiological background and clinical characteristics of sleep disorders in multiple sclerosis. Clin Neurol Neurosurg 2013;115(Suppl 1):S82–5.
7. Patel SR, et al. Correlates of long sleep duration. Sleep 2006;29:881–9.
8. Pokryszko-Dragan A, et al. Sleep disturbances in patients with multiple sclerosis. Neurol Sci 2013;34(8):1291–6.
9. Kaminska M, et al. Sleep disorders and fatigue in multiple sclerosis: evidence for association and interaction. J Neurol Sci 2011;302(1–2):7–13.
10. Kos D, et al. Origin of fatigue in multiple sclerosis: review of the literature. Neurorehabil Neural Repair 2008;22(1):91–100.
11. Krupp LB, et al. Fatigue in multiple sclerosis. Arch Neurol 1998;45:435–7.
12. Simmons RD, et al. Living with multiple sclerosis: longitudinal changes in employment and the importance of symptom management. Neurology 2010;257:926–36.
13. Veauthier C, Paul F. Sleep disorders in multiple sclerosis and their relationship to fatigue. Sleep Med 2014;15:5–14.
14. Ohayon M. Epidemiology of insomnia: what we know and what we still need to learn. Sleep Med Rev 2002;6:97–111.
15. Breslau N, et al. Sleep disturbance and psychiatric disorders: a longitudinal epidemiologic study of young adults. Biol Psychiatry 1996;39:411–18.
16. Achiron A, et al. Sleep disturbance in multiple sclerosis: clinical and neuroradiologic correlations related to disease activity. J Neuroimmunol 1995;56–63(Suppl 1):57.
17. Veauthier C, et al. Fatigue in multiple sclerosis is closely related to sleep disorders: a polysomnographic cross-sectional study. Mult Scler 2011;17:613–22.
18. American Academy of Sleep Medicine. The international classification of sleep disorders, 2nd ed. Westchester, IL: American Academy of Sleep Medicine, 2005.
19. Stanton BR, et al. Sleep and fatigue in multiple sclerosis. Mult Scler 2006;12:481–6.
20. Bamer AM, et al. Prevalence of sleep problems in individuals with multiple sclerosis. Mult Scler 2008;14:1127–30.
21. Beck AT, Steer RA. Internal consistencies of the original and revised Beck Depression Inventory. J Clin Psychol 1984;40:1365–7.
22. Brola W, et al. Symptomatology and pathogenesis of different types of pain in multiple sclerosis. Neurol Neurochir Pol 2014; 48(4):272–9.
23. Osterberg A, et al. Central pain in multiple sclerosis: prevalence and clinical characteristics. Eur J Pain 2005;9:531–42.
24. Kalia LV, O'Connor PW. Severity of chronic pain and its relationship to quality of life in multiple sclerosis. Mult Scler 2005;11:322–7.
25. Onen SH, et al. The effects of total sleep deprivation, selective sleep interruption and sleep recovery on pain tolerance thresholds in healthy subjects. J Sleep Res 2001;10:35–42.
26. Solaro C, et al. Gabapentin is effective in treating nocturnal painful spasms in multiple sclerosis. Mult Scler 2000;6:192–3.
27. Solaro C, et al. Pregabalin for treating paroxysmal painful symptoms in multiple sclerosis: a pilot study. J Neurol 2009;256(10):1773–4.
28. Rog DJ, et al. Randomized, controlled trial of cannabis-based medicine in central pain in multiple sclerosis. Neurology 2005;65:812–19.
29. Koppel BS, et al. Systematic review: efficacy and safety of medical marijuana in selected neurologic disorders: report of the Guideline Development Subcommittee of the American Academy of Neurology. Neurology 2014;82:1556–63.
30. Kalsi V, Fowler CJ. Therapy insight: bladder dysfunction associated with multiple sclerosis. Nat Clin Pract Urol 2005;2:492–501.
31. Amarenco G, et al. Bladder and sphincter disorders in multiple sclerosis. Clinical, urodynamic and neurophysiological study of 225 cases. Rev Neurol (Paris) 1995;151:722–30.
32. Fleming WE, Pollack C. Sleep disorders in multiple sclerosis. Semin Neurol 2005;25:64–8.
33. Valiquette G, et al. Desmopressin in the management of nocturia in patients with multiple sclerosis. A double-blind, crossover trial. Arch Neurol1996;53:1270–5.
34. Adli Oel Y, Corcos J. Botulinum neurotoxin-A treatment of lower urinary tract symptoms in multiple sclerosis. Can Urol Assoc J 2014;8(1–2): E61–7.
35. Patten SB, et al. Major depression in multiple sclerosis: a population-based perspective. Neurology 2003;61:1524–7.
36. Chwastiak L, et al. Depressive symptoms and severity of illness in multiple sclerosis: epidemiologic study of a large community sample. Am J Psychiatry 2002;159:1862–8.
37. McGuigan C, Hutchinson M. Unrecognised symptoms of depression in a community-based population with multiple sclerosis. J Neurol 2006;253:219–23.
38. Mohr DC, et al. Treatment of depression for patients with multiple sclerosis in neurology clinics. Mult Scler 2006;12:204–8.
39. Feinstein A, et al. The link between multiple sclerosis and depression. Nat Rev Neurol 2014;10(9):507–17.
40. Fruehwald S, et al. Depression and quality of life in multiple sclerosis. Acta Neurol Scand 2001;104:257–61.
41. Picchietti D, Winkelman JW. Restless legs syndrome, periodic limb movements in sleep and depression. Sleep 2005;28:891–8.
42. Hoque R, Chesson AL Jr. Pharmacologically induced/exacerbated restless legs syndrome, periodic limb movements of sleep, and REM behavior disorder/REM sleep without atonia: literature review, qualitative scoring, and comparative analysis. J Clin Sleep Med 2010;6(1):79–83.
43. Despault-Duquette PO, et al. Restless legs syndrome in multiple sclerosis. Ann Neurol 2002;52 (Suppl 1):S42.
44. Ferini-Strambi L, et al. Nocturnal sleep study in multiple sclerosis: correlations with clinical and brain magnetic resonance imaging findings. J Neurol Sci 1994;125:194–7.
45. Montplaisir J, Allen R, Walters SA, Ferini-Strambi L. Restless legs syndrome and periodic limb movements during sleep. In: Kryger MH, Roth T, Dement WC, eds. Principles and practice of sleep medicine, 4th ed. Philadelphia: Elsevier-Saunders, 2005:839–52.
46. Coleman RM, Bliwise DL, Sajben N, et al. Epidemiology of periodic limb movements during sleep. In: Guilleinault C, Lugaresi E, eds. Sleep/wake disorders: natural history, epidemiology and long term evolution. New York: Raven Press, 1988:217–29.
47. Schürks M, Bussfeld P. Multiple sclerosis and restless legs syndrome: a systematic review and meta-analysis. Eur J Neurol 2013;20(4):605–15.
48. Manconi M, et al. Restless legs syndrome is a common finding in multiple sclerosis and correlates with cervical cord damage. Mult Scler 2008;14:86–93.
49. Winkelmann J, et al. Periodic limb movements in syringomyelia and syringobulbia. Mov Disord 2000;15(4):752–3.

50. de Mello MT, et al. Treatment of periodic leg movements with a dopaminergic agonist in subjects with total spinal cord lesions. Spinal Cord 1999;37(9):634–7.

51. Lee JS, et al. Periodic limb movements in sleep after a small deep subcortical infarct. Mov Disord 2005;20(2):260–1.

52. Yokota T, et al. Sleep-related periodic leg movements (nocturnal myoclonus) due to spinal cord lesion. J Neurol Sci 1991;104(1):13–18.

53. Hartmann M, et al. Restless legs syndrome associated with spinal cord lesions. J Neurol Neurosurg Psychiatry 1999;66(5):688–9.

54. Bara-Jimenez W, et al. Periodic limb movements in sleep: state-dependent excitability of the spinal flexor reflex. Neurology 2000;54(8):1609–16.

55. Provini F, et al. Motor pattern of periodic limb movements during sleep. Neurology 2001;57(2):300–4.

56. Ondo WG, et al. Clinical correlates of 6-hydroxydopamine injections into A11 dopaminergic neurons in rats: a possible model for restless legs syndrome. Mov Disord 2000;15(1):154–8.

57. Leriche L, et al. The dopamine D3 receptor mediates locomotor hyperactivity induced by NMDA receptor blockade. Neuropharmacology 2003;45(2):174–81.

58. Schattschneider J, et al. Idiopathic restless legs syndrome: abnormalities in central somatosensory processing. J Neurol 2004;251(8):977–82.

59. Ferini-Strambi L, Marelli S. Pharmacotherapy for restless legs syndrome. Expert Opin Pharmacother 2014;15(8):1127–38.

60. Huber S, et al. Multiple sclerosis: therapy with recombinant beta-1b interferon: initial results with 30 multiple sclerosis patients in northwest Switzerland. Schweiz Med Wochenschr 1996;126:1475–81.

61. Born J, et al. Differential effects of hydrocortisone, fluocortolone, and aldosterone on nocturnal sleep in humans. Acta Endocrinol 1987;116:129–37.

62. Chrousos GA, et al. Side effects of glucocorticoid treatment. Experience of the opic neuritis treatment trial. JAMA 1993;269:2110–12.

63. Antonijevic IA, Steiger A. Depression-like changes of the sleep-EEG during high dose corticosteroid treatment in patients with multiple sclerosis. Psychoneuroendocrinology 2003;28:780–95.

64. Vallittu AM, et al. The efficacy of glatiramer acetate in beta-interferon-intolerant MS patients. Acta Neurol Scand 2005;112:234–7.

65. Fox EJ. Management of worsening multiple sclerosis with mitxantrone: a review. Clin Ther 2006;28:461–74.

66. Haas J, et al. Intravenous immunoglobulins in the treatment of relapsing remitting multiple sclerosis: results of a retrospective multicenter observational study over 5 years. Mult Scler 2005;11:562–7.

67. He D, et al. Laquinimod for multiple sclerosis. Cochrane Database Syst Rev 2013;8:CD010475.

68. Auer RN, et al. Multiple sclerosis with medullary plaques and fatal sleep apnea (Ondine's curse). Clin Neuropathol 1996;15:101–5.

69. Howard RS, et al. Respiratory involvement in multiple sclerosis. Brain 1992;115:479–94.

70. Braley TJ, et al. Sleep-disordered breathing in multiple sclerosis. Neurology 2012;79(9):929–36.

71. Kaminska M, et al. Obstructive sleep apnea is associated with fatigue in multiple sclerosis. Mult Scler 2012;18(8):1159–69.

72. Kallweit U, et al. Fatigue and sleep-disordered breathing in multiple sclerosis: a clinically relevant association?. Mult Scler Int 2013;2013:286581.

73. Ferini-Strambi L, et al. Nocturnal sleep study in multiple sclerosis: correlations with clinical and brain magnetic resonance imaging findings. J Neurol Sci 1994;125:194–7.

74. Kaynak H, et al. Fatigue and sleep disturbance in multiple sclerosis. Eur J Neurol 2006;13:1333–9.

75. Veauthier C, et al. Fatigue in multiple sclerosis is closely related to sleep disorders: a polysomnographic cross-sectional study. Mult Scler 2011;17:613–22.

76. Neau JP, et al. Sleep disorders and multiple sclerosis: a clinical and polysomnography study. Eur Neurol 2012;68:8–15.

77. Jacobson E. Fall von narcolepsie. Klin Wochenschr 1926;2:2188.

78. Guillain G, Alajouanine T. La somnolence dans la sclerose en plaques. Les episodes aigus ou subaigus de la sclerose en laques pouvant simuler l'encephalite lethargique. An Med 1928;24:111–18.

79. Bonduelle M, Degos C. Symptomatic narcolepsies: a critical study. In: Guilleminault C, Dement WC, Passouant P, eds. Narcolepsy. New York: Spectrum, 1976:322–5.

80. Peraita-Adrados R, et al. A patient with narcolepsy with cataplexy and multiple sclerosis: two different diseases that may share pathophysiologic mechanisms? Sleep Med 2013;14(7):695–6.

81. Schrader H, et al. Multiple sclerosis and narcolepsy/cataplexy in a monozygotic twin. Neurology 1980;30:105–8.

82. Mignot E. Narcolepsy: pharmacology, pathophysiology and genetics. In: Kryger MH, Roth T, Dement WC, eds. Principles and practice of sleep medicine, 4th ed. Philadelphia: Elsevier Saunders, 2005:761–79.

83. Duquette P, et al. Clinical sub-groups of multiple sclerosis in relation to HLA: DR alleles as possible markers of disease progression. Can J Neurol Sci 1985;12:106–10.

84. Iseki K, et al. Hypersomnia in MS. Neurology 2002;59:2006–7.

85. Kato T, et al. Hypersomnia and low CSF hypocretin-1 (orexin-A) concentration in a patient with multiple sclerosis showing bilateral hypothalamic lesions. Intern Med 2003;42:743–5.

86. Kanbayashi T, et al. Symptomatic narcolepsy in patients with neuromyelitis optica and multiple sclerosis: new neurochemical and immunological implications. Arch Neurol 2009;66(12):1563–6.

87. Scammell TE, et al. Hypothalamic arousal regions are activated during modafinil-induced wakefulness. J Neurosci 2000;20:8620–8.

88. Guilleminault C, Fromherz S. Narcolepsy: diagnosis and treatment. In: Kryger MH, Roth T, Dement WC, eds. Principles and practice of sleep medicine, 4th ed. Philadelphia: Elsevier Saunders, 2005:781–90.

89. Rammohan KW, et al. Efficacy and safety of modafinil (Provigil) for the treatment of fatigue in multiple sclerosis: a two centre phase 2 study. J Neurol Neurosurg Psychiatry 2002;72:179–83.

90. Sheng P, et al. Efficacy of modafinil on fatigue and excessive daytime sleepiness associated with neurological disorders: a systematic review and meta-analysis. PLoS One 2013;8(12):e81802.

91. Ferini Strambi L, et al. REM sleep behavior disorder. Neurol Sci 2005;Suppl 3:186–92.

92. Boeve BF. REM sleep behavior disorder: updated review of the core features, the REM sleep behavior disorder–neurodegenrative diseases association, evolving concepts, controversies, and future directions. Ann NY Acad Sci 2010;1184:15–54.

93. Plazzi G, Montagna P. Remitting REM sleep behavior disorder as the initial sign of multiple sclerosis. Sleep Med 2002;3:437–9.

94. Tippmann-Peikert M, et al. REM sleep behavior disorder initiated by acute brainstem multiple sclerosis. Neurology 2006;66:1277–9.

95. Gomez-Choco MJ, et al. Prevalence of restless legs syndrome and REM sleep behavior disorder in multiple sclerosis. Mult Scler 2007;13:805–8.

96. Nofzinger EA, Reynolds CF. REM sleep behavior disorder. JAMA 1994;271:820.

97. Mahowald MW, Schenck CH. REM sleep parasomnias. In: Kryger MH, Roth T, Dement WC, eds. Principles and practice of sleep medicine, 4th ed. Philadelphia: Elsevier Saunders, 2005:897–916.

98. Winkelman JW, James L. Serotonergic antidepressants are associated with REM sleep without atonia. Sleep 2004;27(2):317–21.

CHAPTER 34

Sleep and dreams
A clinical neurological perspective

Mark Solms

Background

Historically, there has been little systematic investigation of changes in dreaming due to neurological disease, despite numerous clinical reports of marked abnormalities in some patient groups. Accordingly, the topic remains poorly understood. This reflects a lack of development in the field of dream research itself: an understanding of the brain mechanisms of dreaming lagged behind that of other cognitive functions. There are two main reasons for this. First, unlike most cognitive functions that were the focus of nineteenth- and twentieth-century behavioral neuroscience, dreaming is almost entirely subjective. The observable data are retrospective, single-witness qualitative descriptions, only indirectly related to the phenomenon of dreaming itself. This poses special methodological problems.

The second reason for the undeveloped state of this field is closely related to the first. Researchers seeking an objective approach to dreaming eagerly alighted on a physiological state that *correlates* closely with it—namely rapid eye movement (REM) sleep [1–4]. This physiological state was then conflated with dreaming itself, resulting in the development of neuropsychological models of dreaming that were in fact models of REM sleep [5]. This conflation was compounded by the fact that the models were empirically grounded in animal studies (where dream reports are of course precluded) rather than human lesion studies of the kind that classically informed models of other cognitive functions. When the conventional human lesion studies were belatedly performed, it became apparent that dreaming and REM sleep are in fact doubly dissociable states [6].

A traditional neuropsychology or behavioral neurology grounded in the clinico-anatomical method—which was widely applied to other cognitive functions from the mid-nineteenth century—is less than 30 years old in the case of dreaming. Incidental reports of changes in dream phenomenology associated with focal cerebral lesions did nevertheless accumulate in the literature over a long period, albeit without any attempt to synthesize the scattered observations into a coherent picture. Systematic clinico-anatomical studies were first published in the 1980s [7–9], and the available evidence was not comprehensively reviewed before the 1990s [10–12]. The conventional clinico-anatomical studies have since been complemented by a slew of functional brain imaging studies, with strongly convergent findings [13]. Rigorous probes of the neurochemistry of dreaming (as opposed to REM sleep) have surprisingly not yet been conducted [14].

An understanding of the brain mechanisms of dreaming is nevertheless beginning to emerge. Systematic observation of abnormalities of dreaming in neurological disease has contributed fundamentally to this emerging picture. The bewildering array of clinical phenomena may perhaps best be grouped under two headings: (1) deficits of dreaming and (2) excesses of dreaming.

Deficits of dreaming

The earliest clinical observations of changes in dreaming with neurological disease concerned *cessation* of dreaming (or cessation of aspects of dreaming). The terms "Charcot–Wilbrand syndrome" and "anoneira" have been used to describe this abnormality, which is typically seen in the acute phase of posterior cortical pathology.

Charcot–Wilbrand syndrome

The concept of this syndrome, based on two single-case reports by Charcot [15,16] and Wilbrand [17,18], was first articulated by Pötzl, who defined the syndrome as "mind-blindness with disturbance of optic imagination" ([19], p. 306). Nielsen defined it as "visual agnosia plus loss of the ability to revisualize" ([20], p. 74). Critchley's widely cited definition was:

> a patient loses the power to conjure up visual images or memories, and furthermore, ceases to dream during his sleeping hours. ([21], p. 311)

> Reproduced from Critchley, M, The parietal lobes, Copyright (1953), Macmillan.

Critchley described prosopagnosia and topographical agnosia or topographical amnesia as associated features. The localization of the lesion producing this syndrome was never precisely defined, but the occipital cortex (especially area 19) was implicated by most early authors—usually bilaterally. The Charcot–Wilbrand syndrome remained in late twentieth century nosographical usage, although the condition was (until recently) considered rare. A modern definition of the syndrome, by Murri et al., reads:

> the association of loss of the ability to conjure up visual images or memories and the loss of dreaming … [indicates] a lesion in an acute phase affecting the posterior regions. ([8], p. 185)

> Reproduced from Arch Neurol, 41(2), Murri, L., Arena, R., Siciliano, G., Mazzotta, R., & Murarorio, A, Dream recall in patients with focal cerebral lesions, pp. 183–185, Copyright (1984), American Medical Association.

Deficient revisualization (called "irreminiscence" in the nomenclature of Nielsen [20]) was the fundamental deficit in almost all definitions of the syndrome. Cessation of dreaming ("or at least, an alteration in the vivid visual component of the dreaming state"; Critchley [21], p. 311) was seen as a secondary consequence of the visual imagery deficit. The associated visual agnosias, too, were originally attributed to the defective revisualization, since visual agnosia was classically understood as a loss of "visual memory images" [21–23].

Subsequent advances in the agnosia concept, and a misreading of the original French and German case reports, have resulted in considerable nosographic confusion regarding this syndrome [12,24]. It is widely assumed that Wilbrand's case—an elderly female patient with bilateral posterior cerebral artery thrombosis—could not *visualize* familiar places [20,21,25,26]. However, the original report stated only that she was unable to *recognize* familiar places. This symptom (which we would today call topographical *agnosia*) was conceptualized, in accordance with classical theory, as a disorder of "topographical *memory*" (Wilbrand [17], p. 52, emphasis added). This conceptualization was then misconstrued by secondary authors as a disorder of topographical *revisualization*. The original report reveals that Wilbrand's case actually lacked the cardinal feature of the so-called Charcot–Wilbrand syndrome. As the patient herself clearly stated: "With my eyes shut I see my old Hamburg in front of me again" [15,16] (Wilbrand [17], p. 56). Charcot's case [15,16]—an elderly male patient also with a probable posterior cerebral artery thrombosis (autopsy findings were lacking)—was quite different. He described a striking absence of visual mental imagery. The Charcot–Wilbrand syndrome is therefore misconceived.

It is also misnamed. Charcot's [15,16] patient ceased to dream in visual images, but he continued to dream in words. Wilbrand's [17,18] patient, on the other hand, dreamed "almost not at all anymore" ([17], p. 54). The original report is ambiguous as to whether Wilbrand's patient merely dreamed infrequently or actually lost the capacity to dream completely (and then gradually recovered it); but either way, there is no question of an isolated loss of *visual* dream imagery, which is what Charcot's patient unequivocally described. The "Charcot–Wilbrand syndrome" therefore appears to be two different (but related) syndromes, Charcot's variant is characterized by unimodal loss of *visual* dream imagery and Wilbrand's variant by *global* (heteromodal) cessation or suppression of dreaming. This distinction is supported by my review of the world literature [12]. However, the further conclusion drawn from that review, namely, that Charcot's variant occurs with occipital lesions and Wilbrand's variant with parietal lesions, is probably incorrect (see the discussion later in the chapter).

Charcot's variant: unimodal loss of visual dream imagery

At least 10 case reports of unimodal loss of visual dream imagery have been published, together with five further reports of patients who experienced deficits of specific *aspects* of visual dream imagery (eg, color, movement, and faces). Cessation of visual imagery or aspects thereof results from various pathologies, usually of acute onset (thrombosis, hemorrhage, trauma, or CO poisoning), but it has also been described in cases of neoplasm, probable Alzheimer disease, callosal dysgenesis, and Turner syndrome). The lesion is typically localized to the mesial occipitotemporal or lateral occipitoparietal regions, and is usually bilateral, but precise localizing information is lacking in many of the published cases [12,15,26–41].

Defective revisualization (irreminiscence) is a constant feature in these cases, although it is typically restricted to the disordered aspect of vision (eg, color, movement, and faces) in cases where the loss of visual dream imagery is partial (i.e, submodal). This strongly suggests a common underlying image-generation deficit causing the same disorder in both waking and dream cognition. Various forms of visual agnosia are commonly associated features, but agnosia is definitely absent in some cases and therefore cannot be considered integral to the syndrome [12].

Most published reports of deficits in visual dream imagery derive from retrospective accounts in a clinical setting. However such reports have been confirmed by REM awakenings in a sleep-laboratory setting in at least three cases [32–34].

Negative findings

Interestingly, unimodal deficits of dream imagery outside the higher visual sphere have never been demonstrated, nor have unimodal deficits been observed in any modality other than vision. Thus although achromatopsic, akinetopsic, prosopagnosic, and hemineglect disorders are duplicated in dreams, patients with lower visual disorders such as cortical blindness and hemianopia invariably report normal vision (full fields) in their dreams. This, incidentally, has important implications for theories of visual consciousness. Moreover, hemiplegic patients experience normal somatomotor and somatosensory functions in their dream imagery (as do acute-phase paraplegic and quadriplegic patients) [12,42]. The same applies to the extrapyramidal movement disorders. Similarly, nonfluent aphasics claim to speak normally in their dreams [12].

Of related interest, perhaps, is the fact that the dreams of patients with substantial impairments of executive function due to massive dorsolateral prefrontal lesions are indistinguishable from the dreams of controls [43]. This suggests that dreams (apart from their higher visual aspects) do not involve simple activations of the entire cortex, as Hobson and McCarley's [5] activation-synthesis model originally proposed. The clinico-anatomical findings point to a differentiated network of forebrain structures involved in dream cognition, a conclusion that is strongly confirmed by neuroimaging findings (see the discussion later in this chapter).

Wilbrand's variant: global (heteromodal) loss or suppression of dreaming

At least 108 cases of global loss of dreaming have been reported, excluding leucotomy cases, which will be discussed separately (see [12] for a nearly complete tabulation of these cases). A larger number of cases in group studies, where individual case data were lacking and where "loss of dreaming" was defined in variable ways [7–9], have also been reported.

As with Charcot's variant, global loss of dreaming (which I called "anoneira" [12]) is typically—but not invariably—associated with acute-onset, focal cerebral lesions. Thrombosis, hemorrhage, and trauma are the most commonly reported pathologies. The first systematic attempt to identify the lesion site responsible for global cessation of dreaming pointed to the inferior parietal lobule [12]. Unilateral lesions of either hemisphere were shown to be commonplace, with no lateralizing bias. However, at least two cases have since been reported in which the parietal lobe was apparently spared [44,45], as indeed it appears to have been in Wilbrand's original case [18]. Members of my group will shortly be reporting five further cases of this type [46]. However, it is difficult to imagine how a lesion in unimodal cortex can produce a heteromodal disorder. It is therefore worth noting that in Bischof and Bassetti's case [44], as in ours [46], lacunar infarction of the posterolateral thalamus (which modulates parietal functions) was present. Similarly, Poza & Marti's case [45] (ruptured arteriovenous malformation) was not suitable for localizing purposes; there may very well have been a parietal aspect to his extensive lesion. Moreover, a re-analysis of my data by Yu [47] revealed that the lesions in my "parietal" cases almost always extended into adjacent occipitotemporal tissues (especially Brodmann areas 22, 19, and 37). The parietal lobe therefore may or may not have been the constant feature in my clinical series. It is therefore, sadly, still not possible to make a more precise localizing statement than the one offered by Murri et al.: "a lesion in an acute phase affecting the posterior regions" ([8], p. 185). Hopefully future studies will refine this statement.

The reference to an *acute phase* is not superfluous. I observed that almost all cases of global anoneira recover the capacity to dream within 12 months [12]. This fact, which suggests diaschitic effects, may further help explain the imprecise localization of the causal lesion.

Of particular clinical interest is the observation [12] that hydrocephalus is associated with cessation of dreaming, and that dreaming recovers after successful ventriculoperitoneal shunting (or shunt revision) in these cases. Cessation of dreaming might therefore be used as a clinical warning of shunt malfunction.

Defective revisualization (irreminiscence) is a relatively common but by no means invariable feature of the global cases. It was overrepresented in the earlier case reports for the probable reason that patients were only asked about their dreams once irreminiscence had been established. The more recent cases that I reported in [12] were part of an unselected series and are therefore more likely to be representative of the clinical population as a whole. Global anoneira (unlike unimodal visual dream deficits) therefore cannot be reduced to irreminiscence.

Not surprisingly, considering the lesion site, global anoneira is frequently associated with disorders of spatial cognition, including visuospatial short-term memory deficits [12]. The lack of association between cessation of dreaming and *long-term* memory disorder of any kind excludes the possibility that cessation of dreaming is really a memory disorder—i.e., failure to remember dreams as opposed to cessation of dreaming per se [48–50]. This applies also to the various language disorders that were previously thought to explain loss of dreaming [10,51–54]. In my systematic survey of the literature and my own cases [12], I found no relationship between cessation of dreaming and any form of language disorder or amnesia.

The veracity of retrospective reports of absence of dreaming on morning awakening has also been repeatedly confirmed by the REM awakening method [44,45,55,56]. This further supports the assumption that anoneira concerns cessation of dreaming per se, as opposed to loss of memory for dreams. Even severe amnesiacs with bilateral hippocampal lesions report dreams on awakening from REM sleep and at sleep onset (Ramachandran, 2004 personal communication). This is consistent with the reports of Stickgold et al [57] and Torda [58] and also with Corkin's [59] observations upon the celebrated case of "HM."

Cessation or suppression of dreaming following prefrontal leucotomy

In a survey of 200 cases of prefrontal leucotomy, Frank observed that a common result of the procedure was "a poverty or entire lack of dreams" ([60], p. 508). In a later report on the same series of cases, then comprising more than 300 patients, he confirmed this finding [61]. Replication of Frank's findings in prefrontal leucotomy

cases was forthcoming from many other authors [26,62–65] (see also Slater, cited by Humphreys and Zangwill [66]). Moreover, Jus et al. [62] confirmed the absence of morning dream reports following prefrontal leucotomy by the REM awakening method.

In apparent contradiction to these reports, however, Humphrey and Zangwill [66], Cathala et al. [7], Murri et al. [8,9], and Doricchi and Violani [10] all observed a relatively *low* incidence of cessation of dreaming with frontal versus posterior cerebral lesions. The same applies to the observation reported earlier in this chapter to the effect that the dreams of frontal patients are indistinguishable from those of controls [43]. This apparent contradiction was resolved when I reviewed the lesions in the previously reported cases and described nine new cases with cessation of dreaming following naturally occurring bifrontal lesions [12]. My conclusion was that dreaming was entirely spared with *dorsolateral* prefrontal cortical lesions but lost with deep *white matter* lesions in the ventromesial quadrant of the frontal lobes (see Figs. 34.1 and 34.2). The lesion site in these nine cases coincided exactly with the area that was targeted by prefrontal leucotomy: "a circumscribed lesion just anterior to the frontal horns of the ventricle, in the lower medial quadrant of the frontal lobes" ([67], p. 177). A reanalysis of the original data in 35 cases from my series [12] with global cessation of dreaming associated with subcortical lesions revealed that the lesion was located in either the deep frontal white matter (areas F09 and F14 in the classification of Damasio and Damasio [68]; see Fig. 34.3), or the head of the caudate nucleus, or both [69]. The lesion is typically but not exclusively bilateral. Of theoretical importance is the fact that the region defined as the "head of the caudate nucleus" in the latter study [69] included the nucleus accumbens, which is situated immediately beneath it.

It is noteworthy that the psychotropic medications that replaced prefrontal leucotomy as the treatment of choice for psychotic disorders block dopamine (DA) transmission at D_2-type receptors in a mesial forebrain pathway that projects primarily to the nucleus accumbens. Probably related to this is the observation that both prefrontal leucotomy in general and cessation of dreaming in particular, due to lesions in this general area, are associated with reduced motivational incentive [12], as indeed are most antipsychotic medications [70]. Leu-Semenescu et al. [71] recently described strikingly reduced dream frequency and intensity in neurological patients with auto-activation deficits (i.e, adynamia/abulia). Also of interest in this connection are the observations by Piehler [64] and Schindler [65] to the effect that early recovery of dreaming after prefrontal leucotomy typically predicted psychiatric relapse, suggesting that absence of dreaming could serve as an index of the clinical success of the operation. Dreaming is, after all, a psychotic state.

Effects of pontine brainstem lesions

Cessation of dreaming following circumscribed pontine lesions—with or without cessation of REM sleep—has never been demonstrated (for reviews, see [6,12]), despite the longstanding assumption that dreaming is caused by—if not identical with—the cyclical, spontaneous activation of cholinergic (ACh) cell groups in the mesopontine tegmentum during the REM state, together with reciprocal inhibition of serotonergic (5-HT) and noradrenergic (NA) cell groups in the dorsal raphe and locus coeruleus complex [72,73]. Consciousness in general is of course frequently compromised by pontine lesions, but at least eight cases with cessation

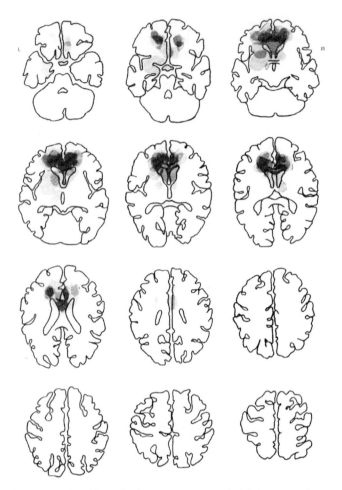

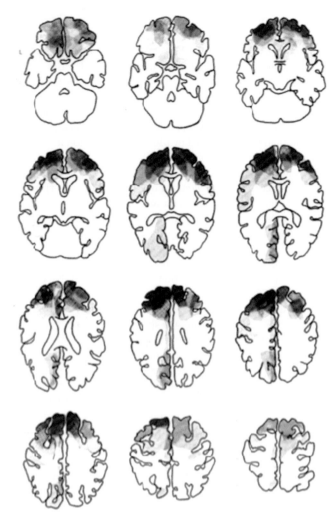

Fig. 34.1 Combined facsimile of scans in nine cases with global cessation of dreaming caused by deep frontal lesions, illustrating the strong involvement of the white matter surrounding the frontal horns of the lateral ventricles.
Reproduced from Solms, M, The Neuropsychology of Dreams: A clinico-anatomical study, Copyright (1997), Taylor & Francis.

Fig. 34.2 Combined facsimile of scans in 14 cases with preserved dreaming with bifrontal lesions, illustrating the relative preponderance of cortical convexity involvement.
Reproduced from Solms, M, The Neuropsychology of Dreams: A clinico-anatomical study, Copyright (1997), Taylor & Francis.

or near-cessation of REM sleep have been reported in which the patients were capable of communicating meaningfully about their dreams [74–77]. Indeed, one such patient did actually report loss of dreaming [74], but the pathology—ruptured traumatic aneurysm of the basilar artery—almost certainly extended beyond the pontine brainstem and included the visual–spatial cortical areas discussed earlier in this chapter. Even this isolated case therefore does not support the old equation of pontine brainstem mechanisms with dream generation [72,73]. This conclusion is buttressed by the fact that drugs that suppress REM sleep do not suppress dreaming [78]; in fact, the opposite is the case [79–85]. There is further discussion of the relationship between dreaming and REM sleep later in this chapter.

Neuroimaging and transcranial magnetic stimulation studies

Neuroimaging studies have determined patterns of regional brain activation and deactivation during REM sleep, the stage of sleep during which dream reports are most frequently obtained [86]. These patterns of activity are highly consistent with the brain areas

linked with dreaming in the clinical lesions studies reviewed above. Significant increases in regional brain activity have been observed in the basal forebrain and other limbic and paralimbic structures, including the hippocampal complex, the anterior cingulate cortex, and the pontine tegmentum, during REM sleep. Also consistent with the lesion studies [43] is the fact that the dorsolateral convexity is strikingly deactivated during REM sleep [87–89].

Braun et al. [90] reported a dissociated pattern of activity between visual association areas (extrastriate cortices—fusiform, inferotemporal, and ventral lateral occipital) and primary visual areas (striate cortices) during REM sleep compared with slow-wave sleep (SWS). Activation within the visual association cortices was also shown to correlate positively with activity within parahippocampal gyri and contiguous portions of the hippocampus, and with deactivation of dorsolateral and orbital prefrontal association areas. Based on these findings, the authors concluded that "during REM sleep, the extrastriate cortices and paralimbic areas to which they project may be operating as a closed system, functionally disconnected from frontal regions in which the highest

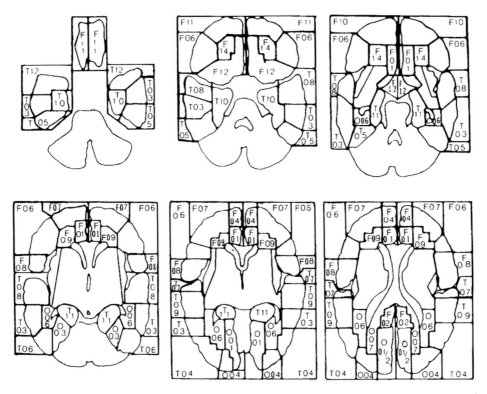

Fig. 34.3 Global cessation of dreaming is associated with subcortical lesions located in the deep frontal white matter.
Reproduced from Damasio, H., & Damasio, A, Lesion analysis in neuropsychology, Copyright (1989), with permission from Oxford University Press.

order integration of visual information takes place. Such a dissociation could explain many of the experiential features of dreams" ([90], p. 94). This notion of a closed loop between certain medial forebrain and limbic regions and higher order visual association areas is consistent with my suggestion [6,12] that dreaming is a product of deep ventromesial frontal (mesocortical–mesolimbic) structures activating higher visual association areas during sleep, instead of the dorsolateral frontal (executive and motor) areas they activate during waking, thereby generating imaginary versus real action.

A recent study, using [^{15}O]H$_2$O positron emission tomography (PET) in healthy subjects with habitually high and low dream recall frequencies, also showed that high dream recallers—compared with low dream recallers—had greater regional cerebral blood flow in the temporoparietal junction during SWS, REM sleep, and waking, as well as greater regional cerebral blood flow in the medial prefrontal cortex during REM sleep and waking [91]. These brain regions are highly consistent with those identified by the lesion studies as being critically related to the dream process. As the temporoparietal junction may facilitate the orientation of attention during sleep to external stimuli, it has been argued that the increase in activation of this region may be responsible for the observed increase in intra-sleep wakefulness in high dream recallers. According to the arousal–retrieval model of dreaming [92], intra-sleep wakefulness may facilitate the encoding of dream content into long-term memory, consequently facilitating dream recall upon awakening in high dream recallers.

Consistent with this model, high dream recallers are more reactive to their external environments during all stages of sleep, as well

as during wakefulness, when compared with low dream recallers [93]. Using a novelty oddball paradigm, high dream recallers were shown to have enhanced P3a and late latency event-related potentials (ERPs) to novel and unexpected auditory stimuli. As the P3a and late latency potentials are associated with complex cognitive processes such as familiarity, episodic memory, and emotional processing [94–96], Eichenlaub et al. [93] have argued that the robust differences in brain responsivity show that the cerebral organization of high recallers is intrinsically different to that of low recallers, and that this difference may potentially facilitate either production or encoding of the dream.

The propensity to be more reactive to the external environment is consistent with enhanced activation of the posterior attentional networks in high dream recallers. Whether increased dream recall in high dream recallers is due to more efficient encoding of the memory trace of the dream into long-term memory, or whether activity within these regions indicates a genuine increase in dream activity, remains inconclusive. However, the latter possibility is supported by a recent set of transcranial magnetic stimulation (TMS) studies, which found that visual dream imagery could be enhanced by inhibiting certain frontal regions while stimulating the right posterior parietal cortex during stage 2 sleep but not during SWS [97,98]. This finding must be understood in relation to the fact that TMS is unable to propagate through connected networks during SWS as efficiently as during lighter NREM sleep [99]. It nevertheless corroborates the notion that activity in the posterior association cortex is responsible for the perceptual construction of dreams, and moreover that activity in these regions during sleep represents an increase in dream activity.

Despite all the strong evidence that *higher* visual association cortices are responsible for the perceptual construction of dreams, it has recently been shown that primary visual areas may also be somehow involved. In an innovative combined electroencephalographic/functional magnetic resonance imaging (EEG/fMRI) study, participants' dream imagery (as verbally reported) was decoded from neural activity measured during sleep onset, by software trained to correlate discrete visual stimuli (i.e, pictures) with brain activity during waking [100]. Horikawa et al. concluded that the "principle of perceptual equivalence, which postulates a common neural substrate for perception and imagery, generalizes to spontaneously generated visual experience during sleep" ([100], p. 642). As lesions to primary visual regions do not result in dream loss, or any visual disturbances in dreams [12], the exact contribution of the primary visual regions to conscious dream imagery remains unclear.

Excesses of dreaming

Dream/reality confusion

In [12], I loosely grouped together 12 case reports in the literature and 10 of my own cases under the heading of dream/reality confusion (or "anoneirognosis"). These patients reported excesses of dreaming, ranging from increased frequency and/or vivacity of dreams to intrusions of dreaming and dream-like thinking into waking cognition. The principal justification for collecting these cases under a unitary nosological heading was the fact that the focal lesions (representing a wide variety of pathologies) that cause "anoneirognosis" are typically located in the transitional zone between the anterior diencephalon and basal forebrain. Kindred phenomena are, however, also observed with visual deafferentation, peduncular hallucinosis, delirium, parkinsonian syndromes or medications (see below), Guillain–Barré syndrome, and a variety of toxic and metabolic conditions, as well as by many psychoactive drugs. The common denominator in these cases may therefore simply be degradation of constraints on consciousness. Certainly, any suggestion on the basis of the currently available evidence that dream/reality confusion may be considered a focal symptom is unjustified.

Dream/reality confusion in parkinsonian syndromes is difficult to interpret. Increased dreaming and hallucinations are frequently seen with Parkinson disease (PD), but this may be iatrogenic. It is well-established that hallucinations and excessive dreaming can be provoked by the administration of L-DOPA, both in PD [101] and in normal subjects, independently of any concomitant changes in REM sleep [102]. Accordingly, it has been shown that both reduction of dopamine agonists and administration of dopamine blockers reduce hallucinations and excessive dreaming in PD [103]. However visual hallucinations in PD may also be an indication of the presence of Lewy body pathology, with involvement of parieto-occipital and limbic regions [104,105]. Apart from the iatrogenic explanation, excessive dreaming in parkinsonian syndromes may also have a different mechanism in cases with and without cortical Lewy bodies. In PD, hallucinations occur late in the course of the disorder, whereas they are an early feature of dementia with Lewy bodies (DLB). All of these phenomena must of course be differentiated from REM behavior disorder (RBD), which may occur early in a variety of parkinsonian diseases (see the subsection later in this chapter).

Hallucinations and dream/reality confusion are also common in narcolepsy [106]. In these cases, hallucinations may accompany or follow attacks of cataplexy and sleep paralysis. Hallucinations of the presence of someone nearby ("sensed presence") or a pressure on the chest with breathing difficulties ("incubus/succubus"), and floating/flying and "out-of-body" experiences, are typical in these cases. Dreams can occur at sleep onset (at night or during daytime naps), as well as on awakening (Rosenthal syndrome). The retention of elements of normal waking mentation, such as volitional control or environmental awareness, is characteristic of narcoleptic dreams.

Various other rare disorders are associated with dream/reality confusion. Idiopathic hypersomnia manifests in excessive daytime sleepiness, prolonged unrefreshing sleep and "sleep drunkenness" on attempting to wake up. Habitual dreaming, hypnagogic hallucinations, and sleep paralysis are common in these cases [106]. Kleine–Levin syndrome (KLS) is a rare disorder characterized by recurrent episodes of hypersomnia, compulsive eating behavior, and various psychopathological changes like hypersexuality, irritability, and apathy. Hallucinations, delusions, and "dreamy states" are reported in 14–24% of patients with KLS [107]. In fatal familial insomnia, a variant of Creutzfeldt–Jakob disease (CJD), progressive insomnia is coupled with an oneiric stuporous state in which patients perform complex, jerky movements that correspond to reported dream content [108]. Dream/reality confusion with hallucinations also occurs in sporadic CJD [109].

In populations without neurological disorders, excessive dreaming has been reported as a primary complaint in certain sleep clinics [110]. A study comparing these patients with controls revealed that complaints of excessive dreaming were related to significant microstructural changes, including increased arousals, intra-sleep awakenings, periodic leg movements, alpha–delta sleep, and REM density; however, no macrostructural changes were noted, and no differences in REM sleep and sleep onset latencies were observed. Excessive dreamers were also found to be significantly more stressed, fatigued, and anxious than controls, and to have more headaches.

Nightmares

Nocturnal seizures (and temporal lobe seizures in particular) sometimes present as recurring nightmares [111,112]. In [12], I identified 24 cases of this type in the literature and 9 in my own clinical series. Of theoretical interest is the fact that such nightmares typically occur during NREM sleep. The content of the nightmares frequently coincides with that of the patient's typical aura or 'dreamy state' seizures [12,113]. Penfield was able to artificially generate a waking aura resembling the recurring nightmare reported in one case by stimulating exposed cortex in the region of the epileptogenic focus [114–116]. Successful pharmacological or surgical treatment of the seizure disorder invariably results in disappearance of the recurring nightmares. These facts further support the interpretation of the nightmares in these cases as seizure equivalents (and indeed as NREM phenomena).

As with dream/reality confusion (which frequently co-occurs with nightmares), increased frequency of nightmares is associated with a wide range of toxic and withdrawal states and metabolic abnormalities. The grounds for detaching these two "excesses of dreaming" from each other are not entirely clear. The common denominator here may therefore, once again, simply be general degradation of constraints on consciousness.

It is important to note that nocturnal panic attacks and sleep terrors are not instances of nightmares. Detailed dream recall is often lacking in such attacks [117,118], although in certain studies dream content has been reported [119].

REM behavior disorder

In this disorder, dreamed behaviors are physically acted out. This is due to disruption of the pontomedullary mechanisms that induce REM atonia [120]. The enacted behaviors may be dramatic or even violent, and usually relate to vivid, frightening dreams. A fair proportion of cases injure their bed partners [121]. The disorder is most common in males, with onset often in the sixth or seventh decade. RBD manifests mainly in the second half of the sleep cycle (where REM is predominant). Increased SWS and periodic limb movements across all sleep stages are also seen [122–125].

Of special interest is the association of RBD with parkinsonian syndromes. The presence of RBD in PD patients is associated with cognitive deficits and appears to predict dementia [126,127]. Disorders with Lewy body pathology often involve RBD. The incidence of RBD in PD is 25–50%, and more than 50% in DLB and multisystem atrophy (MSA). In contrast, disorders without Lewy bodies rarely involve RBD. Notably, idiopathic RBD may present many years prior to the other symptoms of an incipient Parkinsonian process [121,128–133]. The prognostic significance of RBD as a precursor to PD, DLB, and MSA is now well established, resulting in the suggestion that the term "cryptogenic" RBD should replace "idiopathic" RBD [124,134]. The propensity to *instinctual* behaviors in RBD, and in animal models of the disorder, is of distinct theoretical interest, as it suggests that dreams are instinctually motivated mental states (see the section later in the chapter), as Freud [135] classically proposed on the basis of purely psychological investigations.

Pharmacological findings

The neurochemical and pharmacological evidence is extremely difficult to interpret. This is due partly to the dynamic interactions that characterize neurotransmitter systems and to the paucity of rigorous pharmacological studies [14]. Mention will only be made here of recent findings that seem particularly relevant to understanding dream generation and the distinction between dreaming and REM sleep.

The neurochemical signature of the REM state is well established, namely, autochthonous activation of ascending pontine ACh cell groups—which is thought to produce characteristic pontine–geniculate–occipital (PGO) waves—and reciprocal inhibition of pontine aminergic (5-HT and NA) cell groups—which is thought to demodulate the dreaming forebrain [136]. Equally well established is the fact that NREM sleep has the opposite pattern. Less widely known is the fact that, unlike other aminergic brainstem cells, the source cells in the ventral tegmental area (VTA) of the mesocortical–mesolimbic DA pathway described earlier in this chapter in connection with prefrontal leucotomy continue to fire at similar rates during sleeping and waking [137,138]. These cells also fire with far greater interspike variability during REM than NREM sleep [137]. This has recently been shown to indicate prominent burst activity in the REM state [139], resulting in greater terminal DA release in the nucleus accumbens. DA delivery to the nucleus accumbens is in fact maximal during REM sleep when compared with NREM sleep and waking [140].

The REM state is also characterized by minimal prefrontal glutamate release [140], which presumably coincides with the observation reported above to the effect that dorsolateral prefrontal lesions have no obvious effect on dream content (and with the observation that this region is strongly deactivated in PET imaging studies of REM sleep [87]). The chemical signature of the REM state, as regards the neurotransmitter interactions underlying the observed regional patterns of forebrain activation and deactivation, is therefore certainly more complex than was previously assumed [141].

This complexity is underscored by the impenetrable thicket of psychopharmacological evidence. Of particular value is any evidence that could clarify the pathophysiology of dream cessation following deep ventromesial frontal lesions. Since the sleep cycle is unaffected by such lesions [62], it is reasonable to assume that they impair a mechanism that is specific to dream generation (as opposed to REM generation). Two competing hypotheses have been advanced to account for dream cessation following deep ventromesial frontal white matter lesions (and the commensurate hyperactivation of this region in fMRI and PET imaging of dreaming sleep and schizophrenic hallucinations [87,142]). The first hypothesis is that it reflects activation of ACh cells in the basal forebrain; the second is that it reflects activation of DA cells in the VTA.

Against the former hypothesis is the observation that ACh antagonists (like scopolamine), rather than suppressing dreaming and dream-like thinking, have the opposite effect: they produce dream/reality confusion [143]. In fact, in this respect, anticholinergic drugs mirror the effects of lesions in cholinergic basal forebrain nuclei [144]. These and other considerations led Braun [145] to observe that activation of these nuclei during REM sleep may actually reflect *inhibition* of forebrain ACh in dreaming sleep.

In favor of the latter hypothesis is the observation that DA agonists increase dream bizarreness, vivacity, complexity, and emotionality without having any commensurate effects on REM sleep [102]. DA agonists, of course, also provoke other psychotic symptoms. Systematic studies of the effects on dreaming of DA antagonists have not yet been performed. However a preliminary study by Yu (unpublished observation) concerning the effects on dreaming of antipsychotic medications found significant dream-suppressing effects.

Also incompatible with the view that dreaming and REM sleep are generated by the same pontine mechanisms is the accumulating evidence to the effect that 5-HT agonists (selective serotonin reuptake inhibitors, SSRIs), like anticholinergics, have the opposite effect to what the REM-dreaming hypothesis would have predicted. As already noted, SSRIs suppress REM sleep but produce excesses of dreaming, of both types described above [79–85].

The available pharmacological evidence therefore supports the view that dreaming—like other forms of psychosis—is primarily generated by (demodulated) DA mechanisms rather than ACh ones [146]. The role of reward processing in the "drug dreams" of addicts in withdrawal and remission, as it relates to mesocortical–mesolimbic DA activation, has recently been used to further elucidate the dream process [147]. It is likely that interactions between DA and other neurotransmitter systems also affect dreaming, since enhanced dreaming has been shown in populations receiving noradrenergic beta-blockers [148]. However the neurochemical basis of dreaming is likely to be far more complex than demodulated DA activation, the partial conclusion that the limited current evidence reasonably allows.

Reward and motivational processes during sleep and dreaming

DA circuitry is central to reward processing. The mesocortical–mesolimbic DA system is defined as the "system [that] is formed by dopamine neurons located in the ventral tegmental area … which project to the nucleus accumbens, prefrontal cortex, septum, amygdala, and hippocampus" [139]. This system, termed the SEEKING system by Panksepp, is thought to "drive and energize many mental complexities that humans experience as persistent feelings of interest, curiosity, sensation seeking" ([149], p. 145). It is also involved in reward processing, which refers to "an instinctual affective and exploratory drive to seek biologically-important stimuli in the external or internal ('intrapsychic') environment" ([150], p. 1936).

Perogamvros and Schwartz [150] have proposed the reward activation model (RAM) of dreaming, which postulates that reward processing during sleep may contribute to the consolidation of memories with a high motivational/emotional relevance, and to the modulation of REM sleep through projections to REM generating brainstem structures. Owing to the strong interconnections between the hippocampus and the VTA, RAM proposes that activation of the hippocampus during sleep may stimulate the VTA and lead to reward activation; in turn, VTA activity can lead to the reactivation of certain memories in the hippocampus. It is thought that during SWS in particular, the reactivation of the ventral striatum and the hippocampal complex allows for consolidation of "memory–reward associations" [151]. Thereby—as originally proposed by Freud—"the fabric of the dream-thoughts is resolved into its raw material" ([135], p. 543).

In support of motivational theories of dreaming are studies of addiction, which has been associated with dysregulation in this (mesocortical) dopamine system. [152]. It is common for abstinent drug addicts to have dreams related to finding and taking drugs, a phenomenon that Johnson [153] first termed "drug dreams" (see above). As many as 80% of acutely abstinent drug addicts experience such dreams related to drug craving [147,154–157]. Drug craving can be triggered by cues related to drug taking, both conscious and unconscious [158]. These types of drug-related cues have also been shown to be associated with the subsequent occurrence of drug dreams [159,160]. In the absence of drug-related cues, drug dreams tend to dissipate [147]. Drug dreams persist in addicts undergoing pharmacological treatment during abstinence, such as methadone treatment in heroin addicts [161] and nicotine gum in smokers [156] (indicating that drug dreams do not merely result from physical withdrawal, but rather are a psychological withdrawal symptom) [162]. Furthermore, up-regulation of the mesocortical–mesolimbic dopamine system—as measured indirectly by the Limbic System Activity Scale—has been associated with drug dreams [163]. This association with up-regulation of the system provides further evidence for this DA system's role in the motivational aspects of dream genesis [147]. This line of research has been used to argue that not only is the DA system involved in dream genesis, but also the content of drug dreams favors motivational theories of dreaming [153,164].

Conclusion

Despite the minimal attention that physicians typically pay to dreams, their assessment can be of diagnostic interest, as well as having prognostic and management implications. Dreams can also be a major source of distress to patients. There is every reason to expect that systematic studies of clinical dream phenomena will continue to provide valuable new insights into the functions and malfunctions of the human brain and mind. The extension of our understanding of dreams to healthy populations by means of contemporary neuroscientific research methods has been extremely valuable in furthering our knowledge of the dream process. Consistencies in certain neurophysiological models of dreaming in these two populations are providing the field with sound theoretical departures from which the dream process can be better understood.

References

1. Aserinsky E, Kleitman N. Regularly occurring periods of eye motility and concurrent phenomena during sleep. Science, 1953;118:273–4.
2. Aserinsky E, Kleitman N. Two types of ocular motility during sleep. J Appl Physiol 1955;8:1–10.
3. Dement W, Kleitman N. Cyclic variations in EEG during sleep and their relation to eye movements, bodily motility and dreaming. Electroencephalogr Clin Neurophysiol 1957;9:673–90.
4. Dement W, Kleitman N. The relation of eye movements during sleep to dream activity: an objective method for the study of dreaming. J Exp Psychol 1957;53:89–97.
5. Hobson JA, McCarley R. The brain as a dream-state generator: an activation–synthesis hypothesis of the dream process. Am J Psychiatry 1977;134:1335–48.
6. Solms M. Dreaming and REM sleep are controlled by different brain mechanisms. Behav Brain Sci 2000;23:843–50.
7. Cathala H, Laffont F, Siksou M, et al. Sommeil et rêve chez des patients de lesions parietals et frontales [Sleep and dreams in patients with parietal and frontal lesions]. Rev Neurol (Paris) 1983;139:497–508.
8. Murri L, Arena R, Siciliano G, et al. Dream recall in patients with focal cerebral lesions. Arch Neurol 1984;41:183–5.
9. Murri L, Massetani R, Siciliano G, Arena R. Dream recall after sleep interruption in brain-injured patients. Sleep 1985;8:356–62.
10. Doricchi F, Violani C. Dream recall in brain-damaged patients. A contribution to the neuropsychology of dreaming through a review of the literature. In: Antrobus J, Bertini M, eds. The neuropsychology of sleep and dreaming. Hillsdale, NJ: Lawrence Erlbaum Associates, 1992: pp. 99–140.
11. Solms M. Anoneira and the neuropsychology of dreams. Doctoral dissertation, University of the Witwatersrand, Johannesburg, 1991.
12. Solms M. The neuropsychology of dreams: a clinico-anatomical study. Hillsdale, NJ: Lawrence Erlbaum Associates, 1997.
13. Pace-Schott EF, Hobson JA. Review of Mark Solms (1997), The neuropsychology of dreams: a clinico-anatomical study. Trends Cogn Sci 1998;2:199–200.
14. Hobson JA. The dream drugstore: chemically altered states of consciousness. Cambridge, MA: MIT Press, 2001.
15. Charcot J-M. Un cas de suppression brusque et isolée de la vision mentale des signes et des objets, (formes et couleurs). Progrès Médical 1883;11:568–71.
16. Charcot J-M. Clinical lectures on diseases of the nervous system, Vol. 3. (Savill T, trans.). London: The New Sydenham Society, 1889. (Original work published 1883).
17. Wilbrand H. Die Seelenblindheit als Herderscheinung und ihre Beziehung zur Alexie und Agraphie. Wiesbaden: Bergmann, 1887.
18. Wilbrand H. Ein Fall von Seelenblindheit und Hemianopsie mit Sectionsbefund. Dtsch Z Nervenheilkd 1892;2:361–87.
19. Pötzl O. Die Aphasielehre vom Standpunkt der klinischen Psychiatrie, I: Die optisch-agnostischen Storungen (die verschiedenen Formen der Seelenblindheit). Leipzig: Deuticke, 1928.

20. Nielsen J. Agnosia, apraxia, aphasia: their value in cerebral localization, 2nd ed. New York: Hoeber, 1946.
21. Critchley M. The parietal lobes. London: Edward Arnold, 1953.
22. Munk H. Weitere Mittheilungen zur Physiologie des Grosshirnrinde. Arch Anat Physiol 1878;2:161–78.
23. Lissauer H. Ein Fall von Seelenblindheit nebst einen Beitrage zur Theorie derselben. Archiv Psychiatrie, 1890;21:222–70.
24. Solms M, Kaplan-Solms K, Brown, J. Wilbrand's case of "mind-blindness." In: Code C, Wallesch C-W, Joanette Y, Lecours A-R, eds. Classic cases in neuropsychology. Hove, England: Psychology Press, 1996: pp. 89–110.
25. Farah M, Levine D, Calvanio D. A case study of mental imagery deficit. Brain Cogn 1988;8:147–64.
26. Gloning K, Sternbach I. Über das Träumen bei zerebralen Herdläsionen. Wien Z Nervenheilkd 1953;6:302–29.
27. Adler A. Disintegration and restoration of optic recognition in visual agnosia: analysis of a case. Arch Neurol Psychiatry 1944;51:243–59.
28. Adler A. Course and outcome of visual agnosia. J Nerv Ment Dis 1950;111:41–51.
29. Botez M, Olvier M, Vézina J-L, et al. Defective revisualization: dissociation between cognitive and imagistic thought. Case report and short review of the literature. Cortex 1985;21:375–89.
30. Brain R. The cerebral basis of consciousness. Brain 1950;73:465–79.
31. Brain R. Loss of visualization. Proc R Soc Med 1954;47:288–90.
32. Brown JW. Aphasia, apraxia, agnosia: clinical and theoretical aspects. Springfield, IL: Thomas, 1972.
33. Efron R. What is perception? Boston studies in the philosophy of science. New York: Basic Books, 1968.
34. Kerr N, Foulkes D, Jurkovic G. Reported absence of visual dream imagery in a normally sighted subject with Turner's syndrome. J Ment Imagery 1978;2:247–64.
35. Macrae D, Trolle E. The defect of function in visual agnosia. Brain 1956;79:94–110.
36. Sacks, O. The man who mistook his wife for a hat. London: Duckworth, 1985.
37. Sacks O. Neurological dreams. MD 1991;February:29–32.
38. Sacks O. An anthropologist from Mars. London: Picador, 1995.
39. Sacks O, Wasserman R. The case of the colorblind painter. New York Review of Books 1987;34(18):25–34.
40. Sparr S, Jay M, Drislane F, Venna N. A historic case of visual agnosia. Revisited after 40 years. Brain 1991;114:789–900.
41. Tzavaras A. Contribution á l'étude de l'agnosie des physiognomies. Unpublished doctoral dissertation, Faculté de Médecine de Université de Paris, 1967.
42. Saurat M, Agbakou M, Attigui P, et al. Walking dreams in congenital and acquired paraplegia. Conscious Cogn 2011;20:1425–32.
43. Badenhorst T, Solms, M. Dreaming and the dorsolateral frontal lobes. MA research psychology dissertation, University of Cape Town, 2006.
44. Bischof M, Bassetti CL. Total dream loss: a distinct neuropsychological dysfunction after bilateral PCA stroke. Ann Neurol 2004;56:583–6.
45. Poza J, Marti J. Total dream loss secondary to left temporo-occipital brain injury. Neurologia 2006;21:152–4.
46. Hattingh C, Cameron-Dow C, Marchbank G, Solms, M. Cessation of dreaming after posterior cerebral artery infarction. (In preparation.)
47. Yu C. Neuroanatomical correlates of dreaming: The supramarginal gyrus controversy (dream work). Neuro-Psychoanalysis 2001;30:47–59.
48. Feinberg I. REM sleep: desperately seeking isomorphism. Behav Brain Sci 2000;23:931.
49. LaBerge S. Lucid dreaming: evidence and methodology. Behav Brain Sci 2000;23:962–4.
50. Ogilvie RD, Takeuchi T, Murphy TI. Expanding Nielsen's covert REM model, questioning Solm's approach to dreaming and REM sleep, and re-interpreting the Vertes & Eastman view of REM sleep and memory. Behav Brain Sci 2000;23,981–3.
51. Ananev B. Psixologija cuvstvennogo poznanija [The psychology of learning through experience]. Moscow: Academy of Pedagogical Science, 1960.
52. Jakobson R. Towards a linguistic classification of aphasic impairments. In: Goodglass H, Blumstein S, eds. Psycholinguistics & aphasia. Baltimore: Johns Hopkins University Press, 1973: pp. 29–47.
53. Moss CS. Recovery with aphasia: the aftermath of my stroke. Urbana: University of Illinois Press, 1972.
54. Zinkin, N. Psixologiceskaja nauka vSSSR [Psychological science in the USSR]. Moscow: Academy of Pedagogical Science, 1959.
55. Michel F, Sieroff E. Une approche anatomo-clinique des deficits de l'imagerie oneirique, est-elle possible? In: Sleep: proceedings of an international colloquium. Milan: Carlo Erba Formitala, 1981.
56. Schanfald D, Pearlman C, Greenberg R. The capacity of stroke patients to report dreams. Cortex 1985;21:237–47.
57. Stickgold R, Malia A, Maguire D. et al. Replaying the game: hypnagogic images in normals and amnesics. Science 2000;90, 350–3.
58. Torda, C. Dreams of subjects with loss of memory for recent years. Psychophysiology 1969;6:358–65.
59. Corkin S. Permanent present tense. New York: Basic Books, 2013.
60. Frank J. Clinical survey and results of 200 cases of prefrontal leucotomy. J Ment Sci 1946;92:497–508.
61. Frank J. Some aspects of lobotomy (prefrontal leucotomy) under psychoanalytic scrutiny. Psychiatry 1950;13:35–42.
62. Jus A, Jus K, Villeneuve A, et al. Studies on dream recall in chronic schizophrenic patients after prefrontal lobotomy. Biol Psychiatry 1973;6:275–93.
63. Partridge M. Pre-frontal leucotomy: a survey of 300 cases personally followed for 1½–3 years. Oxford: Blackwell, 1950.
64. Piehler R. Über das Traumleben leukotomierter (Vorläufige Mitteilung) [On the dream-life of the leukotomized (preliminary communication)]. Nervenärzt 1950;21:517–21.
65. Schindler R. Das Traumleben der Leukomierten. Wien Z Nervenheilkd 1953;6:330.
66. Humphrey M, Zangwill O. Cessation of dreaming after brain injury. J Neurol Neurosurg Psychiatry 1951;14, 322–5.
67. Walsh K. Neuropsychology: a clinical approach, 3rd ed. Edinburgh: Churchill Livingstone, 1994.
68. Damasio H, Damasio A. Lesion analysis in neuropsychology. New York: Oxford University Press, 1989.
69. Yu C. Neuroanatomical correlates of dreaming. II: the ventromesial frontal region controversy (dream investigation). Neuro-Psychoanalysis 2001;30:193–201.
70. Kapur S. Psychosis as a state of aberrant salience: a framework linking biology, phenomenology, and pharmacology in schizophrenia. Am J Psychiatry 2003;160:13–23.
71. Leu-Semenescu S, Uguccioni G, Golmard, J-L, et al. Can we still dream when the mind is blank? Sleep and dream mentations in auto-activation deficit. Brain 2013;136:3076–84.
72. Hobson JA, McCarley RW, Wyzinki PW. Sleep cycle oscillation: reciprocal discharge by two brainstem neuronal groups. Science 1975;189:55–8.
73. Hobson JA, Lydic R, Baghdoyan H. Evolving concepts of sleep cycle generation: from brain centers to neuronal populations. Behav Brain Sci 1986;9:371–400.
74. Feldman M. Physiological observations in a chronic case of "locked-in" syndrome. Neurology 1971;21:459–78.
75. Lavie P, Pratt H, Scharf B, et al. Localized pontine lesion: nearly total absence of REM sleep. Neurology 1984;34:118–120.
76. Markand O, Dyken M. Sleep abnormalities in patients with brain stem lesions. Neurology 1976;26:769–76.
77. Osorio L, Daroff R. Absence of REM and altered NREM sleep in patients with spino-cerebellar degeneration and slow saccades. Ann Neurol 1980;7:277–80.
78. Oudiette, D, Dealberto MJ, Uguccioni G, et al. Dreaming without REM sleep. Conscious Cogn 2012;21:1129–40.
79. Armitage R, Rochlen A., Fitch T, et al. Dream recall and major depression: a preliminary report. Dreaming 1995:5:189–98.

80. Koponen H, Lepola U, Leiononen E, et al. Citalopram in the treatment of obsessive–compulsive disorder: an open pilot study. Acta Psychiatr Scand 2000;96:343–346.

81. Lepkifker E, Dannon PN, Iancu I, et al. Nightmares related to fluoxetine treatment. Clin Neuropharmacol 1995;18:90–4.

82. Markowitz J. Fluoxetine and dreaming. J Clin Psychiatry 1991;52:432.

83. Pace-Schott EF, Hobson JA, Stickgold R. The fluoxetine-mediated increase in NREM eye movements can be detected in the home setting using the Nightcap. Sleep Res 1994;23:459.

84. Pace-Schott EF, Gersh T, Silvestri R, et al. Enhancement of subjective intensity of dream features in normal subjects by the SSRIs paroxetine and fluvoxamine. Sleep 2000;23(Suppl):A173–4.

85. Pace-Schott EF, Gersh T, Silvestri R, et al. SSRI treatment suppresses dream recall frequency but increases subjective dream intensity in normal subjects. J Sleep Res 2001;10:129–42.

86. Nielsen TA. A review of mentation in REM and NREM sleep: "covert" REM sleep as a possible reconciliation of two opposing models. Behav Brain Sci 2000;23:851–66.

87. Braun AR, Balkin TJ, Wesenten NJ, et al. Regional cerebral blood flow throughout the sleep–wake cycle. An $H_2^{15}O$ PET study. Brain 1997;120:1173–97.

88. Maquet P, Péters J, Aerts J, et al. Functional neuroanatomy of human rapid-eye-movement sleep and dreaming. Nature 1996;383:163–6.

89. Nofzinger EA, Mintun MA, Wiseman M, et al. Forebrain activation in REM sleep: an FDG PET study. Brain Res 1997;770:192–201.

90. Braun AR, Balkin TJ, Wesensten NJ, et al. Dissociated pattern of activity in visual cortices and their projections during human rapid eye movement sleep. Science 1998;279:91–5.

91. Eichenlaub JB, Nicolas A, Daltrozzo J, et al. Resting brain activity varies with dream recall frequency between subjects. Neuropsychopharmacology 2014;39:1594–602.

92. Koulack D, Goodenough DR. Dream recall and dream recall failure: an arousal–retrieval model. Psychol Bull 1976;83:975.

93. Eichenlaub JB, Bertrand O, Morlet D, Ruby P. Brain reactivity differentiates subjects with high and low dream recall frequencies during both sleep and wakefulness. Cereb Cortex 2014;24:1206–15.

94. Eichenlaub J, Ruby P, Morlet D. What is the specificity of the response to the own first-name when presented as a novel in a passive oddball paradigm? An ERP study. Brain Res 2012;1447:65–78.

95. Holeckova I, Fischer C, Giard M, et al. Brain responses to a subject's own name uttered by a familiar voice. Brain Res 2006;1082:142–52.

96. Kissler J, Herbert C, Winkler I, Junghofer M. Emotion and attention in visual word processing—an ERP study. Biol Psychol 2009;80:75–83.

97. Jakobson AJ, Fitzgerald PB, Conduit R. Induction of visual dream reports after transcranial direct current stimulation (tDCS) during stage 2 sleep. J Sleep Res 2012;21:369–79.

98. Jakobson AJ, Conduit R, Fitzgerald PB. Investigation of visual dream reports after transcranial direct current stimulation (tDCS) during REM sleep. Int J Dream Res 2012;5:87–93.

99. Massimini M, Ferrarelli F, Huber R, et al. Breakdown of cortical effective connectivity during sleep. Science 2005;309:2228–32.

100. Horikawa T, Tamaki M, Miyawaki Y, Kamitani Y. Neural decoding of visual imagery during sleep. Science 2013;340:639–42.

101. Moscovitz C, Moses, H, Klawans H. Levodopa-induced psychosis: a kindling phenomenon. Am J Psychiatry 1978;135:669–75.

102. Hartmann E, Russ D, Oldfield M, et al. Dream content: effects of L-DOPA. Sleep Res 1980;9:153.

103. French Clozapine Parkinson Study Group. Clozapine in drug-induced psychosis in Parkinson's disease. Lancet 1999;353:2041–2.

104. Fenelon G, Mahieux F, Huon R, Ziegler M. Hallucinations in Parkinson's disease: prevalence, phenomenology and risk factors. Brain 2000;123:733–45.

105. Williams D, Lees A. Visual hallucinations in the diagnosis of idiopathic Parkinson's disease: a retrospective autopsy study. Lancet Neurol 2005;4:605–10.

106. Bassetti C. Narcolepsy: selective hypocretin (orexin) neuronal loss and multiple signalling deficiencies. Neurology 2005;65:1152–3.

107. Arnulf I, Zeitzer J, File J, et al. Kleine–Levin syndrome: a systematic review of 186 cases in the literature. Brain 2005;128:2763–76.

108. Montagna P. Fatal familial insomnia: a model disease in sleep physiopathology. Sleep Med Rev 2005;9:339–53.

109. Landolt H, Glatzel M, Blatter T, et al. Sleep–wake disturbances in sporadic Creutzfeldt–Jakob disease. Neurology 2006;66:1418–24.

110. Rebocho SB. Hiperonirismo ea microestrutura do sono: análise de microdespertares, movimentos oculares rápidos, sono alfa-delta e movimentos periódicos do sono. Dissertation, University of Lisbon, 2010.

111. Silvestri R, Bromfield E. Recurrent nightmares and disorders of arousal in temporal lobe epilepsy. Brain Res Bull 2004;63:369–76.

112. Vercueil L. Dreaming of seizures. Epilepsy Behav 2005;7:127–8.

113. Reami D, Silva D, Albuquerque M, Campos C. Dreams and epilepsy. Epilepsia 1991;32:51–3.

114. Penfield W. The cerebral cortex in man: I. The cerebral cortex and consciousness. Arch Neurol Psychiatry 1938;40:417–42.

115. Penfield W, Erickson T. Epilepsy and cerebral localization. Springfield, IL: Thomas, 1941.

116. Penfield W, Rasmussen T. The cerebral cortex of man. New York: MacMillan, 1955.

117. Gastaut H, Broughton R. A clinical and polygraphic study of episodic phenomena during sleep. Biol Psychiatry 1965;7:197–221.

118. Jacobson A, Kales A, Lehmann D, Zweizig J. Somnambulism: all-night electroencephalographic studies. Science 1965;148:975–7.

119. Fisher C, Kahn E, Edwards A, et al. A psychophysiological study of nightmares and night terrors: III. Mental content and recall of stage 4 night terrors. J Nerv Ment Dis 1974;158:174–88.

120. Jouvet M, Michel F. Release of the "paradoxical phase" of sleep by stimulation of the brainstem in the intact and chronic mesencephalic cat. C R Hebd Seances Acad Sci 1960;154:636–41.

121. Olsen E, Boeve B, Silber M. Rapid eye movement sleep behaviour disorder: demographic, clinical and laboratory findings in 93 cases. Brain 2000;123:331–9.

122. Eisensehr I, Linke R, Noachtar S, et al. Reduced striatal dopamine transporters in idiopathic rapid eye movement sleep behaviour disorder: comparison with Parkinson's disease and controls. Brain 2000;123:1155–60.

123. Eisensehr I, Linke R, Tatsch K, et al. Increased muscle activity during rapid eye movement sleep correlates with decrease of striatal presynaptic dopamine transporters: IPT and IBZM SPECT in subclinical and clinically manifest idiopathic REM sleep behaviour disorder, Parkinson's disease and controls. Sleep 2003;26:507–12.

124. Fantini M, Gagnon J, Petit D, et al. Slowing of electroencephalogram in rapid eye movement sleep behaviour disorder. Ann Neurol 2003;53:774–80.

125. Ferrini-Strambi L, Di Gioia M, Castronovo V, et al. Neuropsychological assessment in idiopathic REM sleep behaviour disorder (RBD): does the idiopathic form of RBD really exist? Neurology 2004;62:41–5.

126. Marion M, Qurashi M, Marshall G, Foster O. Is REM sleep behaviour disorder (RBD) a risk factor of dementia in idiopathic Parkinson's disease? J Neurol 2008;255:192–6.

127. Vendette M, Gagnon J, Décary A, et al. REM sleep behavior disorder predicts cognitive impairment in Parkinson disease without dementia. Neurology 2007;69:1843–9.

128. Boeve B, Silber M, Ferman T, et al. REM sleep behaviour disorder and degenerative dementia: an association likely reflecting Lewy body disease. Neurology 1998;51:363–70.

129. Comella C, Nardine T, Diederich N, Stebbins G. Sleep-related violence, injury and REM sleep behaviour disorder in Parkinson's disease. Neurology 1998;51:526–9.

130. Gagnon J, Bedard M, Fantini M, et al. REM sleep behaviour disorder and REM sleep without atonia in Parkinson's disease. Neurology 2002;59:585–9.

131. Plazzi G, Cortelli P, Montagna P, et al. REM sleep behavior disorder differentiates pure autonomic failure from multiple systems atrophy with autonomic failure. J Neurol Neurosurg Psychiatry 1998;64:683–5.

132. Scaglione C, Vignatelli L, Plazzi G, et al. REM sleep behaviour disorder in Parkinson's disease: a questionnaire based study. Neurol Sci 2005;25:316–21.

133. Schenck C, Bundlie S, Mahowald M. Delayed emergence of a Parkinsonian disorder in 38% of 29 older men initially diagnosed with idiopathic rapid eye movement sleep behaviour disorder. Neurology 1996;46:388–93.

134. Iranzo A, Molinuevo J, Santamaría J, et al. Rapid-eye-movement sleep behaviour disorder as an early marker for a neurodegenerative disorder: a descriptive study. Lancet Neurol 2006;5:572–7.

135. Freud S. The interpretation of dreams. Standard edition. London: Hogarth, 1900: vols. 4–5.

136. Hobson JA, Pace-Schott EF, Stickgold R. Consciousness: its vicissitudes in waking and sleep—an integration of recent neurophysiological and neuropsychological evidence. In: Gazzangia M, ed. The new cognitive neurosciences, 2nd ed. MIT Press, 2000.

137. Miller JD, Farber J, Gatz P, et al. Activity of mesencephalic dopamine and non-dopamine neurons across stages of sleep and waking in the rat. Brain Res 1983;273:133–41.

138. Trulson ME, Preussler DW. Dopamine-containing ventral tegmental area neurons in freely moving cats: activity during the sleep–waking cycle and effects of stress. Exp Neurol 1984;83:367–77.

139. Dahan L, Astier B, Vautrelle N, et al. Prominent burst firing of dopaminergic neurons in the ventral tegmental area during paradoxical sleep. Neuropsychopharmacology 2007;32:1232–41.

140. Lena I, Muffat S, Deschaux O, et al. Dreaming and schizophrenia have the same neurochemical background. J Sleep Res 2004;13(Suppl 1):141.

141. Gottesmann C. Brain inhibitory mechanisms involved in basic and higher integrated sleep processes. Brain Res Rev 2004;45:230–49.

142. Silbersweig D, Stern E, Frith C, et al. A functional neuroanatomy of hallucinations in schizophrenia. Nature 1995;378:176–9.

143. Cartwright RD. Dream and drug-induced fantasy behavior. A comparative study. Arch Gen Psychiatry 1966;15:7–15.

144. Damasio A, Graff-Radford N, Eslinger P, et al. Amnesia following basal forebrain lesions. Arch Neurol 1985;42:263–71.

145. Braun AR. The new neuropsychology of sleep. Neuro-Psychoanalysis 1999;1:196–201.

146. Solms M. The neurochemistry of dreaming: cholinergic and dopaminergic hypotheses. In: Perry E, Ashton H, Young A, eds. The neurochemistry of consciousness. Amsterdam: John Benjamins Publishing 2002: pp. 123–31.

147. Colace C. Drug dreams: clinical and research implications of dreams about drugs in drug-addicted patients. London: Karnac Books, 2014.

148. Thompson DF, Pierce DR. Drug-induced nightmares. Ann Pharmacother 1999;33:93–8.

149. Panksepp J. Affective neuroscience: the foundations of human and animal emotions. Oxford: Oxford University Press, 1998.

150. Perogamvros L, Schwartz S. The roles of the reward system in sleep and dreaming. Neurosci Biobehav Rev 2012;36:1934–51.

151. Lansink CS, Goltstein PM, Lankelma JV, et al. Hippocampus leads ventral striatum in replay of place-reward information. PLoS Biol 2009;7(8): e1000173.

152. Nestler EJ. Is there a common molecular pathway for addiction? Nat Neurosci 2005;8:1445–9.

153. Johnson B. Drug dreams: a neuropsychoanalytic hypothesis. J Am Psychoanal Assoc 2001;49:75–96.

154. Araujo RB, Oliveira M, Piccoloto LB, Szupszynski KP. Dreams and craving in alcohol addicted patients in the detoxication stage. Rev Psiquiatr Clin 2004;31(2):63–9.

155. Choi SY. Dreams as a prognostic factor in alcoholism. Am J Psychiatry 1973;130:699–702.

156. Christo G, Franey C. Addicts drug-related dreams: their frequency and relationship to six-month outcomes. Subst Use Misuse 1996;31:1–15.

157. Fiss H. Dream content and response to withdrawal from alcohol. Sleep Res 1980;9:152.

158. Childress AR, Ehrman RN, Wang Z, et al. Prelude to passion: limbic activation by "unseen" drug and sexual cues. PLoS One 2008;3(1):e1506.

159. Christensen RL. A multi-level analysis of attentional biases in abstinent and non-abstinent problem drinkers. Dissertation. Florida State University College of Arts and Sciences, 2009.

160. Yee T, Perantie DC, Dhanani N, Brown ES. Drug dreams in outpatients with bipolar disorder and cocaine dependence. J Nerv Ment Dis 2004;192:238–42.

161. Colace C. Drug dreams in mescaline and LSD addiction. Am J Addictions 2010;19:192.

162. Hajek P, Belcher M. Dream of absent-minded transgression: an empirical study of a cognitive withdrawal symptom. J Abnorm Psychol 1991;100:487.

163. Colace C, Claps M, Antognoli A, et al. Limbic system activity and drug dreaming in drug-addicted subjects. Neuro-psychoanalysis 2010;12:201–6.

164. Colace C. Dreaming in addiction: a study on the motivational bases of dreaming processes. Neuro-psychoanalysis, 2004;6;165–79.

CHAPTER 35

Neurological diseases and their effects on the sleep–wake cycle

Paul J. Reading

Introduction

Although the precise reasons why every organism with a brain has an absolute need for sleep are hotly debated, there remains no doubt about the importance of sustained good-quality sleep for optimal cerebral function and mental health. Similarly, it is recognized that virtually every pathological process involving the brain has the potential to adversely affect the sleep–wake cycle, with increasingly defined cognitive and neuropsychiatric consequences. Of note, accumulating evidence from a variety of sources also suggests that a prolonged abnormal sleep–wake cycle may actually fuel irreversible cerebral pathology, particularly in an aging brain that is already at risk of neurodegenerative disease [1,2]. It is therefore imperative that neurologists managing both common and rare brain diseases should have a working knowledge of sleep neurobiology and the main manifestations of identifiable sleep disorders that associate with neurological disease. Although evidence-based treatment pathways for sleep-related symptoms remain relatively poorly defined, improvement of the sleep–wake cycle in affected neurological subjects is likely to have immediate as well as potential long-term benefits.

If the neurological importance of an abnormal sleep–wake cycle is accepted, it is disappointing that exposure to the principles of sleep medicine remains limited in many neurology training programs. This chapter attempts to address the definition of abnormal sleep patterns in neurological disease given our current knowledge of the underlying neurobiological processes. Although clinico-pathological correlations are often speculative, particularly in multisystem neurodegenerative diseases, it will be emphasized that recognizing an abnormal sleep–wake cycle may have important implications for treatment strategies and even provide important diagnostic clues. Furthermore, any improvement in sleep-related symptoms may well have a positive impact on the underlying neurological disorder itself, particularly in progressive disease.

If studied systematically, the effects of normal aging on the sleep–wake cycle are profound, although the underlying neuroanatomical basis for the changes remains largely undefined. These age-related effects will be covered before exploring how the main sleep-related symptoms of insomnia, hypersomnia, and the consequences of abnormal clock mechanisms potentially relate to defined neurological disease. A summary of the main sleep-related symptoms and their relation to neurological disorders is given in Table 35.1.

A variety of neuromuscular diseases have the potential to cause significant adverse effects on breathing, specifically during sleep.

Typically, these involve nocturnal hypoventilation related to respiratory muscle weakness or apnea from upper airway obstruction secondary to palatal or bulbar involvement. This potentially extremely important but indirect consequence of neuromuscular disease on the sleep–wake cycle will not be addressed in detail here.

A brief neuroanatomy of sleep

It is increasingly clear that normal overnight sleep architecture is highly orchestrated. Moreover, the state of sleep should be considered an active process, contingent on neural activity in several key areas, rather than resulting simply from cortical inactivity or the absence of wakefulness [3]. Traditionally, the wakeful or conscious state is considered to be mediated by an ascending arousal system comprising several pathways that course through the brainstem and innervate the cortex in a widespread and relatively nonspecific distribution. There appears to be significant redundancy in the "wake system" such that specific lesions to one area or a single neurochemical system have little observable effects. The key neurochemical components of the ascending reticular system are noradrenergic and serotonergic, comprising a ventral branch, with an additional important dorsal branch that is cholinergic [4]. This latter pathway comprises thalamic projections from predominantly cholinergic areas in the dorsal pons such as the pedunculopontine nucleus, thereby providing an indirect thalamocortical activating input to the cortical mantle. Other important cortical wake "signals" arise from the cholinergic nuclei in the basal forebrain and also from the histaminergic tuberomammillary nucleus (TMN) in the posterior hypothalamus. The precise role of dopamine in generating conscious awareness remains obscure, especially as it has been difficult to demonstrate clear diurnal variation in dopaminergic neuronal activity across the sleep–wake cycle [5]. Furthermore, cortical dopaminergic projections are limited to prefrontal areas and have been presumed to play little overall role in generating alertness. However, the observation that most stimulant drugs are highly dependent on a dopaminergic mechanism of action suggests that dopamine does play a key role, perhaps via a thalamic pathway as with the dorsal cholinergic arousal system [6].

The assumption that a wakeful or conscious brain will always show observable signs of reaction to external stimuli has been challenged by recent functional imaging studies [7]. In a proportion of unfortunate patients exhibiting a persistent vegetative state, often for many years, specific cerebral responses to verbal commands and imagined scenarios have provided convincing evidence of

Table 35.1 Table listing the main sleep-related symptoms and their possible association with defined neurological conditions

Predominant sleep complaint	Associated neurological condition	Proposed pathological correlate or mechanism
Sleep-onset insomnia	Subcortical cerebrovascular disease	Anterior thalamic ischemic change
	Prion disorders, particularly fatal familial insomnia	Thalamic prion pathology at early stage of disease
	Autoimmune or paraneoplastic encephalitides	Autoantibodies (eg, against voltage-gated potassium channels) disrupt thalamocortical generation of EEG sleep oscillations
	Restless legs syndrome and neuropathic pain	Peripheral neuropathies and central inflammatory disease (eg, multiple sclerosis) increase chances of developing symptoms
Sleep-maintenance insomnia	Most neurodegenerative conditions, particularly Alzheimer disease	Increased cortical thinning, particularly medial prefrontal cortex; hypothalamic pathology (particularly SCN)
	Restless legs syndrome and neuropathic pain	Peripheral neuropathies and central inflammatory disease (eg, multiple sclerosis) increase chances of developing symptoms
Excessive daytime sleepiness	Most neurodegenerative conditions, particularly parkinsonian syndromes	Damage to ascending reticular activating systems; hypothalamic pathology
	Lesions in or around hypothalamus	Tumors or cysts in third ventricle may damage posterior hypothalamus; inflammatory lesions, particularly in neuromyelitis optica
	Traumatic brain injury	Transient reduced activity in hypocretin system may contribute
	Myotonic dystrophy	Often a central nervous system component after breathing-related problems have been excluded
Circadian dysrhythmia	Most neurodegenerative conditions, particularly Huntington disease and Alzheimer disease	Blunted circadian rhythms due to direct damage to the SCN or its efferent pathways
	Non-24-hour sleep phase syndrome (usually in blind)	Retinohypothalamic tract absent or dysfunctional

comprehension and presumed conscious awareness. It is a worrying thought that there may be subjects who appear entirely "locked in" to outside observers but who retain some degree of cognitive awareness of their surroundings with the potential to respond appropriately to verbal stimuli or questions.

The discovery in 1999 that full-blown narcolepsy with cataplexy is due to a specific deficiency of the neuropeptide hypocretin (also known as orexin) in the posterolateral hypothalamus has greatly furthered our knowledge of how the brain maintains the wakeful state [8–10]. Activity in this small area of the brain numbering around 40 000 neurons is capable of stimulating all the major "alerting" nuclei via its widespread efferent connectivity. Hypocretin appears to stabilize or consolidate wakefulness, potentially inhibiting the natural homeostatic sleep drive that builds exponentially with the passing of time. The neural origin of sleepiness or the drive to sleep remains largely speculative, although a key component is likely to reflect extracellular levels of adenosine in certain important areas such as the basal forebrain [11]. As a breakdown product of general neuronal activity during wakefulness, extracellular adenosine levels rise with time and potentially may trigger sleep onset.

The perception of sleepiness increases exponentially after significant periods of wakefulness and is mostly contingent on the homeostatic sleep drive, termed "process S," although circadian or "clock" factors, process C, have an important interactive influence [12,13]. The field of chronobiology has made enormous advances over the last two decades, particularly at a subcellular level, where the mechanisms of the clock have been thoroughly dissected at a molecular level [14]. It is clear there is very little fundamental difference between fruit flies and primates at the level of protein expression and genetic control. Significant challenges remain in defining how the clock effectively communicates with the organism

and how it can be influenced by internal or external factors. The suprachiasmatic nucleus (SCN) within the hypothalamus has long been considered the "master clock" and is capable of controlling or entraining the vast majority of processes within the body that have a circadian rhythm [15]. Although there are hundreds of output pathways from the SCN, one of the most important for regulation of the sleep–wake cycle is to the neighboring paraventricular nucleus, which ultimately relays to the pineal gland to cause melatonin release via the intermediolateral cell column in the spinal cord [16]. This pathway involves the sympathetic autonomic nervous system and may be blunted by beta-blockade, for example. Melatonin release normally occurs between 1 and 2 hours before sleep and is thought to facilitate the process of sleep onset. This and other important "rhythms" are potentially controlled by external factors or "zeitgebers," the most important of which is light exposure, although daytime physical activity and food availability are also increasingly recognized [17]. The retinohypothalamic tract is a key input to the SCN, and melanopsin-containing photocells within the retina are key to the process of collecting information on levels of daylight, ultimately helping to coordinate circadian timing with the day–night cycle [18].

Defining sleep onset with precision is difficult, although increased activity of neurons containing gamma-aminobutyric acid (GABA) and the neuropeptide galanin in the anterior hypothalamus plays a key role. The ventrolateral preoptic area (VLPO) can be considered a true "sleep center." It interacts with the arousal system by a process of mutual inhibition, allowing sleep to become initially established and then stabilized [19]. The subsequent generation and particularly the so-called "ultradian" regulation of light and deep sleep, characterized primarily by EEG markers of sleep spindles and slow waves in the delta frequency, are only partly understood. Parts of the thalamus, particular the surrounding reticular nuclei, play a key role in the generation of thalamocortical oscillations that ultimately define the stages of non-rapid eye movement (NREM) sleep as defined neurophysiologically [3]. The tendency to enter the deepest stages of NREM (slow-wave) sleep dissipates through the night, although the neurobiological basis of the homeostatic mechanism to regulate and monitor this sleep drive remains obscure [20].

Rapid eye movement (REM) sleep can be considered an enigmatic state of brain arousal that occurs in discrete phases that increase in length through the night, in the absence of conscious awareness. Largely from animal studies, the concept of "REM-on" centers has evolved that negatively interact with "REM-off" centers in a similar fashion to the sleep–wake switch described by Saper and colleagues [21]. Although some form of "sleep mentation" can occur from any stage of sleep, arousals from REM sleep suggest that this state is most often associated with true dreams or nightmares that contain typically bizarre narrative themes, often involving previous fragments of memory [22]. From a neurochemical perspective, REM sleep is associated with activity in the ascending cholinergic system from dorsal pons to thalamus in the complete absence of equivalent activity in the brainstem noradrenergic and serotonergic systems that are normally associated with wakefulness [3]. The neurobiology of REM sleep homeostasis or regulation is largely unknown. However, suppression of REM sleep pharmacologically by tricyclic agents or alcohol, for example, produces a rebound response of earlier and more intense REM sleep on discontinuation [23].

The effects of normal aging on the sleep–wake cycle

Through the lifespan of a normal individual, there are profound and measurable changes in the nature and quality of sleep, particularly the deep NREM phase [24]. Indeed, a diminution of the amplitude of slow (delta) waves in the early part of the night when sleep is at its deepest can be observed even in young men, potentially reflecting one of the earliest biomarkers of aging. It is clear that the depth of slow-wave sleep (SWS) continues to diminish with age as measured by the parameter of slow-wave activity (SWA). Normal aging is also associated with poorer sleep consolidation and an increasing number of spontaneous arousals through the night, not all of which are necessarily registered consciously. Typically, a 70-year-old will sleep for only 85% of the nocturnal sleep period, whereas a younger subject would expect to achieve a figure of well over 90% [25].

As a subject ages, there is also a tendency to awake earlier in the morning in association with an earlier sleep onset time, reflecting a shift of around 30 minutes for every decade of aging. Cultural factors may well play a role but are not considered the key mechanism. It is not clear whether there are true changes in the circadian timing of sleep with age or whether reduced homeostatic regulation is largely responsible for this observation [26].

The neuroanatomical correlates of the observed age-related changes in sleep patterns remain largely speculative. An obvious candidate is the normal and nonspecific process of cortical neuronal pruning that occurs with age, potentially interfering with the generation of thalamocortical oscillations that define SWS. Of interest, this has been proposed to occur even through cortical maturation in adolescence [27]. A recent study provided interesting evidence that the medial prefrontal cortex, an area particularly prone to age-related atrophy, exhibits neuronal loss that correlates

very well with parameters of reduced SWS quality [28]. Of further note, these changes also predicted mnemonic performance and provided some evidence that minimal cognitive changes in normal aging might result from impaired ability to obtain deep SWS.

The strength of circadian influences on sleep almost certainly also diminish with age and the diurnal variation of melatonin levels, for example, are less robust. The neuroanatomical basis of this is not well established in normal aged subjects, but age-related atrophy of the hypothalamus, including the SCN, has been proposed [29].

Insomnia in neurological conditions

Sleep onset insomnia

The inability to fall asleep when it is both appropriate and desired is clearly an extremely common complaint and most commonly associated with psychological states of increased, presumed cortical, arousal. Rarely, however, discrete neurological pathology, particularly in the anterior thalamus, may directly result in an inability to achieve sleep and might be regarded as a cause of "organic insomnia" [30]. This is not surprising, given the key role of the thalamus in the generation of both sleep spindles and slow oscillations of deeper sleep. The condition most strongly associated with intractable sleep onset insomnia, however, is the extremely rare prion disorder, fatal familial insomnia (FFI), in which thalamic pathology is an early and prominent feature [31]. The term "agrypnia" has been used to describe the persistent state of stuporose wakefulness seen in this disorder [32]. It is likely that other more familiar prion disorders such as sporadic Creutzfeldt–Jacob disease (CJD) are also associated with significant insomnia and sleep–wake disruption as initial or even prodromal features [33].

Thalamic infarction can certainly cause sleep–wake disturbance as a prominent clinical feature, although pure insomnia is rare. Acute onset of severe insomnia with mania and unilateral dyskinesia has been reported following unilateral thalamic strokes [34].

Generalized encephalopathy in the context of significant head injury or certain inflammatory autoimmune disorders may also produce sleep onset insomnia. Regarding the former, it is difficult to be certain whether associated psychological factors are more important than any specific neural damage. In a prospective study, only 5% of brain trauma subjects developed insomnia on objective testing [35]. It is possible that head-injured patients may have a tendency to overestimate their sleep-related difficulties. Autoimmunity, however, particularly when directed against voltage-gated potassium channels, can cause severe insomnia as part of an encephalitic picture [36]. Agitation, hallucinations, seizures, as well as enhanced peripheral neuromuscular excitability (neuromyotonia) may accompany the lack of ability to sleep. The term Morvan's syndrome is often used, and it is tempting to speculate that potassium channels in the thalamus are sensitive to the presence of antibody as a potential pathogenetic mechanism [37]. More rarely, encephalitis due to antibodies against the N-methyl-D-aspartate (NMDA) receptor may cause a very similar picture with profound insomnia [38].

It might be expected that anterior hypothalamic lesions would cause severe insomnia if the VLPO is damaged. Indeed, it is interesting that von Economo in his original neuropathological observations of encephalitis lethargica noted that a small proportion of patients exhibited severe insomnia if anterior hypothalamic changes predominated [39]. However, it is extremely rare for modern imaging techniques to demonstrate specific hypothalamic pathology in cases of suspected "organic" insomnia.

Restless legs syndrome (RLS) is a relatively common treatable cause of significant sleep onset insomnia and has a variety of potential treatment options [40]. RLS is considerably more prevalent in a number of disorders such as peripheral neuropathy and central inflammatory conditions, notably multiple sclerosis [41]. Unless specifically questioned, this potentially treatable or secondary cause of sleep onset insomnia may be missed or interpreted simply as a (neuropathic) pain symptom.

Sleep maintenance insomnia

Numerous factors associated with neurological disease may interfere with sleep continuity either directly or indirectly, producing poor-quality or unrefreshing sleep with negative consequences on daily functioning. In neurological patients, other than sleep disordered breathing, typical "sleep toxins" include neuropathic pain, nocturia, and either excessive or reduced movements at night, usually in the context of an extrapyramidal movement disorder. Even if full arousals from sleep are not observed, pain, such as that seen in diabetic neuropathy or post-herpetic neuralgia, may alter sleep architecture by increasing the proportion of light NREM sleep compared with deep SWS [42]. Reduction of the latter almost certainly produces sleep that is less restorative.

Many neurodegenerative conditions appear to have direct and adverse effects on the sleep–wake cycle, often producing poor-quality sleep that, at face value, may appear to mimic those of an accelerated aging process [43]. Parkinsonian syndromes, particularly when advanced, are associated with sleep that is generally "destructured," with poor sleep maintenance and an abnormal sleep architecture across the night [44]. These changes are seen early, potentially predating clinical motor disease and can be very significant in advanced cases, almost certainly fuelling daytime somnolence and fluctuating cognitive performance. Although there are well-characterized changes in REM sleep associated with Parkinson disease (PD) and other synucleinopathies such as multiple system atrophy, particularly the lack of REM sleep atonia, these do not necessarily impair subjective sleep quality. Correlating any sleep disturbance in PD with pathology in specific brain regions remains speculative, although REM sleep behavior disorder (RBD) is most likely due to Lewy bodies in key brainstem nuclei involved in producing muscle atonia during REM sleep [45]. These include areas caudal to the locus coeruleus (equivalent to the sublaterodorsal nucleus in the rat) and the pedunculopontine nucleus, brainstem locations known to be vulnerable to Lewy body pathology. From primate PD models, it is likely that dopaminergic depletion also directly impairs the sleep–wake cycle, although dissecting the secondary motor consequences on sleep maintenance from any primary effects on sleep regulation remains difficult. Particularly in advanced cases, it also seems likely that hypothalamic pathology plays an increasing role such that the clinical picture from a sleep perspective may mimic narcolepsy in the degree of sleep–wake disruption and poor control of state switching [46].

Given the widespread nature of pathology in advanced cases of dementia such as Alzheimer disease (AD), it is very difficult to determine specific neural substrates to account for the virtually universal sleep–wake disruption. However, hypothalamic pathology is likely to explain some of the major problems with sleep timing [47,48], whereas general cortical pruning may explain the progressive lack of SWS [28]. Similar profiles of profoundly altered sleep continuity and timing can also be seen in Huntington disease [HD], whereas the evidence for altered circadian control of sleep is even stronger [49].

Hypersomnia in neurological conditions

The term "hypersomnia" is often used loosely and simply interpreted as a synonym for excessive daytime sleepiness (EDS). Strictly, it refers to the situation where the total sleep time over a 24-hour period is at least 2 hours more than might normally be expected. As such, some subjects with a longer sleep need than average who are effectively sleep-restricted by a conventional sleep–wake schedule might be considered to have hypersomnia. In this situation, the diagnosis of idiopathic hypersomnia (IH) can be difficult to determine, although there is increasing evidence that there may be a neurochemical correlate in a proportion of IH subjects, and this finding will improve diagnostic precision and allow more focused treatments [50]. In most neurological conditions, troublesome daytime sleepiness stems from impaired or insufficient nocturnal sleep rather than reflecting a primary increased sleep drive per se, although making this distinction can be very difficult and, clinically, be only of academic interest.

Planned daytime napping is usually perceived as an accepted and common feature of normal aging. However, in the absence of a sleep disorder or a "siesta culture," napping probably relates more to general physical inactivity or even boredom, given the increasing evidence that objective or measurable daytime sleepiness actually declines with normal aging [51]. However, excessive or unplanned napping should not be regarded as normal at any age, particularly in the context of neurodegenerative disease. The causes of EDS in significant dementia, typically AD, are nearly always multifactorial, reflecting sleep–wake dysregulation akin to accelerated aging with behavioral and pharmacological factors playing a significant role. Impaired "clock mechanisms" with respect to both timing and amplitude of the circadian rhythm are almost certainly contributory, partly explaining the reversed sleep–wake cycle and potentially the phenomenon of "sundowning" present in many advanced subjects [52]. Pathological changes in the SCN are well documented in AD, although correlating this with the clinical picture of a disturbed sleep–wake cycle is difficult given the widespread nature of any cerebral pathology.

The sleep–wake disturbance in Lewy body disease, whether Lewy body dementia or advanced PD, is particularly complicated. Pathology in the hypothalamus and brainstem nuclei key to sleep regulation such as the pedunculopontine nucleus and subcoerulean area almost certainly contribute to symptoms of EDS directly and indirectly [53]. Despite the absence of cataplexy, the resemblance to classical narcolepsy can be striking given the nature and degree of EDS together with specific disruption of processes underlying REM sleep regulation [54]. In accordance with this, there is some evidence that partial hypocretin deficiency may be an important factor in generating EDS [55].

The concept of "secondary narcolepsy" is increasingly invoked, particularly when structural or inflammatory pathology involving the (posterior) hypothalamus is proposed to produce significant EDS [56]. A variety of pathologies have been reported, including cysts or tumors in the region of the floor of the third ventricle adjacent to the hypothalamus (Fig. 35.1). The clinical similarity of such

(a)

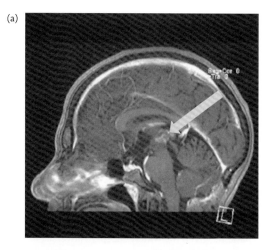

(b)

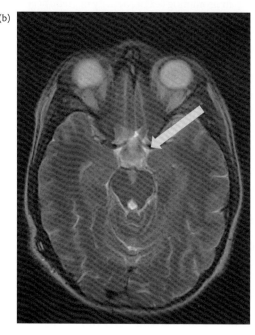

Fig. 35.1 Magnetic resonance imaging brain scans, sagittal (a) and axial (b) views, of a 20-year-old man who developed severe sleepiness resembling a form of narcolepsy after removal of a low-grade tumor (glioma) in the region of the third ventricle. The arrows show abnormal signal indicating postoperative scar tissue (gliosis) predominantly in the posterior hypothalamus.

cases to idiopathic narcolepsy is variable, although some have all the hallmarks of narcolepsy including cataplexy and other REM sleep-related phenomena. For example, inflammatory plaques as a consequence of multiple sclerosis or, more commonly, neuromyelitis optica (NMO), in which there is a predilection for involvement of the hypothalamus, may produce narcoleptic symptomology, occasionally with cataplexy and objective hypocretin deficiency in the cerebrospinal fluid (CSF) [55,56]. Other rarer presumed autoimmune or paraneoplastic conditions with specific antibody markers may also produce recognizable symptom complexes with striking levels of EDS as a main feature. The presence of anti-MA2 antibodies most commonly associated with testicular carcinoma is a well characterized example [57]. Recent post-mortem evidence suggests that this antibody may induce a cytotoxic lymphocytic

response exclusively in the hypothalamus with destruction of hypocretin neurons [58].

True hypersomnia without specific narcoleptic features such as abnormal REM sleep is a recognized consequence of subcortical cerebrovascular disease, particularly in the context of bilateral paramedian thalamic strokes [59]. This may occur with occlusion of the artery of Percheron, an anatomical variant whereby a single trunk from the posterior cerebral artery supplies the mesial aspect of both thalami and the rostral midbrain. The most striking clinical manifestation is profound hypersomnolence and reduced alertness, often with vertical gaze palsy and variable cognitive deficit. Sleep recordings usually demonstrate an abnormal excess of stage 1 sleep with reduced spindle density [60]. Hypersomnia usually improves after a few months despite persistent abnormalities of sleep spindle generation. Recovery is presumed to reflect the integrity and possible adaptation of underlying reticular ascending arousal systems [61].

The effects of traumatic brain injury (TBI) on the sleep–wake cycle have been difficult to elucidate, given the heterogeneous nature of any pathology and the lack of prospective studies addressing sleep in detail. However, the most common significant sleep-related sequela appears to be hypersomnia with increased sleep need over 24 hours seen in over 20% of a nonselected group studied prospectively [62]. Correlations with trauma severity or site of pathological damage have not been established, although transient reduction in CSF hypocretin levels and reduced melatonin rhythms have been proposed as relevant observations in some subjects.

A variety of neuromuscular diseases have the potential to cause significant EDS, which may masquerade clinically as fatigue or lethargy. Most commonly, respiratory or palatal muscle weakness in the context of a progressive myopathic or neuromuscular disorder may fuel sleep disordered breathing as the primary cause of EDS [63]. Indeed, nocturnal hypoventilation with or without obstructive apnea is almost certainly under-diagnosed in progressive conditions such as motor neuron disease. However, other factors, including presumed central nervous system pathology, almost certainly contribute to pathological EDS in certain neuromuscular disorders, notably myotonic dystrophy (MD, types 1 and 2) [64]. MD1, in particular, is associated with increased fatigue and somnolence beyond the potential effects of sleep disordered breathing, including central sleep apnea. In a proportion of subjects, hypocretin deficiency has been documented as a possible underlying mechanism, although this does not appear to be a consistent finding [65]. In MD2, levels of EDS are generally less striking, but a number of sleep-related phenomena such as significant RLS have been identified [66].

Abnormal circadian rhythms in neurological disease

Despite increasing knowledge of the underlying neuroanatomy of central clock mechanisms, identifying or attributing problems of circadian timing to a specific neurological disease or process is difficult. Indeed, with very few exceptions, the underlying pathological processes that might alter a subject's clock to cause a so-called "circadian dysrhythmia" remain obscure. At the subcellular level, genetic factors, including point mutations and polymorphisms of key clock-related genes, are increasingly implicated in abnormal sleep timing in defined sleep disorders, notably, delayed sleep phase syndrome and the far less common condition, advanced sleep phase syndrome

[67]. In neurological disease, however, problems of circadian timing usually stem from a blunted or absent daily rhythm (irregular sleep phase syndrome) or a clock that is not entrained to a 24-hour cycle (non-24-hour sleep phase syndrome) [68,69]. The latter occurs with subjects blind from an early age, typically causing a "free-running" rhythm usually of around 24.4 hours such that the propensity to sleep rarely coincides with a conventional sleep–wake cycle. This lack of light entrainment reflects disruption of the retinohypothalamic tract and may also contribute to sleep-related problems in a variety of conditions associated with acquired severe visual impairment [70]. A totally irregular or chaotic sleep–wake cycle with no discernible rhythm is most often encountered in severe dementia syndromes. Hypothalamic pathology specifically in the region of the SCN is presumed to be the main underlying pathophysiological process [71]. Some patients with frontotemporal dementia (FTD) also exhibit striking abnormalities of the sleep–wake cycle early in the disease course characterized by sleep fragmentation and possible advanced sleep phase syndrome despite normal core body temperature rhythms [72]. This contrasts to the pattern in many subjects with AD, who, if anything, show phase delay [72].

Less striking disruption of circadian rhythms may play an important role in the sleep–wake problems associated with several other neurodegenerative conditions. For example, parkinsonian subjects appear to have blunted melatonin rhythms compared with controls, with particularly severe changes in those patients reporting significant EDS [73,74]. Furthermore, even in newly diagnosed PD patients, reduced circulating melatonin levels and altered clock gene expression have been documented [75]. Given the widespread pathology from retina to cortex in PD, the neuroanatomical basis of any circadian abnormalities remains speculative. In HD and associated animal models, abnormal circadian rhythms may also contribute significantly to sleep-related problems and potentially the cognitive aspects of the disease [76]. As with other neurodegenerative conditions, there is no clear or specific "signature" associated with the sleep disorder in HD, and any problems are typically not readily recognized by the subjects themselves. However, the rest–activity cycles are disrupted in early disease, and biomarkers of clock function are reliably disrupted in mouse animal models [77]. Of interest, in the mouse HD model, pharmacological treatment of the abnormal sleep–wake cycle appeared both to improve performance in cognitive testing and to reverse dysregulation of circadian gene expression [78]. The anatomical basis of clock dysfunction in the HD model is suggested to arise from a dysfunctional output from the central clock, potentially within local circuits, since the subcellular circadian oscillator appears intact [79]. This dysfunctional output from the central clock has interesting peripheral effects, particularly on liver metabolism even though self-sustaining oscillators in liver cells remain intact [80].

Spinal injuries may not be readily associated with altered circadian rhythms, but tetraplegic patients have been shown to have absent melatonin cycles [81]. This reflects disrupted output from the intermediolateral cell column in the upper spinal cord to the superior cervical ganglion, which provides the sympathetic postganglionic output to the pineal gland. This, together with reduced levels of daily physical activity that would be expected in such subjects, potentially contributes significantly to a disturbed sleep–wake cycle.

It is not clear whether other causes of autonomic dysfunction, either in the context of primary disorders such as multiple system atrophy or peripheral neuropathies caused by diabetes, for example, also have blunted melatonin cycles. The few studies that have assessed dysautonomia have focused primarily on the potential adverse effects on nocturnal breathing, including significant central sleep apnea [82,83]. However, it is likely that subjects with primary autonomic failure also have poor sleep efficiency in general and also blunted cardiac responses to any arousals from sleep [84]. The underlying mechanisms causing sleep disruption in such patients remain largely speculative.

Abnormal sleep in epilepsy

A disturbed sleep–wake cycle has particular clinical relevance for epileptic patients, given the widely accepted adverse effects of inadequate sleep in promoting seizure activity in predisposed individuals, particularly in generalized epileptic syndromes [85]. It is well established that certain seizure types are prone to occur at certain times of the day or night. For example, temporal lobe seizures peak in the mid-afternoon both in humans and in rat models [86]. This probably reflects a true circadian effect, given the opposite rest–activity cycles in rodents compared with humans. Frontal lobe seizures are commoner from a state of sleep, particularly the light NREM stage, and myoclonic epilepsies are most noticeable at the sleep–wake transition. Some evidence also suggests that focal epilepsies such as temporal lobe epilepsy may blunt endogenous circadian rhythms, causing reduced melatonin peaks [87] as well as affecting the pulsatile secretion of sex hormones under circadian control [88].

Active epilepsy clearly has the potential for disturbing sleep–wake patterns in a nonspecific manner. Indeed, several studies have commented on the increased incidence of sleep-related symptoms, particularly daytime somnolence, in epileptic populations, with up to twice the level of symptoms [89]. Often, it is assumed that antiepileptic medication is the main culprit, although some evidence suggests that epilepsy itself may disturb sleep quality even during nights that appear seizure-free [90]. Certainly, when nocturnal seizures are recorded early in the night, the subsequent adverse effects on sleep quality through the night are profound, particularly regarding REM sleep [91]. Aside from daytime sleepiness, it is likely that resistant epilepsy might also worsen cognitive functions sensitive to chronic sleep disruption, particularly memory.

Coexisting sleep disorders such as sleep apnea may often be overlooked in sleepy epileptic subjects, and a low threshold for screening is appropriate. The associated weight gain with many antiepileptic agents might well increase the likelihood of sleep-related breathing disorders.

Conclusions

Evidence is emerging from a variety of sources that a disturbed sleep–wake cycle is not only extremely prevalent but also a significant cause of reduced life quality in a significant proportion of those suffering from neurological disease. Furthermore, epidemiological studies, data from animal models of dementia, and analysis of subcellular mechanisms for handling stress such as the unfolded protein response all indicate that chronically impaired sleep may actively contribute or fuel any underlying disease process, particularly in neurodegenerative conditions.

In complex neurological diseases, determining the precise anatomical source for sleep–wake disruption is usually speculative, and the inevitable influence of normal aging on any sleep disorder may complicate the picture. However, strategies, both pharmacological and nonpharmacological, may considerably improve sleep-related symptoms and confer a more normal rest-activity cycle in many subjects. A working knowledge of sleep neurobiology, the likely consequences of its disruption, and the potential beneficial consequences of treating sleep disorders effectively should all be essential core areas of knowledge for general neurologists.

References

1. Jo YE, Lucey BP, Holtzman DM. Sleep and Alzheimer disease pathology—a bidirectional relationship. Nat Rev Neurol 2014;10(2):115–19.
2. Costandi M. Neurodegeneration: amyloid awakenings. Nature 2013;497(7450):S19–20.
3. Brown RE, Basheer R, McKenna JT, Strecker RE, McCarley RW. Control of sleep and wakefulness. Physiol Rev 2012;92(3):1087–187.
4. Rosenwasser AM. Functional neuroanatomy of sleep and circadian rhythms. Brain Res Rev 2009;61(2):281–306.
5. Rye DB. The two faces of Eve: dopamine's modulation of wakefulness and sleep. Neurology 2004;63(8 Suppl 3):S2–7.
6. Freeman A, Ciliax B, Bakay R, et al. Nigrostriatal collaterals to thalamus degenerate in parkinsonian animal models. Ann Neurol 2001;50(3):321–9.
7. Owen AM. Detecting consciousness: a unique role for neuroimaging. Annu Rev Psychol 2013;64:109–33.
8. Lin L, Faraco J, Li R, et al. The sleep disorder canine narcolepsy is caused by a mutation in the hypocretin (orexin) receptor 2 gene. Cell 1999;98(3):365–76.
9. Chemelli RM, Willie JT, Sinton CM, et al. Narcolepsy in orexin knockout mice: molecular genetics of sleep regulation. Cell 1999;98(4):437–51.
10. Mignot E, Taheri S, Nishino S. Sleeping with the hypothalamus: emerging therapeutic targets for sleep disorders. Nat Neurosci 2002;5 Suppl:1071–5.
11. Basheer R, Strecker RE, Thakkar MM, McCarley RW. Adenosine and sleep–wake regulation. Prog Neurobiol 2004;73(6):379–96.
12. Van Dongen HP, Dinges DF. Investigating the interaction between the homeostatic and circadian processes of sleep–wake regulation for the prediction of waking neurobehavioural performance. J Sleep Res 2003;12(3):181–7.
13. Achermann P. The two-process model of sleep regulation revisited. Aviat Space Environ Med 2004;75(3 Suppl):A37–43.
14. Hastings MH, Maywood ES, Reddy AB. Two decades of circadian time. J Neuroendocrinol 2008;20(6):812–19.
15. Ralph MW, Foster RG, Davis FC, Menaker M. Transplanted suprachiasmatic nucleus determines circadian period. Science 1990;247(4945):975–8.
16. Morin LP. Neuroanatomy of the extended circadian rhythm system. Exp Neurol 2013; 243:4–20.
17. Hughes AT, Piggins HD. Feedback actions of locomotor activity to the circadian clock. Prog Brain Res 2012;199:305–36.
18. Roenneberg T, Kantermann T, Juda M, Vetter C, Allebrandt KV. Light and the human circadian clock. Handb Exp Pharmacol 2013;217:311–31.
19. Saper CB, Chou TC, Scammell TE. The sleep switch: hypothalamic control of sleep and wakefulness. Trends Neurosci 2001;24(12):726–31.
20. Dijk DJ. Regulation and functional correlates of slow wave sleep. J Clin Sleep Med. 2009; 5(2 Suppl):S6–15.
21. Fuller PM, Saper CB, Lu J. The pontine REM switch: past and present. J Physiol. 2007; 584(3):735–41.
22. Hobson JA, Pace-Schott EF, Stickgold R. Dreaming and the brain: toward a cognitive neuroscience of conscious states. Behav Brain Sci. 2000;23(6):793–842.
23. Gillin JC, Smith TL, Irwin M, Kripke DF, Schuckit M. EEG studies in "pure" primary alcoholism during subacute withdrawal: relationships to normal controls, age, and other clinical variables. Biol Psychiatry. 1990;27(5):477–88.
24. Dijk DJ, Duffy JF. Circadian regulation of human sleep and age-related changes in its timing, consolidation and EEG characteristics. Ann Med. 1999;31(2):130–40.
25. Dijk DJ, Groeger JA, Stanley N, Deacon S. Age-related reduction in daytime sleep propensity and nocturnal slow wave sleep. Sleep. 2010;33(2):211–23.
26. Yoon IY, Kripke DF, Elliot JA, Youngstedt SD, Rex KM, Hauger RL. Age-related changes of circadian rhythms and sleep–wake cycles. J Am Geriatr Soc. 2003;51(8):1085–91.
27. Tarokh L, Van Reen E, LeBourgeois M, Seifer R, Carskadon MA. Sleep EEG provides evidence that cortical changes persist into late adolescence. Sleep. 2011;34(10):1385–91.
28. Mander BA, Rao V, Lu B, Saletin JM, Lindquist JR, Ancoli-Israel S et al. Prefrontal atrophy, disrupted NREM slow waves and impaired hippocampal-dependent memory in aging. Nat Neurosci. 2013;16(3):357–64.
29. Schmidt C, Peigneux P, Cajochen C. Age-related changes in sleep and circadian rhythms: impact on cognitive performance and underlying neuroanatomical networks. Front Neurol. 2012;3:118.
30. Child ND, Benarroch EE. Anterior nucleus of the thalamus: functional organization and clinical implications. Neurology. 2013;81(21):1869–76.
31. Lugaresi E, Provini F. Fatal familial insomnia and agrypnia excitata. Rev Neurol Dis. 2007;4(3):145–52.
32. Provini F. Agrypnia excitata. Curr Neurol Neurosci Rep. 2013;13(4):341.
33. Landolt HP, Glatzel M, Blättler T, Achermann P, Roth C, Mathis J et al. Sleep–wake disturbances in sporadic Creutzfeldt–Jakob disease. Neurology. 2006;66(9):1418–24.
34. Kulisevsky J, Berthier ML, Pujol J. Hemiballismus and secondary mania following a right thalamic infarction. Neurology. 1993;43(7):1422–44.
35. Baumann CR, Werth E, Stocker R, Ludwig S, Bassetti CL. Sleep–wake disturbances 6 months after traumatic brain injury: a prospective study. Brain. 2007;130(7):1873–83.
36. Thieben MJ, Lennon VA, Boeve BF, Aksamit AJ, Keegan M, Vernino S. Potentially reversible autoimmune limbic encephalitis with neuronal potassium channel antibody. Neurology. 2004;62(7):1177–82.
37. Serratrice G, Serratrice J. Continuous muscle activity, Morvan's syndrome and limbic encephalitis: ionic or non ionic disorders? Acta Myol. 2011;30(1):32–33.
38. DeSena AD, Greenberg BM, Graves D. "Light switch" mental status changes and irritable insomnia are two particularly salient features of anti-NMDA receptor antibody encephalitis. Pediatr Neurol. 2014;51(1):151–3.
39. Triarhou LC. The percipient observations of Constantin von Economo on encephalitis lethargica and sleep disruption and their lasting impact on contemporary sleep research. Brain Res Bull. 2006;69(3):244–58.
40. Garcia-Borreguero D, Kohnen R, Silber MH, Winkelman JW, Earley CJ, Hogl B et al. The long-term treatment of restless legs syndrome/ Willis–Ekbom disease: evidence-based guidelines and clinical consensus best practice guidance: a report from the International Restless Legs Syndrome Study Group. Sleep Med. 2013;14(7):675–84.
41. Schurks M, Bussfiled P. Multiple sclerosis and restless legs syndrome: a systematic review and meta-analysis. Eur J Neurol. 2013;20(4):605–15.
42. Lavigne G, Brousseau M, Kato T, Mayer P, Manzini C, Guitard F et al. Experimental pain perception remains equally active over all sleep stages. Pain. 2004;110(3):646–55.

43. Gagnon JF, Petit D, Latreille V, Montplaisir J. Neurobiology of sleep disturbances in neurodegenerative disorders. Curr Pharm Des. 2008; 14(32):3430–45.

44. Compta Y, Santamaria J, Ratti L, Tolosa E, Iranzo I, Munoz E et al. Cerebrospinal hypocretin, daytime sleepiness, and sleep architecture in Parkinson's disease dementia. Brain. 2009;132(2):3308–17.

45. Iranzo A, Tolosa E, Gelpi E, Molinuevo JL, Valldeoriola F, Serradell M et al. Neurodegenerative disease status and post-mortem pathology in idiopathic rapid-eye-movement sleep behaviour disorder: an observational cohort study. Lancet Neurol. 2013:12(5):443–53.

46. Wienecke M, Werth E, Poryoazova R, Baumann-Vogel H, Bassetti CL, Weller M et al. Progressive dopamine and hypocretin deficiencies in Parkinson's disease: is there an impact on sleep and wakefulness? J Sleep Res. 2012;21(6):710–17.

47. Lim AS, Ellison BA, Wang JL, Yu L, Schneider JA, Buchman AS et al. Sleep is related to neuron numbers in the ventrolateral preoptic/ intermediate nucleus in older adults with and without Alzheimer's disease. Brain. 2014;137(10):2847–61.

48. Sanchez-Espinosa MP, Atienza M, Cantero JL. Sleep deficits in mild cognitive impairment are related to increased levels of plasma amyloid-β and cortical thinning. Neuroimage. 2014;98:395–404.

49. Pallier PN, Maywood ES, Zheng Z, Chesham JE, Inyushkin AN, Dyball R et al. Pharmacological imposition of sleep slows cognitive decline and reverses dysregulation of circadian gene expression in a transgenic model of Huntington's disease. 2007;27(29):7869–78.

50. Rye DB, Bliwise DL, Parker K, Trotti LM, Saini P, Fairley J et al. Modulation of vigilance in the primary hypersomnias by endogenous enhancement of $GABA_A$ receptors. Sci Transl Med. 2012;4(161):161

51. Ohayon MM, Carskadon MA, Guilleminault C, Vitiello MV. Meta-analysis of quantitative sleep parameters from childhood to old age in healthy individuals: developing normative sleep values across the human life span. Sleep. 2004;27(7):1255–73.

52. Hatfield CF, Herbert J, van Someren EJ, Hodges JR, Hastings MH. Disrupted daily activity/rest cycles in relation to daily cortisol rhythms of home-dwelling patients with early Alzheimer's disease. Brain. 2004;127(5):1061–74.

53. Arnulf I, Konofal E, Merino-Andreu M, Houeto JL, Mesnage V, Welter ML et al. Parkinson's disease and sleepiness: an integral part of PD. Neurology. 2002;58(7):1019–24.

54. Baumann C, Ferini-Strambi L, Waldvogel D, Werth E, Bassetti CL. Parkinsonism with excessive daytime sleepiness—a narcolepsy-like disorder? J Neurol. 2005;252(2):139–45.

55. Kanbayashi T, Sagawa Y, Takemura F, Ito SU, Tsutsui K, Hishikawa Y et al. The pathophysiologic basis of secondary narcolepsy and hypersomnia. Curr Neurol Neurosci Rep. 2011;11(2):235–41.

56. Nishino S, Kanabayashi T. Symptomatic narcolepsy, cataplexy and their implications in the hypothalamic hypocretin/orexin system. Sleep Med Rev. 2005;9(4):269–310.

57. Compta Y, Iranzo A, Santamaria J, Casamitjana R, Graus F. REM sleep behaviour disorder and narcoleptic features in anti-Ma2-associated encephalitis. Sleep. 2007;30(6):767–9.

58. Dauvilliers Y, Bauer J, Rigau V, Lalloyer N, Labauge P, Carlander B et al. Hypothalamic immunopathology in anti-Ma-associated diencephalitis with narcolepsy-cataplexy. JAMA Neurol. 2013;70(10):1305–10.

59. Bassetti CL, Mathis J, Gugger M, Lovblad KO, Hess CW. Hypersomnia following paramedian thalamic stroke: a report of 12 patients. Ann Neurol. 1996;39(4):471–80.

60. Fonseca AC, Geraldes R, Pires J, Falcao F, Bentes C, Melo TP. Improvement of sleep architecture in the follow up of a patient with bilateral paramedian thalamic stroke. Clin Neurol Neurosurg. 2011;113(10):911–3.

61. Luigetti M, Di Lazzaro V, Broccolini A, Vollono C, Dittoni S, Frisullo G et al. Bilateral thalamic stroke transiently reduces arousals and NREM sleep instability. J Neurol Sci. 2011;300(1–2):151–4.

62. Sommerauer M, Valko PO, Werth E, Baumann CR. Excessive sleep need following traumatic brain injury: a case-control study of 36 patients. J Sleep Res. 2013;22(6):634–9.

63. Chokroverty S. Sleep and breathing in neuromuscular disorders. Handb Clin Neurol. 2011;99:1087–108.

64. van der Meche FG, Bogaard JM, van der Sluys JC, Schimsheimer RJ, Ververs CC, Busch HF. Daytime sleep in myotonic dystrophy is not caused by sleep apnoea. J Neurol Neurosurg Psychiatry. 1994;57(5):626–8.

65. Ciafaloni E, Mignot E, Sansone V, Hilbert JE, Lin L, Lin X et al. The hypocretin neurotransmission system in myotonic dystrophy type 1. Neurology. 2008;70(3):226–30.

66. Lam EM, Shepard PW, St Louis EK, Dueffert LG, Slocumb N, McCarter SJ et al. Restless legs syndrome and daytime sleepiness are prominent in myotonic dystrophy type 2. Neurology. 2013;81(2):157–64.

67. Jones CR, Huang AL, Ptacek LJ, Fu YH. Genetic basis of human circadian rhythm disorders. Exp Neurol. 2013;243:28–33.

68. Zee PC, Vitiello MV. Circadian rhythm sleep disorder: irregular sleep wake rhythm type. Sleep Med Clin. 2009;4(2):213–8.

69. Emens JS, Laurie AL, Songer JB, Lewy AJ. Non-24-hour disorder in blind individuals revisited: variability and the influence of environmental time cues. Sleep. 2013;36(7):1091–100.

70. Hayakawa T, Uchiyama M, Kamei Y, Shibui K, Tagaya H, Asada T et al. Clinical analyses of sighted patients with non-24-hour sleep phase syndrome: a study of 57 consecutively diagnosed cases. Sleep. 2005;28(8):945–52.

71. Zee PC, Manthena P. The brain's master circadian clock: implications and opportunities for therapy of sleep disorders. Sleep Med Rev. 2007;11(1):59–70.

72. Harper DG, Stopa EG, McKee AC, Satlin A, Harlan PC, Goldstein R et al. Differential circadian rhythm disturbances in men with Alzheimer disease and frontotemporal degeneration. Arch Gen Psychiatry. 2001;58(4):353–60.

73. Videnovic A, Noble C, Reid KJ, Peng J, Turek FW, Marconi A et al. Circadian melatonin rhythm and excessive daytime sleepiness in Parkinson's disease. JAMA Neurol. 2014;71(4):463–9.

74. Videnovic A, Lazar AS, Barker RA, Overeem S. "The clocks that time us"—circadian rhythms in neurodegenerative disorders. Nat Rev Neurol 2014;10:683–93.

75. Breen DP, Vuono R, Nawarathna U, Fisher K, Shneerson JM, Reddy AB et al. Sleep and circadian rhythm regulation in early Parkinson disease. JAMA Neurol. 2014;71(5):589–95.

76. Morton AL. Circadian and sleep disorder in Huntington's disease. Exp Neurol. 2013;243:34–44.

77. Fisher SP, Black SW, Schwartz MD, Wilk AJ, Chen TM, Lincoln WU et al. Longitudinal analysis of the electroencephalogram and sleep phenotype in the R6/2 mouse model of Huntington's disease. Brain. 2013;136(7):2159–72.

78. Pallier PN, Morton AJ. Management of sleep/wake cycles improves cognitive function in a transgenic mouse model of Huntington's disease. Brain Res. 2009;1279:90–98.

79. Kuljis D, Schroeder AM, Kudo T, Loh DH, Willison DL, Colwell CS. Sleep and circadian dysfunction in neurodegenerative disorders: insights from a mouse model of Huntington's disease. Minerva Pneumol. 2012;51(3):93–106.

80. Maywood ES, Fraenkel E, McAllister CJ, Wood N, Reddy AB, Hastings MH et al. Disruption of peripheral circadian timekeeping in a mouse model of Huntington's disease and its restoration by temporally scheduled feeding. J Neurosci. 2010;30(30):10199–204.

81. Verheggen RJ, Jones H, Nyakayiru J, Thompson A, Groothuis JT, Atkinson G et al. Complete absence of evening melatonin increase in tetraplegics. FASEB J. 2012;26(7):3059–64

82. Guilleminault C, Briskin JG, Greenfield MS, Silvestri R. The impact of autonomic nervous system dysfunction on breathing during sleep. Sleep. 1981;4(3):263–78.

83. Gadoth N, Sokol J, Lavie P. Sleep structure and disordered nocturnal breathing in familial dysautonomia. J Neurol Sci. 1983;60(1):117–25.
84. Freilich S, Goff EA, Malaweera AS, Twigg GL, Simonds AK, Mathias CJ, Morrell MJ. Sleep architecture and attenuated heart rate response to arousal from sleep in patients with autonomic failure. Sleep Med. 2010;11(1):87–92.
85. Bazil CW. Epilepsy and sleep disturbance. Epilepsy Behav. 2003;4(Suppl 2):S39–45.
86. Quigg M, Staume M, Menaker M, Bertram EH 3rd. Temporal distribution of partial seizures: comparison of an animal model with human partial epilepsy. Ann Neurol. 1998;43(6):748–55.
87. Bazil CW. Short D, Crispin D, Zheng W. Patients with intractable epilepsy have low melatonin, which increases following seizures. Neurology. 2000;55(11):1746–8.

88. Quigg M, Kiely JM, Johnson ML, Straume M, Bertram EH, Evans WS. Interictal and postictal circadian and ultradian luteinizing hormone secretion in men with temporal lobe epilepsy. Epilepsia. 2006;47(9):1452–9.
89. de Weerd, de Haas S, Otte A, Trenite DK, van Erp G, Cohen A et al. Subjective sleep disturbance in patients with partial epilepsy: a questionnaire-based study on prevalence and impact on quality of life. Epilepsia. 2004;45(11):1397–404.
90. Touchon J, Baldy-Moulinier M, Billiard M, Besset A, Cadilhac J. Sleep organization and epilepsy. Epilepsy Res Suppl. 1991(2):73–81.
91. Bazil CW, Castro LH, Walczak TS. Reduction of rapid eye movement sleep by diurnal and nocturnal sleep in temporal lobe epilepsy. Arch Neurol. 2000;57(3):363–8.

CHAPTER 36

Clinical and neurophysiological aspects of fatigue

Sushanth Bhat and Sudhansu Chokroverty

Introduction

It has long been appreciated that fatigue is a common occurrence in patients with various medical, neurological and primary sleep disorders. The French physician Duchesne [1] first described fatigue in medical disorders in 1857, and Klenner [2] gave an account of fatigue in multiple sclerosis (MS) and myasthenia gravis in 1949. Patients with a variety of medical and neurological disorders also have secondary disturbances of sleep, resulting in both fatigue and excessive daytime sleepiness (EDS). In many cases, fatigue may be attributed to EDS, but it is important for the practitioner to be aware of fatigue and EDS as distinct and independent symptoms, with different etiologies and treatment approaches.

The Multiple Sclerosis Council in 1998 established clinical guidelines and defined fatigue as a "subjective lack of physical and/or mental energy that is perceived by the individual or the caregiver to interfere with usual and desired activities" [3]. Fatigue is often perceived as a pervasive sense of tiredness impacting quality of life. EDS, on the other hand, refers to an inability to stay awake, with the patient often involuntarily closing their eyes, lapsing into episodes of microsleep with inattention, yawning, and succumbing to irresistible attacks of sleepiness. This "pressure to sleep" is not a feature of pure fatigue [4], but the distinction is often fine and patients may not be able to distinguish between them unless very pointed questions are asked and a thorough history elicited. Useful tools in this regard include questionnaires that assess daytime sleepiness, notably the Epworth Sleepiness Scale, where high scores are seen in patients with EDS but not in those with pure fatigue. A number of self-reported fatigue scales with proven validity and reliability are used in clinical practice, including the Fatigue Severity Scale (Box 36.1) [5], the Checklist Individual Strength, and the Abbreviated Fatigue Questionnaire (AFQ) [6,7]. However, they are heavily weighted toward measuring cognitive fatigue, which, as discussed below, may not be the only source of disability in these patients. Nevertheless, these self-reported patient tools may help distinguish fatigue from EDS.

This chapter focuses on the neurophysiological basis of fatigue, and the causes and management of fatigue in a variety of neurological conditions, primary sleep disorders and general medical disorders.

Defining fatigue

The classic meaning of fatigue is, as described above, a feeling of generalized tiredness and trouble initiating and sustaining motor tasks despite intact motor strength, and has both physical and cognitive components. However, from a practical point of view, a patient complaining of fatigue may be experiencing a variety of other symptoms, such as muscle weakness, inability to sustain voluntary activity (muscle fatigability), exercise intolerance, EDS, inability to concentrate and perceived cognitive deficits, apathy, and a loss of motivation. These other symptoms may coexist with the overwhelming lack of energy, making a precise description of the situation difficult for the patient. Nevertheless, each of these symptoms has different clinical implications, and a careful history and physical examination are therefore paramount. In many cases, fatigue is attributable to a previously diagnosed neurological, medical or sleep disorder. In a significant number of cases, however, no apparent cause of the patient's fatigue can be found, and the complaints may be labeled psychosomatic, at great disservice to the patient. Fatigue management is not made easier by the fact that the underlying pathophysiology remains conjectural, and optimal treatment protocols have hardly been optimized.

Chronic fatigue is an extremely common and undertreated problem. Published data suggest that it is present in 21–38% of primary care patients, with up to 18% complaining of fatigue lasting greater than 6 months [8,9]. Despite the significant impact of chronic fatigue on quality of life, studies have shown that more than half of patients often do not report it to their physicians, and only a small

---

Box 36.1 Fatigue severity scale

Patients choose a number from 1 to 7 that shows their degree of agreement with every statement, where 1 indicates strongly disagree and 7 indicates strongly agree.

- My motivation is lower when I am fatigued
- Exercise brings on my fatigue
- I am easily fatigued
- Fatigue interferes with my physical functioning
- Fatigue causes frequent problems for me
- My fatigue prevents sustained physical functioning
- Fatigue interferes with carrying out certain duties and responsibilities
- Fatigue is among my three most disabling symptoms
- Fatigue interferes with my work, family, or social life

minority receive specific treatment for this disabling symptom [10]. These figures emphasize the need for a high level of vigilance for fatigue-related issues in the clinical setting.

Pathophysiological mechanisms for fatigue

Attempts have been made to develop neurophysiological models for fatigue. In this context, it is useful to classify fatigue as being of either a central or peripheral etiology [11]. Peripheral fatigue is due to a failure of the motor unit (the anterior horn cell, the motor axon, the neuromuscular junction, or the muscle fiber itself). A common model for measuring peripheral fatigue involves recording and comparing the force generated by electrical stimulation of muscle before and after exercise. Typically, after a pre-exercise electrical stimulation, the subject performs a maximum voluntary contraction (MVC) for a pre-determined period of time, generally 30 or 60 s, which is measured with a force transducer. A subsequent post-exercise electrical stimulation is then performed and the force generated is compared with the pre-exercise tracing. Lower amplitudes of the waveform and slow relaxation phases are characteristic of peripheral fatigue (Fig. 36.1) [12,13].

On the other hand, central fatigue is generated in the central nervous system (CNS), namely, the brain, spinal cord, and descending central motor pathways. This is assessed by measuring central activation failure (CAF), which suggests suboptimal CNS output to the motor unit. CAF can be measured by analyzing the force generated during MVC and providing superimposed electrical stimulation. The resulting twitch interpolation is then analyzed; the absence of a significant twitch amplitude suggests full voluntary contraction and no central fatigue, whereas a large superimposed twitch suggests significant CAF (Fig. 36.1). Transcranial magnetic

stimulation (TMS) studies of the motor cortex support the concept of central fatigue; patients with CNS lesions have been shown to have prolonged recovery of TMS-induced motor evoked potential amplitudes, which reflect conduction in the CNS, whereas measurements of conduction in the peripheral nervous system (PNS) were no different from controls [14]. Other reports have suggested that central fatigue might be related at least in part to a reduced safety factor of cortical synaptic transmission in the CNS [15]. Recent magnetoencephalographic data suggest that prolonged mental fatigue-inducing tasks cause overactivation of the visual cortex, manifest as decreased alpha power in this brain region [16]. However, in most CNS disorders, both central and peripheral fatigue play a role in the patient's symptomatology; these patients may therefore experience physical fatigue that may not be explainable by clinically demonstrable neurological deficits. Thus, fatigue as a symptom appears to defy localization to a particular site or structure; it involves diffuse as well as multifocal dysfunction across large neuroanatomical pathways and endocrinological feedback systems, with immunological abnormalities playing a role in certain disease processes [17].

Certain sites of dysfunction at the central level have been implicated in fatigue [18]. While voluntary physical activity originates in the motor cortex, feedback control from a number of areas (including cognitive input) must be present to convert intention into action. Such input may be pathologically altered in psychiatric disorders or with certain centrally active medications, contributing to the overall perception of fatigue. The prefrontal cortex, as well as multiple subcortical areas, including the hypothalamus, the brainstem, and the cerebellum, all influence motor output; unsurprisingly, diseases affecting them may result in fatigue in addition to obvious neurological deficits on clinical examination. Neuronal systems subserving arousal and attention (i.e, the ascending reticular activating system and the limbic system) are particular areas of focus inasmuch as their dysfunction would naturally be expected to limit motivation and cognitive drive to work.

Neuroimaging studies in central fatigue, while still largely research tools, have produced interesting results. No single anatomical substrate has been identified, but cortical atrophy of the parietal lobe on magnetic resonance imaging (MRI) in patients with MS was found to have the strongest correlation with fatigue [19]. Another study found that complaints in the physical and cognitive domains of fatigue in patients with MS correlated with MRI findings in different parts of the brain [20], suggesting that lesions in different parts of the brain may be responsible for physical and cognitive central fatigue, even in the same disease. White matter lesion burden and atrophy of the corpus callosum on MRI have been correlated with cognitive impairment and fatigue in MS [21,22]. Functional MRI studies in MS patients with fatigue have shown greater activation of the motor–attentional network when performing a simple motor task [23], as well as greater activation of the contralateral cingulate motor area [24], and more diffuse cervical cord recruitment [25] compared with controls or with MS patients without fatigue. Positron emission tomography (PET) scans, which measure cerebral perfusion, have shown widespread cerebral hypometabolism [26], as well as selective hypometabolism in the bifrontal and basal gangliar regions [27] in fatigued patients with MS. A recent study found no brain atrophy on MRI in patients with post-polio syndrome (PPS) and fatigue, whereas atrophy was present in MS patients [28].

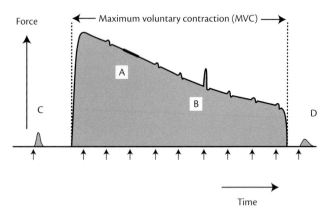

Fig. 36.1 Peripheral fatigue can be studied by measuring the maximum voluntary contraction (MVC) of muscle as recorded by a force transducer. Note the normal linear decrease in force generated attributable to peripheral fatigue. Superimposed tetanic stimulation (denoted by the arrows) is used to detect the presence of central fatigue. Absence of significant twitch amplitude (A) suggests the absence of central activation failure (CAF), whereas a large twitch amplitude (B) suggests the presence of CAF. A pre-MVC tetanic contraction (C) and post-MVC tetanic contraction (D) are compared. The lower amplitude and slower relaxation phase of the post-MVC contraction is suggestive of the development of peripheral fatigue.

Reproduced from Sleep Med Clin., 8(2), Bhat and Chokroverty, Fatigue in neurological disorders, pp. 191–212, Copyright (2013), with permission from Elsevier; Adapted from Clinical neurophysiology, 119(1), Zwarts et al., Clinical neurophysiology of fatigue, pp. 2–10, Copyright (2008), with permission from Elsevier.

Cognition and fatigue

While physical fatigue is at least partly explainable by the concepts of central and peripheral fatigue as discussed above, less well understood is cognitive fatigue, defined as a failure to endure sustained mental tasks in patients with fatigue. There is also a deficit of self-motivation, and overall debilitation not attributable to motor weakness, dyscoordination, or sensory loss. In addition, patients with central fatigue perceive greater expenditure of effort in completing a task, even in the absence of deficits that would limit them from performing the task, and even if the task is completed successfully. This cognitive component of central fatigue can be assessed by cognitive and motor-task processing parameters [29]. The factors leading to the development of cognitive fatigue remain poorly elucidated. Recent data suggest that in patients with depression and insomnia, unhelpful beliefs about sleep and symptom-focused rumination were predictive of both physical and mental fatigue [30], suggesting that at least part of the cognitive aspects of fatigue may be a manifestation of the patient's responses and attitudes toward their underlying illnesses.

Fatigue as a comorbid symptom

Chronic fatigue occurs in a wide variety of medical conditions. These include anemia, autoimmune disorders such as systemic lupus erythematosus (SLE) and sarcoidosis, chronic infectious diseases such as HIV and Lyme disease, cardiopulmonary disorders such as chronic obstructive pulmonary disease (COPD) and congestive heart failure (CHF), rheumatological disorders such as fibromyalgia, and cancers. In addition, it may be a side effect of a wide variety of medications, most commonly beta-blockers, anxiolytics (eg, benzodiazepines and barbiturates), antiepileptics (valproic acid, carbamazepine, and levetiracetam), antipsychotics, dopaminergics, proton pump inhibitors, chemotherapeutic agents, and beta-interferons, to name the most commonly prescribed classes [17]. Fatigue is also a frequent complaint in psychiatric disorders such as major depression, and there is a high correlation between complaints of fatigue and psychological morbidity, suggesting a large overlap [31]. Fatigue occurs in a multitude of neurological disorders, both central (eg, MS, Parkinson disease (PD), and post stroke) and peripheral (neuromuscular junction diseases, Guillain–Barré syndrome (GBS), PPS, and myopathies). As a symptom, it occurs with virtually all known primary sleep disorders and is a major source of disability, impacting the ability of the patient to lead a productive life.

Fatigue in primary sleep disorders

Most patients with sleep disorders complain of fatigue. It is important to differentiate this from EDS. Among patients with sleep disorders, younger age, female sex, and a high number of awakenings and arousals have been shown to be predictive of fatigue [32]. Obstructive sleep apnea (OSA), a disorder in which there is sleep fragmentation due to recurrent episodes of upper airway narrowing and collapse, results in EDS. In addition, fatigue occurs in up to 42% of patients with OSA [33]. However, no correlation between the degrees of reported fatigue and the severity of OSA, or even between fatigue severity scores and objective measures of EDS (such as multiple sleep latency testing, MSLT) have been established, suggesting that in these patients, sleepiness and fatigue

are distinct symptoms [34]. Rather, fatigue in OSA appears to be closely related to co-occurrence of depressive symptoms [35]. Nevertheless, treatment of OSA with continuous positive airway pressure (CPAP) improves both fatigue and EDS [36].

Fatigue is also commonly seen in narcolepsy, a sleep disorder characterized by EDS, fragmented nocturnal sleep, and intrusion of rapid eye movement (REM) sleep phenomena (such as cataplexy, hypnagogic and hypnopompic hallucinations, and sleep paralysis) into non-REM (NREM) and waking states. The prevalence of fatigue may be as high as 63% in patients with narcolepsy, although the degree of EDS does not correlate with the degree of fatigue, again suggesting that these are two independent symptoms [37]. Modafinil has been shown to improve both symptoms [38].

Restless legs syndrome (RLS, recently renamed Willis–Ekbom disease, WED) is characterized by uncomfortable sensations in the legs accompanied by an urge to move them, usually occurring around bedtime and often hampering sleep onset, but improving with movement. It is associated with depression, sleep disruption, and insomnia, and, unsurprisingly, frequently results in fatigue. A recent study suggested that this is particularly true in patients with comorbid diabetes mellitus [39]. Similarly, periodic limb movements of sleep (PLMS), present in over 80% of RLS patients, have been found to correlate with sleep disruption and fatigue [40].

Circadian rhythm disorders are a common cause of sleep disruption and fatigue. In particular, many shift workers (patients who work nontraditional hours such as late evening, early morning, or full nights) complain of EDS and fatigue, independent of mood disorders [41]. Frequency of night shifts correlates positively with the degree of fatigue. The underlying pathophysiology remains speculative, but may be related to lower morning serum cortisol levels in shift workers [42].

Insomnia, either as a primary disorder or as a symptom of another sleep disorder or medical condition, is commonly associated with fatigue. PET scans have demonstrated that, compared with controls, patients with insomnia have increased global cerebral metabolism during sleep and wakefulness, a smaller decline in relative metabolism from waking to sleep states in wake-promoting regions, and reduced relative metabolism in the prefrontal cortex while awake [43]. In addition, studies of spectral electroencephalogram (EEG) patterns in patients with primary insomnia suggest that stress patterns impact neurophysiological systems [44]. The role of mood and anxiety on insomnia and therefore fatigue in these patients is quite convincing. Cognitive–behavioral therapy (CBT) appears to not only improve sleep but also reduce comorbid psychological and fatigue-related symptoms [45]. In any patient with insomnia, of course, a careful evaluation for an underlying comorbid sleep disorder such as OSA or PLMS is warranted.

Fatigue in neurological disorders

Fatigue in CNS disorders

Fatigue in multiple sclerosis

Over 80% of patients with MS complain of fatigue, including cognitive fatigue, as one of their most disabling symptoms [4]. The seminal work on fatigue in MS was published by Krupp et al. [46]. However, the etiology of fatigue in MS remains unclear and is likely multifactorial, with no single area of the brain identifiable as a source of the problem. Hypothalmopituitary axis hyperactivity, elevated adrenocorticotropic hormone levels, and higher levels of circulating proinflammatory cytokines have been implicated [47,48]. Neurophysiologically, fatigue in MS has been associated with more anteriorly widespread event-related desynchronization during a movement (indicating hyperactivity during movement execution), and lower post-movement contralateral event-related synchronization (indicating failure of the inhibitory mechanisms intervening after movement termination) compared with normal subjects and MS patients without fatigue. This is consistent with a central origin of fatigue in MS [49]. While MS is a major cause of chronic fatigue, paradoxically, its treatment may be responsible for fatigue as well. Interferon therapy is generally acknowledged as a major contributor to MS-related fatigue [50]. Glatiramer acetate is effective in treating MS-related fatigue [51]. In addition, sleep dysfunction is a major predictor of fatigue in MS patients [52]. Insomnia is a common complaint, and is strongly associated with fatigue in MS [53]. MS patients with severe fatigue are more likely than controls or those with mild fatigue to have a circadian rhythm disorder [54]. OSA is frequent in MS, seen in up to 40% of patients [55,56], and is associated with fatigue but not EDS, independent of MS-related disability and other covariates [57]. Several studies have consistently shown that moderate to severe RLS is more frequent in MS than in the general population, and this has a significant impact on sleep quality [4]. Another factor that may contribute to daytime fatigue is the carryover effect of the hypnotic agents, particularly over-the-counter diphenhydramine-containing products, that are frequently used by MS patients [58]. Treating comorbid sleep disorders in MS patients has been shown to improve fatigue [59]. Management of fatigue in MS has proven to be quite challenging. Modafinil [60] and amantadine [61], are most commonly prescribed, but have performed unevenly in large trials. On the other hand, nonpharmacological measures for managing fatigue are more consistently beneficial in patients with MS-related fatigue, with exercise programs and CBT showing heartening results and compliance rates, as well as improvement of quality of life [62,63].

Fatigue in Parkinson disease

In patients with PD, sleep disturbances and fatigue have been shown to be the most disabling non-motor symptoms, affecting up to two-thirds of PD patients [64,65]. Functional neuroimaging has suggested that reduced serotonergic function in the basal ganglia and limbic structures, insular dopaminergic dysfunction [66], and frontal lobe dysfunction may be responsible for fatigue [67]. Although sleep disorders are common in PD (including insomnia, circadian rhythm abnormalities, RLS/PLMS, nocturnal bradykinesia and discomfort, complicated sleep apnea, and REM sleep behavior disorder) and worsen with disease progression [68], fatigue in PD seems to be independent of excessive daytime sleepiness [69]. The fatigue may respond to levodopa therapy [70], but the roles of CBT or exercise programs remain to be elucidated.

Post-stroke fatigue

Fatigue plagues nearly half the patients who suffer strokes, and is consistently associated with a poor outcome. Indeed, it was recently shown that fatigue in the acute phase is an independent predictor of poor physical health 18 months after stroke [71] Functional recovery seems to be worsened by concomitant depression [72]. Fatigue impacts post-stroke patients in several dimensions and is a salient feature during the recovery period [73]. Risk factors for the development of post-stroke fatigue appear to be younger age, post-stroke depressive symptoms, and infratentorial infarctions [74]. No neuroimaging findings predict post-stroke fatigue [75], and it does not appear to correlate with degree of neurological deficit, although there appears to be a relationship between fatigue and pain [76]. Unfortunately, at this time, there are no clear guidelines or recommendations for treating post-stroke fatigue. Antidepressants, though commonly prescribed to post-stroke patients, have not been conclusively proven to be helpful [77], and the role of CBT and medications like modafinil or amantadine remain uncertain in this setting.

Fatigue in traumatic brain injury

Patients with traumatic brain injury (TBI) often suffer from a variety of long-term consequences, including sleep complaints such as insomnia and daytime sleepiness, cognitive impairment, mood disorders, and fatigue [78]. Notably, the degree of initial injury does not seem to predict the severity of post-TBI impairment [79]. Fatigue, in particular, is present in nearly half of all patients post TBI, and does not appear to significantly improve with time [80]. It seems to be independent of depression or EDS [81]. The natural history of fatigue in TBI remains unclear, but CBT, lifestyle modification, pharmacological treatments with modafinil and melatonin, and light therapy have been suggested as possible interventional strategies [82].

Fatigue in PNS disorders

Fatigue in post-polio syndrome

The prevalence of significant fatigue has been reported to be as high as 77% among patients with PPS, while polio survivors without PPS have fatigue rates comparable to those of healthy controls [83]. A recent study showed that younger PPS patients who had shorter polio duration, more pain, and higher body mass index were more fatigued and had a lower quality of life [84]. Fatigue seems to worsen as the day progresses in PPS [85]. Both central and peripheral causes seem to be at play; while neurophysiological studies have shown that fatigue in these patients originates at the neuromuscular junction [86], neuropsychological evaluation of patients with PPS has shown defects of attention and information processing, while cognitive abilities and verbal memory were unaffected [87]. White matter hyperintensities in the reticular formation, putamen, medial lemniscus, and white matter tracts were found in more than half of PPS patients with high levels of fatigue and correlated with fatigue severity and subjective problems in attention, concentration, and recent memory [88]. Sleep is commonly adversely affected, and sleep fragmentation due to PLMS is frequent [89]. Hypersomnolence due to sleep-related breathing dysfunction is frequently seen, and these patients may have OSA, hypoventilation, or a combination of both [90]. Medically supervised and graded exercise seems to be beneficial in strength preservation in PPS, although the improvement in fatigue scores, if any, remains to be clarified [91]. From a pharmacological perspective, amantadine, modafinil, and intravenous immunoglobulin (IVIg) have all been studied, but no consistent benefit has been found [17]; a very small trial suggested that bromocriptine, another dopamine agonist used in the treatment of PD, might be efficacious in alleviating all aspects of PPS fatigue, including cognitive fatigue [92].

Fatigue in neuromuscular junction disorders

Neuromuscular junction disorders are characterized by failure of transmission across the neuromuscular junction and may be presynaptic (eg, Lambert–Eaton myasthenic syndrome) or postsynaptic (eg, myasthenia gravis). Models of peripheral fatigue in these disorders have been well studied and well understood, and are easily demonstrated in the electrophysiology laboratory using repetitive nerve stimulation studies. More difficult to explain are the reports of patients with myasthenia gravis experiencing significantly more cognitive fatigue in addition to physical fatigue than control subjects, and their perceptions of this fatigue increasing significantly following completion of demanding cognitive work [93]. It has been suggested that fatigue in neuromuscular junction disorders may be related to autonomic dysfunction [94]. As in most other neurological conditions, there appear to be poorly understood central fatigue mechanisms at play. An interesting recent study suggests that in patients with myasthenia gravis and fatigue, supplementation of low vitamin D levels may be of benefit [95].

Fatigue in amyotrophic lateral sclerosis

The prevalence of fatigue in amyotrophic lateral sclerosis (ALS) has been reported to be as high as 83% in some studies, more frequent in younger patients, and tending to worsen as the disease progresses [96]. Again, both central and peripheral fatigue seem to contribute to the overall decreased quality of life. Patients with ALS show evidence of CAF on MVC studies, as well as less intramuscular phosphocreatine depletion and less fatigue of stimulated tetanic force during exercise compared with controls, suggesting that central fatigue plays a major role in this condition [97]. Maladaptation of cortical processes related to degeneration of inhibitory GABAergic intracortical circuits is a feature of ALS that significantly correlates with development of fatigue and weakness [98]. Peripheral fatigue has been demonstrated in muscles that show no evidence of denervation-related injury, suggesting that motor weakness and fatigue in ALS are distinct entities. As in most other neurological conditions causing fatigue, sleep disruption plays a major role [99].

Fatigue in other neuromuscular diseases

The vast majority of patients with acquired immune-mediated neuropathies (history of GBS, stable chronic inflammatory demyelinating polyradiculoneuropathy, or monoclonal gammopathies) complain of persistent, disabling fatigue years after recovery or stabilization of their neurological deficits [100]. Central sources of fatigue seem to be responsible, as neurophysiological studies show no evidence of residual peripheral nerve dysfunction; similarly, the severity of fatigue does not depend on time between evaluation and recovery from GBS [101]. Medically supervised home exercise programs may be beneficial in these patients [102]. Modafinil has shown some benefit in alleviating fatigue in patients with hereditary motor and sensory neuropathy type 1 (HMSN-1, also known as Charcot–Marie–Tooth disease 1, CMT-1), the most common inherited neuropathy [103]. "Fatigue" in metabolic myopathies is characterized by cramping, painful contractions, and myalgias after exercise, while being asymptomatic at rest. This "exercise intolerance" may occur in the absence of motor weakness or clinical exam abnormalities. Genetic testing is often required for diagnosis. Fatigue has also been described in a large number of patients with a variety of inherited myopathies like facioscapulohumeral dystrophy and myotonic dystrophy [104]. Myotonic dystrophy type 1

(DM-1), a multisystem disorder characterized by muscle weakness and myotonia, cataracts, cardiac conduction defects, frontal balding, and endocrine abnormalities, and caused by an autosomal dominantly inherited triple nucleotide expansion mutation of the CTG sequence of the *DMPK* gene on the long arm of chromosome 19, deserves special mention because of the frequency of sleep dysfunction in these patients; sleep disordered breathing, numerous microarousals, and periodic limb movements are all very common, as are both fatigue and EDS (76% and 52% respectively in one study) [105]. DM1 patients have short sleep latencies on MSLT as well as sleep onset REM periods (SOREMPs), suggesting a narcoleptic phenotype. Periodic paralyses (hypokalemic and hyperkalemic periodic paralysis, myotonia congenita, paramyotonia congenita and Andersen–Tawil syndrome are examples of periodic paralyses) are channelopathies that present with paroxysmal attacks of periodic generalized weakness as well as muscle fatigability brought on by exposure to cold, carbohydrate-rich meals, exercise, or rest, depending on the exact disorder. Except for the first mentioned, these patients also have myotonia on electromyography (EMG) and can be diagnosed by genetic testing. Muscle weakness in these disorders may last from a few minutes to a few hours per attack, with a normal neurological exam, including normal strength testing, in between the attacks. The symptoms are often treated with acetazolamide, although the exact mechanism of action of this agent in these conditions is unknown [17].

Fatigue in general medical conditions

Fatigue in major cardiopulmonary diseases

Fatigue is a common complaint in patients with a wide variety of chronic cardiopulmonary disorders. Fatigue is highly prevalent in sarcoidosis and interstitial lung disease. It also frequently occurs in patients with COPD, a chronic, inflammatory disorder of the airways and lung parenchyma characterized by obstructive pulmonary dynamics, hypoxemia, and hypercapnia. The prevalence of daily fatigue in COPD has been reported to be as high as 68–80% [106], and nearly half of COPD patients describe it as their most disabling symptom, affecting cognitive, physical, and psychosocial well-being [107]. High fatigue scores negatively impact quality of life in COPD [108]. A recent study demonstrated positive correlation between fatigue severity and disease severity in COPD; patients with the most intense fatigue had the higher risk of hospitalization [109].

The etiology of fatigue in COPD is incompletely understood, but is most likely multifactorial. Exercise intolerance is a hallmark feature of COPD that contributes to the pervasive feeling of fatigue and has been shown to be related to pulmonary function and lung hyperinflation [110]. Interesting preliminary data suggest that increased dependence on glycolysis for muscle energy production in COPD may be an explanation for the exercise intolerance [111]. Patients with COPD often have comorbid sleep disorders that are major overall contributors to fatigue. Although OSA has not been demonstrated to occur with greater prevalence in COPD patients, the combination of COPD and OSA, known as the "overlap syndrome," is a common cause of severe nocturnal hypoxemia, sleep disruption, and subsequent EDS and fatigue [112] More severe COPD is also associated with complaints of insomnia and non-restorative sleep [113]. In a small study, Cavalcante et al. recently found that RLS was present in almost 31% of patients with COPD, and these patients complained of sleep fragmentation and high levels of fatigue [114]. Concurrent mood disorders were also predictive of fatigue in COPD [115].

Treatment of fatigue in COPD is challenging and is closely linked to improvement of pulmonary status and comorbid sleep dysfunction. Multidimensional programs that include pharmacotherapy to improve lung function and pulmonary rehabilitation have shown promising results [116]. Patients with COPD and insomnia may benefit from CBT [117].

In addition to orthopnea, peripheral edema, nocturnal cough and exertional dyspnea, fatigue is a significantly distressing symptom in patients with CHF. Prevalence rates are quite high, approximating 70–90% in various studies [118]. A recent small study suggested that fatigue was indicative of a poorer prognosis in CHF [119]. Although there is some evidence that the severity of fatigue may correlate with pulmonary arterial pressures [120], a consistent relationship between fatigue and degree of cardiac dysfunction has not been demonstrated [121]. Nevertheless, there are multiple proposed causes of fatigue in CHF, including impaired peripheral perfusion during exercise, reduced oxidative capacity of skeletal muscle, impaired muscle strength, and possibly reflex mechanisms associated with alterations in the metabolism of skeletal muscle. However, researchers have failed to demonstrate consistent reduction in fatigue even with optimization of cardiac output, oxygen delivery, and blood flow, leading to the hypothesis that a structural abnormality of muscle itself may be the ultimate culprit [122]. As with COPD, comorbid sleep complaints contribute to fatigue in CHF, with sleep disordered breathing, nocturia, and insomnia being the most common [123]. Fatigue and depression appear to occur independently in CHF [124]. In addition, pharmacotherapy of CHF, especially with beta-blockers, has been linked to fatigue and has often necessitated its discontinuation [125]. Unfortunately, optimal management of fatigue in CHF is unclear, and much research obviously needs to be done in this regard. Individualized exercise training programs for all patients with stable CHF have been advocated by some groups [126]

Fatigue in other medical conditions

Patients with chronic renal failure often experience debilitating fatigue. This is likely multifactorial, due to anemia, cachexia, and abnormal calcium and phosphate metabolism. Fatigue is particularly debilitating in patients on dialysis; almost half of patients with end-stage renal disease (ESRD) on hemodialysis complain of major fatigue, which appears to affect both physical and cognitive function and is often associated with depression [127]. In addition, patients on dialysis often have poor sleep quality [128], and frequently have OSA and RLS/PLMS that fragment their sleep, leading to both insomnia and EDS. Optimal treatment of fatigue in ESRD patients on hemodialysis is unclear, but may include strengthening of social support structures [129], exercise programs, erythropoietin supplementation, and L-carnitine supplementation [130].

Fatigue is also very commonly seen in chronic anemia, and often responds to judicious use of erythropoietin-stimulating agents and blood transfusions as necessary. In several autoimmune conditions such as SLE and Sjögren syndrome, fatigue is a prominent syndrome that is resistant to treatment and may be caused by underlying inflammatory states and coexistent fibromyalgia [131]. Endocrinological disorders such as hypothyroidism and hypothalamopituitary axis dysfunction are other causes of chronic fatigue [10].

Cancer-related fatigue

Fatigue is near universal in patients with cancer, and markedly more severe than in controls. It occurs in patients undergoing chemotherapy, radiation therapy, bone marrow transplantation, and treatment with biological response modifiers. There is some evidence that it worsens with age, possibly owing to lower hemoglobin levels [132]. Many factors contribute to cancer-related fatigue. Nutritional status and comorbid mood disorders play a major role. It is often difficult to determine how much of this fatigue is due to the underlying cancer itself and how much to chemotherapy; early data suggest this may depend on the location of the underlying malignancy, but both factors are likely contributory in most patients [133]. In patients with cancer, poor sleep quality correlated positively with fatigue and depression and negatively with quality-of-life indicators [134]; it has been postulated that altered cytokine profiles and circadian rhythm abnormalities may play a role [135]. Treatment of cancer-related fatigue is best individualized, with proper treatment of any comorbid medical or sleep-related conditions forming the cornerstone. Anemia is a major underlying cause of fatigue in cancer patients, and several studies have shown that fatigue responds to improvements in hemoglobin levels in anemic patients with a variety of malignancies, both on and off chemotherapy [136]. Several studies have shown that erythropoietin-stimulating agents improve subjective fatigue, although the exact magnitude of benefit is unclear and needs to be weighed against the risks of thrombosis [137]. Daily exercise appears to have a significant effect on cancer-related fatigue [138]. Early trials of pharmacotherapy with antidepressants, wakefulness-promoting agents, and psychostimulants in cancer-related fatigue have shown encouraging results, but their routine use has yet to be elucidated [139]. Recent data also suggest a role for CBT in cancer patients in improving both sleep quality and perception of fatigue [140].

Fatigue and psychiatric disorders

Fatigue is a prominent symptom in many primary psychiatric disorders, and fatigue or fatigue-like symptoms are described as part of a large number of diagnoses in the Diagnostic and Statistical Manual of Mental Disorders, Fourth Edition (DSM-IV) including attention deficit hyperactivity disorder, major depressive disorder, bipolar disorder, generalized anxiety disorder, substance intoxication and withdrawal, and post-traumatic stress disorder [31]. In addition, the frequent co-occurrence of psychiatric disorders and sleep dysfunction, both of which can cause insomnia, daytime somnolence, and fatigue, makes the exact prevalence of fatigue in psychiatric disorders difficult to estimate. Many patients with chronic fatigue syndrome (CFS) meet the criteria for a mood disorder [141], and even in patients with chronic fatigue not diagnosed with CFS, there is a high likelihood of a concurrent psychiatric disorder [142]. However, fatigue can exist without a comorbid psychiatric disorder [143]. The treatment of fatigue as an individual symptom in patients with depression and other psychiatric disorders has been poorly studied; it is often resistant to treatment with antidepressants. Graded exercise therapy, CBT, dopaminergic therapy, psychostimulants, and wakefulness-promoting agents such as modafinil have all been advocated in the literature, but data are sparse and their routine use remains to be validated with large trials [144].

Chronic fatigue syndrome

CFS is a complex and still somewhat poorly defined entity, with estimates of prevalence varying greatly, from 0.002% to 11.3% in primary care practices [145]. It appears to occur more often in women, minority groups, and lower socioeconomic and educational classes, with a significant comorbidity with psychiatric disorders [17]. Attempts to develop standard diagnostic criteria for CFS have proven challenging; the US Centers for Disease Control (CDC) diagnostic criteria (Box 36.2) are among the most widely accepted, but are highly dependent upon patient self-reporting of symptoms.

Its alternate nomenclature, "myalgic encephalitis" may mistakenly imply that its pathophysiology is clearly defined, but in truth the etiology of CFS remains elusive. The concept of a post-viral cause remains popular, although no particular organism has been consistently identified. Many patients complain of relatively acute onset of fatiguing symptomatology after a flu-like illness, but neither antibody nor immune dysfunction studies have been conclusive [146]. Numerous neurophysiological studies have failed to establish a peripheral cause of fatigue in CFS [147]. While studies have shown that there is a delay in information processing speed in patients with CFS [148], levels of cognitive fatigue are comparable to those in patients with major depression, and twice as many patients with CFS as those with neuromuscular diseases meet criteria for a psychiatric illness [141]. Similarly, MRI and single-photon emission computerized tomography (SPECT) studies have not identified structural or functional markers for CFS [17]. However, in one study of PET scans in patients with CFS, there was significant hypometabolism in the right mediofrontal cortex and brainstem compared with controls; patients with depression who were concurrently studied showed a severe hypometabolism of the medial and upper frontal regions bilaterally, whereas the metabolism of the brainstem was normal [149]. Nevertheless, the significance of these findings, and their clinical relevance, is unclear at this time.

CFS is comorbid with a variety of other conditions that can also cause fatigue. In a recent study, nearly half of patients with CFS had a coexistent primary sleep disorder (mainly OSA, as well as psychophysiologic insomnia and PLMS), and 45% had a psychiatric disorder (mostly mood and anxiety disorder) [150]. Sleep complaints, in particular, are extremely common in patients with CFS, most of whom complain of poor-quality, unrefreshing sleep, EDS, and insomnia. Polysomnography studies have not shown consistent sleep-architectural abnormalities in CFS [151], but a number of small studies have described a variety of nonspecific changes, suggesting that much more work needs to be done in this area. Notably, it has been demonstrated that treatment of any comorbid primary sleep disorder in patients with CFS does not improve fatigue. Thus, the symptoms of CFS do not seem to be due purely to underlying sleep disorders in these patients; the diagnosis of a primary sleep disorder should therefore not be an exclusion criterion for CFS [152]. EDS and fatigue exist as distinct symptoms in this disorder as well.

The optimal treatment of CFS is unclear. High-dose glucocorticoids [153] and IVIg therapy have not been found to be beneficial [154]. More recently, valganciclovir showed promising results in a subset of CFS patients with elevated IgG antibody titers against human herpesvirus- 6 (HHV-6) and Epstein–Barr virus [155]. Another study suggested that hyperbaric oxygen may have a role to play [156]. Intriguing as these results are, they await validation with larger studies. However, several studies have consistently shown the superiority of nonpharmacological interventions in CFS. While CBT is clearly beneficial, patient outcome seems to be dependent on the degree of patients' attribution of symptoms to exclusively physical causes [157]. Low-impact, graded aerobic exercise therapy was also found to be a beneficial strategy [158].

Box 36.2 Centers for Disease Control (CDC) criteria for the diagnosis of chronic fatigue syndrome (CFS)

In order to be diagnosed with chronic fatigue syndrome, a patient must satisfy two criteria:

1. Have severe chronic fatigue for 6 months or longer with other known medical conditions (whose manifestation includes fatigue) excluded by clinical diagnosis

   and

2. Concurrently have four or more of the following symptoms:

   - post-exertional malaise
   - impaired memory or concentration
   - unrefreshing sleep
   - muscle pain
   - multi-joint pain without redness or swelling
   - tender cervical or axillary lymph nodes
   - sore throat
   - headache

The symptoms must have persisted or recurred during 6 or more consecutive months of illness and must not have predated the fatigue.

References

1. Duchesne EA. Des chemins de fer et de leur influence sur la santé des mecaniciens et des chauffers, Paris: Bachelier, Imprimeur-Librairie de l'Ecole Polytechinque et du Bureau des Longitudes; 1857:183–5.
2. Klenner FR. Fatigue, normal and pathological, with special consideration of myasthenia gravis and multiple sclerosis. South Med Surg 1949;111:273–7.
3. Multiple Sclerosis Council for Clinical Practice Guidelines. Fatigue and multiple sclerosis: evidence-based management strategies for fatigue in multiple sclerosis. Washington, DC: Paralyzed Veterans of America, 1998.
4. Veauthier C, Friedmann P. Sleep disorders in multiple sclerosis and their relationship to fatigue. Sleep Med 2014;15(1):5–14.
5. Krupp L, LaRocca N, Muir-Nash, Steinberg AD. The Fatigue Severity Scale: application to patients with multiple sclerosis and systemic lupus erythematosus. Arch Neurol 1989;46(10):1121–3.
6. Albers M, Smets EM, Vercoulen JH, Garssen B, Bleijenberg G. [Abbreviated fatigue questionnaire; a practical tool in the classification of fatigue.] [Article in Dutch.] Ned Tidschr Geneeskd 1997;141:1526–30.
7. Beurskens AJ, Bultmann U, Kant I, et al. Fatigue among working people: validity of a questionnaire measure. Occup Environ Med 2000;57:353–7.
8. Finsterer J, Mahjoub SZ. Fatigue in healthy and diseased individuals. Am J Hosp Palliat Care 2014;31:562–75.

9. Pawlikowska T, Chalder T, Hirsch SR, et al. Population based study of fatigue and psychological distress. BMJ 1994;308:763–6.

10. Krupp LB. Fatigue. Philadephia: Butterworth-Heinemann, 2003.

11. Chaudhuri A, Behan PO. Fatigue and basal ganglia. J Neurol Sci 2000;179(1–2):34–42.

12. Schillings ML, Stegeman DF, Zwarts MJ. Determining central activation failure and peripheral fatigue in the course of sustained maximal voluntary contractions: a model-based approach. J Appl Physiol 2005;98(6):2292–7.

13. Zwarts MJ, Bleijenberg G, van Engelen BGM. Clinical neurophysiology of fatigue. Clin Neurophysiol 2008;119:2–10.

14. Liepert J, Kotterba S, Tegenthoff M, Malin JP. Central fatigue assessed by transcranial magnetic stimulation. Muscle Nerve 1996;19:1429–34.

15. Brasil-Neto JP, Cohen LG, Hallett, M. Central fatigue as revealed by postexercise decrement of motor evoked potentials. Muscle Nerve 1994;17:713–19.

16. Ishii A, Tanaka M, Shigihara Y, et al. Neural effects of prolonged mental fatigue: a magnetoencephalography study. Brain Res 2013;1529:105–12.

17. Bhat S, Chokroverty S. Fatigue in neurological disorders. Sleep Med Clin 2013;8(2):191–212.

18. Chaudhuri A, Behan PO. Fatigue in neurological disorders. Lancet 2004;363(9413):978–88.

19. Pellicano C, Gallo A, Li X. Relationship of cortical atrophy to fatigue in patients with multiple sclerosis. Arch Neurol 2010;67(4):447–53.

20. Calabrese M, Rinaldi F, Grossi P, et al. Basal ganglia and frontal/parietal cortical atrophy is associated with fatigue in relapsing–remitting multiple sclerosis. Mult Scler 2010;16(10):1220–8.

21. Papadopoulou A, Müller-Lenke N, Naegelin Y, et al. Contribution of cortical and white matter lesions to cognitive impairment in multiple sclerosis. Mult Scler 2013;19(10):1290–6.

22. Yaldizli O, Penner IK, Frontzek K, et al. The relationship between total and regional corpus callosum atrophy, cognitive impairment and fatigue in multiple sclerosis patients. Mult Scler 2014;20:356–64.

23. Specogna I, Casagrande F, Lorusso A, et al. Functional MRI during the execution of a motor task in patients with multiple sclerosis and fatigue. Radiol Med 2012;117(8):1398–407.

24. Filippi M, Rocca MA, Colombo B, et al. Functional magnetic resonance imaging correlates of fatigue in multiple sclerosis. Neuroimage 2002;15(3):559–67.

25. Rocca MA, Absinta M, Valsasina P, et al. Abnormal cervical cord function contributes to fatigue in multiple sclerosis. Mult Scler 2012;18(11):1552–9.

26. Bakshi R, Miletich RS, Kinkel PR, Emmet ML, Kinkel WR. High-resolution fluorodeoxyglucose positron emission tomography shows both global and regional cerebral hypometabolism in multiple sclerosis. J Neuroimaging 1998;8:228–34.

27. Roelcke U, Kappos L, Lechner-Scott J, et al. Reduced glucose metabolism in the frontal cortex and basal ganglia of multiple sclerosis patients with fatigue: a ^{18}F-fluorodeoxyglucose positron emission tomography study. Neurology 1997;48:1566–71.

28. Trojan DA, Narayanan S, Francis SJ, et al. Brain volume and fatigue in postpoliomyelitis syndrome patients. PM R 2014;6:215–20.

29. Togo F, Lange G, Natelson BH, Quigley KS. Attention network test: assessment of cognitive function in chronic fatigue syndrome. J Neuropsychol 2015;9:1–9.

30. Carney CE, Moss TG, Lachowski AM, Atwood ME. Understanding mental and physical fatigue complaints in those with depression and insomnia. Behav Sleep Med 2014;12:272–89.

31. Herman J. Psychiatric disorders and fatigue. Sleep Med Clin 2013;8(2):213–20.

32. Veauthier C. Younger age, female sex, and high number of awakenings and arousals predict fatigue in patients with sleep disorders: a retrospective polysomnographic observational study. Neuropsychiatr Dis Treat 2013;9:1483–94.

33. Mills PJ, Kim JH, Bardwell W, Hong S, Dimsdale JE. Predictors of fatigue in obstructive sleep apnea. Sleep Breath 2008;12(4):397–9.

34. Aguillard RN, Riedel BW, Lichstein KL, et al. Daytime functioning in obstructive sleep apnea patients: exercise tolerance, subjective fatigue, and sleepiness. Appl Psychophysiol Biofeedback 1998;23(4):207–17.

35. Stepnowsky CJ, Palau JJ, Zamora T, Ancoli-Israel S, Loredo JS. Fatigue in sleep apnea: the role of depressive symptoms and self-reported sleep quality. Sleep Med 2011;12(9):832–7.

36. Tomfohr LM, Ancoli-Israel S, Loredo JS, Dimsdale JE. Effects of continuous positive airway pressure on fatigue and sleepiness in patients with obstructive sleep apnea: data from a randomized controlled trial. Sleep 2011;34(1):121–6.

37. Droogleever Fortuyn HA, Fronczek R, Smitshoek M, et al. Severe fatigue in narcolepsy with cataplexy. J Sleep Res 2012;21(2):163–9.

38. Becker PM, Schwartz JR, Feldman NT, Hughes RJ. Effect of modafinil on fatigue, mood, and health-related quality of life in patients with narcolepsy. Psychopharmacology (Berl) 2004;171(2):133–9.

39. Cuellar NG, Ratcliffe SJ. A comparison of glycemic control, sleep, fatigue, and depression in type 2 diabetes with and without restless legs syndrome. J Clin Sleep Med 2008;4(1):50–6.

40. Martinez S, Guilleminault C. Periodic leg movements in prepubertal children with sleep disturbance. Dev Med Child Neurol 2004;46(11):765–70.

41. Øyane NM, Pallesen S, Moen BE, Akerstedt T, Bjorvatn B. Associations between night work and anxiety, depression, insomnia, sleepiness and fatigue in a sample of Norwegian nurses. PLoS One 2013;8(8):e70228.

42. Niu SF, Chung MH, Chen CH, et al. The effect of shift rotation on employee cortisol profile, sleep quality, fatigue, and attention level: a systematic review. J Nurs Res 2011;19(1):68–81.

43. Nofzinger EA, Buysse DJ, Germain A, et al. Functional neuroimaging evidence for hyperarousal in insomnia. Am J Psychiatry 2004;161(11):2126–8.

44. Hall M, Buysse DJ, Nowell PD, et al. Symptoms of stress and depression as correlates of sleep in primary insomnia. Psychosom Med 2000;62(2):227–30.

45. Thorndike FP, Ritterband LM, Gonder-Frederick LA, et al. A randomized controlled trial of an internet intervention for adults with insomnia: effects on comorbid psychological and fatigue symptoms. J Clin Psychol 2013;69(10):1078–93.

46. Krupp LB, Alvarez LA, LARocca NG, Scheinberg LC. Fatigue in multiple sclerosis. Arch Neurol 1988;45:435–7.

47. Gold SM, Krüger S, Ziegler KJ, et al. Endocrine and immune substrates of depressive symptoms and fatigue in multiple sclerosis patients with comorbid major depression. J Neurol Neurosurg Psychiatry 2011;82(7):814–18.

48. Melief J, de Wit SJ, van Eden CG, et al. HPA axis activity in multiple sclerosis correlates with disease severity, lesion type and gene expression in normal-appearing white matter. Acta Neuropathol 2013;126(2):237–49.

49. Leocani L, Colombo B, Magnani G, et al. Fatigue in multiple sclerosis is associated with abnormal cortical activation to voluntary movement—EEG evidence. Neuroimage 2001;13(6 Pt 1):1186–92.

50. Nielly L, Goodin D, Goodkin D, Hauser SL. Side effect profile of interferon beta-1b in MS: results of an open label trial. Neurology 1996;46:552–3.

51. Ziemssen T, Hoffman J, Apfel R, Kern S. Effects of glatiramer acetate on fatigue and days of absence from work in first-time treated relapsing-remitting multiple sclerosis. Health Qual Life Outcomes 2008;6:67.

52. Strober LB, Arnett PA. An examination of four models predicting fatigue in multiple sclerosis. Arch Clin Neuropsychol 2005;20(5):631–46.

53. Stanton BR, Barnes F, Silber E. Sleep and fatigue in multiple sclerosis. Mult Scler 2006;12(4):481–6.

54. Najafi MR, Toghianifar N, Etemadifar M, et al. Circadian rhythm sleep disorders in patients with multiple sclerosis and its association with fatigue: a case–control study. J Res Med Sci 2013;18(Suppl 1):S71–3.

55. Dias RA, Hardin KA, Rose H, et al. Sleepiness, fatigue, and risk of obstructive sleep apnea using the STOP-BANG questionnaire in multiple sclerosis: a pilot study. Sleep Breath 2012;16(4):1255–65.

56. Braley TJ, Segal BM, Chervin RD. Obstructive sleep apnea and fatigue in patients with multiple sclerosis. J Clin Sleep Med 2014;10(2):155–62.

57. Kaminska M, Kimoff RJ, Benedetti A, et al. Obstructive sleep apnea is associated with fatigue in multiple sclerosis. Mult Scler 2012;18(8):1159–69.

58. Braley TJ, Segal BM, Chervin RD. Hypnotic use and fatigue in multiple sclerosis. Sleep Med 2015;16:131–7.

59. Veauthier C, Gaede G, Radbruch H, et al. Treatment of sleep disorders may improve fatigue in multiple sclerosis. Clin Neurol Neurosurg 2013;115(9):1826–30.

60. Zifko U, Rupp M, Schwartz S, Zipko HT, Maida EM. Modafinil in treatment of fatigue in multiple sclerosis: results of an open-label study. J Neurol 2002;249(8):983–7.

61. Cohen R, Fisher M. Amantadine treatment of fatigue associated with multiple sclerosis. Arch Neurol 1989;46(6):676–80

62. Bjarnadottir OH, Konradsdottir AD, Reynisdottir K, Olafsson E. Multiple sclerosis and brief moderate exercise: a randomised study. Mult Scler 2007;13(6):776–82.

63. van Kessel K, Moss-Morris R, Willoughby E, et al. A randomized controlled trial of cognitive behavior therapy for multiple sclerosis fatigue. Psychosom Med 2008;70(2):205–13.

64. Freidman J, Friedman H. Fatigue in Parkinson's disease. Neurology 1993;43(10):2016–18.

65. Song W, Guo X, Chen K, et al. The impact of non-motor symptoms on the Health-Related Quality of Life of Parkinson's disease patients from Southwest China. Parkinsonism Relat Disord 2014;20:149–52.

66. Pavese N, Metta V, Bose S, Chaudhuri KR, Brooks DJ. Fatigue in Parkinson's disease is linked to striatal and limbic serotonergic dysfunction. Brain 2010;133(1):3434–43.

67. Abe K, Takanashi M, Yanagihara T. Fatigue in patients with Parkinson's disease. Behav Neurol 2000;12(3):103–6.

68. Zhang L, Dong J, Liu W, Zhang Y. Subjective poor sleep quality in Chinese patients with Parkinson's disease without dementia. J Biomed Res 2013;27(4):291–5.

69. Havlikova E, van Dijk JP, Rosenberger J, et al. Fatigue in Parkinson's disease is not related to excessive sleepiness or quality of sleep. J Neurol Sci 2008;270(1):107–13.

70. Lou JS, Kearns G, Benice T, et al. Levodopa improves physical fatigue in Parkinson's disease: a double-blind, placebo-controlled, crossover study. Mov Disord 2003;18(10):1108–14.

71. Lerdal A, Gay CL. Fatigue in the acute phase after first stroke predicts poorer physical health 18 months later. Neurology 2013;81(18):1581–7.

72. Christensen D, Johnsen SP, Watt T, et al. Dimensions of post-stroke fatigue: a two-year follow-up study. Cerebrovasc Dis 2008;26:134–41.

73. Young CA, Mills RJ, Gibbons C, Thornton EW. Poststroke fatigue: the patient perspective. Top Stroke Rehabil 2013;20(6):478–84.

74. Snaphaan L, van der Werf S, de Leeuw FE. Time course and risk factors of post-stroke fatigue: a prospective cohort study. Eur J Neurol 2011;18:611–17.

75. Kutlubaev MA, Shenkin SD, Farrall AJ, et al. CT and clinical predictors of fatigue at one month after stroke. Cerebrovasc Dis Extra 2013;3(1):26–34.

76. Hoang CL, Salle JY, Mandigout S, et al. Physical factors associated with fatigue after stroke: an exploratory study. Top Stroke Rehabil 2012;19(5):369–76.

77. Choi-Kwon S, Choi J, Kwon SU, Kang DW, Kim JS. Fluoxetine is not effective in the treatment of poststroke fatigue: a double-blind, placebo-controlled study. Cerebrovasc Dis 2007;23:103–8.

78. Farrell-Carnahan L, Franke L, Graham C, McNamee S. Subjective sleep disturbance in veterans receiving care in the Veterans Affairs Polytrauma System following blast-related mild traumatic brain injury. Mil Med 2013;178(9):951–6.

79. Wäljas M, Lange R, Hakulinen U, et al. Biopsychosocial outcome after uncomplicated mild traumatic brain injury. J Neurotrauma 2014;31:108–24.

80. Belmont A, Agar N, Hugeron C, Gallais B, Azouvi P. Fatigue and traumatic brain injury. [Article in English, French.] Ann Readapt Med Phys 2006;49(6):283–8, 370–4.

81. Schönberger M, Herrberg M, Ponsford J. Fatigue as a cause, not a consequence of depression and daytime sleepiness: a cross-lagged analysis. J Head Trauma Rehabil 2014;29:427–31.

82. Ponsford JL, Ziino C, Parcell DL, et al. Fatigue and sleep disturbance following traumatic brain injury—their nature, causes, and potential treatments. J Head Trauma Rehabil 2012;27(3):224–33.

83. On AY, Oncu J, Atamaz F, Durmaz B. Impact of post-polio fatigue on quality of life. J Rehabil Med 2006;38:329–32.

84. Östlund G, Wahlin Å, Sunnerhagen KS, et al. Post polio syndrome: fatigued patients a specific subgroup? J Rehabil Med 2011;43(1):39–45.

85. Viana CF, Pradella-Hallinan M, Quadros AA, Marin LF, Oliveira AS. Circadian variation of fatigue in both patients with paralytic poliomyelitis and post-polio syndrome. Arq Neuropsiquiatr 2013;71(7):442–5.

86. Trojan DA, Genrdon D, Cashman NR. Anticholinesterase-responsive neuromuscular junction transmission defects in post-poliomyelitis fatigue. J Neurol Sci 1993;114(2):170–7.

87. Ostlund G, Borg K, Wahlin A. Cognitive functioning in post-polio patients with and without general fatigue. J Rehabil Med 2005;37(3):147–51.

88. Bruno RL, Cohen JM, Frick NM. The neuroanatomy of post-polio fatigue. Arch Phys Med Rehabil 1994;75:498–504.

89. Araujo MAD, de Silva TM, Moreira GA, et al. Sleep disorders frequency in post-polio syndrome patients caused by periodic limb movements. Arq Neuropsiquiatr 2010;68(1):35–8.

90. Hsu AA, Staats BA. "Postpolio" sequelae and sleep-related disordered breathing. Mayo Clin Proc 1998;73(3):216–24.

91. Chan KM, Amirjani N, Sumrain M, Clarke A, Strohschein FJ. Randomized controlled trial of strength training in post-polio patients. Muscle Nerve 2003;27:332–8.

92. Bruno R, Zimmerman J, Creange S, et al. Bromocriptine in the treatment of post-polio fatigue: a pilot study with implications for the pathophysiology of fatigue. Am J Phys Med Rehabil 1996;75(5):340–7.

93. Paul RH, Cohen RA, Goldstein JM, Gilchrist JM. Fatigue and its impact on patients with myasthenia gravis. Muscle Nerve 2000;23:1402–6.

94. Elsais A, Wyller VB, Loge JH, Kerty E. Fatigue in myasthenia gravis: is it more than muscular weakness? BMC Neurol 2013;13(1):132.

95. Askmark H, Haggård L, Nygren I, Punga AR. Vitamin D deficiency in patients with myasthenia gravis and improvement of fatigue after supplementation of vitamin D_3: a pilot study. Eur J Neurol 2012;19(12):1554–60.

96. Ramirez C, Piemonte MEP, Callegaro D, Da Silva HC. Fatigue in amyotrophic lateral sclerosis: frequency and associated factors. Amyotroph Lateral Scler 2008;9(2):75–80.

97. Kent-Braun JA, Miller RG. Central fatigue during isometric exercise in amyotrophic lateral sclerosis. Muscle Nerve 2000;23:909–14.

98. Vucic S, Cheah BC, Kiernan MC. Maladaptation of cortical circuits underlies fatigue and weakness in ALS. Amyotroph Lateral Scler 2011;12(6):414–20.

99. Lo Coco D, La Bella V. Fatigue, sleep, and nocturnal complaints in patients with amyotrophic lateral sclerosis. Eur J Neurol 2012;19(5):760–3.

100. Merkies ISJ, Schmitz PIM, Samijn JPA, van der Meché FG, van Doorn PA. Fatigue in immune-mediated polyneuropathies. Neurology 1999;53(8):1648–54.

101. Garssen MPG, van Koningsveld R, Van Doorn PA. Residual fatigue is independent of antecedent events and disease severity in Guillain-Barré syndrome. J Neurol 2006;253(9):1143–6.

102. Ruhland JL, Shields RK. The effects of a home exercise program on impairment and health-related quality of life in persons with chronic peripheral neuropathies. Phys Ther 1997;77(10):1026–39.

103. Carter G, Han J, Mayadev A. Modafinil reduces fatigue in Charcot–Marie–Tooth disease type 1A: a case series. Am J Hosp Palliat Care 2006;23(5):412–16.

104. Kalkman S, Schillings ML, van der Werf SP, et al. Experienced fatigue in facioscapulohumeral dystrophy, myotonic dystrophy, and HMSN-1. J Neurol Neurosurg Psychiatry 2005;76(10):1406–9.

105. Salva MQ, Blumen M, Jacquette A, et al. Sleep disorders in childhood-onset myotonic dystrophy type 1. Neuromuscul Disord 2006; 16(9–10):564–70.

106. Sharafkhaneh A, Melendez J, Akthar F, Lan C. Fatigue in cardiopulmonary conditions. Sleep Med Clin 2013;8(2):221–7.

107. Theander K, Unosson M. Fatigue in patients with chronic obstructive pulmonary disease. J Adv Nurs 2004;45(2):172–7.

108. Akinci AC, Yildirim E. Factors affecting health status in patients with chronic obstructive pulmonary disease. Int J Nurs Pract 2013;19(1):31–8.

109. Paddison JS, Effing TW, Quinn S, Frith PA. Fatigue in COPD: association with functional status and hospitalisations. Eur Respir J 2013;41(3):565–70.

110. Zhang Y, Sun XG, Yang WL, Tan XY, Liu JM. Inspiratory fraction correlates with exercise capacity in patients with stable moderate to severe COPD. Respir Care 2013;58(11):1923–30.

111. Saey D, Lemire BB, Gagnon P, et al. Quadriceps metabolism during constant workrate cycling exercise in chronic obstructive pulmonary disease. J Appl Physiol 2011;110(1):116–24.

112. McNicholas WT, Verbraecken J, Marin JM. Sleep disorders in COPD: the forgotten dimension. Eur Respir Rev 2013;22(129):365–75.

113. Hynninen MJ, Pallesen S, Hardie J, et al. Insomnia symptoms, objectively measured sleep, and disease severity in chronic obstructive pulmonary disease outpatients. Sleep Med 2013;14(12):1328–33.

114. Cavalcante AG, de Bruin PF, de Bruin VM, et al. Restless legs syndrome, sleep impairment, and fatigue in chronic obstructive pulmonary disease. Sleep Med 2012;13(7):842–7.

115. Doyle T, Palmer S, Johnson J, et al. Association of anxiety and depression with pulmonary-specific symptoms in chronic obstructive pulmonary disease. Int J Psychiatry Med 2013;45(2):189–202.

116. Lewko A, Bidgood PL, Jewell A, Garrod R. Evaluation of multidimensional COPD-related subjective fatigue following a pulmonary rehabilitation programme. Respir Med 2014;108(1):95–102.

117. Kapella MC, Herdegen JJ, Perlis M, et al. Cognitive behavioral therapy for insomnia comorbid with COPD is feasible with preliminary evidence of positive sleep and fatigue effects. Int J Chron Obstruct Pulmon Dis 2011;6:625–35.

118. Fini A, de Almeida Lopes Monteiro da Cruz D. Characteristics of fatigue in heart failure patients: a literature review. Rev Lat Am Enfermagem 2009;17(4):557–65.

119. Fink AM, Gonzalez RC, Lisowski T, et al. Fatigue, inflammation, and projected mortality in heart failure. J Card Fail 2012;18(9):711–16.

120. Guglin M, Patel T, Darbinyan N. Symptoms in heart failure correlate poorly with objective haemodynamic parameters. Int J Clin Pract 2012;66(12):1224–9.

121. Shah AB, Udeoji DU, Baraghoush A, et al. An evaluation of the prevalence and severity of pain and other symptoms in acute decompensated heart failure. J Palliat Med 2013;16(1):87–90.

122. Drexler H, Coats AJ. Explaining fatigue in congestive heart failure. Annu Rev Med 1996;47:241–56.

123. Broström A, Strömberg A, Dahlström U, Fridlund B. Sleep difficulties, daytime sleepiness, and health-related quality of life in patients with chronic heart failure. J Cardiovasc Nurs 2004;19(4):234–42.

124. Smith OR, Kupper N, Schiffer AA, Denollet J. Somatic depression predicts mortality in chronic heart failure: can this be explained by covarying symptoms of fatigue? Psychosom Med 2012;74(5):459–63.

125. Kalra PR, Morley C, Barnes S, et al. Discontinuation of beta-blockers in cardiovascular disease: UK primary care cohort study. Int J Cardiol 2013;167(6):2695–9.

126. Chung CJ, Schulze PC. Exercise as a nonpharmacologic intervention in patients with heart failure. Phys Sportsmed 2011;39(4):37–43.

127. Bossola M, Di Stasio E, Antocicco M, Tazza L. Qualities of fatigue in patients on chronic hemodialysis. Hemodial Int 2013;17(1):32–40.

128. Masoumi M, Naini AE, Aghaghazvini R, Amra B, Gholamrezaei A. Sleep quality in patients on maintenance hemodialysis and peritoneal dialysis. Int J Prev Med 2013;4(2):165–72.

129. Karadag E, Kilic SP, Metin O. Relationship between fatigue and social support in hemodialysis patients. Nurs Health Sci 2013;15:164–71.

130. Horigan A, Rocchiccioli J, Trimm D. Dialysis and fatigue: implications for nurses—a case study analysis. Medsurg Nurs 2012;21(3):158–75.

131. Iannuccelli C, Spinelli FR, Guzzo MP, et al. Fatigue and widespread pain in systemic lupus erythematosus and Sjögren's syndrome: symptoms of the inflammatory disease or associated fibromyalgia? Clin Exp Rheumatol 2012;30(6 S74):117–21.

132. Butt Z, Rao AV, Lai JS, Abernethy AP, Rosenbloom SK, Cella D. Age-associated differences in fatigue among patients with cancer. J Pain Symptom Manage 2010;40(2):217–23.

133. Butt Z, Rosenbloom SK, Abernethy AP, et al. Fatigue is the most important symptom for advanced cancer patients who have had chemotherapy. J Natl Compr Canc Netw 2008;6(5):448–55.

134. Sanford SD, Wagner LI, Beaumont JL, et al. Longitudinal prospective assessment of sleep quality: before, during, and after adjuvant chemotherapy for breast cancer. Support Care Cancer 2013;21(4):959–67.

135. Balachandran DD, Faiz S, Bashoura L, Manzullo E. Cancer-related fatigue and sleep disorders. Sleep Med Clinics 2013;8(2); 229–234.

136. Cella D, Kallich J, McDermott A, Xu X. The longitudinal relationship of hemoglobin, fatigue and quality of life in anemic cancer patients: results from five randomized clinical trials. Ann Oncol 2004;15(6):979–86.

137. Eton DT, Cella D. Do erythropoietic-stimulating agents relieve fatigue? A review of reviews. Cancer Treat Res 2011;157:181–94.

138. Schwartz AL, Mori M, Gao R, Nail LM, King ME. Exercise reduces daily fatigue in women with breast cancer receiving chemotherapy. Med Sci Sports Exerc 2001;33(5):718–23.

139. Barsevick AM, Irwin MR, Hinds P, et al. Recommendations for high-priority research on cancer-related fatigue in children and adults. J Natl Cancer Inst 2013;105(19):1432–40.

140. Vargas S, Antoni MH, Carver CS, et al. Sleep quality and fatigue after a stress management intervention for women with early-stage breast cancer in southern Florida. Int J Behav Med 2014;21:971–81.

141. Wessely S, Powell R. Fatigue syndromes: a comparison of chronic "postviral" fatigue with neuromuscular and affective disorders. J Neurol Neurosurg Psychiatry 1989;52:940–8.

142. Wessely S, Chalder T, Hirsch S, Wallace P, Wright D. Psychological symptoms, somatic symptoms, and psychiatric disorder in chronic fatigue and chronic fatigue syndrome: a prospective study in the primary care setting. Am J Psychiatry 1996;153(8):1050–9.

143. Harvey SB, Wessely S, Kuh D, Hotopf M. The relationship between fatigue and psychiatric disorders: evidence for the concept of neurasthenia. J Psychosom Res 2009;66(5):445–54.

144. Marin H, Menza MA. Specific treatment of residual fatigue in depressed patients. Psychiatry (Edgmont) 2004;1(2):12–18.

145. Wessely S, Chalder T, Hirsch S, Wallace P, Wright D. The prevalence and morbidity of chronic fatigue and chronic fatigue syndrome: a prospective primary care study. Am J Public Health 1997;87(9):1449–55.

146. Moss-Morris R, Deary V, Castell B. Chronic fatigue syndrome. Handb Clin Neurol 2013;110:303–14.

147. Schillings ML, Kalkmanb JS, van der Werf SP, et al. Diminished central activation during maximal voluntary contraction in chronic fatigue syndrome. Clin Neurophysiol 2004;115:2518–24.

148. Cockshell SJ, Mathias JL. Cognitive deficits in chronic fatigue syndrome and their relationship to psychological status, symptomatology, and everyday functioning. Neuropsychology 2013;27(2):230–42.

149. Tirelli U, Chierichetti F, Tavio M, et al. Brain positron emission tomography (PET) in chronic fatigue syndrome: preliminary data. Am J Med 1998;105(3s1):54S–58S.

150. Mariman A, Delesie L, Tobback E, et al. Undiagnosed and comorbid disorders in patients with presumed chronic fatigue syndrome. J Psychosom Res 2013;75(5):491–6.

151. Jackson M, Bruck D. Sleep abnormalities in chronic fatigue syndrome/myalgic encephalomyelitis: a review. J Clin Sleep Med 2012;8(6):719–28.

152. Le Bon O, Fischler B, Hoffmann G, et al. How significant are primary sleep disorders and sleepiness in the chronic fatigue syndrome? Sleep Res Online 2000;3(2):43–8.

153. McKenzie R, O'Fallon A, Dale J, et al. Low-dose hydrocortisone for treatment of chronic fatigue syndrome: a randomized controlled trial. JAMA 1998;280(12):1061–6.

154. Vollmer-Conna U, Hickie I, Hadzi-Pavlovic D, et al. Intravenous immunoglobulin is ineffective in the treatment of patients with chronic fatigue syndrome. Am J Med 1997;103(1):38–43.

155. Montoya JG, Kogelnik AM, Bhangoo M, et al. Randomized clinical trial to evaluate the efficacy and safety of valganciclovir in a subset of patients with chronic fatigue syndrome. J Med Virol 2013;85(12):2101–9.

156. Akarsu S, Tekin L, Ay H, et al. The efficacy of hyperbaric oxygen therapy in the management of chronic fatigue syndrome. Undersea Hyperb Med 2013;40(2):197–200.

157. Butler S, Chalder T, Ron M, Wessely S. Cognitive behaviour therapy in chronic fatigue syndrome. J Neurol Neurosurg Psychiatry 1991;54(2):153–8.

158. Fulchera K, White P. Randomised controlled trial of graded exercise in patients with the chronic fatigue syndrome. BMJ 1997;314(7095):1647–52.

CHAPTER 37

Role of positive pressure therapy on sleep disordered breathing and cognition in the elderly

Molly E. Zimmerman and Mark S. Aloia

Sleep disordered breathing in older adults

Prevalence rates of sleep disordered breathing (SDB) in the elderly have been reported to reach as high as 62%, considerably greater than those of middle- and younger-aged adults [1,2]. Several theories have been proposed for these staggering rates, including age-related changes in the upper airway musculature and age-related changes in sleep architecture [3]. SDB is a general term that describes the presence of abnormal respiratory events in sleep. Sleep apnea syndrome is diagnosed when apneas (complete breathing pauses) and hypopneas (partial breathing pauses) are present during sleep in conjunction with other symptoms (eg, excessive daytime sleepiness). Breathing events must last at least 10 s to be characterized as a breathing abnormality. These breathing events may occur up to several hundred times per night and frequently result in variable arterial oxygen desaturations (hypoxemia) and involuntary arousals that lead to sleep fragmentation. SDB is related to cognitive dysfunction as well as changes in brain structure and function [4–6]. SDB is also associated with a wide range of cardiovascular and cerebrovascular conditions (eg, hypertension and stroke), depression, anxiety, obesity, metabolic syndrome, and motor vehicle accidents [7–10]. There are three primary types of sleep apnea events: obstructive sleep apnea (OSA), central sleep apnea, and mixed sleep apnea. OSA is typically diagnosed when breathing events number at least 5 (apneas or hypopneas) per hour of sleep. If the patient has fewer than 15 events per hour of sleep, then associated daytime symptoms or cardiovascular comorbidities are required to make the diagnosis. The International Classification of Sleep Disorders (ICSD) diagnostic criteria currently do not have age-specific definitions for OSA, although different age-based thresholds have been proposed, given the prominent prevalence differences between younger and older adults [11,12]. CSA is characterized by the presence of apneas and hypopneas associated with a patent upper airway and reduced respiratory muscle effort. Individuals sleeping at high altitudes, with stroke, or with Cheyne–Stokes respiration commonly experience central sleep apnea events [13]. Mixed sleep apnea refers to a combination of obstructive and central features, such as the presence of upper airway collapse at the end of a central apnea event. Obstructive, central, and mixed respiratory events cause both sleep fragmentation and intermittent drops in arterial oxygenation that are quantified

using the apnea–hypopnea index (AHI: the number of apneas and hypopneas per hour of sleep) and the respiratory disturbance index (RDI: the number of apneas and hypopneas associated with arousals from sleep). An effective treatment for OSA is nightly use of a positive airway pressure (PAP) device, such as a continuous positive airway pressure (CPAP) machine. PAP functions as a pneumatic splint for the upper airway through use of an external air pump and a nasal mask. Although studies have shown that proper use of PAP significantly reduces behavioral and biological sequelae associated with OSA (eg, excessive daytime sleepiness, impaired driving performance, depressed mood, and hypertension), long-term adherence is often poor owing to mask discomfort, claustrophobia, and general aversions to nightly use of the machine in bed [14–17]. Several studies have shown dose–response relationships between exposure to PAP and various behavioral outcomes, with "optimal" levels of adherence varying as a function of outcome [17,18]. Efforts to improve PAP adherence include device design enhancements (eg, heated humidification of the mask and pressure ramp settings) and behavioral interventions (eg, motivational interviewing and cognitive–behavioral therapy) [19–22].

SDB and cognition in older adults

The identification of both age and SDB as risk factors for cognitive decline in the elderly has led researchers to focus on relationships between SDB and cognition among older adults (for a review, see [23]). Table 37.1 summarizes characteristics of these studies and their major findings. Study samples are largely drawn from three populations: community-dwellers, sleep or general medical clinics, and memory disorders clinics or nursing homes. Herein, we summarize extant findings and highlight key studies.

Community-based studies

Community-based studies of SDB provide observations that are applicable to the general population, particularly older adults who may experience abnormal respiratory events during sleep but have never been formally diagnosed with a clinical sleep disorder. Some community-based studies have been largely negative, reporting no significant relationships between SDB and cognition [24–27]. Others have reported relationships between abnormal nocturnal respiratory events and poorer performance on tests of

Table 37.1 Sleep disordered breathing and cognition in elderly adults

Authors, year reference	Sample setting, design	Subjects				Major findings
		N	Age	Gender	SDB severity	
Yamout et al., 2012 [43]	Memory clinic, cross-sectional	108 (65 MCI, 43 dementia)	74 (9)	49 M 59 W	DI = 7 (11)	◆ ↑DI associated with attention and executive function ◆ Strength of association influenced by cardiovascular disease
Yaffe et al., 2011 [35]	Community, longitudinal	105 SDB 193 NC	83 (3) SDB 82 (3) NC	Women	AHI N = 298: median=10; interquartile range = 5–20	◆ SDB: ↑hypoxemia had ↑risk of developing MCI or dementia over 5 years of follow-up ◆ Sleep fragmentation and duration not associated with cognition
Kim et al., 2011 [39]	Clinic, cross-sectional	30 MCI 30 NC	68 (4) MCI 67 (4) NC	42 M 18 W	AHI: 13 (12) MCI; 15 (14) NC	◆ ↑AHI associated with ↓language in MCI
Blackwell et al., 2011 [28]	Community, cross-sectional	2909	76 (6)	Men	43% had AHI ≥ 15	◆ ↑hypoxemia associated with ↓vigilance
Sforza et al., 2010 [27]	Community, cross-sectional	827	68 (2)	343 M 484 W	AHI: 20 (15); 53% had AHI ≥ 15	◆ No relationships
Cooke et al., 2009 [59]	Clinical trial follow-up	10 (5 CPAP+, 5 CPAP−) with dementia	76 (6)	7 M 3 M	N/A	◆ CPAP+ showed less cognitive decline with sustained use (mean 13.3 months) following completion of previous clinical trial [60]
Ancoli-Israel et al., 2008 [60]	Clinical trial	52 (27 CPAP, 25 placebo) with dementia	79 (7) CPAP; 78 (8) placebo	39 M 13 W	Baseline AHI: 30 (16) CPAP; 27 (16) placebo	◆ 3 weeks of therapeutic CPAP in both groups associated with ↑ executive function and memory
Spira et al., 2008 [32]	Community, cross-sectional	448	83 (3)	Women	AHI: 16 (15); 13% had AHI ≥ 30	◆ ↑AHI and ↑hypoxemia& ↑ central apnea associated with ↓global cognition ◆ APOE4+ associated with 5× risk of cognitive impairment
Alchanatis et al., 2008 [36]	Sleep clinic, cross-sectional	58 OSAS 41 NC	Range = 32–65 OSAS; Range = 33–63 NC	N/A	AHI: range 31–137 OSAS; range 1–7 NC	◆ OSAS patients ≥ 50 years had ↓reaction time compared with age-matched controls and younger OSAS and controls
Mathieu et al., 2008 [40]	Sleep clinic, cross-sectional	28 OSAS 30 NC	38 (2) OSAS younger; 62 (2) OSAS older	26 M 2 W	AHI: 51 (4) OSAS younger; 43 (4) OSAS older	◆ No group-by-age interaction for cognitive performance ◆ Main effects for both group and age
O'Hara et al., 2005 [33]	Community, cross-sectional	36	70(6) APOE4+ 72 (10) APOE4−	12 M 24 W	AHI: 9 (8) APOE4+; 6 (7) APOE4−	◆ ↑AHI associated with ↓verbal delayed recall memory in APOE4+ only ◆ Hypoxemia not associated with cognition
Kim et al., 2007 [31]	Community, cross-sectional	611	Range = 35–74	346 M 265 W	AHI: median = 2.8; range = 0–121	◆ SDB associated with ↓vigilance in older adults
Aloia et al., 2003 [37]	Clinic, cross-sectional	12	65 (6) OSAS compliant; 65 (3) noncompliant	N/A	RDI: 51 (20) OSAS compliant; 46 (22) OSAS noncompliant	◆ ↑RDI associated with verbal delayed recall memory ◆ ↑hypoxemia associated with verbal delayed recall memory and construction
Foley et al., 2003 [25]	Community, cross-sectional	718	Range = 79–97	Men	71% had AHI ≥ 5; 19% had AHI ≥ 30	◆ No relationships
Boland et al., 2002 [24]	Community, cross-sectional	1700	62; range = 52–75	837 M 923 W	RDI median range: 0.4–23	◆ No relationships
Cohen-Zion et al., 2001 [34]	Community, longitudinal	46	80 (3)	7 M 39 W	RDI: 10 (9)	◆ ↑ EDS associated with ↓ global cognitive decline over 3 years of follow-up ◆ Hypoxemia and RDI not associated with cognition

(continued)

Table 37.1 Continued

Authors, year reference	Sample setting, design	Subjects				Major findings
		N	Age	Gender	SDB severity	
Dealberto et al., 1996 [29]	Community, cross-sectional	1389	65 (3)	574 M 815 W	Questionnaire: breathing stoppage and snoring	◆ Breathing stoppage and snoring associated with ↓ attention
Hayward et al., 1992 [30]	Community, cross-sectional	96	78 (4)	21 M 75 W	RDI: 6 (6)	◆ RDI associated with "cerebral efficiency" factor (attention and executive function measures) at baseline assessment
Phillips et al., 1992 [26]	Community, cross-sectional	92	64 (9)	44 M 48 W	AHI:3 (4)	◆ No relationships
Ancoli-Israel et al., 1991 [42]	Nursing home, cross-sectional	235	Median age 80 M, 84 W	83 M 152 W	70% had RDI ≥ 5	◆ Severe SDB associated with ↓ attention, executive function, and memory
Berry et al., 1990 [38]	Sleep clinic, cross-sectional	8 OSAS 12 HC	67 (5) OSAS 68 (2) HC	Men	AHI: 28 (12) OSAS; 3 (3) NC	◆ OSAS: ↓ nonverbal IQ and nonverbal memory delayed recall
Yesavage et al., 1985 [41]	Sleep clinic, cross-sectional	41	70 (6)	Men	RDI: 26 (30); 73% had RDI > 5	◆ RDI associated with ↓ attention and executive function

Age and symptom severity presented as mean (standard deviation) unless otherwise specified; M: men; W: women; DI: desaturation index (number of drops of oxygen saturation ≥4% per hour recording; AHI: apnea–hypopnea index; RDI: respiratory disturbance index; EDS: excessive daytime sleepiness; MCI : mild cognitive impairment; NC: normal control; OSAS: obstructive sleep apnea syndrome; CPAP: continuous positive airway pressure; APOE4: apolipoprotein E ε4 allele; IQ: intelligence quotient.

vigilance, attention, and executive function [28–31]. The possible contributing role of the apolipoprotein E ε4 (*APOE4*) allele, a genetic risk factor for late-onset Alzheimer disease, was highlighted in two studies that found associations between SDB and general cognitive impairment [32] or impaired memory [33] that were unique to older adults who were *APOE4*+. Two notable longitudinal community-based studies distinguished between the negative impacts of excessive daytime sleepiness (EDS), sleep fragmentation, and/or hypoxemia on cognitive function in the elderly. Cohen-Zion and colleagues [34] found that EDS, but not hypoxemia or RDI, was associated with decline on a global cognition measure over a 3-year period. However, Yaffe and colleagues [35] found that it was hypoxemia associated with SDB, and not sleep fragmentation, that was the strongest contributor to the development of dementia or cognitive impairment in older women. In addition to providing some etiological specificity, these studies are noteworthy because they provide valuable information on the directionality of the relationship between SDB and cognitive function, suggesting that SDB may lead to cognitive decline in community-dwelling older adults.

Sleep or general medical clinic studies

Sleep clinic-based studies have the advantage of being able to examine detailed measures of SDB using overnight polysomnography (PSG) in study participants with the most severe respiratory events. Many of these studies show significant relationships between SDB and cognitive performance, with the most consistent findings being in the memory domain, although reaction time, attention, executive function, visuospatial construction, and language have also been reported [36–41]. Three notable studies will be highlighted here. In 1985, Yesavage and colleagues [41] conducted the first clinic-based study of SDB and cognition in 41 older men. They found that more severe SDB was associated with poorer performance

on tests of attention and executive function. In the first study to include a healthy control comparison group, Berry and colleagues [38] reported that SDB was associated with overall cognitive abilities and memory in eight older men with OSA compared with 12 healthy controls. Finally, the first study to examine cognition as a function of PAP adherence in older adults [37] found that RDI was associated with memory performance, while hypoxemia measures were associated with memory and construction abilities. Other clinic-based studies have conducted direct comparisons between older and younger adults with OSA in order to specifically address the possible compounding effect of age on cognition and SDB relationships. While one study [40] reported that younger adults with OSA may be more vulnerable to the effects of hypoxemia on cognition because they are unable to adapt to the intermittent oxygen desaturations, another study [36] reported an opposing finding that it is actually older adults with OSA who are more vulnerable to the effects of hypoxemia on cognition owing to the availability of fewer neural resources to support compensatory efforts.

Memory disorders clinic or nursing home studies

Studies of SDB that draw their samples from memory disorders clinics or nursing homes are important because they are able to focus on individuals whose primary presentation is clinically significant cognitive impairment. This provides a comparison for samples drawn from sleep clinics and indirect cross-sectional evidence for possible bidirectionality of the relationship between SDB and cognition in older adults. That is, while it is commonly proposed that SDB may cause brain dysfunction that may be clinically expressed as cognitive impairment, it is also possible that brain dysfunction associated with dementia may lead to the development of abnormal breathing events. Such causal attributions, however, can only be determined through longitudinal study designs. A seminal investigation by Ancoli-Israel and colleagues

[42] conducted cognitive assessment and portable sleep studies in 235 nursing home patients. They found that 70% demonstrated an RDI ≥ 5 and 96% displayed cognitive impairments consistent with a diagnosis of dementia. Older adults with more severe SDB had poorer scores on subscales measuring attention, executive function, and memory. These findings support the notion that SDB and dementia are strongly associated, but do not provide evidence of directionality or outcomes associated with treatment. A more recent study by Yamout and colleagues [43] used ambulatory nocturnal pulse oximetry screening to report that more severe levels of hypoxemia were associated with poorer performance on tests of attention and executive function among 108 older adults with dementia and mild cognitive impairment (MCI: a term used to describe individuals at high risk for developing dementia). These findings persisted after accounting for age, sex, education, and depressive symptoms. In addition, they were most prominent among individuals with a history of cardiovascular disease, consistent with other literature that suggests that vascular disease has a critical moderating or mediating effect on these relationships in the elderly.

Role of PAP with regard to cognitive function in middle-aged adults with SDB

PAP is the treatment of choice for OSA because it effectively reduces the sleep fragmentation and hypoxemia that define the disorder. Given that longitudinal community-based studies [34,35] have shown that subclinical SDB is a strong predictor of the development of cognitive impairment and dementia, much research has focused on PAP with the hope that it may mitigate or even reverse the deleterious effects of SDB on cognition. Findings from many of these studies, largely carried out in middle-aged adults, have been positive. Reviewed in detail most recently by Ferini-Strambi and colleagues [44], studies vary by design (eg, case–control or within-subjects), inclusion/exclusion criteria, adherence to PAP, and length of PAP treatment. Nonetheless, reports provide support for improvements in vigilance, attention, psychomotor speed, executive function, and memory following PAP treatment [18,45–51]. However, it is important to note that some studies found only modest cognitive gains of uncertain clinical significance in a small number of cognitive domains relative to the total number surveyed (eg, [46,51]). The Apnea Positive Pressure Long-Term Efficacy Study (APPLES) [52–54] was the first large-scale randomized, double-blind, sham-controlled, multicenter trial to examine whether PAP improved cognitive function in middle-aged adults within a 6-month follow-up period. Baseline data [54] were essentially negative and did not survive adjustment for demographic confounders. Follow-up data [53] were also negative for cognitive improvement, revealing a small improvement in executive function at 2 months that did not persist at a 6-month follow-up visit. The authors concluded that "CPAP use resulted in mild, transient improvement in the most sensitive measures of executive and frontal-lobe function for those with severe disease, which suggests the existence of a complex OSA-neurocognitive relationship." Bliwise [55,56] commented in detail on several aspects of the APPLES study design that may have influenced findings, including the primary emphasis on cardiovascular outcomes and the exclusion of individuals with mild cognitive impairment and dementia. In addition, as Bliwise has argued, the individuals in the

APPLES study demonstrated intact cognitive performance on specific cognitive tests and overall high general intellectual functioning at baseline (for example, the average IQ score was nearly one standard deviation *above* the standard population mean); therefore it is inherently clinically and statistically unlikely that such individuals would demonstrate a cognitive gain in response to *any* type of intervention. It may also be that these high-functioning individuals have some genetic protective factor against apnea. This is an important but subtle issue that should be a critical consideration for any future investigation that seeks to study cognitive performance.

Role of PAP with regard to cognitive function in older adults with SDB

Randomized clinical trials focused on older adults are necessary to fully explicate the complex relationship among aging, SDB, and cognitive function. An important series of randomized, double-blind, placebo-controlled clinical trials from Ancoli-Israel and colleagues examined the effect of PAP on a range of neurobehavioral outcomes in older adults with SDB and dementia. Although the generally small sample size varied slightly across studies (i.e, 39–52), the overall design included community-dwelling older adults with mild–moderate Alzheimer disease and SDB who were randomly assigned to either (1) 6 weeks of therapeutic PAP or (2) 3 weeks of sham PAP followed by 3 weeks of therapeutic PAP. Initial studies demonstrated that dementia patients were able to tolerate PAP treatment [57], reported a reduction in excessive daytime sleepiness in response to PAP treatment [58], and demonstrated improvements in sleep architecture associated with PAP use [59]. When cognitive function was examined as an outcome [60], the results indicated that cognitive performance improved after 3 weeks of therapeutic PAP, particularly in the domains of memory and executive function. This finding was particularly exciting, as it suggested that cognitive dysfunction could be reversed in those older adults who stand to benefit the most from interventions, namely, those with dementia. Finally, a preliminary study from the same research group [59] examined sustained PAP use among a subset of study participants from the parent randomized clinical trial who continued to use PAP by their own choice following the completion of the study. Although the sample sizes were small (five who continued PAP versus five who discontinued PAP), after an average 13-month follow-up period, those dementia patients who continued to use PAP demonstrated less cognitive decline, an improvement in sleep quality, and stabilization of depressive symptoms and daytime sleepiness compared with dementia patients who discontinued PAP. This was an important contribution to the literature, as it provided additional evidence supporting the role of PAP in the alleviation of cognitive decline in a highly prevalent and clinically devastating neurodegenerative disease.

Conclusions and future directions

Epidemiological and community-based studies have convincingly shown that SDB is common among the elderly and is associated with a wide range of neurobehavioral and psychosocial outcomes that include cognitive dysfunction. Although PAP is an effective treatment for SDB, its impact on SDB-associated cognitive sequelae in the elderly requires further systematic examination. Guided by the previously reviewed studies, the following considerations for future work are provided:

1. Additional randomized clinical trials of PAP use in older adults with SDB are needed. Prior work is lauded for seminal findings in an understudied population. Although sample sizes were modest, future studies may benefit from identification to barriers to treatment in this vulnerable population in order to increase study enrollment and generalizability of findings.

2. Studies of cognitive change in response to PAP intervention should include individuals with a wide range of cognitive function, particularly those who are cognitively impaired. Individuals performing at or above the population mean are unlikely to show cognitive gains, because they have little to no room for improvement. In addition, future studies would benefit from differentiation between clinically significant cognitive changes versus statistically significant cognitive changes. Psychometric properties of neurocognitive tests should also be reviewed, as some tests are more sensitive to changes than others owing to their measurement properties.

3. Dose–response relationships between exposure to PAP and various behavioral outcomes may exist, with "optimal" levels of adherence varying as a function of outcome. Elucidation of such thresholds would have important implications for the development of treatment guidelines and motivational practices, particularly for individuals struggling with PAP adherence.

4. The effects of SDB disease severity and potential contributing roles of hypoxemia, sleep fragmentation, and/or EDS to cognitive function should prospectively be differentiated.

5. Particularly relevant to the study of older adults, onset and length of SDB exposure should be estimated and considered in analyses and the interpretation of findings as appropriate.

6. Given the prominent role of *APOE4+* genotype to risk for both SDB and dementia, future studies should examine its potential moderating role as well as the contribution of other candidate genotypes. Such genotypes might also represent a protection against the cognitive effects of SDB.

7. It is important to examine potential moderating or mediating roles of cardiovascular and cerebrovascular disease with regard to the relationships among aging, PAP use, cognitive function, and SDB.

8. PAP use characteristics should be reported and explicitly studied. For instance, what is the optimal length of PAP treatment? What is the optimal level of PAP adherence? Does this vary in older adults compared with younger and middle-aged adults?

References

1. Ancoli-Israel S, Kripke DF, Klauber MR, et al. Sleep-disordered breathing in community-dwelling elderly. Sleep 1991;14(6):486–95.
2. Young T, Palta M, Dempsey J, et al. The occurrence of sleep-disordered breathing among middle-aged adults. N Engl J Med 1993;328(17):1230–5.
3. Launois SH, Pepin JL, Levy P. Sleep apnea in the elderly: a specific entity? Sleep Med Rev 2007;11(2):87–97.
4. Aloia MS, Arnedt JT, Davis JD, et al. Neuropsychological sequelae of obstructive sleep apnea–hypopnea syndrome: a critical review. J Int Neuropsychol Soc 2004;10(5):772–85.
5. Bucks RS, Olaithe M, Eastwood P. Neurocognitive function in obstructive sleep apnoea: a meta-review. Respirology 2013;18(1):61–70.
6. Zimmerman ME, Aloia MS. A review of neuroimaging in obstructive sleep apnea. J Clin Sleep Med 2006;2(4):461–71.
7. Babson KA, Del Re AC, Bonn-Miller MO, et al. The comorbidity of sleep apnea and mood, anxiety, and substance use disorders among obese military veterans within the Veterans Health Administration. J Clin Sleep Med 2013;9(12):1253–8.
8. Kabir A, Ifteqar S, Bhat A. Obstructive sleep apnea in adults. Hosp Pract 2013;41(4):57–65.
9. Logan AG, Perlikowski SM, Mente A, et al. High prevalence of unrecognized sleep apnoea in drug-resistant hypertension. J Hypertens 2001;19(12):2271–7.
10. Silverberg DS, Oksenberg A, Iaina A. Sleep-related breathing disorders as a major cause of essential hypertension: fact or fiction? Curr Opin Nephrol Hypertens 1998;7(4):353–7.
11. Berry DT, Webb WB, Block AJ. Sleep apnea syndrome. A critical review of the apnea index as a diagnostic criterion. Chest 1984;86(4):529–31.
12. American Academy of Sleep Medicine. International classification of sleep disorders: diagnostic and coding manual, 2nd ed. Westchester, IL: American Academy of Sleep Medicine, 2005.
13. De Backer WA. Central sleep apnea, pathogenesis and treatment: an overview and perspective. Eur Respir J 1995;8(8):1372–83.
14. Aloia MS, Arnedt JT, Stepnowsky C, et al. Predicting treatment adherence in obstructive sleep apnea using principles of behavior change. J Clin Sleep Med 2005;1(4):346–53.
15. Mazza S, Pepin JL, Naegele B, et al. Driving ability in sleep apnoea patients before and after CPAP treatment: evaluation on a road safety platform. Eur Respir J 2006;28(5):1020–8.
16. McMahon JP, Foresman BH, Chisholm RC. The influence of CPAP on the neurobehavioral performance of patients with obstructive sleep apnea hypopnea syndrome: a systematic review. WMJ 2003;102(1):36–43.
17. Weaver TE, Grunstein RR. Adherence to continuous positive airway pressure therapy: the challenge to effective treatment. Proc Am Thorac Soc 2008;5(2):173–8.
18. Zimmerman ME, Brickman AM, Paul RH, et al. Normalization of memory performance and positive airway pressure adherence in memory-impaired patients with obstructive sleep apnea. Chest 2006;130(6):1772–8.
19. Aloia MS, Arnedt JT, Riggs RL., et al. Clinical management of poor adherence to CPAP: motivational enhancement. Behav Sleep Med 2004;2(4):205–22.
20. Aloia MS, Arnedt JT, Strand M, et al. Motivational enhancement to improve adherence to positive airway pressure in patients with obstructive sleep apnea: a randomized controlled trial. Sleep 2013;36(11):1655–62.
21. Richards D, Bartlett DJ, Wong K, et al. Increased adherence to CPAP with a group cognitive behavioral treatment intervention: a randomized trial. Sleep 2007;30(5):635–40.
22. Weaver TE. Predicting adherence to continuous positive airway pressure—the role of patient perception. J Clin Sleep Med 2005;1(4):354–6.
23. Zimmerman ME, Aloia MS. Sleep-disordered breathing and cognition in older adults. Curr Neurol Neurosci Rep 2012;12(5):537–46.
24. Boland LL, Shahar E, Iber C, et al. Measures of cognitive function in persons with varying degrees of sleep-disordered breathing: the Sleep Heart Health Study. J Sleep Res 2002;11(3):265–72.
25. Foley DJ, Masaki K, White L, et al. Sleep-disordered breathing and cognitive impairment in elderly Japanese-American men. Sleep 2003;26(5):596–9.
26. Phillips BA, Berry DT, Schmitt FA, et al. Sleep-disordered breathing in the healthy elderly. Clinically significant? Chest 1992;101(2):345–9.
27. Sforza E, Roche F, Thomas-Anterion C, et al. Cognitive function and sleep related breathing disorders in a healthy elderly population: the SYNAPSE study. Sleep 2010;33(4):515–21.
28. Blackwell T, Yaffe K, Ancoli-Israel S, et al. Associations between sleep architecture and sleep-disordered breathing and cognition in older

community-dwelling men: the Osteoporotic Fractures in Men Sleep Study. J Am Geriatr Soc 2011;59(12):2217–25.

29. Dealberto MJ, Pajot N, Courbon D, Alperovitch A. Breathing disorders during sleep and cognitive performance in an older community sample: the EVA Study. J Am Geriatr Soc 1996;44(11):1287–94.

30. Hayward L, Mant A, Eyland A, et al. Sleep disordered breathing and cognitive function in a retirement village population. Age Ageing 1992;21(2):121–8.

31. Kim H, Dinges DF, Young T. Sleep-disordered breathing and psychomotor vigilance in a community-based sample. Sleep 2007;30(10):1309–16.

32. Spira AP, Blackwell T, Stone KL, et al. Sleep-disordered breathing and cognition in older women. J Am Geriatr Soc 2008;56(1):45–50.

33. O'Hara R, Schroder CM, Kraemer HC, et al. Nocturnal sleep apnea/hypopnea is associated with lower memory performance in APOE ε4 carriers. Neurology 2005;65(4):642–4.

34. Cohen-Zion M, Stepnowsky C, Marler M, et al. Changes in cognitive function associated with sleep disordered breathing in older people. J Am Geriatr Soc 2001;49(12):1622–7.

35. Yaffe K, Laffan AM, Harrison SL, et al. Sleep-disordered breathing, hypoxia, and risk of mild cognitive impairment and dementia in older women. JAMA 2011;306(6):613–19.

36. Alchanatis M, Zias N, Deligiorgis N, et al. Comparison of cognitive performance among different age groups in patients with obstructive sleep apnea. Sleep Breath 2008;12(1):17–24.

37. Aloia MS, Ilniczky N, Di Dio P, et al. Neuropsychological changes and treatment compliance in older adults with sleep apnea. J Psychosom Res 2003;54(1):71–6.

38. Berry DT, Phillips BA, Cook YR, et al. Geriatric sleep apnea syndrome: a preliminary description. J Gerontol 1990;45(5):M169–74.

39. Kim SJ, Lee JH, Lee DY, et al. Neurocognitive dysfunction associated with sleep quality and sleep apnea in patients with mild cognitive impairment. Am J Geriatr Psychiatry 2011;19(4):374–81.

40. Mathieu A, Mazza S, Decary A, et al. Effects of obstructive sleep apnea on cognitive function: a comparison between younger and older OSAS patients. Sleep Med 2008;9(2):112–20.

41. Yesavage J, Bliwise D, Guilleminault C, et al. Preliminary communication: intellectual deficit and sleep-related respiratory disturbance in the elderly. Sleep 1985;8(1):30–3.

42. Ancoli-Israel S, Klauber MR, Butters N, et al. Dementia in institutionalized elderly: relation to sleep apnea. J Am Geriatr Soc 1991;39(3):258–63.

43. Yamout K, Goldstein FC, Lah JJ, et al. Neurocognitive correlates of nocturnal oxygen desaturation in a memory clinic population. J Clin Exp Neuropsychol 2012;34(3):325–32.

44. Ferini-Strambi L, Marelli S, Galbiati A, Castronovo C. Effects of continuous positive airway pressure on congnitition and neuroimaging data in sleep apnea. Int J Psychophysiol 2013;89(2):203–12.

45. Antic NA, Catcheside P, Buchan C, et al. The effect of CPAP in normalizing daytime sleepiness, quality of life, and neurocognitive function in patients with moderate to severe OSA. Sleep 2011;34(1):111–19.

46. Bardwell WA, Ancoli-Israel S, Berry CC, Dimsdale JE. Neuropsychological effects of one-week continuous positive airway pressure treatment in patients with obstructive sleep apnea: a placebo-controlled study. Psychosom Med 2001;63(4):579–84.

47. Engleman HM, Kingshott RN, Wraith PK, et al. Randomized placebo-controlled crossover trial of continuous positive airway pressure for mild sleep apnea/hypopnea syndrome. Am J Respir Crit Care Med 1999;159(2):461–7.

48. Ferini-Strambi L, Baietto C, Di Gioia MR, et al. Cognitive dysfunction in patients with obstructive sleep apnea (OSA): partial reversibility after continuous positive airway pressure (CPAP). Brain Res Bull 2003;61(1):87–92.

49. Lim W, Bardwell WA, Loredo JS, et al. Neuropsychological effects of 2-week continuous positive airway pressure treatment and supple-mental oxygen in patients with obstructive sleep apnea: a randomized placebo-controlled study. J Clin Sleep Med 2007;3(4):380–6.

50. Munoz A, Mayoralas LR, Barbe F, et al. Long-term effects of CPAP on daytime functioning in patients with sleep apnoea syndrome. Eur Respir J 2000;15(4):676–81.

51. Ryan CM, Bayley M, Green R, et al. Influence of continuous positive airway pressure on outcomes of rehabilitation in stroke patients with obstructive sleep apnea. Stroke 2011;42(4):1062–7.

52. Kushida CA, Nichols DA, Quan SF, et al. The Apnea Positive Pressure Long-term Efficacy Study (APPLES): rationale, design, methods, and procedures. J Clin Sleep Med 2006;2(3):288–300.

53. Kushida CA, Nichols DA, Holmes TH, et al. Effects of continuous positive airway pressure on neurocognitive function in obstructive sleep apnea patients: the Apnea Positive Pressure Long-Term Efficacy Study (APPLES). Sleep 2012;35(12):1593–602.

54. Quan SF, Chan CS, Dement WC, et al. The association between obstruc-tive sleep apnea and neurocognitive performance—the Apnea Positive Pressure Long-Term Efficacy Study (APPLES). Sleep 2011;34(3):303–14.

55. Bliwise DL, Greenaway MC. Will APPLES hit a ceiling? Sleep 2011;34(3):249–50.

56. Bliwise DL. Alzheimer's disease, sleep apnea, and positive pressure therapy. Curr Treat Options Neurol 2013;15(6):669–76.

57. Ayalon L, Ancoli-Israel S, Stepnowsky C, et al. Adherence to continuous positive airway pressure treatment in patients with Alzheimer's disease and obstructive sleep apnea. Am J Geriatr Psychiatry 2006;14(2):176–80.

58. Chong MS, Ayalon L, Marler M, et al. Continuous positive airway pressure reduces subjective daytime sleepiness in patients with mild to moderate Alzheimer's disease with sleep disordered breathing. J Am Geriatr Soc 2006;54(5):777–81.

59. Cooke JR, Ayalon L, Palmer BW, et al. Sustained use of CPAP slows deterioration of cognition, sleep, and mood in patients with Alzheimer's disease and obstructive sleep apnea: a preliminary study. J Clin Sleep Med 2009;5(4):305–9.

60. Ancoli-Israel S, Palmer BW, Cooke JR, et al. Cognitive effects of treating obstructive sleep apnea in Alzheimer's disease: a randomized controlled study. J Am Geriatr Soc 2008;56(11):2076–81.

SECTION 8

Parasomnias

CHAPTER 38

REM sleep behavior disorder

Ronald B. Postuma

Introduction

Rapid eye movement (REM) sleep behavior disorder (RBD) is caused by loss of the normal atonia of REM sleep, allowing patients to "act out their dreams." Manifestations range from mild occasional sleep-talking and transient movements to severe yelling, kicking, and thrashing. The primary differential diagnoses are non-REM (NREM) parasomnia and pseudo-RBD due to obstructive sleep apnea (OSA). Usually a careful history can accurately distinguish the two, but only a polysomnogram (PSG) to document loss of REM atonia and rule out mimics can confirm the diagnosis. The goal of treatment is mainly to reduce injury. In addition to bed safety measures, melatonin and clonazepam are generally effective, although surveillance for side effects of somnolence, falls and cognitive impairment is required. In its idiopathic form, RBD occurs in just over 1% of the population over 60. RBD also can be triggered by medications, particularly antidepressants. However, RBD is most commonly associated with neurological disease, in particular neurodegenerative synucleinopathy: Parkinson disease (PD), dementia with Lewy bodies (DLB), and multiple system atrophy (MSA). In this case, it is related to neurodegeneration of pontine (subcoeruleus) and/or medullary (ventromedial medulla) structures that regulate REM atonia. Most cases of "idiopathic" RBD are in fact in early prodromal stages of neurodegeneration, and are at over 70% risk of eventually developing parkinsonism or dementia. This has profound implications for patient counseling and management, as well as for the understanding and eventual treatment of neurodegenerative disease.

Epidemiology of RBD

Few comprehensive studies of idiopathic RBD prevalence have been performed, mainly because proper study requires conducting PSG in the general population. The only true population-based PSG study was recently performed in Korean men and women aged 60 and over [1]. PSGs were evaluated for abnormal REM tone, and all those with increased tone were assessed for dream enactment behavior. This produced a prevalence estimate of 1.2%. Asymptomatic loss of REM atonia was diagnosed in an additional 5%. This estimate is consistent with population-based estimates of 0.4% and 0.5% for severe RBD (i.e, only assessing cases that have resulted in injury) [2,3]. The great majority of patients never present to sleep clinics, so RBD is vastly underdiagnosed.

In sleep clinics, the majority of patients are male, and most are over 50. The age distribution likely reflects the demographics of neurodegenerative synucleinopathy in the population. The reason for the sex difference is less clear. Although neurodegenerative synucleinopathies are more common in men, selection bias is also possible. Men may be more likely to present to medical attention with dream enactment behavior, owing to potential differences in aggressivity of dream content and consequent need for medical attention, different levels of awareness or concern of bed partners, and a lower likelihood of being widowed, owing to sex-specific mortality rates. A second demographic cluster occurs among psychiatric patients, mainly because of antidepressant-induced RBD (perhaps better termed antidepressant-triggered RBD, since many patients show signs of prodromal neurodegeneration [4]). Among medication-associated RBD, demographics are skewed younger and there is no longer a clear male predominance [5].

Risk factors for idiopathic RBD are somewhat similar to those of PD and DLB. Patients with RBD are more likely to have had occupational pesticide exposure and to have experienced head trauma [6]. They may be more likely to report a family history of dream enactment; this may either reflect differential recognition of dream enactment (patients with RBD are more likely to ask family members about similar symptoms) or could point to a true genetic component to RBD [7]. Family history of dementia also increased risk of conversion to defined neurodegenerative disease [8]. Like dementia, patients with idiopathic RBD also have lower levels of education than controls. Strikingly unlike PD, patients with RBD are more likely to smoke, and do not have lower exposure to caffeine (and neither caffeine nor smoking affected risk of conversion to neurodegenerative disease [8]). RBD patients are also more likely than controls to report a history of ischemic heart disease, as well as a history of depression (the latter association is probably consistent with antidepressant-triggered RBD) [9].

Clinical diagnosis of RBD

Rigorous and careful history taking is key in making a diagnosis. The majority of RBD patients in sleep clinics present with a complaint of dream enactment behavior. Typically, the bed partner first becomes aware of the problem, and bed partners remain the key to obtaining accurate history. Patients without bed partners may present with injuries from falls out of bed or from striking objects, or may have noticed items from the bed table knocked over. Often, especially among patients with neurodegenerative synucleinopathy, the history is subtler, and must be actively elicited. For example, any PD patient who falls from bed while asleep probably has RBD. They may also present with isolated sleep-talking/laughing, or minor movements that have not concerned the bed partner.

The range of manifestations of dream enactment in RBD is very broad, and reflects the diversity of dream content. Generally, most bed partners will be able to identify the movement as "acting out of their dreams," particularly if patients waken soon after an episode. Although many patients will mumble, sleep-talking can also be clearly articulated, often sounding like "one half of a conversation." Movements in the limbs can be minor, sometimes confined to myoclonic twitches (note that occasional myoclonic twitches can be a normal phenomenon of REM sleep). When of larger amplitude, there is often a subtle limb ataxia [10]. Hands are often limp, and held in a wrist-flexion posture. Movements related to aggressive dream content are notably common in idiopathic RBD; this may reflect a true change in dream content, or may be an artifact of selection bias (those with disturbing dream enactment are more likely to seek out medical attention). Of note, movements can be quite brisk in parkinsonian patients who are unable to perform these rapid movements during wakefulness [11].

Dating the onset of RBD can be particularly problematic. Most patients without a medication trigger will have noticed a gradual onset of symptoms. In many cases, bed partners can recall a very long history of milder symptoms, dating from the beginning of the relationship. It is unclear whether these symptoms were a true prodrome of RBD, a general susceptibility to sleep movements unrelated to degeneration of REM atonia nuclei, or variations of normal behavior. Mild symptoms of dream enactment can occur in up to 15% of normal controls [12]; in most of these cases, there is no loss of REM atonia, and, given a 3–5% lifetime prevalence of synucleinopathies, most presumably do not have an underlying neurodegenerative cause.

In evaluating a complaint of dream enactment behavior, there are two critical differential diagnoses; NREM parasomnia and OSA (a.k.a. pseudo-RBD [13]). A third alternate diagnosis is of frontal lobe seizures, which can also occasionally appear like dream enactment with bizarre behavior, yelling, and posturing; for this reason, epileptic abnormalities on the sleep electroencephalogram (EEG) should be ruled out. Other, very different sleep movements (periodic limb movements of sleep, hypnic myoclonus, etc.) can usually be readily distinguished on history. OSA is often more prominent during REM sleep, because the normal REM atonia exacerbates apnea. Episodes probably reflect arousals from REM sleep rather than true dream enactment. In many cases, patients will be hypoxic or will waken incompletely, resulting in prolonged episodes of confused or bizarre behavior. It should be recognized that OSA is common, and so many patients with true RBD may have OSA that is unrelated to their RBD. If REM atonia is clearly abnormal on PSG, and if manifestations continue despite successful treatment with continuous positive airway pressure (CPAP), then idiopathic RBD can still be diagnosed.

Usually, the most difficult differential diagnosis is between RBD and NREM parasomnia. The following clues can help distinguish these conditions:

1. Unlike NREM parasomnia, RBD patients cannot walk during an episode; if they leave the bed, they might take one or two steps, but will soon fall.

2. During RBD episodes, eyes are closed. This limits contact with the environment; for example, they cannot deliberately reach for an object that is not in their immediate vicinity. They may grab objects that happen to touch their hands or may hit partners because of random thrashing, but will not deliberately reach.

3. Since patients with NREM parasomnia are "half awake," they may interact with their environment during an episode. For

example, they may talk back when addressed, use objects appropriately, open doors, etc. RBD patients will not generally respond to the environment in a meaningful way, unless woken.

4. Unlike NREM parasomnia, if woken during an episode, RBD patients often become rapidly alert and appropriate. They may be able to provide an explanation for the movements, related to their recent dream content. In contrast, NREM parasomnia patients usually have a gradual emergence from episodes, or will quickly return to sleep.

5. The nature of sleep-talking differs. Although both groups may mumble or yell out, the characteristic sustained "one half of a conversation" (like being in a room with a person speaking on the telephone) does not occur in NREM parasomnia.

6. Demographics differ—NREM parasomnia patients have a younger onset and often have a family history. Idiopathic RBD patients are usually older and male, or, in the case of medication-induced RBD, have a history of psychiatric disease and antidepressant use.

7. The time of behavior differs. NREM parasomnia episodes emerge from slow-wave sleep, which predominates early in the night. RBD episodes predominate later, in the early morning hours.

It should be noted that patients can have both RBD and NREM parasomnia, the "parasomnia overlap" syndrome [14]. These patients are generally younger, and the NREM parasomnia component is most prominent in the clinical presentation. Psychiatric disease and antidepressant exposure occur in some, but associated neurodegenerative disease is uncommon.

PSG diagnosis of RBD

In cases of idiopathic RBD, PSG is essential for making the diagnosis. Diagnostic criteria for RBD (according to the International Classification of Sleep Disorders, Second Edition, ICSD-2 as well as ICSD-3 [15]) primarily center on two features:

1. Loss of the normal atonia associated with REM sleep;

2. Dream enactment behavior—this can be diagnosed either on history or on direct observation during the PSG.

By definition, patients presenting to sleep clinics with complaints of dream enactment behavior have already met criterion 2. So, observation of dream enactment behavior during PSG is not required for diagnosis. The main purpose of PSG in this setting is to document loss of REM atonia.

The gold standard method for tone evaluation is manual scoring during REM sleep (see Figs. 38.1 and 38.2 for examples of PSG findings in RBD). There is no universally agreed upon standard for what constitutes abnormal REM atonia. The Montplaisir method quantifies both phasic and tonic REM in the chin (mentalis) [16]. If tonic REM (defined as amplitude 2 times baseline) exceeds 30% of REM epochs, or phasic activity (defined as amplitude 4 times baseline) exceeds 15%, then tone is defined as abnormal. Using this method, sensitivity was 89% and specificity 83% (compared with the gold standard of final clinical impression). The SINNBAR method combines phasic and tonic REM in a combined "any" tone measure, and a cut-off of 18% in the mentalis is defined as abnormal [17] (with >90% sensitivity and 100% specificity in the original publication). Addition of limb muscles (particularly the flexor

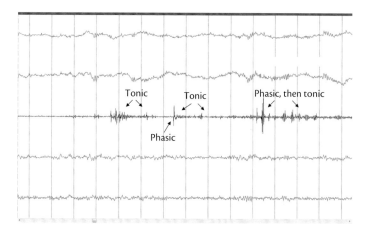

Fig. 38.1 Illustration of abnormal tonic and phasic REM in a patient with RBD. Measurements are taken from the mentalis muscle.

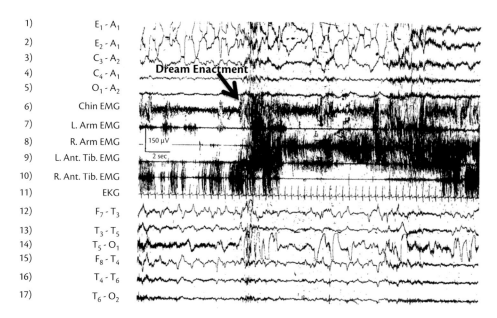

Fig. 38.2 Illustration of a severe RBD episode on PSG. Electromyography (EMG) leads show severe loss of REM atonia, followed by an episode of dream enactment (arrow) with generalized EMG activity related to vigorous movements.

digitorum superficialis) can further increase sensitivity without sacrificing specificity. For this, the combined cut-off is 32%. Neither of the methods has perfect sensitivity, so it is possible that some true cases of RBD are missed with current quantification methods. For practical reasons, most centers use a single-night recording, as night-to-night variability is relatively modest. However, a second night can be useful in the case of equivocal results on the first night.

Manual scoring is time-consuming and requires specialized training, limiting real-world applicability. Recently, automated scoring techniques to quantitate REM atonia have been developed [18,19]. These techniques still require manual correction to eliminate artifacts and arousals. Although currently confined to research contexts, these may eventually be used as an alternative to manual scoring in non-specialized centers.

In the absence of a history of dream enactment, criterion 2 can also be met by direct observation of dream enactment movements during REM sleep on overnight video. There are no clear criteria for what constitutes dream enactment. Clinicians must be aware that

transitory myoclonic movements can be observed during normal REM sleep. In addition, care must be taken to distinguish dream enactment from movements during arousals. Moreover, it has been suggested that occasional apparent dream enactment movements (termed "REM behavioral events") may occur normally (among 15% of controls in one single-night study [12]). Therefore, caution must be used in diagnosing RBD in patients with no dream enactment history. In fact, the ICSD-3 draft criteria require repeated episodes of sleep-talking or movements; this prevents RBD from being diagnosed in asymptomatic patients based only upon a single-night PSG.

Screening for RBD

PSG is time-consuming and expensive, and especially given the importance of RBD as a prodromal marker of neurodegeneration, it is important to develop methods to screen for RBD. To this end, several screening questionnaires have been developed. The simplest are single-question screens; the Mayo Sleep Questionnaire (which queries bed partners), and the RBD1Q (which queries patients). Both are very similar questions (although independently designed), and are simple to administer. Sensitivity and specificity are good, and the Mayo Sleep Questionnaire has the advantage of being the only RBD questionnaire tested in the general population (with sensitivity 98% and specificity 74%) [20]. The Mayo sleep question is as follows:

Have you ever seen the patient appear to 'act out his or her dreams' (punched or flailed arms in the air, shouted, or screamed) while sleeping?

Follow-up questions are provided in the case of a positive response. The RBD1Q has been tested in sleep center patients, with 94% sensitivity and 87% specificity (sensitivity assessments must be taken with caution, as sleep center patients are already aware of having RBD) [21]. It is free for use, and has been translated into eight languages. It is as follows:

Have you ever been told, or suspected yourself, that you seem to 'act out your dreams' while asleep (for example, punching, flailing your arms in the air, making running movements, etc.)?

Other screening alternatives include the 14-item RBDSQ (96% sensitivity but only 56% specificity) [22], the 13-item RBDQ-HK (82% sensitivity and 87% specificity) [23], and the simpler 5-item Innsbruck Questionnaire (91% sensitivity and 86% specificity) [24]. The RBDQ-HK queries the frequencies of mild to severe manifestations of dream enactment; therefore, with minimal modification, it can be used as a severity scale.

It is essential to realize that idiopathic RBD is uncommon, so the positive predictive value of even an excellent-specificity tool is low. Assuming 1% prevalence, with a 90% specificity screen, only 9% of screen positives will actually have the condition. Therefore, PSG remains essential for diagnosis in the general population. Within neurodegenerative synucleinopathy, the prevalence of RBD can exceed 50%, so the positive predictive value approximates the specificity, and PSG may be less essential in making at least an empirical diagnosis.

Treatment of RBD

The goal of treatment is primarily to reduce the risk of injury to bed partners and patients. There is no clear evidence that dream enactment itself causes substantial impairment of sleep in most cases; therefore, specific pharmacological RBD treatment to improve sleep quality or reduce somnolence is probably not warranted. Nonpharmacological bed safety measures must always be considered; simple measures like placing a soft mattress beside the bed, having a pillow barrier between bed partners, and clearing the night table of glass or sharp objects can help improve safety. Spouses often elect to sleep apart to prevent bed partner injury.

The next step in treatment is to look for reversible triggers. Primary among these are antidepressant medications. If no longer clearly necessary, they can be stopped. If medications are needed, bupropion may be an option, as there have been suggestions that it causes less REM atonia loss [25]. Paradoxically, in severe treatment-resistant cases of idiopathic RBD, antidepressants can be used to reduce REM sleep, and thereby reduce episode frequency (in this case, caution must be used when withdrawing the antidepressant—the only known fatality due to RBD occurred in the context of antidepressant withdrawal). Selegiline, cholinesterase inhibitors and bisoprolol have also been reported to trigger RBD, although only in small series or case reports.

If pharmacological treatment is required, there are two primary options: melatonin and clonazepam. Clonazepam (0.5–2 mg at bedtime) was the first medication used for RBD, and can help up to 90% of patients. Clonazepam does not appear to directly influence tonic REM, but may reduce phasic REM and alter dream content. Melatonin (3–12 mg at bedtime) also helps to reduce RBD, although perhaps less effectively. Observational studies have suggested that melatonin directly increases REM tone. Melatonin also has a small randomized trial supporting its utility [26].

The choice of first-line agent is not straightforward. There have been suggestions that clonazepam is more effective—in a recent observational study, clonazepam resulted in at least moderate improvement in 78% of users, compared with 48% of melatonin users [27]. On the other hand, melatonin is generally better tolerated: 33% of patients on melatonin reported side effects, compared with 61% of clonazepam users. Of concern, the primary side effects of clonazepam (falls, somnolence, and impaired cognition) are also common symptoms of neurodegenerative synucleinopathy; therefore, patients with idiopathic RBD may be at especially high risk. We have recently observed that idiopathic RBD patients taking clonazepam at baseline were more likely to develop a "dementia-first" neurodegenerative synucleinopathy than patients with melatonin. Although alternate explanations are possible (eg, confounding by indication), it may also suggest that clonazepam is causing substantial cognitive impairment. Given these considerations, melatonin may be a safer first-line option.

If monotherapy with clonazepam or melatonin is ineffective, then the next step is probably combined therapy with both agents. If this fails, options may be limited. There have been reports that dopamine agonists may reduce RBD symptoms—this is not consistently observed, but remains a reasonable third-line option. As mentioned above, antidepressants can reduce RBD episode frequency. Other possible options, which have been supported only with case report evidence, include levodopa, cholinesterase inhibitors (also reported by others to trigger RBD), sodium oxybate, and zopiclone [28].

Pathophysiology and disease associations

During normal REM sleep, skeletal muscles (except for the eyes and diaphragm) are essentially paralyzed, via hyperpolarization of spinal neurons. The control of REM atonia relies upon several brain regions and several neurotransmitters. The most critical of these are located in the tegmental pons and medial medulla. In 1965 (before the description of RBD as a clinical syndrome), Jouvet produced RBD-like symptoms in cats by lesioning the pons, in areas corresponding to the subcoeruleus area in humans [29]. Selective loss of REM atonia has also been produced by lesioning rodents in the analogous sublaterodorsal tegmental nucleus, where the existence of a REM atonia flip-flop switch has been proposed [3]0. The subcoeruleus area projects both to spinal cord motor neurons and/or spinal interneurons via a direct pathway, and to the ventromedial medulla via an indirect pathway [31]. The direct and indirect pathways both inhibit muscle tone via glycinergic and GABAergic innervation of spinal motor neurons and interneurons. The different pathways may differentially regulate phasic versus tonic REM.

In humans, there are several case reports documenting that lesions of the pons and medulla can induce RBD, consistent with predictions from animal models. There are reported cases of RBD secondary to pontine/medullary strokes, hemorrhages, brain tumors, and demyelinating lesions. Autoimmune causes, including voltage-gated potassium channel encephalitis, other limbic encephalitides, and a newly described parasomnia overlap syndrome with antibodies against the neural cell adhesion molecule IgLON5, have been clearly documented [32]. There are also reports of RBD occurring in progressive supranuclear palsy, spinocerebellar ataxias (especially type III), and the Guam PD–dementia–ALS complex [33]. Many of these syndromes are associated with brainstem pathology. Apparent dream enactment behavior has also been frequently described in Huntington disease, although a recent detailed PSG analysis has suggested that this is not true RBD.

However, RBD may also occur without apparent pontine/medullary lesions. An animal model with generalized motor activation during sleep, including RBD, has been created by selective reduction of GABA and glycine transmission [34]. There are also examples of human RBD not associated with focal neurological damage. Antidepressants commonly trigger RBD, possibly by increasing the direct serotoninergic activation of lower motor and cranial nerves (an activation that normally turns off during REM sleep) [10]. RBD is also commonly seen with narcolepsy, suggesting a role of the hypocretin system in REM atonia; RBD in narcolepsy is part of a general dysregulation of sleep state and sleep stage instability, suggesting potential for a different mechanism. Increased tone (and potentially dream enactment) in narcoleptic RBD may be related to frequent and often partial intrusions of wakefulness during REM sleep. Reported cases of RBD in Guillain–Barré syndrome [35] and in limbic encephalitis without evident brainstem involvement have not been completely explained. Finally, post-traumatic stress has commonly been associated with dream enactment behavior [36]; this might suggest that severe nightmares in the context of general stress can "override" otherwise functioning REM atonia systems. This mechanism may also underlie the occasional dream enactment behavior that can occur in otherwise normal young persons.

Although many conditions are associated with RBD, the large majority of patients have a specific underlying neurodegenerative etiology. This is arguably the most critical feature of RBD, and is discussed in detail in the next section.

RBD and neurological disease

By far, the most common association with RBD is neurodegenerative synucleinopathies. Synucleinopathies refer to diseases associated with deposition of alpha-synuclein in the form of Lewy bodies, Lewy neurites, or glial cytoplasmic inclusions. The three principal synucleinopathies are PD, DLB, and MSA. Combined, they occur in 3–5% of persons over 70. All three conditions have extensive degeneration in pontine structures, consistent with the patho-anatomy of RBD. This synucleinopathy association dwarfs all other associations with neurological disease; in a recent neuropathological study, 94% of patients with probable RBD and neurodegenerative disease (mostly dementia) had synuclein deposition at autopsy [37]. Restricting analysis to those with PSG confirmation (i.e, excluding possible false positives) increased this proportion to 98%. If 94–98% of neurological patients with RBD have underlying synucleinopathy, this is of clinical diagnostic importance in

neurology; for example, documentation of RBD in any patient with amnestic dementia implies that the patient almost certainly has a neurodegenerative synucleinopathy (i.e, DLB/PD dementia), and not Alzheimer disease.

Within established neurodegenerative synucleinopathies, RBD is common. Approximately 75% of DLB patients, 70–90% of MSA patients, and 35–50% of PD patients have RBD. Within PD, the presence of RBD is associated with features of cognitive and autonomic dysfunction (i.e, the primary features of DLB and MSA) [38] and, similarly, DLB patients with PD are more likely to present with early parkinsonism [39]. This highlights the interconnected nature of the synucleinopathies (of note, a recent task force of the Movement Disorders Society concluded that DLB and PD should no longer be considered mutually exclusive diagnostic conditions [40]). RBD also has prognostic implications: PD patients with associated RBD are at much higher risk of dementia [41] and have a worse overall prognosis [42], and DLB patients with RBD have higher mortality [39].

Of profound interest to the neurological community is the time course of the RBD/synucleinopathy connection. In 1996, Schenck et al. described the follow-up of their initial cohort of idiopathic RBD; over a 5-year period, 38% of their patients had developed PD or dementia [43]. Over the subsequent 10 years, 81% of these patients had developed neurodegenerative disease [44]. In the Barcelona cohort of idiopathic RBD patients, 82% had developed either defined neurodegenerative disease or mild cognitive impairment [45] (see Fig. 38.3). An autopsy study of one of these "still-idiopathic" patients documented moderately advanced synucleinopathy [46], and a recent study in this cohort has documented synuclein deposition in submandibular gland needle biopsies in the majority (suggesting the exciting possibility of in vivo pathological diagnosis) [47]. In our cohort, we have seen over 70% of our idiopathic RBD patients develop neurodegeneration [8,48]. Moreover, in all these cohorts, disease conversion rates will continue to climb over time. This has profound implications for our understanding of RBD and of synucleinopathy in general; the large majority of patients with a diagnosis of "idiopathic" RBD are in fact in prodromal stages of a neurodegenerative disease.

The ability of RBD to anticipate PD, DLB, and MSA has a pathological correlate. This has been best encapsulated in the six-stage PD staging system of Braak [49]. Based upon a large series of autopsies stained for synuclein deposition, Braak hypothesized that PD first starts in the dorsal motor nucleus of the vagus, peripheral autonomic nerves, and olfactory structures. At stage II, pontine and medullary structures are affected, including the structures associated with RBD in humans and animal models. This implies that idiopathic RBD probably corresponds to stage II PD. Only at stage III does the dopaminergic substantia nigra become involved (and because of redundancy of the dopaminergic system, patients may not present until stages IV or V). The last three stages are characterized by spread of synuclein to the cortex, resulting in PD dementia. Although the model remains incomplete (eg, DLB is incompletely explained), and with numerous exceptions to this pattern (i.e, many PD patients present with relatively "pure" motor PD), it nonetheless illustrates why RBD is a prodromal feature of PD.

Recognizing that most idiopathic RBD patients are in prodromal stages of neurodegenerative synucleinopathy has immediate clinical relevance. First, a duty of disclosure by the sleep clinician exists. This can range in detail according to the patient's values and

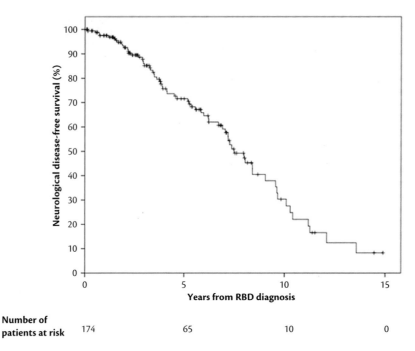

Fig. 38.3 Kaplan–Meier analysis of risk of neurodegenerative disease in a cohort of 174 patients followed in Barcelona. It can be seen that less than 25% of patients remain free of neurodegenerative synucleinopathy at 10 years.

Reproduced from PLoS One, 9, Iranzo A, Fernandez-Arcos A, Tolosa E, et al., Neurodegenerative disorder risk in idiopathic REM sleep behavior disorder: study in 174 patients, pp. e89741, Copyright (2014), PLOS ONE, reproduced under the Creative Commons Attribution License 4.0.

preferences; although patients have the absolute right to know all the details of their condition, they also have the right "not to know." Deciphering the degree of information that is desired requires a great deal of judgment and subtlety. At a minimum, patients need to be aware that their disorder may be an early sign of other neurological problems and so ongoing follow-up is important. Second, there may be treatment opportunities. Currently, there are no clear neuroprotective (or disease-modifying) therapies available for synucleinopathy. So, idiopathic RBD does not imply automatic treatment implications. However, there are numerous excellent symptomatic treatments for DLB, MSA, and especially PD, even in their prodromal stages. These can range from dopamine replacement therapy for motor problems to cholinesterase inhibitors for cognitive impairment and hallucinations (from personal experience particularly effective in this population), as well as effective medications for orthostatic hypotension, constipation, urinary dysfunction, psychiatric symptoms, etc. Therefore, all patients with idiopathic RBD should be offered regular follow-up with neurologists equipped to diagnose and treat these conditions as they emerge. This regular follow-up also provides the opportunity to provide neuroprotective therapy when it becomes available (given the profoundly high risk and early stage of neurodegeneration in idiopathic RBD, these patients may be the ideal candidates for neuroprotective therapy to prevent parkinsonism and dementia) [50].

The ability of RBD to anticipate neurodegenerative synucleinopathy has attracted considerable interest from the PD and DLB community. There is no other marker of prodromal synucleinopathy with anywhere close to the predictive value of RBD. For example, olfactory loss, another well-established prodromal marker, is associated with a two- to fourfold increased risk of PD compared, with a more than 100-fold increase with RBD [51]. In the new prodromal MDS criteria, in any male over 70, RBD alone can suffice to make a diagnosis of prodromal PD; something that no other marker can do [52]. Studying patients with idiopathic RBD can provide a "test-lab" to assess whether other prodromal markers of neurodegeneration can predict disease. Using RBD, the predictive values of abnormal olfaction [53], color vision, quantitative motor testing [54], autonomic function [55], dopaminergic functional neuroimaging [56], substantia nigra ultrasound [56], PD-related network patterns of glucose utilization on PET scanning [57], hippocampal perfusion [58], and electroencephalographic slowing [59] have been directly confirmed. Moreover, following patients with idiopathic RBD allows one to directly witness the evolution of neurodegenerative disease from its prodromal stages; this has led to studies directly observing the pace of evolution of quantitative motor slowing, cardinal parkinsonian signs, dopaminergic denervation [60], olfactory loss, color vision loss, and autonomic dysfunction before fully defined neurodegenerative disease. Finally, and most critically, RBD patients offer the ideal group in which to test future neuroprotective therapies against neurodegenerative disease. In idiopathic RBD, one can intervene early in the disease course (when disease-modifying agents are most likely to be effective), and before symptomatic therapies for parkinsonism and dementia make the reliable assessment of outcome impossible. Stratification of patients by documenting other prodromal features can identify patients with conversion rates exceeding 90% over 5 years, and 60% over 3 years, well within the required parameters for neuroprotective trials [61].

Conclusions

RBD is an intriguing parasomnia, with symptoms that are readily treatable. However, its underlying pathology is not treatable. In addition to insights into the mechanisms of sleep regulation, study of RBD provides a means to study neurodegenerative disease in general. The opportunity to intervene early in a neurodegenerative process is unique, making RBD an especially compelling research target.

References

1. Kang SH, Yoon IY, Lee SD, et al. REM sleep behavior disorder in the Korean elderly population: prevalence and clinical characteristics. Sleep 2013;36:1147–52.
2. Ohayon MM, Caulet M, Priest RG. Violent behavior during sleep. J Clin Psychiatry 1997;58:369–76.
3. Chiu HF, Wing YK, Lam LC, et al. Sleep-related injury in the elderly—an epidemiological study in Hong Kong. Sleep 2000;23:513–17.
4. Postuma RB, Gagnon JF, Tuineaig M, et al. Antidepressants and REM sleep behavior disorder: isolated side effect or neurodegenerative signal? Sleep 2013;36:1579–85.
5. Ju YE, Larson-Prior L, Duntley S. Changing demographics in REM sleep behavior disorder: possible effect of autoimmunity and antidepressants. Sleep Med 2011;12:278–83.
6. Postuma RB, Montplaisir JY, Pelletier A, et al. Environmental risk factors for REM sleep behavior disorder: a multicenter case-control study. Neurology 2012;79:428–34.
7. Dauvilliers Y, Postuma RB, Ferini-Strambi L, et al. Family history of idiopathic REM behavior disorder: a multicenter case–control study. Neurology 2013;80:2233–5.
8. Postuma RB, Iranzo A, Hogl B, et al. Risk factors for neurodegeneration in idiopathic rapid eye movement sleep behavior disorder: a multicenter study. Ann Neurol 2015;77:830–9.
9. Frauscher B, Jennum P, Ju YE, et al. Comorbidity and medication in REM sleep behavior disorder: a multicenter case–control study. Neurology 2014;82:1076–9.
10. Arnulf I. REM sleep behavior disorder: motor manifestations and pathophysiology. Mov Disord 2012;27:677–89.
11. De Cock VC, Vidailhet M, Leu S, et al. Restoration of normal motor control in Parkinson's disease during REM sleep. Brain 2007;130:450–6.
12. Sixel-Doring F, Trautmann E, Mollenhauer B, Trenkwalder C. Rapid eye movement sleep behavioral events: a new marker for neurodegeneration in early Parkinson disease? Sleep 2014;37:431–8.
13. Iranzo A, Santamaria J. Severe obstructive sleep apnea/hypopnea mimicking REM sleep behavior disorder. Sleep 2005;28:203–6.
14. Dumitrascu O, Schenck CH, Applebee G, Attarian H. Parasomnia overlap disorder: a distinct pathophysiologic entity or a variant of rapid eye movement sleep behavior disorder? A case series. Sleep Med 2013;14:1217–20.
15. American Academy of Sleep Medicine. The international classification of sleep disorders, 2nd ed. Diagnostic and coding manual. Westchester, IL: American Academy of Sleep Medicine, 2007.
16. Montplaisir J, Gagnon JF, Fantini ML, et al. Polysomnographic diagnosis of idiopathic REM sleep behavior disorder. Mov Disord 2010;25:2044–51.
17. Frauscher B, Iranzo A, Gaig C, et al. Normative EMG values during REM sleep for the diagnosis of REM sleep behavior disorder. Sleep 2012;35:835–47.
18. Ferri R, Manconi M, Plazzi G, et al. A quantitative statistical analysis of the submentalis muscle EMG amplitude during sleep in normal controls and patients with REM sleep behavior disorder. J Sleep Res 2008;17:89–100.
19. Frauscher B, Gabelia D, Biermayr M, et al. Validation of an integrated software for the detection of rapid eye movement sleep behavior disorder. Sleep 2014;37:1663–71.
20. Boeve BF, Molano JR, Ferman TJ, et al. Validation of the Mayo Sleep Questionnaire to screen for REM sleep behavior disorder in an aging and dementia cohort. Sleep Med 2011;12:445–53.
21. Postuma RB, Arnulf I, Hogl B, et al. A single-question screen for rapid eye movement sleep behavior disorder: a multicenter validation study. Mov Disord 2012;27:913–16.
22. Stiasny-Kolster K, Mayer G, Schafer S, et al. The REM sleep behavior disorder screening questionnaire—a new diagnostic instrument. Mov Disord 2007;22:2386–93.
23. Li SX, Wing YK, Lam SP, et al. Validation of a new REM sleep behavior disorder questionnaire (RBDQ-HK). Sleep Med 2010;11:43–8.
24. Frauscher B, Ehrmann L, Zamarian L, et al. Validation of the Innsbruck REM Sleep Behavior Disorder Inventory. Mov Disord 2012;27:1673–8.
25. Schenck CH, Montplaisir JY, Frauscher B, et al. Rapid eye movement sleep behavior disorder: devising controlled active treatment studies for symptomatic and neuroprotective therapy—a consensus statement from the International Rapid Eye Movement Sleep Behavior Disorder Study Group. Sleep Med 2013;14:795–806.
26. Kunz D, Mahlberg R. A two-part, double-blind, placebo-controlled trial of exogenous melatonin in REM sleep behaviour disorder. J Sleep Res 2010;19:591–6.
27. McCarter SJ, Boswell CL, St Louis EK, et al. Treatment outcomes in REM sleep behavior disorder. Sleep Med 2013;14:237–42.
28. Schenck CH, Mahowald MW. REM sleep behavior disorder: clinical, developmental, and neuroscience perspectives 16 years after its formal identification in SLEEP. Sleep 2002;25:120–38.
29. Jouvet M, Delorme F. Locus coeruleus et sommeil paradoxal. C R Soc Biol 1965;159:895–9.
30. Lu J, Sherman D, Devor M, Saper CB. A putative flip-flop switch for control of REM sleep. Nature 2006;441:589–94.
31. Luppi PH, Clement O, Sapin E, et al. The neuronal network responsible for paradoxical sleep and its dysfunctions causing narcolepsy and rapid eye movement (REM) behavior disorder. Sleep Med Rev 2011;15:153–63.
32. Sabater L, Gaig C, Gelpi E, et al. A novel non-rapid-eye movement and rapid-eye-movement parasomnia with sleep breathing disorder associated with antibodies to IgLON5: a case series, characterisation of the antigen, and post-mortem study. Lancet Neurol 2014;13:575–86.
33. Gagnon JF, Postuma RB, Mazza S, Doyon J, Montplaisir J. Rapid-eye-movement sleep behaviour disorder and neurodegenerative diseases. Lancet Neurol 2006;5:424–32.
34. Brooks PL, Peever JH. Impaired GABA and glycine transmission triggers cardinal features of rapid eye movement sleep behavior disorder in mice. J Neurosci 2011;31:7111–21.
35. Cochen V, Arnulf I, Demeret S, et al. Vivid dreams, hallucinations, psychosis and REM sleep in Guillain–Barré syndrome. Brain 2005;128:2535–45.
36. Manni R, Ratti PL, Terzaghi M. Secondary "incidental" REM sleep behavior disorder: do we ever think of it? Sleep Med 2011;12(Suppl 2):S50–3.
37. Boeve BF, Silber MH, Ferman TJ, et al. Clinicopathologic correlations in 172 cases of rapid eye movement sleep behavior disorder with or without a coexisting neurologic disorder. Sleep Med 2013;14:754–62.
38. Romenets SR, Gagnon JF, Latreille V, et al. Rapid eye movement sleep behavior disorder and subtypes of Parkinson's disease. Mov Disord 2012;27:996–1003.
39. Dugger BN, Boeve BF, Murray ME, et al. Rapid eye movement sleep behavior disorder and subtypes in autopsy-confirmed dementia with Lewy bodies. Mov Disord 2012;27:72–8.
40. Berg D, Postuma RB, Bloem B, et al. Time to redefine PD? Introductory statement of the MDS Task Force on the definition of Parkinson's disease. Mov Disord 2014;29:454–62.
41. Postuma RB, Bertrand JA, Montplaisir J, et al. Rapid eye movement sleep behavior disorder and risk of dementia in Parkinson's disease: a prospective study. Mov Disord 2012;27:720–6.
42. Fereshtehnejad SM, Romenets SR, Anang JB, et al. New clinical subtypes of Parkinson disease and their longitudinal progression: a prospective cohort comparison with other phenotypes. JAMA Neurol 2015;72:863–73.

43. Schenck CH, Bundlie SR, Mahowald MW. Delayed emergence of a parkinsonian disorder in 38% of 29 older men initially diagnosed with idiopathic rapid eye movement sleep behaviour disorder. Neurology 1996;46:388–93.

44. Schenck CH, Boeve BF, Mahowald MW. Delayed emergence of a parkinsonian disorder or dementia in 81% of older males initially diagnosed with idiopathic REM sleep behavior disorder: a 16-year update on a previously reported series. Sleep Med 2013;14:744–8.

45. Iranzo A, Fernandez-Arcos A, Tolosa E, et al. Neurodegenerative disorder risk in idiopathic REM sleep behavior disorder: study in 174 patients. PLoS One 2014;9:e89741.

46. Iranzo A, Gelpi E, Tolosa E, et al. Neuropathology of prodromal Lewy body disease. Mov Disord 2014;29:410–15.

47. Vilas D, Iranzo A, Tolosa E, et al. Assessment of α-synuclein in submandibular glands of patients with idiopathic rapid-eye-movement sleep behaviour disorder: a case-control study. Lancet Neurol 2016;15:708–18.

48. Postuma RB, Gagnon JF, Vendette M, et al. Quantifying the risk of neurodegenerative disease in idiopathic REM sleep behavior disorder. Neurology 2009;72:1296–300.

49. Braak H, Del TK. Nervous system pathology in sporadic Parkinson disease. Neurology 2008;70:1916–25.

50. Postuma RB, Gagnon JF, Montplaisir JY. REM sleep behavior disorder: from dreams to neurodegeneration. Neurobiol Dis 2012;46:553–8.

51. Postuma RB, Aarsland D, Barone P, et al. Identifying prodromal Parkinson's disease: pre-motor disorders in Parkinson's disease. Mov Disord 2012;27:617–26.

52. Berg D, Postuma RB, Adler CH, et al. MDS research criteria for prodromal Parkinson's disease. Mov Disord 2015;30:1600–11.

53. Postuma RB, Gagnon JF, Vendette M, Desjardins C, Montplaisir J. Olfaction and color vision identify impending neurodegeneration in REM behavior disorder. Ann Neurol 2011;69:811–18.

54. Postuma RB, Lang AE, Gagnon JF, Pelletier A, Montplaisir JY. How does parkinsonism start? Prodromal parkinsonism motor changes in idiopathic REM sleep behaviour disorder. Brain 2012;135:1860–70.

55. Postuma RB, Gagnon JF, Pelletier A, Montplaisir J. Prodromal autonomic symptoms and signs in Parkinson's disease and dementia with Lewy bodies. Mov Disord 2013;28:597–604.

56. Iranzo A, Lomena F, Stockner H, et al. Decreased striatal dopamine transporters uptake and substantia nigra hyperechogenicity as risk markers of synucleinopathy in patients with idiopathic rapid-eye-movement sleep behaviour disorder: a prospective study. Lancet Neurol 2010;9:1070–7.

57. Holtbernd F, Gagnon JF, Postuma RB, et al. Abnormal metabolic network activity in REM sleep behavior disorder. Neurology 2014;82:620–7.

58. Dang-Vu TT, Gagnon JF, Vendette M, et al. Hippocampal perfusion predicts impending neurodegeneration in REM sleep behavior disorder. Neurology 2012;79:2302–6.

59. Iranzo A, Isetta V, Molinuevo JL, et al. Electroencephalographic slowing heralds mild cognitive impairment in idiopathic REM sleep behavior disorder. Sleep Med 2010;11:534–9.

60. Iranzo A, Valldeoriola F, Lomena F, et al. Serial dopamine transporter imaging of nigrostriatal function in patients with idiopathic rapid-eye-movement sleep behaviour disorder: a prospective study. Lancet Neurol 2011;10:797–805.

61. Postuma RB, Gagnon JF, Bertrand JA, Genier Marchand D, Montplaisir JY. Parkinson risk in idiopathic REM sleep behavior disorder: preparing for neuroprotective trials. Neurology 2015;84:1104–13.

CHAPTER 39

NREM and other parasomnias

Caterina Ferri, Maria Turchese Caletti,
and Federica Provini

Introduction

Parasomnias are undesirable, but not always pathological, events. They consist of abnormal behaviors during sleep due to an inappropriate activation of cognitive processes or physiological systems such as the motor and/or autonomic nervous systems. Parasomnias may occur during sleep or during the transition from wake to sleep and vice versa. According to the International Classification of Sleep Disorders, parasomnias are distinguished on the basis of the stage of sleep in which they appear: (1) parasomnias arising from non-rapid eye movement (NREM) sleep, which comprise arousal disorders and sleep-related eating disorders; (2) parasomnias associated with rapid eye movement (REM) sleep; (3) "other parasomnias" occurring in any sleep stage [1]. Most parasomnias constitute unusual but physiological manifestations, occurring especially during childhood; they can become pathological if they appear or continue at an inappropriate age or when they are very frequent, associated with a significant impairment of nocturnal sleep or daytime alertness. Nevertheless, parasomnias may also manifest themselves in a violent way with tragic consequences; this is especially true for REM behavior disorder (RBD), which is an REM sleep parasomnia (see Chapter 38 of this volume). In this chapter, we will describe the NREM parasomnias and the "other parasomnias."

NREM parasomnias: arousal disorders

Arousal disorders (ArDs) are motor behaviors arising from deep sleep, usually only once per night and in the first part of the night when deep sleep is prominent. They are most common in children—probably because of the abundance of slow-wave sleep (SWS). ADs include a spectrum of manifestations with overlapping features and increasing complexity, from confusional arousal to sleep terror to sleepwalking [2,3]. They are dissociated states in which awakening and sleeping features coexist [4]. During the episode, the patient seems to be alert, but is sleeping, appearing confused, disoriented, and unresponsive to environmental stimuli. The patient should not be awakened, because this would be counterproductive, prolonging the episode and resulting in resistant or even violent behavior [5]. Usually, there is no recollection of the event the following morning. During ADs, a wide range of behaviors can be seen: inconsolable crying, moaning, screaming, stereotyped and complex actions such as dressing, playing an instrument, or driving a car, or aggressive and injurious behavior, which may have forensic implications. An autonomic activation can also be present.

The pathophysiology of ADs is unknown. It has been proposed that a dysfunctional and independent action of the system involved in NREM sleep and wakefulness is at the basis of these disorders [6,7]. It has been suggested that the occurrence of ADs is due to the association between an abnormal deep sleep and a high SWS fragmentation [8]. Patients with ADs show a normal sleep macrostructure, even though they may present a high arousal index and an increased number of awakenings during sleep, with reduced sleep efficiency [8–10]. An intracerebral EEG study has reported the persistence of delta activity in the hippocampal and frontal associative cortices, accompanied by a local activation of the motor, cingulate, insular and temporopolar cortices, and amygdala during episodes of confusional arousals in a young boy [11].

Loss of the inhibitory function of the frontoparietal cortices, together with activation of the motor and cingulate cortices, could explain the appearance of innate, complex motor patterns [12,13].

Many other factors have been involved in determining ADs, such as developmental, genetic, psychological, and organic ones. In most cases, as the child grows up, ADs become less frequent and intense until they disappear altogether. Genetic influence has been seen in many studies: the concordance between twins is high and the prevalence in first-degree relatives of individuals with ADs is higher than in the general population [14]; however, the transmission mode is still unknown. Psychological factors are sometimes involved, since an association has been found between ADs (especially sleep terrors and sleepwalking) and anxiety level [15–17]. It seems that vulnerability to stress and inadequate coping strategies are common factors predisposing to parasomnias. Stress is related to AD frequency, and experiences like hospitalization, parental divorce, and traumatic events may aggravate the disorder. In susceptible individuals, some stimuli such as deepening sleep factors can precipitate or influence the frequency of ADs: fever, sleep deprivation, intense physical activity, hyperthyroidism, alcohol, and use of central nervous system (CNS) depressant drugs. Also, forced arousals during SWS, such as those induced by auditory stimulation and by intrinsic sleep disorders like obstructive sleep apnea (OSA), periodic limb movements in sleep (PLMS), and restless legs syndrome (RLS), may trigger ADs, inducing repeated arousals [18–20]. Children with neurodevelopmental disorders, like cerebral palsy or Down syndrome, are more likely to have upper airway obstruction, and therefore their prevalence of ADs is higher than that in healthy children.

It is important to differentiate ADs from other parasomnias and from nocturnal frontal lobe epilepsy (NFLE) because of their specific and different management [21]. A detailed description of AD episodes (better if accompanied by home videos) generally facilitates the diagnosis [4]. Attention should be paid to the time of occurrence during the night, the duration of the episodes, and the condition of the patient immediately after the episode [22]. Features supporting the diagnosis of NFLE are the presence of stereotyped and bizarre motor behavior or sustained dystonic–dyskinetic postures, several attacks per night, brief duration of the attacks, onset or persistence into adulthood, and response to antiepileptic medication [21,23–25]. A physical and neurological examination should be done to identify any signs of possible associated sleep disorders [4]. Nocturnal video-polysomnography (VPSG) is useful in the case of frequent attacks or atypical manifestations or when other sleep disorders are associated. If nocturnal seizures are suspected, multiple EEG channels should be included in the VPSG recording montage, even though the EEG presentation of NFLE is often without abnormalities. Rarely, seizures emerge from REM sleep; most such seizures appear during stage 2 NREM. Seizures may occur throughout the night, whereas ADs usually occur during the first hours of sleep. A simple and validated clinical scale called the Frontal Lobe Epilepsy and Parasomnia (FLEP) scale or a structured interview (SINFLE) may be useful for the differential diagnosis [24–26].

Pharmacological treatment is not usually necessary in ADs: the child's parents must be reassured about the benignity of the disorder, which is in most cases self-limiting [3]. Some behavioral advice should be followed, particularly in case of complex motor attacks, to ensure the child's safety. Medications like benzodiazepines and tricyclic drugs should be reserved for children with severe and frequent episodes, when other measures have failed. Adults more often than children require pharmacological treatment—also because of the frequent association of ADs with other disorders. This is shown in Table 39.1.

Confusional arousals

Confusional arousals (CAs) are a less severe form of AD and are defined as "mental confusion or confusional behavior during or following arousals from sleep" [1]. They are generally characterized by incomplete and confused awakenings from deep sleep. This is shown in Fig. 39.1.

Isolated CAs are a common experience also in normal subjects and may affect both children and adults, but in a different way [5]. *CAs in childhood* are almost ubiquitous, rare, or confined to a period of life, and they are not always considered pathological. CAs affect primarily infants and toddlers, arising in almost all cases before the age of 5 years [22]. Their exact prevalence is unknown: detailed epidemiological studies are lacking and the information is largely anecdotal [5,17]. Clinically, during the episode, the child may open his or her eyes, seeming to be alert but appearing confused and unresponsive to environmental stimuli. Movements, moaning, vocalization, and autonomic activation may be present during the episodes, but the attacks are usually quite mild. The episodes can have different durations, from seconds to 15 minutes, subsequently resolving in restful sleep [4]. Usually, on awakening in the morning, the child does not remember the episode, even though the recall ability depends on child's age. Usually, only one episode occurs during the night, within the first 2 hours after going to sleep [5]. Multiple episodes of confusional arousal, however, are not uncommon, although this

Table 39.1 Behavioral advice and management for arousal disorders

	Confusional arousals	Sleep terrors	Sleepwalking
Reassure parents	+	+	+
Avoid precipitating factors	+	+	+
Avoid waking the patient up	+	+	+
Remove obstructions in the bedroom	−	−	+
Cover windows with heavy curtains	−	−	+
Secure windows	−	−	+
Install locks or alarms on outside doors	−	−	+
Use a nightlight	−	−	+
Place barriers in stairways	−	−	+
Sleep on the ground floor	−	−	+
Scheduled awakenings	−	±	±
Pharmacological treatment	±	±	±
Psychotherapy	±	±	±
Hypnosis	−	±	±

fact has not received sufficient emphasis in the research literature or in textbooks. The EEG during a CA shows a mixture of brief episodes of delta activity with theta rhythms and poorly reactive alpha waves intermixed with muscle and movement artifacts [22]. The diagnosis is primarily based on clinical features: a detailed description is sufficient in most cases to identify a CA. Generally, additional information can be obtained by a homemade video recording of the episodes [4], but if the diagnosis remains unclear or if other sleep disorders are suspected, nocturnal VPSG is mandatory. CAs do not require medical treatment, since in most cases the disorder is self-limiting, remitting spontaneously [5].

CAs in adulthood are clinically more heterogeneous than those of childhood, they are more often associated with other sleep or psychiatric disorders and with violent behaviors, and they may consequently lead to legal complications.

The prevalence of CAs in the adult population is about 3–4% [15], with no gender influence. CAs in adulthood may present as typical CAs similar to those of childhood or as sleep drunkenness, sleep inertia, or "automatic episodes." Sleep drunkenness, also known as Elpenor syndrome (from Homer's Odyssey), was formerly considered a synonym of CA. Actually, sleep drunkenness is not strictly a CA: it is defined as a prolonged transition from sleep to waking, with partial alertness, disorientation, poor coordination, instability, and sometimes excited or violent behavior; excessive daytime sleepiness is usually present [5]. Some authors also consider sleep inertia as a CA, even though it is a state of impaired vigilance with confusion and disorientation occurring immediately after awakening in the morning or after a prolonged daytime nap and not during the night [22]. Sleep inertia has a variable and sometimes long duration. The only common feature between sleep

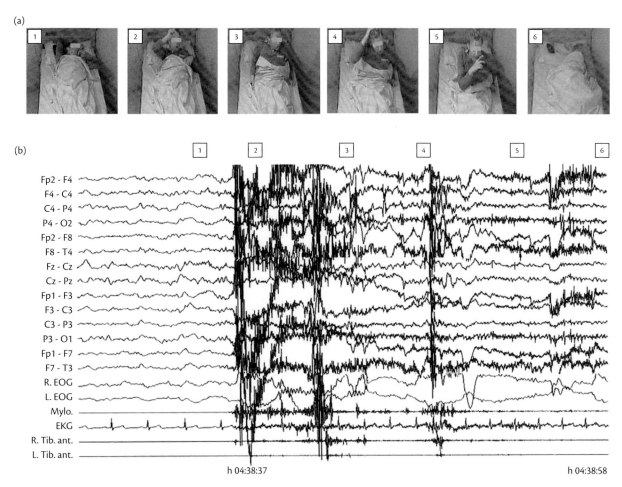

Fig. 39.1 Confusional arousals (CAs). (a) Photo-sequence of a CA episode: (1) the patient is sleeping; (2) he opens his eyes and raises his head and his right arm; (3) he then sits up in bed looking to his left; (4) he scratches his head, appearing confused; (5) he utters some nonsense words while staring into space; (6) he then falls asleep again.

(b) PSG excerpt of the episode. There is an abrupt and brief arousal from deep sleep (note the movement artifacts on the EEG tracing), which is associated with a slight increase in heart rate. EOG: electro-oculogram; Mylo.: mylohyoideus; EKG: electrocardiogram; Tib. Ant.: tibialis anterior muscle; R.: right; L.: left.

inertia and CAs is the presence of mental confusion. In adulthood, motor behavior during a CA can be more vigorous, and violent acts or sleep-related sexual behavior have been reported, with possible legal consequences [27–30]. As in children, CAs may be triggered by sleep deprivation (due both to recreational activities and to shift or night work), but they are more often associated with other sleep disorders like OSA, sleep bruxism, and CNS hypersomnias [15]. It should be emphasized that in adulthood, CAs can be related to the presence of psychological disorders such as adjustment disorder, depression, and bipolar and anxiety disorders. Other medical conditions predisposing to CAs are endocrine disorders, heavy sedation, alcoholism or substance abuse, viral infection, and CNS lesions. More often than children, adults require VPSG in order to clarify the clinical features of the episodes and the possibly associated sleep disorders.

The medical treatment depends on the etiology and the relationship with other sleep disorders: pharmacological therapy with clonazepam or with antidepressants such as imipramine, paroxetine, and trazodone may be useful, while if OSA is present, continuous positive airway pressure (CPAP) is needed [5]. If an underlying psychiatric problem is suspected, an appropriate psychiatric evaluation could be useful.

Sleep terrors

Sleep terrors, also called "pavor nocturnus," are the most dramatic form of AD [1,31]. For a long time, sleep terrors and nightmares were considered synonymous; however, in 1949, Jones was the first to differentiate these two disorders. Later, some studies demonstrated that sleep terrors occurred during SWS and were quite different from nightmares, a typical REM sleep parasomnia [32,33]. Broughton first suggested the hypothesis that sleep terrors were disorders of arousal [34].

Sleep terror emerges in a sudden and unexpected way: the child wakes up, sometimes also opening his or her eyes, cries and screams exaggeratedly and inconsolably, and does not respond to external stimuli like parents' voices. This state of intense agitation and fear is reflected in the patient's facial expression, which appears terrified. Sleep terrors are also accompanied by a "fight or flight response," which implies a considerable autonomic activation characterized by tachycardia, tachypnea, and increased respiratory tidal volume, flushing of the skin, diaphoresis, and mydriasis [4,35]. Patients usually tend to stay in bed during sleep terrors; nevertheless, they sometimes get out of bed and walk or run around the house, with the risk of injuring themselves or other people [29]. The episode ends in a few minutes, most often from 1 to 5, but it can last up to 20 minutes. As the attack stops, the patient simply continues to sleep and generally the next morning does not remember the episode although sometimes remembers feeling completely isolated and frightened [19]. These attacks occur often only once per night. Patients suffering from sleep terrors are usually prepubertal children: the peak prevalence is between 5 and 7 years, but the disorder may appear as early as 2–3 years and may continue up to adolescence [31]. Usually, the child outgrows sleep terrors spontaneously before adolescence [4,15]. The prevalence is not influenced by sex, race, or cultural background, but heredity may play a role since more than one family member may be affected [15,16]. When sleep terrors arise during adulthood, it may be symptomatic of a neurological disease, like a brainstem lesion or a thalamic tumor.

During the episode, the EEG records a diffuse and hypersynchronous delta rhythm with intermixed faster frequencies (alpha or theta) or prominent alpha and beta activity; there are also associated increases in muscle tone, respiratory and heart rate.

The diagnosis of sleep terrors may be suspected on the basis of a clinical evaluation which must include a detailed description of the nocturnal episodes from a witness and also a physical, neurological, and developmental examination [3]. If doubt remains, it is necessary to perform a nocturnal VPSG. The VPSG is useful especially for the differential diagnosis between sleep terrors and other disorders like sleep-related epilepsy (Table 39.2), nightmares, confusional arousal, RBD, nocturnal delirium, and nocturnal panic attacks. VPSG also allows determination of the presence of comorbid sleep disorders such as OSA [4].

Differential diagnosis between sleep terrors and nightmares is based mainly on clinical features. Nightmares are not usually associated with vocalization, major motor activity, or autonomic symptoms, and patients are more easily aroused, do not appear confused after being awakened, and can describe their dream. CAs overlap with less severe sleep terror episodes, but they do not present terror,

intense autonomic arousal and ambulation. RBD is characterized by loss of REM sleep atonia, resulting in dream enacting behavior (DEB). This may be associated with violent behavior, vocalization, and walking during sleep, but the autonomic response is usually absent or mild; nevertheless, some patients have elements of both sleep terrors and RBD with an overlap syndrome. Patients with nocturnal panic attacks frequently show associated psychopathology and present similar episodes during daytime. Psychogenic dissociative episodes can be distinguished by the presence of a waking EEG pattern during the attack.

Management of sleep terrors includes adoption of safety measures to protect patient during the attack, although pharmacological treatment is not usually necessary. The patient should be counseled to prevent sleep deprivation and avoid other triggering factors [3,4]. When the episodes are frequent and occur at a particular time, scheduled awakenings, 15–30 minutes before the attack, may curtail the episode [3,5]. Drug therapy is rarely indicated, and is used only when sleep terrors are very frequent or when the patient's violent behavior puts themself or other family members in danger. Benzodiazepines (eg, clonazepam or diazepam), tricyclic antidepressants (imipramine), and paroxetine or trazodone have been used successfully [5]. Attention must be paid to the appearance of daytime sedation when using benzodiazepines, especially those with long half-life (diazepam): the dose must be increased slowly. In children, satisfactory results have been reported also with L-5-hydroxytryptophan and melatonin [36]. Specific treatment is required when sleep disordered breathing or other neurological diseases are associated. Hypnosis has been found to be effective in both children and adults [37]. The coexistence of psychopathology, in adults, may be treated with psychotherapy and progressive relaxation.

Sleepwalking

Sleepwalking (SW) is a series of complex behaviors, initiated during an arousal from SWS, such as changes in body position, turning and resting on one's hand, staring with open "glassy" eyes, playing with the sheets, sitting up in bed, and resting on the knees [1], which may culminate in walking behavior [20,35]. Both in a scientific and a literary context, different descriptions have been given of a typical sleepwalker; perhaps the best one was given by Roger in 1932: "The sleeper performs various acts with a certain degree of dexterity and can avoid obstacles. But his behavior is characterized by a rigidity, which gives him the appearance of an automation. He can answer questions correctly and is quite receptive to suggestions. At the end of 15–30 minutes of activity, he goes back to bed, sometimes fully clothed, and wakes up the next morning quite surprised to find himself dressed" [38]. Episodes occur rarely, on a weekly or even monthly frequency, usually in the first third of the night [39]. Somnambulistic episodes can last from a few seconds to more than 30 minutes [20,35], and subjects are typically completely or partially amnestic of the event, with little or no recall [40].

Because SW is coupled with an altered state of consciousness and impaired judgment [1], during the episode, sleepwalkers are difficult to awaken and generally confused upon forced awakening. Agitation and aggressive behavior occur rarely, usually when prompted by people attempting to restrain the subject [39]. Nevertheless, there have been isolated reports of sleep-related violence, homicide, and suspected suicide [41], raising fundamental questions about the medico-forensic implications of these acts

Table 39.2 Several differentiating features to establish the correct diagnosis of arousal disorders (ArDs) or nocturnal frontal lobe epilepsy (NFLE)

	ADs	NFLE
Age/gender	Childhood	Any age
	Any gender	Male predominance
Episodes' time of occurrence and frequency	One per night	Several per night
	First third of the night	Any time
Clinical course throughout life	Sporadic episodes	Many episodes every night
	Tendency to disappear	Increasing frequency
Triggering factors	Usually present (fever, sleep deprivation)	Absent
Motor pattern	Heterogeneous	Stereotyped
	Absence of abnormal movements	Dystonic–dyskinetic postures

and the neurophysiological and cognitive states that characterize patients during such episodes [20,35]. Although only few studies have investigated the mental content of sleepwalkers during episodes, some thought-like mentation or fragmentary images have been described [42]. The prevalence of SW in the general population is 1–11% [43] and, more specifically, it has a prevalence of around 3% in toddlers [17], increasing to about 13.5% at 10 years [24], before falling significantly after age 25 [15]. Adults who sleepwalk almost invariably report a history of childhood somnambulism or other ADs previously in life [3]. SW can also arise de novo in adults [24], posing some problems of differential diagnosis with organic, neurological, or psychiatric disorders. Even if there is no evidence suggesting that SW during adulthood is associated with the subsequent development of neuropathological disorders [24], there is a high prevalence of AD in some neurological disorders [39]. Antiarrhythmic medications, cocaine and alcohol abuse, benzodiazepines, and tricyclic agents have been reported as possible triggering factors for SW. Recently, zolpidem has been specifically implicated as a possible inducer of SW episodes in people with sleep-related eating disorder (SRED) [44].

A detailed history of the episode is necessary for the diagnosis; homemade video-recordings can be useful to capture events closest to real-life episodes. If events are stereotypic or repetitive and occur frequently, the patient should be considered for video-EEG monitoring in a sleep laboratory [45]. VPSG is also required in the presence of simultaneous sleep pathologies to establish the precise relationship with these events, and to differentiate SW from NFLE, especially in adults [21,23,46]. Usually, medications are not necessary to treat SW [3] and the "first aid" treatment involves providing a safe sleep environment [39] (Table 39.1). Precipitating factors, such as sleep deprivation or bladder fullness, should be avoided, as should certain medications known to exacerbate SW, including thioridazine, fluphenazine, perphenazine, desipramine, chloral hydrate, and lithium. If SW episodes are very frequent, or when a child or others are in danger because of the related behaviors, imipramine 25–150 mg, diazepam 2–5 mg, or clonazepam 0.5 mg at bedtime can be used [47]. Alternatively, trazodone and selective serotonin reuptake inhibitors (SSRIs) have been successfully employed [48]. Treatment of all related sleep disorders seen as possible precipitating factors should also be addressed [39]. In particular, children with respiratory sleep disorders should be referred for specialist treatment, such as adenotonsillectomy for OSA [19]. Alternative therapies such as hypnosis have proven helpful and safe in several cases [37].

Sexsomnia

Sexsomnia, also called somnambulistic sexual behavior, or sleepsex, is a particular form of parasomnia, usually occurring in NREM sleep, characterized by atypical sexual behavior during sleep [49]. Although not classified as a unique parasomnia, sexsomnia is mentioned in the ICSD-3 as a variant of confusional arousal [1].

The frequency of sexsomnia is underestimated, since most afflicted individuals do not seek therapeutic intervention [50], because of ignorance of the condition [51]. The majority of reports in the literature concern male patients. Common features of sexsomnia include sexual arousal with autonomic activation (eg, nocturnal erection, vaginal lubrication, ejaculation, sweating, and cardiorespiratory response), explicit sexual vocalizations, masturbation, and complex sexual activities [52]. Sexsomnia without

sexual arousal, however, has also been reported: sexual behavior in sleep may arise from either a dreamlike experience, arising from NREM sleep, or from dreams with sexual content (a feature of REM sleep). Complete amnesia on waking occurs in all reported cases of sexsomnia [28]. The exact cause of sexsomnia has not yet been identified, although several precipitating factors have been reported, including stress, sleep deprivation, alcohol use, and drug abuse [28,50,51]. Sexsomnia has been described in association with REM parasomnias, RLS, and narcolepsy [28]. A particular psychological history of major trauma during childhood, namely, sexual abuse, and rape of the mother, as well as particular psychiatric conditions, such as depressive disorder, obsessive personality trait, and generalized anxiety, have also been reported [51,52].

In order to differentiate voluntary violence from sexual behavior provoked by an automatism during sleep, the history must include a detailed description of the event and the degree of amnesia of the patient, as well as his or her attitude when fully awake after the event [49]. A collateral history from the bed partner or a family member is also helpful. Diagnosis of sexsomnia usually relies on neurological and psychiatric evaluation in order to detect particular personality traits, anxiety, or depressive disorders, early dementia, or Kleine–Levin syndrome, all of which can be responsible for abnormal behavior during sleep. This clinical examination must be completed by EEG and VPSG recordings, to rule out the presence of other sleep-related disorders [52]. According to PSG findings, sleep structure is usually normal, but sudden arousals from SWS are frequently observed.

As with other parasomnias, sleep hygiene measures reduce the negative effect of the precipitating factors. Psychotherapy may be helpful, especially in the case of associated anxiety or depression. In patients with other sleep disorders, treatment should be aimed at the main disorder [50]. Positive therapeutic responses to benzodiazepines, especially clonazepam from 0.5 to 2 mg at bedtime, antidepressant medications such as SSRIs, valproic acid, and lamotrigine have been observed [50,51].

Sleep-related eating disorder

SRED, first described by Schenck and colleagues in 1991 [53], is a parasomnia characterized by recurrent episodes of involuntary compulsive eating during sleep, with morning anorexia and frequent comorbid sleep disorders [1]. Episodes typically arise from NREM sleep, mostly stage N3, but there are cases of episodes occurring during REM sleep [1,53].

During an SRED episode, patients usually get out of bed to eat and drink after having fallen asleep normally. Eating is compulsive, unassociated with any feeling of hunger, and chewing starts right after awakening (eating latency is less than 30 s in about half of the episodes) [54]. Once food is ingested, the feeling abates and the patient is able to resume sleep [1,55]. The spectrum of the substances ingested is wide, varying from ordinary to unusual substances, generally with high-caloric nutrients [1,53]. More than 65% of SRED patients ingest unpalatable substances, such as frozen food or buttered cigarettes [56]. Alcohol consumption during nocturnal episodes is rare. Eating may occur up to eight times nightly, although one or two episodes nightly are more common, lasting an average of 3–5 minutes [54]. Episodes are associated with variable degrees of awareness, ranging from dense unawareness, typical of parasomnias like somnambulism, to partial awareness [57]. Ninety percent of patients report being half or fully asleep [58], although impaired consciousness is not a universal finding [54,59,60]. Morning amnesia for the event may be present [61].

The onset of SRED can be sudden, associated with precipitating factors, such as major life stresses, medical, neurological, sleep, or psychiatric disorders, administration of medications [62], including triazolam, amitriptyline, olanzapine, risperidone, and zolpidem [44,62–64] or cessation of cigarette smoking, alcohol abuse, or marijuana use. SRED can also develop gradually, without any identified precipitant.

Obesity and daytime sleepiness are the most important consequences of SRED; weight gain may precipitate or aggravate pre-existing diabetes mellitus, hyperlipidemia, hypercholesterolemia, hypertension, and OSA. Furthermore, injuries from careless food preparation, such as burns and lacerations, seem to occur in almost one-third of patients [63]. As initially described by Schenck and colleagues, SRED is often associated with other sleep-related motor disorders, such PLMS, RLS, SW, and, to a lesser extent, OSA, bruxism, and circadian rhythm disorders [54,58,63,65,66]. SRED is not associated with daytime eating disturbances, and behaviors such as self-induced vomiting or excessive exercise, typical of bulimic/anorexic disorders, are absent [61].

There are no current prevalence data on SRED in the general population, and the reported prevalence results are inconsistent (0.5–4.7%) [53]. Although SRED can affect both sexes and all ages, it is more common in young adult women [55]; the average age of onset of SRED is approximately 22–27 years [55,57]. A familial relationship has been described, suggesting a role of genetic factors. The pathophysiology of SRED remains largely unknown. In patients with concomitant sleep disorders, it has been suggested that arousals may provoke varying levels of consciousness, prompting SW and sleep-related eating in predisposed individuals [58]. The association of SRED with dopaminergic responsive disorders such as PLMS and RLS [53,55], its clinical response to dopaminergic drugs [55], and the major role of dopamine as a mediator of the mesolimbic reward mechanism support a link between SRED and dopaminergic dysfunction.

A thorough sleep history is essential for the recognition and diagnosis of SRED. The timing, frequency, and description of food ingested during eating episodes should be elicited. A complete medication history, including when medications were started, is required [56]. If drugs have been implicated in the initiation of SRED, their cessation will stop eating episodes. If other sleep disorders are suspected, or if the episodes are stereotypical or have resulted in injury, VPSG should be performed, ideally with food placed at the bedside [54–56,58]. The most frequent PSG findings are an increased number of arousals, most of which occur during NREM sleep or exclusively during SWS [59], together with chewing and swallowing movements during stage 2 (Fig. 39.2).

SRED shares some clinical features with night eating syndrome (NES), such as a chronic course, familial association, comorbid neuropsychiatric diseases, and a frequent association with weight gain and obesity [56,60,67]. There is a debate as to whether SRED and NES should be classified as independent entities or whether they should be considered as a continuum of a single condition involving eating urges and sleep disorders. In fact, NES is best characterized as a circadian delay in meal timing [60], associated with insomnia, rather than as a parasomnia [56].

Treatment of SRED usually involves the management of concomitant sleep disorders if present. For patients with SW, PLMS, and RLS, clonazepam, codeine, and carbidopa/levodopa or bromocriptine are often effective [63]. Dopaminergic agonists, such as low doses of pramipexole, are also effective (0.18–0.36 mg at bedtime), especially in patients with RLS [63,67]. Success with combinations of dopaminergic and opioid drugs, with the occasional addition of sedatives, has also been described in a small series of patients without associated sleep disorders [60]. In those for whom opioids and sedatives are relatively contraindicated (eg, those with a history of substance abuse), a combination of bupropion, levodopa, and trazodone has been suggested [68]. Fluoxetine may also help, either alone or in combination with dopaminergic agonists, especially in patients with depression and a history of substance abuse [63]. SSRIs, especially sertraline, have been shown effective in the treatment of both SRED and NES [69]. Topiramate, given at a dose range of 100–400 mg at night, can reduce night eating, improving nocturnal sleep and producing weight loss in patients with SRED [60].

Other parasomnias

This section describes parasomnias that are independent of sleep stage, appearing during both REM and NREM sleep [1]. These consist of the following:

1. Sleep enuresis.

2. Exploding head syndrome (EHS).

3. Sleep-related hallucinations, hallucinatory experiences, principally visual, that occur at sleep onset (hypnagogic hallucinations) or on awakening from sleep (hypnopompic hallucinations).

4. Parasomnias due to drug or substance or medical condition, behaviors emerging with a close temporal relationship between exposure to a drug medication or biological substance or as a manifestation of an underlying neurological or medical condition.

Sleep enuresis

Sleep enuresis is one of the most common and distressing parasomnias of childhood, consisting of involuntary micturition during sleep in children after the age of 5 years [70]. Sleep enuresis includes primary enuresis, meaning that the child has never achieved urinary control, which represents most cases in early childhood (75–80%), and secondary enuresis, which implies that the child has had at least 6 months of dryness before bedwetting. The prevalence of sleep enuresis in 5-year-old children is between 15% and 25%, with a decrease with age of 15% per year and with a prevalence of up to 1% in 15-year-old patients. The prevalence is influenced by many factors, such as male gender, low socioeconomic status, institutionalization, and black race. Even if it is no longer believed that enuresis is mainly a psychiatric disorder, psychosocial factors may have a role: children with post-traumatic stress or bullied children are more likely to have sleep enuresis [70]. Enuresis can also have psychological consequences such as low self-esteem, which disappears with dryness. Several studies have shown the important role of genetic and familial factors in determining sleep enuresis; children whose parents have a history of sleep enuresis are more frequently affected, and in some patients, it has been seen to have an autosomal dominant inheritance with high penetrance [70]. Finally, a more important factor involved in the pathogenesis of sleep enuresis is

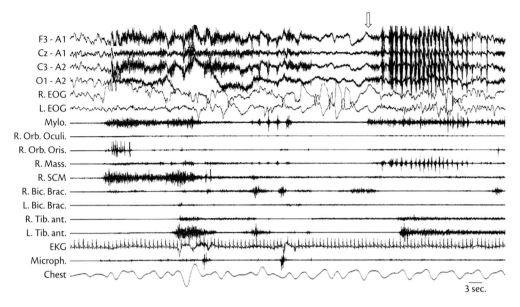

Fig. 39.2 Sleep-related eating disorder (SRED). The PSG excerpt shows an eating episode occurring some seconds after a complete awakening from stage 3 NREM sleep. During the episode, the 45-year-old woman consumes some crackers. The episode is characterized by rhythmic masticatory-muscle activity, chewing and swallowing movements on EEG, and masseter muscle traces. EOG: electro-oculogram; Mylo.: mylohyoideus; Orb.: orbicularis; Mass.: masseter; SCM: sternocleidomastoideus; Bic.Brac: biceps brachii; Tib. ant.: tibialis anterior; EKG: electrocardiogram; Microph.: microphone; Chest: chest respirogram; R.: right; L.: left.

the developmental delay in the brain areas involved in micturition control network [71,72].

Enuretic episodes can occur from once a week to every night, usually in the first half of the night. The sleep pattern of enuretic children is not significantly different from that of non-enuretic children; it can be characterized by an increased number of sleep cycles and by a longer time spent in bed. Enuretic children are considered "deep sleepers," showing decreased arousability, and, during the night, they present more parasympathetic activity and less sympathetic activity than controls [70].

Primary enuresis can be monosymptomatic (without other clinical manifestations referable to the urogenital or gastrointestinal tracts) or polysymptomatic (associated with daytime symptoms like urgency, chronic constipation, or encopresis). Polysymptomatic enuresis has been associated with a polymorphism in the gene encoding 5-hydroxytryptamine receptor 2A [73]; the etiopathogenesis of monosymptomatic enuresis is uncertain.

Basing on clinical and pathogenetic features, two different forms of sleep enuresis can be distinguished: diuresis-dependent and detrusor-dependent enuresis [70]. Diuresis-dependent enuresis is characterized by nocturnal polyuria that may be due to polydipsia or to a reduced ability to concentrate urine. In these cases, enuretic children show a decreased vasopressin peak during sleep, with a high overnight urine production exceeding the functional bladder capacity. It has been proposed that a defect at the central arginine vasopressin receptor level or in the signal transduction pathway causes deficiency in arginine vasopressin in these patients. Detrusor-dependent enuresis is associated with detrusor overactivity. In these cases, enuretic children, usually non-responders to antidiuretic therapy, show frequently uninhibited detrusor contractions during sleep that fail to awake the child and result in bedwetting [74]. These children may also have daytime symptoms such as urgency and incontinence or may be constipated. Children may

present signs of both forms of enuresis and consequently require combined therapy with antidiuretic and detrusor-relaxant drugs. Secondary enuresis may be caused by a variety of disorders, such as diabetes mellitus, diabetes insipidus, epilepsy, neurogenic bladder, urinary tract infection, and ureteral malformations. Other diseases may facilitate sleep enuresis, including, for example, attention-deficit hyperactivity disorder, sickle cell anemia, and other sleep disorders such as OSA [70,75]. From 8% to 47% of children with OSA have nocturnal enuresis, which improves with adenotonsillectomy.

If sleep enuresis is monosymptomatic, then only urinalysis and urine cultures are needed [76]. When other symptoms coexist, further investigations should be performed: ultrasonography, vesical sphincter electromyography, cystometry, cystoscopy, and MRI of the spine to exclude spinal malformations.

Sleep enuresis usually resolves spontaneously; treatment options include lifestyle modification, medications, and alternative therapies. Behavioral techniques are nowadays preferred to medications and consist of behavior modifications such as evening fluid limitation and caffeine avoidance, wetness alarms, and retention control exercises. The bell-and-pad method is based on the use of a urine detector, with an alarm sounding and waking the child as voiding starts; its success rate is 65–80%, with relapses occurring in 10–15% of cases. Drug therapy includes desmopressin for patients with vasopressin deficiency with a diuresis-dependent enuresis, coupled with anticholinergic drugs if needed, such as oxybutynin and the newer tolterodine, in therapy-resistant patients [70,76–79]. Desmopressin side effects like hyponatremia and water intoxication are possible but rare. Tricyclic antidepressants, especially imipramine, may also be used; however, because of their high relapse rate and risk of fatal overdose, they are not considered as a primary treatment. Reboxetine may be used as an alternative to imipramine. Medications usually provide a decrease in the frequency of episodes, but only a few patients reach complete dryness and the treatment effect is not sustained once the medication is stopped. Psychotherapy, hypnotherapy, and electro-acupuncture are alternative therapies, but their effectiveness is not so clear.

Exploding head syndrome

EHS is a rare parasomnia characterized by a violent sense of explosion in the head [80], which arises abruptly and awakes the patient from sleep. The syndrome is confined to sleep and occurs predominantly when the patient is falling asleep, as well as during daytime naps [80]. Patients experience a tremendously loud imagined noise originating from within their head and described as a gunshot noise, waves crashing against rocks, loud voices, or the sound of electrical buzzing [81]. A simultaneous flash of light may accompany the sound and a myoclonic jerk may sometimes occur [1]. The condition appears to be a sensory variant of the better known transient motor phenomenon of sleep starts, or hypnic jerks. Although the event is typically painless [1], patients are often so alarmed that they first describe it as a pain. Some patients report a sensation as if they had stopped breathing [82], along with cold sweating. The attack is very brief, typically lasting only a few seconds [81], and by the time the patient is wide awake, it has gone [80], although it may recur on further sleep attempts [81].

The prevalence of EHS is unknown [1], but it is reported to have a slight female preponderance [81]. The median age of onset is 58 years [1], although in few cases it may start in childhood [80]. The pathophysiology of EHS is unknown; preceding events or precipitating factors are usually unremarkable, but many patients report an increase in the number of attacks that coincides with personal stress or overtiredness [80]. EHS has also been linked to rapid withdrawal from benzodiazepines and SSRIs.

According to the International Classification of Sleep Disorders, for the diagnosis, it is necessary to meet all three of the following criteria: (A) the patient complains of a sudden loud noise or sense of explosion in the head either at the wake–sleep transition or upon waking during the night; (B) the experience is not associated with significant pain complaints; (C) the patient arises immediately after the event, usually with a sense of fright [1].

PSG findings are not specific, indicating a normal sleep structure [1,81].

Differential diagnoses includes thunderclap headache and icepick headache, which can occur at sleep onset but are more common during wakefulness [1,81]. Furthermore, EHS can mimic nocturnal headache syndromes, including sleep-related migraines, cluster headaches, hypnic headaches, and nocturnal paroxysmal hemicrania. All of these headache disorders usually cause the patient to awaken with an actual headache, in contrast to EHS, which is painless [81]. EHS is usually a self-limiting phenomenon [1,80], so no treatment is generally required and reassurance to the patient is often all that is needed [81]. However in a small subgroup of patients, medications, like nifedipine, flunarizine, topiramate, or clomipramine, have been found to be effective [81].

Conclusions

Parasomnias are a heterogeneous group of manifestations that accompany sleep. In some cases, they can result in sleep disruption and injuries, with adverse health or psychosocial consequences for patients, bed partners, or both. The complex and goal-directed behavior observed during the episodes is usually disconnected from conscious awareness.

To date, the nature and mechanisms of many parasomnias, as well as their effective and specific treatment, remain largely unknown. In recent years, many significant advances have been made in understanding the clinical features of parasomnias and elucidating their pathophysiology. A full comprehension of these mechanisms will also constitute an invaluable tool for the comprehension of the mechanisms that regulate sleep.

References

1. American Academy of Sleep Medicine. International Classification of Sleep Disorders, 3rd ed.: Diagnostic and coding manual. Darien, IL: American Academy of Sleep Medicine, 2014.
2. Mahowald MW, Schenck CH. NREM sleep parasomnias. Neurol Clin 1996;14:675–96.
3. Provini F, Tinuper P, Bisulli F, et al. Arousal disorders. Sleep Med 2011; 2:S22–6.
4. Mason TB, Pack AI. Pediatric parasomnias. Sleep 2007;30:141–51.
5. Stores G. Confusional arousals. In: Thorpy MJ, Plazzi G, eds. The parasomnias and other sleep-related movement disorders. New York: Cambridge University Press, 2010:99–108.
6. Mahowald MW, Schenck CH. Insights from studying human sleep disorders. Nature 2005;437:1279–85.
7. Nobili L, Ferrara M, Moroni F, et al. Dissociated wake-like and sleep-like electro-cortical activity during sleep. Neuroimage 2011;58:612–19.
8. Espa F, Ondze B, Deglise P, et al. Sleep architecture, slow wave activity, and sleep spindles in adult patients with sleepwalking and sleep terrors. Clin Neurophysiol 2000;111:929–39.
9. Zucconi M, Oldani A, Ferini-Strambi L, et al. Arousal fluctuations in non-rapid eye movement parasomnias: the role of cyclic alternating pattern as a measure of sleep instability. J Clin Neurophysiol 1995;12:147–54.
10. Bruni O, Ferri R, Novelli L, et al. NREM sleep instability in children with sleep terrors: the role of slow wave activity interruptions. Clin Neurophysiol 2008;119:985–92.
11. Terzaghi M, Sartori I, Tassi L, et al. Dissociated local arousal states underlying essential clinical features of non-rapid eye movement arousal parasomnia: an intracerebral stereo-electroencephalographic study. J Sleep Res 2012;21:502–6.
12. Bassetti C, Vella S, Donati F, et al. SPECT during sleepwalking. Lancet 2000;356:484–5.
13. Tassinari CA, Rubboli G, Gardella E, et al. Central pattern generators for a common semiology in fronto-limbic seizures and in parasomnias. A neuroethologic approach. Neurol Sci 2005;26:225–32.
14. Kales A, Soldatos CR, Bixler EO, et al. Hereditary factors in sleepwalking and night terrors. Br J Psychiatry 1980;137:111–18.
15. Ohayon MM, Guilleminault C, Priest RG. Night terrors, sleepwalking, and confusional arousals in the general population: their frequency and relationship to other sleep and mental disorders. J Clin Psychiatry 1999;60:268–76.
16. Laberge L, Tremblay RE, Vitaro F, et al. Development of parasomnias from childhood to early adolescence. Pediatrics 2000;106:67–74.
17. Petit D, Touchette E, Tremblay RE, et al. Dyssomnias and parasomnias in early childhood. Pediatrics 2007;119:e1016–25.
18. Fisher C, Kahn E, Edwards A, et al. A psychophysiological study of nightmares and night terrors. I. Physiological aspects of the stage 4 night terror. J Nerv Ment Dis 1973;157:75–98.
19. Guilleminault C, Palombini L, Pelayo R, et al. Sleepwalking and sleep terrors in prepubertal children: what triggers them? Pediatrics 2003;111:e17–25.
20. Zadra A, Desautels A, Petit D, et al. Somnambulism: clinical aspects and pathophysiological hypotheses. Lancet Neurol 2013;12:285–94.
21. Tinuper P, Provini F, Bisulli F, et al. Movement disorders in sleep: guidelines for differentiating epileptic from non-epileptic motor phenomena arising from sleep. Sleep Med Rev 2007;11:255–67.
22. Chokroverty S. Confusional arousals. In: Kushida C, ed. Encyclopedia of sleep. San Diego, CA: Elsevier, 2013:199–201.

23. Provini F, Plazzi G, Tinuper P, et al. Nocturnal frontal lobe epilepsy. A clinical and polygraphic overview of 100 consecutive cases. Brain 1999;122:1017–31.

24. Bisulli F, Vignatelli L, Provini F, et al. Parasomnias and nocturnal frontal lobe epilepsy (NFLE): lights and shadows—controversial points in the differential diagnosis. Sleep Med 2011;12:S27–32.

25. Bisulli F, Vignatelli L, Naldi I, et al. Diagnostic accuracy of a structured interview for nocturnal frontal lobe epilepsy (SINFLE): a proposal for developing diagnostic criteria. Sleep Med 2012;13:81–7.

26. Derry C. Nocturnal frontal lobe epilepsy vs parasomnias. Curr Treat Options Neurol 2012;14:451–63.

27. Bornemann MA, Mahowald MW, Schenck CH. Parasomnias: clinical features and forensic implications. Chest 2006;130:605–10.

28. Schenck CH, Arnulf I, Mahowald MW. Sleep and sex: what can go wrong? A review of the literature on sleep related disorders and abnormal sexual behaviors and experiences. Sleep 2007;30:683–702.

29. Ohayon MM, Schenck CH. Violent behavior during sleep: prevalence, comorbidity and consequences. Sleep Med 2010;11:941–6.

30. Mahowald MW, Cramer Bornemann MA, Schenck CH. State dissociation, human behavior, and consciousness. Curr Top Med Chem 2011;11:2392–402.

31. Mason TB. Sleep terrors. In: Kushida C, ed. Encyclopedia of sleep. San Diego, CA: Elsevier; 2013:205–8.

32. Gastaut H, Broughton RJ. A clinical and polygraphic study of episodic phenomena during sleep. Recent Adv Biol Psychiatry 1965;7:197–223.

33. Fisher C, Byrne J, Edwards A, et al. A psychophysiological study of nightmares. J Am Psychoanal Assoc 1970;18:747–82.

34. Broughton RJ. Sleep disorders: disorders of arousal? Science 1968;159:1070–8.

35. Zadra A, Pilon M. NREM parasomnias. Handb Clin Neurol 2011;99:851–68.

36. Bruni O, Ferri R, Miano S, et al. L-5-Hydroxytryptophan treatment of sleep terrors in children. Eur J Pediatr 2004;163:402–7.

37. Hauri PJ, Silber MH, Boeve BF. The treatment of parasomnias with hypnosis: a 5-year follow-up study. J Clin Sleep Med 2007;3:369–73.

38. Roger H. Les troubles du sommeil—hypersomnies, insomnies, parasomnies. Paris: Masson, 1932:180–3.

39. Silvestri R. Somnambulism, Somniloquy and Sleep Terrors. In: Culebras A, ed. Sleep disorders and neurologic diseases. New York: Informa Healthcare, 2007:255–62.

40. Meltzer LJ, Mindell JA. Sleep and sleep disorders in children and adolescents. Psychiatr Clin North Am 2006;29:1059–76.

41. Mahowald MW, Schenck CH, Goldner M, et al. Parasomnia pseudo-suicide. J Forensic Sci 2003;48:1158–62.

42. Oudiette D, Leu S, Pottier M, et al. Dreamlike mentations during sleepwalking and sleep terrors in adults. Sleep 2009;32:1621–7.

43. Partinen M, Hublin C. Epidemiology of sleep disorders. In: Kryger MH, Roth T, Dement WC, eds. Principles and practice of sleep medicine. Philadelphia: WB Saunders, 2000:558–79.

44. Morgenthaler TI, Silber MH. Amnestic sleep-related eating disorder associated with zolpidem. Sleep Med 2002;3:323–7.

45. Kushida CA, Littner MR, Morgenthaler T, et al. Practice parameters for the indications for polysomnography and related procedures: an update for 2005. Sleep 2005;28:499–521.

46. Lugaresi E, Provini F. Seizures versus parasomnias. In: Overeem S, Reading P, eds. Sleep disorders in neurology, a practical approach. Hoboken, NJ: Wiley-Blackwell, 2010:189–204.

47. Schenck CH, Mahowald MW. Long-term, nightly benzodiazepine treatment of injurious parasomnias and other disorders of disrupted nocturnal sleep in 170 adults. Am J Med 1996;100:333–7.

48. Balon R. Sleep terror disorder and insomnia treated with trazodone: a case report. Ann Clin Psychiatry 1994;6:161–3.

49. Fenwick P. Sleep and sexual offending. Med Sci Law 1996;36:122–34.

50. Andersen ML, Poyares D, Alves RS, et al. Sexsomnia: abnormal sexual behavior during sleep. Brain Res Rev 2007;56:271–82.

51. Béjot Y, Juenet N, Garrouty R, et al. Sexsomnia: an uncommon variety of parasomnia. Clin Neurol Neurosurg 2010;112:72–5.

52. Guilleminault C, Moscovitch A, Yuen K, et al. Atypical sexual behavior during sleep. Psychosom Med 2002;64:328–36.

53. Schenck CH, Hurwitz TD, Bundlie SR, et al. Sleep-related eating disorders: polysomnographic correlates of a heterogeneous syndrome distinct from daytime eating disorders. Sleep 1991;14:419–31.

54. Spaggiari MC, Granella F, Parrino L, et al. Nocturnal eating syndrome in adults. Sleep 1994;17:339–44.

55. Schenck CH, Mahowald MW. Review of nocturnal sleep-related eating disorders. Int J Eat Disord 1994;15:343–56.

56. Auger RR. Sleep-related eating disorders. Psychiatry (Edgmont) 2006;3:64–70.

57. Winkelman JW, Johnson EA, Richards LM. Sleep-related eating disorder. Handb Clin Neurol 2011;98:577–85.

58. Winkelman JW. Clinical and polysomnographic features of sleep-related eating disorder. J Clin Psychiatry 1998;59:14–19.

59. Vetrugno R, Manconi M, Ferini-Strambi L, et al. Nocturnal eating: sleep-related eating disorder or night eating syndrome? A videopolysomnographic study. Sleep 2006;29:949–54.

60. Howell MJ, Schenck CH. Treatment of nocturnal eating disorders. Curr Treat Options Neurol 2009;11:333–9.

61. Perogamvros L, Baud P, Hasler R, et al. Active reward processing during human sleep: insights from sleep-related eating disorder. Front Neurol 2012;3:168.

62. Lu M, Shen W. Sleep-related eating disorder induced by risperidone. J Clin Psychiatry 2004;65:273–4.

63. Schenck CH, Hurwitz TD, O'Connor KA, Mahowald MW. Additional categories of sleep-related eating disorders and the current status of treatment. Sleep 1993;16:457–66.

64. Paquet V, Strul J, Servais L, et al. Sleep-related eating disorder induced by olanzapine. J Clin Psychiatry 2002;63:597.

65. Ekbom KA. Restless legs syndrome. Neurology 1960;10:868–73.

66. Howell MJ, Schenck CH. Restless nocturnal eating: a common feature of Willis–Ekbom syndrome (RLS). J Clin Sleep Med 2012;8:413–19.

67. Provini F, Albani F, Vetrugno R, et al. A pilot double-blind placebo-controlled trial of low-dose pramipexole in sleep-related eating disorder. Eur J Neurol 2005;12:432–6.

68. Schenck CH, Mahowald MW. Combined bupropion–levodopa–trazodone therapy of sleep-related eating and sleep disruption in two adults with chemical dependency. Sleep 2000;23:587–8.

69. Stunkard AJ, Allison KC. Two forms of disordered eating in obesity: binge eating and night eating. Int J Obes Relat Metab Disord 2003;27:1–12.

70. Nevéus T. Sleep enuresis. Handb Clin Neurol 2011;98:363–9.

71. Freitag CM, Röhling D, Seifen S, et al. Neurophysiology of nocturnal enuresis: evoked potentials and prepulse inhibition of the startle reflex. Dev Med Child Neurol 2006;48:278–84.

72. Lei D, Ma J, Shen X, et al. Changes in the brain microstructure of children with primary monosymptomatic nocturnal enuresis: a diffusion tensor imaging study. PLoS One 2012;7:e31023.

73. Wei CC, Wan L, Lin WY, et al. Rs 6313 polymorphism in 5-hydroxytryptamine receptor 2A gene association with polysymptomatic primary nocturnal enuresis. J Clin Lab Anal 2010;24:371–5.

74. Yeung CK, Chiu HN, Sit FK. Bladder dysfunction in children with refractory monosymptomatic primary nocturnal enuresis. J Urol 1999;162:1049–54.

75. Jeyakumar A, Rahman SI, Armbrecht ES, et al. The association between sleep-disordered breathing and enuresis in children. Laryngoscope 2012;122:1873–7.

76. Kiddoo DA. Nocturnal enuresis. CMAJ 2012;184:908–11.

77. Cohen-Zrubavel V, Kushnir B, Kushnir J, et al. Sleep and sleepiness in children with nocturnal enuresis. Sleep 2011;34:191–4.

78. Moffatt ME. Nocturnal enuresis: a review of the efficacy of treatments and practical advice for clinicians. J Dev Behav Pediatr 1997;18:49–56.

79. Mathew JL. Evidence-based management of nocturnal enuresis: an overview of systematic reviews. Indian Pediatr 2010;47:777–80.

80. Pearce JM. Clinical features of the exploding head syndrome. J Neurol Neurosurg Psychiatry 1989;52:907–10.

81. Ganguly G, Mridha B, Khan A, et al. Exploding head syndrome: a case report. Case Rep Neurol 2013;5:14–17.

82. Oswald I. Sleeping and waking. Amsterdam: Elsevier, 1962.

SECTION 9

Sleep and medical disorders

CHAPTER 40

Sleep and the heart

Winfried J. Randerath and Shahrokh Javaheri

Introduction

There is a bidirectional relationship between sleep and the heart. Normal non-rapid eye movement (NREM) sleep is peaceful for the cardiovascular system, since favorable autonomic changes occur that result in a decrease in heart rate and blood pressure. Therefore, cardiac workload and oxygen consumption decrease. On the other hand, sleep pathology such as sleep apnea or periodic limb movements can adversely affect cardiac function and structure, while cardiac pathology such as heart failure disrupts sleep architecture, which in turn adversely affects the heart. In this chapter, we review some of these disorders in detail.

Sleep-related breathing disorders

The main two phenotypes of sleep-related breathing disorders (SRBDs) that are the focus of this review are obstructive and central sleep apnea [1]. While there is some overlap between the mechanisms underlying these two sleep breathing disorders, the sine qua non of obstructive sleep apnea (OSA) (Fig. 40.1) is occlusion of the upper airway, while central sleep apnea (CSA) (Fig. 40.2) is of diverse etiology, with varying underlying mechanisms. Among these are increased loop gain, explaining periodic breathing in heart failure, and failure of the breathing rhythm generator, the pre-Bötzinger complex, in opioid-induced CSA.

Also, since this review is focused mostly on sleep apnea and the heart, we emphasize the bidirectional relationship of sleep apnea and heart disease such that, when comorbid, a vicious circle ensues.

Obstructive sleep apnea

OSA is characterized by increased collapsibility and obstruction of the upper airways leading to complete cessation (apnea) or partial reduction of airflow (hypopnea). Predispositions include male gender, obesity, old age, family history, and altered upper airway anatomy (eg, macroglossia, retrognathia, large tonsils, or adenoids) resulting in a narrow airway. The last of these, along with increasing prevalence of obesity, accounts for the increased prevalence of childhood OSA.

The Wisconsin cohort longitudinal studies [2,3] are the most systematic epidemiological data on the prevalence of OSA in the general population, and the most recent updated data indicate increasing prevalence of OSA in the USA [3]. Using a definition for OSA of an apnea–hypopnea index (AHI) ≥ 5 per hour of sleep, the current estimates are 34% in adult males and 17% in adult females aged 30–70 years. The prevalence of moderate to severe OSA, defined as an AHI ≥ 15/h is 13% in men and 6% in women aged 30–70 years [3].

OSA remains greatly underdiagnosed [4,5]. A telephone survey in Great Britain showed that 31% of 5000 participants had contacted a physician more than 6 times within the preceding year because of symptoms of SRBD during sleep. Surveys in practices of general practitioners revealed that 32% of the patients with high probability for OSA were not diagnosed [4,5]. Undiagnosed OSA may result in a variety of cardiocerebrovascular disorders such as hypertension, coronary artery disease, neurocognitive dysfunction, transient ischemic attack, and stroke.

OSA syndrome (OSAS)—that is, an AHI ≥ 5/h plus excessive daytime sleepiness (EDS)—remains among the most prevalent sleep disorders. Patients present with diurnal and nocturnal symptoms such as EDS (hence the syndrome), fatigue, loud and irregular snoring, nocturia, waking up not refreshed, and morning headache. Partners often report breathing cessations during sleep [6]. EDS may result in crashes, lack of attention, and poor performance. The current estimates of the syndrome in US adults are 14% in males and 5% in females aged 30–70 years [3].

Obstructive breathing disturbances are associated with repetitive oxygen desaturations, increases in $PaCO_2$ (the arterial partial pressure of carbon dioxide, PCO_2), and arousals. Futile ventilatory efforts of the diaphragm and the thoracic muscles against a closed upper airway may result in a paradoxical breathing pattern of thorax and abdomen (Fig. 40.1). Obstructive disturbances terminate abruptly, often in association with arousals, which are themselves associated both with increased sympathetic activity resulting in high arterial blood pressure and with decreased parasympathetic activity causing tachycardia. The level of pleural pressure generated by respiratory effort, seems to be one potential trigger of arousals from NREM sleep [7]. Nevertheless, any causal relationship between these phenomena is ambiguous. One important question that has therapeutic implication is the role of the arousals in perpetuating obstructive breathing disorders. Younes et al. found that inspiratory flow increased in 22% of events before arousal and was restored in 70% without an arousal [8]. In these situations, combinations of stimuli, such as elevated levels of carbon dioxide and negative pressure reflexes, can activate upper airway dilator muscles, and delaying the arousal may be beneficial to restore pharyngeal patency. The limited flow through the narrowed airways during hypopneas and the abrupt reopening at the end of an apnea represents the correlate of the typical loud and irregular snoring sound [9–11].

Central sleep apnea

CSA is characterized by recurrent cessations (central apnea) (Fig. 40.2), or reduction of airflow with a simultaneous proportional reduction of the breathing effort (central hypopnea). Ventilatory

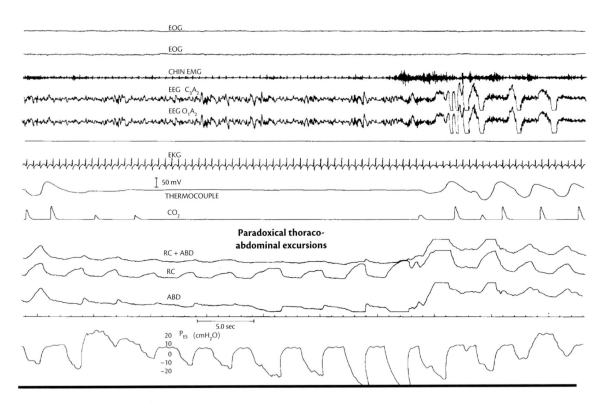

Fig. 40.1 A 30-second epoch of obstructive sleep apnea.

Reproduced from Javaheri S, Heart Failure. In: Kryger M, Roth T, Dement W, [eds], Principles and Practices of Sleep Medicine, pp. 1400–15, Copyright (2011), with permission from Elsevier.

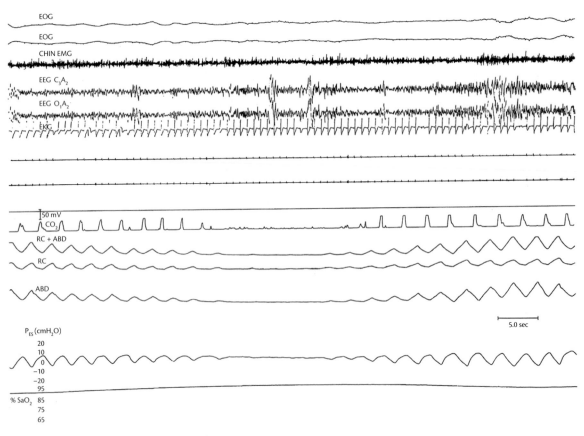

Fig. 40.2 A 30-second epoch showing central sleep apnea [13].

Reproduced from Am Rev Respir Dis., 141(4 Pt 1), Dowdell WT, Javaheri S, McGinnis W, Cheyne-Stokes respiration presenting as sleep apnea syndrome. Clinical and polysomnographic features, pp. 871–9, Copyright (1990), with permission from American Thoracic Society.

impulses generated by the brainstem respiratory centers are limited or lacking. In contrast to OSA, the upper airways are not necessarily narrowed, although passive closure of the pharyngeal airways may occur [12]. This was shown in patients with heart failure in whom an esophageal balloon was in place, who exhibited frequent upper airway occlusions at the end of central apneas [13]. These events were considered mixed apneas.

CSA as a polysomnographic (PSG) finding is associated with a large number of clinical conditions, including Cheyne–Stokes breathing (hereinafter referred to as Hunter–Cheyne–Stokes breathing, HCSB, as John Hunter, a Scottish surgeon, described this unique pattern of breathing almost four decades before John Cheyne; see [14]), exposure to high altitude, brainstem lesions, stroke, endocrine disorders, and opioids [14–19]. Similar to OSA, CSA can—but does not necessarily has to—be associated with daytime sleepiness, frequent nocturnal awakenings, and decreased sleep insufficiency and insomnia [18].

HCSB is characterized by recurrent central apneas and hypopneas and a crescendo–decrescendo pattern of flow and effort (Fig. 40.2) [13]. Although these events are characterized by central apneas, upper airway obstruction has been documented at the end of the events before resumption of breathing, as noted above [13].

Cardiocerebrovascular disorders, especially atrial fibrillation, heart failure, and stroke, predispose to the development of CSA [14,15,20–24]. HCSB describes a pattern of periodic breathing in patients with heart failure [23]. The mechanisms underlying HCSB will be discussed in detail later.

Opioid-induced sleep apnea presents with mixed SRBD consisting of both obstructive and central apneas and hypopneas, and at times sustained oxygen desaturations, due to hypoventilation. These SRBD occur in the background of Biot and cluster breathing [17,18,25]. This pattern of breathing characterized by irregular respiratory pauses and gasping without periodicity (Fig. 40.3) is the most typical PSG finding in opioid-induced sleep apnea and is distinguished from periodic breathing (HCSB) in heart failure (Fig. 40.2). The mechanism of opioid-associated sleep apnea is beyond the scope of this chapter, and is reviewed here only briefly (for reviews, see [17,18,25]). Opioid receptors are prevalent in carotid bodies, brainstem, and respiratory-related neurons. The pre-Bötzinger complex, the site of breathing rhythm generation, is inhibited by opioids and underlies the mechanism of central apneas. In addition, opioids inhibit hypoglossal neuronal pool, diminishing genioglossal muscle activity and promoting upper airway occlusion.

In recent years, additional phenotypes have been described, such as central disturbances emerging under therapy with continuous positive airway pressure (CPAP). Moreover, several patients suffer not only from one type, but from coexisting obstructive and central disturbances [14,15,25–27]. This hybrid breathing pattern was first recognized in early studies of patients with heart failure [14,15,25] and is also well recognized in patients taking opioids [16–18].

A clear separation of the different entities is not feasible, owing to limitations of standard PSG on the one hand and overlap of the pathophysiologies on the other [28].

Pathophysiology of OSA

The pharyngeal region, which is not stiffened by bony or cartilaginous structures, represents an unstable, collapsible part of the

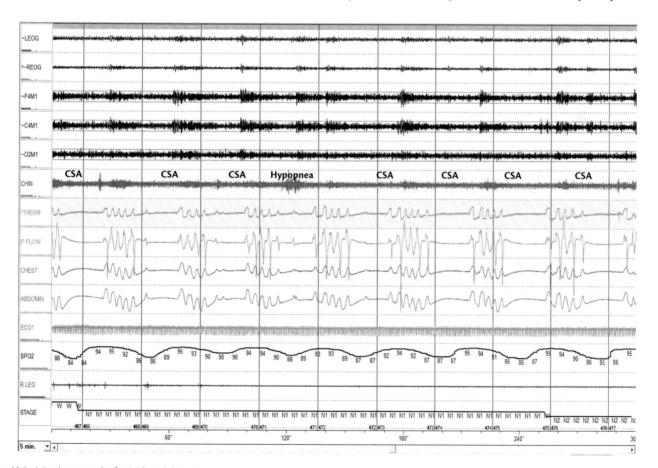

Fig. 40.3 A 5-minute epoch of opioids and sleep apnea.
Reproduced from Compr Physiol., 3(1), Javaheri S, Dempsey JA, Central sleep apnea, pp. 141–63, Copyright (2013), American Physiological Society.

airways. Its width depends, among other things, on morphological factors, namely, the volume of the surrounding soft tissue and the structure and position of the tongue and mandible into which it inserts. The degree of upper airway collapse varies continuously according to sleep stage or body position. It can be quantified by the critical closing pressure, which represents the pressure of the surrounding collapsible segment when it collapses [29,30].

Obesity, via multiple mechanisms, is the major risk factor for OSA [31]. One such mechanism is narrowing of the upper airway by excess fatty tissue. There is growing evidence that, in the supine position, fluid shifts from the lower to the upper body compartments and accumulates in the soft tissue of the upper airways, promoting upper airway closure during sleep. The extent of this fluid shift correlates with the number of respiratory disturbances [32].

Under normal circumstances and in most individuals, the activity of dilating upper airway muscles counterbalances these unfavorable predispositions. Several muscles show phasic activity depending on inspiration, although tonic activity of some decreases during sleep. Local reflex mechanisms additionally contribute to the muscle tone [33]. The tonic muscular activity is increased in sleep apnea patients during wakefulness as a compensation for the mechanical load—a mechanism that fails during sleep [34–36]. It has been hypothesized that the continuous stress on the muscles or the long-term vibrational trauma of snoring might change the ultrastructure and integrity of the muscle bundles [6,37]. Moreover, impairment of the sensory characteristics of the upper airway mucosa [38] might interrupt the reflex mechanisms that counterbalance negative intraluminal pressure (negative pressure reflex).

Cardiovascular consequences of OSA

The complete (apnea) or partial (hypopnea) obstruction of the upper airways leads to oxygen desaturation, arousals, and neuro-hormonal activation and excretion of catecholamines during sleep [39–47]. The frequent changes between hypoxia and reoxygenation seem to be the most relevant factor contributing to the development of cardiovascular consequences via reactive oxygen species [41]. Altered blood gas chemistry increases muscle sympathetic nerve activity, blood pressure, and vascular resistance. The oxidative stress leads to endothelial dysfunction and atherosclerosis [39,48]. Several studies have shown that OSA is an independent risk factor for the development of arterial hypertension, heart failure, and stroke [45,46,49–51].

Most studies on the prevalence of SRBD in heart failure focus on patients with systolic dysfunction, which is characterized by a reduction of the left ventricular ejection fraction. In contrast, isolated diastolic heart failure is pathophysiologically due to a non-compliant, stiff left ventricle. The left-ventricular end-diastolic pressure increases and leads to pulmonary congestion and edema. However, the left-ventricular ejection fraction is commonly preserved [44,52]. Both OSA and diastolic dysfunction are common disorders of the elderly population. The pathophysiological effects of OSA, including sympathetic activity, arterial hypertension, and intermittent hypoxia, may contribute to the development of diastolic heart failure [40,45,46]. Although the body of evidence is still limited, the coherence between OSA and diastolic dysfunction is supported by the finding that PAP therapy may reverse the remodeling of the myocardial structure [44–46].

In addition, coronary artery disease is also adversely influenced by OSA. Major cardiac events, restenosis of coronary vessels, and mortality are associated with greater respiratory disturbance during sleep [53–58].

The association of SRBD and cerebrovascular events has been studied intensively. A cross-sectional analysis showed a fourfold increased risk of stroke in patients with an AHI ≥ 20/h. Moreover, an AHI ≥ 20/h also increased the risk of developing stroke in the next 4 years which failed to reach statistical significance after adjustment of confounders [49]. A meta-analysis of studies on sleep apnea and stroke showed a strong correlation with OSA [51]. The relative risk of stroke in sleep apnea may differ between the genders. While there is a continuous increase of the risk by 6% per AHI unit in men, the risk increases in women with an AHI ≥ 25/h [50]. These data need to be reconfirmed.

OSA also adversely affects the prognosis of patients, mainly owing to cardiovascular consequences [56–58]. Survival is reduced in OSA patients in a dose-dependent manner, with AHI as the metric; however, mortality becomes significant in those with an AHI ≥ 30/h [56–58]. Observational studies show that survival improves with CPAP therapy [56], even in the those with less severe OSA [59]. The latter observation is consistent with dose-dependent association of OSA with mortality. If this observation is further confirmed, it has major implications, since most patients with sleep apnea fall in the category of mild to moderate disorder. OSA-related mortality is primarily due to cardiovascular disease [58].

Pathophysiology of CSA

The pathophysiology of CSA is complex, as it is associated with many conditions, as noted earlier [14,15]. Below, we discuss the mechanisms underlying development of CSA in heart failure, the most common cause of CSA in the general population. We discuss the loop gain, which is the ratio of the ventilatory response to internal or external stimuli, the proximity of the prevailing $PaCO_2$ to the apnea threshold PCO_2 during sleep, referred to as PCO_2 reserve, and the instability of the respiratory control system during transition to sleep, shift in sleep stages and arousals. All of these collectively increase the likelihood of developing periodic breathing and central apneas during sleep.

We also briefly discuss the mechanism of CSA associated with opioids, since this category of drugs is among the most commonly used, and central apneas are prevalent in chronic opioid users.

During wakefulness, ventilation is mainly regulated by behavioral, non-chemical factors. As these factors become irrelevant during NREM sleep, owing to withdrawal of the wakefulness drive to breathe, ventilation is influenced mainly by $PaCO_2$ level. For the same reason, small changes in $PaCO_2$ level have profound influence on ventilation [15,60]. Furthermore, the apnea threshold, which defines the $PaCO_2$ level below which breathing ceases, is unmasked during NREM sleep. Third, if the difference between the actual prevailing $PaCO_2$ and the apnea threshold is narrowed, as is in some patients with heart failure, the likelihood of developing CSA is increased [61]. With these powerful mechanisms exposed in NREM sleep, small variations in ventilation may either lower the $PaCO_2$ below or elevate it above the apnea threshold, a self-sustaining mechanism for recurring central apneas.

Central apneas are prevalent during NREM sleep, but are rare during REM sleep, as the difference between the prevailing $PaCO_2$ and the apnea threshold is wide (for reviews, see [15,60]).

Loop gain is an engineering term and when applied to the negative feedback system controlling breathing, it defines the ratio of ventilatory response to a disturbance in ventilation, for example an

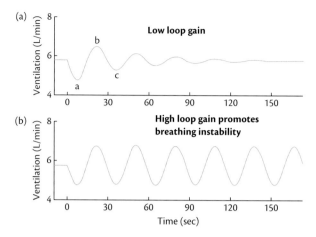

Fig. 40.4 The ventilatory response (at B) to a reduction in ventilation (at A), for example a hypopnea. In (a), the magnitude of the compensatory ventilator response, i.e, the amount of hyperventilation, is less than the disturbance. In this case, the loop gain is less than 1 and shortly the ventilation returns to normal level (at C). In (b), the loop gain is more than 1. Consequently, the disturbance elicits periodic breathing [85].

Adapted from Comprehensive Physiology, 3(1), Javaheri S, Dempsey JA, Central sleep apnea, pp. 141–163, Copyright (2013), with permission from John Wiley and Sons.

apnea or hypopnea [15, 62]. The higher the loop gain, the greater the tendency toward breathing instability (Fig. 40.4). When the magnitude of the increase in ventilation is greater than or equal to the magnitude of the preceding apnea or hypopnea (i.e, loop gain ≥ 1), the respiratory system is unstable and periodic breathing occurs in NREM sleep. The three major components of the loop gain are increased in some patients with heart failure, and these are the patients who suffer from periodic breathing. These three components (gains) are increased chemosensitivity (increased controller gain), decreased functional residual capacity (increased plant gain: a large change in PCO_2 for a given change in ventilation), and increased circulation time (mixing gain). The longer the circulation time, the time it takes for the changes in pulmonary capillary blood PCO_2 and partial pressure of oxygen (PO_2) to reach the sites of chemoreceptors, the longer the cycle of periodic breathing. This increased circulation time converts a negative feedback system to a positive one. It follows that the greater the magnitude of chemosensitivity to PCO_2 and PO_2, and the lower the functional residual capacity, the higher the loop gain. The three gains discussed above describe the characteristics of the loop gain under steady -state conditions, whereas the loop gain is dynamic and more complex during sleep, while periodic breathing is occurring [62].

$PaCO_2$ is chronically reduced in some patients with heart failure and pulmonary congestion [20,62–64]. In these patients, increased pulmonary capillary pressure stimulates juxtacapillary receptors, causing hyperventilation. Pulmonary capillary wedge pressure (PCWP), normally measured by insertion of a Swan–Ganz catheter through the jugular vein into the pulmonary artery, is a measure of mean left-atrial pressure and left-ventricular end-diastolic pressure (in the absence of mitral valve disease), and it correlates significantly with $PaCO_2$ [20]. Medical therapy of heart failure reduces the PCWP, $PaCO_2$, and respiratory disturbances during sleep [20].

At this point, however, we need to emphasize that although an awake low steady-state $PaCO_2$ is highly predictive of CSA [63], a low steady-state $PaCO_2$ by itself is protective against CSA [65], unless it

is accompanied by a low PCO_2 reserve (see [15,60]). In the absence of a low PCO_2 reserve, a low $PaCO_2$ is protective against developing central apnea as dictated by the alveolar ventilation equation [65].

As noted earlier, heart failure patients with CSA/HCSB exhibit an augmented hypercapnic ventilatory response while awake [66,67]. This results in an overshoot in ventilation even in the face of a small rise in PCO_2 that may occur after a short pause in breathing, or as PCO_2 rises in the course of an apnea or hypopnea. This overshoot in ventilation transiently lowers the prevailing PCO_2 toward or below apneic threshold, causing another hypopnea or apnea. The cycle is maintained, as central apnea begets central apnea.

The reactivity of *cerebral blood flow* response to hyper- and hypocapnia differs between healthy persons and heart failure patients with CSA. Normally, the homeostatic response of the cerebral vascular bed to changes in $PaCO_2$ is an important protector of brain extracellular fluid $PCO_2/[H^+]$. Specifically, when $PaCO_2$ increases, cerebral vessels dilate, and if the mean arterial blood pressure remains unchanged, then cerebral blood flow increases, washing out CO_2 from the brain, maintaining brain PCO_2 as close to normal as possible. The reverse occurs when $PaCO_2$ decreases. Therefore, this homeostatic regulation of cerebral blood flow in response to changes in $PaCO_2$ (either increases or decreases) reduces the impact of arterial hypercapnia and hypocapnia on brain and central chemoreceptor $PCO_2/[H^+]$. It has been shown that in heart failure patients with CSA, the physiological increase in cerebral blood flow following elevation of $PaCO_2$ is diminished (for details, see [15]). As an example, therefore, with a central apnea, for a given rise in $PaCO_2$, the brain and central chemoreceptor $PCO_2/[H^+]$ will be higher, resulting in overshoot and breathing instability.

The instability of ventilation becomes aggravated by *arousals* from sleep. Arousals stimulate ventilatory drive and reduce the CO_2 level, as the sleeping PCO_2 is excessive when the brain arouses from sleep. Furthermore, the CO_2 hypersensitivity of the chemoreceptors in some heart failure patients, discussed earlier, augments hyperventilation during transient arousals, resulting in PCO_2 falling below the apneic threshold, with consequent central apnea.

CSA in cardiac diseases

CSA is quite rare in the general population, but occurs frequently in a number of cardiovascular disorders, including heart failure with either reduced or preserved ejection fraction, atrial fibrillation, and pulmonary hypertension [14,15]. In this section, we concentrate on heart failure with reduced ejection fraction, which has been most systematically investigated.

Several studies have consistently shown high prevalence of CSA in patients with reduced left-ventricular ejection fraction (LVEF) (for reviews, see [23,66], even in the absence of symptoms of heart failure [21]. Central apneas and hypopneas are interspersed between long cycles of waxing and waning of ventilation, a unique pattern of breathing that, as already mentioned, is referred to as HCSB [66,68]. It is of crucial clinical relevance that many of these patients do not present with the classical symptoms of habitual snoring or with subjective daytime sleepiness [14,15,18]. Furthermore, heart failure patients with CSA are normally not obese [14,18]. The absence of these risk factors for sleep apnea was recognized in early studies of heart failure [14,15,18], and therefore we have referred to sleep apnea as an occult sleep disorder [15]. These findings have subsequently been confirmed by others [69]. This lack of subjective daytime sleepiness may contribute to under-diagnosis of CSA in heart failure, particularly since these patents are generally not obese or hypertensive and do not snore much [24].

Heart failure patients with CSA have higher levels of brain natriuretic peptide as compared with those without breathing disturbances [70]. Moreover, the urinary norepinephrine (noradrenaline) concentration—a measure of integrated overnight sympathetic activity—is increased in heart failure with CSA as compared with heart failure without breathing disturbances [71]. Moreover, CSA significantly increases malignant cardiac arrhythmias [72,73] and cardioverter–defibrillator therapies [72] as compared with heart failure patients without breathing disturbances. Importantly, effective treatment of CSA decreases the number of nocturnal ventricular arrhythmias [74] and the associated mortality [75] when effectively treated [76].

The mechanism underlying arrhythmias is in part due to the increased sympathetic activity already discussed. It is therefore not surprising that heart failure patients who smoke have an excess probability of nocturnal ventricular arrhythmias [73] and perhaps sudden cardiac death. Nicotine, the active chemical in tobacco, increases efferent sympathetic activity through stimulating the nicotinic receptors in peripheral arterial chemoreceptors in the carotid bodies. Active discussion regarding cessation of smoking needs to be part of any physician visit, and is critical in patients with cardiovascular disease and heart failure.

So far, we have concentrated on heart failure with reduced LVEF, but in passing we also note a high prevalence of CSA and OSA in isolated diastolic heart failure and in heart failure with preserved ejection fraction (HFpEF). Isolated diastolic heart failure is pathophysiologically due to a noncompliant, stiff left ventricle. This altered remodeling of the left ventricle causes increased left-ventricular end-diastolic pressure and consequent pulmonary congestion and edema.

In spite of the large number of studies in heart failure with reduced ejection fraction, there has been only one large, though excellent, study in HFpEF [52]. In a prospective study, Bitter et al. evaluated 244 consecutive patients with HFpEF who were on optimal therapy and were well characterized, including by right-heart catheterization. Similar to the prevalence in patients with reduced ejection fraction, using an AHI ≥ 15 per hour of sleep, the prevalence of moderate to severe sleep apnea was close to 50%, with almost half of these patients suffering from OSA and half from CSA. Randomized controlled therapeutic trials are needed to delineate the causation and whether treatment of either OSA or CSA influences outcomes of HFpEF.

In conclusion, SRBDs, both OSA and CSA, are prevalent in patients with cardiovascular disorders, including asymptomatic left-ventricular dysfunction, atrial fibrillation, coronary artery disease, and heart failure, both with normal and with reduced ejection fraction. Biomarkers of poor heart function and mortality or severe cardiac events are increased in patients with cardiovascular disease comorbid with sleep apnea. These patients may not present with daytime sleepiness, but suffer from reduced quality of life and excess mortality. Taking these aspects together, we recommend routine screening for SRBDs in patients with cardiovascular diseases and appropriate treatment in order to improve outcome.

Treatment options for sleep apnea

Treatment options of sleep apnea, both OSA and CSA, in heart disease have been reviewed elsewhere [23,26–28,44,66,68,77–80]. In general, in the presence of cardiovascular comorbidities such as hypertension, coronary artery disease, atrial fibrillation, and heart failure, the best treatment option for OSA is CPAP therapy. Treatment of CSA is more difficult than that of OSA, and multiple options are available as discussed below.

Treatment of OSA

The pathophysiology of OSA is characterized by an imbalance between dilating and obstructing factors in the upper airways. Mechanical properties and neuromuscular control of the upper airway muscles are the key factors contributing to upper airway occlusion. In some patients, a high loop gain also plays a role.

Intensive education and advice of patients and relatives, coupled with reduction of body weight in obese patients, is generally recommended [81,82]. However, weight loss as a single procedure is insufficient in most cases. Therefore, frequently, additional therapy is offered, particularly in patients with preexisting cardiovascular disease. In these patients, we invariably recommend treatment with positive airway pressure devices, for which there are multiple options available [83–86].

CPAP for treatment of OSA

Since its first description in the early 1980s, CPAP treatment has become the therapy of choice for OSA [87]. The positive airway pressure is provided by a flow generator device and applied to the patient via a tube and a mask, usually placed on the nose. Thus, the intraluminal pressure of the upper airways is increased enough to counterbalance the obstructive tissue pressure. The device also provides humidity to prevent nasobuccal dryness [88].

The optimal treatment pressure is individually adjusted by manual or automatic titration, aiming at complete resolution of apneas, hypopneas, snoring, and flow limitations. CPAP stabilizes the upper airways independent of the localization of the obstruction, which makes it the most effective treatment option. It normalizes respiratory disturbances and sleep quality, daytime performance, neurocognitive deficits, and the ability to drive cars and operate machines safely. In addition, CPAP has been shown to reduce the risk of cardiovascular comorbidities. Kohler et al. found significant reductions in the augmentation index and the mean arterial blood pressure in effectively treated patients [89]. There are contradictory findings in terms of arterial hypertension, and this is mostly due to inclusion of patients with "hypertension" whose blood pressure (BP) was not that elevated (they were on antihypertensive medications) at the time of CPAP therapy; another issue has been lack of efficacy in CPAP non-adherent patients. We should, however, expect improvement in hypertension in OSA patients who are truly hypertensive as defined by blood pressure measurement (not simply being on medication with normal or near normal blood pressure) and in those with uncontrolled hypertension. Those with severe OSA are most likely to gain the greatest hemodynamic benefit from CPAP treatment. Campos-Rodriguez et al. found a significant improvement after 24 months of CPAP in patients with insufficiently controlled hypertension and in those who used their devices for more than 3.5 hours a day [90]. However, in the subgroup analysis of 35 patients with incompletely controlled hypertension at entry, a significant decrease in the 24-hour mean systolic and diastolic BP ranging from 4.2 to 5.1 mmHg was noted. Similarly, in the subgroup analysis of 27 patients who used CPAP for more than 5.3 hours a day, the range in BP drop varied from 4.3 to 6.7 mmHg. Linear regression analysis showed that baseline systolic BP and hours of CPAP were independent predictors of reductions in BP with CPAP. In a randomized controlled trial, use of CPAP significantly decreased the

BP of patients with moderate to severe hypertension by about 10 mmHg within a few weeks [91]. There is also evidence showing a reduction of coronary artery disease in patients treated optimally by CPAP [90]. In addition, CPAP improves the prognosis of OSA patients. Marin et al. showed significantly more fatal and nonfatal cardiovascular events in untreated patients with severe OSAS (AHI ≥ 30/h) as compared with untreated patients with lesser degrees of the disease, simple snorers, healthy controls, and also patients effectively treated with CPAP [56]. Büchner et al. followed 449 OSA patients for 72 months, including 364 effectively treated and adherent patients and 85 patients who refused treatment. While both groups presented with similar cardiovascular comorbidities and risk factors, OSA was more severe in the adherent group [59]. In spite of this, effective therapy with CPAP was associated with a substantial reduction in fatal and nonfatal cardiovascular events. Although limited by low treatment adherence, a most recently published RCT did not show a significant difference between CPAP and usual care on cardiovascular endpoints but found improvements of daytime symptoms. However, the number of cerebrovascular events was significantly improved in those patients with good adherence [92].

There are limited studies of patients with heart failure and OSA treated with CPAP. Overnight application of nasal CPAP has been shown to eliminate obstructive disordered breathing events, desaturation and the large negative swings in juxtacardiac pressure that occur during upper airway occlusion [74]. As a result of these favorable physiological changes, treatment of OSA with CPAP may increase LVEF, as reported in three [93,94] of the four randomized controlled trials. In one trial, which was the only one with a placebo arm (i.e, a CPAP device with minimal pressure) [95], there was no change in BP, but adherence to the device was less than the other studies [93,94] in which adherence was reported.

Javaheri et al. [96] analyzed more than 30 000 files of a cohort of Medicare beneficiaries with newly diagnosed heart failure. Normally, such patients are 65 years or older with a high prevalence of heart failure. Based on the data in the literature and reviewed above, all such patients should have been referred for sleep study as 15 000 of them are likely to suffer from moderate to severe sleep apnea. However, only 4% were suspected of suffering from SRBDs, most probably OSA, which is easier to suspect clinically based on obesity, hypertension, and snoring. However, only 2% underwent diagnosis and treatment. In multiple regression analysis, after accounting for a number of covariates, there was a significant improvement in survival of those patients diagnosed and treated for sleep apnea, compared with the rest of the patients.

A small observational study from Japan [97] showed significantly improved survival in heart failure patients with OSA who were adherent to CPAP compared with those who were not.

The principle of positive airway pressure treatment has not been changed since its first description. However, several modifications, such as automatic expiratory positive airway pressure (EPAP) and bilevel and expiratory pressure relief, have been introduced. These algorithms may be preferred in individual cases and therefore extend the therapeutic portfolio available to the patients and sleep physician.

CPAP therapy is not associated with severe adverse effects, but may be limited by local side effects and inconvenience. The long-term efficacy of CPAP depends primarily on adherence by the patient [98–100].The main symptom of OSA, namely, EDS, normally improves with CPAP use; however, the amount of improvement is dose-dependent with average nightly use [100]. This correlation with dose dependence of CPAP use has also been demonstrated with

improvements in inflammation, hypertension, LVEF, and mortality. The minimum acceptable adherence criterion for Medicare and other insurance companies to pay for the device is an average daily use of 4 or more hours, at least 70% of nights. Positive airway pressure compliance depends on several factors, including the patient's awareness of symptoms and their improvement, and optimal education and support in the first days of the adaptation, but also the social and economic situation of the patient [100]. In patients with cardiovascular disease, the better the adherence, the greater is the improvement in outcome, as already eluded to.

Mandibular advancement devices for treatment of OSA
Mandibular advancement devices (MADs) widen the diameter of the upper airways and counterbalance their collapse during sleep by protruding the mandible and the tongue [101]. Unfortunately, the efficacy of treatment cannot be predicted in individual patients. Data from prospective and controlled studies show a reduction of respiratory disturbances in about half of patients by 50–60% of the baseline AHI [102]. Current guidelines recommend adjustable, two-piece devices custom-made by a specialized dental specialist. Itzhaki et al. demonstrated in a case–control study a reduction of respiratory disturbances by 40–50% after 1 year of treatment as compared with untreated patients. Notably, this limited effect was associated with an improvement in parameters of endothelial function and oxidative stress [103]. In addition, Phillips et al. [104] compared CPAP with MAD in a prospective, randomized cross-over trial over 1 month each. Although CPAP was more effective in terms of respiratory disturbances, the authors did not find a difference in arterial hypertension or symptoms of sleep apnea. However, during the short treatment period, neither method improved arterial hypertension.

There has been only one observational study of an MAD in patients with heart failure. Eskafi [105,107] studied 11 patients with heart failure with reduced ejection fraction (mean LVEF = 34%) and moderate sleep apnea, presumably a combination of both OSA and CSA. Mandibular advancement was found to result in a significant reduction in AHI from 25 to 15 per hour. After 6 months of therapy, brain natriuretic peptide also decreased significantly; there was, however, no significant change in ejection fraction. This is an area that needs further research.

Alternatives
There is limited evidence for the use of alternative treatment options [106]. Tonsillectomy can be recommended in children and adults in the case of tonsillar hypertrophy [107,108]. Maxillomandibular osteotomy has proven to be as effective as CPAP and may be suitable in individual patients who cannot accept the latter [109]. Distraction osteogenesis may be useful in patients with congenital micrognathia and midface hypoplasia [110].

Most recently, hypoglossal nerve stimulation by an implanted device has been tried in a prospective observational (nonrandomized) trial [111] in which 126 individuals who had difficulty in either accepting or tolerating CPAP were implanted. The mean BMI was 28.4 kg/m^2 and patients with AHI ≥ 50/h were excluded. The mean AHI was 32/h and decreased to 15.2/h at 12 months. Two secondary outcomes also improved significantly. The Epworth Sleepiness Scale score decreased from 11.6 to 7. Disease-specific quality of life was assessed by the Functional Outcomes of Sleep Questionnaire (FOSQ) score, which increased by 2.9 points—typically, a 2-point increase is clinically significant. Stimulation resulted in tongue soreness and abrasions in 40% and 21%, respectively. In the latter group, the device had to be reprogrammed, and some required a mouthpiece. About 18% of the participants complained of tongue weakness, which resolved within a month. Two participants required reoperation to reposition the stimulator. This was considered a serious device-related adverse complication. No favorable cardiometabolic changes were reported.

Treatment options for CSA

The treatment options for CSA are evolving (for reviews, see [23,62,68]). In general, CSA is more difficult to treat than OSA. Both positive airway pressure devices and multiple medications have been tried. With virtually all of these therapeutic options, significant residual events remain, as discussed below.

Optimization of cardiopulmonary function

Aggressive treatment of heart failure may improve or even eliminate periodic breathing. Several mechanisms may be invoked, including decreasing wedge pressure, increasing stroke volume, decreasing arterial circulation time, and normalizing functional residual capacity [23,62,68], all of which should stabilize periodic breathing. Both pharmacological (eg, angiotensin-converting enzyme (ACE) inhibitors and beta-blockers) [112,113] and nonpharmacological device [114,115] therapy of heart failure have been shown to improve CSA. In spite of these findings, the prevalence of sleep apnea has not changed with the introduction of beta-blockers into the armamentarium of therapy for heart failure [23,68], as heart failure is a progressive disease and with progression sleep apnea either develops or worsens.

A study of 45 patients showed that CSA is virtually eliminated after cardiac transplantation [116]. The results of this study therefore indicate that heart failure is a cause of CSA. Many cardiac transplant recipients develop OSA owing to weight gain, and those who gain the most are most prone to develop OSA. Cardiac transplant patients with OSA also developed hypertension and had poor quality of life compared with those without OSA [116]. For reasons that are not well known, restless legs syndrome (RLS) and periodic limb movements in sleep (PLMS) are also prevalent after cardiac transplantation [116]. Approximately 31% of patients had PLMS with an index of 55 per hour of sleep, and 45% of these patents suffered from RLS.

Nocturnal supplemental nasal oxygen

Systematic studies (reviewed in [23]) of patients with systolic heart failure have shown that nocturnal administration of supplemental nasal oxygen improves CSA and desaturation. In the largest study [117] of 36 subjects with systolic heart failure (mean LVEF about 22%), it was observed that the central apnea index decreased significantly from 28/h to 10/h.

Supplemental nasal oxygen improves CSA by multiple mechanisms [118] (reviewed in [23]), such as decreasing hypoxic and hypercapnic ventilatory drives and decreasing sympathetic activity. In addition, oxygen administration may also widen the PCO_2 reserve, i.e, the difference between the prevailing PCO_2 and the apneic threshold PCO_2 [119].

The long-term effects of administration of nocturnal oxygen on the mortality of patients with heart failure need to be studied. In a randomized parallel-design open trial of 56 patients with systolic heart failure, Sasayama et al. [120] reported that the use of nocturnal supplemental nasal oxygen resulted in significant improvements in LVEF and New York Heart Association (NYHA) functional class. Such changes were not observed in the control group.

With regard to potential adverse effects of supplemental oxygen, it has been reported that in patients with congestive heart failure, hyperoxia may be associated with adverse hemodynamic effects [121]. However, this has been shown primarily with a high fractional concentration of oxygen, at doses that are beyond what is necessary to treat desaturation due to CSA [117,120]. Furthermore, the results of these studies are not applicable to patients with heart failure and CSA, since supplemental oxygen is used to prevent desaturation, not to increase it above normal, the way this study [121] was designed.

Other medications

The respiratory stimulant *theophylline* has been shown to reduce CSA in heart failure [3,122,123]. Javaheri et al. studied oral theophylline in 15 stable patients with systolic heart failure in a randomized double-blind placebo-controlled design. They showed a reduction of the AHI by 50% associated with an improvement of oxygen saturation [123]. However, long-term data on the use of theophylline are lacking. Due to potential pro-arrythmogenic potency of theophylline and the limited evidence in CSA/HCSB, theophylline should be only used in selected cases under close supervision.

Acetazolamide is a mild diuretic and respiratory stimulant, which has been used to prevent and treat periodic breathing at high altitude, as well as idiopathic CSA [124,125]. A randomized double blind placebo-controlled crossover study in 12 heart failure patients showed a significant reduction of CSA under acetazolamide. Although patients reported improvements in parameters of sleep quality and quality of life, respiratory disturbances were only reduced by about 40% [126]. More data are needed to allow general recommendations to be made.

CPAP in the treatment of CSA/HCSB

Application of positive airway pressure in patients with impaired cardiac function seems to be reasonable, as it might improve oxygen supply, reduce oxygen requirement, and unload the heart mechanically. CPAP reduces ventilation–perfusion mismatch by recruiting poorly/non-ventilated portions of the lungs. Consecutively, oxygen levels in the blood and oxygen delivery to the organs increase. Positive airway pressure decreases venous return to the right heart, which may then decrease right-ventricular stroke volume and consequently pulmonary capillary volume and pressure. Pulmonary capillary pressure may also decrease with reduction in left-ventricular end-diastolic pressure, as CPAP unloads the left ventricle. Decreased pulmonary capillary pressure is critical in improving periodic breathing and CSA.

These pathophysiological considerations are in accordance with the findings of clinical trials. A post-hoc analysis of CanPAP data showed that CPAP improved the prognosis of those patients with a substantial reduction of SRBDs [76]. No benefit was observed in those whose CSA was not suppressed by CPAP. In fact, CPAP might be harmful in this group [127]. Therefore, we begin our therapeutic approach with a one-night CPAP trial, and if AHI decreases below 15/h, the patient is considered CPAP-responsive. Otherwise, we proceed with the adaptive servoventilation (ASV) therapy described below.

Adaptive servoventilation devices

These are the most advanced of positive airway pressure devices [83,84,128]. They interfere most precisely with the pathophysiology of HCSB. The algorithms apply variable inspiratory pressure support (defined as the pressure difference between inspiratory and expiratory pressures) according to the actual requirements of the patient on a breath-by-breath base (Fig. 40.5). The pressure support is increased during periods of hypoventilation and reduced during hyperventilation. Additionally, mandatory breaths are applied to avoid central apneas. The most advanced algorithms also apply variable expiratory pressure to adapt to changing levels of upper airway obstruction. This automatic variable pressure is in contrast to CPAP devices, and should provide the greatest comfort for patients.

ASV has been proven to effectively suppress CSA/HCSB [129], and observational studies show improved survival of heart failure patients who used the device compared with those who refused or were intolerant [130–133]. These devices are also effective in coexisting obstructive and central disturbances in cardiac patients [27] and in patients with opioid-induced sleep apnea [25,134]. However, the recently published SERVE-HF study [135] investigated the effects of ASV in addition to optimal cardiac treatment as compared with optimal cardiac treatment alone in patients with symptomatic systolic heart failure (NYHA II with previous hospitalization, NYHA III, and NYHA IV), LVEF ≤ 45%, and predominant CSA. While the study failed to show a significant difference in the primary outcome parameter of the composite of cardiac events, secondary analyses showed an increased rate of cardiac death and death from any cause in the ASV group. We have discussed some potential reasons for the failure of this trial [136]. One of these, among multiple issues, is the use of an old-generation ASV device with outdated algorithms that (1) were unable to adjust the expiratory pressure to the changing dynamic of upper airway and

(2) provided an aggressive inspiratory pressure support that rose rapidly and declined slowly. As a result, some patients were under-pressurized and some over-pressurized by the device. In either case, the consequences could have been fatal. These deficiencies were modified significantly in a new-generation device [85]. Unfortunately, the results are also affected by a low adherence rate (40% of patients with daily use for less than 3 hours), a high crossover between the treatment arms (23%), and differences in the baseline therapies (higher use of anti-arrhythmic drugs in the ASV group). Subgroup analysis suggests that patients with a very low ejection fraction < 30% and patients using anti-arrhythmic drugs represent the groups at risk for cardiac death. More detailed data from per-protocol analyses and subgroup studies of the SERVE-HF trial are required. In addition, results from another multicenter study (ADVENT-HF) are expected. At present, ASV should not be prescribed to patients with systolic, symptomatic heart failure with LVEF ≤ 45% and predominant CSA/HCSB.

Phrenic nerve stimulation
A new device has been introduced into the therapeutic armamentarium for CSA. This phrenic nerve pacemaker is placed intravenously into a thoracic vein where the phrenic nerve overlaps the vein. The unilateral phrenic nerve can be stimulated during sleep at a set frequency to prevent the development of central apnea. In an early study, overnight stimulation resulted in virtual elimination of central apneas, with consequent improvements in desaturation and arousals [137]. A multicenter randomized clinical trial with a control arm has begun.

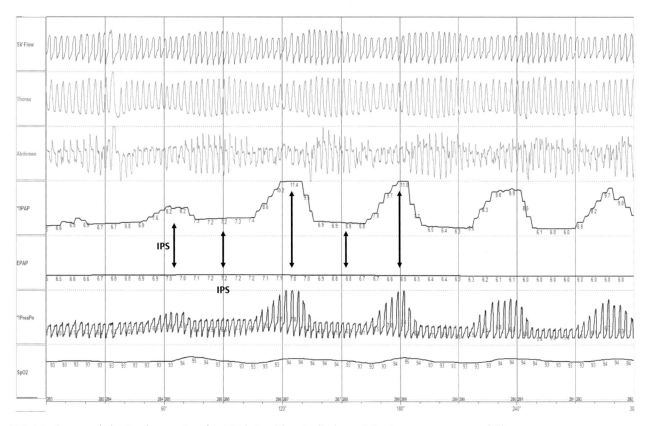

Fig. 40.5 A 5-minute epoch showing the operation of an ASV device with anticyclic changes in inspiratory pressure support (IPS).
Reproduced from Chest, 146(2), Javaheri S, Brown LK, Randerath WJ, Positive airway pressure therapy with adaptive servoventilation: part 1: operational algorithms, pp. 514–23, Copyright (2014), with permission from Elsevier.

Periodic limb movements

Since the introduction of PSG to study SRBDs in heart failure, few studies [24,129,138,139] have reported on the prevalence of PLMS in heart failure patients. Hanly and Zuberi-Khokhar [139] are credited with the first report. In their study of 23 patients with severe heart failure and reduced ejection fraction, the prevalence of PLMS was 53%, with an average PLMS index of 73 per hour of sleep. In a later study of 14 patients with left-heart failure, Teschler group [129] reported an index of 12/h. It is not clear how to reconcile such huge differences between the two studies, although the number of patients was small in both. In the largest study of 55 patients [24], also in patients with systolic heart failure, 20% had PLMS (index ≥ 5/h), with an average index of 35/h. In another study from Brazil [138], a prevalence of 20% was confirmed.

It is critical to emphasize a potential misclassification of PLMS, where a leg movement is not part of PLMS, but rather a consequence of sleep apneas and hypopneas. If arousals occur as a result of an SRBD, then, if the leg movement occurs after the arousals, it should not cause misclassification. However, frequently, there may be no arousals in association with an SRBD, but there is leg movement. Under such circumstances, misclassification may occur, inflating the PLMS index.

The mechanisms of PLMS in heart failure are not known. One risk factor could be iron-deficiency anemia, which is more common in severe chronic heart failure and could be due to several mechanisms, including reduced intestinal iron absorption. Another possibility is increased sympathetic activity, which has been suggested to play a primary role in the generation of idiopathic PLMS [140]. Since increased sympathetic activity is the hallmark of heart failure with reduced ejection fraction, it could be the link with PLM.

We must emphasize here that there has been no study on RLS in heart failure. However, in spite of this, in the setting of congestive heart failure, PLMS may have adverse hemodynamic consequences, and the question arises whether PLMS should be treated.

Hemodynamic consequences of PLMS, particularly with arousals, are increased heart rate and blood pressure. Pennestri and colleagues [141] studied patients with RLS without known cardiovascular disease, who underwent PSG simultaneously with noninvasive, beat-to-beat blood pressure monitoring. The systolic blood pressure increased by an average of 22 mmHg and the diastolic blood pressure by 11 mmHg with PLMS and arousals. The increments were less in the absence of arousals. Although the long-term effects of these alterations due to PLMS remain to be established in a randomized controlled trial, the rises in blood pressure and heart rate could have deleterious effects on cardiovascular functions, particularly in patients with established cardiovascular disease. Meanwhile three studies [142–144] have investigated the long-term association of PLMS and cardiovascular disease. In the first observational study in a large cohort of men older than 65 years, Koo and colleagues [143] followed 2911 men for 4 years. Participants had PSG at home. The authors reported a significant association between PLMS and incident all-cause cardiocerebrovascular disease plus peripheral arterial disease, but not coronary heart disease or cerebrovascular disease in isolation. In another observational study, Yumino and colleagues [142] followed 218 consecutive patients with heart failure and reduced ejection fraction from 1997 to 2004. The mean follow-up was about 40 months. After adjusting for a number of covariates, PLMS index ≥ 5/h remained a significant independent risk factor for mortality. The hazard ratio was 2.42, with a 95% confidence interval of 1.16–5.02, $p = 0.018$.

The third study [144] was a retrospective chart review suggesting an association between PLMS and left-ventricular hypertrophy.

These associations [142–144] do not prove causality, and, as already noted, the difficulty of recognizing PLMS accurately remains a concern.

In contrast to CSA, which is eliminated after cardiac transplantation, PLMS is not. As noted earlier, in a study of 45 cardiac transplant patients, about 30% suffered from severe PLMS, and almost half of them had RLS [116].

Insomnia, poor sleep efficiency, and the heart

In this section, we briefly review the effects of sleep on the cardiovascular system and the effects of cardiac pathology on sleep. A more detailed review of these interactions can be found in [145].

As NREM sleep deepens from stage N1 to stage N3, there is a progressive diminution in sympathetic activity and an increase in parasympathetic activity. Consequently, arterial blood pressure and heart rate decrease by approximately 10–20% relative to the mean daytime values. Therefore, NREM sleep, which occupies about 80% of total sleep time, is associated with cardiovascular quiescence as the cardiac workload decreases. In contrast, during REM sleep, in association with pontogeniculo-occipital (PGO) waves, sympathetic activity increases, with concomitant increases in heart rate, blood pressure, and myocardial oxygen demand. In this period of sleep, the heart is vulnerable to ischemia, arrhythmias, and potentially sudden death.

Also, the normal dipping and decrease in heart rate may not occur in the presence of sleep disorders such as sleep apnea or PLMS, potentially resulting in deleterious long-term consequences.

Sleep in patients with heart failure is quite disturbed. In the study of patients with systolic heart failure who underwent habituation in the sleep laboratory and had full-night PSG on the second night, sleep efficiency was decreased and architecture was disrupted. Stage N1 occupied 34% of total sleep time, stage N3 was not achieved, and arousals were excessive [17,24]. There was objective evidence of insomnia, with a sleep efficiency of about 72%, though sleep onset was not increased. As noted, patients had been habituated to the environment of the laboratory, and in the morning they invariably felt that they had slept as usual. Historically, this kind of insomnia has been referred to as secondary (i.e, secondary to heart failure). In these patients, awakenings and insomnia are multifactorial. Some of the symptoms of heart failure, such as nocturia, paroxysmal nocturnal dyspnea, orthopnea, and cough, are disruptive. In addition, melatonin synthesis and secretion may be impaired owing to administration of certain beta-blockers, as the synthesis and secretion of melatonin are regulated through the β-adrenergic signal transduction system [145,146].

Finally, we should note that insomnia may be due to depression, which is frequently comorbid with heart failure. The impact of insomnia comorbid with heart failure and its consequences for the morbidity and mortality of the latter are not clear. Being insomniac and/or awake, in contrast to being asleep, can be associated with increased sympathetic and decreased parasympathetic activity. Not surprisingly, a number of studies have shown that patients with insomnia have elevated heart rate, blood pressure, whole-body and cerebral metabolic rate, interleukin-6, and catecholamines [147–151]. It is possible, however, that the biomarkers of primary insomnia, a hyperarousal state, are different from those of being awake after sleep onset as it occurs in patients with heart failure. Prolonged wakefulness, excess stage N1 and arousals, and absence of deep sleep stages collectively could result in increased sympathetic activity, with deleterious cardiovascular effects. Furthermore, research studies show that acute sleep deprivation in the laboratory is associated with activation of proinflammatory pathways [149], and increased ghrelin and decreased leptin [150]. The ratio of these latter two hormones is increased, promoting hunger and weight gain associated with short sleep duration. It is notable that the prevalence of obesity is about 43% among patients with heart failure [152], in contrast to a 35% prevalence in the US general population.

One question is whether there is a bidirectional relationship between short sleep and heart failure. Reinhard and colleagues [153] have studied 188 consecutive patients with heart failure and have concluded that PSG-documented short sleep and reduced sleep efficiency are associated with excess mortality in patients with heart failure. On the other hand, Laugsand and colleagues [154] followed a large cohort of patients with *symptoms* of insomnia and, in Cox proportional hazard models, insomnia was associated with incident heart failure and there was a dose-dependent association between the number of insomnia symptoms and the risk of heart failure. In patients with three symptoms of insomnia (difficulty falling asleep, maintaining sleep, and having nonrestorative sleep), compared with those without symptoms of insomnia, the hazard ratio was 4.53, with a 95% confidence interval of 1.99–10.31, $p = 0.021$. Randomized controlled trails are needed to elucidate the bidirectional relationship of insomnia and heart failure and to determine its impact. In the absence of such data, the use of ramelteon, a melatonin receptor agonist, is appropriate, particularly in patients who are receiving beta-blockers, which may impair melatonin synthesis and secretion. Ramelteon is an M_1 and M_2 receptor agonist acting on the suprachiasmatic nucleus promoting sleep. Ramelteon is not habit-forming and does not promote SRBDs. However, it is only appropriate for sleep onset insomnia. Because sleep-related breathing disorders are common in patients with heart failure, and some hypnotics may promote sleep apnea, PSG is recommended if γ-aminobutyric acid (GABA) receptor agonists are used to treat insomnia in patients with heart failure.

Summary

Sleep disorders are highly prevalent in patients with heart failure. Both OSA and CSA are associated with arterial oxyhemoglobin desaturation and arousals. In the long run, these pathological consequences result in functional and structural cardiac alterations. Observational studies show that effective treatment of sleep apnea improves cardiac function and survival. Large-scale randomized controlled trials are in progress.

PLMS are also observed by PSG in heart failure patients, but the prevalence of RLS is not known. Randomized clinical trials are needed to determine the impact of PLMS on survival in heart failure.

Patients with heart failure have poor sleep, which could be due to multiple reasons. Studies suggest a bidirectional relationship between heart failure and insomnia. However, surprisingly, there are no trials on insomnia in heart failure to determine the impact of this bidirectional relationship.

References

1. Javaheri S. Sleep and cardiovascular disease: present and future. In: Kryger M, Roth T, Dement W, eds. Principles and practice of sleep medicine, 5th ed. Philadelphia: WB Saunders, 2011:1349–52.
2. Young T, Palta M, Dempsey J, et al. The occurrence of sleep-disordered breathing among middle-aged adults. N Engl J Med 1993;328(17):1230–5.
3. Peppard PE, Young T, Barnet JH, et al. Increased prevalence of sleep-disordered breathing in adults. Am J Epidemiol 2013;177(9):1006–14.
4. Netzer NC, Hoegel JJ, Loube D, et al. Prevalence of symptoms and risk of sleep apnea in primary care. Chest 2003;124(4):1406–14.
5. Ohayon MM, Guilleminault C, Priest RG, Caulet M. Snoring and breathing pauses during sleep: telephone interview survey of a United Kingdom population sample. BMJ 1997;314(7084):860–3.
6. Randerath W. Continuous positive airway pressure. Minerva Pneumol 2011;50(1):5–16.
7. Eckert DJ, Malhotra A. Pathophysiology of adult obstructive sleep apnea. Proc Am Thorac Soc 2008;5(2):144–53.
8. Younes M. Role of arousals in the pathogenesis of obstructive sleep apnea. Am J Respir Crit Care Med 2004;169(5):623–33.
9. Schwab RJ, Pasirstein M, Pierson R, et al. Identification of upper airway anatomic risk factors for obstructive sleep apnea with volumetric magnetic resonance imaging. Am J Respir Crit Care Med 2003;168(5):522–30.
10. Schwab RJ, Gefter WB, Hoffman EA, Gupta KB, Pack AI. Dynamic upper airway imaging during awake respiration in normal subjects and patients with sleep disordered breathing. Am Rev Respir Dis 1993;148(5):1385–400.
11. De Backer W. Obstructive sleep apnea–hypopnea syndrome: definitions and pathophysiology. In: Randerath WJ, Sanner BM, Somers VK, eds. Sleep apnea. Basel: Karger, 2006:90–6.
12. Badr MS, Toiber F, Skatrud JB, Dempsey J. Pharyngeal narrowing/occlusion during central sleep apnea. J Appl Physiol 1995;78(5):1806–15.
13. Dowdell WT, Javaheri S, McGinnis W. Cheyne–Stokes respiration presenting as sleep apnea syndrome. Clinical and polysomnographic features. Am Rev Respir Dis 1990;141(4 Pt 1):871–9.
14. Javaheri S. Central sleep apnea. Clin Chest Med 2010;31(2):235–48.
15. Javaheri S, Dempsey JA. Central sleep apnea. Compr Physiol 2013;3(1):141–63.
16. Cao M, Javaheri S. Chronic opioid use: effects on respiration and sleep. In: Tvildiani D, Gegechkori K, eds. Opioids pharmacology, clinical uses and adverse effects. New York: Nova Science, 2012:1–13.
17. Javaheri S, Cao M. Opioid induced central sleep apnea. In: Fabiani M, ed. Proceedings of the 10th World Congress on Sleep Apnea, Section: respiratory disorders and snoring. Turin: Edizioni Minerva Medica, 2012:133–7.
18. Javaheri S, Parker TJ, Liming JD, et al. Sleep apnea in 81 ambulatory male patients with stable heart failure. Types and their prevalences, consequences, and presentations. Circulation 1998;97(21):2154–9.
19. Javaheri S, Parker TJ, Wexler L, et al. Occult sleep-disordered breathing in stable congestive heart failure. Ann Intern Med 1995;122(7):487–92.
20. Solin P, Bergin P, Richardson M, et al. Influence of pulmonary capillary wedge pressure on central apnea in heart failure. Circulation 1999;99(12):1574–9.
21. Lanfranchi PA, Somers VK, Braghiroli A, et al. Central sleep apnea in left ventricular dysfunction: prevalence and implications for arrhythmic risk. Circulation 2003;107(5):727–32.
22. Nopmaneejumruslers C, Kaneko Y, Hajek V, Zivanovic V, Bradley TD. Cheyne–Stokes respiration in stroke: relationship to hypocapnia and occult cardiac dysfunction. Am J Respir Crit Care Med 2005;171(9):1048–52.
23. Javaheri S. Heart failure. In: Kryger M, Roth T, Dement W, eds. Principles and practice of sleep medicine, 5th ed. Philadelphia: WB Saunders, 2011:1400–15.

24. Javaheri S. Sleep disorders in systolic heart failure: a prospective study of 100 male patients. The final report. Int J Cardiol 2006;106(1):21–8.

25. Javaheri S, Randerath W. Opioids-induced central sleep apnea: mechanisms and therapies. Sleep Med Clin 2014;9:49–56.

26. Randerath WJ, Galetke W, Kenter M, Richter K, Schafer T. Combined adaptive servo-ventilation and automatic positive airway pressure (anticyclic modulated ventilation) in co-existing obstructive and central sleep apnea syndrome and periodic breathing. Sleep Med 2009;10(8):898–903.

27. Randerath WJ, Nothofer G, Priegnitz C, Anduleit N, Treml M, Kehl V, Galetke W. Long-term auto-servoventilation or constant positive pressure in heart failure and coexisting central with obstructive sleep apnea. Chest 2012;142(2):440–7.

28. Randerath W. Therapy in central and mixed sleep breathing disorders. In: Barkoukis T, Matheson J, Ferber R, Doghramji K, eds. Therapy in sleep medicine. Philadelphia: Elsevier Saunders, 2012:243–53.

29. Patil SP, Schneider H, Schwartz AR, Smith PL. Adult obstructive sleep apnea: pathophysiology and diagnosis. Chest 2007;132(1):325–37.

30. Gleadhill IC, Schwartz AR, Schubert N, et al. Upper airway collapsibility in snorers and in patients with obstructive hypopnea and apnea. Am Rev Respir Dis 1991;143(6):1300–3.

31. Almoosa K, Javaheri S. Obesity and the control of breathing. In: Ward D, Dahan A, Teppema L, eds. Pharmacology and pathophysiology of the control of breathing. Boca Raton, FL: Taylor & Francis, 2005:383–412.

32. Redolfi S, Yumino D, Ruttanaumpawan P, et al. Relationship between overnight rostral fluid shift and obstructive sleep apnea in nonobese men. Am J Respir Crit Care Med 2009;179(3):241–6.

33. Fogel RB, Malhotra A, Shea SA, Edwards JK, White DP. Reduced genioglossal activity with upper airway anesthesia in awake patients with OSA. J Appl Physiol 2000;88(4):1346–54.

34. Mezzanotte WS, Tangel DJ, White DP. Waking genioglossal electromyogram in sleep apnea patients versus normal controls (a neuromuscular compensatory mechanism). J Clin Invest 1992;89(5):1571–9.

35. Remmers JE, deGroot WJ, Sauerland EK, Anch AM. Pathogenesis of upper airway occlusion during sleep. J Appl Physiol 1978;44(6):931–8.

36. Katz ES, White DP. Genioglossus activity during sleep in normal control subjects and children with obstructive sleep apnea. Am J Respir Crit Care Med 2004;170(5):553–60.

37. Friberg D, Ansved T, Borg K, et al. Histological indications of a progressive snorers disease in an upper airway muscle. Am J Respir Crit Care Med 1998;157(2):586–93.

38. Nguyen AT, Jobin V, Payne R, et al. Laryngeal and velopharyngeal sensory impairment in obstructive sleep apnea. Sleep 2005;28(5):585–93.

39. McNicholas WT, Javaheri S. Pathophysiologic mechanisms of cardiovascular disease in obstructive sleep apnea. Sleep Med Clin 2007;2:539–47.

40. Somers V, Javaheri S. Cardiovascular effects of sleep-related breathing disorders. In: Kryger M, Roth T, Dement W, eds. Principles and practice of sleep medicine, 5th ed. Philadelphia: WB Saunders, 2011: 1370–80.

41. Gilmartin GS, Lynch M, Tamisier R, Weiss JW. Chronic intermittent hypoxia in humans during 28 nights results in blood pressure elevation and increased muscle sympathetic nerve activity. Am J Physiol Heart Circ Physiol 2010;299(3):H925–31.

42. Peppard PE, Young T, Palta M, Skatrud J. Prospective study of the association between sleep-disordered breathing and hypertension. N Engl J Med 2000;342(19):1378–84.

43. Young T, Nieto J, Javaheri S. Systemic and pulmonary hypertension in obstructive sleep apnea. In: Kryger M, Roth T, Dement W, eds. Principles and practice of sleep medicine, 5th ed. Philadelphia: WB Saunders, 2011:1381–92.

44. Javaheri S. Sleep dysfunction in heart failure. Curr Treat Options Neurol 2008;10(5):323–35.

45. Arias MA, Garcia-Rio F, Alonso-Fernandez A, et al. Obstructive sleep apnea syndrome affects left ventricular diastolic function: effects of nasal continuous positive airway pressure in men. Circulation 2005;112(3):375–83.

46. Shivalkar B, Van de Heyning C, Kerremans M, et al. Obstructive sleep apnea syndrome: more insights on structural and functional cardiac alterations, and the effects of treatment with continuous positive airway pressure. J Am Coll Cardiol 2006;47(7):1433–9.

47. Nieto FJ, Young TB, Lind BK, et al. Association of sleep-disordered breathing, sleep apnea, and hypertension in a large community-based study. Sleep Heart Health Study. JAMA 2000;283(14):1829–36.

48. Garvey JF, Taylor CT, McNicholas WT. Cardiovascular disease in obstructive sleep apnoea syndrome: the role of intermittent hypoxia and inflammation. Eur Respir J 2009;33(5):1195–205.

49. Arzt M, Young T, Finn L, Skatrud JB, Bradley TD. Association of sleep-disordered breathing and the occurrence of stroke. Am J Respir Crit Care Med 2005;172(11):1447–51.

50. Redline S, Yenokyan G, Gottlieb DJ, et al. Obstructive sleep apnea–hypopnea and incident stroke: the sleep heart health study. Am J Respir Crit Care Med 2010;182(2):269–77.

51. Johnson KG, Johnson DC. Frequency of sleep apnea in stroke and TIA patients: a meta-analysis. J Clin Sleep Med 2010;6(2):131–7.

52. Bitter T, Faber L, Hering D, et al. Sleep-disordered breathing in heart failure with normal left ventricular ejection fraction. Eur J Heart Fail 2009;11(6):602–8.

53. Duran J, Esnaola S, Rubio R, Iztueta A. Obstructive sleep apnea–hypopnea and related clinical features in a population-based sample of subjects aged 30 to 70 yr. Am J Respir Crit Care Med 2001;163(3 Pt 1):685–9.

54. Peker Y, Hedner J, Kraiczi H, Loth S. Respiratory disturbance index: an independent predictor of mortality in coronary artery disease. Am J Respir Crit Care Med 2000;162(1):81–6.

55. Yumino D, Tsurumi Y, Takagi A, Suzuki K, Kasanuki H. Impact of obstructive sleep apnea on clinical and angiographic outcomes following percutaneous coronary intervention in patients with acute coronary syndrome. Am J Cardiol 2007;99(1):26–30.

56. Marin JM, Carrizo SJ, Vicente E, Agusti AG. Long-term cardiovascular outcomes in men with obstructive sleep apnoea–hypopnoea with or without treatment with continuous positive airway pressure: an observational study. Lancet 2005;365(9464):1046–53.

57. Punjabi NM, Caffo BS, Goodwin JL, et al. Sleep-disordered breathing and mortality: a prospective cohort study. PLoS Med 2009;6(8):e1000132.

58. Young T, Finn L, Peppard PE, et al. Sleep disordered breathing and mortality: eighteen-year follow-up of the Wisconsin sleep cohort. Sleep 2008;31(8):1071–8.

59. Buchner NJ, Sanner BM, Borgel J, Rump LC. Continuous positive airway pressure treatment of mild to moderate obstructive sleep apnea reduces cardiovascular risk. Am ZJ Respir Crit Care Med 2007;176(12):1274–80.

60. Javaheri S, Dempsey J. Mechanisms of sleep apnea and periodic breathing in systolic heart failure. Sleep Med Clin 2007;2:623–30.

61. Xie A, Skatrud JB, Puleo DS, Rahko PS, Dempsey JA. Apnea–hypopnea threshold for CO_2 in patients with congestive heart failure. Am J Respir Crit Care Med 2002;165(9):1245–50.

62. Javaheri S, Sands SA, Edwards BA. Acetazolamide attenuates Hunter–Cheyne–Stokes breathing but augments the hypercapnic ventilatory response in patients with heart failure. Ann Am Thorac Soc 2014;11(1):80–6.

63. Javaheri S, Corbett WS. Association of low $PaCO_2$ with central sleep apnea and ventricular arrhythmias in ambulatory patients with stable heart failure. Ann Intern Med 1998;128(3):204–7.

64. Randerath W. Central and mixed sleep-related breathing disorders. In: Barkoukis T, Matheson J, Ferber R, Doghramji K, Blumer J, eds. Therapy in sleep medicine. Philadelphia: Elsevier, 2012:243–53.

65. Javaheri S, Almoosa KF, Saleh K, Mendenhall CL. Hypocapnia is not a predictor of central sleep apnea in patients with cirrhosis. Am J Respir Crit Care Med 2005;171(8):908–11.

66. Javaheri S. A mechanism of central sleep apnea in patients with heart failure. N Engl J Med 1999;341(13):949–54.

67. Wilcox I, McNamara SG, Dodd MJ, Sullivan CE. Ventilatory control in patients with sleep apnoea and left ventricular dysfunction: comparison of obstructive and central sleep apnoea. Eur Respir J 1998;11(1):7–13.

68. Javaheri S. Sleep-related breathing disorders in heart failure. In: Douglas L, Mann F, eds. Heart failure: a companion to Braunwald's heart disease. Philadelphia: WB Saunders, 2011:471–87.

69. Arzt M, Young T, Finn L, et al. Sleepiness and sleep in patients with both systolic heart failure and obstructive sleep apnea. Arch Intern Med 2006;166(16):1716–22.

70. Carmona-Bernal C, Quintana-Gallego E, Villa-Gil M, et al. Brain natriuretic peptide in patients with congestive heart failure and central sleep apnea. Chest 2005;127(5):1667–73.

71. Solin P, Kaye DM, Little PJ, et al. Impact of sleep apnea on sympathetic nervous system activity in heart failure. Chest 2003;123(4):1119–26.

72. Bitter T, Westerheide N, Prinz C, et al. Cheyne-Stokes respiration and obstructive sleep apnoea are independent risk factors for malignant ventricular arrhythmias requiring appropriate cardioverter-defibrillator therapies in patients with congestive heart failure. Eur Heart J 2011;32(1):61–74.

73. Javaheri S, Shukla R, Wexler L. Association of smoking, sleep apnea, and plasma alkalosis with nocturnal ventricular arrhythmias in men with systolic heart failure. Chest 2012;141(6):1449–56.

74. Javaheri S. Effects of continuous positive airway pressure on sleep apnea and ventricular irritability in patients with heart failure. Circulation 2000;101(4):392–7.

75. Javaheri S, Shukla R, Zeigler H, Wexler L. Central sleep apnea, right ventricular dysfunction, and low diastolic blood pressure are predictors of mortality in systolic heart failure. J Am Coll Cardiol 2007;49(20):2028–34.

76. Arzt M, Floras JS, Logan AG, et al. Suppression of central sleep apnea by continuous positive airway pressure and transplant-free survival in heart failure: a post hoc analysis of the Canadian Continuous Positive Airway Pressure for Patients with Central Sleep Apnea and Heart Failure Trial (CANPAP). Circulation 2007;115(25):3173–80.

77. Javaheri S. Treatment of obstructive and central sleep apnea in heart failure: practical options. Eur Respir Rev 2007;16:183–8.

78. Javaheri S, Somers V. Sleep and cardiovascular disease. Handb Clin Neurol 2011;98:327–45.

79. Javaheri S. Heart failure. In: Kushida C, ed. The encyclopedia of sleep. Waltham, MA: Academic Press, 2013:374–86.

80. Brack T, Randerath W, Bloch KE. Cheyne–Stokes respiration in patients with heart failure: prevalence, causes, consequences and treatments. Respiration 2012;83(2):165–76.

81. Harman EM, Wynne JW, Block AJ. The effect of weight loss on sleep-disordered breathing and oxygen desaturation in morbidly obese men. Chest 1982;82(3):291–4.

82. Johansson K, Neovius M, Lagerros YT, et al. Effect of a very low energy diet on moderate and severe obstructive sleep apnoea in obese men: a randomised controlled trial. BMJ 2009;339:b4609.

83. Harris N, Javaheri S. Advanced PAP therapies. In: Mattice C, Brooks R, Lee-Chiong T, eds. Fundamentals of sleep technology. Philadelphia: Lippincott, Williams & Wilkins, 2012:444–52.

84. Javaheri S, Goetting MG, Khayat R, et al. The performance of two automatic servo-ventilation devices in the treatment of central sleep apnea. Sleep 2011;34(12):1693–8.

85. Javaheri S, Brown LK, Randerath WJ. Positive airway pressure therapy with adaptive servoventilation: part 1: operational algorithms. Chest 2014;146(2):514–23.

86. Randerath W, Javaheri S. Adaptive servo-ventilation in central sleep apnea. Sleep Med Clin 2014(9):69–85.

87. Sullivan CE, Issa FG, Berthon-Jones M, Eves L. Reversal of obstructive sleep apnoea by continuous positive airway pressure applied through the nares. Lancet 1981;1(8225):862–5.

88. Randerath WJ, Meier J, Genger H, Domanski U, Ruhle KH. Efficiency of cold passover and heated humidification under continuous positive airway pressure. Eur Respir J 2002;20(1):183–6.

89. Kohler M, Pepperell JC, Casadei B, et al. CPAP and measures of cardiovascular risk in males with OSAS. Eur Respir J 2008;32(6):1488–96.

90. Campos-Rodriguez F, Perez-Ronchel J, Grilo-Reina A, et al. Long-term effect of continuous positive airway pressure on BP in patients with hypertension and sleep apnea. Chest 2007;132(6):1847–52.

91. Kaneko Y, Floras JS, Usui K, et al. Cardiovascular effects of continuous positive airway pressure in patients with heart failure and obstructive sleep apnea. N Engl J Med 2003;348(13):1233–41.

92. McEvoy RD, et al. NEJM 2016;375:919–31.

93. Mansfield DR, Gollogly NC, Kaye DM, et al. Controlled trial of continuous positive airway pressure in obstructive sleep apnea and heart failure. Am J Respir Crit Care Med 2004;169(3):361–6.

94. Egea CJ, Aizpuru F, Pinto JA, et al. Cardiac function after CPAP therapy in patients with chronic heart failure and sleep apnea: a multicenter study. Sleep Med 2008;9(6):660–6.

95. Smith LA, Vennelle M, Gardner RS, et al. Auto-titrating continuous positive airway pressure therapy in patients with chronic heart failure and obstructive sleep apnoea: a randomized placebo-controlled trial. Eur Heart J 2007;28(10):1221–7.

96. Javaheri S, Caref EB, Chen E, Tong KB, Abraham WT. Sleep apnea testing and outcomes in a large cohort of Medicare beneficiaries with newly diagnosed heart failure. Am J Respir Crit Care Med 2011;183(4):539–46.

97. Kasai T, Narui K, Dohi T, et al. Prognosis of patients with heart failure and obstructive sleep apnea treated with continuous positive airway pressure. Chest 2008;133(3):690–6.

98. Budhiraja R, Parthasarathy S, Drake CL, et al. Early CPAP use identifies subsequent adherence to CPAP therapy. Sleep 2007;30(3):320–4.

99. Simon-Tuval T, Reuveni H, Greenberg-Dotan S, et al. Low socioeconomic status is a risk factor for CPAP acceptance among adult OSAS patients requiring treatment. Sleep 2009;32(4):545–52.

100. Weaver TE, Maislin G, Dinges DF, et al. Relationship between hours of CPAP use and achieving normal levels of sleepiness and daily functioning. Sleep 2007;30(6):711–19.

101. Randerath WJ, Heise M, Hinz R, Ruehle KH. An individually adjustable oral appliance vs continuous positive airway pressure in mild-to-moderate obstructive sleep apnea syndrome. Chest 2002;122(2):569–75.

102. Ferguson KA, Cartwright R, Rogers R, Schmidt-Nowara W. Oral appliances for snoring and obstructive sleep apnea: a review. Sleep 2006;29(2):244–62.

103. Itzhaki S, Dorchin H, Clark G, et al. The effects of 1-year treatment with a Herbst mandibular advancement splint on obstructive sleep apnea, oxidative stress, and endothelial function. Chest 2007;131(3):740–9.

104. Phillips CL, Grunstein RR, Darendeliler MA, et al. Health outcomes of continuous positive airway pressure versus oral appliance treatment for obstructive sleep apnea: a randomized controlled trial. Am J Respir Crit Care Med 2013;187(8):879–87.

105. Eskafi M. Sleep apnoea in patients with stable congestive heart failure an intervention study with a mandibular advancement device. Swed Dent J Suppl 2004(168):1–56.

106. Randerath WJ, Verbraecken J, Andreas S, et al. Non-CPAP therapies in obstructive sleep apnoea. Eur Respir J 2011;37(5):1000–28.

107. Nakata S, Miyazaki S, Ohki M, et al. Reduced nasal resistance after simple tonsillectomy in patients with obstructive sleep apnea. Am J Rhinol. 2007;21(2):192–5.

108. Tauman R, Gulliver TE, Krishna J, et al. Persistence of obstructive sleep apnea syndrome in children after adenotonsillectomy. J Pediatr 2006;149(6):803–8.

109. Bettega G, Pepin JL, Veale D, et al. Obstructive sleep apnea syndrome. Fifty-one consecutive patients treated by maxillofacial surgery. Am J Respir Crit Care Med 2000;162(2 Pt 1):641–9.

110. Molina F. Mandibular distraction osteogenesis: a clinical experience of the last 17 years. J Craniofac Surg 2009;20 Suppl 2:1794–800.

111. Strollo PJ Jr, Soose RJ, Maurer JT, et al. Upper-airway stimulation for obstructive sleep apnea. N Engl J Med 2014;370(2):139–49.

112. Tamura A, Kawano Y, Kadota J. Carvedilol reduces the severity of central sleep apnea in chronic heart failure. Circulation 2009;73(2):295–8.

113. Walsh JT, Andrews R, Evans A, Cowley AJ. Failure of "effective" treatment for heart failure to improve normal customary activity. Br Heart J 1995;74(4):373–6.

114. Gabor JY, Newman DA, Barnard-Roberts V, et al. Improvement in Cheyne–Stokes respiration following cardiac resynchronisation therapy. Eur Respir J 2005;26(1):95–100.

115. Kara T, Novak M, Nykodym J, et al. Short-term effects of cardiac resynchronization therapy on sleep-disordered breathing in patients with systolic heart failure. Chest 2008;134(1):87–93.

116. Javaheri S, Abraham WT, Brown C, et al. Prevalence of obstructive sleep apnoea and periodic limb movement in 45 subjects with heart transplantation. Eur Heart J 2004;25(3):260–6.

117. Javaheri S, Ahmed M, Parker TJ, Brown CR. Effects of nasal O_2 on sleep-related disordered breathing in ambulatory patients with stable heart failure. Sleep 1999;22(8):1101–6.

118. Javaheri S. Pembrey's dream: the time has come for a long-term trial of nocturnal supplemental nasal oxygen to treat central sleep apnea in congestive heart failure. Chest 2003;123(2):322–5.

119. Chowdhuri S, Sinha P, Pranathiageswaran S, Badr MS. Sustained hyperoxia stabilizes breathing in healthy individuals during NREM sleep. J Appl Physiol (1985) 2010;109(5):1378–83.

120. Sasayama S, Izumi T, Seino Y, Ueshima K, Asanoi H. Effects of nocturnal oxygen therapy on outcome measures in patients with chronic heart failure and Cheyne–Stokes respiration. Circulation 2006;70(1):1–7.

121. Kaye DM, Mansfield D, Aggarwal A, Naughton MT, Esler MD. Acute effects of continuous positive airway pressure on cardiac sympathetic tone in congestive heart failure. Circulation 2001;103(19):2336–8.

122. Hu K, Li Q, Yang J, Hu S, Chen X. The effect of theophylline on sleep-disordered breathing in patients with stable chronic congestive heart failure. Chin Med J (Engl) 2003;116(11):1711–16.

123. Javaheri S, Parker TJ, Wexler L, et al. Effect of theophylline on sleep-disordered breathing in heart failure. N Engl J Med 1996;335(8):562–7.

124. DeBacker WA, Verbraecken J, Willemen M, et al. Central apnea index decreases after prolonged treatment with acetazolamide. Am J Respir Crit Care Med 1995;151(1):87–91.

125. Verbraecken J, Willemen M, De Cock W, et al. Central sleep apnea after interrupting long term acetazolamide therapy. Respir Physiol 1998;112(1):59–70.

126. Javaheri S. Acetazolamide improves central sleep apnea in heart failure: a double-blind, prospective study. Am J Respir Crit Care Med 2006;173(2):234–7.

127. Javaheri S. CPAP should not be used for central sleep apnea in congestive heart failure patients. J Clin Sleep Med 2006;2(4):399–402.

128. Javaheri S, Brown L, Randerath W. Positive air way pressure therapy with adaptive servo-ventilation: part 1: operational algorithms. Chest 2014;146:514–23.

129. Teschler H, Dohring J, Wang YM, Berthon-Jones M. Adaptive pressure support servo-ventilation: a novel treatment for Cheyne–Stokes respiration in heart failure. Am J Respir Crit Care Med 2001;164(4):614–19.

130. Koyama T, Watanabe H, Igarashi G, et al. Short-term prognosis of adaptive servo-ventilation therapy in patients with heart failure. Circ J 2011;75(3):710–12.

131. Pepperell JC, Maskell NA, Jones DR, et al. A randomized controlled trial of adaptive ventilation for Cheyne–Stokes breathing in heart failure. Am J Respir Crit Care Med 2003;168(9):1109–14.

132. Jilek C, Krenn M, Sebah D, et al. Prognostic impact of sleep disordered breathing and its treatment in heart failure: an observational study. Eur J Heart Fail 2011;13(1):68–75.

133. Takama N, Kurabayashi M. Effect of adaptive servo-ventilation on 1-year prognosis in heart failure patients. Circ J 2012;76(3):661–7.

134. Javaheri S, Harris N, Howard J, Chung E. Adaptive servoventilation for treatment of opioid-associated central sleep apnea. J Clin Sleep Med 2014;10(6):637–43.

135. Cowie MR, Woehrle H, Wegscheider K, et al. Adaptive servo-ventilation for central sleep apnea in systolic heart failure. N Engl J Med 2015;373(12):1095–105.

136. Javaheri S, Brown L, Randerath W, Khayat R. SERVE-HF: more questions than answers. Chest 2016;149:900–4.

137. Ponikowski P, Javaheri S, Michalkiewicz D, et al. Transvenous phrenic nerve stimulation for the treatment of central sleep apnoea in heart failure. Eur Heart J 2012;33(7):889–94.

138. Skomro R, Silva R, Alves R, Figueiredo A, Lorenzi-Filho G. The prevalence and significance of periodic leg movements during sleep in patients with congestive heart failure. Sleep Breath 2009;13(1):43–7.

139. Hanly PJ, Zuberi-Khokhar N. Periodic limb movements during sleep in patients with congestive heart failure. Chest 1996;109(6):1497–502.

140. Guggisberg AG, Hess CW, Mathis J. The significance of the sympathetic nervous system in the pathophysiology of periodic leg movements in sleep. Sleep 2007;30(6):755–66.

141. Pennestri MH, Montplaisir J, Colombo R, Lavigne G, Lanfranchi PA. Nocturnal blood pressure changes in patients with restless legs syndrome. Neurology 2007;68(15):1213–18.

142. Yumino D, Redolfi S, Ruttanaumpawan P, et al. Nocturnal rostral fluid shift: a unifying concept for the pathogenesis of obstructive and central sleep apnea in men with heart failure. Circulation 2010;121(14):1598–605.

143. Koo BB, Blackwell T, Ancoli-Israel S, et al. Association of incident cardiovascular disease with periodic limb movements during sleep in older men: Outcomes of Sleep Disorders in Older Men (MrOS) study. Circulation 2011;124(11):1223–31.

144. Mirza M, Shen WK, Sofi A, et al. Frequent periodic leg movement during sleep is associated with left ventricular hypertrophy and adverse cardiovascular outcomes. J Am Soc Echocardiogr 2013;26(7):783–90.

145. Javaheri S. Sleep in cardiovascular disease. In: Kushida C, ed. The encyclopedia of sleep. Waltham, MA: Academic Press, 2013:557–62.

146. Arendt J, Bojkowski C, Franey C, Wright J, Marks V. Immunoassay of 6-hydroxymelatonin sulfate in human plasma and urine: abolition of the urinary 24-hour rhythm with atenolol. J Clin Endocrinol Metab 1985;60(6):1166–73.

147. Lanfranchi PA, Pennestri MH, Fradette L, et al. Nighttime blood pressure in normotensive subjects with chronic insomnia: implications for cardiovascular risk. Sleep 2009;32(6):760–6.

148. Stoschitzky K, Sakotnik A, Lercher P, et al. Influence of beta-blockers on melatonin release. Eur J Clin Pharmacol 1999;55(2):111–15.

149. Grandner MA, Sands-Lincoln MR, Pak VM, Garland SN. Sleep duration, cardiovascular disease, and proinflammatory biomarkers. Nat Sci Sleep 2013;5:93–107.

150. Van Cauter E, Spiegel K, Tasali E, Leproult R. Metabolic consequences of sleep and sleep loss. Sleep Med 2008;9 Suppl 1:S23–8.

151. Bonnet M, Arand D. Cardiovascular implications of poor sleep. Sleep Med Clin 2007;2:529–38.

152. Wong CY, Chaudhry SI, Desai MM, Krumholz HM. Trends in comorbidity, disability, and polypharmacy in heart failure. Am J Med 2011;124(2):136–43.

153. Reinhard W, Plappert N, Zeman F, et al. Prognostic impact of sleep duration and sleep efficiency on mortality in patients with chronic heart failure. Sleep Med 2013;14(6):502–9.

154. Laugsand LE, Strand LB, Platou C, Vatten LJ, Janszky I. Insomnia and the risk of incident heart failure: a population study. Eur Heart J 2014;35(21):1382–93.

CHAPTER 41

Pulmonary disorders and sleep

Sandrine H. Launois and Patrick Lévy

Sleep is commonly disrupted in pulmonary disorders, either by symptoms of the lung disease or by an associated sleep disorder. This situation is, however, under-recognized and therefore untreated. Our goal in this chapter is to broadly underline the close association between pulmonary disorders and sleep disturbances, rather than provide an exhaustive compilation of studies on sleep and pulmonary disorders. In some cases, this association is fortuitous and simply reflects the impact of a chronic, serious medical condition on sleep quality, with patients complaining of nonrestorative sleep, daytime fatigue, and sleepiness. However, in other instances, specific sleep-related phenomena may adversely affect the pulmonary disorder (eg, restrictive lung diseases and REM-related hypoventilation). A sleep disorder can coexist with a pulmonary disorder and worsen pulmonary outcome or quality of life—for example, chronic obstructive pulmonary disease (COPD) and restless legs syndrome (RLS). Lastly, a sleep disorder, namely obstructive sleep apnea (OSA), has been implicated as a risk factor for pulmonary hypertension and pulmonary embolism. Overall, discounting the possibility of a chance occurrence, the following ICSD-3 disorders are found in association with various pulmonary diseases [1]: chronic insomnia disorder, sleep-related breathing disorders, and restless leg syndrome (RLS) (Table 41.1).

Chronic insomnia disorder

In pulmonary disorder patients, insomnia is common [2–7], often multifactorial, with anxiety, depression, nocturnal respiratory symptoms and hypoxemia, treatment, and associated sleep disorders all potentially contributing to poor sleep. Although prevalence varies from one study to the other, one-third to two-thirds of COPD patients suffer from insomnia or nonrestorative sleep [8,9], a fact that is underestimated by physicians [10]. The prevalence of sleep disturbances does not appear to be closely correlated with objective severity of airway obstruction, but rather with the severity of symptoms, the exacerbation rate, and the presence of sleep disordered breathing (SDB) [2,8,10–12].

Nocturnal wheezing, nasal congestion due to allergies, esophageal reflux, and some asthma medications (see Table 41.2) induce sleep disruption. Indeed, patients suffering from asthma, particularly from nocturnal or allergic asthma, often complain about sleep quality, insomnia, and nonrestorative sleep [13].

While life-saving for end-stage pulmonary disease patients, lung transplantation is a long and stressful process, while the patient is on a waiting list as well as while recovering from the procedure. Sleep may therefore be disrupted by anxiety and depression, in addition to respiratory symptoms due to the underlying disease, medication, or associated SDB and RLS (see below) [14]. Some disturbances may disappear after lung transplant, leading to sleep improvement, but insomnia may persist after the transplant (Fig. 41.1).

While the most commonly acknowledged sleep disorder in patients with chest wall and respiratory muscle diseases is sleep-related hypoventilation (see below), sleep studies in these patients demonstrate poor sleep efficiency, fragmented sleep, and decreased slow-wave and REM sleep [15,16] (Fig. 41.2). These findings are likely to be multifactorial and, at least in part, caused by SDB, as sleep is improved by nocturnal noninvasive ventilation [15].

Adverse consequences of chronic insomnia have been studied only in COPD patients, but are likely to also occur in other lung diseases. Not surprisingly, poor sleep strongly affects quality of life [8,10,12,17] and cognitive function [12], but excessive daytime sleepiness (EDS) is uncommon [10,11]. In a recent longitudinal study, poor sleep quality was associated with an increased exacerbation and emergency hospitalization rate and with a trend toward increased mortality in the more severe patients [12]. However, increased morbidity/mortality may result from adverse consequences of SDB and sleep hypoxemia, which are likely to play a role in more severe COPD patients, rather than insomnia alone [9,11].

Sleep-related breathing disorders

Obstructive sleep apnea

OSA is a highly prevalent disorder in the general population and can therefore coexist with any chronic pulmonary disorder. OSA further deteriorates sleep quality in patients whose sleep may already be disrupted (see above). In some diseases such as asthma [18–20] and interstitial lung disease (ILD) [21], the prevalence of OSA is even higher than in the general population. The underlying pathophysiological mechanism for this relationship, however, is not clear. Patients with end-stage lung disease waiting for a lung transplant also have an increased prevalence of OSA, often associated with mixed and/or central apneas [22-23]. Resolution of SDB is not constant following the transplant, and some patients may even develop sleep apneas after the procedure [23,24].

In asthma patients, poor disease control, as evidenced by emergency admission rate or steroid treatment, is a risk factor for OSA [19,20]. Consequently, screening for sleep apnea is recommended in patients with uncontrolled asthma or in those who are overweight or obese [25]. Indeed, continuous positive airway pressure (CPAP) treatment has a beneficial impact not only on sleep quality [26] but also on bronchial reactivity [27]. In addition, treating OSA with CPAP is likely to improve esophageal reflux [28], which may contribute to poor sleep and arousals in asthma [20] and ILD [21].

SDB may have a direct deleterious impact on the associated lung disease outcomes. The most illustrative example is that of the

Table 41.1 Occurrence of sleep disorders in patients with pulmonary diseases

	Chronic insomnia disorders			Sleep-related breathing disorders		Restless leg syndrome
	Insomnia due to nocturnal symptoms	Insomnia due to anxiety and/or depression	Insomnia due to medication	Sleep-related hypoventilation and hypoxemia	Sleep apnea	
Asthma	x	x	x		x	
Chronic obstructive pulmonary disease	x	x	x	x	x	x
Cystic fibrosis	x	x		x	x	
Lung transplant	x	x	x		x	x
Pulmonary embolism					x	
Pulmonary hypertension					x	
Interstitial lung diseases		x	x	x		
Chest wall and neuromuscular disorders		x		x		
Chronic respiratory failure	x	x	x	x		

Table 41.2 Role of medication in sleep disorders associated with pulmonary diseases

Sleep disorder	Medications commonly used in pulmonary disorder patients
Restless leg syndrome	Antidepressants
	Beta-blockers
Insomnia	Corticosteroids
	Antibiotics: quinolones, isoniazid
	Salbutamol, terbutaline
	Theophylline
	PDE4 inhibitors
Sleep-related hypoventilation and hypoxemia	Opiates
	Benzodiazepines
	Buspirone
	Myorelaxants

"overlap syndrome" (OS), the fortuitous association of OSA and COPD [11,29]. Compared with patients with COPD alone, patients with OS have more frequent exacerbations requiring hospitalization and a higher mortality rate [30]. Several potential interactions have been proposed to account for this finding, such as more severe OSA-induced intermittent hypoxia [11] and greater systemic inflammation and oxidative stress in patients with OS compared with COPD patients [31]. In OS patients who accept CPAP treatment, mortality is reduced compared with patients who decline treatment and is comparable to mortality in COPD alone [30,32], with CPAP compliance being an independent factor for this improvement [32]. CPAP also has a beneficial effect on COPD exacerbation rate [30], but does not improve either pulmonary function tests or supplemental oxygen requirements [32]. Surprisingly, the

Global Initiative for Chronic Obstructive Lung Disease guidelines updated in January 2015 do not suggest any recommendation for performing sleep studies in COPD patients. Yet sleep clinical evaluation of COPD patients is crucial, and if it leads to a suspicion of OSA, a full polysomnography (PSG) should be performed, rather than a portable monitoring study [33].

OSA is an independent risk factor for deep venous thrombosis and pulmonary embolism (PE) [34]. This is not surprising, as platelet activation and increases in procoagulant factors, resulting in hypercoagulability, have been demonstrated in apneic patients [35]. These abnormalities are correlated with the severity of nocturnal hypoxemia [36] and are reversible following CPAP treatment [34]. While intermittent hypoxia and the consequent oxidative stress and inflammation are likely to be the main contributors to hypercoagulability [35,37], the role of comorbid systemic hypertension has also been suggested [38]. Although there are no guidelines to systematically assess patients with acute PE for sleep apnea [39], one could argue that patients with recurrent PE and no obvious risk factors should undergo a sleep evaluation.

OSA patients are subjected to chronic intermittent hypoxia, and severe patients are therefore at risk for developing pulmonary hypertension (PH) [40,41]. Although the prevalence of PH in OSA is not clearly established, a systematic assessment of sleep apnea is recommended in PH patients [41,42]. Treatment of OSA with CPAP significantly reduces elevated pulmonary pressures [40].

Sleep-related hypoventilation due to a medical disorder

During sleep, patients with diseases that affect the chest wall or the respiratory muscles may develop alveolar hypoventilation [16,43]. Several mechanisms account for this common complication: the physiological decrease in respiratory drive is superimposed on already-weakened respiratory muscles and decreased lung volumes, as well as impaired respiratory control. Patients are

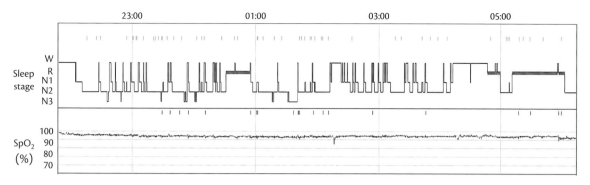

Fig. 41.1 Hypnogram and pulse oximetry (SpO$_2$) extracted from overnight PSG in a 40-year-old woman performed 3.5 years following lung transplantation for end-stage emphysema. The patient complained of unrefreshing sleep and daytime fatigue. The PSG showed poor sleep efficiency and architecture with repeated arousals, 74 minutes of wake after sleep onset and 16 minutes of slow-wave sleep. There was no respiratory disturbance; the apnea–hypopnea index was 0.7/h. The mean oxygen saturation during the night was 94%.

particularly vulnerable in REM sleep, as can be seen in Fig. 41.2, and during the course of the disease, REM sleep-related alveolar hypoventilation often precedes NREM and daytime hypoventilation. Associated obstructive or central sleep apneas worsen sleep hypoventilation [16,43]. Although the overnight oximetry pattern can be evocative of sleep-related alveolar hypoventilation, measurement of CO$_2$ level, through noninvasive means during sleep or arterial blood gases measurement upon morning awakening, is required to confirm the diagnosis [1]. Treatment of the underlying chest wall or neuromuscular disease is often limited, but nocturnal noninvasive ventilation is effective in alleviating sleep hypoventilation [16,43,44] and sleep difficulties [15]. However, there is still a lack of large controlled trials to demonstrate a long-term effect on symptoms, quality of life, and survival [44].

Sleep-related hypoxemia disorders

While physiological changes in ventilation during sleep do not result in significant hypoxemia in individuals with healthy lungs, reduction in functional residual capacity, worsening of ventilation/perfusion mismatch, and decreased ventilatory responses to chemical and mechanical stimuli may lead to isolated hypoxemia during sleep in patients with chronic pulmonary lung diseases. Oxygenation during sleep has been extensively studied in COPD patients [9,11,45], in whom the severity of sleep-related hypoxemia is closely related to the severity of airway obstruction and the presence of daytime hypoxemia. Sleep hypoxemia is likely to contribute to poor sleep, cardiovascular morbidity, and increased mortality [45], but its relationship to pulmonary hypertension and

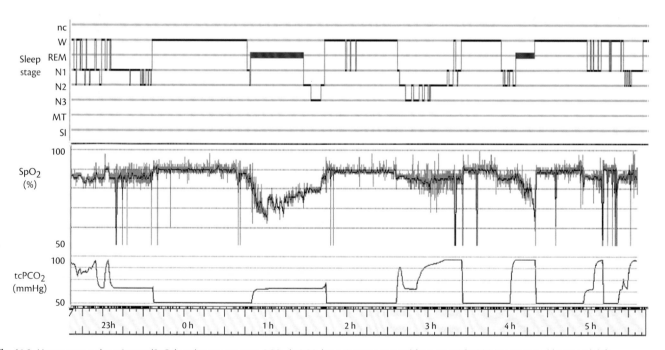

Fig. 41.2 Hypnogram, pulse oximetry (SpO$_2$), and transcutaneous PCO$_2$ (tcPCO$_2$) monitoring extracted from overnight PSG in a 49-year-old man with left-diaphragmatic paralysis and severe obesity (body mass index 44 kg/m^2). Pulmonary function testing showed a restrictive syndrome with mild daytime hypoxemia but no alveolar hypoventilation. The patient complained of severe insomnia. The PSG showed prolonged awakenings due to breathlessness, fragmented sleep, and central sleep hypopneas in NREM sleep with an apnea–hypopnea index of 58/h and REM alveolar hypoventilation. Owing to the patient's agitation throughout the night, the quality of both oximetry and CO$_2$ monitoring was poor.

polycythemia is less clear [9,45]. Sleep-related hypoxemia may also present in patients with cystic fibrosis [46], neuromuscular diseases [16], or ILD [47].Associated apneas and/or alveolar hypoventilation, particularly during REM sleep, are common in these patients, and will obviously contribute to and worsen sleep hypoxemia. Simple overnight pulse oximetry is inadequate to properly assess the nature of sleep-induced hypoxemia in pulmonary disorders, and a complete evaluation, including CO_2 monitoring, should be performed in these patients. Determining the mechanisms responsible for sleep hypoxemia is crucial to select treatment options (supplemental oxygen, noninvasive ventilation, etc.).

Restless legs syndrome

Like OSA, RLS is a common disorder and can be associated by chance with any pulmonary disorder. However, the prevalence of RLS is increased in some pulmonary diseases. An observational study in lung transplant recipients showed that the prevalence of RLS in these patients was more than double that in the general population, with a rate of 48% [48]. Although subjective or objective sleep variables were not recorded in the study, 80% of patients had moderate (25%) or severe (55%) RLS and were likely to suffer from sleep difficulties. One recent study suggests that the prevalence of RLS is increased in COPD patients and contributes to difficulty initiating and/or maintaining sleep and to daytime fatigue [49]. Although RLS prevalence has not been studied in other pulmonary disorders, patients should be questioned on possible RLS symptoms. Low blood iron level is a known causal factor for RLS, and ferritin level should be tested and corrected by iron supplementation if necessary. Some drugs used for the treatment of pulmonary diseases can worsen or cause RLS (Table 41.2), but may not always be discontinued. When considering drug treatment for severe RLS, the adverse effects of opiates should be kept in mind, as they can cause sleep-related hypoventilation and hypoxemia.

Miscellaneous situations and considerations

Acute pulmonary disorders

So far, we have only considered *chronic* pulmonary disorders. Sleep is also disrupted in *acute* pulmonary disorders (eg, bronchitis, pneumonia, and acute respiratory failure) because of symptoms such as fever, cough, pain, dyspnea, and anxiety. Furthermore, treatment itself may disrupt sleep: medication (Table 41.2), nocturnal noninvasive ventilation, and oxygen therapy may delay sleep onset and/or cause repeated arousals. Finally, intensive care unit hospitalization is known to disturb sleep [50]. However, to date, there have been no studies regarding the potential adverse consequences on acute pulmonary disease outcome.

Sleep and tobacco use or withdrawal

Even more than other smokers, patients with lung diseases are strongly and repeatedly advised to stop smoking. Nicotine is a wakefulness-promoting substance, and may cause difficulties in initiating sleep and sleep fragmentation [51], therefore contributing to chronic insomnia in patients who continue smoking [52]. On the other hand, smoking cessation may also be associated with poor sleep, whether because of withdrawal symptoms (craving, insomnia, anxiety, and depressive symptoms) or because of use of smoking cessation aids [52]. When selecting nicotine substitutes, taking

pharmacokinetics over the 24-hour period into consideration may help patients sleep better [52,53]. Following smoking cessation, weight gain is common and should be closely monitored, as it may worsen pre-existing OSA.

Pulmonary rehabilitation

This plays a central role in the management of patients with COPD, but may also benefit patients with other pulmonary diseases, such as asthma, ILD or cystic fibrosis [54]. Exercise is the key component of rehabilitation programs. Sleep quality and duration play an important role in motivation, performance, and post-exercise recovery [55]. Therefore, improving sleep in patients enrolled in a pulmonary rehabilitation program may help them complete the exercise regimen more easily. In addition, there is a reciprocal effect between sleep and exercise, as exercise is a well-established nonpharmacological treatment option for insomnia and poor sleep quality [55].

Conclusions

Sleep disorders and pulmonary diseases are closely associated, but their relationship is underestimated in routine patient care. Yet, the occurrence of sleep disorders in pulmonary disorder patients results in poor quality of life and may worsen morbidity and mortality. This relationship has implications for both pulmonary and sleep specialists. Pulmonary physicians should systematically assess sleep complaints in patients with pulmonary disorders, particularly COPD and restrictive lung diseases, and, if warranted, order further investigations (Box 41.1), with the goal of improving quality of life and, in some cases, the outcome of the pulmonary disease itself. Sleep physicians should be aware that while general guidelines for sleep disorder management apply to patients with pulmonary disorders, there are specific diagnostic and therapeutic features to take into consideration. We have stressed, for instance, the importance of documenting sleep alveolar hypoventilation in these patients, and noninvasive CO_2 monitoring is essential in pulmonary disorder patients. Because of their potential respiratory-depressant effect, sedative medications and muscle relaxants should be avoided, and insomnia in patients with compromised respiratory function should be managed through nonpharmacological options.

In spite of the abundant literature on the topic, many questions remain unanswered, such as the long-term negative outcomes of sleep disruption and chronic insomnia in pulmonary disorder patients, and these need to be addressed by future studies.

Box 41.1 Evaluation tools in pulmonary disorder patients with sleep complaints

Clinical evaluation

Pittsburg Sleep Quality Index
Insomnia Severity Scale
Hospital Anxiety and Depression Scale
Epworth Sleepiness Scale

Investigations

Sleep log/actimetry
Overnight oximetry and capnography
Iron workup
Polysomnography with capnography

References

1. American Association of Sleep Medicine. International classification of sleep disorders, 3rd ed. Westchester, IL: American Association of Sleep Medicine, 2014.

2. Hynninen MJ, Pallesen S, Hardie J, et al. Insomnia symptoms, objectively measured sleep, and disease severity in chronic obstructive pulmonary disease outpatients. Sleep Med 2013;14(12):1328–33.

3. Bosse-Henck A, Wirtz H, Hinz A. Subjective sleep quality in sarcoidosis. Sleep Med 2015;16(5):570–6.

4. Jankelowitz L, Reid KJ, Wolfe L, et al. Cystic fibrosis patients have poor sleep quality despite normal sleep latency and efficiency. Chest 2005;127(5):1593–9.

5. Dean GE, Redeker NS, Wang YJ, et al. Sleep, mood, and quality of life in patients receiving treatment for lung cancer. Oncol Nurs Forum 2013;40(5):441–51.

6. Milioli G, Bosi M, Poletti V, et al. Sleep and respiratory sleep disorders in idiopathic pulmonary fibrosis. Sleep Med Rev 2015;26:57–63.

7. Krishnan V, McCormack MC, Mathai SC, et al. Sleep quality and health-related quality of life in idiopathic pulmonary fibrosis. Chest 2008;134(4):693–8.

8. Agusti A, Hedner J, Marin JM, et al. Night-time symptoms: a forgotten dimension of COPD. Eur Respir Rev 2011;20(121):183–94.

9. Budhiraja R, Siddiqi TA, Quan SF. Sleep disorders in chronic obstructive pulmonary disease: etiology, impact, and management. J Clin Sleep Med 2015;11(3):259–70.

10. Price D, Small M, Milligan G, et al. Impact of night-time symptoms in COPD: a real-world study in five European countries. Int J Chron Obstruct Pulmon Dis 2013;8:595–603.

11. Sanders MH, Newman AB, Haggerty CL, et al. Sleep and sleep-disordered breathing in adults with predominantly mild obstructive airway disease. Am J Respir Crit Care Med 2003;167(1):7–14.

12. Omachi TA, Blanc PD, Claman DM, et al. Disturbed sleep among COPD patients is longitudinally associated with mortality and adverse COPD outcomes. Sleep Med 2012;13(5):476–83.

13. Shigemitsu H, Afshar K. Nocturnal asthma. Curr Opin Pulm Med 2007;13(1):49–55.

14. Reilly-Spong M, Park T, Gross CR. Poor sleep in organ transplant recipients: self-reports and actigraphy. Clin Transplant 2013;27(6):901–13.

15. Contal O, Janssens JP, Dury M, et al. Sleep in ventilatory failure in restrictive thoracic disorders. Effects of treatment with non invasive ventilation. Sleep Med 2011;12(4):373–7.

16. Bourke SC, Gibson GJ. Sleep and breathing in neuromuscular disease. Eur Respir J 2002;19(6):1194–201.

17. Scharf SM, Maimon N, Simon-Tuval T, et al. Sleep quality predicts quality of life in chronic obstructive pulmonary disease. Int J Chron Obstruct Pulmon Dis 2011;6:1–12.

18. Prasad B, Nyenhuis SM, Weaver TE. Obstructive sleep apnea and asthma: associations and treatment implications. Sleep Med Rev 2014;18(2):165–71.

19. Teodorescu M, Polomis DA, Teodorescu MC, et al. Association of obstructive sleep apnea risk or diagnosis with daytime asthma in adults. J Asthma 2012;49(6):620–8.

20. Shen TC, Lin CL, Wei CC, et al. Risk of obstructive sleep apnea in adult patients with asthma: a population-based cohort study in Taiwan. PLoS One 2015;10(6):e0128461.

21. Lancaster LH, Mason WR, Parnell JA, et al. Obstructive sleep apnea is common in idiopathic pulmonary fibrosis. Chest 2009;136(3):772–8.

22. Romem A, Iacono A, McIlmoyle E, et al. Obstructive sleep apnea in patients with end-stage lung disease. J Clin Sleep Med 2013;9(7):687–93.

23. Malouf MA, Milrose MA, Grunstein RR, et al. Sleep-disordered breathing before and after lung transplantation. J Heart Lung Transplant 2008;27(5):540–6.

24. Naraine VS, Bradley TD, Singer LG. Prevalence of sleep disordered breathing in lung transplant recipients. J Clin Sleep Med 2009;5(5):441–7.

25. National Asthma Education and Prevention Program. Expert Panel Report 3 (EPR-3): Guidelines for the diagnosis and management of asthma—summary report 2007. J Allergy Clin Immunol 2007;120(5 Suppl):S94–138.

26. Ciftci TU, Ciftci B, Guven SF, Kokturk O, Turktas H. Effect of nasal continuous positive airway pressure in uncontrolled nocturnal asthmatic patients with obstructive sleep apnea syndrome. Respir Med 2005;99(5):529–34.

27. Busk M, Busk N, Puntenney P, et al. Use of continuous positive airway pressure reduces airway reactivity in adults with asthma. Eur Respir J 2013;41(2):317–22.

28. Zanation AM, Senior BA. The relationship between extraesophageal reflux (EER) and obstructive sleep apnea (OSA). Sleep Med Rev 2005;9(6):453–8.

29. Flenley DC. Sleep in chronic obstructive lung disease. Clin Chest Med 1985;6(4):651–61.

30. Marin JM, Soriano JB, Carrizo SJ, Boldova A, Celli BR. Outcomes in patients with chronic obstructive pulmonary disease and obstructive sleep apnea: the overlap syndrome. Am J Respir Crit Care Med 2010;182(3):325–31.

31. McNicholas WT. Chronic obstructive pulmonary disease and obstructive sleep apnea: overlaps in pathophysiology, systemic inflammation, and cardiovascular disease. Am J Respir Crit Care Med 2009;180(8):692–700.

32. Stanchina ML, Welicky LM, Donat W, et al. Impact of CPAP use and age on mortality in patients with combined COPD and obstructive sleep apnea: the overlap syndrome. J Clin Sleep Med 2013;9(8):767–72.

33. Collop NA, Anderson WM, Boehlecke B, et al. Clinical guidelines for the use of unattended portable monitors in the diagnosis of obstructive sleep apnea in adult patients. Portable Monitoring Task Force of the American Academy of Sleep Medicine. J Clin Sleep Med 2007;3(7):737–47.

34. Lippi G, Mattiuzzi C, Franchini M. Sleep apnea and venous thromboembolism. A systematic review. Thromb Haemost 2015;114:958–63.

35. Liak C, Fitzpatrick M. Coagulability in obstructive sleep apnea. Can Respir J 2011;18(6):338–48.

36. Rahangdale S, Yeh SY, Novack V, et al. The influence of intermittent hypoxemia on platelet activation in obese patients with obstructive sleep apnea. J Clin Sleep Med 2011;7(2):172–8.

37. von Kanel R, Loredo JS, Powell FL, Adler KA, Dimsdale JE. Short-term isocapnic hypoxia and coagulation activation in patients with sleep apnea. Clin Hemorheol Microcirc 2005;33(4):369–77.

38. von Kanel R, Le DT, Nelesen RA, et al. The hypercoagulable state in sleep apnea is related to comorbid hypertension. J Hypertens 2001;19(8):1445–51.

39. Konstantinides SV. 2014 ESC Guidelines on the diagnosis and management of acute pulmonary embolism. Eur Heart J 2014;35(45):3145–6.

40. Arias MA, Garcia-Rio F, Alonso-Fernandez A, Martinez I, Villamor J. Pulmonary hypertension in obstructive sleep apnoea: effects of continuous positive airway pressure: a randomized, controlled cross-over study. Eur Heart J 2006;27(9):1106–13.

41. Jilwan FN, Escourrou P, Garcia G, et al. High occurrence of hypoxemic sleep respiratory disorders in precapillary pulmonary hypertension and mechanisms. Chest 2013;143(1):47–55.

42. Atwood CW Jr, McCrory D, Garcia JG, Abman SH, Ahearn GS. Pulmonary artery hypertension and sleep-disordered breathing: ACCP evidence-based clinical practice guidelines. Chest 2004;126(1 Suppl): 72S–77S.

43. Aboussouan LS. Sleep-disordered breathing in neuromuscular disease. Am J Respir Crit Care Med 2015;191(9):979–89.

44. Annane D, Orlikowski D, Chevret S. Nocturnal mechanical ventilation for chronic hypoventilation in patients with neuromuscular and chest wall disorders. Cochrane Database Syst Rev 2014;12:CD001941.

45. Weitzenblum E, Chaouat A. Sleep and chronic obstructive pulmonary disease. Sleep Med Rev 2004;8(4):281–94.

46. Milross MA, Piper AJ, Dobbin CJ, Bye PT, Grunstein RR. Sleep disordered breathing in cystic fibrosis. Sleep Med Rev 2004;8(4):295–308.

47. Agarwal S, Richardson B, Krishnan V, et al. Interstitial lung disease and sleep: what is known? Sleep Med 2009;10(9):947–51.

48. Minai OA, Golish JA, Yataco JC, et al. Restless legs syndrome in lung transplant recipients. J Heart Lung Transplant 2007;26(1):24–9.

49. Cavalcante AG, de Bruin PF, de Bruin VM, et al. Restless legs syndrome, sleep impairment, and fatigue in chronic obstructive pulmonary disease. Sleep Med 2012;13(7):842–7.

50. Drouot X, Cabello B, d'Ortho MP, Brochard L. Sleep in the intensive care unit. Sleep Med Rev 2008;12(5):391–403.

51. Jaehne A, Unbehaun T, Feige B, et al. How smoking affects sleep: a polysomnographical analysis. Sleep Med 2012;13(10):1286–92.

52. Jaehne A, Loessl B, Barkai Z, Riemann D, Hornyak M. Effects of nicotine on sleep during consumption, withdrawal and replacement therapy. Sleep Med Rev 2009;13(5):363–77.

53. Staner L, Luthringer R, Dupont C, Aubin HJ, Lagrue G. Sleep effects of a 24-h versus a 16-h nicotine patch: a polysomnographic study during smoking cessation. Sleep Med 2006;7(2):147–54.

54. Bolton C, Bevan-Smith E, Blakey J, et al. BTS guideline on pulmonary rehabilitation in adults. Thorax 2013;68(Suppl 2):ii1–30.

55. Chennaoui M, Arnal PJ, Sauvet F, Leger D. Sleep and exercise: a reciprocal issue? Sleep Med Rev 2015;20:59–72.

CHAPTER 42

Gastrointestinal functioning during sleep

William C. Orr

INTRODUCTION

A more complete understanding of how sleep influences gastrointestinal (GI) functioning has only been realized in the past decade or so. Much of this lack of understanding can be attributed to the relative inaccessibility of the GI tract to physiological monitoring in the conscious human. Careful monitoring of pH changes and GI tract motility during the waking state and polysomnographically (PSG) determined sleep have revealed significant changes during sleep, as well as very different physiological responses to endogenous or exogenous stimuli. For example, responses to esophageal acid–mucosal contact are substantially altered during sleep compared with the waking state. This chapter provides an overview of this research as well as a recent proposal that nighttime heartburn combined with sleep-related gastroesophageal reflux (GER) is a distinct clinical entity apart from daytime reflux and conventional heartburn.

Acid-related diseases

Gastric acid secretion

The earliest studies of gastric acid and its digestive function were carried out by Dr. William Beaumont around 1830. Beaumont was a US Army surgeon attending Alexis St. Martin, who had sustained an accidental shotgun wound to the abdomen. St. Martin developed a gastric fistula through which Beaumont could observe the effects of a variety of stimuli on gastric functioning. These observations led to the important discovery that stomach acid was essential for digestion. Beaumont also observed the relationship between gastric function and emotional state, as the gastric mucosa would become engorged with blood in relation to St. Martin being upset or stressed [1]. Almost a century later, Johnston and Washeim [2] studied gastric acid secretion during sleep in normal subjects and described a rise in acidity, a decrease in volume, and delayed gastric emptying. Later studies described a circadian rhythm of gastric acid secretion in healthy subjects characterized by a peak in acid secretion between 10 pm and 2 am, and minimal acid secretion during wake [3]. These studies established that gastric acid secretion was very labile and altered not only by emotional state, but also by state of consciousness and time of day. These observations laid the groundwork for our understanding of the pathogenesis of gastroesophageal reflux disease (GERD) and duodenal ulcer (DU) disease.

Duodenal ulcer and vagotomy

Prior to the discovery of the important role of *Helicobacter pylori* in the pathogenesis of DU disease, it was felt to be purely an acid-related disease, and the healing of DU was felt to be closely related to the suppression of gastric acid secretion. The differential diagnosis and treatment of DU disease was detailed by Moynihan, noting that many patients had symptoms of nocturnal abdominal pain that were alleviated by food [4]. Vagotomy was introduced by Dragstedt in the late 1940s as an effective strategy for treating chronic DU disease theoretically caused by excessive vagal stimulation [5]. Initially, the procedure was believed to reduce excessive nocturnal acid secretion in DU patients [6]. This is most likely due to a larger parietal cell mass producing a larger acid output in response to stimuli that provoke gastric secretion. Thus, the greater resting secretion in patients with DU compared with controls is thought to be caused by a normal basal drive acting upon a larger number of normally sensitive parietal cells [7,8].

Other investigators were not able to support Dragstedt's reasoning that vagotomy reduces basal secretions; instead, it was revealed that the procedure reduces histamine-stimulated secretion [9,10]. Nevertheless, Dragstedt's work served to stimulate much further research that lead to a more comprehensive understanding of acid secretion during waking and sleep and the relationship of acid secretion to the pathogenesis of DU. His hypothesis related to the importance of nocturnal acid secretion in the pathogenesis of DU was particularly significant in bringing sleep into the critical thinking related to the diagnosis and treatment of a major medical condition.

Esophagitis and nighttime heartburn

The regurgitation of "peptic juice and its stagnation" was demonstrated as the cause for esophagitis in the absence of comorbidities by Selye in 1938 [11]. Subsequent observations have demonstrated that the condition of esophagitis is much more complex than simple occurrence of acid contact with the esophageal mucosa. The pattern of esophageal acid contact has now been shown to be markedly different during the daytime compared with that during sleep, and the notion that sleep-related GER played a role in the development of esophagitis and other complications of GER emerged in the 1970s by the pioneering work of Johnson and DeMeester [12,13]. Their work, which incorporated the new technology of 24-hour esophageal pH monitoring, encouraged further investigation of the effect of sleep on GER and acid contact time. Indeed, these investigators noted that episodes of reflux occurring in the upright position, presumably during the waking state, are rapidly cleared. Episodes of reflux occurring in the recumbent position, presumably during sleep, are associated with markedly prolonged acid clearance. These studies effectively demonstrated the link between prolongation of acid clearance during the sleeping interval and the occurrence of esophagitis. During the same time period, Atkinson and Van Gelder also showed a relationship between the severity of esophagitis and the duration of nocturnal periods of high esophageal acidity [14]. Collectively, these studies suggested acid clearance is prolonged during sleep; however, none monitored sleep via PSG, and thus could not confirm this notion.

Orr and colleagues [15] conducted the first PSG study on patients with esophagitis and confirmed that acid clearance from the distal esophagus is prolonged during sleep in both healthy participants and patients with esophagitis, but more so in the esophagitis group. They also provided the additional insight that acid clearance is dependent on a brief awakening from sleep. Thus, patients who reflux during sleep were at greater risk to develop esophagitis. A later study by Robertson and colleagues [16] in which patients were monitored with a 24-hour pH probe demonstrated that those with complications of esophagitis have more severe acid reflux than those with simple uncomplicated disease, and they concluded that this was likely due to prolonged periods of nighttime acid reflux. With this deeper understanding of the significance of prolonged acid contact time during sleep and its more complicated disease progression, a need for clinically differentiating sleep-related reflux and nighttime heartburn from daytime heartburn has become apparent.

Recognizing nighttime heartburn and associated sleep-related GER as a distinct clinical entity has been suggested in a review by Orr [17]. Data are reviewed to support the notion that recognizing the presence of nighttime heartburn suggests a more aggressive treatment approach for GERD patients. Nighttime heartburn and sleep-related GER are considered a distinct clinical entity due to several factors, including the following: the association of sleep-related GER with prolonged acid–mucosal contact, which promotes mucosal injury,; the greater risk of developing esophagitis among patients with nighttime heartburn; the higher incidence of extra-esophageal symptoms such as chest pain and cough among patients with nighttime heartburn; and the significantly poorer quality of life of patients with nighttime heartburn. Two epidemiological studies have provided similar data suggesting that nighttime heartburn is a common symptom [18,19], and that the majority of patients with nighttime heartburn (approximately 70% in both studies) indicated that this symptom disrupted their sleep.

Acid reflux is due to the failure of the lower esophageal sphincter (LES) to prevent the retrograde flow of acid from the stomach into the esophagus. This may occur as a result of decreased pressure in the LES or what is called a spontaneous relaxation of the LES, where the pressure suddenly decreases to the intragastric baseline. Responses to acid–mucosal contact are quite different during sleep compared with responses that characterize acid–mucosal contact during the waking state. Normal acid–mucosal contact produces the waking sensation of heartburn, enhances salivary flow and bicarbonate concentration, and stimulates a higher frequency of swallowing. These responses prevent prolonged acid–mucosal contact by effectively removing the refluxate from the distal esophagus and neutralizing the mucosa. However, these responses are suppressed during sleep, resulting in prolonged acid–mucosal contact [15,20]. The subsequent back-diffusion of hydrogen ions into the esophageal mucosa is related to the duration of acid–mucosal contact [21]. Prolonged acid contact with the esophageal mucosa disrupts the normal barrier to the submucosa by increasing intercellular spaces, allowing easier access of hydrogen ions [22]. Thus, the longer reflux episodes noted during sleep carry a greater risk of producing mucosal damage compared with the more rapidly cleared reflux episodes during the waking state. Thus, clinicians may find it useful to assess symptoms of nighttime heartburn in differentiating patients who have a more serious form of GERD and experience more daytime sleepiness and a decline in work productivity and quality of life [23]. Much of the literature related to nighttime heartburn and sleep-related GER has been reviewed by Orr, who has postulated that nighttime heartburn constitutes a distinct clinical entity that merits a more aggressive approach to treatment, focusing on the suppression of sleep-related acid reflux [17].

Intestinal motility

The small bowel and the colon are difficult to monitor because of the invasive techniques that must be employed to obtain direct measurements. This is especially challenging during sleep. Characterizing intestinal motility using advanced telemetry or electrodes in conjunction with PSG has yielded a more comprehensive description of intestinal motor activity in general, and more specifically during sleep. Electromyographic (EMG) recording of duodenal muscle activity during the various stages of sleep revealed an inhibition of duodenal EMG activity associated with rapid eye movement (REM) sleep and an increase in activity with changes from one sleep stage to another [24]. Deep sleep is associated with decreased motility compared with light sleep, and the motility index for REM sleep is similar to that for light sleep [25], similar to the findings of Tassinari and colleagues [26], who demonstrated stage 1 sleep to have more duodenal contractions compared with stages 2, 3, 4, and REM. An overall greater motility found during REM sleep compared with deep sleep is similar to findings that have been reported in the colon [27].

Cyclic motor activity, referred to as the migrating motor complex (MMC), has been observed in the human GI tract in the fasting state with a periodicity of 90 minutes and with significant alterations during sleep compared with wake [28]. The physiological significance of the MMC is related to propulsion of intraluminal contents and intestinal absorption of nutrients. Because the human REM/non-REM (NREM) sleep cycle also has a periodicity of 90 minutes, hypotheses of the MMC and REM/NREM cycles being linked initiated several investigations. However, several subsequent studies have been unable to document a correlation between sleep stages and MMC cycling [25,28], thus providing support for the notion that the MMC cycle is separately regulated by the peripheral enteric nervous system, whereas sleep cycling is modulated within the central nervous system (CNS). These studies confirmed that sleep does indeed influence GI motility, but further research is needed to confirm the details of exactly how intestinal motility is modulated by sleep.

Irritable bowel syndrome

Irritable bowel syndrome (IBS) is a functional disorder of intestinal motility that affects women considerably more frequently than men [29]. The definition of IBS relates to three distinguishing characteristics: intermittent abdominal pain, altered bowel habit (constipation or diarrhea), and no obvious organic cause. In the absence of organic abdominal disease, IBS is characterized by abdominal distension and pain, relief of pain with a bowel movement, more frequent and looser stools at the onset of pain, the presence of mucus in the stool, and feelings of incomplete evacuation. Miniature pressure transducers allow long-term manometric recording in ambulatory patients, including during sleep, in order to identify abnormal bowel motility. Substantial differences in small-bowel motor activity have been observed between waking and sleeping in IBS patients [30]. A marked increase in contractility recorded in the daytime is notably absent during sleep. Comparatively, patients with IBS experience pain accompanied by propulsive clusters of small-bowel contractions with short MMC intervals during the day, and normal MMC propagation velocity during sleep [31]. Although abnormalities associated with IBS are confined to the waking state, sleep disturbances are frequently reported in IBS patients.

Nonspecific symptoms of insomnia, nonrestorative sleep, and fatigue have been reported in women with IBS symptoms [32]. This population also reports significantly more awakenings compared with controls and has been noted to have a significantly longer REM onset latency compared to controls. However, these results have not been confirmed by other studies [33,34]. Another study by Buchanan et al. studied women diagnosed with IBS who reported sleep symptoms and symptoms of abdominal pain over an entire menstrual cycle. They noted that disturbed sleep predicted the presence of abdominal pain, anxiety, and fatigue the following day (35). Disturbed sleep in IBS patients could also play a role in lowering the visceral sensory threshold, similar to the findings of Schey and colleagues in which esophageal hyperalgesia was documented in GERD patients after three nights of disturbed sleep [36].

Increased sympathetic nervous system activity among IBS patients was documented in a study of catecholamine and cortisol levels as measures of physiological arousal [37]. Autonomic abnormalities associated with sleep have been highlighted by a study by Heitkemper and colleagues demonstrating significantly lower levels of vagal tone during the sleeping interval in women with IBS compared with women without IBS [38]. Autonomic abnormalities have also been documented by patient subgroup. Decreased vagal tone (i.e, cholinergic abnormality) was characteristic of patients experiencing constipation-predominant IBS symptoms, whereas patients experiencing diarrhea-predominant IBS symptoms had sympathetic adrenergic dysfunction [39]. Following these observations, Orr and colleagues coupled PSG and autonomic monitoring in IBS patients with alternating symptoms subgroups (i.e, diarrhea- and constipation-predominant patients) to reveal differences in autonomic functioning during sleep [40]. Greater sympathetic activity during wake and greater overall sympathetic dominance during REM sleep were found in patients with IBS. Taken together, these studies support the notion of altered autonomic nervous system activation subserving the pathophysiology of IBS, thus sensitizing the gut to waking stimulation in patients with IBS.

Conclusions

Sleep is associated with substantial changes in GI functioning that have considerable clinical relevance. Acid secretion during sleep and its inhibition plays an important role in the pathogenesis of DU and its effective treatment. Sleep-related GER is now accepted as an important, if not the most important, phenomenon in the pathophysiology of reflux esophagitis. GI motility differs not only between waking and sleeping states, but also between REM and NREM stages of sleep. Further research is needed to better understand the effects of sleep on GI motility and, in turn, the effects of functional disorders of GI motility on sleep. This chapter has provided an overview of evidence-based reasons for the gastroenterologists to address sleep symptoms as well as sleep-related changes in physiological functioning that may have considerable relevance to the pathophysiology of GI diseases.

References

1. Beaumont W. Experiments and observations on the gastric juice and the physiology of digestion. Edinburgh: Maclachlan and Stewart, 1838.
2. Johnston RL, Washeim H. Studies in gastric secretion. Am J Physiol 1924;70:247–53.
3. Moore JG, Englert E. Circadian rhythm of gastric acid secretion in man. Nature 1970;226:1261–62.
4. Moynihan BG. A discussion on "The diagnosis and treatment of duodenal ulcer." Proc R Soc Med 1910;3:69–87.
5. Dragstedt LR. Section of vagus nerves to the stomach in the treatment of peptic ulcer. Surgery 1947;21:144.
6. Dragstedt LR. Excerpta Medical Section IX: Surgery Vol. 10, 1956. In: Garnott Allen JG. The physiology and treatment of peptic ulcer. Chicago: University of Chicago Press, 1959:231.
7. Hobsley M. Dragstedt, gastric acid and duodenal ulcer. Yale J Biol Med 1994;67:173–80.
8. Hobsley M. Pyloric reflux: a modification of the two-component hypothesis of gastric secretion. Clin Sci Mol Med 1974; 47:131–41.
9. Roxburgh JC, Whitfield P, Hobsley M. Parietal cell sensitivity in man: control and duodenal ulcer subjects, somkers and nonsmokers. Euro J Gastroenterol Hepatol 1994;6:235–40.
10. Faber RG, Hobsley M. Basal gastric secretion: reproducibility and relationships with duodenal ulcers. Gut 1977;18:57–63.
11. Selye H. The experimental production of peptic haemorrhagic oesophagitis. Can Med Assoc J 1938;39:447–8.
12. Johnson LF, DeMeester TR. Twenty-four hour pH monitoring of the distal esophagus: a quantitative measure of gastroesophageal reflux. Am J Gastroenterol 1974;62:325–32.
13. Johnson LF, Harmon JW. Experimental esophagitis in a rabbit model. Clinical relevance. J Clin Gastroenterol 1986;8:S26–44.
14. Atkinson M, Van Gelder A. Esophageal intraluminal pH recording in the assessment of gastroesophageal reflux and its consequences. Am J Dig Dis 1977;22:365–70.
15. Orr WC, Robinson MG, Johnson LF. Acid clearance during sleep in the pathogenesis of reflux esophagitis. Dig Dis Sci 1981;26:423–7.
16. Robertson D, Aldersley M, Shepherd H, Smith CL. Patterns of acid reflux in complicated oesophagitis. Gut 1987;28:1484–8.
17. Orr WC. Review article: sleep-related gastro-oesophageal reflux as a distinct clinical entity. Aliment Pharmacol Ther 2010;31:47–56.
18. Farup C, Kleinman L, Sloan S, et al. The impact of nocturnal symptoms associated with gastroesophageal reflux disease on health-related quality of life. Arch Intern Med 2001;161:45–52.
19. Shaker R, Castell DO, Schoenfeld PS, Spechler SJ. Nighttime heartburn is an under-appreciated clinical problem that impacts sleep and daytime function: the results of a Gallup survey conducted on behalf of the American Gastroenterological Association. Am J Gastroenterol 2003;98:1487–93.
20. Orr WC, Johnson LF, Robinson. Effect of sleep on swallowing, esophageal peristalsis, and acid clearance. Gastroenterology 1984;86:814–19.

21. Johnson LF, Harmon JW. Experimental esophagitis in a rabbit model. Clinical relevance. J Clin Gastroenterol 1986;8:S26–44.

22. Caviglia R, Ribolsi M, Maggiano N, et al. Dilated intercellular spaces of esophageal epithelium in nonerosive reflux disease patients with physiological esophageal acid exposure. Am J Gastroenterol 2005;100:543–8.

23. Dubois RW, Aguilar D, Fass R, et al. Consequences of frequent nocturnal gastro-oesophageal reflux disease among employed adults: symptom severity, quality of life and work productivity. Aliment Pharmacol Ther 2007;25:487–500.

24. Spire JP, Tassinari CA. Duodenal EMG activity during sleep. Electroencephalogr Clin Neurophysiol 1971;31:179–83.

25. Gorard DA, Vesselinova-Jenkins CK, Libby GW, Farthing MJ. Migrating motor complex and sleep in health and irritable bowel syndrome. Dig Dis Sci 1995;40:2383–9.

26. Tassinari CA, Coccagna G, Mantovani M, et al. Duodenal EMG activity during sleep in man. In: Jovanovic UJ, ed. The nature of sleep. Stuttgart: Fischer, 1973.

27. Furukawa Y, Cook IJ, Panagopoulos V, et al. Relationship between sleep patterns and human colonic motor patterns. Gastroenterology 1994;107:1372–81.

28. Kumar D, Idzikowski C, Wingate DL, et al. Relationship between enteric migrating motor complex and the sleep cycle. Am J Physiol 1990;259:983–90.

29. Harvey RF, Salih SY, Read AE. Organic and functional disorders in 2000 gastroenterology outpatients. Lancet 1983;1:632–4.

30. Kellow JE, Gill RC, Wingate DL. Prolonged ambulant recordings of small bowel motility demonstrate abnormalities in the irritable bowel syndrome. Gastroenterology 1990;98:1208–18.

31. Kellow JE, Phillips SF. Altered small bowel motility in irritable bowel syndrome is correlated with symptoms. Gastroenterology 1987;92:1885–93.

32. Heitkemper M, Charman ABD, Shaver J, Lentz MJ, Jarrett ME. Self-report and polysomnographic measures of sleep in women with irritable bowel syndrome. Nurs Res 1998;47:270–7.

33. Kumar D, Thompson PD, Wingate DL, Vesselinova-Jenkins CK, Libby G. Abnormal REM sleep in the irritable bowel syndrome. Gastroenterology 1992;103:12–17.

34. Orr WC, Crowell MD, Lin B, Harnish MJ, Chen JD. Sleep and gastric function in irritable bowel syndrome: derailing the brain-gut axis. Gut 1997;41:390–3.

35. Buchanan DT, Cain K, Heitkemper M, et al. Sleep measures predict next-day symptoms in women with irritable bowel syndrome. J Clin Sleep Med 2014;10:1003–9.

36. Schey R, Dickman R, Parthasarathy S, et al. Sleep deprivation is hyperalgesic in patients with gastroesophageal reflux disease. Gastroenterology 2007;133:1787–95.

37. Heitkemper M, Jarrett M, Cain K, et al. Increased urine catecholamines and cortisol in women with irritable bowel syndrome. Am J Gastroenterol 1996;91:906–13.

38. Heitkemper M, Burr RL, Jarrett M, et al. Evidence for autonomic nervous system imbalance in women with irritable bowel syndrome. Dig Dis Sci 1998;43:2093–8.

39. Aggarwal A, Cutts TF, Abell TL, et al. Predominant symptoms in irritable bowel syndrome correlate with specific autonomic nervous system abnormalities. Gastroenterology 1994;106:945–50.

40. Orr WC, Elsenbruch S, Harnish MJ. Autonomic regulation of cardiac function during sleep in patients with irritable bowel syndrome. Am J Gastroenterol 2000;95:2865–71.

CHAPTER 43

Sleep in chronic renal insufficiency

Giorgos K. Sakkas and Christoforos D. Giannaki

Introduction

Chronic kidney disease (CKD) is a significant and growing medical and public health problem, responsible for a substantial burden of illness and premature mortality. More than 26 million American adults have being diagnosed with CKD, while at least a millions more are at high risk. The Centers for Disease Control estimates that over 15% of the US population over 20 years of age may have some form of CKD. Diabetes continue to be the leading cause of renal failure, accounting for 44% of new cases, while uncontrolled or poorly controlled hypertension is the second leading cause, accounting for 28% of all cases [1]. Sleep disorders are remarkably prevalent in end-stage renal disease (ESRD) patients, affecting 80% of the population, especially in those receiving some type of replacement therapy such as hemodialysis (HD). Renal disease has a dramatic impact on patients' quality of life (QoL), while sleep disorders contribute significantly towards impaired QOL [2]. Sleep disorders seem to be a major and potentially treatable component of the low QoL and poor health, with implications for mortality [3–5].

Sleep disorders in patients with kidney diseases

The most common sleep complains in CKD patients are discussed in this section. Briefly, up to 80% of HD patients report symptoms of disturbed sleep, including 69% insomnia, 24% sleep apnea, 18–30% restless legs syndrome (RLS), and 12% daytime sleepiness and fatigue [6,7]. It is notable, however, that a high prevalence of renal insufficiency (approximately 30%) was also observed among patients with sleep apnea, indicating further a relation between sleep disorders and renal disease [8].

Patients with ESRD are characterized by low quantity and quality of restorative sleep, low score in sleep efficiency, disordered breathing during sleep, increased leg activity during sleep, sleep fragmentation, impaired daytime functioning, tiredness, and fatigue. All these symptoms will finally cause a significant reduction in QoL and everyday activity [7,9–11], leading to fatigue and further to inactivity, with the result that patients end up in a mode of permanent weakness and disability [12]. It is not surprising, therefore, that sudden cardiac death and heart failure are the two leading causes of death in these patients [13].

Restless legs syndrome (Willis–Ekbom disease)

RLS is very common among the CKD population [14,15]. This type of secondary RLS, called uremic RLS, appears to provoke further impairments in the already-diminished QoL and health status of uremic patients [16].The prevalence of uremic RLS is significantly higher than that of RLS in the general population, reaching approximately 30% among the CKD population (range 7–45%) [14–17]. RLS symptoms can also appear during HD therapy. Symptoms can be both sensory [18, 19] and motor [20], significantly disturbing patients' relaxation and leading to increased anxiety and finally to a premature discontinuation of HD therapy [21]. It is known that RLS symptoms begin or worsen during rest or inactivity, making HD procedures one of the main triggers of RLS [22].

Periodic limb movements in sleep

Periodic limb movements in sleep (PLMS) represent another very common sleep complaint in patients receiving HD therapy, affecting almost 80% of patients with uremic RLS [23]. PLMS has been recognized as an independent predictor of mortality in renal patients [24]. It has been recently reported that uremic RLS patients with severe PLMS experienced further detrimental alterations in cardiac structure, including an increased left-ventricular internal diameter in diastole (LVIDd), which lead to a significantly increased left-ventricular (LV) mass compared with their PLMS-free counterparts [5]. Similar results were reported in non-uremic patients, where PLMS was independently associated with severe LV hypertrophy leading to an increased risk for cardiovascular morbidity and mortality [25].

Sleep-related breathing disorders

The prevalence of sleep-related breathing disorders in HD patients is at least 10 times higher [26] than the values reported in the otherwise-healthy population [27]. Patients with severe apnea during sleep (apnea–hypopnea index AHI > 30) are characterized by insufficient quantity and quality of restorative sleep, impaired daytime functioning, tiredness, and general fatigue, leading to a significant reduction in QoL [2,9,28]. A strong body of evidence suggests that uremia-related factors are responsible for the prevalence of sleep apnea disorders in hemodialysis patients [29–31], since a substantial reduction of symptoms occurs after renal transplantation [32] or nocturnal dialysis [33]. The presence of sleep apnea is also associated with elevated blood pressure, LV hypertrophy, and increased mortality [30]. In addition, HD patients with a high AHI were found to have reduced functional capacity and altered muscle composition favoring fat deposition and increased visceral adiposity compared with HD patients with normal AHI index [2]. Body mass index (BMI) and the percentage of total body fat, however, do not seem to predispose to sleep apnea—it is rather the increased fat deposition in the abdominal area that plays the pivotal role [34].

Daytime sleepiness and fatigue

More than 50% of CKD patients are subject to daytime sleepiness [35,36], while the majority of ESRD patients have experienced some symptoms of excessive daytime sleepiness. This daytime drowsiness often leads to excessive sleep during the HD session and an increased risk of fall accidents during the day or of car accidents during the journey home after HD therapy [37]. Fragmented sleep due to sleep apnea or nocturnal sleep disruptions due to PLMS has been implicated in the pathophysiology of daytime sleepiness [36]. HD patients with a high score on the Epworth Sleepiness Scale have been found to suffer from severe sleep apnea syndrome, and these are the patients with the higher reported levels of general fatigue [2,12]. The lack of restorative sleep [3], excess pre-dialysis weight [38], poor nutritional status [39], RLS [16], and the overall mental status of the patients [39] are some of the other factors that contribute to excessive daytime fatigue. Evidently, all these factors can contribute to a self-exacerbating process, a vicious circle, of fatigue due to inactivity and further inactivity due to fatigue that leads to a significant reduction of physical activity and functional capacity. This inactivity in turn contributes to the increased cardiovascular mortality in ESRD patients [40].

Insomnia

Daytime dysfunction that accompanies various sleep disorders has a direct effect on all aspects of QoL, such as fatigue, poor cognitive function, mood disturbance, and distress or interference with personality [41]. Insomnia is a common complaint in patients with chronic renal disease and is characterized by insufficient quantity and quality of restorative sleep, low sleep efficiency, sleep fragmentation, impaired daytime functioning, tiredness, and fatigue. The prevalence in renal patients varies from 25% to 50%, depending on the patient's emotional distress related to a different lifestyle during the initial years of HD treatment and treatment of their renal disease for many years [42].

Factors affecting sleep in CKD patients

In kidney diseases, various causative factors have been involved in the development of sleep disorders. The most important factors are presented in this section.

Cardiovascular diseases

The Dialysis Outcomes and Practice Patterns Study (DOPPS) reported that patients with low quality of sleep were those with high comorbidity index, especially patients with diabetes, coronary artery disease, congestive heart failure, hypertension, and peripheral arterial disease [10]. It is important to investigate further whether therapies targeting cardiovascular diseases would improve sleep quality and quantity.

Uremic toxicity

Uremic toxicity is an "unknown" condition used to describe the harmful situation resulting from the accumulation of substances that are not efficiently removed from the failing kidney or the dialysis filter, causing inflammation and oxidative injury to organs or to the whole body. Based on the removal pattern, uremic toxins are subdivided into three major classes: (i) small water-soluble compounds, (ii) larger middle molecules, and (iii) protein-bound molecules. These substances are mostly waste products of protein catabolism and are collectively called "uremic toxins."

Uremic toxicity has been involved in sleep disturbances in CKD patients. Patients in the early stages of CKD where their kidneys maintained some function were less prone to sleep disturbances compared with HD patients [11]. Serum phosphorus levels above 7 mg/dL and calcium–phosphorus product above 80 mg^2/dL^2 were linked to poor sleep quality in DOPPS [10]. Other small protein-bound uremic toxins such as p-cresol sulfate and indoxyl sulfate have been linked to cardiovascular disease and oxidative injury that could lead to sleep disordered breathing syndromes [43]. However, the data linking the dialysis efficiency index Kt/V and sleep disorders in patients on HD are still not clear [2,44]. In kidney transplant patients, the prevalences of both insomnia and RLS are reduced to those observed in the general population; however, the prevalence of sleep apnea is still very high, reaching almost 30% [45,46]. More research is required to examine different modalities such as nocturnal HD to fully elucidate the contribution of uremic toxins in the development of sleep problems.

Blood pressure

The majority of ESRD patients suffer from renal hypertension. In addition, hypertension has been linked to sleep disturbances [47], while low blood pressure (hypotension) is one of the main reason for napping or dozing during the day or after HD sessions, disturbing the normal sleep cycle of the patient. The large fluctuations in patients' blood pressure during the day, the inability to maintain adequate control, and the lack of a dipping effect during the night [5] affect physical and mental health as well as disturbing the normal sleep cycle. In addition, antihypertensive medication increases the risk for fragmented sleep and daytime sleepiness [48].

Adequacy of hemodialysis

Efficient elimination of uremic toxins has been associated with a reduction in sleep disturbances [49]. On the other hand, inadequate HD may be associated with increased severity of uremic RLS symptoms [22]. Nocturnal dialysis significantly reduces the sleep apnea–hypopnea syndrome and the duration of nocturnal hypoxemia, possibly as a result of more efficient dialysis, since this modality has been shown to more effectively control uremia [50,51]. Another parameter that seems to influence sleep quality is the temperature of the dialysate solution during nocturnal HD. The reduction of the temperature by 2°C (from 37°C to 35°C) improves sleep by decreasing sympathetic activation and sustaining a constant skin temperature [52].

Fluid overload

In patients with ESRD, fluid overload may contribute to their high prevalence of obstructive sleep apnea by increasing the amount of fluid displaced from the legs into the neck overnight, and possibly compressing the upper airway compartments. It has been shown that the amount of overnight rostral fluid displacement from the legs is related to the frequency of apneas and hypopneas per hour of sleep [53].

Conclusions

Sleep disturbances have emerged as a problem for both CKD and ESRD patients, affecting up to 80% of these patients [7,54]. Low quality of sleep has a remarkable effect on patients' QoL, jeopardizing also the quality of their medical care. Many patients with sleep disorders remain underdiagnosed, since many of the signs and symptoms related to poor sleep are thought to be an unavoidable consequence of renal failure or inadequate dialysis. Effective management of sleep disorders could improve patients' QoL and mortality. A growing body of evidence suggests significant advantages of nocturnal hemodialysis for control of uremia and therefore for improving sleep quality and daytime sleepiness. Screening for sleep disorders should be part of a patient's routine checkup, especially when signs and symptoms of sleepiness are overwhelming. It is clear that more research is needed to investigate the mechanism of sleep disturbance in renal diseases and to explore alternative treatments.

Acknowledgements

We would like to thank Dr. C. Karatzaferi (University of Thessaly) for her comments during the preparation of this chapter.

References

1. USRDS. Annual data report: atlas of chronic kidney disease and end-stage renal disease in the United States, National Institutes of Health, National Institute of Diabetes and Digestive and Kidney Diseases. Bethesda, National Institutes of Health, 2013.
2. Sakkas GK, Gourgoulianis KI, Karatzaferi C, et al. Haemodialysis patients with sleep apnoea syndrome experience increased central adiposity and altered muscular composition and functionality. Nephrol Dial Transplant 2008;23(1):336–44.
3. Sakkas GK, Karatzaferi C, Zintzaras E, et al. Liver fat, visceral adiposity, and sleep disturbances contribute to the development of insulin resistance and glucose intolerance in nondiabetic dialysis patients. Am J Physiol Regul Integr Comp Physiol 2008;295(6):R1721–9.
4. Giannaki CD, Karatzaferi C, Hadjigeorgiou GM, et al. Periodic limb movements in sleep and cardiovascular disease: time to act. Front Neurol 2013;4:97.
5. Giannaki CD, Zigoulis P, Karatzaferi C, et al. Periodic limb movements in sleep contribute to further cardiac structure abnormalities in hemodialysis patients with restless legs syndrome. J Clin Sleep Med 2013;9(2):147–53.
6. Casey KR. Sleep disorders in chronic kidney disease. Sleep Med 2010;11(3):231–2.
7. Merlino G, Piani A, Dolso P, et al. Sleep disorders in patients with end-stage renal disease undergoing dialysis therapy. Nephrol Dial Transplant 2006;21(1):184–90.
8. Iseki K, Tohyama K, Matsumoto T, Nakamura H. High prevalence of chronic kidney disease among patients with sleep related breathing disorder (SRBD). Hypertens Res 2008;31(2):249–55.
9. Sanner BM, Tepel M, Esser M, et al. Sleep-related breathing disorders impair quality of life in haemodialysis recipients. Nephrol Dial Transplant 2002;17(7):1260–5.
10. Elder SJ, Pisoni RL, Akizawa T, et al. Sleep quality predicts quality of life and mortality risk in haemodialysis patients: results from the Dialysis Outcomes and Practice Patterns Study (DOPPS). Nephrol Dial Transplant 2008;23(3):998–1004.
11. Barmar B, Dang Q, Isquith D, Buysse D, Unruh M. Comparison of sleep/wake behavior in CKD stages 4 to 5 and hemodialysis populations using wrist actigraphy. Am J Kidney Dis 2009;53(4):665–72.
12. Sakkas GK, Karatzaferi C. Hemodialysis fatigue: just "simple" fatigue or a syndrome on its own right? Front Physiol 2012;3:306.
13. Covic A, Siriopol D, Voroneanu L. Dialysis-induced segmental wall motion abnormalities, post-dialysis fatigue and cardiovascular mortality: the new Bermuda triangle? Nephrol Dial Transplant 2013;28(10):2404–6.
14. Murtagh FE, Addington-Hall J, Higginson IJ. The prevalence of symptoms in end-stage renal disease: a systematic review. Adv Chronic Kidney Dis 2007;14(1):82–99.
15. Stefanidis I, Vainas A, Dardiotis E, et al. Restless legs syndrome in hemodialysis patients: an epidemiologic survey in Greece. Sleep Med 2013;14(12):1381–6.
16. Giannaki CD, Sakkas GK, Karatzaferi C, et al. Evidence of increased muscle atrophy and impaired quality of life parameters in patients with uremic restless legs syndrome. PLoS One 2011;6(10):e25180.
17. Schormair B, Plag J, Kaffe M, et al. MEIS1 and BTBD9: genetic association with restless leg syndrome in end stage renal disease. J Med Genet 2011;48(7):462–6.
18. Merlino G, Lorenzut S, Romano G, et al. Restless legs syndrome in dialysis patients: a comparison between hemodialysis and continuous ambulatory peritoneal dialysis. Neurol Sci 2012;33(6):1311–18.
19. Araujo SM, de Bruin VM, Nepomuceno LA, et al. Restless legs syndrome in end-stage renal disease: clinical characteristics and associated comorbidities. Sleep Med 2010;11(8):785–90.
20. Giannaki CD, Sakkas GK, Hadjigeorgiou GM, et al. Non-pharmacological management of periodic limb movements during hemodialysis session in patients with uremic restless legs syndrome. Asaio J 2010;56(6):538–42.
21. Winkelman JW, Chertow GM, Lazarus JM. Restless legs syndrome in end-stage renal disease. Am J Kidney Dis 1996;28(3):372–8.
22. Giannaki CD, Hadjigeorgiou GM, Karatzaferi C, et al. Epidemiology, impact, and treatment options of restless legs syndrome in end-stage renal disease patients: an evidence-based review. Kidney Int 2014;85(6):1275–82.
23. Parker KP. Sleep disturbances in dialysis patients. Sleep Med Rev 2003;7(2):131–43.
24. Benz RL, Pressman MR, Hovick ET, Peterson DD. Potential novel predictors of mortality in end-stage renal disease patients with sleep disorders. Am J Kidney Dis 2000;35(6):1052–60.
25. Mirza M, Shen WK, Sofi A, et al. Frequent periodic leg movement during sleep is associated with left ventricular hypertrophy and adverse cardiovascular outcomes. J Am Soc Echocardiogr 2013;26(7):783–90.
26. Kraus MA, Hamburger RJ. Sleep apnea in renal failure. Adv Perit Dial 1997;13:88–92.
27. Young T, Palta M, Dempsey J, et al. The occurrence of sleep-disordered breathing among middle-aged adults. N Engl J Med 1993;328(17):1230–5.
28. Kales A, Vela-Bueno A, Kales JD. Sleep disorders: sleep apnea and narcolepsy. Ann Intern Med 1987;106(3):434–43.
29. Novak M, Mendelssohn D, Shapiro CM, Mucsi I. Diagnosis and management of sleep apnea syndrome and restless legs syndrome in dialysis patients. Semin Dial 2006;19(3):210–16.
30. Zoccali C, Benedetto FA, Tripepi G, et al. Nocturnal hypoxemia, night-day arterial pressure changes and left ventricular geometry in dialysis patients. Kidney Int 1998;53(4):1078–84.
31. Beecroft J, Duffin J, Pierratos A, et al. Enhanced chemo-responsiveness in patients with sleep apnoea and end-stage renal disease. Eur Respir J 2006;28(1):151–8.

32. Auckley DH, Schmidt-Nowara W, Brown LK. Reversal of sleep apnea hypopnea syndrome in end-stage renal disease after kidney transplantation. Am J Kidney Dis 1999;34(4):739–44.

33. Hanly PJ, Pierratos A. Improvement of sleep apnea in patients with chronic renal failure who undergo nocturnal hemodialysis. N Engl J Med 2001;344(2):102–7.

34. Sakkas GK, Karatzaferi C, Liakopoulos V, et al. Polysomnographic evidence of sleep apnoea disorders in lean and overweight haemodialysis patients. J Ren Care 2007;33(4):159–64.

35. Parker KP, Bliwise DL, Bailey JL, Rye DB. Daytime sleepiness in stable hemodialysis patients. Am J Kidney Dis 2003;41(2):394–402.

36. Hanly PJ, Gabor JY, Chan C, Pierratos A. Daytime sleepiness in patients with CRF: impact of nocturnal hemodialysis. Am J Kidney Dis 2003;41(2):403–10.

37. Drake C, Roehrs T, Breslau N, et al. The 10-year risk of verified motor vehicle crashes in relation to physiologic sleepiness. Sleep 2010;33(6):745–52.

38. Sklar A, Newman N, Scott R, et al. Identification of factors responsible for postdialysis fatigue. Am J Kidney Dis 1999;34(3):464–70.

39. Jhamb M, Pike F, Ramer S, et al. Impact of fatigue on outcomes in the hemodialysis (HEMO) study. Am J Nephrol 2011;33(6):515–23.

40. Sarnak MJ, Levey AS, Schoolwerth AC, et al. Kidney disease as a risk factor for development of cardiovascular disease. Hypertension 2003;42(5):1050–65.

41. Buysse DJ. Insomnia. JAMA 2013;309(7):706–16.

42. Ginieri-Coccossis M, Theofilou P, Synodinou C, Tomaras V, Soldatos C. Quality of life, mental health and health beliefs in haemodialysis and peritoneal dialysis patients: investigating differences in early and later years of current treatment. BMC Nephrol 2008;9:14.

43. Raff AC, Meyer TW, Hostetter TH. New insights into uremic toxicity. Curr Opin Nephrol Hypertens 2008;17(6):560–5.

44. Masuda T, Murata M, Honma S, et al. Sleep-disordered breathing predicts cardiovascular events and mortality in hemodialysis patients. Nephrol Dial Transplant 2011;26(7):2289–95.

45. Molnar MZ, Lazar AS, Lindner A, et al. Sleep apnea is associated with cardiovascular risk factors among kidney transplant patients. Clin J Am Soc Nephrol 2010;5(1):125–32.

46. Molnar MZ, Novak M, Mucsi I. Sleep disorders and quality of life in renal transplant recipients. Int Urol Nephrol 2009;41(2):373–82.

47. Sabbatini M, Minale B, Crispo A, et al. Insomnia in maintenance haemodialysis patients. Nephrol Dial Transplant 2002;17(5):852–6.

48. De Santo RM, Lucidi F, Violani C, Di Iorio BR. Sleep disorders in hemodialyzed patients—the role of comorbidities. Int J Artif Organs 2005;28(6):557–65.

49. Unruh ML, Buysse DJ, Dew MA, et al. Sleep quality and its correlates in the first year of dialysis. Clin J Am Soc Nephrol 2006;1(4):802–10.

50. Tang SC, Lam B, Ku PP, et al. Alleviation of sleep apnea in patients with chronic renal failure by nocturnal cycler-assisted peritoneal dialysis compared with conventional continuous ambulatory peritoneal dialysis. J Am Soc Nephrol 2006;17(9):2607–16.

51. Chan CT, Hanly P, Gabor J, et al. Impact of nocturnal hemodialysis on the variability of heart rate and duration of hypoxemia during sleep. Kidney Int 2004;65(2):661–5.

52. Parker KP, Bailey JL, Rye DB, Bliwise DL, Van Someren EJ. Insomnia on dialysis nights: the beneficial effects of cool dialysate. J Nephrol 2008;21 Suppl 13:S71–7.

53. Elias RM, Chan CT, Paul N, et al. Relationship of pharyngeal water content and jugular volume with severity of obstructive sleep apnea in renal failure. Nephrol Dial Transplant 2013;28(4):937–44.

54. De Santo RM, Bartiromo M, Cesare MC, Di Iorio BR. Sleeping disorders in early chronic kidney disease. Semin Nephrol 2006;26(1):64–7.

CHAPTER 44

Sleep in endocrine disorders

Axel Steiger

Introduction

During sleep, various endocrine systems are distinctly active. A bidirectional interaction exists between the electrophysiological component that corresponds to the rapid eye movement (REM)–non-REM (NREM) cycle and the endocrine component of sleep corresponding to the nocturnal secretion pattern of various hormones. Sleep–endocrine activity in healthy volunteers and patients with various disorders, including endocrine disorders, is assessed by simultaneous polysomnographic (PSG) recordings and collection of blood by long catheters for later analysis of plasma hormone concentrations. Sleep–endocrine studies in female and male healthy volunteers from young adulthood to senescence are performed under baseline conditions, after manipulation of the sleep–wake pattern (eg, by sleep deprivation), and after administration of synthetic and endogenous compounds influencing the central nervous system (CNS), particularly neuropeptides and steroids. In addition, animal models are used, involving administration of hormones, sleep deprivation, surgery on endocrine glands, and transgenic animals. Such studies have shown a specific role of certain hormones in sleep regulation. Changes in the activity of these hormones in endocrine disorders result in changes in sleep.

In young healthy male subjects, the major portion of slow-wave sleep (SWS) and the major amount of slow-wave activity (SWA) in quantitative electroencephalogram (EEG) analysis are found during the first half of the night. Most of the growth hormone (GH) secretion during 24 hours occurs at this time [1,2], in most male subjects as a single large peak, but in women as a pre-sleep GH surge followed by one or more additional GH peaks [3]. During this period, the concentration of the hormones of the hypothalamic–pituitary–adrenocortical (HPA) system—corticotropin (ACTH) and cortisol—are low. During the second half of the night, REM sleep preponderates, and ACTH and cortisol are secreted in several pulses until they reach their acrophase near to awakening in the morning, whereas the amounts of SWS and GH are low [4]. During normal aging and episodes of depression, similar changes in sleep–endocrine activity are well documented, including increases in SWS and GH (Fig. 44.1). These patterns in young and older healthy subjects and in depressed patients point to the existence of common regulating factors of the electrophysiological sleep pattern and the nocturnal secretion of GH, ACTH, and cortisol. Indeed, there are many hints of a reciprocal interaction of the key hormones of the hypothalamic–pituitary–somatotropic (HPS) and HPA systems,—GH-releasing hormone (GHRH) and corticotropin-releasing hormone (CRH)—at least in men [5]. In short, animal models show that GHRH promotes NREM sleep [6,7], whereas CRH enhances wakefulness [6] and REM sleep [8]. Similarly, in healthy male volunteers, pulsatile injections of GHRH near to sleep onset resulted in increases in SWS and GH and blunted cortisol secretion [9], whereas after CRH secretion, SWS and GH are reduced and cortisol is elevated [10]. It is thought that in young healthy men during the first half of the night, the influence of GHRH preponderates, resulting in the peak activity of GH and SWS. When CRH dominates during the second half of the night, the major amounts of ACTH, cortisol, and REM sleep occur. The balance between GHRH and CRH is changed in favor of CRH during aging (reduced GHRH activity) and depression (CRH overactivity) (Fig. 44.2).

Sleep in disorders of the HPS system

All components of the HPS system—GH, GHRH, ghrelin, somatostatin, and insulin-like growth factor 1—participate in sleep regulation.

Isolated GH deficiency was initially diagnosed in eight patients by slowing of their growth, an abnormal insulin hypoglycemia test, and retarded bone age. Possibly, the GH deficiency was related to reduced GHRH activity. In these patients, SWS was reduced in comparison with healthy volunteers. The total sleep time and the time spent in sleep stages 1 and 2 were elevated [11]. Furthermore, in these patients, a decrease in SWA was found [12]. A small sample of children with psychosocial dwarfism was investigated by Guilhaume et al. [13]. When these previously neglected young patients were transferred to a new environment, after several weeks during recovery of growth, their sleep quality improved and SWS increased. Patients with acquired GH deficiency related to therapy of pituitary tumors frequently report fatigue during daytime. In a sample of these patients, the multiple sleep latency test (MSLT) performed to examine daytime sleepiness was in the normal range. Nocturnal sleep did not differ in these patients between baseline and the end of 1 year with GH replacement [14].

In patients with acromegaly, GH levels are excessive. Obstructive sleep apnea (OSA) syndrome (OSAS) develops frequently in these patients owing to hyperplasia of their upper airway soft tissue [15]. In patients with acromegaly without sleep apnea, an abnormal sleep structure and daytime sleepiness were also observed. In a sample of these patients, the time spent in REM sleep and SWS increased 1 year after therapy by adenomectomy. In this study, sleep energy was calculated by quantitative EEG analysis. REM sleep and SWS energy were higher at baseline than after adenomectomy [16].

Besides GHRH, ghrelin stimulates the release of GH. Furthermore, ghrelin is a strong stimulus of appetite [17] and, in men, of sleep [18]. Nocturnal sleep is disrupted in night-eating disorder owing to nocturnal hunger and the resulting food intake.

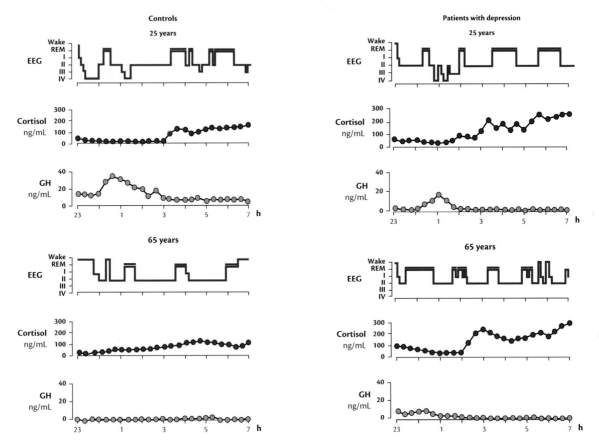

Fig. 44.1 Hypnograms and patterns of secretion of cortisol and GH of four male subjects (young and older patients with depression and healthy volunteers). REM: rapid eye movement sleep; I–IV: non-REM sleep stages 1–4.

Reproduced from D'haenen H, den Boer JA, Westenberg H, and Willner P, Neuroendocrinology of sleep disorders. In: Steiger A, (ed.), Textbook of Biological Psychiatry, pp. 1229–1246, Copyright (2002) with permission from John Wiley and Sons.

Distinctly enhanced ghrelin levels were found in a patient with this disorder [19].

Reduced nocturnal GH secretion was reported in obese patients by several studies [20]. Nocturnal sleep and GH secretion were compared in obese patients without OSA in a longitudinal study before and after weight loss due to a hypocaloric diet. As control group, lean healthy volunteers were used. Sleep variables did not differ between groups. A nearly total absence of GH secretion was found in the obese patients before weight loss. The mean body mass index of the patients decreased after weight loss from 37.1 to 31.4 (healthy volunteers 22.3). Whereas sleep architecture remained unchanged after weight loss, GH levels increased. This finding suggests a partial restoration of GH secretion [20].

Sleep in disorders of the HPA system

The HPA system is also called the stress axis. It mediates the reaction to acute physical and psychological stress. This is a prerequisite for the individual's survival. After release of CRH from the parvocellular neurons of the paraventricular nucleus of the hypothalamus, ACTH is secreted from the anterior pituitary. Finally, cortisol is secreted from the adrenal cortex.

The production of corticosteroids by the adrenal glands is distinctly reduced in Addison's disease. There are only a few case reports on sleep EEGs in these patients. No major sleep disturbances were observed [21,22]. In one study, patients with Addison's disease were compared under two conditions: either continuous hydrocortisone replacement or short-term hydrocortisone withdrawal. In comparison with withdrawal after hydrocortisone replacement, REM latency (the interval between sleep onset and the first REM period) was shortened and REM time and intermittent wakefulness were increased. These data suggest a role for cortisol in the initiation and maintenance of REM sleep [23].

In Cushing's disease, excessive cortisol levels occur, of either peripheral or central origin. In these patients, SWS is reduced compared with healthy volunteers [22,24]. In addition, in one study, increases in sleep latency and in intermittent wake time and disinhibition of REM sleep (shortened REM latency and elevated REM density) were found [24]. In particular, the latter study points to similarities of sleep-EEG changes in Cushing's disease and depression. Beside similar sleep-EEG changes (for a review, see [25]), HPA overactivity [26] and HPS dysfunction [27] are well documented. The dysregulation of the HPA system is more subtle in affective disorders than in Cushing's disease, with elevated cortisol levels being found throughout the night and elevated ACTH levels throughout 24 hours in comparison with healthy volunteers [27–29]. Nocturnal GH secretion in depressed patients was reduced in most [27,30,31] but not all [28] reports. A longitudinal study showed persistence of pathological sleep EEG and low GH levels between acute depression and recovery. In contrast, cortisol decreased after recovery [27].

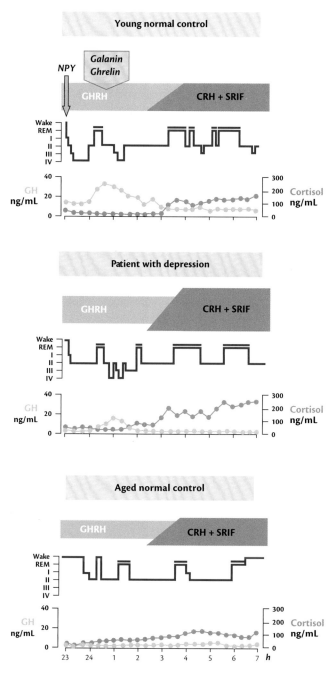

Fig. 44.2 (See colour plate section) Model of peptidergic sleep regulation. A reciprocal interaction between the neuropeptides growth hormone-releasing hormone (GHRH) and corticotropin-releasing hormone (CRH) appears likely, at least in male subjects. GHRH is thought to preponderate during the first half of the night, whereas CRH (and SRIF, somatostatin) dominate during the second half of the night. Neuropeptide Y (NPY) influences the time of sleep onset. Ghrelin and galanin are cofactors to GHRH. The balance between GHRH and CRH is changed during aging (reduced GHRH activity) and during depression (CRH overactivity). Therefore, similar sleep–endocrine changes are found during aging and in patients with depression.

Reproduced from Der Nervenarzt, 66, Steiger A, Schlafendokrinologie, pp. 15–27, Copyright (1995), with permission from Springer.

The persistence of most sleep-EEG changes [32] and blunted GH secretion [30] after recovery were confirmed over a period of 3 years. Obviously elevated cortisol secretion was eliminated during sleep in remitted patients. It appears likely that elevated HPA activity contributes to the sleep-EEG changes in depression and in Cushing's disease. As mentioned earlier, depression-like sleep–endocrine changes occur after CRH administration to healthy controls [10]. Furthermore, after high-dose glucocorticoid therapy of patients with multiple sclerosis for 10 days, sleep-EEG alterations occurred resembling those in depressed patients [33]. It is thought that the endocrine changes during acute depression cause a biological stigma resulting in the persisting changes of sleep EEG and GH secretion in remitted patients. This view is supported by similar findings in male survivors of severe brain injury. Several months later, the cortisol concentrations of these patients did not differ from those of healthy volunteers. However, their GH levels and the amounts of stage 2 sleep were diminished, whereas the cortisol concentrations were in the normal range at the time of the study. It appears likely that elevated HPA activity due to stress associated with brain injury or treatment with glucocorticoids in a subgroup of patients contributes to changes in sleep and GH secretion [34].

In patients with OSAS, during an episode of apnea, progressive hypoxemia due to asphyxia and upper airway constriction, autonomic activation, and sleep-EEG arousal occur. It is thought that OSA results in activation of the HPA system by autonomic hyperactivity [35]. This HPA activation may contribute to the development of metabolic syndrome in untreated OSA. In addition, it is suggested [35] that HPA hyperactivity may contribute to the pathophysiology of hypertension in OSAS.

Sleep fragmentation and reduced SWS are associated with sleep apnea [36]. Sleep apnea is eliminated by nasal continuous positive airway pressure (CPAP) therapy [37]. The effect of nasal CPAP therapy on sleep–endocrine activity was examined in obese patients with OSAS. At baseline, the amounts of SWS and REM sleep were low, the number of apneas was enhanced, and the arterial oxygen saturation was diminished. All these variables were normalized after one night of nasal CPAP therapy. GH secretion, which was blunted at baseline, increased during the CPAP night, whereas cortisol secretion did not differ between baseline and the post-CPAP period [38]. Cessation of nasal CPAP therapy in patients who used this device regularly resulted in an immediate recurrence of sleep apnea. ACTH and cortisol levels remained unchanged, however [39]. Sleep, plasma renin activity, and aldosterone levels were compared in patients with OSAS between baseline and 1 night after CPAP therapy [40]. At baseline, frequent awakenings, lack of SWS, and few short REM periods were observed. CPAP therapy induced improvements in sleep depth and REM sleep. In some of these patients, regular REM–NREM cycles occurred, whereas in others, the sleep structure remained irregular. As is known from healthy volunteers [41], plasma renin activity profiles reflect the pattern of REM–NREM cycles, with increasing plasma renin activity during NREM periods and declining activity during REM sleep. Normalization of the sleep cycles in some of the investigated patients resulted in regular oscillating plasma renin activity, whereas irregular sleep patterns in other patients led to a general non-oscillatory pattern of plasma renin activity. After CPAP therapy, the mean concentrations of plasma renin activity and aldosterone were enhanced [40].

Sleep in hypothyroidism and hyperthyroidism

Changes in sleep–wake behavior are well known in disorders of the thyroid gland. It is well established from clinical practice that insomnia is a characteristic symptom of hyperthyroidism. On the other hand, fatigue is frequent in patients with hypothyroidism. Therefore, it is astonishing that there is a paucity of sleep-EEG studies in these disorders. In one study, reduced SWS was reported in patients with hypothyroidism when compared with healthy volunteers, and after treatment these changes normalized [42].

Insulin, diabetes mellitus, and sleep

Insulin is a stimulus for glucose uptake in adipocytes and skeletal muscles. Circadian rhythmicity and sleep influence the profiles of glucose and insulin secretion rate, resulting in higher mean concentrations during nocturnal sleep [43]. After administration of insulin in rats, either systemic [44] or intracerebroventricular administration for 3 days [45], NREM sleep increased. Reduced amounts of NREM and REM sleep were observed in rats with experimentally induced diabetes mellitus, but their sleep normalized after insulin infusion [46].

Sleep–endocrine activity was investigated in non-hypoglycemic type 1 diabetic patients and matched healthy controls. The patients spent slightly less time in SWS during the first half of the night. Stage 2 sleep was increased throughout the night in comparison with the controls. As expected, plasma glucose and serum insulin levels were consistently higher in patients throughout the night. Furthermore, GH and epinephrine (adrenaline) were elevated during the night. In the first half of the night, higher levels of ACTH and cortisol (nonsignificant) occurred in the patients [47], compared with levels in the second half of the night.

Sleep in prolactinoma

Prolactin is a neuroprotein and a circulating hormone. Exogenous prolactin administration enhances REM sleep in cats, rabbits, and rats [48]. SWS is increased selectively in patients with hyperprolactinemia (Fig. 44.3) [49]. Compared with other endocrine disorders, the symptoms appear to be unique as they are related to impaired sleep. Studies on the effect of a moderate exogenous enhancement of prolactin levels in humans are lacking. Such investigations could clarify whether REM sleep is enhanced in this condition similar to the preclinical studies mentioned before.

Sleep in disorders related to gonadal hormones

After administration of gonadal hormones to adult animals, only minimal effects on sleep or on sex differences in sleep were found

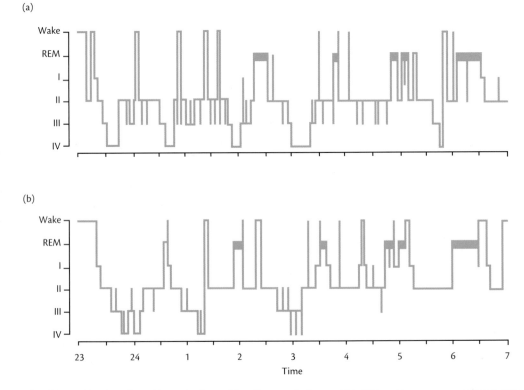

Fig. 44.3 Sleep patterns in a 25-year-old male patient with a prolactinoma (a) and in a matched control (b). REM: rapid eye movement sleep; I–IV, non-REM sleep stages 1–4.

Reproduced from Journal of Clinical Endocrinology & Metabolism, 83, Frieboes RM, Murck H, Stalla GK, Antonijevic IA, Steiger A, Enhanced slow wave sleep in patients with prolactinoma, pp. 2706–2710, Copyright (1998), with permission from The Endocrine Society.

[50]. Similarly, after high chronic dosages of estradiol in transsexual men who had undergone cross-gender therapy, only slight sleep-EEG changes were observed. In these patients, sleep stage 1 increased [51].

In men with reduced libido, blunted sleep-related testosterone concentrations were found when compared with healthy volunteers [52].

Disturbed endocrine rhythms related to environmental influences

The sleep–wake schedule of millions of people throughout the world is influenced by modern civilization. Intercontinental flights, shift work, and prolonged wake time due to artificial light influence sleep–endocrine activity distinctly.

Light is a major environmental factor influencing the timing of neuroendocrine rhythms via the suprachiasmatic nucleus. In one study [53], 24-hour hormone profiles were sampled in healthy volunteers on two separate occasions: (i) after chronic exposure to simulated short (8-hour) "summer nights" and (ii) after chronic exposure to simulated long (14-hour) "winter nights." During the "winter nights," the duration of active melatonin secretion, rising cortisol concentrations, and high prolactin secretion was longer than during the "summer nights".

In shift workers, long-lasting resistance of cortisol rhythm to total adaptation to an inverted sleep–wake schedule was observed in one study [54]. Young male night workers had been on night shift permanently for at least 2 years. They were compared with day-active healthy controls. Sleep and hormone secretion were investigated in each group during the usual sleep time (07:00–15:00 in the night workers and 23:00–07:00 in the controls) and during the usual work time. No major differences in sleep-EEG variables were found between the groups. However, cortisol concentrations were elevated and thyroid-stimulating hormone (TSH) concentrations were reduced in the night workers during their usual sleep time. During work hours cortisol levels were blunted in night workers. In another study from the same laboratory [55], a more random distribution of GH pulses during sleep in the daytime sleep of night workers was found than in controls.

Sleep EEG and hormone secretion were investigated in healthy volunteers before and after a transmeridian flight from Europe to North America. GH secretion adapted quickly to the new sleep schedule, but it took 2 weeks for the cortisol pattern to be totally adjusted [56]. The dissociation of sleep and cortisol rhythm during the first few days after transmeridian travel may contribute to the symptoms of jet lag.

Conclusions

Hormones play a major role in sleep regulation. Reduced and enhanced hormone levels in endocrine disorders result frequently in sleep changes. In most endocrine disorders, sleep is impaired. Only in patients with prolactinoma is SWS elevated.

References

1. Quabbe HJ, Schilling E, Helge H. Pattern of growth hormone secretion during a 24-hour fast in normal adults. J Clin Endocrinol Metab 1966;26:1173–7.
2. Takahashi Y, Kipnis DM, Daughaday WH. Growth hormone secretion during sleep. J Clin Invest 1968;47:2079–90.
3. Antonijevic IA, Murck H, Frieboes RM, Holsboer F, Steiger A. On the gender differences in sleep-endocrine regulation in young normal humans. Neuroendocrinology 1999;70:280–7.
4. Weitzman ED. Circadian rhythms and episodic hormone secretion in man. Annu Rev Med 1976;27:225–43.
5. Steiger A. Neurochemical regulation of sleep. J Psychiatric Res 2007;41:537–52.
6. Ehlers CL, Reed TK, Henriksen SJ. Effects of corticotropin-releasing factor and growth hormone-releasing factor on sleep and activity in rats. Neuroendocrinology 1986;42:467–74.
7. Obál F Jr, Krueger JM. GHRH and sleep. Sleep Med Rev 2004;8:367–77.
8. Kimura M, Müller-Preuss P, Lu A, et al. Conditional corticotropin-releasing hormone overexpression in the mouse forebrain enhances rapid eye movement sleep. Molec Psychiatry 2010;15:154–65.
9. Steiger A, Guldner J, Hemmeter U, et al. Effects of growth hormone-releasing hormone and somatostatin on sleep EEG and nocturnal hormone secretion in male controls. Neuroendocrinology 1992;56:566–73.
10. Holsboer F, von Bardeleben U, Steiger A. Effects of intravenous corticotropin-releasing hormone upon sleep-related growth hormone surge and sleep EEG in man. Neuroendocrinology 1988;48:32–8.
11. Åström C, Lindholm J. Growth hormone-deficient young adults have decreased deep sleep. Neuroendocrinology 1990;51:82–4.
12. Åström C, Jochumsen PL. Decrease in delta sleep in growth hormone deficiency assessed by a new power spectrum analysis. Sleep 1989;12:508–15.
13. Guilhaume A, Benoit O, Gourmelen M, Richardet JM. Relationship between sleep stage IV deficit and reversible hGH deficiency in psychosocial dwarfism. Pediatr Res 1982;16:299–303.
14. Schneider HJ, Oertel H, Murck H, et al. Night sleep EEG and daytime steep propensity in adult hypopituitary patients with growth hormone deficiency before and after six months of growth hormone replacement. Psychoneuroendocrinology 2005;30:29–37.
15. Hart TB, Radow SK, Blackard WG, Tucker HSG, Cooper KR. Sleep apnea in active acromegaly. Arch Int Med 1985;145:865–6.
16. Åström C, Trojaborg W. Effect of growth hormone on human sleep energy. Clin Endocrinol 1992;36:241–5.
17. Tschöp M, Smiley DL, Heiman ML. Ghrelin induces adiposity in rodents. Nature 2000;407:908–13.
18. Steiger A, Dresler M, Schüssler P, Kluge M. Ghrelin in mental health, sleep, memory. Molec Cell Endocrinol 2011;340:88–96.
19. Rosenhagen MC, Uhr M, Schüssler P, Steiger A. Elevated plasma ghrelin levels in night-eating syndrome. Am J Psychiatry 2005;162:813.
20. Ferini-Strambi L, Franceschi M, Cattaneo AG, et al. Sleep-related growth hormone secretion in human obesity: effect of dietary treatment. Neuroendocrinology 1991;54:412–15.
21. Gillin JC, Jacobs LS, Snyder F, Henkin RI. Effects of ACTH on the sleep of normal subjects and patients with Addison's disease. Neuroendocrinology 1974;15:21–31.
22. Krieger DT, Glick SM. Sleep EEG stages and plasma growth hormone concentration in states of endogenous and exogenous hypercortisolemia or ACTH elevation. J Clin Endocrinol Metab 1974;39:986–1000.
23. Garcia-Borreguero D, Wehr TA, Larrosa O, et al. Glucocorticoid replacement is permissive for rapid eye movement sleep and sleep consolidation in patients with adrenal insufficiency. J Clin Endocrinol Metab 2000;85:4201–6.
24. Shipley JE, Schteingart DE, Tandon R, Starkman MN. Sleep architecture and sleep apnea in patients with Cushing's disease. Sleep 1992;15:514–18.
25. Steiger A, Kimura M. Wake and sleep EEG provide biomarkers in depression. J Psychiatr Res 2010;44:242–52.
26. Holsboer F. The rationale for corticotropin-releasing hormone receptor (CRH-R) antagonists to treat depression and anxiety. J Psychiatr Res 1999;33:181–214.

27. Steiger A, von Bardeleben U, Herth T, Holsboer F. Sleep EEG and nocturnal secretion of cortisol and growth hormone in male patients with endogenous depression before treatment and after recovery. J Affect Disord 1989;16:189–95.

28. Linkowski P, Mendlewicz J, Kerkhofs M, et al. 24-hour profiles of adrenocorticotropin, cortisol, and growth hormone in major depressive illness: effect of antidepressant treatment. J Clin Endocrinol Metab 1987;65:141–52.

29. Antonijevic IA, Murck H, Frieboes RM, Steiger A. Sexually dimorphic effects of GHRH on sleep-endocrine activity in patients with depression and normal controls—part II: hormone secretion. Sleep Res Online 2000;3:15–21.

30. Jarrett DB, Miewald JM, Kupfer DJ. Recurrent depression is associated with a persistent reduction in sleep-related growth hormone secretion. Arch Gen Psychiatry 1990;47:113–18.

31. Voderholzer U, Laakmann G, Wittmann R, et al. Profiles of spontaneous 24-hour and stimulated growth hormone secretion in male patients with endogenous depression. Psychiatry Res 1993;47:215–27.

32. Kupfer DJ, Ehlers CL, Frank E, et al. Electroencephalographic sleep studies in depressed patients during long-term recovery. Psychiatry Res 1993;49:121–38.

33. Antonijevic IA, Steiger A. Depression-like changes of the sleep-EEG during high dose corticosteroid treatment in patients with multiple sclerosis. Psychoneuroendocrinology 2003;28:780–95.

34. Frieboes RM, Müller U, Murck H, et al. Nocturnal hormone secretion and the sleep EEG in patients several months after traumatic brain injury. J Neuropsychiatry Clin Neurosci 1999;11:354–60.

35. Buckley TM, Schatzberg AF. On the interactions of the hypothaloamic–pituitary–adrenal (HPA) axis and sleep: normal HPA axis activity and circadian rhythm, exemplary sleep disorders. J Clin Endocrinol Metab 2005;90:3106–14.

36. Bradley TD, Phillipson EA. Pathogenesis and pathophysiology of the obstructive sleep apnea syndrome. Med Clinic N Am 1985;69:1169–85.

37. Sullivan CE, Issa FG, Berthon-Jones M, Eves L. Reversal of obstructive sleep apnoea by continuous positive airway pressure applied through the nares. Lancet 1981;1:862–5.

38. Cooper BG, White JE, Ashworth LA, Alberti KG, Gibson GJ. Hormonal and metabolic profiles in subjects with obstructive sleep apnea syndrome and the acute effects of nasal continuous positive airway pressure (CPAP) treatment. Sleep 1995;18:172–9.

39. Grunstein RR, Stewart DA, Lloyd H, et al. Acute withdrawal of nasal CPAP in obstructive sleep apnea does not cause a rise in stress hormones. Sleep 1996;19:774–82.

40. Krieger J, Follenius M, Sforza E, Brandenberger G. Effects of treatment with nasal continuous positive airway pressure on atrial natriuretic peptide and arginine vasopressin release during sleep in patients with obstructive sleep apnoea. Clin Sci 1991;80:443–9.

41. Brandenberger G, Charifi C, Muzet A, et al M. Renin as a biological marker of the NREM–REM sleep cycle: effect of REM sleep suppression. J Sleep Res 1994;3:30–5.

42. Kales A, Heuser G, Jacobson A, et al. All night sleep studies in hypothyroid patients, before and after treatment. J Clin Endocrinol Metab 1967;27:1593–9.

43. Van Cauter E, Blackman JD, Roland D, et al. Modulation of glucose regulation and insulin secretion by circadian rhythmicity and sleep. J Clin Invest 1991;88:934–42.

44. Sangiah S, Caldwell DF, Villeneuve MJ, Clancy JJ. Sleep: sequential reduction of paradoxical (REM) and elevation of slow-wave (NREM) sleep by a non-convulsive dose of insulin in rats. Life Sci 1982;31:763–9.

45. Danguir J, Nicolaidis S. Chronic intracerebroventricular infusion of insulin causes selective increase of slow wave sleep in rats. Brain Res 1984;306:97–103.

46. Danguir J. Sleep deficits in diabetic rats: restoration following chronic intravenous or intracerebroventricular infusions of insulin. Brain Res Bull 1984;12:641–5.

47. Jauch-Chara K, Schmid SM, Hallschmid M, Born J, Schultes B. Altered neuroendocrine sleep architecture in patients with type 1 diabetes. Diabetes Care 2008;31:1183–8.

48. Roky R, Valatx JL, Paut-Pagano L, Jouvet M. Hypothalamic injection of prolactin or its antibody alters the rat sleep–wake cycle. Physiol Behav 1994;55:1015–19.

49. Frieboes RM, Murck H, Stalla GK, Antonijevic IA, Steiger A. Enhanced slow wave sleep in patients with prolactinoma. J Clin Endocrinol Metab 1998;83:2706–10.

50. Manber R, Armitage R. Sex, steroids and sleep: a review. Sleep 1999;22:540–55.

51. Künzel HE, Murck H, Korali Z, et al. Impaired sleep in male to female transsexual patients treated with estrogens. Exp Clin Endocrinol Diabetes 2000;108(Suppl 1):S93.

52. Schiavi RC, Fisher C, White D, Beers P, Szechter R. Pituitary-gonadal function during sleep in men with erectile impotence and normal controls. Psychosom Med 1984;46:239–54.

53. Wehr TA. Effect of seasonal changes in daylength on human neuroendocrine function. Horm Res 1998;49:118–24.

54. Weibel L, Brandenberger G. Disturbances in hormonal profiles of night workers during their usual sleep and work times. J Biol Rhythm 1998;13:202–8.

55. Weibel L, Follenius M, Spiegel K, Gronfier C, Brandenberger G. Growth hormone secretion in night workers. Chronobiol Int 1997;14:49–60.

56. Desir D, Van Cauter E, Fang VS, et al. Effects of "jet lag" on hormonal patterns. I. Procedures, variations in total plasma proteins, and disruption of adrenocorticotropin-cortisol periodicity. J Clin Endocrinol Metab 1981;52:628–41.

CHAPTER 45

Sleep disturbances in critically ill patients

Gerald L. Weinhouse

Introduction

The intensive care unit (ICU) is an almost uniquely hostile environment for sleep. Bright lights throughout the day and night, loud noises, frequent interruptions, numerous medications known to suppress deep sleep, mechanical support devices, pain, anxiety, stress, and severe medical illnesses themselves influence and restrict the amount and quality of sleep attainable by the sickest patients. In fact sleep, as defined by the established criteria of Rechtschaffen & Kales (R & K), may be unrecognizable in some critically ill patients.

ICU sleep studies

The challenges of performing systematic sleep studies in the critically ill are formidable; however, there have been many studies over the past 40 years using polysomnography, still considered the gold standard, to measure the sleep of critically ill patients. Most of the studies have included small numbers of patients, but the results have been consistent across different types of ICU. Critically ill patients, especially those supported on mechanical ventilators, often have severely fragmented sleep, deprived of the deep, restorative stages of sleep [1–7]. These patients have a correspondingly poor perceived sleep quality [3,8]. The total number of hours a critically ill patient may sleep in the 24 hours of a day ultimately may be normal, but they are distributed in short periods throughout the day and night, with no single extended (consolidated) period as is considered normal. Their circadian rhythm, as measured by core body temperature and levels of 6-sulfatoxymelatonin, is abnormal [9,10]. And survivors of a critical illness often report that they recall having slept poorly while in the ICU and that it was very stressful for them [6,11–14].

Studies of the sleep of mechanically ventilated patients have also been consistent in demonstrating electrophysiological anomalies. These studies have found that some critically ill patients have sleep that cannot be classified with standard scoring criteria [2,6,15–17]. For example, what has been described in critically ill patients as "atypical sleep" is characterized by alpha and/or theta activity without sleep spindles or K-complexes and may have high-amplitude continuous, irregular delta activity. "Pathological wakefulness," as described in these patients, is characterized by EEG frequency exclusive of alpha and beta activity in patients with behavioral characteristics of wakefulness. These anomalies appear to be more prevalent in patients on sedative medications than those who are not, but they have been described in both. The clinical relevance of these

electrophysiological abnormalities is uncertain, but one interpretation is that a subset of critically ill patients may be in a dissociative state where the line between sleep and wakefulness is blurred.

There has been some interest in using additional strategies, such as spectral analysis and clinical observations of arousal, as an adjunct to interpreting the results of polysomnography in the critically ill [15,16]. However, an improved understanding of (1) the significance of these deviations from the R & K criteria, (2) the relationship between this altered state of consciousness and normal, restorative sleep, and (3) the impact of this altered state of consciousness on patients' recovery from critical illness may only come from an integrative approach incorporating data from neuroimaging and other measures of brain physiology.

The abnormal EEG patterns of some ICU patients and their relationship with critical illness is potentially important. ICU delirium, for example, is highly prevalent among patients supported by mechanical ventilation, and it is an independent risk factor for six-month mortality, longer length of hospital stay, and higher cost [18,19]. Sleep loss and ICU delirium both share common clinical and neurophysiological features. Both conditions are associated with poor thought processing, memory and attention deficits, and fluctuating mental status, and have been found to have altered brain activity in the prefrontal and nondominant parietal cortices. In one small study, critically ill patients with a more severe reduction in REM sleep were more likely to develop ICU delirium [20]. If the observed deviations from normal sleep patterns experienced by critically ill patients have a relationship with ICU delirium, then it may be reasonable to hypothesize that improving the sleep of these patients could also reduce the incidence of delirium and improve the associated outcomes.

Effect of critical illness on sleep

Sepsis

Between 20% and 40% of admissions to a medical ICU are for sepsis [21,22]. Sepsis itself has been associated with altered sleep, possibly by an effect on the neurohormonal environment of the central nervous system (CNS) or by a more direct effect on the electrical system of the CNS as manifested by changes in the EEG. These patients have been found to have low-voltage, mixed-frequency waves with variable amounts of theta and delta waves [6,23]. This pattern has been referred to as "septic encephalopathy" and, similar to those patients with "pathological wakefulness" or "atypical sleep," the state of consciousness cannot be determined by the EEG alone. This pattern has been reported to appear prior to the clinical manifestations of sepsis [6]. Along with this EEG pattern is a reduction in the percentage of time in REM sleep and loss of normal circadian melatonin secretion.

Acute cardiovascular syndromes

Acute cardiovascular events necessitating critical care have been associated with a high incidence of sleep-disordered breathing. Between 40% and 70% of patients presenting to a coronary care unit may have sleep apnea–hypopnea syndrome [24,25]. Obstructive events predominate, although central respiratory events may be detected in a minority of patients. A significant number of these cases may be transient and improve or resolve with resolution of the acute event.

Respiratory failure

Respiratory failure of any cause and its treatments all may be associated with a disruption of sleep. Mechanically ventilated patients face a particularly difficult challenge due to the discomfort of the endotracheal tube and lack of synchrony with mechanically supported breaths. Several studies have been done to investigate the relationship between the ventilator mode and the frequent arousals from sleep observed in these patients. In one such study, patients with congestive heart failure had fewer central apneas and associated arousals while supported on assist control ventilation as compared with pressure support ventilation [26]. Other studies have compared proportional assist ventilation with pressure support ventilation and suggested that optimizing patient–ventilator synchrony can lead to improved sleep [27,28]. Similarly, Delisle et al [29] found that patients ventilated with NAVA (neurally adjusted ventilatory assist) had more slow-wave sleep and REM sleep, most likely as a result of better patient comfort through better neuromechanical coupling. In aggregate, these studies suggest that the mode of ventilation (in some circumstances), improved patient comfort, and optimal patient-ventilator synchrony may all lead to improved sleep.

Medications used in the ICU

Numerous medications have been demonstrated to affect sleep in healthy individuals, although they have not been tested in critically ill patients.

1. **Benzodiazepines**. Although there has been a movement away from routinely using sedatives in ICU patients because of their association with the development of ICU delirium [30], they continue to be widely prescribed, especially for those supported by mechanical ventilation. Benzodiazepines interact with the GABA receptors of the central nervous system, leading to anxiolysis, muscle relaxation, and altered consciousness at higher doses. This altered consciousness differs from "natural" sleep neurophysiologically, lacks circadian rhythmicity, is not readily reversible like natural sleep, and has an unknown relationship with the essential functions of sleep [31]. In healthy adults, benzodiazepines suppress slow-wave and REM sleep and increase and alter the morphology of sleep spindles [32].

2. **Alpha agonists**, such as dexmedetomidine, also may suppress REM sleep. The sedation produced by this drug is thought to

more closely mimic natural sleep [33]. Regardless, its theoretical advantages have not been realized clinically in this regard [34].

3. **Analgesics**. Opioids are a mainstay in the treatment of pain in critically ill and postoperative patients. These medications potently suppress both slow wave and REM sleep [35–37]. If pain is the primary cause of sleep disturbance, however, they would likely improve sleep efficiency.

4. **Vasopressors**. Adrenergic receptor agonists, such as epinephrine and norepinephrine, and dopamine are all associated with insomnia and the suppression of slow-wave and REM sleep [38].

Treatment

There is no protocol that has been demonstrated to improve the sleep of critically ill patients. One recent protocol, however, was designed to improve sleep by controlling noise and light and increasing daytime activities [39]. An effort was made to engage patients in activities during the day and minimize napping in order to restore circadian rhythms and increase the pressure for nighttime sleep. Notably, this protocol did lead to a significant reduction in the incidence of delirium but not to a demonstrable improvement in perceived sleep quality.

It seems most likely that only through a conscious effort to provide a safe, quiet, comfortable, and restful environment for sleep combined with the judicious use of medications will "natural" (non-chemically induced) sleep be preserved.

References

1. Aurell J, Elmqvist D. Sleep in the surgical intensive care unit: continuous polygraphic recording of sleep in nine patients receiving postoperative care. BMJ 1985;290:1029–32.
2. Cooper AB, Thornley KS, Young GB, et al. Sleep in critically ill patients requiring mechanical ventilation. Chest 2000;117:809–18.
3. Richards KC, Bairnsfather L. A description of night sleep patterns in the critical care unit. Heart Lung 1988;17:35–42.
4. Broughton R, Baron R. Sleep patterns in the intensive care unit on the ward after acute myocardial infarction. Electroencephalogr Clin Neurophysiol 1978;45:348–60.
5. Orr WC, Stahl ML. Sleep disturbances after open heart surgery. Am J Cardiol 1977;39:196–201.
6. Freedman NS, Gazendam J, Levan L, et al. Abnormal sleep/wake cycles and the effect of environmental noise on sleep disruption in the intensive care unit. Am J Respir Crit Care Med 2001;163:451–7.
7. Gabor J, Cooper A, Crombach S, et al. Contribution of the intensive care unit environment to sleep disruption in mechanically ventilated patients and healthy subjects. Am J Respir Crit Care Med 2003;167:708–15.
8. Friese RS, Diaz-Arrastia R, McBride D, et al. Quantity and quality of sleep in the surgical intensive care unit: are our patients sleeping? J Trauma 2007;63:1210–14.
9. Gehlbach BK, Chapotot F, Leproult R, et al. Temporal disorganization of circadian rhythmicity and sleep–wake regulation in mechanically ventilated patients receiving continuous intravenous sedation. Sleep 2012;35:1105–14.
10. Gazendam J, Van Dongen H, Grant DA, et al. Altered circadian rhythmicity in patients in the ICU. Chest 2013;144:483–89.
11. Rotondi AJ, Lakshmipathi C, Sirio C, et al. Patients' recollections of stressful experiences while receiving prolonged mechanical ventilation in an intensive care unit. Crit Care Med 2002;30:746–52.
12. Novaes MA, Knobel E, Bork AM, et al. Stressors in ICU: perception of the patient, relatives and health care team. Intensive Care Med 1999;25:1421–6.

13. Simini B. Patients' perceptions of intensive care. Lancet 1999;354:571–2.

14. Nelson JE, Meier DE, Oei EJ, et al. Self-reported symptom experience of critically ill cancer patients receiving intensive care. Crit Care Med 2001;29:277–82.

15. Ambrogio C, Koebnick J, Quan SF, et al. Assessment of sleep in ventilator-supported critically ill patients. Sleep 2008;31:1559–68.

16. Watson PL, Pandharipande P, Gehlbach BK, et al. Atypical sleep in ventilated patients: empirical electroencephalography findings and the path toward revised ICU sleep scoring criteria. Crit Care Med 2013;41:1958–67.

17. Drouot X, Roche-Campo F, Thille AW, et al. A new classification for sleep analysis in critically ill patients. Sleep Med 2012;13:7–14.

18. Ely EW, Shintani A, Truman B, et al. Delirium as a predictor of mortality in mechanically ventilated patients in the intensive care unit. JAMA 2004;291:1753–62.

19. Lin S, Liu C, Wang C, et al. The impact of delirium on the survival of mechanically ventilated patients. Crit Care Med 2004;32:2254–59.

20. Trompeo AC, Vidi Y, Locane MD, et al. Sleep disturbances in the critically ill patients: role of delirium and sedative agents. Minerva Anesthesiol 2011;77:604–12.

21. Harrison DA, Welch CA, Eddleston JM. The epidemiology of severe sepsis in England, Wales and Northern Ireland, 1996 to 2004: secondary analysis of a high quality clinical database, the ICNARC case mix programme database. Crit Care 2006;10:R42.

22. Vincent JL, Sakr Y, Sprung CL, et al. Sepsis in European intensive care units: results of the SOAP study. Crit Care Med 2006;34:344–53.

23. Bolton C, Young G, Zochodne D. The neurologic complications of sepsis. Ann Neurol 1993;33:94–100.

24. Areias V, Romero J, Cunha K, et al. Sleep apnea–hypopnea syndrome and acute coronary syndrome—an association not to forget. Rev Port Pneumol 2012;18:22–8.

25. Skinner MA, Choudhury MS, Homan S, et al. Accuracy of monitoring for sleep-related breathing disorders in the coronary care unit. Chest 2005;127:66–71.

26. Parthasarathy S, Tobin M. Effect of ventilator mode on sleep quality in critically ill patients. Am J Respir Crit Care Med 2002;166:1423–9.

27. Bosma K, Ferreyra G, Ambrogio C, et al. Patient–ventilator interaction and sleep in mechanically ventilated patients: pressure support versus proportional assist ventilation. Crit Care Med 2007;35:1048–54.

28. Alexopoulou C, Kondili E, Vakouti E, et al. Sleep during proportional-assist ventilation with load-adjustable gain factors in critically ill patients. Intensive Care Med 2007;33:1139–47.

29. Delisle S, Ouellet P, Bellemare P, et al. Sleep quality in mechanically ventilated patients: comparison between NAVA and PSV modes. Ann Int Care 2011;1:42.

30. Pandharipande P, Shintani A, Peterson J, et al. Lorazepam is an independent risk factor for transitioning to delirium in intensive care unit patients. Anesthesiology 2006;104:21–6.

31. Weinhouse GL, Schwab RJ. Sleep in the critically ill patient. Sleep 2006;29:707–16.

32. Feshchenko VA, Veselis RA, Reinsel RA. Comparison of the EEG effects of midazolam, thiopental, and propofol: the role of underlying oscillatory systems. Neuropsychobiology 1997;35:211–20.

33. Nelson LE, Lu J, Guo T, et al. The α_2-adrenoceptor agonist dexmedetomidine converges on an endogenous sleep-promoting pathway to exert its sedative effect. Anesthesiology 2003;98:428–36.

34. Oto J, Yamamoto K, Koike S, et al. Sleep quality of mechanically ventilated patients sedated with dexmedetomidine. Intensive Care Med 2012;38:1982–9.

35. Shaw IR, Gilles L, Mayer P, et al. Acute intravenous administration of morphine perturbs sleep architecture in healthy pain-free young adults: a preliminary study. Sleep 2005;28:677–82.

36. Dimsdale JE, Norman D, DeJardin D, et al. The effects of opioids on sleep architecture. J Clin Sleep Med 2007;3:33–6.

37. Cronin A, Keifer JC, Baghdoyan HA, et al. Opioid inhibition of rapid eye movement sleep by a specific mu receptor agonist. Br J Anaesth 1995;74:188–92.

38. Bourne RS, Mills GH. Sleep disruption in critically ill patients—pharmacological considerations. Anaesthesia 2004;59:374–84.

39. Kamdar BB, King LM, Collop NA, et al. The effect of a quality improvement intervention on perceived sleep quality and cognition in a medical ICU. Crit Care Med 2013;41:800–9.

CHAPTER 46

Sleep and pain
Interactions and syndromes

Gilles J. Lavigne, Samar Khoury, Caroline Arbour, and Nadia Gosselin

Pain is classically defined as an unpleasant sensory experience that may be felt in the presence or absence of injury and can even persist after the original injury has healed. Pain is considered chronic when persistent or recurrent episodes (eg, interspersed with pain-free periods) are experienced for more than 3 months. At the physiological level, pain occurs when sensory and emotional brain pathways are activated, generating an adapted or non-adapted response. This pain response is dependent on mood, past exposures, expectations of pain relief, placebo influences, and many other factors [1]. In Europe and North America, about 20% of adults report chronic pain, and this prevalence increases with age [2–4]. Pain may be associated with unstable sleep, disruption of NREM to REM sleep cycle continuity, and excessive sleep fragmentation (i.e, interruptions by overly frequent and powerful arousals, body movements, or sleep stage shifts), which may in turn increase perceptions of unrefreshing or nonrestorative sleep (NRS) [5].

Sleep characteristics associated with pain

NRS refers to the subjective experience of sleep as insufficiently refreshing, or the feeling that sleep is restless, light, or of poor quality, even though traditional objective sleep parameters (eg, total sleep duration, sleep stage distribution) may appear normal [6]. The prevalence of NRS in the general European population is estimated at 10.8%, and more than 40% of individuals with insomnia suffer from at least one chronic painful physical condition [4,7]. Having either less than 6 hours or more than 9 hours of sleep appears to be critical to predict current day's pain [8,9]. Reduced total sleep time is associated with more moderate and severe pain, and more specifically, a reduction in total slow wave is associated with more pain only in men. Poor sleep in pain patients may result from a common environmental and genetic background; however, data are emerging only slowly, and specific sleep and pain markers are difficult to identify [10]. Diurnal fatigue, mood alteration, and work shift schedule have been less often documented as causes of NRS in chronic pain patients. Fortunately, NRS is reversible, which can potentially benefit most chronic pain patients as the return of restorative sleep appears to predict, with an odds ratio (OR) of 2.0, the resolution of chronic widespread pain (CWP) [11].

Insomnia (i.e, difficulty falling asleep or an incapacity to resume sleep after awakening during the sleep period) is a sleep disorder that is frequently reported by chronic pain patients [4,12]. The classical association of pain and insomnia with hyperarousal, both considered a hypervigilance state, may help explain complaints of fatigue, anxiety and other associated co-morbidities in chronic pain patients. In addition, the influence of mood on sleep quality in pain patients seems critical [12–17]. In fact, in patients with insomnia, the endogenous pain inhibitory system that naturally induces analgesia is dysfunctional. In other words, because of the steady hypervigilance state associated with insomnia, the descending inhibitory analgesic system is already at its ceiling effect, and consequently cannot provide further pain relief when required. The net result is that more pain is felt in patients with insomnia than those without insomnia [18].

Other sleep parameters associated with an increased likelihood of pain exacerbation or reports are short sleep duration and presence of frequent sleep awakening, periodic limb movements in sleep, and breathing disorders [5].

The pain–sleep interaction

The classical notion of an interrelated negative affect between pain and sleep cannot be applied to all pain syndromes and conditions. It is not a case of "one size fits all" [5,15]. Accordingly, the interaction between pain and sleep has been conceptualized in various models.

In the "linear model," sleep interacts with acute pain in situations such as postoperative or post-traumatic pain. A few days of pain are accompanied by poor sleep, but everything returns to normal when the pain disappears [19]. The "circular model" fits better with the pain–sleep interaction idea for most chronic pain conditions, but it does not exclusively explain the deleterious effect of pain on poor sleep and vice versa [5,20]. Thus, the pain may not necessarily be more intense on the next day after poor sleep. Instead, after a poor night's sleep, a wider range of pain severity is reported [21]. While pre-sleep pain is a weak predictor of sleep quality, level of arousal before sleep appears to be more critical for predicting poor sleep quality (again, the awake time hyperarousal state may be a risk factor), which in turn predicts pain for only the first half of the following day [15]. Again, this model cannot be generalized to all patients as the variability could be explained by other predisposing risk factors (eg, mood, insomnia, hyperarousal–hypervigilance, and previous pain history) as well as by hyper-reactivity in the hypothalamic–pituitary–adrenal stress (HPA) axis, by a protective immune or genetic mechanism, the exact nature of which remains open to debate [22–24]. To better understand the strength of the pain–sleep interaction, it is also worth noting that good sleep quality is associated with better musculoskeletal health (with an OR of 3.4). In other words, the risk of pain is lower [25].

Several other factors may contribute to a patient's risk of experiencing an interaction between pain and poor sleep, including: (1) the patient's lifestyle and fitness level; (2) their beliefs and attitudes toward disease and healthcare, including expectations of relief; and (3) the presence of sleep comorbidities such as insomnia, periodic limb movement disorder (PLMD), or sleep disordered breathing (apnea/hypopnea or obstructive apnea syndrome, respiratory effort-related arousal (RERA), or upper airway resistance syndrome (UARS)). Regarding sleep comorbidities, PLMD and sleep apnea have been reported in patients with fibromyalgia (a musculoskeletal pain subcondition of chronic widespread pain) or with temporomandibular disorders (TMDs: jaw, muscle, and joint problems)—these can contribute to increasing the likelihood of sleep fragmentation and influences on perception of sleep quality [26–28].

Clinical recognition

When assessing chronic pain, the clinician should consider a history of fatigue, depression, anxiety, sleep habits, sleepiness, risk factors for the sleep disorders mentioned in the previous section, and the presence of psychological or physical trauma. Many validated assessment questionnaires are available, but this topic is beyond the scope of this chapter. Well-known instruments include the Epworth Sleepiness Scale, the Berlin Questionnaire to assess apnea, the Pittsburgh Sleep Quality Index, and the Beck Anxiety and Depression Inventory. Polysomnographic recordings are performed on pain patients mainly to rule out comorbidities such as insomnia, sleep movement disorders (PLMD, bruxism, and REM behavior disorder), and breathing disorders (see Chapters 7 & 10 and Section 8 of this volume) [29,30].

Among the types of chronic pain reported to interfere with sleep are musculoskeletal pain (eg, arthritis, fibromyalgia/widespread pain, and temporomandibular pain), neuropathic pain (herpes zoster and trigeminal neuralgia), and headaches. In this chapter, we will also introduce a prospective model of minor traumatic brain injury (mTBI), with which we investigate new onset of pain and sleep problems and consider the sequence and roles of various risk factors in the transition from acute to chronic pain after trauma.

Chronic widespread musculoskeletal pain, fibromyalgia, and temporomandibular disorders

CWP is characterized by muscle and joint pain in many body sites. Its prevalence is higher than that of what is referred to as fibromyalgia, which is a syndrome that includes, aside from muscle and joint stiffness, mood, sleep, and gastrointestinal disorders, as described in the next paragraph [31,32]. Adult patients with CWP have a higher risk (OR > 3) of fatigue, headaches, gastrointestinal problems, and sleep disturbances [33]. Patients with CWP who are seen in family medicine practice report complaints of daytime sleepiness, dozing off during daily activities, frequent awakenings during the night, and/or restless leg syndrome (i.e, uncomfortable sensations associated with an urge to move and frequent periodic limb movements in sleep). In addition, they report more signs of sleep-disordered breathing,

such as loud snoring or repeated breathing cessations (OR 1.4–2.7) [34]. We found that CWP patients tend to have three NREM to REM sleep cycles instead of five, lose about 60 minutes of total sleep time, and experience intermediate numbers of periodic limb movements per hour of sleep: more than healthy subjects and less than PLMD patients. Furthermore, their EEGs show no alpha–delta sleep, but instead a loss of slow-wave activity in the first and second NREM cycles (observed in female subjects only) [35,36] Gender predisposition to pain and poor sleep is an issue that deserves more attention.

Patients with fibromyalgia have diffuse and widespread muscle pain and tenderness in numerous body sites, along with complaints of unrefreshing sleep, somatic and cognitive symptoms, mood alterations, and fatigue [37]. Studies have identified a causal sequence involving sleep problems, pain, poor physical functioning, and depression, which strongly suggests that poor sleep in fibromyalgia patients can predict pain over a one-year period [38]. Furthermore, past history of pain, sleep quality, and delay from onset of fibromyalgia symptoms explained 22% of the pain variance in these patients at a one-year follow-up. Only a few controlled sleep studies have compared the strength of this relationship between fibromyalgia patients and control subjects using quantitative analysis of sleep variables (polysomnography). From these studies, several distinctions between these two populations have been made. Specifically, compared with controls, fibromyalgia patients were shown to have (1) fewer EEG sleep spindles during light sleep (stage 2 or N2) after controlling for age, depression, and psychiatric conditions in females [39], (2) shorter stage 2 sleep duration (with females having more sleep stage shifts), (3) more cyclic alternating pattern (CAP) cycles, scored by measuring the balance between sleep maintenance and sleep arousal pressure, and (4) clustering and/or phasic alpha EEG activity in female patients [40,41]. It was also suggested that the sleep regulatory process differs between chronic fatigue syndrome and fibromyalgia, although the two conditions may overlap in some individuals [42].

TMDs consist of pain in the jaw joint and muscles; the causes are unknown and several psychosocial, genetic, inflammatory and hormonal/gender factors are candidates [43,44]. They are reported by about 7% of the general population [45]. An individual may have both chronic orofacial pain and widespread pain/fibromyalgia, and this comorbidity is often associated with fatigue, mood, and self-regulatory deficits [46,47]. A case–control experimental sleep laboratory study revealed that one-third of patients with myofascial TMD experience insomnia and sleep apnea and that poor sleep quality increases progressively the risk of painful TMD [26,48]. However, no causal relationship was observed between the frequency of sleep bruxism motor activity and TMD-related pain complaints, although a higher frequency of mild sleep disturbances causing arousal (RERA) was observed [25,49].

Sleep and headaches

The clinical classification of headaches was updated in 2004 by a consensus statement entitled the International Classification of Headache Disorders (ICHD; http://www.i-h-s.org). In this classification, primary headaches were grouped into four main categories: (1) migraine (with or without nausea and vomiting); (2) tension-type headache; (3) cluster headache; and (4) other trigeminal autonomic cephalalgia [50]. In this chapter, we will focus exclusively on sleep-related headaches.

In the latest ICHD Classification (ICHD-3), primary headaches are classified into four main categories: (1) migraine; (2) tension-type headache; (3) trigeminal autonomic cephalalgias; and (4) other primary headache disorders [51]. Sleep-related headaches, as defined by the International Classification of Sleep Disorders [52], include headaches such as migraine, cluster headaches (related to circadian rhythms and REM sleep stage), chronic paroxysmal hemicranias, and hypnic headache, a rare condition occurring upon awakening from REM sleep and possibly from deep sleep, stage N3 [31,50,52–62]. Recent studies on morning headache (MHA) have focused on the most prevalent types: tension-type and migraine headaches *without* aura, nausea, or vomiting. Morning headache is empirically defined as a recurrent, bilateral, and pressing pain that is present at awakening three or more times a week [63,64]. MHA is most frequently a tension-type or migraine headache, with reports both of pressing (over 60% of cases) and of throbbing (at least 11–46%) sensation [53,65–68]. Episodic MHA is a good indicator of major depressive and insomnia disorders, and has been found to affect 5–8% of the general population [63,64].

It has now been recognized that tension-type and migraine headaches have different pathophysiologies [69–73]. Tension-type headache is described by patients as a tight band-like or pressing sensation that is bilateral, with no nausea or vomiting. It is a benign but highly prevalent condition in the general population. In the USA, the one-year prevalence of the episodic type of tension-type headache is 38%. Worldwide, this prevalence varies from 11 to 60%, depending on the data collection method (interviews, clinical assessments, or lifestyle questionnaires) and country (lower in Norway and Switzerland than in the USA) [70,71,74–76]. Women are slightly more at risk (OR ≥ 1.16), and complaints of tension headache frequency peak between ages 30 and 39 years (OR = 1.2) [76]. MHA is reported by close to 70% of sleep bruxism patients, but the tension-type headaches are not strongly associated with sleep bruxism motor activity—a subject of debate [77,78].

Migraine is a common episodic unilateral headache with or without aura, sensitivity to light (photophobia) or sound (phonophobia), nausea, and vomiting. The population prevalence of migraine with aura is about 1%, and in Canada it is 26% for all types of migraine [52,72,74,79,80]. The one-year prevalence of migraine without aura is 5–15% in the general population, but is twice as high in females. [74,75]. Attacks may be triggered by a vast array of conditions, including sleep problems (such as sleep apnea), and jaw disorders.

Migraine and tension headaches may overlap with TMDs, bruxism, and neck pain [81–84]. Tension-type headache is reported by 4.6–32% of diagnosed PLMD patients and by almost 50% of sleep bruxism patients, again without any relationship to frequency of jaw muscle activity [68,78,85,86].

Another frequent sleep-related headache is sleep apnea headache. Based on an etiologic classification, the International Headache Society (2004) suggests the following diagnostic criteria for sleep apnea headache [50]:

A. Recurrent headache with at least one of the following characteristics and fulfilling criteria C and D: 1. occurs on >15 days per month; 2. bilateral, pressing quality and not accompanied by nausea, photophobia or phonophobia; 3. each headache resolves within 30 minutes. B. Sleep apnea (Respiratory Disturbance Index > 5) is demonstrated by overnight polysomnography. C. Headache is present upon awakening; and D. headache ceases within 72 hours, and does not recur after effective treatment of sleep apnea.

Recent evidence indicates that MHA can last up to 1–4 hours in more than 55–74% of subjects with or without sleep-apnea-related HA [53,66].

The daily functioning of an MHA patient is associated with stress, anxiety, and depressive mood, plus irritability, fatigue, and a feeling of inefficiency, in addition to oversensitivity to sound, touch, and light [63]. The frequency of sleep complaints in MHA patients is similar to that for all headaches. Complaints of difficulty initiating or maintaining sleep, feeling unrefreshed in the morning, disturbed sleep, and tossing and turning are 2–4 times higher than in controls [64]. Risk factors include gender (OR for women is 1.1), age (worse in the 20s and 40s, and lower after age 60), regular alcohol or medication use, and, in some cases, overuse of medications (also known as medication-overuse headache or rebound headache) [63,64].

Sleep and pain in mild traumatic brain injury patients

Sleep disruptions following mTBI are commonly reported and are part of the symptoms that make up chronic traumatic encephalopathy. Sleep disruptions can be as high as 44% in the year following an mTBI, making it an interesting model for the study of sleep [87,88]. Specifically, several sleep disorders have been reported in mTBI victims, including (1) post-traumatic hypersomnia, (2) insomnia, (3) periodic limb movements in sleep, (4) narcolepsy, (5) REM behavior disorder, and (6) obstructive sleep apnea [89–93]. The causes of these sleep disturbances are unknown, and quantitative polysomnographic studies have not provided much helpful evidence. Indeed, findings on sleep stage duration, sleep efficiency, and REM sleep duration were either inconsistent or showed no significant differences from healthy controls [94–97]. Still, studies using EEG spectral power analysis have reported lower delta and higher alpha and beta power during NREM sleep in mTBI patients compared with controls at one week post-trauma [98]. Similarly, a significant power reduction in low EEG frequency bands (0.5–9.75 Hz) during NREM sleep was found in adolescents post-mTBI [98]. Conversely, no differences in quantitative sleep EEG were reported in mTBI patients or in athletes with mTBI compared with healthy subjects and control athletes [99,100].

Pain is a highly prevalent post-concussion symptom in mTBI patients, occurring in more than 75% of cases [101]. In fact, patients with mTBI report more pain compared with patients with severe TBI [101,102]. The presence of pain exacerbates complaints of insomnia twofold in mTBI patients [102]. In previous studies, mTBI patients with sleep complaints reported more headaches [103] and about one-third of mTBI patients progress to chronic pain [104,105].

In a study using high-density spectral analysis, we found that, compared with mTBI without pain and healthy controls, mTBI patients with pain reported poorer sleep quality on the Pittsburgh Sleep Quality Index (PSQI), which was correlated to higher predominance of beta and gamma EEG activity during all sleep stages, including the N3 deep sleep stage [106]. Also, it should be noted that treating one condition may not contribute to reverse the second, and vice versa.

Management of the pain–sleep interaction

Management is a broad term that covers the management of both pain and sleep, with a particular focus on balancing the predominant factors in the etiology of patient complaints. As a general rule, patients should be advised about lifestyle factors and sleep hygiene, cognitive–behavioral therapies (CBTs), manual therapies (eg, physical therapy), and medications (see Box 46.1).

Napping is a strategy used by many chronic pain patients to cope with fatigue and the effects of poor sleep. Naps should not last more than 20–30 minutes (the exact duration is debated) to avoid the

---

Box 46.1 Strategies to manage the pain–sleep interaction

The supporting evidence in the literature for most of the items presented below is low to moderate. Some of these medications are off-label; clinicians should refer to the guidelines provided by the appropriate government agencies.

1. Establish a strong differential diagnosis to assess roles or exclude comorbidities such as sleep breathing disorders, periodic limb movement disorder, depression, and anxiety

2. Review lifestyle and sleep behavior patterns and beliefs

3. Assess the patient's expectations: pain relief or improved sleep or both in relation to his or her definition of quality of life

4. Suggest the use of relaxation therapy, yoga, mild exercise, etc

5. Review whether the patient uses complementary alternative medicine (CAM) approaches or other methods to self-manage their pain and sleep problems (melatonin, valerian, cannabis, etc.)

6. Guide their choice of *over-the-counter (OTC) medications* such as anti-inflammatories (aspirin, ibuprofen) or acetaminophen (paracetamol) alone or in combination with a muscle relaxant or sleep aid (antihistamine)

7. Refer the patient to a sleep medicine clinic if sleep disordered breathing or periodic limb movement disorder is suspected

8. Cognitive–behavioral therapy (CBT) is indicated if insomnia and/or anxiety mood are concomitant

9. Physical therapy or massage may help patients restore functionality

10. Prescribe clonazepam (if sleep arousal and anxiety predominate), cyclobenzaprine (if muscle pain predominates), or trazodone (if sleep arousal/fragmentation predominates) given PRN and for short periods. Be alert for side effects and risks (eg, sleepiness, habituation)

11. Based on pain intensity and impacts on sleep, consider the following medications: antidepressants (eg, duloxetine or amitriptyline), pregabalin (in the evening to reduce daytime sleepiness), opioids (earlier during the day if there is a risk of sleep breathing disorders; assess risks for misuse and addiction)

12. Sleep medications may help, but in the short term only, during the transition to CBT (see point 8)

13. Sleep disordered breathing or periodic limb movement disorders should be managed according to standard medical practice (CPAP, oral devices, or dopaminergic medications)

---

influence of sleep inertia on performance and mood disturbance (grogginess). Reliable studies are lacking on the benefits of this simple strategy, for instance, the identification of the best time of day to nap or its effectiveness on the pain–sleep interaction [107]. Furthermore, because mTBI patients also tend to nap longer, some sleep behavioral changes would probably be concomitant with mood alterations, pain, and poor sleep [108]. Exercise, yoga, meditation, and meditative movement are other simple strategies that could benefit individuals suffering from the pain–sleep interaction. Solid complementary and alternative study designs are emerging to corroborate these findings. In addition, the benefits appear to persist over time [109–112]. CBTs constitute a well-established approach to managing insomnia. However, more recent studies have indicated that these approaches need to be customized in order to effectively manage the pain–sleep interaction and insomnia [113–115].

Among the medications prescribed to manage the pain–sleep interaction, the first-line recommendation is a nonsteroidal analgesic alone or in combination with a muscle relaxant. Patients who use aspirin, ibuprofen, or acetaminophen (paracetamol) should be advised to continue using these medications, but physicians should be alert for signs of abuse. Nonsteroidal analgesics can actually induce headache if overused. Stronger medications include low-dose anticonvulsants such as clonazepam or pregabalin at bedtime (daytime use should be avoided if possible to reduce sleepiness), low-dose antidepressive medications such as amitriptyline or trazodone, and finally opioids, as long as sleep apnea or addiction risk is not suspected (see Chapter 19 of this volume for insomnia and Chapter 20 for a general review) [116–121] Note that some of these medications are off-label, i.e, not authorized as sleep or pain–sleep medication.

In the presence of breathing disorders, it is mandatory to initially exclude adenoid and large tonsil or nasal obstruction. If the condition is mild, such as RERA or UARS, a mandibular advancement appliance can be used after performing a polysomnographic sleep test. For more severe cases, a continuous positive airway pressure system (CPAP) is an alternative that appears to help some patients, although, again, not all patients will benefit from breathing therapy (see Chapter 17 for more information on CPAP treatment) [122–124].

Phenotyping each case for risk factors and possible causative vectors is a difficult task that requires specialized expertise. The same challenge applies to the selection of the best nonpharmacological or pharmacological treatment. To date, no simple algorithms have been developed, owing to the modest concordance between sleep and pain treatment outcomes [125].

Conclusions

Pain poses a critical obstacle to restful sleep. Although never welcome, pain is nevertheless a reminder that something is not normal. Patients should be made aware that pain is a signal that their body homeostasis is under threat, and that pain is part of a protective reaction that prevents future action. Therefore, it is not surprising that acute and chronic pain have been associated with hypervigilance, sleep disruption with excessive sleep fragmentation, and insomnia with hyperarousal. Acute pain may affect sleep for short periods, after which the pain intensity lessens and sleep resumes as normal. Adequate pain management is critical in this transitional period. The problem arises when pain becomes chronic and consequently disrupts sleep. To prevent this critical situation, which can occur in at least 1–15% of patients, depending on the type of surgery or post-traumatic state [106,126], it is mandatory to identify the risks for sleep disorders (breathing, movement, insomnia/dyssomnia) and to manage the pain with medications that are less harmful to sleep homeostasis (see Box 46.1). However, when pain becomes persistent or overly recurrent (also called pain chronification), effective management of the pain and the impacts on sleep calls for a major reassessment of the differential diagnosis and a determination of the role of comorbidities, since associated conditions such as mood changes, anxiety, and depression may obscure the clinical picture. One of the challenges for clinicians is to assess whether the pain is driving the complaints of poor sleep or whether poor sleep is exacerbating the pain. Unfortunately, there are no simple answers. The risk of suicide in pain patients is well recognized and suicidal ideation increases fivefold if the patient has a history of illicit drug use [127]. The patient's individual vulnerability to pain and sleep disruption should be assessed by considering a number of critical variables, including age, gender, concomitant or history of depression and anxiety, past experience with pain, expectations of treatment, use of medications or complementary alternative medicine or illicit drugs, risk of misuse or addiction to medication, history of chronic fatigue syndrome, and any other conditions that could explain the variance in the pain–sleep interaction. Clinicians should also take into account the discrepancies in their perceptions of management success and failure.

Acknowledgements

The research conducted by the principal author (GJL) is supported by the Canada Research Chair Program, the CIHR, a CFI grant from the Canadian Government, and the Quebec Pain Research Network of the FRQS, Quebec Government. SK was funded by a CIHR Frederick Banting and Charles Best doctoral fellowship.

References

1. Tracey I. Getting the pain you expect: mechanisms of placebo, nocebo and reappraisal effects in humans. Nat Med 2010;16:1277–83.
2. Boulanger A, Clark AJ, Squire P, et al. Chronic pain in Canada: have we improved our management of chronic noncancer pain? Pain Res Manag. 2007;12:39–47.
3. Reitsma ML, Tranmer JE, Buchanan DM, Vandenkerkhof EG. The prevalence of chronic pain and pain-related interference in the Canadian population from 1994 to 2008. Chronic Dis Inj Can 2011;31:157–64.
4. Ohayon MM. Relationship between chronic painful physical condition and insomnia. J Psychiatr Res 2005;39:151–9.
5. Lavigne GJ, Nashed A, Manzini C, Carra MC. Does sleep differ among patients with common musculoskeletal pain disorders? Curr Rheumatol Rep 2011;13:535–42.
6. Wilkinson K, Shapiro C. Nonrestorative sleep: symptom or unique diagnostic entity? Sleep Med 2012;13:561–9.
7. Ohayon MM. Prevalence and correlates of nonrestorative sleep complaints. Arch Intern Med 2005;165):35–41.
8. Edwards RR, Almeida DM, Klick B, et al. Duration of sleep contributes to next-day pain report in the general population. Pain 2008;137:202–7.
9. Weingarten JA, Dubrovsky B, Basner RC, et al. Polysomnographic measurement of sleep duration and bodily pain perception in the sleep heart health study. Sleep 2016;39(8):1583–9.
10. Zhang J, Lam SP, Li SX, et al. Insomnia, sleep quality, pain, and somatic symptoms: sex differences and shared genetic components. Pain 2012;153:666–73.
11. Davies KA, Macfarlane GJ, Nicholl BI, et al. Restorative sleep predicts the resolution of chronic widespread pain: results from the EPIFUND study. Rheumatology 2008;47:1809–13.
12. Sutton DA, Moldofsky H, Badley EM. Insomnia and health problems in Canadians. Sleep 2001;24:665–70.
13. Bonnet MH, Arand DL. Hyperarousal and insomnia: state of the science. Sleep Med Rev 2010;14:9–15.
14. Tang NK, Wright KJ, Salkovskis PM. Prevalence and correlates of clinical insomnia co-occurring with chronic back pain. J Sleep Res 2007;16:85–95.
15. Tang NK, Goodchild CE, Sanborn AN, et al. Deciphering the temporal link between pain and sleep in a heterogeneous chronic pain patient sample: a multilevel daily process study. Sleep 2012;35:675–87A.
16. Lautenbacher S, Huber C, Kunz M, et al. Hypervigilance as predictor of postoperative acute pain: its predictive potency compared with experimental pain sensitivity, cortisol reactivity, and affective state. Clin J Pain 2009;25:92–100.
17. Zautra AJ, Fasman R, Parish BP, Davis MC. Daily fatigue in women with osteoarthritis, rheumatoid arthritis, and fibromyalgia. Pain 2007;128:128–35.
18. Haack M, Scott-Sutherland J, Santangelo G, et al. Pain sensitivity and modulation in primary insomnia. Eur J Pain 2012;16:522–33.
19. Vanini G. Sleep deprivation and recovery sleep prior to a noxious inflammatory insult influence characteristics and duration of pain. Sleep 2016;39(1):133–42.
20. Lavigne G, Smith MT, Denis R, Zucconi M. Pain and sleep. In: Kryger HM, Roth T, Dement WC, eds. Principles and practice of sleep medicine, 5th ed. St Louis, MO: Elsevier Saunders, 2011:1442–51.
21. Liszka-Hackzell JJ, Martin DP. Analysis of nighttime activity and daytime pain in patients with chronic back pain using a self-organizing map neural network. J Clin Monit Comput 2005;19:411–14.
22. Holliday KL, McBeth J, Macfarlane G, et al. Investigating the role of pain-modulating pathway genes in musculoskeletal pain. Eur J Pain 2013;17:28–34.
23. Holliday KL, Nicholl BI, Macfarlane GJ, et al. Genetic variation in the hypothalamic-pituitary-adrenal stress axis influences susceptibility to musculoskeletal pain: results from the EPIFUND study. Ann Rheum Dis 2010;69:556–60.
24. McBeth J, Silman AJ, Gupta A, et al. Moderation of psychosocial risk factors through dysfunction on the hypothalamic–pituitary–adrenal stress axis in the onset of chronic widespread musculoskeletal pain: findings of a population-based prospective cohort study. Arthritis Rheum 2007;56:360–71.
25. Jones EA, McBeth J, Nicholl B, et al. What characterizes persons who do not report musculoskeletal pain? Results from a 4-year population-based longitudinal study (the Epifund study). J Rheumatol 2009;36:1071–7.
26. Smith MT, Wickwire EM, Grace EG, et al. Sleep disorders and their association with laboratory pain sensitivity in temporomandibular joint disorder. Sleep 2009;32:779–90.
27. Dubrovsky B, Raphael KG, Lavigne GJ, et al. Polysomnographic investigation of sleep and respiratory parameters in women with temporomandibular pain disorders. J Clin Sleep Med 2014;10:195–201.
28. Moldofsky H, Inhaber NH, Guinta DR, Alvarez-Horine SB. Effects of sodium oxybate on sleep physiology and sleep/wake-related symptoms in patients with fibromyalgia syndrome: a double-blind, randomized, placebo-controlled study. J Rheumatol 2010;37:2156–66.
29. Walters AS, Lavigne G, Hening W, et al. The scoring of movements in sleep. J Clin Sleep Med 2007;3:155–67.
30. Lavigne GJ, Khoury S, Laverdure-Dupont D, et al. Tools and methodological issues in the investigation of sleep and pain interactions. In: Lavigne GJ, Sessle BJ, Choinière M, Soja P, eds. Sleep and pain. Seattle, WA: IASP Press, 2007:235–66.

31. Von Korff M, Leresche L. Epidemiology of pain. In: Merskey H, Loeser JD, Dubner R, eds. The paths of pain 1975–2005. Seattle, WA: IASP Press, 2005:339–52.

32. Wolfe F, Walitt BT, Katz RS, Häuser W.. Symptoms, the nature of fibromyalgia, and Diagnostic and Statistical Manual 5 (DSM-5) defined mental illness in patients with rheumatoid arthritis and fibromyalgia. PLoS One 2014;9(2):e88740.

33. Rohrbeck J, Jordan K, Croft P. The frequency and characteristics of chronic widespread pain in general practice: a case–control study. Br J Gen Pract 2007;57:109–15.

34. Alattar M, Harrington JJ, Mitchell CM, Sloane P. Sleep problems in primary care: a North Carolina Family Practice Research Network (NC-FP-RN) study. J Am Board Fam Med 2007;20:365–74.

35. Okura K, Lavigne GJ, Huynh N, et al. Comparison of sleep variables between chronic widespread musculoskeletal pain, insomnia, periodic leg movements syndrome and control subjects in a clinical sleep medicine practice. Sleep Med 2008;9:352–61.

36. Lavigne GJ, Okura K, Abe S, et al. Gender specificity of the slow wave sleep lost in chronic widespread musculoskeletal pain. Sleep Med 2011;12:179–85.

37. Wolfe F, Clauw DJ, Fitzcharles MA, et al. The American College of Rheumatology preliminary diagnostic criteria for fibromyalgia and measurement of symptom severity. Arthritis Care Res 2010;62:600–10.

38. Bigatti SM, Hernandez AM, Cronan TA, Rand KL. Sleep disturbances in fibromyalgia syndrome: relationship to pain and depression. Arthritis Rheum 2008;59:961–7.

39. Landis CA, Lentz MJ, Rothermel J, et al. Decreased sleep spindles and spindle activity in midlife women with fibromyalgia and pain. Sleep 2004;27:741–50.

40. Burns JW, Crofford LJ, Chervin RD. Sleep stage dynamics in fibromyalgia patients and controls. Sleep Med 2008;9:689–96.

41. Rizzi M, Sarzi-Puttini P, Atzeni P, et al. Cyclic alternating pattern: a new marker of sleep alteration in patients with fibromyalgia? J Rheumatol 2004;31:1193–9.

42. Kishi A, Natelson BH, Togo F, et al. Sleep-stage dynamics in patients with chronic fatigue syndrome with or without fibromyalgia. Sleep 2011;34:1551–60.

43. Maixner W, Diatchenko L, Dubner R, et al. Orofacial pain prospective evaluation and risk assessment study—the OPPERA study. J Pain 2011;12(11 Suppl):T4–11.e1–2.

44. Fillingim RB, Ohrbach R, Greenspan JD, et al. Psychological factors associated with development of TMD: the OPPERA prospective cohort study. J Pain 2013;14(12 Suppl):T75–90.

45. Goulet JP, Lavigne GJ, Lund JP. Jaw pain prevalence among French-speaking Canadians in Quebec and related symptoms of temporomandibular disorders. J Dent Res 1995;74:1738–44.

46. Solberg Nes L, Carlson CR, Crofford LJ, et al. Self-regulatory deficits in fibromyalgia and temporomandibular disorders. Pain 2010;151:37–44.

47. da Silva LA, Kazyiama HH, de Siqueira JT, et al. High prevalence of orofacial complaints in patients with fibromyalgia: a case–control study. Oral Surg Oral Med Oral Pathol Oral Radiol 2012;114(5):e29–34.

48. Sanders AE, Akinkugbe AA, Bair E, et al. Subjective sleep quality deteriorates before development of painful temporomandibular disorder. J Pain 2016;17(6):669–77.

49. Raphael KG, Sirois DA, Janal MN, et al. Sleep bruxism and myofascial temporomandibular disorders: a laboratory-based polysomnographic investigation. J Am Dent Assoc 2012;143:1223–31.

50. Olesen J, Lipton RB. Headache classification update 2004. Curr Opin Neurol 2004;17:275–82.

51. Olesen J. ICHD-3 beta is published. Use it immediately. Cephalalgia 2013;33:627–8.

52. AASM. International classification of sleep disorders, 3rd ed. Darien, IL: American Academy of Sleep Medicine, 2014.

53. Alberti A, Mazzotta G, Gallinella E, Sarchielli P. Headache characteristics in obstructive sleep apnea syndrome and insomnia. Acta Neurol Scand 2005;111:309–16.

54. Russell MB. Epidemiology and genetics of cluster headache. Lancet Neurol 2004;3:279–83.

55. Culebras A. Other neurological disorders. In: Kryger MH, Roth T, Dement WC, eds. Principles and practice of sleep medicine, 5th ed. St Louis, MO: Elsevier Saunders, 2011:1064–74.

56. Lavigne G, Blanchet P, Khoury S, et al. Céphalées et sommeil: un survol diagnostique et un guide pour le clinicien [Headache and sleep: guidance in recognition]. Douleur analg 2010;23:175–80.

57. Poceta JS. Sleep-related headache. Curr Treat Options Neurol 2002;4:121–8.

58. Scher AI. Migraine and headache: a meta-analytic approach. In: Crombie IK, ed. Epidemiology of pain. Seattle, WA: IASP Press, 1999:159–70.

59. Greenough GP, Nowell PD, Sateia MJ. Headache complaints in relation to nocturnal oxygen saturation among patients with sleep apnea syndrome. Sleep Med 2002;3:361–4.

60. Jennum P, Jensen R. Sleep and headache. Sleep Med Rev 2002;6:471–9.

61. Malow BA. Impact, presentation, and diagnosis. In: Kryger HM, ed. Principles and practice of sleep medicine. Philadelphia: Elsevier Saunders, 2005:589–93.

62. Lavigne GJ, Morisson F, Khoury S, Mayer P. Sleep-related pain complaints: morning headaches and tooth grinding. Insomnia 2006;7:4–11.

63. Ohayon MM. Prevalence and risk factors of morning headaches in the general population. Arch Intern Med 2004;164:97–102.

64. Seidel S, Klösch G, Moser D, et al. Morning headaches, daytime functioning and sleep problems--a population-based controlled study. Wien Klin Wochenschr 2010;122:579–83.

65. Chen PK, Fuh JL, Lane HY, et al. Morning headache in habitual snorers: frequency, characteristics, predictors and impacts. Cephalalgia 2011;31:829–36.

66. Goksan B, Gunduz A, Karadeniz D, et al. Morning headache in sleep apnoea: clinical and polysomnographic evaluation and response to nasal continuous positive airway pressure. Cephalalgia 2009;29:635–41.

67. Sand T, Hagen K, Schrader H. Sleep apnoea and chronic headache. Cephalalgia 2003;23:90–5.

68. Loh NK, Dinner DS, Foldvary N, et al. Do patients with obstructive sleep apnea wake up with headaches? Arch Intern Med 1999;159:1765–8.

69. Manzoni GC, Stovner LJ. Epidemiology of headache. In: Aminoff MJ, Boller F, Swaab DF, eds. Handbook of clinical neurology, Vol 97. Amsterdam: Elsevier, 2010:3–22.

70. Stovner LJ, Andree C. Prevalence of headache in Europe: a review for the Eurolight project. J Headache Pain 2010;11:289–99.

71. Fumal A, Schoenen J. Tension-type headache: current research and clinical management. Lancet Neurol 2008;7:70–83.

72. Alberti A. Headache and sleep. Sleep Med Rev 2006;10:431–7.

73. Rains JC, Poceta JS. Headache and sleep disorders: review and clinical implications for headache management. Headache 2006;46:1344–63.

74. Merikangas KR, Cui L, Richardson AK, et al. Magnitude, impact, and stability of primary headache subtypes: 30 year prospective Swiss cohort study. BMJ 2011;343:d5076.

75. Kristiansen HA, Kværner KJ, Akre H, et al. Tension-type headache and sleep apnea in the general population. J Headache Pain 2011;12:63–9. .

76. Schwartz BS, Stewart WF, Simon D, Lipton RB. Epidemiology of tension-type headache. JAMA 1998;279:381–3.

77. Abe S, Carra MC, Huynh NT, et al. Females with sleep bruxism show lower theta and alpha electroencephalographic activity irrespective of transient morning masticatory muscle pain. J Orofac Pain 2013;27:123–34.

78. Yachida W, Castrillon EE, Baad-Hansen L, et al. Craniofacial pain and jaw-muscle activity during sleep. J Dent Res 2012;91:562–7.

79. Aguggia M, Cavallini M, Divito N, et al. Sleep and primary headaches. Neurol Sci 2011;32 Suppl 1:S51–4.

80. Cooke LJ, Becker WJ. Migraine prevalence, treatment and impact: the canadian women and migraine study. Can J Neurol Sci 2010;37:580–7.

81. Blumenfeld A, Schim J, Brower J. Pure tension-type headache versus tension-type headache in the migraineur. Curr Pain Headache Rep 2010;14:465–9.

82. Hoffmann RG, Kotchen JM, Kotchen TA, et al. Temporomandibular disorders and associated clinical comorbidities. Clin J Pain 2011;27:268–74.

83. Kaniecki RG. Migraine and tension-type headache: an assessment of challenges in diagnosis. Neurology 2002;58(9 Suppl 6):S15–20.

84. Evans RW, Bassiur JP, Schwartz AH. Bruxism, temporomandibular dysfunction, tension-type headache, and migraine. Headache. 2011;51:1169–72.

85. Huynh N, Khoury S, Rompré PH, et al. Prevalence of headache and neck pain in a sleep bruxism population investigated in a sleep laboratory. Sleep 2006;29(Abst Suppl):A282.

86. Chen PK, Fuh JL, Chen SP, Wang SJ. Association between restless legs syndrome and migraine. J Neurol Neurosurg Psychiatry 2010;81:524–8.

87. McKee AC, Cantu RC, Nowinski CJ, et al. Chronic traumatic encephalopathy in athletes: progressive tauopathy after repetitive head injury. J Neuropathol Exp Neurol 2009;68:709–35.

88. Hartvigsen J, Boyle E, Cassidy JD, Carroll LJ. Mild traumatic brain injury after motor vehicle collisions: what are the symptoms and who treats them? A population-based 1-year inception cohort study. Arch Phys Med Rehabil 2014;95(3 Suppl):S286–94.

89. Castriotta RJ, Murthy JN. Sleep disorders in patients with traumatic brain injury: a review. CNS Drugs 2010;25:175–85.

90. Theodorou AA, Rice SA. Is the silent epidemic keeping patients awake? J Clin Sleep Med. 2007;3:347–8.

91. Masel BE, Scheibel RS, Kimbark T, Kuna ST. Excessive daytime sleepiness in adults with brain injuries. Arch Phys Med Rehabil 2001;82:1526–32.

92. Webster JB, Bell KR, Hussey JD, et al. Sleep apnea in adults with traumatic brain injury: a preliminary investigation. Arch Phys Med Rehabil 2001;82:316–21.

93. Castriotta RJ, Wilde MC, Lai JM, et al. Prevalence and consequences of sleep disorders in traumatic brain injury. J Clin Sleep Med 2007;3:349–56.

94. Verma A, Anand V, Verma NP. Sleep disorders in chronic traumatic brain injury. J Clin Sleep Med. 2007;3:357-62.

95. Prigatano GP, Stahl ML, Orr WC, Zeiner HK. Sleep and dreaming disturbances in closed head injury patients. J Neurol Neurosurg Psychiatry 1982;45:78–80.

96. Ouellet MC, Morin CM. Subjective and objective measures of insomnia in the context of traumatic brain injury: a preliminary study. Sleep Med 2006;7:486–97.

97. Rao V, Bergey A, Hill H, et al. Sleep disturbance after mild traumatic brain injury: indicator of injury? J Neuropsychiatry Clin Neurosci 2011;23:201–5.

98. Parsons LC, Crosby LJ, Perlis M, et al. Longitudinal sleep EEG power spectral analysis studies in adolescents with minor head injury. J Neurotrauma 1997;14:549–59.

99. Gosselin N, Lassonde M, Petit D, et al. Sleep following sport-related concussions. Sleep Med 2009;10:35–46.

100. Williams BR, Lazic SE, Ogilvie RD. Polysomnographic and quantitative EEG analysis of subjects with long-term insomnia complaints associated with mild traumatic brain injury. Clin Neurophysiol 2008;119:429–38.

101. Nampiaparampil DE. Prevalence of chronic pain after traumatic brain injury: a systematic review. JAMA 2008;300:711–19.

102. Beetar JT, Guilmette TJ, Sparadeo FR. Sleep and pain complaints in symptomatic traumatic brain injury and neurologic population. Arch Phys Med Rehabil 1996;77:1298–302.

103. Chaput G, Giguère JF, Chauny JM, et al. Relationship among subjective sleep complaints, headaches, and mood alterations following a mild traumatic brain injury. Sleep Med 2009;10:713–16.

104. Lahz S, Bryant RA. Incidence of chronic pain following traumatic brain injury. Arch Phys Med Rehabil 1996;77:889–91.

105. Beetar JT, Guilmette TJ, Sparadeo FR. Sleep and pain complaints in symptomatic traumatic brain injury and neurologic populations. Arch Phys Med Rehabil 1996;77:1298–302.

106. Khoury S, Chouchou F, Amzica F, et al. Rapid EEG activity during sleep dominates in mild traumatic brain injury patients with acute pain. J Neurotrauma 2013;30:633–41.

107. Werth E, Diijk DJ, Achermann P, Borbely AA. Dynamics of the sleep EEG after an early evening nap: experimental data and simulations. Am J Physiol 1996;271(3 Pt 2):R501–10.

108. Ponsford JL, Parcell DL, Sinclair KL, et al. Changes in sleep patterns following traumatic brain injury: a controlled study. Neurorehabil Neural Repair 2013;27:613–21.

109. Mork PJ, Vik KL, Moe B, et al. Sleep problems, exercise and obesity and risk of chronic musculoskeletal pain: the Norwegian HUNT study. Eur J Public Health 2014;24:924–9.

110. Sherman KJ, Wellman RD, Cook AJ, et al. Mediators of yoga and stretching for chronic low back pain. Evid Based Complement Alternat Med 203;2013:130818.

111. Langhorst J, Klose P, Dobos GJ, et al. Efficacy and safety of meditative movement therapies in fibromyalgia syndrome: a systematic review and meta-analysis of randomized controlled trials. Rheumatol Int 2013;33:193–207.

112. Sawynok J, Lynch M, Marcon D. Extension trial of qigong for fibromyalgia: a quantitative and qualitative study. Evid Based Complement Alternat Med 2013;2013:726062.

113. Tang NK. Cognitive-behavioral therapy for sleep abnormalities of chronic pain patients. Curr Rheumatol Rep. 2009;11:451–60.

114. Vitiello MV, McCurry SM, Shortreed SM, et al. Cognitive–behavioral treatment for comorbid insomnia and osteoarthritis pain in primary care: the lifestyles randomized controlled trial. J Am Geriatr Soc 2013;61:947–56.

115. Mendoza ME, Capafons A, Gralow JR, et al. Randomized controlled trial of the Valencia model of waking hypnosis plus CBT for pain, fatigue, and sleep management in patients with cancer and cancer survivors. Psychooncol. 2016 Jul 28. doi: 10.1002/pon.4232. [Epub ahead of print].

116. Hindmarch I, Dawson J, Stanley N. A double-blind study in healthy volunteers to assess the effects on sleep of pregabalin compared with alprazolam and placebo. Sleep 2005;28:187–93.

117. Doufas AG, Tian L, Padrez KA, et al. Experimental pain and opioid analgesia in volunteers at high risk for obstructive sleep apnea. PLoS One 2013;8(1):e54807.

118. Carette S, Oakson G, Guimont C, Steriade M. Sleep electroencephalography and the clinical response to amitriptyline in patients with fibromyalgia. Arthritis Rheum 1995;38:1211–17.

119. Saletu B, Prause W, Anderer P, et al. Insomnia in somatoform pain disorder: sleep laboratory studies on differences to controls and acute effects of trazodone, evaluated by the Somnolyzer 24 x 7 and the Siesta database. Neuropsychobiology 2005;51:148–63.

120. Russell IJ, Crofford LJ, Leon T, et al. The effects of pregabalin on sleep disturbance symptoms among individuals with fibromyalgia syndrome. Sleep Med 2009;10:604–10.

121. Russell IJ, Mease PJ, Smith TR, et al. Efficacy and safety of duloxetine for treatment of fibromyalgia in patients with or without major depressive disorder: results from a 6-month, randomized, double-blind, placebo-controlled, fixed-dose trial. Pain 2008;136:432–44.

122. Franco L, Rompre PH, de Grandmont P, et al. A mandibular advancement appliance reduces pain and rhythmic masticatory muscle activity in patients with morning headache. J Orofac Pain 2011;25:240–9.

123. Onen SH, Onen F, Albrand G, et al. Pain tolerance and obstructive sleep apnea in the elderly. J Am Med Dir Assoc 2010;11:612–16.

124. Khalid I, Roehrs TA, Hudgel DW, Roth T. Continuous positive airway pressure in severe obstructive sleep apnea reduces pain sensitivity. Sleep 2011;34:1687–91.

125. Doufas AG, Panagiotou OA, Ioannidis JP. Concordance of sleep and pain outcomes of diverse interventions: an umbrella review. PLoS One 2012;7(7):e40891.

126. Kehlet H, Jensen TS, Woolf CJ. Persistent postsurgical pain: risk factors and prevention. Lancet 2006;367:1618–25.

127. Racine M, Choiniere M, Nielson WR. Predictors of suicidal ideation in chronic pain patients: an exploratory study. Clin J Pain 2014;30:371-8.

SECTION 10

Sleep and psychiatric disorders

CHAPTER 47

Depression and anxiety disorders

Susan Mackie and John W. Winkelman

Depression and anxiety disorders are common conditions, frequently encountered throughout the practice of clinical medicine. The lifetime prevalence in the United States is approximately 17% and 29%, respectively [1]. These conditions are commonly comorbid with each other. In one recent survey, 75% of those with depression met criteria for an anxiety disorder in their lifetime, and 79% of those with an anxiety disorder met criteria for lifetime major depressive disorder [2]. These disorders are also markedly over-represented in a wide array of medical and neurological conditions.

Patients with depression and anxiety disorders frequently demonstrate disturbances in sleep architecture, sleep quality, and sleep quantity. There is also a marked over-representation of many common sleep disorders in these conditions. Although in the past these abnormalities of sleep were often viewed merely as symptoms of the psychiatric condition, understanding in recent years has shifted. We now recognize that there are frequently complex bidirectional relationships between sleep disturbances and depression and anxiety disorders.

This chapter will address several of the most common mood and anxiety disorders associated with abnormalities in sleep: major depressive disorder, post-traumatic stress disorder, obsessive–compulsive disorder, and panic disorder. Changes in objective and subjective sleep parameters associated with each psychiatric disorder will be addressed, followed by a discussion of the most common sleep disorders comorbid with these conditions.

Major depressive disorder

Major depressive disorder (MDD) is a disorder characterized by discrete episodes (lasting at least 2 weeks) with characteristic changes in mood, cognition, and neurovegetative function [3]. Either depressed mood or anhedonia (decreased interest or pleasure) is required for this diagnosis. Other common features include changes in appetite, psychomotor functioning, and energy; feelings of worthlessness or guilt; decreased concentration; and recurrent thoughts of death. The fifth edition of the Diagnostic and Statistical Manual (DSM-5) includes insomnia or hypersomnia as an additional category of symptoms, though the latter more likely represents increased time in bed (due to decreased energy, interest, etc.) without true excessive need for sleep or inability to maintain wakefulness. When true hypersomnia is identified, a separate primary sleep disorder should be suspected.

Abnormalities in sleep characteristic of MDD

Even in the absence of a comorbid sleep disorder, several changes in polysomnographic (PSG) patterns of sleep exist in patents with MDD. The most consistent abnormalities are related to REM sleep: shortened REM latency (time from sleep onset to the first episode of REM), prolongation of the first REM period, and increased density of eye movements during REM. These observations have led to the hypothesis that "disinhibition" of REM sleep may play a role in the pathophysiology of depression. There is also evidence that REM abnormalities may constitute a biomarker that predicts incident episodes of depression and increased vulnerability to relapse in remitted patients. Thus, the abnormalities of sleep observed in depressed patients are closely tied to the precipitation and perpetuation of the mood disorder and may be important as novel treatment targets.

Insomnia in MDD: epidemiology and clinical features

The relationship between insomnia and MDD is perhaps the most well studied and complex topic in the study of sleep and mood disorders.

As already mentioned, insomnia is a common symptom of MDD However, frequently insomnia symptoms are sufficiently severe to warrant diagnosis as a primary sleep disorder. Such patients may be most appropriately conceptualized as suffering from comorbid depression and insomnia. This approach recognizes that the two diagnoses, albeit inter-related, carry distinct symptoms and may follow different courses. It should not be assumed that sleep problems will inevitably resolve with appropriate treatment of the mood disorder, or vice versa.

Estimates of the prevalence of insomnia among depressed patients vary widely. Most studies agree that sleep problems affect the majority. In a large epidemiological study including nearly 4000 unipolar MDD patients in the US (the STAR*D study), 85% of the depressed participants met criteria for insomnia, and sleep symptoms correlated with more severe depression [4]. Because insomnia may be either a cause or a consequence of depression, longitudinal studies may provide additional insight beyond that afforded by such cross-sectional descriptions. One recent meta-analysis included 21 studies examining the incidence of new-onset depression in insomniacs without baseline depression. The mean sample size was 3200 and included a mean follow-up of 6 years. The meta-analysis concluded that the overall odds ratio of new onset depression in those with insomnia compared with those without was 2.6 (confidence interval (CI) = 1.98–3.42) [5].

One of the most consistently observed and clinically important features of comorbid insomnia and depression is the association with increased risk of suicidality. A majority of attempted and completed suicides occur in depressed patients [6]. Within this group, insomnia is a consistent predictor of suicidal thoughts and actions.

This has been demonstrated in cross-sectional as well as longitudinal population-based studies, and within the context of clinical trials of MDD. This association persists after adjustment for depression severity and other psychiatric comorbidity [7]. In some studies, insomnia appears to be a better predictor of suicidality than the severity of the depression itself.

Special treatment considerations in patients with comorbid insomnia and depression

Many medications used in the treatment of depression have well-established effects on sleep (Table 47.1). Selective serotonin reuptake inhibitors (SSRIs) and serotonin–norepinephrine (noradrenaline) reuptake inhibitors (SNRIs) are frequently first-line medications. These agents markedly suppress REM sleep, increase sleep onset latency (SOL: the time from bedtime to first onset of sleep), increase arousal index (AI: the number of awakenings per hour of sleep), increase wake after sleep onset (WASO), and decrease total sleep time. Despite these PSG observations, the experience of patients is often different in that sleep often improves subjectively. Nevertheless, these agents can produce hypersomnia in some individuals and insomnia in others.

Treatment of insomnia also has the potential to affect the course of MDD. Although it is unlikely to be clear whether the sleep disorder is a cause or a symptom of depression, it is clear that treatment of insomnia in this group improves both sleep and quality of life [8,9]. However, data are mixed regarding the effect of insomnia treatment on the mood disorder itself. The most commonly used drugs in the treatment of insomnia are the benzodiazepine receptor agonists (BZRAs). Although in the past there was concern that these drugs may adversely affect mood, recent data suggest that this is unlikely. In fact, pharmacological treatment of insomnia has been studied adjunctively with antidepressants as initial therapy for MDD with comorbid insomnia. Fava and colleagues compared zolpidem extended-release in combination with escitalopram versus escitalopram alone [9]. Zolpidem extended-release improved total sleep time, morning energy, concentration, and next-day functioning. However, zolpidem did not significantly improve mood. In contrast, another similarly designed study compared eszopiclone

in combination with fluoxetine versus fluoxetine alone [8]. In addition to improvement in sleep, the eszopiclone group showed a faster onset of antidepressant response and a greater magnitude of the antidepressant effect. Furthermore, both depression and insomnia remained significantly improved in the combination-therapy group during the 2-week run-out period after discontinuation of eszopiclone [10]. This suggests that patients with MDD can be safely treated with an adjunctive hypnotic without concern for rebound or withdrawal and with possible persistent benefits for mood and sleep even after cessation of the drug.

Behavioral treatment of insomnia is also appropriate in depressed patients.

Cognitive–behavioral therapy for insomnia (CBT-i) improves sleep acutely with an effect size comparable or superior to pharmacological treatment, often with a more sustained benefit [11–13]. CBT-i is often used adjunctively with medications, and the most effective approach may be a combined treatment. The aspects of CBT-i with established efficacy include stimulus control and sleep restriction. Depressed patients may have difficulty implementing these techniques owing to amotivation, low energy, and psychomotor slowing. Despite these theoretical barriers, there is evidence that depressed patients are able to benefit from CBT-i. In a study by Manber et al., over 300 patients referred for treatment of insomnia underwent seven group CBT-i treatment sessions [12]. The authors examined differences between depressed and non-depressed individuals in terms of treatment efficacy and adherence. Despite somewhat reduced adherence to CBT-i principles, improvement in insomnia severity, perceived energy, productivity, and self-esteem did not differ based on the presence of depression. Although this study was not placebo-controlled, another study [14] compared CBT-i with a sham treatment in depressed patients, demonstrating improvement in both sleep and mood in the CBT-i group. These data indicate that CBT-i is effective in depressed insomniacs and should be considered an important component of treatment.

Benzodiazepine receptor agonists have also been studied for residual insomnia during otherwise successful treatment of MDD. Asnis and colleagues randomized nearly 200 subjects with persistent insomnia despite remitted depression to zolpidem 10 mg or placebo for 4 weeks [15]. Compared with placebo, zolpidem was associated with improved subjective sleep quality, fewer awakenings, less daytime sleepiness, and improved concentration. As with eszopiclone, there was no evidence of dependence or withdrawal during a wash-out placebo substitution.

MDD and obstructive sleep apnea

Depression is common among patients with obstructive sleep apnea (OSA). In the National Health and Nutrition Examination Survey, snoring/stopping breathing ≥ 5 nights/week compared with never was strongly associated with probable major depression in men (OR = 3.1; CI = 1.8–5.2) and women (OR = 3.0; CI = 1.6–5.4) [16]. Conversely, in one cross-sectional telephone survey, 18% of individuals with a diagnosis of MDD also reported symptoms consistent with probable OSA [17]. After controlling for shared risk factors, the OR of sleep-disordered breathing was 5.26 (CI = 4.29–6.47) for those with MDD compared with those without MDD. Although most of the available data—including those summarized here—are limited by the absence of rigorous identification of either OSA or MDD, the consistent over-representation of MDD among OSA patients and vice versa is clear.

Table 47.1 Effects of antidepressant medications on sleep

Drug class	Effect on sleep			
	Continuity	Slow-wave sleep	REM %	REM latency
Tricyclic antidepressants	+	0	−	+
SSRIs	+/−	0	−	+
SNRIs	−	0	−	+
Bupropion	0	0	+	−
Mirtazapine	+	+	0	0
Trazodone	+	+	−	+

+ indicates that the drug increases this parameter; − indicates that the drug decreases this parameter; +/− indicates inter-drug or inter-individual variation; 0 indicates no effect.

Adapted from Harv Rev Psychiatry, 8(6), Gursky JT, Krahn LE, The effects of antidepressants on sleep: a review, pp. 298–306, Copyright (2000), with permission from Wolters Kluwer Health, Inc.

In patients with comorbid depression and OSA, the presence of each disorder affects treatment of the other. Several studies have shown that sleep apnea interferes with the response of MDD to both CBT [18] and antidepressants [19]. This effect was demonstrated in a study of patients with coronary heart disease who were being treated with sertraline for MDD [19]. Moderate to severe OSA was detected in approximately 30%. This subset had a significantly poorer response to the antidepressant effect of sertraline compared with those without OSA. This difference remained significant after controlling for baseline depression, demographic variables, and serum inflammatory markers. It is important to emphasize that sleep apnea was untreated in this study. It remains uncertain whether this effect would persist if OSA were appropriately treated.

Continuous positive airway pressure (CPAP) is the mainstay of treatment for OSA. The effect of CPAP therapy on mood in patients with MDD has been the topic of considerable investigation and debate. Schwartz et al. examined a group of patients with a pretreatment respiratory disturbance index (RDI) >15 and confirmed a significant response to CPAP (>50% drop in RDI) [20]. In this group, nearly all experienced a decrease in depressive symptoms. The mean Beck Depression Inventory fell from 7.2 (moderate depression) to 1.8 (normal) after CPAP. An analysis of variance showed no effect of gender or baseline RDI, and the improvement was unaffected by current antidepressant treatment. Despite these and other impressive data, [21–23], others have failed to show any effect of CPAP on mood [24–27]. Inconsistencies may be related to the variable use of a control group and incomplete (and usually unmeasured) compliance with CPAP treatment.

Effects of antidepressants on motor activity in sleep (RLS, PLMS, RBD)

In addition to the aforementioned effects of antidepressants on sleep continuity and architecture, these agents also frequently alter motor activity during sleep. This effect is most pronounced in individuals with pre-existing restless legs syndrome (RLS) or periodic limb movements in sleep (PLMS), but both disorders may also emerge de novo with antidepressant treatment. Most SSRIs, as well as the atypical antidepressant mirtazapine, tend to worsen RLS symptoms [28,29], and the consequent compromise in sleep quality may hinder successful treatment of depression. In addition, SSRIs are associated with abnormal muscle activity during REM sleep and dream enactment behavior, a secondary form of REM sleep behavior disorder (RBD). Dream enactment may be associated with significant injury to the patient or bed partner and should prompt consideration of down-titrating or changing antidepressants. In contrast to SSRIs, the norepinephrine–dopamine reuptake inhibitor (NDRI) bupropion appears to be free of adverse effects on motor activity in sleep [29,30] and may be an appropriate alternative for patients who experience problematic nocturnal movements due to an SSRI.

Anxiety disorders

Anxiety disorders are the most frequently occurring type of psychiatric disorder, with a lifetime prevalence of 29% in the general population [1]. Sleep disturbances are highly prevalent in this group. One survey of primary-care patients with anxiety disorders found that 74% reported subjective complaints about sleep, including

difficulty falling asleep, waking during the night, or restless sleep. Predictors of sleep difficulties in this group of patient with anxiety disorders were similar to those reported in the general population: minority populations; those who were divorced, separated, or widowed; and older individuals all tended toward higher rates of sleep disturbances [31].

There are high rates of comorbidity between MDD and anxiety disorders. Because of the close relationship between depressive disorders and sleep, many of the data about anxiety disorders are complicated by the presence of comorbid depressive symptoms in a (frequently unreported) segment of study participants. Despite this confound, most clinicians and researchers agree that there is likely a relationship between anxiety disorders per se and sleep disturbances. Mechanisms of this association may vary between anxiety disorders. However, it is clear that sleep deprivation potentiates anxiety, and the arousal response due to anxiety impairs sleep. This vicious cycle may provide a common mechanism to explain the strong association between nearly every type of anxiety disorder and sleep problems.

This review will focus on three anxiety disorders with a clearly established relationship to sleep problems: obsessive–compulsive disorder (OCD) post-traumatic stress disorder (PTSD), and panic disorder.

Obsessive–compulsive disorder

OCD is an anxiety disorder characterized by obsessions (distressing and recurrent thoughts, impulses, or images) and compulsions (excessive action taken to relieve the anxiety caused by the obsessions, often ritualistic in nature). Although OCD is a chronic illness, symptoms may wax and wane over time. Similar to MDD, patients with OCD appear to experience increased prevalence of various sleep abnormalities, some inherent to the anxiety disorder and others representing comorbid sleep disorders.

Abnormalities in sleep characteristic of OCD

Several authors have shown that total sleep time (TST) and sleep efficiency are reduced in patients with OCD compared with healthy adults. In one large study using self-reported sleep time, Park et al. found that OCD was associated with sleep duration of 5h or less compared with control subjects [32]. After controlling for sociodemographic and other variables, the OR of sleep duration less than 5 hours was 3.88 (CI = 1.63–9.23) compared with control subjects. Several PSG studies also found reduced TST [33,34], an abnormality that seems to be particularly prominent in women. On the other hand, a recent study by Marcks et al. found no correlation between OCD and sleep duration [31]. Such inconsistencies may be connected with the complex relationship with OCD and depression. Bobdey et al. found that OCD patients with depression were considerably more likely to have decreased sleep time and increased sleep latency compared with those in whom depression was rigorously excluded [35].

There are also characteristic changes in sleep architecture in OCD. Similar to the pattern seen in MDD, REM sleep is often abnormal. Insel et al. compared the polysomnographically recorded sleep of patients with depression, OCD, and normal controls [36]. The most striking difference was a marked reduction in latency to REM sleep in OCD patients compared with controls (48.4 minutes, CI = 40.4–57.2 in OCD versus 80.5 minutes, CI = 75.3–86.3 in controls). In this respect, the OCD group was similar to the MDD group

(REM latency 47.3 minutes, CI = 42.2–52.4). A more recent study has demonstrated an even more striking result. Ten patients with OCD without comorbid MDD were compared with controls [37]. Three of the ten with OCD (compared with zero controls) exhibited sleep onset REM periods (SOREMPs), defined as REM latency < 10 minutes. OCD symptom severity was significantly associated with SOREMs.

Delayed sleep phase disorder and OCD

Distinct from other psychiatric disorders, the most consistently over-represented sleep disorder among OCD patients is delayed sleep phase disorder. Mukhopadhyay et al. conducted a retrospective case review of 187 OCD patients in an inpatient unit. In this sample, 33 of the 187 (17.6%) OCD patients fulfilled criteria for DSPD [38]. This seemed to be linked to OCD as opposed to any comorbid depression, since the presence of DSPD correlated with age of onset of OCD ($p = 0.005$), with a trend to correlation between OCD severity and DSPD. Consistent with this trend, another retrospective analysis by Turner et al. found a remarkably high prevalence of DSPD among patients with severe, treatment-resistant OCD [39]. In a sample of 31 inpatients who had failed outpatient psychotherapy and medical management, 13 (42%) met criteria for DPSD (defined as regularly falling asleep after 1 am and awakening after 10 am). Phase-shifted patients were significantly younger and had more severe OCD compared with OCD patients without DSPD. Consistent with the aforementioned data, levels of depression were not significantly different between the groups.

The cause of increased prevalence of DSPD in OCD is unknown. One intriguing case report described a 54-year-old woman with severe OCD who kept sleep and symptom logs as an adjunct to conventional CBT [40]. Owing to compulsive praying behavior, she routinely went to sleep around 5 am, sleeping until 1 pm. Her therapist worked with her to advance her sleep–wake schedule, and this was associated with a decrease in time spent on compulsions from 8 hours per day to 2 hours. The authors suggest that patients who perform compulsions late at night may inadvertently perpetuate the OCD as homeostatic and circadian mechanisms interact to produce fatigue and cognitive deficits that exacerbate OCD symptoms and perpetuate the sleep disorder.

The mainstay of pharmacological treatment of OCD is SSRIs. Effects of these drugs on sleep have been discussed earlier in this chapter. When SSRIs and psychotherapy are not adequate, augmentation therapy generally consists of low-dose atypical antipsychotics. In addition, recent uncontrolled studies have suggested that agomelatine, a combined melatonin-1 (MT_1), MT_2, and serotonin-2C ($5\text{-}HT_{2C}$) receptor agonist, may be a promising new approach for pharmacologic augmentation in OCD [41–44]. Several mechanisms have been proposed to explain this benefit. Given the prominence of DSPD among OCD patients, the benefit may be due to the phase-shifting effects of melatonin agonism. (All subjects for whom the data are provided in these reports suffered from comorbid DSPD.) Another possible mechanism involves serotonin, which may be involved in the pathogenesis of OCD. Serotonin transmission exhibits circadian variation [43]. Resynchronization of circadian serotonergic patterns and/or the direct effect of agomelatine to increase serotonergic transmission at the $5\text{-}HT_{2C}$ receptor may explain the benefit of this drug.

Post-traumatic stress disorder

PTSD is a condition occurring in individuals exposed to actual or threatened death or serious injury. A subset of such patients (ranging between 3% and 15%) will go on to develop symptoms characteristic of PTSD, including intrusion (recurrent, involuntary memories or traumatic nightmares), avoidance (effortful avoidance of distressing trauma-related stimuli), negative alterations in cognition or mood, and alterations in arousal and reactivity (hypervigilance, exaggerated startle response, etc.) [3]. Two of these four diagnostic sets of symptoms often include sleep symptoms: nightmares as a manifestation of intrusion, and insomnia as a manifestation of arousal. These features highlight the centrality of sleep disturbance in this disorder (Box 47.1).

PSG differences characteristic of PTSD have been a matter of considerable investigation, with conflicting conclusions. Given the frequency of nightmares in this disorder, some have hypothesized that REM sleep may be abnormal. Indeed, some studies have reported increased REM density and percentage of REM sleep [45]. However, others have shown contrasting patterns, characterized by decreased percentage of REM sleep [43]. Still others detected no differences in REM sleep parameters between subjects with PTSD compared with control subjects.

Breslau et al. performed PSG of 292 subjects, including 71 with lifetime PTSD [46]. On standard measures of sleep disturbance, PTSD subjects did not differ from controls. Those with PTSD did, however, have higher rates of brief arousals from REM sleep. The authors proposed that sleep complaints in PTSD may represent amplified perception of these arousals rather than objectively

---

Box 47.1 Diagnostic criteria for PTSD

Stressor: exposure to actual or perceived serious injury or death. At least one symptom in each of four symptom clusters must be present:

- Intrusion:
  - Recurrent and unwanted remembering
  - **Nightmares***
  - Dissociation
- Avoidance
  - Of external stimuli
  - Of related feelings
- Negative alteration of cognition or mood
- Increased arousal
  - Irritability
  - Increased startle response
  - Hypervigilance
  - **Sleep disturbance***

* Symptoms overlapping between PTSD and sleep disorders.

Source data from American Psychiatric Association, Diagnostic and Statistical Manual of Mental Disorders, 5th Edition DSM-5, Copyright (2013), American Psychiatric Association.

decreased total sleep time. Alternatively, as Woodward et al. have suggested, "it is possible that most or all PTSD-related sleep changes are substantially ameliorated in the 'guarded' context of the laboratory, and there fall prey, in a statistical sense, to the large underlying normative variation in sleep architecture" [47]. Thus, the lack of a detectable difference may be more a consequence of the limitations of our tools rather than the true absence of a difference.

OSA in PTSD

Sleep disordered breathing (SDB) is common among patients with PTSD. It is possible that SDB is responsible for a portion of the disrupted sleep continuity in this group. However, the causal relationship may also be in the other direction: disruption of any cause may destabilize the upper airway and led to SDB events. Although many PSG studies of PTSD patients have not included respiratory assessment technology designed to rigorously monitor breathing, Krakow and colleagues found that 40 out of 44 patients presenting for CBT for PTSD met criteria for SDB [48]. Although many of these cases were considered mild OSA based on the apnea–hypopnea index (AHI), nearly all were reclassified as moderate to severe when flow limitation was measured and respiratory-effort-related arousals were factored in. The authors concluded that the previous lack of recognition of SDB as an important comorbidity of PTSD may be due to the absence of such advanced measurements.

Given this close relationship, the treatment of SDB has the potential to affect PTSD symptoms. Krakow and colleagues retrospectively examined the effect of CPAP treatment of SDB on sleep and PTSD symptoms in a group of trauma survivors [49]. Whereas all of the untreated patients ($n = 9$) experienced worsening or no change in self-reported symptoms, 13 of the 15 CPAP-treated individuals reported improvement in sleep, and 7 of the 9 treated PTSD patients showed improvement in PTSD-related stress. Regardless of the direction of causality between SDB and PTSD, when approaching the patient with PTSD. it is appropriate to test for and treat comorbid SDB.

Nightmare disorder in PTSD

Recurrent and troubling nightmares are unusual in adults without psychiatric illness. However, this problem is common among PTSD patients. One recent longitudinal, observational study followed 80 veterans with recent combat exposure and at least subthreshold PTSD [50]. Among this group, 61% reported distressing nightmares, and the presence of nightmares was associated with significantly higher PTSD severity at both baseline and 6-month follow-up. Other studies have reported up to 80% prevalence of nightmares among PTSD sufferers. Because of this marked increase in risk for nightmares in PTSD, it is essential that all patients presenting with nightmare complaints be queried regarding trauma exposure and PTSD symptoms.

Although nightmares are frequently considered to be a symptom of PTSD, there are also data to suggest that nightmares prior to trauma exposure predispose exposed individuals to later develop PTSD. Van Liempt and colleagues collected reports about sleep symptoms in 453 Dutch service members prior to military deployment to Afghanistan [51]. PTSD symptoms were assessed at 6 months post-deployment. Self-reported pre-deployment nightmares predicted PTSD symptoms at 6 months (OR = 2.992, CI =1.096–8.551, $p < 0.05$). Because unsuccessful fear extinction may play a role in the development of PTSD, the authors suggested that

poor sleep could contribute to the pathogenesis of PTSD by disrupting the beneficial process of sleep on fear extinction. However, because this effect was not observed in those with insomnia, it seems more likely that pre-exposure nightmares in this group were a marker of impaired fear extinction—and therefore increased vulnerability to PTSD—rather than a mechanism contributing to the development of such impairment.

Treatment of sleep disturbance in nightmares in PTSD

Treatment for nightmares in patients with PTSD may include behavioral and/or pharmacological approaches. Prazosin, an α_1-adrenergic antagonist, has been shown in both retrospective [52] and prospective [53] studies to reduce both PTSD symptoms and nightmares. It should be noted that prazosin doses likely to be beneficial in PTSD may be considerably higher than those commonly used for other indications. Required doses are generally significantly higher in men compared with women. One recent study titrated to an average total daily dose of approximately 20 mg in men compared with 10 mg in woman, without any increased incidence of adverse events compared with placebo [53]. Prazosin's benefit may be mediated by suppression of adrenergic mechanisms that lead to excessive CNS hyperarousal. Whether other adrenergic antagonists may have similar benefits has not been well established.

Behavioral treatment of nightmares is also helpful in PTSD patients. The most well-studied behavioral approach is image rehearsal therapy (IRT). During IRT, the patient is asked to recount the nightmare, create a modified, more positive version of the story, and practice image rehearsal with the new scenario. In one study, a group of 114 patients with moderate to severe PTSD were randomized to three sessions of IRT or a waitlist control group. The IRT treatment group showed significantly reduced nights per week with nightmares, number of nightmares per week, and subjective sleep quality, all highly significant changes with medium to large effect sizes. Waitlist control participants showed no significant improvement over the same time period [54].

Panic disorder

Panic disorder is an anxiety disorder that includes recurrent and unanticipated panic attacks, often characterized by intense fear that reaches a peak within minutes. Patients with panic disorder experience frequent somatic symptoms such as palpitations, shortness of breath, diaphoresis, and nausea. The diagnostic criteria specify that there must be persistent concern about additional panic attacks and/or maladaptive behavioral changes related to the attacks [3].

Nocturnal panic attacks have been reported in 58% of panic disorder patients, with 30–45% experiencing repeated nocturnal panic attacks [55]. The majority of those with nocturnal panic also suffer from daytime attacks, although a small subset experiences predominantly nocturnal symptoms.

Patients who frequently experience sleep disturbance due to panic attacks may be considered to suffer from both a sleep disorder and an anxiety disorder. It has been hypothesized that those with nocturnal symptoms may have a more severe form of the disease [56] but this association has been inconsistent [57]. There is evidence that acute sleep deprivation increases anxiety and fear response to a CO_2 challenge, a common paradigm for modeling the development of panic attacks [58]. Thus, rather than merely a marker of disease severity, it may be that the presence of nocturnal panic attacks has a causative effect to exacerbate panic disorder symptoms.

Nocturnal panic attacks usually occur from stage II or stage III NREM sleep. The symptom profile of nocturnal attacks does not differ significantly from daytime panic attacks. Among those with repeated nocturnal panic symptoms, one survey reported an average of 11.4 attacks per month, rarely more than 1 per night [55]. Most patients report that nocturnal panic attacks occur 1–3 hours after sleep onset and last 2–8 minutes. There is frequently difficulty returning to sleep.

Sleep problems in panic disorder are not limited to those with nocturnal panic attacks. One survey compared 70 panic disorder patients with healthy controls on a variety of subjective sleep characteristics. Of the panic disorder patients, 67% reported sleep complaints, compared with 20% of the controls. As expected, a large majority of panic disorder patients with nocturnal panic attacks (77%) reported some difficulty sleeping, but 53% of the panic disorder patients without nocturnal panic also reported sleep difficulties, which were no less severe [59]. The authors concluded that the sleep difficulties observed in panic disorder cannot be attributed primarily to the presence of nocturnal attacks.

Differential diagnosis of nocturnal panic attacks

Nocturnal panic attacks must be distinguished from other causes of distressing nocturnal arousals from sleep. The primary differential diagnosis is likely to include nightmares, night terrors, and obstructive events in the setting of sleep apnea. Night terrors are more common in children and are distinguished by decreased or absent recollection of the episode. Nightmares should be accompanied by vivid recollection of frightening imagery. Obstructive respiratory events causing arousal may share with panic attacks a sensation of difficulty breathing and palpitations. If OSA is suspected based on other clinical parameters, appropriate screening and treatment should take place prior to establishing a diagnosis of nocturnal panic attacks.

Treatment considerations in nocturnal panic attacks

Due to the contention that panic disorder with nocturnal symptoms may represent a more severe form of the disease, there has been interest in determining whether alternative treatments are necessary. One uncontrolled study enhanced typical CBT for panic disorder with cognitive restructuring to address misconceptions about sleep and maladaptive sleep habits [60]. The intervention effectively reduced panic disorder severity, frequency of daytime and nocturnal panic attacks, and worry about nocturnal panic in people with panic disorders compared with controls. However, as noted in the accompanying editorial, this study was limited in its discernment of specific individual treatments that might be effective, since the treatment provided was so comprehensive.

More recent data have provided further insight into the need for treatment specific to nocturnal panic disorder. Marchand et al. conducted a study of panic disorder patients comparing two treatment arms—conventional CBT for panic disorder compared versus CBT adapted to nocturnal symptoms [61]. In both groups, nocturnal panic attacks decreased faster than daytime attacks, and significant clinical changes persisted in all measures of self-report and clinician ratings for up to a year after treatment. Because these improvements appeared similar in the two groups, the authors concluded that conventional strategies to address panic disorder are likely sufficient for nocturnal panic attacks as well.

References

1. Kessler RC, Berglund P, Demler O, et al. Lifetime prevalence and age-of-onset distributions of DSM-IV disorders in the National Comorbidity Survey Replication. Arch Gen Psychiatry 2005;62(6):593–602.
2. Lamers F, van Oppen P, Comijs HC, et al. Comorbidity patterns of anxiety and depressive disorders in a large cohort study: the Netherlands Study of Depression and Anxiety (NESDA). J Clin Psychiatry 2011;72(3):341–8.
3. American Psychiatric Association. Diagnostic and statistical manual of mental disorders: DSM-5. Washington, DC: American Psychiatric Association, 2013.
4. Sunderajan P, Gaynes BN, Wisniewski SR, et al. Insomnia in patients with depression: a STAR*D report. CNS Spectr 2010;15(6):394–404.
5. Baglioni C, Battagliese G, Feige B, et al. Insomnia as a predictor of depression: a meta-analytic evaluation of longitudinal epidemiological studies. J Affect Disord 2011;135(1–3):10–19.
6. Asnis GM, Friedman TA, Sanderson WC, et al. Suicidal behaviors in adult psychiatric outpatients. I: Description and prevalence. Am J Psychiatry 1993;150(1):108–12.
7. Pigeon WR, Pinquart M, Conner K. Meta-analysis of sleep disturbance and suicidal thoughts and behaviors. J Clin Psychiatry 2012;73(9):e1160–7.
8. Fava M, McCall WV, Krystal A, et al. Eszopiclone co-administered with fluoxetine in patients with insomnia coexisting with major depressive disorder. Biol Psychiatry 2006;59(11):1052–60.
9. Fava M, Asnis GM, Shrivastava RK, et al. Improved insomnia symptoms and sleep-related next-day functioning in patients with comorbid major depressive disorder and insomnia following concomitant zolpidem extended-release 12.5 mg and escitalopram treatment: a randomized controlled trial. J Clin Psychiatry 2011;72(7):914–28.
10. Krystal A, Fava M, Rubens R, et al. Evaluation of eszopiclone discontinuation after cotherapy with fluoxetine for insomnia with coexisting depression. J Clin Sleep Med 2007;3(1):48–55.
11. Morin CM, Vallières A, Guay B, et al. Cognitive behavioral therapy, singly and combined with medication, for persistent insomnia: a randomized controlled trial. JAMA 2009;301(19):2005–15.
12. Manber R, Bernert RA, Suh S, et al. CBT for insomnia in patients with high and low depressive symptom severity: adherence and clinical outcomes. J Clin Sleep Med 2011;7(6):645–52.
13. Mitchell MD, Gehrman P, Perlis M, Umscheid CA. Comparative effectiveness of cognitive behavioral therapy for insomnia: a systematic review. BMC Fam Pract 2012;13:40.
14. Manber R, Edinger JD, Gress JL, et al. Cognitive behavioral therapy for insomnia enhances depression outcome in patients with comorbid major depressive disorder and insomnia. Sleep 2008;31(4):489–95.
15. Asnis GM, Chakraburtty A, DuBoff EA, et al. Zolpidem for persistent insomnia in SSRI-treated depressed patients. J Clin Psychiatry 1999;60(10):668–76.
16. Wheaton AG, Perry GS, Chapman DP, Croft JB. Sleep disordered breathing and depression among U.S. adults: National Health and Nutrition Examination Survey, 2005–2008. Sleep 2012;35(4):461–7.
17. Ohayon MM. The effects of breathing-related sleep disorders on mood disturbances in the general population. J Clin Psychiatry 2003;64(10):1195–200, 1274–6.
18. Freedland KE, Carney RM, Hayano J, et al. Effect of obstructive sleep apnea on response to cognitive behavior therapy for depression after an acute myocardial infarction. J Psychosom Res 2012;72(4):276–81.
19. Roest AM, Carney RM, Stein PK, et al. Obstructive sleep apnea/hypopnea syndrome and poor response to sertraline in patients with coronary heart disease. J Clin Psychiatry 2012;73(1):31–6.
20. Schwartz DJ, Karatinos G. For individuals with obstructive sleep apnea, institution of CPAP therapy is associated with an amelioration of symptoms of depression which is sustained long term. J Clin Sleep Med 2007;3(6):631–5.

21. Schwartz DJ, Kohler WC, Karatinos G. Symptoms of depression in individuals with obstructive sleep apnea may be amenable to treatment with continuous positive airway pressure. Chest 2005;128(3):1304–9.

22. Millman RP, Fogel BS, McNamara ME, Carlisle CC. Depression as a manifestation of obstructive sleep apnea: reversal with nasal continuous positive airway pressure. J Clin Psychiatry 1989;50(9):348–51.

23. Derderian SS, Bridenbaugh RH, Rajagopal KR. Neuropsychologic symptoms in obstructive sleep apnea improve after treatment with nasal continuous positive airway pressure. Chest 1988;94(5):1023–7.

24. Yu BH, Ancoli-Israel S, Dimsdale JE. Effect of CPAP treatment on mood states in patients with sleep apnea. J Psychiatr Res 1999;33(5):427–32.

25. Borak J, Cieślicki JK, Koziej M, Matuszewski A, Zieliński J. Effects of CPAP treatment on psychological status in patients with severe obstructive sleep apnoea. J Sleep Res 1996;5(2):123–7.

26. Lee I-S, Bardwell W, Ancoli-Israel S, Loredo JS, Dimsdale JE. Effect of three weeks of continuous positive airway pressure treatment on mood in patients with obstructive sleep apnoea: a randomized placebo-controlled study. Sleep Med 2012;13(2):161–6.

27. Muñoz A, Mayoralas LR, Barbé F, Pericás J, Agusti AG. Long-term effects of CPAP on daytime functioning in patients with sleep apnoea syndrome. Eur Respir J 2000;15(4):676–81.

28. Hoque R, Chesson AL. Pharmacologically induced/exacerbated restless legs syndrome, periodic limb movements of sleep, and REM behavior disorder/REM sleep without atonia: literature review, qualitative scoring, and comparative analysis. J Clin Sleep Med 2010;6(1):79–83.

29. Yang C, White DP, Winkelman JW. Antidepressants and periodic leg movements of sleep. Biol. Psychiatry 2005;58(6):510–14.

30. Bayard M, Bailey B, Acharya D, et al. Bupropion and restless legs syndrome: a randomized controlled trial. J Am Board Fam Med 2011;24(4):422–8.

31. Marcks BA, Weisberg RB, Edelen MO, Keller MB. The relationship between sleep disturbance and the course of anxiety disorders in primary care patients. Psychiatry Res 2010;178(3):487–92.

32. Park S, Cho MJ, Chang SM, et al. Relationships of sleep duration with sociodemographic and health-related factors, psychiatric disorders and sleep disturbances in a community sample of Korean adults. J Sleep Res 2010;19(4):567–77.

33. Voderholzer U, Riemann D, Huwig-Poppe C, et al. Sleep in obsessive compulsive disorder: polysomnographic studies under baseline conditions and after experimentally induced serotonin deficiency. Eur Arch Psychiatry Clin Neurosci 2007;257(3):173–82.

34. Armitage R, Debus J, Kiger B, et al. Polysomnogram in major depressive and obsessive compulsive disorders. Depression. 1994;2:297e302.

35. Bobdey M, Fineberg N, Gale TM. Reported sleep patterns in obsessive compulsive disorder (OCD). Int J Psychiatry Clin Pract 2002;6:15–21.

36. Insel TR, Gillin JC, Moore A, et al. The sleep of patients with obsessive-compulsive disorder. Arch Gen Psychiatry 1982;39(12):1372–7.

37. Kluge M, Schüssler P, Dresler M, Yassouridis A, Steiger A. Sleep onset REM periods in obsessive compulsive disorder. Psychiatry Res 2007;152(1):29–35.

38. Mukhopadhyay S, Fineberg NA, Drummond LM, et al. Delayed sleep phase in severe obsessive-compulsive disorder: a systematic case-report survey. CNS Spectr 2008;13(5):406–13.

39. Turner J, Drummond LM, Mukhopadhyay S, et al. A prospective study of delayed sleep phase syndrome in patients with severe resistant obsessive–compulsive disorder. World Psychiatry 2007;6(2):108–11.

40. Coles ME, Sharkey KM. Compulsion or chronobiology? A case of severe obsessive–compulsive disorder treated with cognitive-behavioral therapy augmented with chronotherapy. J Clin Sleep Med 2011;7(3):307–9.

41. De Berardis D, Serroni N, Campanella D, et al. A case of obsessive-compulsive disorder successfully treated with agomelatine monotherapy. J Clin Psychopharmacol 2012;32(2):289–90.

42. De Berardis D, Serroni N, Marini S, et al. Agomelatine augmentation of escitalopram therapy in treatment-resistant obsessive–compulsive disorder: a case report. Case Rep Psychiatry 2012;2012:642752.

43. Lange KW, Lange KM, Hauser J, Tucha L, Tucha O. Circadian rhythms in obsessive–compulsive disorder. J Neural Transm 2012;119(10):1077–83.

44. da Rocha FF, Correa H. Is circadian rhythm disruption important in obsessive–compulsive disorder (OCD)? A case of successful augmentation with agomelatine for the treatment of OCD. Clin Neuropharmacol 2011;34(4):139–40.

45. Ross RJ, Ball WA, Dinges DF, et al. Rapid eye movement sleep disturbance in posttraumatic stress disorder. Biol Psychiatry 1994;35(3):195–202.

46. Breslau N, Roth T, Burduvali E, et al. Sleep in lifetime posttraumatic stress disorder: a community-based polysomnographic study. Arch Gen Psychiatry 2004;61(5):508–16.

47. Woodward SH, Arsenault NJ, Murray C, Bliwise DL. Laboratory sleep correlates of nightmare complaint in PTSD inpatients. Biol Psychiatry 2000;48(11):1081–7.

48. Krakow B, Melendrez D, Pedersen B, et al. Complex insomnia: insomnia and sleep-disordered breathing in a consecutive series of crime victims with nightmares and PTSD. Biol Psychiatry 2001;49(11):948–53.

49. Krakow B, Lowry C, Germain A, et al. A retrospective study on improvements in nightmares and post-traumatic stress disorder following treatment for co-morbid sleep-disordered breathing. J Psychosom Res 2000;49(5):291–8.

50. Pigeon WR, Campbell CE, Possemato K, Ouimette P. Longitudinal relationships of insomnia, nightmares, and PTSD severity in recent combat veterans. J Psychosom Res 2013;75(6):546–50.

51. van Liempt S, van Zuiden M, Westenberg H, Super A, Vermetten E. Impact of impaired sleep on the development of PTSD symptoms in combat veterans: a prospective longitudinal cohort study. Depress Anxiety 2013;30(5):469–74.

52. Raskind MA, Thompson C, Petrie EC, et al. Prazosin reduces nightmares in combat veterans with posttraumatic stress disorder. J Clin Psychiatry 2002;63(7):565–8.

53. Raskind MA, Peterson K, Williams T, et al. A trial of prazosin for combat trauma PTSD with nightmares in active-duty soldiers returned from Iraq and Afghanistan. Am J Psychiatry 2013;170(9):1003–10.

54. Krakow B, Hollifield M, Johnston L, et al. Imagery rehearsal therapy for chronic nightmares in sexual assault survivors with posttraumatic stress disorder: a randomized controlled trial. JAMA 2001;286(5):537–45.

55. Craske MG, Tsao JCI. Assessment and treatment of nocturnal panic attacks. Sleep Med Rev 2005;9(3):173–84.

56. Craske MG, Barlow DH. Nocturnal panic. J Nerv Ment Dis 1989;177(3):160–7.

57. Craske MG, Lang AJ, Mystkowski JL, et al. Does nocturnal panic represent a more severe form of panic disorder? J Nerv Ment Dis 2002;190(9):611–18.

58. Babson KA, Trainor CD, Feldner MT, Blumenthal H. A test of the effects of acute sleep deprivation on general and specific self-reported anxiety and depressive symptoms: an experimental extension. J Behav Ther Exp Psychiatry 2010;41(3):297–303.

59. Overbeek T, van Diest R, Schruers K, Kruizinga F, Griez E. Sleep complaints in panic disorder patients. J Nerv Ment Dis 2005;193(7):488–93.

60. Overbeek T, Schruers K. Cognitive behavioural therapy reduces nocturnal panic in people with panic disorder. Evid Based Ment Health 2006;9(1):13.

61. Marchand L, Marchand A, Landry P, Letarte A, Labrecque J. Efficacy of two cognitive–behavioral treatment modalities for panic disorder with nocturnal panic attacks. Behav Modif 2013;37(5):680–704.

CHAPTER 48

Sleep in other psychiatric disorders

Sara Dallaspezia and Francesco Benedetti

Psychiatric patients often complain of their sleep and present sleep abnormalities that increase with the severity of the illness. During the past few decades, different sleep investigations have been performed in psychiatric patients with the aim of identifying specific sleep patterns associated with psychiatric disorders and, although the majority of these studies have focused on major depression, sleep abnormalities have also been reported in other psychiatric disorders. Moreover, epidemiological studies indicate that about half of the patients complaining of chronic insomnia may have some psychiatric condition or may develop it within 1 year [1]. Indeed, the emerging view is that the relationship between psychiatric and sleep disorders is complex and bidirectional: not only are sleep abnormalities symptoms of psychiatric disorders, but also some sleep disorders increase the risks of developing episodes of psychiatric disorders. Moreover, some disturbances of sleep are generated by drug treatment for psychiatric disorders, and some drugs used in the treatment of sleep disorders may increase the risks for psychiatric diseases [2].

Bipolar Disorder

Since the early descriptions of manic depressive insanity by Kraepelin, sleep disturbances were considered a core characteristic of bipolar disorder, being common features of both the manic and depressive phases of the disease [3]. Sleep dysfunction is frequently observed in euthymic bipolar patients, who do not currently fulfill the criteria for major mood episodes [4]. Sitaram et al. found increased REM density and percentage of REM sleep in remitted bipolar patients relative to healthy comparison subjects, as well as an increased sensitivity to the REM-latency-reducing effects of arecoline (an acetylcholine agonist) [5]. These abnormalities have often been interpreted as the result of a reduced homeostatic process, with abnormally reduced slow-wave sleep (SWS) in the early part of the night. In one more recent study, the majority of interviewed euthymic bipolar patients showed poor sleep quality according to the Pittsburgh Sleep Quality Index assessment [6]. Moreover, different actigraphic studies showed that, compared with controls, euthymic bipolar patients had longer sleep onset latency, lower average daily activity, and more fragmentation of the sleep–wake cycle and more night-to-night variability [4].

Maintaining stable sleep–wake cycles is of central importance to the maintenance of stability in bipolar disorder. A clear temporal relation between sleep and mood has been described in bipolar disorder, with mood changes occurring on the day following a change in sleep [7]. Prospective studies have demonstrated that insomnia is an important predictor of depressive episodes and it is associated with higher chances of recurrences in bipolar depression [8]. Moreover, self-monitoring of sleep duration has been proven useful to recognize prodromal symptoms early and predict mood changes [9]. Retrospective studies have consistently showed that insomnia, hypersomnia, and early awakening are frequent symptoms during depressive episodes, with rates between 77% and 90% [4].

Polysomnographic (PSG) studies of sleep in bipolar depression have generally found similar abnormalities in unipolar and bipolar depression. For instance, bipolar patients have a tendency for more early morning awakenings and more fragmented REM sleep periods, but greater total REM sleep density than unipolar patients [10]. Some clinicians believe that hypersomnia, rather than insomnia, is more indicative of bipolar than unipolar depression [11], but clinically significant sleepiness has not been found using the multiple sleep latency test (MSLT) [12].

Not only can sleep loss trigger mania, but also the reduction of sleep duration was found to be a good predictor of hypomania or mania the next day in rapid-cycling bipolar patients [13]. There is a bidirectional causal relationship between sleep loss and mania: the capacity of sleep reduction to cause mania and mania to reduce sleep is a self-reinforcing mechanism that could explain the tendency of mania to escalate out of control [14]. This relationship seems to be important mostly at the beginning of a manic episode [15]. The ability of sleep loss to elevate mood in bipolar disorder has been extensively exploited to develop antidepressant treatments based on a combination of total and partial sleep deprivation and light therapy [16].

Since PSG examinations are very difficult to carry out in patients affected by mania, only a few studies concerning sleep and mania have been published It is unclear whether the PSG abnormalities seen in mania are caused by the manic state per se or are secondary to other features of mania. In healthy subjects, sleep architecture was found to be influenced by increased daytime activity [17]. Thus, in manic patients, PSG measures could be affected by motor hyperactivity during the day. In unmedicated manic patients, shortened total sleep time and increased time awake in bed were found [18]. REM sleep latency was found to be both normal [19] and shorter than normal, while REM density sleep was found to be higher in unmedicated manic patients compared with healthy subjects [18]. Moreover, Linkowski and colleagues [19] found that although manic patients spent less time asleep during the day and took longer to fall asleep than healthy subjects, they showed time spent in any stage of sleep similar to that of unaffected people.

Nevertheless, the clear cut disruption of circadian rhythms in bipolar disorder allows a correct diagnosis in more than 80% of remitted patients based on quantitative and qualitative measures of sleep [20], with sleep disturbance becoming evident soon after the beginning of bipolar disorder and even in high-risk offspring of bipolar patients.

Schizophrenia

Even if it is seldom the predominant complaint, insomnia is a common symptom in schizophrenia, with up to 55% of medicated patients reporting sleep alteration [21]. To be considered as a symptom related to the disease, sleep disturbance must last for at least 1 month and be associated with impaired daytime functioning or daytime fatigue. Patients mainly complain of difficulty in both initiating and maintaining sleep, and poor subjective sleep quality is associated with a reduced quality of life [22]. Although alterations in sleep seem to be a characteristic feature of the disorder regardless of the phase of the clinical course (acute or chronic), severe insomnia is often seen during exacerbation of schizophrenia and may precede the appearance of other symptoms of relapse [23]. On the contrary, chronic stable patients may appear as having long periods of uninterrupted sleep. Different PSG studies focused on sleep architecture in patients affected by schizophrenia have found several differences from healthy controls. The majority of studies indicate that stage 4 sleep and REM latency are reduced, whereas REM sleep duration tends to remain unchanged. Moreover, increased latency to sleep onset, increase wake time during the night, and decreased total sleep time were found [2].

Some studies have also identified associations between PSG findings and specific subsets of symptoms. Both negative and positive symptoms were found to be associated with reduced REM sleep latency, a greater number of positive symptoms were found to be associated with decreased sleep efficacy and higher sleep onset latency, and a greater number of negative symptoms were reported to be linked to lower non-REM (NREM) sleep EEG slow-wave activity (SWA). Moreover, REM sleep duration and density were correlated to a greater likelihood of suicidal ideation. Many of these sleep disturbances in schizophrenia appear to be caused by abnormalities of the circadian system, as indicated by misalignments of the endogenous circadian cycle and the sleep–wake cycle, ranging from delayed and advanced sleep phase, to free-running rest–activity patterns, to irregular sleep–wake patterns [24–26]. Furthermore, different studies have shown alterations in melatonin profiles, with a change in the circadian phase angle often having been found in these patients [27].

In addition, patients affected by schizophrenia are reported to have periodic limb movements of sleep (PLMS), sleep-related breathing disorders, and night-eating syndrome at a higher rate than the general population [28]. These disorders are considered to be possible adverse effects of antipsychotic drugs [29]. Since antipsychotic treatments were found to influence sleep characteristics in healthy subjects, different studies have focused on the possible influence of treatments on patient sleep characteristics. The use of typical antipsychotics (haloperidol, thiothixene, and flupentixol) in patients is consistently associated with an increase in total sleep time, sleep efficiency, and REM latency, whereas the influence on specific sleep stages is variable. On the other hand, a deterioration in sleep quality was found with the suspension of such treatment. As in healthy subjects, second-generation antipsychotics seem to influence sleep continuity in schizophrenic patients, with an increase in either total sleep time or sleep efficiency, and a decrease in wakefulness [29]. In contrast, clozapine was shown to decrease SWS. Moreover, while patients treated with classical neuroleptics were found to have a variety of abnormalities in the circadian rest–activity cycle, patients administered clozapine were showed to have an highly regular and reproducible circadian rest–activity cycle, synchronized at the appropriate phase to external social zeitgebers, and to have fewer nocturnal disturbances [24]. Thus, clozapine increased circadian amplitude (perhaps through its high affinity to dopamine D_4 and serotonin 5-HT$_7$ receptors in the suprachiasmatic nucleus (SCN), thereby improving entrainment.

Alcohol-related Disorders

Several sleep disturbances have been described in alcoholic patients. Although insomnia is the most common complaint, with an estimated prevalence ranging from 36% to 72%, hypersomnia, parasomnia, and circadian disturbances have also been described.

The impact of ethanol on human sleep was first studied in the late 1930s by Kleitman and described in his book *Sleep and Wakefulness* [30]. Since then, a large number of studies have focused on the effect of ethanol on sleep and, in particular, on the sleep of alcoholics.

During heavy periods of drinking, alcoholic patients show a relatively rapid sleep onset, but they have sleep onset difficulties if they do not take alcohol before bedtime. Alcohol intake before bedtime increases NREM sleep during the first part of the night, while sleep during the second part of the night is fragmented, with an increase of awakenings and reduced amount and disruption of REM sleep [31]. Elevated high-frequency activity and reduced SWA (< 4 Hz) during sleep were found in chronic alcoholic men.

Further support for a potential impact of alcoholism on SWA comes from a study by Colrain and colleagues of sleep evoked potentials in alcoholic patients compared with healthy subjects. The incidence and amplitude of the evoked δ frequency responses during stage 2 sleep were found to be significantly reduced in the alcoholic subjects, with the amplitude reduction being apparent only over prefrontal and frontal scalp sites [32].

During wakefulness, ethanol is a mild respiratory depressant, but during sleep, it can exacerbate sleep-related breathing disorders. Indeed, different studies have indicated that patients affected by alcoholism are more likely than control subjects to develop sleep apnea, even during abstinence [33].

Sleep abnormalities are present not only during periods of alcohol abuse but also during withdrawal and abstinence. During acute withdrawal from alcohol, patients take a long time to fall asleep and show very small amount of delta (stages 3 and 4) sleep and poor sleep efficiency [34]. PSG studies performed in patients affected by primary alcoholism after 2 weeks of abstinence have found increased sleep latency, decreased total sleep time and delta sleep time, and increased REM density [34]. Disturbances in sleep continuity (prolonged sleep latency and reduced sleep efficiency) and sleep architecture (reduced total sleep time, NREM sleep, and SWS or delta sleep) may persist months or even years after abstinence and may be associated with the clinical course [35], with different studies finding a relationship between disturbed sleep during abstinence and relapse to drinking. In primary alcoholic patients, REM sleep measures obtained at the time of admission to an inpatient alcohol treatment program have been shown to predict abstinence or relapse during a period of 3 months after discharge. Significantly shortened REM latency and increased percentage of REM sleep were observed in relapsing patients when compared with abstainers [36]. Other PSG variables that have been found to predict a negative outcome are longer sleep onset latency, decreased sleep efficiency, and decreased percentage of SWS [2].

Drug Abuse

Not only is sleep disturbance often a complaint by drug abusers during both their use of substances and their withdrawal from these, but it is also found to predispose to developing a substance use disorder [37].

Trouble sleeping is a frequently cited adverse effect of cocaine intake. PSG studies have confirmed the stimulant properties of cocaine, demonstrating longer sleep latency, reduced total sleep time, and suppression of REM sleep after acute cocaine administration [38]. Both hypersomnia and insomnia have been observed during cocaine withdrawal [39]. Sleep disorders during abuse of amphetamine and methylphenidate are similar to those found in cocaine users [40]. 3,4-Methylenedioxymethamphetamine (MDMA, "ecstasy") users commonly report restless, disturbed sleep during the 48 hours following MDMA intake [41], and an increase in wakefulness and an almost complete suppression of REM sleep were found in a PSG study after intake of MDMA [42].

There is some evidence indicating that cannabis reduces stage 3 but increases stage 4 and total SWS [43,44], but contradictory effects have also been observed. Moreover, the use of Δ^9-tetrahydrocannabinol (THC) was found to be linked to decreased total REM sleep and REM density [44]. In a few studies with high THC doses or marijuana-naive subjects, findings were suggestive of increment in sleep onset latency [45], but the sleep-inducing [46] and SWS-enhancing [47] effects showed tolerance during chronic marijuana administration. The vast majority of studies confirmed the presence of sleep difficulties during withdrawal. They generally occur within 24–72 hours of discontinuation of cannabis use and persist for 6–7 weeks [48].

Subjective reports of opioid effects on sleep vary among patients. Sleep and laboratory studies suggest a different influence depending on whether they are drug abusers or taking opioids for chronic pain. Moreover, the use of opioids seems to cause central sleep apnea in up to 30% of chronic users [49] in a dose-dependent fashion [50]. Reduced SWS, frequent awakening, and reduced sleep efficacy were found in subjects on methadone maintenance treatment [51]. Early studies on prolonged methadone abstinence suggested an improvement in sleep [52].

Borderline Personality Disorder

About 50% of patients affected by borderline personality disorder (BPD) complain of disturbed sleep, such as a reduced sleep quality and reduced restorative effect of sleep [53]. Conflicting results are shown by PSG studies. Prolonged sleep latency, reduced sleep efficiency, heightened number of wake periods, and reduced amount of SWS were initially found in BPD patients when compared with

healthy subjects [54,55], but some recent studies have not confirmed these results [56]. A reduced REM latency, a prolonged first REM period, and increased REM density were found in some studies [54,57] but not others [55,58]. These sleep abnormalities similar to those found in depression were confirmed even when comorbid major depression was excluded [59].

Finally, recent findings have confirmed sleep abnormalities in patients affected by BPD without comorbid major depression or post-traumatic stress disorder. Patients exhibited increased sleep fragmentation, increased REM sleep density, and reduced REM sleep latency compared with healthy controls [60].

Eating Disorders

Despite the significant influence of nutrition on sleep regulation, complaints about disturbed nocturnal sleep are rare in patients affected by anorexia nervosa or bulimia nervosa. Indeed, in most of the controlled PSG-monitored sleep studies that have been performed, sleep continuity measures were similar in patients with eating disorders and age-matched healthy subjects [61]. Conflicting results in REM sleep were found in anorexia nervosa. REM sleep density was shown to be normal [62], increased, or decreased [63], while mean REM latencies were prolonged [64], normal [62], or shortened [63]. In patients with bulimia nervosa, SWS, REM sleep latency, and density were consistently similar to those in healthy subjects [62,65].

Conclusions

Alterations in sleep are an important dimension of the clinical picture of different psychiatric disorders, although they are not considered diagnostic criteria for these disorders. There is growing experimental evidence that the relationship between psychiatric disorders and sleep is complex and involves bidirectional causation. The study of this relationship might be useful in the future to discover the biological underpinning of psychiatric disorders and to find effective new treatments.

References

1. Ford DE, Kamerow DB. Epidemiologic study of sleep disturbances and psychiatric disorders. An opportunity for prevention? JAMA 1989;262:1479–84.
2. Krystal AD. Psychiatric disorders and sleep. Neurol Clin 2012;30:1389–413.
3. Plante DT, Winkelman JW. Sleep disturbance in bipolar disorder: therapeutic implications. Am J Psychiatry 2008;165:830–43.
4. Rocha PM, Neves FS, Corrêa H. Significant sleep disturbances in euthymic bipolar patients. Compr Psychiatry 2013;54:1003–8.
5. Sitaram N, Nurnberger JI Jr, Gershon ES, Gillin JC. Cholinergic regulation of mood and REM sleep: potential model and marker of vulnerability to affective disorder. Am J Psychiatry 1982;139:571–6.
6. Harvey AG, Schmidt DA, Scarna A, Semler CN, Goodwin GM. Sleep-related functioning in euthymic patients with bipolar disorder, patients with insomnia, and subjects without sleep problems. Am J Psychiatry 2005;162:50–7.
7. Bauer M, Grof P, Rasgon N, et al. Temporal relation between sleep and mood in patients with bipolar disorder. Bipolar Disord 2006;8:160–7.
8. Perlman CA, Johnson SL, Mellman TA. The prospective impact of sleep duration on depression and mania. Bipolar Disord 2006;8:271–4.
9. Bauer M, Glenn T, Grof P, et al. Comparison of sleep/wake parameters for self-monitoring bipolar disorder. J Affect Disord 2009;116:170–5.

10. Riemann D, Voderholzer U, Berger M. Sleep and sleep–wake manipulations in bipolar depression. Neuropsychobiology 2002;45 Suppl 1:7–12.

11. Bowden CL. A different depression: clinical distinctions between bipolar and unipolar depression. J Affect Disord 2005;84:117–25.

12. Nofzinger EA, Thase ME, Reynolds CF 3rd, et al. Hypersomnia in bipolar depression: a comparison with narcolepsy using the multiple sleep latency test. Am J Psychiatry 1991;148:1177–81.

13. Leibenluft E, Albert PS, Rosenthal NE, Wehr TA. Relationship between sleep and mood in patients with rapid-cycling bipolar disorder. Psychiatry Res 1996;63:161–8.

14. Wehr TA, Sack DA, Norman E. Sleep reduction as a final common pathway in the genesis of mania. Am J Psychiatry 1987;144:201–4.

15. Barbini B, Bertelli S, Colombo C, Smeraldi E. Sleep loss, a possible factor in augmenting manic episode. Psychiatry Res 1996;Nov 15:121–5.

16. Dallaspezia S, Benedetti F. Chronobiological therapy for mood disorders. Expert Rev Neurother 2011;11:961–70.

17. Horne JA, Moore VJ. Sleep EEG effects of exercise with and without additional body cooling. Electroencephalogr Clin Neurophysiol 1985;60:33–8.

18. Hudson JI, Lipinski JF, Frankenburg FR, Grochocinski VJ, Kupfer DJ. Electroencephalographic sleep in mania. Arch Gen Psychiatry 1988;45:267–73.

19. Linkowski P, Kerkhofs M, Rielaert C, Mendlewicz J. Sleep during mania in manic-depressive males. Eur Arch Psychiatry Neurol Sci 1986;235:339–41.

20. Geoffroy PA, Boudebesse C, Bellivier F, et al. Sleep in remitted bipolar disorder: a naturalistic case–control study using actigraphy. J Affect Disord 2014;158:1–7.

21. Haffmans PM, Hoencamp E, Knegtering HJ, van Heycop ten Ham BF. Sleep disturbance in schizophrenia. Br J Psychiatry 1994;165:697–8.

22. Ritsner M, Kurs R, Ponizovsky A, Hadjez J. Perceived quality of life in schizophrenia: relationships to sleep quality. Qual Life Res 2004;13:783–91.

23. Monti JM, Monti D. Sleep disturbance in schizophrenia. Int Rev Psychiatry 2005;17:247–53.

24. Wirz-Justice A, Haug HJ, Cajochen C. Disturbed circadian rest–activity cycles in schizophrenia patients: an effect of drugs? Schizophr Bull 2001;27:497–502.

25. Wulff K, Dijk DJ, Middleton B, Foster RG, Joyce EM. Sleep and circadian rhythm disruption in schizophrenia. Br J Psychiatry 2012;200:308–16.

26. Bromundt V, Koster M, Georgiev-Kill A, et al. Sleep–wake cycles and cognitive functioning in schizophrenia. Br J Psychiatry 2011;198:269–76.

27. Monti JM, BaHammam AS, Pandi-Perumal SR, et al. Sleep and circadian rhythm dysregulation in schizophrenia. Prog Neuropsychopharmacol Biol Psychiatry 2013;43:209–16.

28. Benson BE, Zarcone VP. Sleep abnormalities in schizophrenia and other psychotic disorders. Rev Psychiatry 1994;13:677–705.

29. Cohrs S. Sleep disturbances in patients with schizophrenia: impact and effect of antipsychotics. CNS Drugs 2008;22:939–62.

30. Kleitman N. Sleep and wakefulness. Chicago: University of Chicago Press, 1939.

31. Roehrs T, Roth T. Sleep, sleepiness, sleep disorders and alcohol use and abuse. Sleep Med Rev 2001;5:287–97.

32. Colrain IM, Crowley KE, Nicholas CL, Padilla M, Baker FC. The impact of alcoholism on sleep evoked Delta frequency responses. Biol Psychiatry 2009;66:177–84.

33. Tan ET, Lambie DG, Johnson RH, Robinson BJ, Whiteside EA. Sleep apnoea in alcoholic patients after withdrawal. Clin Sci (Lond) 1985;69:655–61.

34. Gillin JC, Smith TL, Irwin M, Kripke DF, Schuckit M. EEG sleep studies in "pure" primary alcoholism during subacute withdrawal: relationships to normal controls, age, and other clinical variables. Biol Psychiatry 1990;27:477–88.

35. Drummond SP, Gillin JC, Smith TL, DeModena A. The sleep of abstinent pure primary alcoholic patients: natural course and relationship to relapse. Alcohol Clin Exp Res 1998;22:1796–802.

36. Gillin JC, Smith TL, Irwin M, et al. Increased pressure for rapid eye movement sleep at time of hospital admission predicts relapse in nondepressed patients with primary alcoholism at 3-month follow-up. Arch Gen Psychiatry 1994;51:189–97.

37. Wallander MA, Johansson S, Ruigomez A, Garcia Rodriguez LA, Jones R. Morbidity associated with sleep disorders in primary care: a longitudinal cohort study. Prim Care Companion J Clin Psychiatry 2007;9:338–45.

38. Johanson CE, Roehrs T, Schuh K, Warbasse L. The effects of cocaine on mood and sleep in cocaine-dependent males. Exp Clin Psychopharmacol 1999;7:338–46.

39. Schierenbeck T, Riemann D, Berger M, Hornyak M. Effect of illicit recreational drugs upon sleep: cocaine, ecstasy and marijuana. Sleep Med Rev 2008;12:381–9.

40. Gossop MR, Bradley BP, Brewis RK. Amphetamine withdrawal and sleep disturbance. Drug Alcohol Depend 1982;10:177–83.

41. Huxster JK, Pirona A, Morgan MJ. The sub-acute effects of recreational ecstasy (MDMA) use: a controlled study in humans. J Psychopharmacol 2006;20:281–90.

42. Gouzoulis E, Steiger A, Ensslin M, Kovar A, Hermle L. Sleep EEG effects of 3,4-methylenedioxyethamphetamine (MDE; "eve") in healthy volunteers. Biol Psychiatry 1992;32:1108–17.

43. Barratt ES, Beaver W, White R. The effects of marijuana on human sleep patterns. Biol Psychiatry 1974;8:47–54.

44. Feinberg I, Jones R, Walker JM, Cavness C, March J. Effects of high dosage delta-9-tetrahydrocannabinol on sleep patterns in man. Clin Pharmacol Ther 1975;17:458–66.

45. Cousens K, DiMascio A. $(-)\delta^9$ THC as an hypnotic. An experimental study of three dose levels. Psychopharmacologia 1973;33:355–64.

46. Karacan I, Fernandez-Salas A, Coggins WJ, et al. Sleep electroencephalographic-electrooculographic characteristics of chronic marijuana users: part I. Ann N Y Acad Sci 1976;282:348–74.

47. Pranikoff K, Karacan I, Larson EA, et al. Effects of marijuana smoking on the sleep EEG. Preliminary studies. J Fla Med Assoc 1973;60:28–31.

48. Copersino ML, Boyd SJ, Tashkin DP, et al. Gorelick. Cannabis withdrawal among non-treatment-seeking adult cannabis users. Am J Addict 2006;15:8–14.

49. Teichtahl H, Wang D. Sleep-disordered breathing with chronic opioid use. Expert Opin Drug Saf 2007;6:641–9.

50. Walker JM, Farney RJ, Rhondeau SM, et al. Chronic opioid use is a risk factor for the development of central sleep apnea and ataxic breathing. J Clin Sleep Med 2007;3:455–61.

51. Staedt J, Wassmuth F, Stoppe G, et al. Effects of chronic treatment with methadone and naltrexone on sleep in addicts. Eur Arch Psychiatry Clin Neurosci 1996;246:305–9.

52. Martin WR, Jasinski DR, Haertzen CA, et al. Methadone—a reevaluation. Arch Gen Psychiatry 1973;28:286–95.

53. Semiz UB, Basoglu C, Ebrinc S, Cetin M. Nightmare disorder, dream anxiety, and subjective sleep quality in patients with borderline personality disorder. Psychiatry Clin Neurosci 2008;62:48–55.

54. Reynolds CF 3rd, Soloff PH, Kupfer DJ, et al. Depression in borderline patients: a prospective EEG sleep study. Psychiatry Res 1985;14:1–15.

55. Benson KL, King R, Gordon D, Silva JA, Zarcone VP Jr. Sleep patterns in borderline personality disorder. J Affect Disord 1990;18:267–73.

56. Philipsen A, Feige B, Al-Shajlawi A, et al. Increased delta power and discrepancies in objective and subjective sleep measurements in borderline personality disorder. J Psychiatr Res 2005;39:489–98.

57. Asaad T, Okasha T, Okasha A. Sleep EEG findings in ICD-10 borderline personality disorder in Egypt. J Affect Disord 2002;71:11–18.

58. De la Fuente JM, Bobes J, Vizuete C, Mendlewicz J. Sleep-EEG in borderline patients without concomitant major depression: a

comparison with major depressives and normal control subjects. Psychiatry Res 2001;105:87–95.

59. Battaglia M, Ferini Strambi L, Bertella S, Bajo S, Bellodi L. First-cycle REM density in never-depressed subjects with borderline personality disorder. Biol Psychiatry 1999;45:1056–8.

60. Schredl M, Paul F, Reinhard I, et al. Sleep and dreaming in patients with borderline personality disorder: a polysomnographic study. Psychiatry Res 2012;200:430–6.

61. Lauer CJ, Krieg JC. Sleep in eating disorders. Sleep Med Rev 2004;8:109–18.

62. Levy AB, Dixon KN, Schmidt H. REM and delta sleep in anorexia nervosa and bulimia. Psychiatry Res 1987;20:189–97.

63. Neil JF, Merikangas JR, Foster FG, et al. Waking and all-night sleep EEG's in anorexia nervosa. Clin Electroencephalogr 1980;11:9–15.

64. Katz JL, Kuperberg A, Pollack CP, et al. Is there a relationship between eating disorder and affective disorder? New evidence from sleep recordings. Am J Psychiatry 1984;141:753–9.

65. Lauer C, Zulley J, Krieg JC, Riemann D, Berger M. EEG sleep and the cholinergic REM induction test in anorexic and bulimic patients. Psychiatry Res 1988;26:171–81.

Sleep in children, older adults, and women

CHAPTER 49

Childhood sleep–wake disorders

Suresh Kotagal and Julie M. Baughn

Introduction

Sleep disorders found in adults can also be encountered in children; sleep in children differs from that of adults, however, in several important aspects—there are significant changes in timing, duration, and architecture that evolve from infancy through adolescence. Disordered sleep can impact the development of the child, and, conversely, developmental stages can influence sleep. The sleep of parents may also be affected when the child's sleep is disrupted. Sleep disorders are fairly common in children—a survey of parental reported sleep problems in children from birth to 3 years revealed a 10% prevalence [1]. Other studies have shown that one-third of children 6 months to 5 years have difficulty going to sleep or have nighttime awakenings[2]. The prevalence range for obstructive sleep apnea (OSA) in children is 1.2 to 5.7%[3]. Restless legs syndrome (RLS) in children has a prevalence of about 2% [4] Developmental changes in childhood sleep, common pediatric sleep disorders, and those affecting special populations of children will be addressed in this chapter.

Sleep through development

There are many changes in infant sleep with development. Initially, sleep becomes distinguishable from wakefulness by 26–27 weeks' gestation by the appearance of a discontinuous pattern. Minimal electrical activity may be seen for periods up to several minutes, with intermittent bursts of rhythmic alpha, theta, and delta activity. This is called *tracé discontinue* [5]. By 32 weeks, the bursts of EEG activity and the intervals between them have shortened, and this is called *tracé alternant*. This *tracé alternant* trace is characteristic of "quiet sleep," which is analogous to NREM sleep of later infancy. A continuous, low-voltage, irregular pattern termed "active sleep" also becomes visible and is the precursor to mature REM sleep. Sleep state may at times be difficult to determine at term; thus, "indeterminate sleep" may be present in some instances. High-amplitude slow waves of 0.5–2 Hz develop during NREM sleep around 1 month of age. At 32 weeks' conceptional age, the ratio of active to quiet sleep is 80:20; this drops to 50:50 by full term or 40 weeks' conceptional age. By the age of 3 years, NREM sleep comprises 75–80% of total sleep time, with the remainder being REM sleep. Sleep spindles appear by 2–3 months of age [6]. K-complexes appear between 2 and 3 months of age. Mature NREM sleep stages (N1, N2, and N3) are recognizable by 6 months of age.

The newborn shows ultradian sleep–wake patterns, with 2–3 hours of sleep interrupted by brief periods of wakefulness. It is not until 3–6 months of age that a more mature pattern develops, with the majority of sleep shifting into the night. Prior to 3 months of age, the transition from wakefulness tends to be directly into REM sleep, subsequent to which the mature pattern of wakefulness→NREM sleep→ is established. As infants develop, the sleep cycle lengthens and approaches 90 minutes in preschool children. The amount of N3 (slow-wave) sleep declines as adolescence is approached [7]. Sleep duration decreases across ages from an average of 14.2 hours in a 24-hour period at 6 months of age to an average of 8.1 hours at 16 years of age. Most children give up daytime napping by 4–5 years of age [8].

Sleep-related history

The diagnosis of a sleep disorder in children may be challenging because of their inability to verbalize symptoms. Significant reliance is placed therefore on parental/caregiver history. In contrast to adults, children with sleep disordered breathing (SDB) may not desaturate, owing to their relatively healthy lungs. Snoring may be subtle. Further, the absence of snoring does not exclude the possibility of obstructive sleep apnea (OSA). Children may present with hyperactivity, impulsivity, and inattention when they become sleepy. They may not be able to verbalize their discomfort if suffering from restless legs syndrome (RLS). Key features of the pediatric sleep history can be found in Table 49.1.

Sleep-related examination

Height, weight, and body mass index are recorded because OSA can be associated with poor weight gain in infants and with obesity during adolescence. OSA patients may have a small jaw, dental malocclusion, large tongue, facial muscle weakness, shallow cheek bones, deviated nasal septum, swollen lining of the nasal passages, enlarged tonsils or adenoids, and mouth breathing. Consultation with a pediatric otolaryngologist is required to exclude adenoidal hypertrophy. Inattentiveness, irritability, and mood swings can be clues to daytime sleepiness. OSA related to brainstem abnormalities like the Chiari type I or II malformations can lead to hoarseness of voice, decreased gag reflex, and abnormal tendon reflexes. Muscle diseases like myotonic dystrophy may be associated with upper airway collapse combined with shallow chest and abdominal wall movement (obstructive hypoventilation). The parent–child interaction should be observed for clues toward parental anxiety and insufficient limit setting of behaviors that can perpetuate insomnia in toddlers. Home videos, if available, are invaluable in the assessment of abnormal movement patterns seen in RLS, parasomnias, and nocturnal seizures.

Table 49.1 Key features of the pediatric sleep history

Chief sleep complaint
Sleep–wake patterns
◆ School
◆ Weekends
◆ Vacations/summer break
◆ Regular/irregular
Bedtime routine
◆ Length
◆ Use of electronics
◆ Sleep onset association
Sleep onset time
Morning waking time (spontaneous or with alarm)
Night wakings
◆ Length
◆ Parental involvement
Sleep environment
◆ Bedroom
◆ Own/shared
◆ Electronics
◆ Nightlight
◆ Co-sleeping
Snoring, mouth breathing, breathing pauses, diaphoresis, sleep position
Restless sleep
Leg complaints or discomfort
Secondary nocturnal enuresis
Daytime sleepiness, hyperactivity, or behavioral problems
Age-appropriate napping
Sleepwalking
Sleep terrors
Medications
Caffeine/energy drink use
Family history of obstructive sleep apnea, restless legs syndrome, sleepwalking

Table 49.2 Key principles in pediatric sleep hygiene

Bedtime and wake time should be regular and consistent between weekdays and weekends
A consistent bedtime routine should be maintained
Bedtime routines should be relaxing and brief (20–30 minutes)
A nighttime bath may be activating for some children
Electronics should not be used prior to bedtime or be in the bedroom
The child should learn to fall asleep on his/her own without parental interference
A transitional object (blanket, stuffed animal) may be used
Bedroom environment should be dark and quiet (night lights may be beneficial)
Napping should occur appropriate to developmental age
Fluids prior to bedtime can increase arousals due to bladder distension
A small protein-containing snack may be appropriate before bed
Caffeine-containing beverage intake should be limited

Sleep hygiene measures

Besides specific therapeutic measures, attention to sleep hygiene is extremely important in the management of many sleep disorders in children. Key principles in this regard are listed in Table 49.2.

Specific sleep–wake disorders

Primary central sleep apnea of infancy

Primary central sleep apnea of infancy consists of both *apnea of prematurity* (occurring in an infant < 37 weeks' conceptional age) and *apnea of infancy* (occurring in an infant > 37 weeks' conceptional age). It consists of prolonged central respiratory pauses of ≥ 20 s or of shorter pauses that are associated with decreased heart rate, hypoxemia, clinical changes such as pallor, cyanosis and limpness, or need for intervention. Shorter-duration events

may be obstructive or mixed respiratory apneas [9]. Primary central sleep apnea of infancy needs to be differentiated from normal infant breathing, which includes both periodic breathing and respiratory pauses. Periodic breathing is a pattern of regular respiration for 10–18 s cycled with pauses of ≥3 s in length that occur without clinically significant hypoxemia or heart rate change [9]. It can occur in up to 94.5% of infants of low birth weight [10] and can persist in normal infants through infancy. Infants can have brief (<10 s) respiratory pauses that are self-limited and, if not associated with significant desaturation or heart rate change, can be normal [11]. There is a blunted arousal response to both hypercapnia and hypoxemia in neonates that is exaggerated in those with apnea of infancy [12]. Caffeine citrate is useful as a respiratory stimulant and has been shown to have improved neurocognitive outcomes in very low-birth-weight infants [13].

Brief Resolved Unexplained Events (BRUE)

Brief resolved unexplained events (BRUE) [14] and sudden infant death syndrome (SIDS) are two distinct disorders that can be considered together. While there are risk factors in common between the two entities (maternal smoking, male gender, gestational age, and very low birth weight), other predisposing factors diverge, so they should be considered distinct entities [15]. A BRUE is an event that is frightening to the observer and includes an apnea, color change, decreased muscle tone, or choking/gagging. A BRUE should not be considered as a precursor to SIDS. The differential diagnosis of BRUE is extremely broad; a careful history and exam are needed, with additional focused testing based on the clinical picture. The most common etiologies identified in a large review were gastroesophageal reflux, seizures, and lower respiratory tract infections [16]. Polysomnography (PSG) may be useful in the evaluation of BRUE when there is a concern for upper airway obstruction or other concerns for SDB. A normal PSG does not rule out future BRUE events; many children with BRUE will have a normal sleep study [17].

SIDS is defined as the sudden unexplained death of an infant that remains unexplained after a thorough investigation [18] that includes evaluation of clinical history, complete autopsy, and examination of the death scene. While the cause of SIDS remains unknown, a "triple-risk" model has been suggested that includes the vulnerable infant, a critical developmental period, and exogenous stressors [19]. Infant sleep position is an important consideration in SIDS. When infants sleep in the prone position, the auto-resuscitation reflex to hypoxemia and hypercarbia may not get activated; startle and arousal followed by gasping may be absent, leading to asphyxiation [20]. Prone sleep position is associated with a decreased arousal response [21]. In addition, a critical developmental period occurs between 2 and 5 months of age when the infant transitions from subcortical to cortical arousal. Consequent disorganization of arousal development during this critical period increase the risk of SIDS [22]. The prevalence of SIDS has significantly decreased following the "Back to Sleep" campaign that was introduced in the United States in the 1990s. This recommends supine sleep until 12 months of age. The decline in SIDS incidence has now leveled off, underscoring the persistence of other risk factors such as bed sharing, maternal smoking, and upper respiratory tract infections [23]. In 2011 the American Academy of Pediatrics (AAP) expanded its recommendations to promote safe sleep in infants and target other preventable causes of sleep-related deaths in addition to SIDS. A summary of these recommendations for safe sleep in infants can be found in Table 49.3 [24].

Sleep disordered breathing

Obstructive sleep apnea

OSA is the most common form of sleep disordered breathing (SDB) in children. As defined by the International Classification

Table 49.3 Summary of recommendations for infant safe sleep

Infant should be placed supine for every sleep
A firm sleep surface is recommended
Loose bedding and soft objects should not be used in the crib
Sleep positioners, wedges, and special mattresses are not recommended
Room-sharing is recommended
Bed-sharing is not recommended
Breastfeeding is recommended
The offering of a pacifier at sleep onset may be beneficial
Avoid overheating of the infant (no more than one layer more than an adult would wear)
Regular prenatal care is recommended
Smoke exposure, alcohol, and illicit drug use should be avoided during and after pregnancy
Infants should be immunized
Home cardiorespiratory monitors have not been shown to reduce the risk of SIDS

Source data from Pediatrics, 128(5), Moon RY, SIDS and other sleep-related infant deaths: expansion of recommendations for a safe infant sleeping environment, pp. 1030–9, Copyright (2011), American Academy of Pediatrics.

of Sleep Disorders, Third Edition (ICSD-3), OSA is prolonged or intermittent, partial or complete, upper airway obstruction that impairs ventilation and/or causes sleep disruption [9]. The etiology includes adenotonsillar hypertrophy, craniofacial anomalies (eg, micrognathia, macroglossia, maxillary hypoplasia), neuromuscular disorders (eg, muscular dystrophies), and obesity [25].

The parent may report snoring, labored breathing, and/or obstructed breathing. Additional observations may include the following: paradoxical respiratory effort; restless sleep with frequent movement, diaphoresis, and airway-protective maneuvers such as neck extension; poor weight gain; early morning headache; and secondary enuresis. Symptoms of daytime sleepiness may be present, but hyperactivity or behavior changes can be also be seen. Children are more likely to have partial airway obstruction, in contrast to adults, who are more likely to have complete airway obstruction [9].

On PSG, there are one or more scorable respiratory events per hour [9]. A scorable respiratory event, according to the 2012 American Academy of Sleep Medicine (AASM) Manual for the Scoring of Sleep and Associated Events, includes obstructive apneas or hypopneas. An obstructive apnea is defined by a decrease in amplitude of the oronasal thermal sensor recording by $\geq 90\%$ of baseline for at least two breaths with continued respiratory effort throughout the event. A hypopnea is scored if there is a decrease in nasal pressure signal by $\geq 30\%$ for at least two breaths and there is either an associated oxygen desaturation of $\geq 3\%$ or an associated arousal [26].

First-line treatment for most children with OSA is adenotonsillectomy. The gold standard for diagnosis of OSA in children is attended PSG in the sleep laboratory. Recent guidelines from the AAP and the AASM recommend PSG for diagnosing OSA prior to adenotonsillectomy in children when there is a clinical suspicion of sleep disordered breathing [3,27]. The American Academy of Otolaryngology–Head and Neck Surgery Foundation recommends a sleep study in patients with complex medical conditions or in the uncomplicated patient in whom the diagnosis of SDB is not clear [28]. Children at high risk for complications from adenotonsillectomy should be monitored postoperatively in the hospital setting. They include those with age < 3 years, severe OSA (apnea–hypopnea index (AHI) ≥ 10 or oxygen desaturation < 80%), cardiac complications from OSA, failure to thrive or obesity, craniofacial anomalies or genetic disorder, neuromuscular disorder, or current respiratory infection [28, 29]. Overnight oximetry as a screening test is less useful in children than it is in the adult population. An abnormal oximetry in an uncomplicated child with enlarged tonsils is highly suggestive of OSA (with a positive predictive value of 97%); however, a negative oximetry does not rule out OSA. In a sleep center referred population, children with a negative oximetry still had a 47% chance of OSA on PSG [30]. Children can have severe OSA and maintain normal oxygen saturations.

Continuous positive airway pressure (CPAP) is also used to treat OSA in children, particularly if there is significant residual disease after adenotonsillectomy and/or the child is obese or has other medical comorbidities. While adherence can be a challenge, treatment of OSA with CPAP in children has been associated with improvement in attention, sleepiness, behavior, and quality of life [31]. There are published guidelines for manual titration in the sleep laboratory [32,33].

There are alternative medical therapies to be used in children with mild OSA to avoid adenotonsillectomy or if residual mild OSA persists after adenotonsillectomy. Leukotriene and glucocorticoid receptors have been shown to be present on adenoidal tissue, and treatment with both montelukast and intranasal steroids (intranasal budesonide or fluticasone) has shown a decrease in AHI during treatment that likely persists after the medication is discontinued [34–38]. These medical therapies are likely beneficial in mild OSA (AHI < 5). Optimal treatment length has not been established, but at least 6 weeks is likely needed for benefit. These patients should have close follow-up.

Central sleep apnea, sleep-related hypoventilation, and sleep-related hypoxemia

Less common forms of SDB in children include central sleep apnea (CSA), sleep-related hypoventilation, and sleep-related hypoxemia. There are no clear data on the frequency of CSA in children. If present, it may be associated with neurological issues such as Arnold–Chiari malformation [39]. Children can also have CSA associated with OSA that may resolve after adenotonsillectomy [40]. Brief (<10 s) central apneas can be present in REM sleep or post-sigh/post-arousal, and are likely normal if not associated with significant oxygen saturation. Periodic breathing is also common in normal infants [41].

Sleep-related hypoventilation can occur in association with neuromuscular disorders due to weakness of the chest wall. It can also occur in other restrictive lung diseases such as scoliosis. A rare form of sleep-related hypoventilation is seen with congenital central hypoventilation syndrome (CCHS), which is due to mutations in the *PHOX2B* gene and typically presents in infancy or early childhood [42].

Insomnia

Older children and adolescents can have psychophysiological insomnia similar to adults. *Behavioral insomnia of childhood* is specific to infants, toddlers, and young children. It has been reported in 20–30% of young children [43]. There are similarities with psychophysiological insomnia in that there are likely predisposing, precipitating, and perpetuating factors; however, in behavioral insomnia of childhood, the caregiver may be impacting these factors and is the person verbalizing the impact of the insomnia to the provider. There are two types of behavioral insomnia of childhood: *sleep onset association disorder* and *limiting-setting disorder*. Sleep onset association disorder is characterized by an extended process with special conditions to fall asleep, demanding or problematic sleep onset associations (eg, a need for rocking or patting), delayed or disrupted sleep if associations are absent, and nighttime awakenings that require intervention by the caregiver. The limit-setting type includes difficulty initiating or maintaining sleep, stalling or bedtime refusal at night, increased frequency of awakenings, and insufficient or inappropriate limit setting by the caregiver [9]. Children with chronic medical problems and neurodevelopmental issues such as autism may be particularly vulnerable. The child should also be evaluated for comorbid sleep disorders such as RLS, periodic limb movement disorder, and OSA.

Anticipatory guidance/preventative care and a variety of behavioral treatments have been found to be effective treatments of behavioral insomnia of childhood [43,44]. There are no FDA-approved medications for childhood insomnia, and trials are limited [45].

Behavioral methods that have been suggested include unmodified extinction (commonly referred to as the "cry-it-out" method) and extinction with parental presence. Both involve placing the child in bed without reacting to any behavior, no matter how long the child is upset. This may not be well tolerated by the caregiver. Other methods include graduated extinction, whereby the caregiver responds to the child over varying and increasing intervals. Delaying bedtime and removing the child from the bed have also been suggested. The use of scheduled awakenings is another method. The pattern of awakenings is established, then the parent awakens the child preemptively and the awakenings are faded over time. No single behavioral intervention has been shown to be superior to another [43,44]. Sleep hygiene also plays a role in behavioral insomnia of childhood and should be addressed [46].

Restless legs syndrome (Willis–Ekbom disease)

The diagnosis of RLS (also now known as Willis–Ekbom disease, WED) in adults is made if the patient has an urge to move his or her legs, usually associated with an uncomfortable sensation that is worsened by inactivity and partially relieved by movement. The symptoms are worse or only occur in the evening. In children, besides these diagnostic criteria, additional evidence is required to establish a diagnosis. This includes a description of the discomfort in the child's own words, such as *"owwies ouchies, bugs crawling on the legs, …"*. Since not all children are able to adequately describe the discomfort and urge to move the limbs, at least two of the following should be present: sleep disturbance, a first-degree relative with RLS, elevated periodic limb movements of sleep (periodic limb movement index ≥ 5) on PSG [9]. The pediatric RLS diagnostic criteria have recently been updated [47]. The prevalence of RLS is about 1.9% in children and 2% in adolescents [4]. In a population of patients referred to a sleep disorders center, the prevalence was found to be 5.9% [48].

RLS can impact sleep initiation and maintenance. There is an association with attention-deficit hyperactivity disorder (ADHD), anxiety, and depression [4,49]. Initial treatment should focus on improving sleep hygiene, having a consistent sleep–wake pattern, getting sufficient sleep, and (if possible) eliminating exacerbating factors such as caffeine, alcohol, nicotine, and medications such as sedating antihistamines, serotonergic antidepressants, and certain neuroleptics [49]. Oral iron has been shown to be effective in treating RLS in children, particularly if the serum ferritin is <50 µg/L [50,51]. Use of intravenous iron sucrose may be considered in patients who are unresponsive or intolerant to oral iron [52]. A repeat serum ferritin should be obtained 3–4 months after initiation of oral iron therapy. There are no FDA-approved medications for RLS in children. In severe cases, medication can be used with close follow-up for improvement and monitoring for side effects. Clonidine, gabapentin, sedative–hypnotics, and dopaminergics have all been suggested as possible pharmacological therapy in children [49].

Delayed sleep phase syndrome

Delayed sleep phase syndrome (DSPS) is defined as a delay in the phase of the major sleep period compared with the desired wake time, with the chronic complaint of difficulty falling asleep and awakening at the desired times. If the individual is allowed to choose his or her schedule, there is normal sleep quality and duration for age [9]. A stable delay in the sleep period is demonstrated in sleep logs or actigraphy. While this can occur at any age, this delay in preferred sleep time is a particular problem for adolescents, and the prevalence of DSPS in this age group has been has been reported at 7–16% [53,54]. This may be due to both social and biological factors [55]. Biological factors may include a genetic component: for example, polymorphisms in the *PER* and *CLOCK* genes have been associated with DSPS [54]. Behavioral factors may include increased schoolwork, extracurricular activities, and jobs that may also delay bedtime. Poor sleep hygiene with use of electronic devices may also impact sleep. An early school start time may further contribute to sleep deprivation and daytime sleepiness. Adolescents should be screened for school avoidance and mood disorders. Diagnosis of DSPS is based on a careful history, with sleep logs and actigraphy used as adjunctive aids in diagnosis [56]. A typical pattern involves difficulty falling asleep (i.e, midnight or later) and difficulty arising for school during the week, and "sleeping-in" to late morning/early afternoon at the weekend. PSG is only indicated if an additional sleep disorder (eg, OSA) is suspected. When on vacation or summer break and allowed to revert to his or her natural pattern, the adolescent has no complaint of sleepiness.

Treatment includes good sleep hygiene. Parental-set bedtimes have been shown to be beneficial to adolescent sleep [57]. Phase advancing (shifting sleep onset time to an earlier hour) with adjunctive use of melatonin (0.5 mg about 5–6 hours prior to the desired bedtime) can be tried [56]. Bright light therapy (2500–10 000 lux) timed to be given after the nadir in core body temperature (typically about 2 hours prior to the preferred wake time) may also help advance the sleep phase. Once an earlier sleep onset time has been established, behavioral adherence is key, as relapse to a later sleep onset time can easily occur during vacations and holidays. Along with the above measures, phase advancing (moving backwards) the sleep onset time can be conducted in 15-minute increments every 3–4 days. This is typically most effective if the desired bedtime is less than 3 hours from the actual bedtime. Phase delay (chronotherapy) can be tried by shifting the bedtime forwards 3 hours daily until the desired bedtime is reached. This is better suited if the actual sleep time is in the early morning hours. It also requires vigilance in keeping the adolescent up until the new bedtime and may require time off from school. Both melatonin and bright light therapy should be administered carefully, as inappropriate timing may worsen the phase delay [7,54].

Narcolepsy

Narcolepsy is characterized by excessive daytime sleepiness (EDS), hypnagogic/hypnopompic hallucinations, sleep paralysis, and cataplexy. It is a lifelong neurological disorder. Disrupted nocturnal sleep is often present [9]. These symptoms are caused by an intrusion of REM sleep into wakefulness, together with an overall dysregulation of the sleep and wake states [58]. Not all characteristics may be present in all children. In addition, a cataplexy history may be difficult to elicit, depending on age. This may contribute to a reported delay in diagnosis from symptom onset of 10 years or more [59]. Narcolepsy is increasingly recognized in the pediatric population; however, diagnosis of narcolepsy in children may still be delayed as a result of misdiagnosis [60]. Children may be misdiagnosed with attention difficulties, mood disorders, and/ or behavioral problems. Increased prevalence of obesity and precocious puberty has been observed in childhood narcolepsy with

cataplexy. This may be related to central nervous system hypocretin deficiency [61]. There is a strong association of narcolepsy with cataplexy and *HLA-DQB1*0602*, although this haplotype is found in up to 25% of the normal population and so assay per se is not useful. In addition, cerebrospinal fluid (CSF) levels of hypocretin-1 (also known as orexin A) are low or absent in most patients with narcolepsy with cataplexy [58]. The autoantigen tribbles homolog 2 (Trib2) has been found to be elevated in individuals with recent onset of narcolepsy with cataplexy [62]. An association has also been found between H1N1 influenza exposure and diagnosis of narcolepsy with cataplexy [63].

Diagnosis of narcolepsy is made using a combination of nocturnal PSG and the multiple sleep latency test (MSLT). The PSG should be obtained on the night immediately preceding the MSLT [64]. One to two weeks of sleep logs and actigraphy prior to PSG and MSLT are useful in documenting sleep wake patterns and adequate sleep for age. Children should be free of medications such as stimulants, hypnotics, anxiolytics, and antidepressants for 2–3 weeks prior to sleep studies, as these agents can alter sleep architecture, especially REM sleep. The most common medications in children are stimulants and selective serotonin reuptake inhibitors (SSRIs). Guidelines for the MSLT in childhood have recently been published [64,65]. The MSLT is invalid prior to age of 5 years because napping is still physiological at this age. Most children with narcolepsy will have a mean sleep latency of <8 minutes with ≥2 sleep onset REM periods (SOREMPs) [64]. Some children, however, may require repeat testing over time to make the diagnosis. For children who are not eligible for MSLT because of age <5 years or the use of medications that cannot be safely stopped (eg, SSRIs), testing for low CSF hypocretin levels is useful.

The treatment of narcolepsy in children includes good sleep hygiene, maintaining regular sleep wake patterns, exercise, and scheduled napping. This is rarely effective in isolation. There are no FDA-approved medications for treatment of EDS or cataplexy in children <16 years of age, so all medication use is off-label. Central stimulants are commonly needed. Methylphenidate in the short- or long-acting form can be used, as can dextroamphetamine, modafinil, and armodafinil. Fluoxetine and venlafaxine can be used for cataplexy. Sodium oxybate has also been reported to be beneficial in treating cataplexy in children [7,66,67]. The maintenance of wakefulness test (MWT) may be used to assess treatment efficacy [68].

Parasomnias

Partial arousal parasomnias can arise from both NREM and REM sleep. NREM parasomnias (i.e, sleepwalking, sleep terrors, and confusional arousals) are common in children owing to the increased portion of the night spent in NREM 3 sleep, from which these parasomnias typically arise. Children typically do not recollect the event. One study showed prevalences in children 2.5–6 years of sleep terrors at 39.8% and sleep walking at 14.5% [2]. Because of the predilection to arise out of NREM 3 sleep, these events typically occur in the first third of the night. While parasomnias can be benign, there might be an increased risk of injury, such as during sleepwalking. Exacerbating factors include anxiety, OSA, and RLS, as these disorders may trigger arousals that evolve into a parasomnia episode [69]. If the events described are atypical (highly stereotyped with rhythmic motor behavior or occurring multiple times throughout the night), nocturnal seizures should be considered.

PSG is indicated in the diagnosis of parasomnias if the event is atypical or potentially injurious or there is a concern for seizures. In this case, a 16-channel EEG montage should be utilized [64]. In contrast to parasomnias, epileptiform events typically occur out of N1 or N2 sleep [70]. The PSG should be examined for exacerbating factors such as OSA or periodic limb movements. Parents should not attempt to awaken the child during the episode or discuss the event in the morning, as both may exacerbate the occurrence. For parasomnias that are disruptive or potentially injurious, a small dose of a short-acting benzodiazepine such as clonazepam at bedtime can be considered, with treatment continuing for 3–6 months and then slowly tapered [7].

Parasomnias may also occur out of REM sleep. These include nightmares and REM sleep behavior disorder (RBD). The presence of nightmares has been associated with anxiety in children[71]. While rare, the presence of RBD in children has been reported and may be related to conditions such as narcolepsy, structural brainstem lesions, use of SSRIs, and neurodevelopmental disorders such as autism and Smith–Magenis syndrome [72].

Sleep in specific populations

Certain populations of children have specific sleep disorders or complaints that are unique to their disorder. This section highlights some sleep issues common to specific populations. A summary of the common sleep issues by population can be found in Table 49.4.

Trisomy 21

Children with trisomy 21 (Down syndrome) show a higher prevalence of OSA than the general pediatric population, with rates reported at greater than 50% [73]. Children with trisomy 21 are at risk for sleep disordered breathing as a result of clinical features that include hypotonia, midface hypoplasia, relative macroglossia, posteriorly placed tongue, lymphoid hyperplasia, and being overweight [73]. Additional comorbidities such as congenital heart disease, pulmonary hypertension, airway abnormalities, chronic lung disease, and scoliosis can be impacted by or can impact SDB. Parental reports of sleep symptoms in this population may be unreliable. In a longitudinal study of children with trisomy 21, of those whose parents reported no sleep concerns, 54% had abnormal sleep study results [74]. Unlike other children, the risk of OSA in Down syndrome may not directly correlate with weight, owing to the added risk for upper airway collapse from hypotonia that is typical of this disorder [75]. Children with trisomy 21 may sleep in unusual positions (eg, sitting), which does not correlate with likelihood of OSA [76]. Recent guidelines suggest referral to a pediatric sleep laboratory for PSG in all children with trisomy 21 prior to the age of 4 years. Children should be screened yearly from the age of 5 years up to 21 years for concern for SDB [77]. Because of the inaccuracy of parental reporting in this population, a high index of suspicion for OSA should be present throughout the lifetime of patients with trisomy 21.

Autism spectrum disorder

There is increased prevalence of a variety of sleep disorders in children with autism spectrum disorder (ASD), with parental report as high as 50% to 80% [78–80], independent of intellectual ability [80]. Of particular concern is difficulty with sleep initiation and maintenance of which the causes are likely multifactorial. As

Table 49.4 Summary of sleep disorders found in specific populations

Disorder	Common sleep problems	Evaluation/treatment
Trisomy 21 (Down syndrome)	OSA	PSG recommended prior to age 4 years; yearly screening Adenotonsillectomy CPAP
Autism spectrum disorder	Difficulty with sleep initiation and maintenance	Behavioral treatment for insomnia Melatonin
Angelman syndrome	Difficulty with sleep initiation and maintenance Circadian rhythm disorders May require less sleep than peers	Identify circadian rhythm disorder if present Behavioral treatment of insomnia Melatonin
Prader–Willi syndrome	OSA (risk even greater on growth hormone) CSA Hypoventilation EDS SOREMPs	PSG prior to initiation of GH and yearly after Treatment of SDB can include: ◆ Adenotonsillectomy for OSA ◆ CPAP for OSA ◆ Oxygen for CSA ◆ Bilevel PAP for hypoventilation
Achondroplasia	OSA CSA (cervicomedullary junction compression) Hypoventilation due to restrictive lung disease	Treatment of OSA: ◆ Adenotonsillectomy ◆ CPAP Treatment of CSA: ◆ Spinal cord decompression Treatment of hypoventilation: ◆ Bilevel PAP

OSA: obstructive sleep apnea; PSG: polysomnography; CSA: central sleep apnea; CPAP: continuous positive airway pressure; PAP: positive airway pressure; SOREMPs: sleep onset REM periods.

in typically developing children, behavioral insomnia of childhood can be present. Behavioral deficits specific to ASD can contribute to sleep disruption, including difficulty with emotional regulation, difficulty with transitions, and tendency to perseverate. Parental communication about bedtime expectations may be more difficult for the child with ASD to incorporate. They may not respond typically to environmental clues [81]. Mood disorders such as anxiety and depression can also affect sleep. Medications used to treat autism can further impact sleep [82]. The presence of comorbid epilepsy may also contribute to sleep disruption [83].

There may be biological reasons for sleep difficulties in ASD. The major sleep-promoting neurotransmitter in the brain is γ-aminobutyric acid (GABA). The GABAergic interneurons may be affected in ASD, causing disruption to this pathway [84,85]. Abnormalities in melatonin have also been implicated, with low levels noted in children with ASD. This low level of melatonin may negatively impact the percentage of NREM 3 sleep in these children [86].

A practice pathway has been suggested for the treatment of insomnia in children with ASD [87]. After the impact of other comorbidities and sleep disorders have been addressed, the recommendation for first-line treatment includes behavioral interventions for insomnia. Melatonin is suggested as adjunctive therapy and has been shown to be safe, tolerable, and effective at low doses (1–3 mg) [88]. Other pharmacological therapies should be reserved for refractory cases, and there is limited evidence supporting their use [87].

Angelman syndrome

Angelman syndrome is a genetic disorder with developmental delay, seizures, ataxia, speech delay, and a happy demeanor [89]. An association with a notched delta pattern on EEG has been described [90]. Sleep problems are common and have been described in 20–80% of children with Angelman syndrome [89]. The syndrome is caused by an abnormality in chromosome 15q11–q13 that causes lack of expression of ubiquitin protein ligase E3A (UBE3A) [91]. This protein may also have an effect on circadian rhythm, as shown by a *Drosophila* model of Angelman syndrome [92]. Individuals with Angelman syndrome have been found to have lower levels of nighttime serum melatonin than controls [93]. These factors may be a cause of the increased sleep complaints in individuals with Angelman syndrome. Patients often have difficulty with sleep initiation and maintenance and may require less sleep than typically developing peers. Circadian rhythm disorders have also been described, including DSPS, free-running type and irregular sleep–wake type [93]. Sleep disorders in this population have been shown to impact parental stress [94]. The peak age for sleep problems is between 2 and 6 years [94,95]; some children may have improvement in their sleep as they become adolescents and adults [96]. Key to treatment of children with Angelman syndrome are identification of circadian rhythm disorders if present, behavioral modification, and melatonin. Small clinical trials have shown that both behavioral interventions and melatonin up to 5 mg at bedtime can lead to improvement in sleep symptoms [97–99].

Prader–Willi syndrome

Individuals with Prader–Willi syndrome (PWS) have a risk of both SDB and EDS independent of SDB. PWS is a genetic disorder that is due to a lack of expression of genes from the paternally inherited imprinted region of chromosome 15q11–q13 that causes neurocognitive deficits, hypothalamic dysfunction, and specific behaviors. There is no gender preference. Infants with PWS present with hypotonia, feeding difficulties, and failure to thrive. As individuals with PWS develop, this changes into a pattern of hyperphagia and obesity [100]. Individuals with PWS have many risk factors for SDB and may develop OSA, alveolar hypoventilation, or central apnea. Obesity, craniofacial features that include micrognathia, a small naso/oropharynx, and hypotonia can all contribute to their risk of OSA. In addition, their obesity contributes to an increased load on relatively weak respiratory muscles and a risk of restrictive lung disease, which can lead to alveolar hypoventilation. Scoliosis can also contribute. An abnormal response to both hypercapnia and hypoxia has been demonstrated in children with PWS. They may also have a failure of arousal with respiratory events. These factors may contribute to SDB and may be related to the hypothalamic dysfunction seen in this disorder [101]. Increased central apneas have been observed in infants with PWS [102].

Treatment of OSA should include evaluation for adenotonsillectomy and CPAP therapy if indicated; those with PWS may be at increased risk of residual OSA post-surgery [103]. In those with hypoventilation, bilevel PAP may be indicated. Oxygen has been proposed for infants with central apnea and may improve the SDB in addition to the hypoxemia [102]. Symptoms of SDB should be assessed at least yearly. PSG should be performed prior to initiation of growth hormone therapy, 6–10 weeks after initiation, and then yearly [100]. Growth hormone therapy may increase the risk of OSA, particularly in the initial treatment phase, and may also increase adenotonsillar hypertrophy [104–106]. There have been reports of sudden death associated with growth hormone therapy [107], but this correlation has not been definitively established.

Independent of SDB and obesity, individuals with PWS can have EDS that may be due to hypothalamic dysfunction[101]. This can significantly disrupt quality of life. Increased nocturnal sleep and behavioral problems may be present. SOREMPs can be observed, as can cataplexy. Behavioral problems intrinsic to the disorder can also contribute. Modafinil has been suggested as an effective treatment for enhancing alertness with minimal side effects [108].

Achondroplasia

There are over 100 different forms of dwarfism, of which achondroplasia is the most common. It is related to an autosomal dominant mutation in the fibroblast growth factor receptor 3 gene (*FGFR3*) [109]. Individuals with achondroplasia are short-statured, with enlarged head, mid-face hypoplasia, long narrow trunk, shortened proximal limbs, and hypotonia. They are at risk for OSA from their craniofacial abnormalities. Further, the skull base dysplasia increases the risk for cervicomedullary junction compression and CSA. Coexisting restrictive lung disease may add to the risk of sleep-related hypoventilation, although this may be infrequent in patients less than 3 years of age [110–114]. The prevalence of SDB is unknown, but it occurs in 95% of preschool children with achondroplasia, with the frequency of OSA being 10–35% [110]. The risk of obesity, and upper-airway muscle dysfunction due to jugular foramen or hypoglossal canal stenosis, can also further increase the risk of SDB in an individual with achondroplasia [110]. Sudden unexpected death has been reported in achondroplasia, particularly during infancy, and is thought to be due to the impact on central respiratory drive of compression of the cervicomedullary junction [114]. In addition, infants with achondroplasia may have a decreased arousal response overall, as well as a decreased arousal response to SDB events, which can impact their risk of sudden death [111]. PSG is recommended in the newborn period and subsequently based upon symptoms [114]. A high suspicion should be maintained for SDB throughout the individual's lifetime. Treatment for SDB in achondroplasia may include surgical relief of spinal cord compression, adenotonsillectomy, and CPAP.

Future opportunities in pediatric sleep medicine

Much has been learned about sleep in childhood, but many opportunities remain for future research and exploration. This field would benefit from further prospective randomized controlled pharmacological trials. Many opportunities exist to further our knowledge in the management and long-term consequences of childhood sleep disorders. The assessment of arousals from sleep needs further study, as both cortical and subcortical arousals need to be included. Cyclic alternating patterns in the EEG also need to be considered as a marker for sleep fragmentation. The incorporation of metabolomics, proteomics, and molecular medicine into mainstream pediatric sleep medicine may also provide new insight into mechanisms and open up avenues for treatment.

References

1. Byars KC, Yolton K, Rausch J, Lanphear B, Beebe DW. Prevalence, patterns, and persistence of sleep problems in the first 3 years of life. Pediatrics 2012;129(2):e276–84.
2. Petit D, Touchette E, Tremblay RE, Boivin M, Montplaisir J. Dyssomnias and parasomnias in early childhood. Pediatrics 2007;119(5):e1016–25.
3. Marcus CL, Brooks LJ, Draper KA, et al. Diagnosis and management of childhood obstructive sleep apnea syndrome. Pediatrics 2012;130(3):576–84.
4. Picchietti D, Allen RP, Walters AS, et al. Restless legs syndrome: prevalence and impact in children and adolescents—the Peds REST study. Pediatrics 2007;120(2):253–66.
5. Scher MS. Ontogeny of EEG-sleep from neonatal through infancy periods. Sleep Med 2008;9(6):615–36.
6. Sheldon SH, Ferber R, Kryger M, eds. Principles and practice of pediatric sleep medicine. Philadelphia: Elsevier Saunders, 2005.
7. Mindell JA, Owens J. A clinical guide to pediatric sleep: diagnosis and management of sleep problems, 2nd ed. New York: Lippincott Williams & Wilkins, 2010.
8. Iglowstein I, Jenni OG, Molinari L, Largo RH. Sleep duration from infancy to adolescence: reference values and generational trends. Pediatrics 2003;111(2):302–7.
9. Sateia MJ, ed. The international classification of sleep disorders, 3rd ed. Darien, IL: American Academy of Sleep Medicine, 2014.
10. Fenner A, Schalk U, Hoenicke H, Wendenburg A, Roehling T. Periodic breathing in premature and neonatal babies: incidence, breathing pattern, respiratory gas tensions, response to changes in the composition of ambient air. Pediatr Res 1973;7(4):174–83.
11. Kelly DH, Stellwagen LM, Kaitz E, Shannon DC. Apnea and periodic breathing in normal full-term infants during the first twelve months. Pediatr Pulmonol 1985;1(4):215–19.
12. van der Hal AL, Rodriguez AM, Sargent CW, Platzker AC, Keens TG. Hypoxic and hypercapneic arousal responses and prediction of subsequent apnea in apnea of infancy. Pediatrics 1985;75(5):848–54.
13. Schmidt B, Roberts RS, Davis P, et al. Long-term effects of caffeine therapy for apnea of prematurity. N Engl J Med 2007;357(19):1893–902.
14. Tieder JS, Bonkowsky JL, Etzel RA, et al. Brief Resolved Unexplained Events (formerly Apparent Life-Threatening Events) and evaluation of lower risk infants: executive summary. Pediatrics 2016;137(5): doi/10.1542/peds.2016-0590.
15. Esani N, Hodgman JE, Ehsani N, Hoppenbrouwers T. Apparent life-threatening events and sudden infant death syndrome: comparison of risk factors. J Pediatr 2008;152(3):365–70.
16. McGovern MC, Smith MB. Causes of apparent life threatening events in infants: a systematic review. Arch Dis Child 2004;89(11):1043–8.
17. Wise MS, Nichols CD, Grigg-Damberger MM, et al. Executive summary of respiratory indications for polysomnography in children: an evidence-based review. Sleep 2011;34(3):389–98.
18. National Institutes of Health Consensus Development Conference on Infantile Apnea and Home Monitoring, Sept 29 to Oct 1, 1986. Pediatrics 1987;79(2):292–9.
19. Filiano JJ, Kinney HC. A perspective on neuropathologic findings in victims of the sudden infant death syndrome: the triple-risk model. Biol Neonate 1994;65(3–4):194–7.
20. Tomori Z, Donic V, Benacka R, et al. Reversal of functional disorders by aspiration, expiration, and cough reflexes and their voluntary counterparts. Front Physiol 2012;3:467.
21. Groswasser J, Simon T, Scaillet S, Franco P, Kahn A. Reduced arousals following obstructive apneas in infants sleeping prone. Pediatr Res 2001;49(3):402–6.
22. Franco P, Kato I, Richardson HL, et al. Arousal from sleep mechanisms in infants. Sleep Med 2010;11(7):603–14.
23. Trachtenberg FL, Haas EA, Kinney HC, Stanley C, Krous HF. Risk factor changes for sudden infant death syndrome after initiation of Back-to-Sleep campaign. Pediatrics 2012;129(4):630–8.
24. Moon RY. SIDS and other sleep-related infant deaths: expansion of recommendations for a safe infant sleeping environment. Pediatrics 2011;128(5):1030–9.
25. Tan HL, Gozal D, Kheirandish-Gozal L. Obstructive sleep apnea in children: a critical update. Nat Sci Sleep 2013;5:109–23.
26. Berry RBB, Gamaldo CE, Harding SM, Marcus CL, Vaughn BV, eds. The AASM manual for the scoring of sleep and associated events: rules, terminology, and technical specifications. Version 2.0: www.aasmnet. org. Darien, IL: American Academy of Sleep Medicine, 2012.
27. Aurora RN, Zak RS, Karippot A, et al. Practice parameters for the respiratory indications for polysomnography in children. Sleep 2011;34(3):379–88.
28. Roland PS, Rosenfeld RM, Brooks LJ, et al. Clinical practice guideline: polysomnography for sleep-disordered breathing prior to tonsillectomy in children. Otolaryngol Head Neck Surg 2011;145(1 Suppl):S1–15.
29. Marcus CL, Brooks LJ, Draper KA, et al. Diagnosis and management of childhood obstructive sleep apnea syndrome. Pediatrics 2012;130(3):e714–55.
30. Brouillette RT, Morielli A, Leimanis A, et al. Nocturnal pulse oximetry as an abbreviated testing modality for pediatric obstructive sleep apnea. Pediatrics 2000;105(2):405–12.
31. Marcus CL, Radcliffe J, Konstantinopoulou S, et al. Effects of positive airway pressure therapy on neurobehavioral outcomes in children with obstructive sleep apnea. Am J Respir Crit Care Med 2012;185(9):998–1003.
32. Kushida CA, Chediak A, Berry RB, et al. Clinical guidelines for the manual titration of positive airway pressure in patients with obstructive sleep apnea. J Clin Sleep Med 2008;4(2):157–71.
33. Marcus CL. Concerns regarding the pediatric component of the AASM clinical guidelines for the manual titration of positive airway pressure in patients with obstructive sleep apnea. J Clin Sleep Med 2008;4(6):607; author reply 8–9.
34. Brouillette RT, Manoukian JJ, Ducharme FM, et al. Efficacy of fluticasone nasal spray for pediatric obstructive sleep apnea. J Pediatr 2001;138(6):838–44.
35. Goldbart AD, Goldman JL, Veling MC, Gozal D. Leukotriene modifier therapy for mild sleep-disordered breathing in children. Am J Respir Crit Care Med 2005;172(3):364–70.
36. Goldbart AD, Greenberg-Dotan S, Tal A. Montelukast for children with obstructive sleep apnea: a double-blind, placebo-controlled study. Pediatrics 2012;130(3):e575–80.
37. Kheirandish L, Goldbart AD, Gozal D. Intranasal steroids and oral leukotriene modifier therapy in residual sleep-disordered breathing after tonsillectomy and adenoidectomy in children. Pediatrics 2006;117(1):e61–6.
38. Kheirandish-Gozal L, Gozal D. Intranasal budesonide treatment for children with mild obstructive sleep apnea syndrome. Pediatrics 2008;122(1):e149–55.
39. Dhamija R, Wetjen NM, Slocumb NL, Mandrekar J, Kotagal S. The role of nocturnal polysomnography in assessing children with Chiari type I malformation. Clin Neurol Neurosurg 2013;115(9):1837–41.
40. Baldassari CM, Kepchar J, Bryant L, Beydoun H, Choi S. Changes in central apnea index following pediatric adenotonsillectomy. Otolaryngol Head Neck Surg 2012;146(3):487–90.
41. Brockmann PE, Poets A, Poets CF. Reference values for respiratory events in overnight polygraphy from infants aged 1 and 3months. Sleep Med 2013;14(12):1323–7.
42. Healy F, Marcus CL. Congenital central hypoventilation syndrome in children. Paediatr Respir Rev 2011;12(4):253–63.

43. Mindell JA, Kuhn B, Lewin DS, Meltzer LJ, Sadeh A. Behavioral treatment of bedtime problems and night wakings in infants and young children. Sleep 2006;29(10):1263–76.

44. Morgenthaler TI, Owens J, Alessi C, et al. Practice parameters for behavioral treatment of bedtime problems and night wakings in infants and young children. Sleep 2006;29(10):1277–81.

45. Mindell JA, Emslie G, Blumer J, et al. Pharmacologic management of insomnia in children and adolescents: consensus statement. Pediatrics 2006;117(6):e1223–32.

46. Mindell JA, Meltzer LJ, Carskadon MA, Chervin RD. Developmental aspects of sleep hygiene: findings from the 2004 National Sleep Foundation Sleep in America Poll. Sleep Med 2009;10(7):771–9.

47. Picchietti DL, Bruni O, de Weerd A, et al. Pediatric restless legs syndrome diagnostic criteria: an update by the International Restless Legs Syndrome Study Group. Sleep Med 2013;14(12):1253–9.

48. Kotagal S, Silber MH. Childhood-onset restless legs syndrome. Ann Neurol 2004;56(6):803–7.

49. Picchietti MA, Picchietti DL. Advances in pediatric restless legs syndrome: iron, genetics, diagnosis and treatment. Sleep Med 2010;11(7):643–51.

50. Wang J, O'Reilly B, Venkataraman R, Mysliwiec V, Mysliwiec A. Efficacy of oral iron in patients with restless legs syndrome and a low-normal ferritin: a randomized, double-blind, placebo-controlled study. Sleep Med 2009;10(9):973–5.

51. Mohri I, Kato-Nishimura K, Kagitani-Shimono K, et al. Evaluation of oral iron treatment in pediatric restless legs syndrome (RLS). Sleep Med 2012;13(4):429–32.

52. Grim K, Lee B, Sung AY, Kotagal S. Treatment of childhood-onset restless legs syndrome and periodic limb movement disorder using intravenous iron sucrose. Sleep Med 2013;14:1100–4.

53. Saxvig IW, Pallesen S, Wilhelmsen-Langeland A, Molde H, Bjorvatn B. Prevalence and correlates of delayed sleep phase in high school students. Sleep Med 2012;13(2):193–9.

54. Zhu L, Zee PC. Circadian rhythm sleep disorders. Neurol Clin 2012;30(4):1167–91.

55. Carskadon MA, Wolfson AR, Acebo C, Tzischinsky O, Seifer R. Adolescent sleep patterns, circadian timing, and sleepiness at a transition to early school days. Sleep 1998;21(8):871–81.

56. Morgenthaler TI, Lee-Chiong T, Alessi C, et al. Practice parameters for the clinical evaluation and treatment of circadian rhythm sleep disorders. An American Academy of Sleep Medicine report. Sleep 2007;30(11):1445–59.

57. Short MA, Gradisar M, Wright H, et al. Time for bed: parent-set bedtimes associated with improved sleep and daytime functioning in adolescents. Sleep 2011;34(6):797–800.

58. Viorritto EN, Kureshi SA, Owens JA. Narcolepsy in the pediatric population. Curr Neurol Neurosci Rep 2012;12(2):175–81.

59. Morrish E, King MA, Smith IE, Shneerson JM. Factors associated with a delay in the diagnosis of narcolepsy. Sleep Med 2004;5(1):37–41.

60. Kauta SR, Marcus CL. Cases of pediatric narcolepsy after misdiagnoses. Pediatr Neurol 2012;47(5):362–5.

61. Poli F, Pizza F, Mignot E, et al. High prevalence of precocious puberty and obesity in childhood narcolepsy with cataplexy. Sleep 2013;36(2):175–81.

62. Cvetkovic-Lopes V, Bayer L, Dorsaz S, et al. Elevated Tribbles homolog 2-specific antibody levels in narcolepsy patients. J Clin Invest 2010;120(3):7138–9.

63. Dauvilliers Y, Montplaisir J, Cochen V, et al. Post-H1N1 narcolepsy-cataplexy. Sleep 2010;33(11):1428–30.

64. Aurora RN, Lamm CI, Zak RS, et al. Practice parameters for the non-respiratory indications for polysomnography and multiple sleep latency testing for children. Sleep 2012;35(11):1467–73.

65. Kotagal S, Nichols CD, Grigg-Damberger MM, et al. Non-respiratory indications for polysomnography and related procedures in children: an evidence-based review. Sleep 2012;35(11):1451–66.

66. Morgenthaler TI, Kapur VK, Brown T, et al. Practice parameters for the treatment of narcolepsy and other hypersomnias of central origin. Sleep 2007;30(12):1705–11.

67. Mansukhani MP, Kotagal S. Sodium oxybate in the treatment of childhood narcolepsy-cataplexy: a retrospective study. Sleep Med 2012;13(6):606–10.

68. Zandieh S, Ramgopal S, Khatwa U, et al. The maintenance of wakefulness test in pediatric narcolepsy. Pediatr Neurol 2013;48(6):443–6.

69. Guilleminault C, Palombini L, Pelayo R, Chervin RD. Sleepwalking and sleep terrors in prepubertal children: what triggers them? Pediatrics 2003;111(1):e17–25.

70. Nunes ML, Ferri R, Arzimanoglou A, et al. Sleep organization in children with partial refractory epilepsy. J Child Neurol 2003;18(11):763–6.

71. Mindell JA, Barrett KM. Nightmares and anxiety in elementary-aged children: is there a relationship. Child Care Health Dev 2002;28(4):317–22.

72. Lloyd R, Tippmann-Peikert M, Slocumb N, Kotagal S. Characteristics of REM sleep behavior disorder in childhood. J Clin Sleep Med 2012;8(2):127–31.

73. Churchill SS, Kieckhefer GM, Landis CA, Ward TM. Sleep measurement and monitoring in children with Down syndrome: a review of the literature, 1960-2010. Sleep Med Rev 2012;16(5):477–88.

74. Shott SR, Amin R, Chini B, et al. Obstructive sleep apnea: Should all children with Down syndrome be tested? Arch Otolaryngol Head Neck Surg 2006;132(4):432–6.

75. Shires CB, Anold SL, Schoumacher RA, et al. Body mass index as an indicator of obstructive sleep apnea in pediatric Down syndrome. Int J Pediatr Otorhinolaryngol 2010;74(7):768–72.

76. Senthilvel E, Krishna J. Body position and obstructive sleep apnea in children with Down syndrome. J Clin Sleep Med 2011;7(2):158–62.

77. Bull MJ. Health supervision for children with Down syndrome. Pediatrics 2011;128(2):393–406.

78. Krakowiak P, Goodlin-Jones B, Hertz-Picciotto I, Croen LA, Hansen RL. Sleep problems in children with autism spectrum disorders, developmental delays, and typical development: a population-based study. J Sleep Res 2008;17(2):197–206.

79. Couturier JL, Speechley KN, Steele M, et al. Parental perception of sleep problems in children of normal intelligence with pervasive developmental disorders: prevalence, severity, and pattern. J Am Acad Child Adolesc Psychiatry 2005;44(8):815–22.

80. Richdale AL, Schreck KA. Sleep problems in autism spectrum disorders: prevalence, nature, & possible biopsychosocial aetiologies. Sleep Med Rev 2009;13(6):403–11.

81. Reynolds AM, Malow BA. Sleep and autism spectrum disorders. Pediatr Clin North Am 2011;58(3):685–98.

82. Hollway JA, Aman MG. Sleep correlates of pervasive developmental disorders: a review of the literature. Res Dev Disabil 2011;32(5):1399–421.

83. Giannotti F, Cortesi F, Cerquiglini A, et al. An investigation of sleep characteristics, EEG abnormalities and epilepsy in developmentally regressed and non-regressed children with autism. J Autism Dev Disord 2008;38(10):1888–97.

84. Levitt P, Eagleson KL, Powell EM. Regulation of neocortical interneuron development and the implications for neurodevelopmental disorders. Trends Neurosci 2004;27(7):400–6.

85. Sgado P, Dunleavy M, Genovesi S, Provenzano G, Bozzi Y. The role of GABAergic system in neurodevelopmental disorders: a focus on autism and epilepsy. Int J Physiol Pathophysiol Pharmacol 2011;3(3):223–35.

86. Leu RM, Beyderman L, Botzolakis EJ, et al. Relation of melatonin to sleep architecture in children with autism. J Autism Dev Disord 2011;41(4):427–33.

87. Malow BA, Byars K, Johnson K, et al. A practice pathway for the identification, evaluation, and management of insomnia in children and adolescents with autism spectrum disorders. Pediatrics 2012;130 Suppl 2:S106–24.

88. Malow B, Adkins KW, McGrew SG, et al. Melatonin for sleep in children with autism: a controlled trial examining dose, tolerability, and outcomes. J Autism Dev Disord 2012;42(8):1729–37; author reply 38.

89. Williams CA, Beaudet AL, Clayton-Smith J, et al. Angelman syndrome 2005: updated consensus for diagnostic criteria. Am J Med Genet A 2006;140(5):413–18.

90. Korff CM, Kelley KR, Nordli DR Jr. Notched delta, phenotype, and Angelman syndrome. J Clin Neurophysiol 2005;22(4):238–43.

91. Lehman NL. The ubiquitin proteasome system in neuropathology. Acta Neuropathol 2009;118(3):329–47.

92. Wu Y, Bolduc FV, Bell K, et al. A Drosophila model for Angelman syndrome. Proc Natl Acad Sci U S A 2008;105(34):12399–404.

93. Takaesu Y, Komada Y, Inoue Y. Melatonin profile and its relation to circadian rhythm sleep disorders in Angelman syndrome patients. Sleep Med 2012;13(9):1164–70.

94. Goldman SE, Bichell TJ, Surdyka K, Malow BA. Sleep in children and adolescents with Angelman syndrome: association with parent sleep and stress. J Intellect Disabil Res;56(6):600–8.

95. Clayton-Smith J. Clinical research on Angelman syndrome in the United Kingdom: observations on 82 affected individuals. Am J Med Genet 1993;46(1):12–15.

96. Smith JC. Angelman syndrome: evolution of the phenotype in adolescents and adults. Dev Med Child Neurol 2001;43(7):476–80.

97. Allen KD, Kuhn BR, DeHaai KA, Wallace DP. Evaluation of a behavioral treatment package to reduce sleep problems in children with Angelman Syndrome. Res Dev Disabil 2013;34(1):676–86.

98. Braam W, Didden R, Smits MG, Curfs LM. Melatonin for chronic insomnia in Angelman syndrome: a randomized placebo-controlled trial. J Child Neurol 2008;23(6):649–54.

99. Zhdanova IV, Wurtman RJ, Wagstaff J. Effects of a low dose of melatonin on sleep in children with Angelman syndrome. J Pediatr Endocrinol Metab 1999;12(1):57–67.

100. McCandless SE. Clinical report-health supervision for children with Prader–Willi syndrome. Pediatrics 2011;127(1):195–204.

101. Nixon GM, Brouillette RT. Sleep and breathing in Prader–Willi syndrome. Pediatr Pulmonol 2002;34(3):209–17.

102. Urquhart DS, Gulliver T, Williams G, et al. Central sleep-disordered breathing and the effects of oxygen therapy in infants with Prader–Willi syndrome. Arch Dis Child 2013;98(8):592–5.

103. Meyer SL, Splaingard M, Repaske DR, et al. Outcomes of adenotonsillectomy in patients with Prader–Willi syndrome. Arch Otolaryngol Head Neck Surg 2012;138(11):1047–51.

104. Berini J, Spica Russotto V, Castelnuovo P, et al. Growth hormone therapy and respiratory disorders: long-term follow-up in PWS children. J Clin Endocrinol Metab 2013;98(9):E1516–23.

105. Al-Saleh S, Al-Naimi A, Hamilton J, et al. Longitudinal evaluation of sleep-disordered breathing in children with Prader-Willi Syndrome during 2 years of growth hormone therapy. J Pediatr 2013;162(2):263–8.

106. Vandeleur M, Davey MJ, Nixon GM. Are sleep studies helpful in children with Prader–Willi syndrome prior to commencement of growth hormone therapy? J Paediatr Child Health 2013;49(3):238–41.

107. Craig ME, Cowell CT, Larsson P, et al. Growth hormone treatment and adverse events in Prader–Willi syndrome: data from KIGS (the Pfizer International Growth Database). Clin Endocrinol (Oxf) 2006;65(2):178–85.

108. De Cock VC, Diene G, Molinas C, et al. Efficacy of modafinil on excessive daytime sleepiness in Prader–Willi syndrome. Am J Med Genet A 2011;155A(7):1552–7.

109. Horton WA, Hall JG, Hecht JT. Achondroplasia. Lancet 2007;370(9582):162–72.

110. Afsharpaiman S, Saburi A, Waters KA. Respiratory difficulties and breathing disorders in achondroplasia. Paediatr Respir Rev 2013;14:250–5.

111. Ednick M, Tinkle BT, Phromchairak J, et al. Sleep-related respiratory abnormalities and arousal pattern in achondroplasia during early infancy. J Pediatr 2009;155(4):510–15.

112. Julliand S, Boule M, Baujat G, et al. Lung function, diagnosis, and treatment of sleep-disordered breathing in children with achondroplasia. Am J Med Genet A 2012;158A(8):1987–93.

113. Mogayzel PJ Jr, Carroll JL, Loughlin GM, et al. Sleep-disordered breathing in children with **acho**ndroplasia. J Pediatr 1998;132(4):667–71.

114. Trotter TL, Hall JG. Health **sup**ervision for children with achondroplasia. Pediatrics 2005;116(3):771–83.

CHAPTER 50

Sleep in older adults

Rosalia Silvestri

Introduction

Several sleep modifications occur in elderly people, including EEG and circadian alterations and variations in the distribution of sleep stages (Box 50.1). The hypnogram of an elderly subject compared with that of a young adult (Fig. 50.1) shows increased wake after sleep onset (WASO), a steep decrease in the amount of slow-wave sleep (SWS) already in the first cycle, and, to a lesser extent, a decrease of REM sleep. REM density is also diminished with increased REM fragmentation. Furthermore, there is a rise in phase shifts/transitions and an increased number of arousals throughout the night (Box 50.2), leading to a substantial total sleep time (TST) reduction, more pronounced as intermediate insomnia. In addition, circadian and ultradian modifications also occur, leading to progressive phase advancement that may be erroneously diagnosed as early morning insomnia. A polyphasic sleep rhythm with several naps occurring during the day time is linked to altered body temperature, showing an earlier acrophase and changes in endocrine rhythms including those of melatonin, growth hormone (GH), thyroid-stimulating hormone (TSH), and cortisol [1].

Sleep complaints of the elderly include nocturnal awakenings, superficial and fragmented sleep, early awakening, and daytime involuntary napping (Box 50.3). All of these alterations are often more pronounced in community-dwelling and chronically hospitalized or demented elderly people. Daytime somnolence is also linked to loss of prefrontal cortex restoration during NREM sleep in aging [2].

Melatonin decreases with aging owing to neurodegeneration of the suprachiasmatic nucleus (SCN) [3], as well as alterations of the afferent cholinergic projections from the brainstem and nucleus basalis of Meynert (NBM) [4].

Most human studies suggest a decline in the amplitude of the circadian rhythm due to decreased amplitude of the endogenous relationships between several physiological functions. Early studies by Czeisler et al. [5,6] and Monk [7] in a constant routine protocol to avoid external confounding interference yielded contrasting results, suggesting a 90-minute phase advance with a 30% decrease in amplitude of body temperature rhythm [6] or a less pronounced

difference in the constant routine notwithstanding consistent differences between young and elderly subjects in the entrained conditions, probably due to diminished sensitivity or potency of the normal zeitgebers.

There seems to be a reduced circadian modulation of REM sleep and spindle frequency, with a phase advance relative to the circadian melatonin profile.

Circadian alteration in the expression of the clock genes BMAL1, CRY1, and PER1 [8] are observed in elderly subjects with mild cognitive impairment (MCI) and may represent a risk factor for MCI conversion to Alzheimer dementia (AD) [9].

Circadian alterations, including morning sleepiness and absence of the afternoon dip, in MCI could represent early manifestations of the behavioral and psychological signs of dementia (BPSD) and early expression of later sundowning.

On the other hand, although differences in performance after sleep deprivation (SD) often reflect genetic variances, with subjects possessing a longer version of PER3 showing a significant cognitive decline during SD around the circadian nadir, healthy older people usually tolerate SD better than younger subjects. This is probably due to a less-pronounced reduction of SWS compared with younger people [10]. There are also some gender differences in sleep alterations that occur with age, which reflect the prevalence of insomnia in women rather than in men. In fact, in women, sleep efficiency (SE) declines and WASO and phase shift increase with age compared with men, even if SWS reduction and flattening of the slow-wave activity (SWA) decay curve occur in elderly women 5 years later than in men [11]. Sleep circadian control has a greater role in women [12]. Therefore, manipulation of the circadian timing system may offer more therapeutic approaches in women than in men to alleviate excessive daytime sleepiness (EDS) and insufficient nighttime sleep.

Insomnia prevalence in older women, compared with men, confirms the overall data regarding gender-related expression of insomnia. In a meta-analysis of 29 studies, not only was the incidence of insomnia considerably higher in women compared with men, but gender differences in the population also showed that the overall risk ratio of women to men (F:M) progressively increased from 1.28 in young adults (15–30 years old) to 1.73 in subjects over 65 years of age [13]. Insomnia persistence appears to be both gender- and age-related, with a decreased remission rate in subjects over the age of 65 [14]. Poor sleep is associated with poorer physical performance and greater functional limitations in older women, significantly affecting measures such as gait speed and grip strength [15].

Midlife insomnia has been a significant predictor of all cause-mortality, with hazard ratio (HR) 2.74 (95% confidence interval

---

Box 50.1 Sleep modifications in the elderly

- ◆ EEG alterations
- ◆ Sleep stages and cycle alterations
- ◆ Circadian rhythm alterations

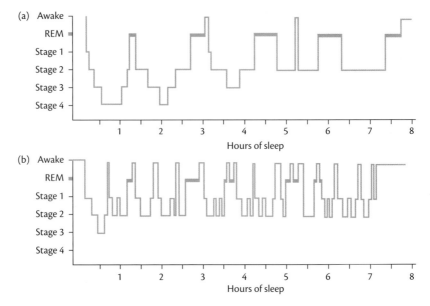

Fig. 50.1 Hypnograms of a (a) a young adult and (b) an elderly subject.

Box 50.2 Summary of major sleep alterations in older subjects

- ↓ S3–S4
- ↓ REM ↓ REM density
- ↑ REM fragmentation, ↑ WASO
- ↑ phase shifts, ↑ number of arousals
- ↑ naps

Box 50.3 Sleep complaints of the elderly

- Nocturnal awakenings (central insomnia)
- Superficial sleep (↓ awareness of the environment)
- Early awakening
- Involuntary daytime napping

(CI) 1.75–4.30), the mortality risk being high only for insomnia associated with short sleep duration, and stronger in men than in women, although still significant in the latter.

Sleep in elderly patients with dementia

BPSD, including sleep–wake rhythm alterations, anxiety, depression, restlessness, and oral and sexual disinhibition, have a severe and frequent (approximately 64%) impact on demented subjects and their families [16]. Among these, sleep disturbance represents a major clinical problem and a consistent burden for caregivers, often leading to patient hospitalization [17]. Among the noncognitive symptoms, sleep disorders and nocturnal agitation in patients with dementia are reported with a variable frequency of 19–54% [18,19].

In particular, AD patients show a progressive TST reduction in parallel with the evolution of the neurodegenerative disease [20]. Sleep is marked by several awakenings with psychomotor agitation and restlessness. Physical and verbal aggression, including complex hallucinations and vocalizations, obscene utterances, delirious wandering, anxiety, rage, and fear usually starts in the late afternoon. This aggression may last for the entire night, characterizing the so-called "sundowning" syndrome that affects up to 28% of patients [21].

EDS is also a prominent feature of demented patients, presenting as a progressive increase in parallel with the advance of the disease [22]. Most recent studies, however, show early EDS independently of previous night sleep, especially during the morning, with a loss of normal vigilance rhythm [23]. Similarly, actigraphic studies demonstrated a loss of physiological sleep propensity in the early afternoon [24]. The loss of circadian rhythmicity in demented subjects is evidenced by both melatonin and body temperature rhythm alterations [3,25]. In fact, although the pineal gland is substantially intact in AD, the SCN is typically affected by early neurodegeneration, even preclinically [26]. The rhythmic expression of *BMAL1*, *CRY1*, and *PER1* in the pineal gland appears to be both preclinically and clinically affected [8], influencing the rhythmicity of cognitive performances and accelerating the progression from MCI to AD.

Recent evidence suggests a role for orexin (hypocretin, HCRT) in driving amyloid plaque formation in AD. Experimental studies indicate that sleep disruption leads to amyloid-beta (Aβ) deposition in mice, whereas, in the presence of an orexin antagonist or in orexin gene knockout mice, the amount of amyloid deposition decreases in parallel with longer periods of both nocturnal and diurnal sleep [27]. In humans, amyloid deposition relates more to sleep quality in terms of reduced SE rather than TST duration [28]. There is a pathological interaction between Aβ42 and HCRT-1 levels, with higher cerebrospinal fluid (CSF) HCRT-1 levels in early disease [29]. Moreover, sleep plays a scavenger role, not only promoting synaptic pruning, but also disposing of neurotoxins by increasing the interstitial space, thereby favoring an increased exchange of CSF with interstitial fluid [30].

There appear to be gender differences in the expression of orexinergic mechanisms via dimorphic modulation of the HCRT-1 receptor driven by steroid hormones in females. This results in a more pronounced gender-related sleep impairment [31].

Gender differences have also been observed in the clinical epidemiology of AD, depending on the extent of the cognitive reserve, which is higher in men, and on the specificity of the affected brain circuitry, with women showing higher cerebral blood flow and connectivity in the parietal association cortices versus the visual and motor cortices in men [32]. Furthermore, environmental and behavioral aspects such as lifestyle, exercise and smoking affect cognitive decline differently in the two genders [33].

The role of gender distribution of specific sleep disorders such as insomnia, sleep apnea and Willis–Ekbom disease/restless legs syndrome (RLS) will be addressed in their respective sections.

Insomnia

Approximately 40% of the American adult population suffers from occasional insomnia, and this is chronic in 15%, with women, older adults, and depressed subjects being most at risk. Considering the recent extension of life expectancy in Western countries, roughly 17% of subjects 65 years or older are potentially at risk. The prevalence of insomnia ranges from 15% to 35% in elderly subjects [34], prevailing in women, is highly comorbid with depression, and may be secondary to coexisting diseases [35]. This remains true for different geographic environments [36,37], with differing gender specificity. Depression and chronic pain-related conditions (eg, arthritis) are the comorbid disorders that are seen more frequently in women, whereas cardiovascular and respiratory disorders are more prevalent in men. Sleep loss reduces not only quality of life but also life expectancy [38], induces hypertension [39,40], increases sustained sympathetic activity, alters cytokine activity, and augments secretion of C-reactive protein (CRP), a marker of systemic inflammation. Furthermore, sleep loss also lowers the pain threshold, thus perpetuating the detrimental mechanism of insomnia. Chronic insomnia is an inherent tendency of aging, and several therapeutic approaches, including cognitive–behavioral therapy (CBT), may be attempted in cognitively fit older patients to treat short- and mid-term insomnia, often consolidating pharmacological therapy [41,42]. The goal of insomnia-specific CBT is to reassess realistic sleep needs and goals, encouraging sleep restriction therapy and improving sleep hygiene through stimulus control procedures.

In addition, relaxation therapy has proven to be exquisitely helpful in tense or anxious patients. Mindfulness-based sleep therapy, involving medication and a variety of relaxation techniques, is particularly promising in chronic patients [43]. Pharmacological therapy includes the use of over-the-counter medicines, including antioxidants, vitamins, valerian, and a variety of herbal products, usually in combination with melatonin or prescription hypnotics. The latter include benzodiazepines (BDZs: temazepam, estazolam, and triazolam) and BDZ receptor agonists (zolpidem, zaleplon, zopiclone, and eszopiclone). When choosing an agent, several factors should be considered, including the patient's cognitive ability, potential for abuse and dependence, and comorbid psychiatric/organic illnesses. Short versus longer half-life will address different

types of insomnia complaints: sleep onset or maintenance problems, and daytime emotional profiles (anxious or depressed subjects with some kind of pain-related syndromes).

Sedative antidepressants such as amitriptyline, trazodone, sertraline, and mirtazapine can be safely used, with the caveat of prescribing selective serotonin reuptake inhibitors (SSRIs) only in the morning, given their known effect in fragmenting sleep and altering REM sleep and dreaming.

Antihistamines should be avoided in elderly people because of their anticholinergic properties and the risk for delirium, besides the deleterious effects on sleep apnea, which is also a potential risk for BDZ users. Typical (haloperidol and phenothiazines) or atypical antipsychotics (quetiapine and risperidone) are often used to control sundowning symptoms, delirium and agitation, whereas $\alpha_2\delta$ drugs, such as gabapentin and pregabalin, may prove helpful in controlling both anxiety and neuropathic pain.

Melatonin is an endogenous night hormone influencing sleep induction (MT_1 receptor) as well as circadian rhythmicity and mood (MT_2 receptor). It also exerts anti-inflammatory and anti-cancer qualities by via the immune system (MT_3 receptor). Melatonin diminishes progressively with age [44] and may be administered with different dosages and timing in the elderly either to shorten sleep latency or to delay an anticipated sleep phase via morning administration [45]. Melatonin agonists such as ramelteon have been used in the USA for long-term treatment of sleep onset insomnia [46], with improvement of latency to persistent sleep [47]. Antidepressants are of no use in the treatment of RLS-related insomnia and in fact may trigger RLS symptoms [48].

Excessive daytime sleepiness

EDS in the elderly stems from reduced SE without reduction in overall sleep need. This can result from a specific sleep disorder (eg, obstructive sleep apnea syndrome (OSAS) or RLS) or from comorbid clinical conditions such as diabetes, hypertension, or chronic pain syndrome. Circadian alteration also induces sleep at inappropriate time, such as 7 pm (forbidden zone) or in the morning with elimination of postprandial dip.

Sleep disordered breathing in the elderly

Sleep disordered breathing (SBD) in the elderly includes several nosological entities ranging from obstructive (OSA) or central (CSA) sleep apnea to chronic obstructive pulmonary disease (COPD), overlap syndrome, and CSA with periodic breathing or Cheyne–Stokes respiration (CSR) in chronic heart failure (Table 50.1).

Table 50.1 SDB in the elderly

Obstructive sleep apnea (OSA)
Central sleep apnea (CSA)
Chronic obstructive pulmonary disease (COPD)
COPD + OSA (overlap syndrome)
CSA with Cheyne–Stokes respiration (periodic breathing) (CSA–CSR) in chronic heart failure

In older populations aged 65–90 years, 81% suffered from OSA with an apnea–hypopnea index (AHI) > 5 events/h (cut-off value), but only 24% presented severe OSA with an AHI > 30 events/h [49]. Elderly patients tend to have stable SDB that may show improvement [50]. This could be due to reduced obesity and different fat distribution, in addition to different chemoreceptor responses. Depression, sleepiness, and cognitive impairment are more prominent in the elderly than in younger subjects. Gender differences in SBD may disappear by old age. Voxel-based morphometry and fractional anisotropy may detect both the gray and white matter alterations induced by hypoxemia and sleep fragmentation in areas crucial to memory and executive functions [51,52]. These changes are responsible for increased cognitive deterioration in OSA patients. The risk of falling in older community-dwelling men may be due to OSA-related EDS and sleep disturbances [53].

There is an increased risk of developing cardiovascular disease in older OSA patients [54], but carotid arteriosclerosis depends on arterial stiffness [55]. Noninvasive continuous positive airway pressure (CPAP) therapy improves sleepiness and reduces cardiovascular mortality in elderly patients with OSA [56].

CSA alone significantly increases the risk of all-cause and cardiovascular mortality by more than twofold in community-dwelling elderly individuals [57], whereas OSA-related risks in the elderly are less than in middle age owing to the decreased severity of AHI and related desaturation. Adherence to CPAP in the elderly is generally similar to that of young adults [58], but may require lower CPAP titration pressure [59]. CPAP in this age group may prevent or delay cognitive dysfunction [60] and car accidents [61].

The pattern of CSA–CSR is most common in older men with low ejection fraction (EF) and atrial fibrillation, and may contribute to the deterioration of cardiac function.

Sleep related changes in COPD or in COPD–OSA overlap syndrome benefit from bilevel positive airway pressure (BiPAP), which is able to rectify both hypoxemia and hypercapnia. Sleep quality is severely affected in these patients, who experience a higher prevalence of insomnia, nightmares, and EDS than the general population [62]. Nighttime oxygen therapy [63] and long-acting inhaled anticholinergic agents [64] have been shown to be improve nocturnal arterial oxygen saturation in elderly COPD subjects, whereas hypnotics may cause serious adverse effects in elderly patients suffering from SDB [65].

Willis–Ekbom disease/restless legs syndrome

Both sleep onset and maintenance symptoms of insomnia prevail in elderly patients with RLS, along with restlessness, nocturnal agitation, and confusion. Iron metabolism or other comorbidities like diabetes mellitus or end-stage renal disease did not differ significantly between subjects with and without RLS in a Korean elderly population [66]. RLS is, however, extensively associated with depression and reduced Mini Mental State Examination (MMSE) scores in elderly subjects. Sympathetic overstimulation overnight may be a potential risk factor for increased association of cardiovascular disease with RLS. Treatment with opioids or dopaminergic agents may induce behavioral alterations and hallucinations in the elderly population.

Parasomnias

NREM parasomnias are exceedingly rare in elderly patients, with some exceptions, such as patients with Parkinson disease (PD) or diffuse Lewy body dementia (DLBD). Several complex REM and NREM sleep enactment behaviors [67], including REM sleep behavior disorder (RBD), may occur in PD and DLBD patients. RBD is often found in middle aged or elderly patients (see also Chapter 38 of this volume), who frequently become symptomatic of neurodegenerative rather than cryptogenic disease, the latter being more common in younger age groups [68].

Conclusions

Sleep is profoundly altered in older adults in terms of its structure and its circadian and ultradian control. These alterations may herald later neurodegenerative processes, further modifying sleep consolidation. Both insomnia and EDS are highly prevalent in this age group, affecting these elderly people both cognitively and emotionally, besides constituting risk factors for cardiovascular diseases (including stroke) and cancer. Preventive efforts to address sleep disturbance before it adversely affect quality of life in this elderly population will be an important contribution.

References

1. Sherman B, Wysham W, Pfoh B. Age-related changes in the circadian rhythm of plasma cortisol in man. J Clin Endocrinol Metab 1985;61(3):439–43.
2. Nofzinger EA. What can neuroimaging findings tell us about sleep disorders? Sleep Med 2004;5(Suppl 1):S16–22.
3. Skene D, Swaab B. Melatonin rhythmicity: effect of age and Alzheimer's disease. Exp Gerontol 2003;38(1–2):199–206.
4. Wisor J, Edgar D, Yesavage J, et al. Sleep and circadian abnormalities in a transgenic mouse model of Alzheimer's disease: a role for cholinergic transmission. Neuroscience 2005;131(2):375–85.
5. Czeisler CA, Kronauer RE, Ríos CD, Sánchez R, Rogacz S. Attenuated output of the endogenous circadian oscillator (X) in an 85 year old man: a case study. Sleep Res 1986a;15:267.
6. Czeisler C, Rios C, Sanchez R, et al. Phase advance and reduction in amplitude of the endogenous circadian oscillator correspond with systemic changes in sleep–wake habits and daytime functioning in the elderly. Sleep Res 1986b;15:268.
7. Monk, T. Circadian rhythm. Clin Geriatr Med 1989;5:331–46.
8. Wu Y, Zhou J, Heerikhuize JV, Jockers R, Swaab DF. Decreased MT1 melatonin receptor expression in the suprachiasmatic nucleus in aging and Alzheimer's disease. Neurobiol Aging 2007;28(8):1239–47.
9. Landry GJ, Liu-Ambrose T. Buying time: a rationale for examining the use of circadian rhythm and sleep interventions to delay progression of mild cognitive impairment to Alzheimer's disease. Front Aging Neurosci 2014;6:325.
10. Duffy JF, Willson HJ, Wang W, Czeisler CA. Healthy older adults better tolerate sleep deprivation than young adults. J Am Geriatr Soc 2009;57(7):1245–51.
11. Ehlers CL, Kupfer DJ, Buysse DJ, et al. The Pittsburgh study of normal sleep in young adults: focus on the relationship between waking and sleeping EEG spectral patterns. Electroencephalogr Clin Neurophysiol 1998;106(3):199–205.
12. Cajochen C, Münch M, Knoblauch V, Blatter K, Wirz-Justice A. Age-related changes in the circadian and homeostatic regulation of human sleep. Chronobiol Int 2006;23(1–2):461–74.
13. Zhang B, Wing YK. Sex differences in insomnia: a meta-analysis. Sleep 2006;29(1):85–93.

14. Morphy H, Dunn KM, Lewis M, Boardman HF, Croft PR. Epidemiology of insomnia: a longitudinal study in a UK population. Sleep 2007;30:274–80.

15. Goldman SE, Stone KL, Ancoli-Israel S, et al. Poor sleep is associated with poorer physical performance and greater functional limitations in older women. Sleep 2007;30(10):1317–26.

16. Finkel SI, Costa e Silva J, Cohen G, et al. Behavioral and psychological signs and symptoms of dementia: a consensus statement on current knowledge and implications for research and treatment. Int Psychogeriatr 2006;8(Suppl 3):497–500.

17. Gaugler JE, Davey A, Pearlin LI, Zarit SH. Modeling caregiver adaptation over time: the longitudinal impact of behavior problems. Psychol Aging 2000;15(3):437–50.

18. McCurry SM, Logsdon RG, Teri L, Vitiello MV. Evidence-based psychological treatments for insomnia in older adults. Psychol Aging 2007;22(1):18–27.

19. Guarnieri B, Adorni F, Musicco M, et al. Prevalence of sleep disturbances in mild cognitive impairment and dementing disorders: a multicenter Italian clinical cross-sectional study on 431 patients. Dement Geriatr Cogn Disord 2012;33(1):50–8.

20. Vitiello M, Bliwise D, Prinz P. Sleep in Alzheimer's disease and the sundown syndrome. Neurology 1992; 42(7 Suppl 6):83–93; discussion 93–4.

21. Bliwise DL. Sleep disorders in Alzheimer's disease and other dementias. Clin Cornerstone 2004;6(1):S16–28.

22. Montplaisir J, Petit D, Lorrain D, et al. Sleep in Alzheimer's disease: further considerations on the role of brainstem and forebrain cholinergic populations in sleep-wake mechanisms. Sleep 1995;18:145–8.

23. Bonanni E, Maestri M, Tognoni G, et al. Daytime sleepiness in mild and moderate Alzheimer's disease and its relationship with cognitive impairment. J Sleep Res 2005;14(3):311–17.

24. Schlosser Covell GES, Dhawan PS, Iannotti JKL, et al. Disrupted daytime activity and altered sleep–wake patterns may predict transition to mild cognitive impairment or dementia. Neurologist 2012;18(6):426–9.

25. Volicer L, Harper DG, Manning BC, Goldstein R, Satlin A. Sundowning and circadian rhythms in Alzheimer's disease. Am J Psychiatry 2001;158(5):704–11.

26. Wu Y, Fischer D, Kalsbeek A, et al. Pineal clock gene oscillation is disturbed in Alzheimer's disease, due to functional disconnection from the "master clock." FASEB J 2006;20(11):1874–6.

27. Kang J-E, Lim MM, Bateman RJ, et al. Amyloid-β dynamics are regulated by orexin and the sleep–wake cycle. Science (NY) 2009;326(5955):1005–7.

28. Ju YS, McLeland JS, Toedebusch CD, et al. Sleep quality and preclinical Alzheimer disease. JAMA Neurol 2013;70(5):587593.

29. Dauvilliers Y, Lehmann S, Jaussent I, Gabelle A. Hypocretin and brain β-amyloid peptide interactions in cognitive disorders and narcolepsy. Front Aging Neurosci 2014;6:119.

30. Xie L, Kang H, Xu Q, et al. Sleep drives metabolite clearance from the adult brain. Science 2013;342(6156):373–7.

31. Schmidt FM, Kratzsch J, Gertz H-J, et al. Cerebrospinal fluid melanin-concentrating hormone (MCH) and hypocretin-1 (HCRT-1, orexin-A) in Alzheimer's disease. PLoS ONE 2013;8(5):e63136.

32. Mielke MM, Vemuri P, Rocca WA. Clinical epidemiology of Alzheimer's disease: assessing sex and gender differences. Clin Epidemiol 2014;6:37–48.

33. Lambiase M, Gabriel K, Kuller L, Matthews K. Sleep and executive function in older women: the moderating effect of physical activity. J Gerontol A Biol Sci Med Sci 2014;69(9):1170–6.

34. Ohayon MM. Epidemiology of insomnia: what we know and what we still need to learn. Sleep Med Rev 2002;6:97–111.

35. Foley D, Ancoli-Israel S, Britz P, Walsh J. Sleep disturbances and chronic disease in older adults: results of the 2003 National Sleep Foundation Sleep in America Survey. J Psychosom Res 2004;56(5):497–502.

36. Su T, Huang S, Chou P. Prevalence and risk factors of insomnia in community-dwelling Chinese elderly: a Taiwanese urban area survey. Aust N Z J Psychiatry 2004;38(9):706–13.

37. Quan SF, Zee P. Evaluating the effects of medical disorders on sleep in the older patient. Geriatrics 2004;59:37–42.

38. Jensen E, Dehlin O, Hagberg B, Samuelsson G, Svensson T. Insomnia in an 80-year-old population: relationship to medical, psychological and social factors. J Sleep Res 1998;7(3):183–9.

39. Bonnet MH. Evidence for the pathophysiology of insomnia. Sleep 2009;32:441–2.

40. Lanfranchi PA, Pennestri M-H, Fradette L, et al. Nighttime blood pressure in normotensive subjects with chronic insomnia: implications for cardiovascular risk. Sleep 2009;32(6):760–6.

41. Morin CM, Colecchi C, Stone J, Sood R, Brink D. Behavioral and pharmacological therapies for late-life insomnia: a randomized controlled trial. JAMA 1999;281(11):991–9.

42. Castronovo V, Kuo T, Giarolli L, et al. W-D-005 clinical outcomes of group cognitive behavioral therapy for insomnia (CBT-I). Sleep Med 2011;12.

43. Mahowald MJ, Bornemann MA. Sleep complaints in the geriatric patient. Minn Med 2007;90:45–7.

44. Dijk D, Lockley S. Integration of human sleep–wake regulation and circadian rhythmicity. J Appl Physiol 2002;92(2):852–62.

45. Saper CB, Cano G, Scammell TE. Homeostatic, circadian, and emotional regulation of sleep. J Comp Neurol 2005;493(1):92–8.

46. Roth T, Seiden D, Sainati S, et al. Effects of ramelteon on patient-reported sleep latency in older adults with chronic insomnia. Sleep Med 2006;7(4):312–18.

47. Erman M, Seiden D, Zammit G, Sainati S, Zhang J. An efficacy, safety, and dose–response study of ramelteon in patients with chronic primary insomnia. Sleep Med 2006;7(1):17–24.

48. Rottach KG, Schaner BM, Kirch MH, et al. Restless legs syndrome as side effect of second generation antidepressants. J Psychiatr Res 2008;43(1):70–5.

49. Roepke S, Ancoli-Israel S. Sleep disorders in the elderly. Indian J Med Res 2010;131:302–10.

50. Sforza E, Gauthier M, Crawford-Achour E, et al. A 3-year longitudinal study of sleep disordered breathing in the elderly. Eur Resp J 2012;40(3):665–72.

51. Canessa N, Castronovo V, Cappa SF, et al. Obstructive sleep apnea: brain structural changes and neurocognitive function before and after treatment. Am J Resp Crit Care Med 2011;183(10):1419–26.

52. Castronovo V, Scifo P, Castellano A, et al. White matter integrity in obstructive sleep apnea before and after treatment. Sleep 2014;37(9):1465–75.

53. Stone KL, Blackwell TL, Ancoli-Israel S, et al. Sleep disturbances and risk of falls in older community-dwelling men: the outcomes of Sleep Disorders in Older Men (MrOS Sleep) study. J Am Geriatr Soc 2014;62:299–305.

54. Wang X, Ouyang Y, Wang Z, et al. Obstructive sleep apnea and risk of cardiovascular disease and all-cause mortality: a meta-analysis of prospective cohort studies. Int J Cardiol 2013;169(3):207–14.

55. Bortolotto LA, Hanon O, Franconi G, et al. The aging process modifies the distensibility of elastic but not muscular arteries. Hypertension 1999;34(4):889–92.

56. Ge X, Han F, Huang Y, et al. Is obstructive sleep apnea associated with cardiovascular and all-cause mortality? PLoS One 2013;8(7):e69432.

57. Johansson P, Alehagen U, Svanborg E, Dahlstrom U, Brostrom A. Clinical characteristics and mortality risk in relation to obstructive and central sleep apnoea in community-dwelling elderly individuals: a 7-year follow-up. Age Ageing 2012;41(4):468–74.

58. Russo-Magno P, O'Brien A, Panciera T, et al. Compliance with CPAP therapy in older men with obstructive sleep apnea. J Am Geriatr Soc 2001;49(9):1205–11.

59. Weaver TE, Chasens ER. Continuous positive airway pressure treatment for sleep apnea in older adults. Sleep Med Rev 2007;11(2):99–111.

60. Sforza E, Roche F. Sleep apnea syndrome and cognition. Front Neurol 2012;3.

61. Ward KL, Hillman DR, James A, et al. Excessive daytime sleepiness increases the risk of motor vehicle crash in obstructive sleep apnea. J Clin Sleep Med 2013;9:1013–21.

62. Klink M, Quan S. Prevalence of reported sleep disturbances in a general adult population and their relationship to obstructive airways diseases. Chest 1987;91(4):540–6.

63. Moloney ED, Kiely JL, Mcnicholas WT. Controlled oxygen therapy and carbon dioxide retention during exacerbations of chronic obstructive pulmonary disease. Lancet 2001;357(9255):526–8.

64. McNicholas W, Calverley P, Lee A, Edwards J. Long-acting inhaled anticholinergic therapy improves sleeping oxygen saturation in COPD. Eur Resp J 2004;23(6):825–31.

65. Steens R, Pouliot Z, Millar T, Kryger M, George C. Effects of zolpidem and triazolam on sleep and respiration in mild to moderate chronic obstructive pulmonary disease. Sleep 1993;16(4):318–26.

66. Kim KW, Yoon I, Chung S, et al. Prevalence, comorbidities and risk factors of restless legs syndrome in the Korean elderly population— results from the Korean Longitudinal Study on Health and Aging. J Sleep Res 2010;19(1-Part-I):87–92.

67. Ratti P, Terzaghi M, Minafra B, et al. REM and NREM sleep enactment behaviors in Parkinson's disease, Parkinson's disease dementia, and dementia with Lewy bodies. Sleep Med 2012;13(7):926–32.

68. Schenck CH, Boeve BF, Mahowald MW. Delayed emergence of a parkinsonian disorder or dementia in 81% of older men initially diagnosed with idiopathic rapid eye movement sleep behavior disorder: a 16-year update on a previously reported series. Sleep Med 2013;14(8):744–8.

CHAPTER 51

Sleep and its disorders in women

Milena Pavlova

Reproductive hormones are among a variety of factors that influence sleep and its disorders. As a result, some common sleep disorders may have a different frequency, presentation, or treatment needs in women than in men. This chapter describes a number of specific disorders. As these disorders are described in more detail in the respective chapters elsewhere in the book, we will concentrate here on the characteristics that are unusual or demand specific attention when treating women.

Insomnia

Table 51.1 lists common presentations of insomnia, together with some that are potential emergencies and some that are rare syndromes. Complaints of difficulty with sleep initiation and/or maintenance are common. Epidemiological reviews indicate that worldwide, women of all age groups are more likely to report symptoms of insomnia [1–3]. The current International Classification of Sleep Disorders (ICSD-2) [4] lists 11 disorders, at least 3 of which are more common in women: insomnia due to mental disorder, psychophysiological insomnia, and presumably paradoxical insomnia. Since depression is also more frequent in women, a recent study was performed to evaluate whether insomnia is truly more prevalent in women or is due to a confounding effect from the higher rate of depressive symptoms. Voderholzer et al. [5] performed polysomnography (PSG) on 86 patients with primary insomnia (without

depression) and 86 age- and sex-matched controls and found no difference in frequency of objectively diagnosed insomnia or subjective sleep complaints in women. They therefore hypothesized that the observed female predominance of insomnia symptoms may be due to the higher frequency of mood disorders or other comorbidities.

A woman who reports insomnia should be evaluated carefully for comorbid disorders, particularly depressive disorders. A cross-sectional study from 10 countries reported that insomnia was present in most patients with depression. Other important comorbidities include obstructive sleep apnea (OSA) and effects of medication. Insomnia is about twice as common in individuals who have a comorbid disorder [6]. Specific comorbidities include heart disease, hypertension, stomach ulcers, migraine, chronic obstructive pulmonary disease (COPD), asthma, and arthritis, as well as menstrual problems. Effects of antidepressants (some reported to have insomnia as a side effect) and self-medication with various over-the-counter substances, should be considered as well (Table 51.2). Circadian rhythm disorders should also be considered, although there is no established sex predominance.

Treatment

Treatment of insomnia should start with a careful review of potential comorbidities and lifestyle factors, and this is particularly important when treating women, for the following reasons:

1. Comorbidities are common, especially of mental health problems. Some comorbidities (eg, hyperthyroidism) require additional evaluations and early treatment.

Table 51.1 Insomnia

Common disorders	Primary insomnia
	Psychophysiological insomnia
	Insomnia due to medication effects
	Insomnia due to mental or medical disorders or as a symptom of another sleep disorder
	Poor sleep hygiene
	Adjustment insomnia
	Circadian rhythm disorders leading to insomnia
Potential emergencies	Depression
	Medical disorders, endocrine abnormalities (thyroid, other endocrine, cardiac, pulmonary, or others)
Rare syndromes	Fatal familial insomnia
	Paradoxical insomnia

Table 51.2 Medications with potential sleep-disruptive effects

Medication	Cause of sleep disruption
Headache medicines	May contain caffeine
Steroids	Primary stimulating effect
Wake-promoting medications (daytime)— given for attention-deficit disorder, adjunct treatment of depression, etc.	Residual stimulating effect
Antidepressants (eg, selective serotonergic–noradrenergic inhibitors)	

2. Women of reproductive age may be considering pregnancy, and many of the commonly used hypnotics are not safe for use in pregnancy.

3. Multiple substances may lead to insomnia. Simplifying the medication regimen and counseling the patient about the effects of over-the-counter substances may be an efficient way to resolve insomnia

Case

A 24-year-old woman presented with complaints of difficulty initiating and maintaining sleep. She described onset in childhood and no obvious provoking factors. For some time, she had been using zolpidem as needed with some success, but was considering potential long-term effects as well as future pregnancy, and wanted to know whether there are safer and/or nonpharmacological methods to treat her symptoms.

On detailed questioning, she reported highly variable bed and wake times, with a tendency to be go to bed at about 3 am and wake up at about 11 am when on vacation or at weekends. During a work week, she had to wake up at 7 am. Her difficulty falling asleep was particularly pronounced on Sunday night.

After a detailed discussion about the effects of a stable circadian rhythm on sleep, she decided to attempt more stable wake and bed times. Formal bright or blue light therapy was not used, but she included a morning routine with an abundant ambient light exposure (morning jog), as well as an evening routine with lower light levels. The initial steps were difficult and required discipline, and she had mixed feelings about her success as it resulted in a somewhat less intense social life. She was encouraged, however, by finding out that she was more concentrated during the times when she had to work, even though she had not appreciated any deficits before. After about 8 months of consistent effort, she had succeeded in balancing her social life with a more regular sleep schedule, and zolpidem was very rarely needed.

Teaching points

- Circadian rhythm disturbances are a common cause of insomnia, especially in young women.
- Nonpharmacological treatments for insomnia are feasible in many cases.

- Treatment includes gradual schedule shifts, light therapy, and, in some cases, melatonin
- Hypnotic medications may have a teratogenic risk.
- Considerations of whether and when any pregnancy is planned should be brought up when evaluating women of reproductive age.

Insomnia is discussed in greater detail in the chapters in Section 5 of this volume.

A particular challenge is the choice of a pharmacological agent for women who are pregnant or considering pregnancy in the near future. As can be seen in Tables 51.3 and 51.4, most prescription medications used for the treatment of insomnia are not considered safe in pregnancy. On the other hand, treatment of insomnia in the third trimester of pregnancy may decrease the risk of postpartum depression. A recent study by Khazaie et al. [7] examined the effect of treating insomnia in 54 women randomly assigned to diphenhydramine, trazodone, or placebo, and found that both medications improved sleep. Moreover, depressive symptoms were reduced at 2 and 6 weeks postpartum with both medications. Thus, careful treatment of insomnia during pregnancy may have important implications for subsequent health. Generally, antihistamines are considered safe in pregnancy [8], and the FDA has recently approved the use of doxylamine (Unisom; Diclegis when combined with pyridoxine) for use in pregnant women. Although antihistamines are not typically the first-line treatment for insomnia, their relative safety makes them a potential pharmacological solution for pregnant women with insomnia who do not respond to nonpharmacological measures.

Hypersomnia

When approaching a woman who presents with hypersomnia, it is paramount to consider comorbid conditions and the use of sedating substances. Primary disorders of sleep–wake regulation are relatively rare disorders (Table 51.5).

There is no known sex predominance of narcolepsy or idiopathic hypersomnia [4]. However, some of the rare hypersomnia syndromes have a sex predominance. Kleine–Levin syndrome is about four times *less* common in women than in men. Recurrent hypersomnia in women may sometimes occur in a pattern, consistent

Table 51.3 Medications used to treat insomnia and corresponding pregnancy and lactation categories (classic hypnotics)

Medication	Also known as	Mechanism of action	Half-life	Pregnancy category	Lactation category
Clonazepam	Klonopin	Benzodiazepine	30–40 h	D (FDA)	Thomson: Infant risk cannot be ruled out
Lorazepam	Ativan	Benzodiazepine	(Oral), about 12 h (mean)	D (FDA)	AAP: Drugs for which the effect on nursing infants is unknown but may be of concern
Oxazepam	Serax	Benzodiazepine	5.7–10.9 h	D (FDA)	WHO: Compatible with breastfeeding / Thomson: Infant risk cannot be ruled out
Temazepam	Restoril	Benzodiazepine	3.5–18.4 h	D (FDA)	Thomson: Infant risk cannot be ruled out
Zaleplon	Sonata	GABA receptor agonist	1 h	C (FDA)	Thomson: Infant risk is minimal
Zolpidem tartrate	Ambien, AmbienCR, Edluar	GABA$_A$ receptor agonist	Varies with formulation, 2.5–2.8 h with immediate-release	C (FDA)	Thomson: Infant risk is minimal

Table 51.4 Medications used to treat insomnia and corresponding pregnancy and lactation categories (other)

Medication	Also known as	Mechanism of action	Half-life	Pregnancy category	Lactation category
Trazodone	Desyrel Desyrel Dividose Oleptro	Related to potentiation of serotonergic activity in the CNS	Immediate-release: 7 h Extended-release: 10 h	C (FDA)	Thomson: Infant risk cannot be ruled out
Diphenhydramine	Benadryl	Histamine receptor blocker		B (FDA)	
Mirtazapine	Remeron	Enhance central noradrenergic and serotonergic activity	37 h (females)	C (FDA)	Thomson: Infant risk cannot be ruled out
Quetiapine	Seroquel, Seroquel XR	Antagonist to serotonin 5-HT$_{1A}$ and 5-HT$_2$, dopamine D$_1$ and D$_2$, histamine H$_1$, and adrenergic α_1 and α_2 receptors.	Immediate-release: 6 h Extended-release: 7 h N-desalkylquetiapine, extended-release tablet: 9–12 h	C (FDA)	Thomson: Infant risk cannot be ruled out

Table 51.5 Hypersomnia

Common disorders	Poor sleep hygiene Obstructive sleep apnea Hypersomnia dues to substance or to medical or psychiatric condition
Potential emergencies	Depression Medical disorders (consider hypothyroidism, toxic/ metabolic encephalopathy, or central nervous system infection)
Rare syndromes	Menstrual-related hypersomnia Narcolepsy Idiopathic hypersomnia Recurrent hypersomnia (Kleine–Levin syndrome in women)

with the menstrual cycle, a rare condition called menstrual-related hypersomnia This condition usually manifests in adolescence, within the first months of menarche. Episodes usually last about one week. Oral contraceptives may lead to prolonged remission [9,10]. Hypersomnia is discussed in more detail in Section 4 of this volume.

Sleep disordered breathing, obstructive sleep apnea

Although many clinicians consider sleep apnea a "man's disease," sleep apnea symptoms are frequently reported by women as well. Kapsimalis et al. [11] performed an analysis of 1254 women in the United States, with an oversample of pregnant and postpartum women, using the Berlin Questionnaire, and found that 25% of the participants reported symptoms that indicate a high risk for sleep apnea syndrome. These women had common symptoms of OSA, such as habitual snoring (61%), observed apneas (7%), and daytime sleepiness (24%). They also frequently reported sleep onset insomnia (32%) or maintenance insomnia symptoms (19%) and restless legs syndrome (RLS) symptoms (33%) or body movements (60%). The risk of OSA increased with age ($p < 0.05$), obesity ($p <$

0.001), and menopause ($p < 0.001$). Women at high risk also had medical disorders more frequently.

Some women with OSA do not present with the classic symptoms of loud snoring and hypersomnolence, yet may have a significantly severe disease. Studies have found that women with OSA frequently report insomnia, morning headaches, fatigue, and mood disturbance [12]. On PSG, women may have more clustering of REM-related and positional events [13]. Particular attention should be paid to older women, as, even in asymptomatic individuals, the frequency of sleep disordered breathing increases with age [14]. A particularly sharp increase in OSA frequency is seen after menopause. In a study of 589 women evaluated with PSG, Young et al. [15] reported an odds ratio of 3.5 for OSA in postmenopausal women, after controlling for age, smoking, body habitus, and other confounding factors. OSA should be considered particularly in women who are overweight or obese, have micro- or retrognathia, have polycystic ovary disease, or are menopausal. Identifying the condition early may be important not only for symptom relief, but also for preventative health reasons. At present, OSA is a recognized risk factor for cardiovascular disease [16,17] and stroke [18].

Treatment

The treatment of OSA depends on severity, presenting symptoms, and comorbid disorders. First-line treatment is considered continuous positive airway pressure (CPAP), based on its effectiveness from randomized controlled trials [19]. Alternatives include oral appliance treatments and surgical interventions. Another recently developed nonsurgical treatment method uses an expiratory nasal pressure device called Provent. OSA is discussed in more detail in Chapter 16 of this volume.

Restless legs syndrome

RLS is another sleep disorder that is more common in women. The overall prevalence is 5–10% of the general population, and it is about 1.5 times more frequent in women [4], and a recent population study [20] reported an incidence of 1.7% per year. Use of estrogen and history of obstructive lung disease were associated with a significantly higher incidence of RLS, which, in turn, was associated with insomnia and increased sleepiness. More than half of the patients report a familial pattern. The symptoms may appear without any apparent comorbidity (primary RLS) or in association with anemia, renal disease, or pregnancy. About 80–90% of patients with RLS have periodic limb movements of sleep (PLMS) noted on a single-night PSG.

RLS is particularly common in pregnant women, possibly in relation to decreased iron stores. In most of these cases, the symptoms abate after delivery, though in some rarer cases they may persist.

Treatment

There is a strong association of RLS and iron metabolism (discussed in Chapter 24 of this volume), and the patient should have an evaluation of ferritin levels. In cases where ferritin is below 50 ng/mL, iron supplementation should be considered. Some authors have also reported a low folate level in pregnant women with RLS and a beneficial effect from folate supplementation.

In a woman of childbearing age, pharmacological treatment should consider pregnancy status. Table 51.6 shows the pregnancy/lactation category of commonly used agents. As most are not confirmed harmless, in a woman who is pregnant it is best to start with nonpharmacological treatments [21]. Measurement of ferritin level and replacement of iron, if appropriate, is indicated. Many advocate using more aggressive supplementation (until ferritin reaches 150 ng/mL, not 100 ng/mL as in non-pregnant women). Gentle exercise and avoidance of caffeine may also be helpful.

For non-pregnant women, after an evaluation of ferritin, and potential comorbid conditions, dopamine agonists are usually used as a starting treatment, starting at the lowest dose (0.125–0.25 mg for pramipexole and 0.25–0.5 mg for ropinirole). Follow-up is indicated to evaluate efficacy, as well as any side effects, some of which may not be recognized by the patient as such. For example, compulsive behaviors are often not easily recognized by patients, but on a questionnaire 23% of patients treated with dopamine agonists for RLS had compulsive eating, 10% compulsive shopping, and another 7% compulsive gambling [22]. In patients who do not respond, gabapentin or in some instances opiates can be considered.

Parasomnias

Several parasomnias have a reported female predominance. Exploding head syndrome is a sensation of a sudden loud noise, often described as cymbals, occasionally associated with a sense of a flashing light. Occasionally, the disorder may be associated with a myoclonic jerk [4] and to some may be terrifying. PSG recordings indicated that most patients are actually in relaxed wakefulness when the sensation occurred [23]. Women may also have a higher risk for sleep-related dissociative disorders and to some extent sleep-related hallucinations.

Some parasomnias have a different sex ratio in different age groups. Nocturnal enuresis in childhood is more common in boys. In older adults, however, enuresis has a female predominance [4]. Nightmares have no established sex ratio in children, but among adults are more common in women. A study of sleep complaints of 2782 young adults suggested that women were more likely to have nightmares, along with multiple awakenings [24]. In another study of 5622 subjects, nightmares were twice more commonly reported by women, and were frequently associated with depressive symptoms [25].

On the other hand, REM sleep behavior disorder (RBD) in association with violence is relatively uncommon in women [26]. There have been suggestions that women may have a less violent, and thus much less visible, presentation. As a result, the disorder may be under-diagnosed in women.

With all parasomnias, an adequate differential diagnosis is key (Table 51.7). Of particular importance is the need to distinguish parasomnias from seizures, especially frontal lobe seizures (which often occur from sleep), as often the behaviors may appear similar.

Case

A 23-year-old woman with a recent diagnosis of depression presented to the sleep clinic with complaints suggestive of dream

---

Table 51.6 Medications used for the treatment of RLS and corresponding pregnancy and lactation categories

Medication	Also known as	Mechanism of action	Pregnancy category	Lactation category
Acetaminophen (paracetamol)/ oxycodone			Oxycodone: C (FDA)	Acetaminophen: Thomson: Infant risk is minimal Oxycodone: Thomson: Infant risk has been demonstrated
Carbidopa/levodopa	Sinemet	Levodopa: triatal dopaminergic neurotransmission is enhanced by exogenous supplementation of dopamine through administration of dopamine's precursor, levodopa Carbidopa: Inhibits the peripheral decarboxylation of levodopa	C (FDA)	WHO: Avoid breastfeeding if possible. May inhibit lactation. Thomson: Infant risk cannot be ruled out.
Gabapentin	Neurontin, Gabarone	Mechanism of action is unknown	C (FDA)	Thomson: Infant risk cannot be ruled out
Pramipaxole.	Mirapex, MirapexER	Non-ergot dopamine agonist	C (FDA)	Thomson: Infant risk cannot be ruled out
Ropinirole	Requip, RequipXL	Non-ergoline dopamine agonist	C (FDA)	Thomson: Infant risk cannot be ruled out

Table 51.7 Parasomnia

Common disorders	Sleepwalking
	REM sleep behavior disorder (RBD)
	Sleep-eating
	Other NREM parasomnias
Potential emergencies	Undiagnosed seizures that have been misdiagnosed as parasomnia
	Injuries from sleepwalking
Rare syndromes	Recurrent isolated sleep paralysis
	Exploding head syndrome
	Rhythmic movement disorder

enactment. She described variable behaviors that occurred in sleep and also had some nightmares and sleep fragmentation. The events were particularly frequent around her menstrual period. Since she had also recently started treatment with a selective serotonin reuptake inhibitor (SSRI), it was concluded that she was most likely to have symptomatic RBD due to this medication. After a change in her depression treatment, the events became rarer and were not so clearly associated with a dream, but did not stop, and sleep fragmentation continued. Her mother also noted rare subtle, but stereotypic 1-minute episodes of speech impairment. The patient was referred to a neurologist, who ordered a further evaluation with a PSG and requested sufficient EEG coverage to assess for the possibility of focal nocturnal seizures. The overnight technologist did not report any abnormal behaviors. The PSG revealed a 20 s focal electrographic seizure, as well as very rare left temporal interictal discharges. Review of the video at the time of the seizure revealed only a brief turn in bed, which was not visually distinguishable from an arousal (i.e, without the supportive evidence from EEG, the seizure would have been missed). A subsequent evaluation revealed a structural left-sided MRI abnormality that likely served as a seizure focus.

Teaching points

- Similarly to insomnia, dysphoria, and other disorders, seizures can have a higher frequency around the menstrual period (catamenial epilepsy).

- Seizures should be carefully considered when evaluating a patient with abnormal nocturnal behaviors.

- Adequate evaluation is key in determining the correct diagnosis.

Sleep through different stages of a woman's life

Sleep architecture is influenced by reproductive hormones. This is reflected through many changes seen in relation to the menstrual cycle, at different times of pregnancy, and in menopause.

Childhood and adolescence

A study of 78 healthy children using logs and actigraphy reported that adolescent girls tend to sleep a little longer, but the evidence is indirect [27]. Complaints of difficulty sleeping are slightly less prevalent in girls than in boys [4]. The major differences in sleep disorder frequency are more evident later in life.

The childbearing woman—the effects of the menstrual cycle

Sleep is influenced by gonadal hormones. The circadian rhythm amplitude may vary with the menstrual cycle [28,29]. Generally, there is some blunting or decrease of the amplitude of multiple circadian regulated functions, including temperature, melatonin secretion, and cortisol secretion, during the luteal phase. Specifically, during the mid-luteal phase, there is increase in the overall value of the core body temperature and a decrease in its circadian variation amplitude, compared with the mid-follicular phase. There is also a reduction in REM sleep during the mid-luteal phase at the time of the temperature minimum [30]. Stage 2 sleep may be significantly increased in the mid-luteal phase compared with the early follicular phase.

The menstrual cycle may affect sleep. A relatively small study from Baker et al. [31] examined the association between sleep and the menstrual cycle in 26 healthy women with a mean age of 21 years and reported a lower sleep quality over the 3 premenstrual days and 4 days during menstruation, compared with the mid-follicular and early/mid-luteal phases.

Menstrual disturbances affect sleep and the circadian rhythms in various ways. For example, slow-wave sleep was significantly increased and melatonin significantly decreased in a study of patients with premenstrual dysphoric disorder compared with controls [32]. Strine et al. [33] examined the associations of menstrual-related problems with mental health and health behaviors. They included an analysis of computer-assisted personal interviews from 11 648 women aged 18–55 years and found that 19% reported menstrual-related problems (eg, heavy bleeding, bothersome cramping, or premenstrual syndrome). These women were significantly more likely than those without menstrual-related problems to report anxiety, depression, sleep problems, and pain. Women with menstrual-related problems were also significantly more likely to report feeling sad, nervous, restless, hopeless, or worthless. Cigarette smoking, heavy alcohol consumption, and being overweight or obese were also more frequently reported among women with menstrual-related problems than those without. The menstrual cycle may even affect upper airway resistance as well [34]. Thus, sleep is affected by the normal menstrual cycle and by menstrual disturbances, and these effects are modified by lifestyle factors and comorbid conditions.

Premenopausal women with an irregular menstrual cycle are reported to be more likely to report sleep difficulties [35]. These women also reported increased light sleep stages and awakenings. Premenstrual complaints were also reported more frequently by women who had periodic limb movements or nocturnal desaturation. Some evidence suggests that circadian disruption may increase the risk of breast cancer [29]

Teaching points

- Gonadal hormones influence sleep.

- During the luteal phase, there is "blunting" of the circadian signal of multiple hormones, including melatonin.

- Irregular menstrual cycles may be associated with more sleep difficulties.

Pregnancy

Sleep normally evolves throughout the duration of pregnancy. In a survey from a questionnaire administered to 325 women [36], sleep duration increased during pregnancy, starting with early pregnancy, and decreased thereafter, being shortest during the first 3 months after delivery. However, during pregnancy, sleep became gradually more fragmented and restless.

Studies that use objective evaluation of sleep indicate changes in sleep architecture. A longitudinal study performed by Driver et al. [37] consisted of serial PSGs performed in five healthy primiparous women, starting in early pregnancy (8–16 weeks of gestational age), repeated every 2 months thereafter, and then again 1 month after delivery. The authors reported an increase in the percentage of slow-wave sleep with advancing pregnancy, mostly after 17 weeks of gestational age (36% in the last trimester versus 26% in the first). A modestly shorter REM latency was noted during the first and second trimesters, compared with the third (65 minutes versus 79 minutes). In the third trimester, slow-wave sleep may be decreased [38].

Sleep deprivation has been linked to multiple adverse endocrine consequences [39–41]. As a result, adverse pregnancy-related outcomes have been hypothesized. Further studies have posed the question whether circadian misalignment may increase the risk of preeclampsia. Animal studies suggest that estradiol may modulate not only sleep structure, but also recovery sleep [42].

A significant health concern is the potential association of poor sleep and adverse pregnancy outcomes. A study on maternal blood pressure reported a higher risk of pregnancy-induced hypertension and preeclampsia with short and long sleep duration [43]. To examine whether sleep deprivation may increase the risk for preeclampsia, preterm delivery, or other complications, Bonzini et al. [44] performed a meta-analysis of 23 relevant studies and found a slightly increased risk of low birth weight with poor sleep. Of particular importance is the adequate diagnosis and treatment of any sleep disordered breathing. Some studies suggest that treatment of any sleep apnea, when present, may reverse the risk of hypertension and preeclampsia [45].

Teaching points

♦ Sleep normally changes during pregnancy.

♦ Poor sleep during pregnancy may increase the risk of hypertension and even preeclampsia.

♦ Identification and treatment of common sleep disorders may improve outcome.

Menopause

Menopause itself probably does not change sleep as an independent factor. Young et al. [46] reported PSG-acquired sleep data from 589 participants: premenopausal, perimenopausal, and postmenopausal women. They reported that sleep quality was not worse in perimenopausal or postmenopausal women compared with premenopausal women. On the contrary, postmenopausal woman had more deep sleep (16% versus 13% stages 3/4, $p < 0.001$) and significantly longer total sleep time (388 minutes versus 374 minutes, $p = 0.05$). Menopausal status was moderately related to self-reported dissatisfaction with sleep, but was not consistently associated with symptoms of insomnia or sleepiness.

Some of the common symptoms of menopause, such as hot flashes, can disrupt sleep. A population-based cohort of 436 women from the USA, ages 35–47 years, who had regular menstrual cycles at enrollment and were followed for an 8-year period,

reported that menopausal status was not significantly associated with sleep quality. In the subsequent analyses in an adjusted model, however, independent predictors of sleep quality were hot flashes ($p < 0.0001$), depressive symptoms (Center for Epidemiological Studies Depression Scale scores) ($p < 0.0001$), and levels of the reproductive hormone inhibin B ($p = 0.05$). Another large community-based study performed in Taiwan [47] reported that almost half of the participating middle-aged women felt dissatisfied with their sleep and that these symptoms correlated strongly with symptoms of depression and anxiety. A large cross-sectional study of 639 women (ages 45–54) reported an elevated depression rating score in association with frequent nocturnal hot flashes, irritability, and other menopausal symptoms such as vaginal discharge, as well as nausea, headaches, weakness, visual problems, muscle stiffness, and incontinence [48].

Frequent nighttime awakenings among menopausal women often appear as part of a cluster of symptoms that also include joint ache, hot flashes, mood changes, and concentration problems [49]. Other factors that contribute to insomnia include vulvovaginal atrophy [50]. Surveys of the prevalence of various sleep symptoms in menopause suggested that 56.6% of surveyed women suffered from either insomnia or poor sleep quality, or both, and that these were often associated with vasomotor symptoms, depressed mood, and anxiety [51]. Women presenting sleep disturbances had a twofold increase in the severity of menopausal symptoms (higher total Menopause Rating Scale (MRS) scores), and a six to eight times higher risk of impaired quality of life. Higher educational level was associated with fewer complaints of insomnia and better sleep quality [51].

Treatment options

Symptomatic treatment of insomnia can be achieve with standard hypnotics. Various studies have reported efficacy of zolpidem at 10 mg [52] and trazodone [53], as well as other frequently used medications, as already discussed under treatment of insomnia.

The decision to use hormone replacement should be individualized for the patient and depends on multiple factors. There may be beneficial effects of variable estrogen preparations on subjective sleep [54,55]. There have also been reports that combined estrogen–progestin regimens may lead to improved markers of information processing and attention [56]. A recent randomized, double-blind, placebo-controlled study of either 300 mg of progesterone or placebo taken in the evening for 3 weeks indicated that, objectively evaluated, sleep was improved [57]. Another study reported improved hot flashes and sleep with a transdermal gel containing 0.75 mg estradiol, which was well tolerated [58].

On the other hand, the use of estrogen replacement should be considered with caution because of its potential role in cerebrovascular events [59]. Alternatives to medication may include nonpharmacological treatment such as psychotherapy, either alone or in combination with hormone replacement therapy [60].

Summary

♦ Sleep is affected by gonadal hormones.

♦ Sleep complaints may vary with the menstrual cycle.

♦ Sleep may also change with the menstrual cycle, during pregnancy, and in menopause.

◆ Some sleep disorders are more common in women, while others may have a different presentation in women.

◆ Lifestyle factors and comorbidities modify the effects of any menstrual irregularities on sleep.

◆ Treatment of sleep disorders in women should consider pregnancy plans, especially when medications with potential teratogenic effects are prescribed.

References

1. Morin CM, LeBlanc M, Bélanger L, et al. Prevalence of insomnia and its treatment in Canada. Can J Psychiatry 2011;56(9):540–8.

2. Ford DE, Cooper-Patrick L. Sleep disturbances and mood disorders: an epidemiologic perspective. Depress Anxiety 2001;14(1):3–6.

3. Kim WH, Kim BS, Kim SK, et al. Prevalence of insomnia and associated factors in a community sample of elderly individuals in South Korea. Int Psychogeriatr 2013;25(10):1729–37.

4. American Academy of Sleep Medicine. International classification of sleep disorders: diagnostic and coding manual, 2nd ed. Darien, IL: American Academy of Sleep Medicine, 2005.

5. Voderholzer U, Al-Shajlawi A, Weske G, Feige B, Riemann D. Are there gender differences in objective and subjective sleep measures? A study of insomniacs and healthy controls. Depress Anxiety 2003;17(3):162–72.

6. Budhiraja R, Roth T, Hudgel DW, Budhiraja P, Drake CL. Prevalence and polysomnographic correlates of insomnia comorbid with medical disorders. Sleep 2011;34(7):859–67.

7. Khazaie H, Ghadami MR, Knight DC, Emamian F, Tahmasian M. Insomnia treatment in the third trimester of pregnancy reduces postpartum depression symptoms: a randomized clinical trial. Psychiatry Res 2013;210(3):901–5.

8. Gilboa SM, Strickland MJ, Olshan AF, et al. Use of antihistamine medications during early pregnancy and isolated major malformations. Birth Defects Res A Clin Mol Teratol 2009;85(2):137–50.

9. Billiard M, Guilleminault C, Dement WC. A menstruation-linked periodic hypersomnia. Kleine–Levin syndrome or new clinical entity? Neurology 1975;25(5):436–43.

10. Billiard M, Jaussent I, Dauvilliers Y, Besset A. Recurrent hypersomnia: a review of 339 cases. Sleep Med Rev 2011;15(4):247–57.

11. Kapsimalis F, Kryger M. Sleep breathing disorders in the U.S. female population. J Womens Health (Larchmt) 2009;18(8):1211–19.

12. Ye L, Pien GW, Ratcliffe SJ, Weaver TE. Gender differences in obstructive sleep apnea and treatment response to continuous positive airway pressure. J Clin Sleep Med 2009;5(6):512–18.

13. O'Connor C, Thornley KS, Hanly PJ. Gender differences in the polysomnographic features of obstructive sleep apnea. Am J Respir Crit Care Med 2000;161(5):1465–72.

14. Pavlova MK, Duffy JF, Shea SA. Polysomnographic respiratory abnormalities in asymptomatic individuals. Sleep 2008;31(2):241–8.

15. Young T, Evans L, Finn L, Palta M. Estimation of the clinically diagnosed proportion of sleep apnea syndrome in middle-aged men and women. Sleep 1997;20:705–6.

16. Nieto FJ, Young TB, Lind BK, et al. Association of sleep-disordered breathing, sleep apnea, and hypertension in a large community-based study. Sleep Heart Health Study. JAMA 2000;283(14):1829–36.

17. Shahar E, Whitney CW, Redline S, et al. Sleep-disordered breathing and cardiovascular disease: cross-sectional results of the Sleep Heart Health Study. Am J Respir Crit Care Med 2001;163(1):19–25.

18. Redline S, Yenokyan G, Gottlieb DJ, et al. Obstructive sleep apnea–hypopnea and incident stroke: the sleep heart health study. Am J Respir Crit Care Med 2010;182(2):269–77.

19. McDaid C, Durée KH, Griffin SC, et al. A systematic review of continuous positive airway pressure for obstructive sleep apnoea–hypopnoea syndrome. Sleep Med Rev 2009;13(6):427–36.

20. Budhiraja P, Budhiraja R, Goodwin JL, et al. Incidence of restless legs syndrome and its correlates. J Clin Sleep Med 2012;8(2):119–24.

21. Aurora RN, Kristo D, Bista SR, et al. The treatment of restless legs syndrome and periodic limb movement disorder in adults—an update for 2012: practice parameters with an evidence-based systematic review and meta-analyses. An American Academy of Sleep Medicine Clinical Practice Guideline. Sleep 2012;35:1039–62.

22. Cornelius JR, Tippmann-Peikert M, Slocumb NL, Frerichs CF, Silber MH. Impulse control disorders with the use of dopaminergic agents in restless legs syndrome: a case-control study. Sleep 2010;33(1):81–7.

23. Sachs C, Svanborg E. The exploding head syndrome: polysomnographic recordings and therapeutic suggestions. Sleep 1991;14(3):263–6.

24. Coren S. The prevalence of self-reported sleep disturbances in young adults. Int J Neurosci 1994;79(1–2):67–73.

25. Ohayon MM, Morselli PL, Guilleminault C. Prevalence of nightmares and their relationship to psychopathology and daytime functioning in insomnia subjects. Sleep 1997;20(5):340–8.

26. Ohayon M, Caulet M, Priest R. Violent behavior during sleep. J Clin Psychiatr 1997;58:369–376.

27. Fallone G, Seifer R, Acebo C, Carskadon MA. How well do school-aged children comply with imposed sleep schedules at home? Sleep 2002;25(7):739–45.

28. Shibui K, Uchiyama M, Okawa M, et al. Diurnal fluctuation of sleep propensity and hormonal secretion across the menstrual cycle. Biol Psychiatry 2000;48(11):1062–8.

29. Baker FC, Driver HS. Circadian rhythms, sleep, and the menstrual cycle. Sleep Med 2007;8(6):613–22.

30. Shechter A, Varin F, Boivin DB. Circadian variation of sleep during the follicular and luteal phases of the menstrual cycle. Sleep 2010;33(5):647–56.

31. Baker FC, Driver HS. Self-reported sleep across the menstrual cycle in young, healthy women. J Psychosom Res 2004;56(2):239–43.

32. Shechter A, Lespérance P, Ng Ying Kin NM, Boivin DB. Nocturnal polysomnographic sleep across the menstrual cycle in premenstrual dysphoric disorder. Sleep Med 2012;13(8):1071–8.

33. Strine TW, Chapman DP, Ahluwalia IB. Menstrual-related problems and psychological distress among women in the United States. J Womens Health (Larchmt) 2005;14(4):316–23.

34. Driver HS, McLean H, Kumar DV, et al. The influence of the menstrual cycle on upper airway resistance and breathing during sleep. Sleep 2005;28(4):449–56.

35. Hachul H, Andersen ML, Bittencourt LR, et al. Does the reproductive cycle influence sleep patterns in women with sleep complaints. Climacteric 2010;13:594–603.

36. Hedman C, Pohjasvaara T, Tolonen U, Suhonen-Malm AS, Myllylä VV. Effects of pregnancy on mothers' sleep. Sleep Med 2002;3(1):37–42.

37. Driver HS, McLean H, Kumar DV, et al. The influence of the menstrual cycle on upper airway resistance and breathing during sleep. Sleep 2005;28(4):449–56.

38. Ursavaş A, Karadağ M. Sleep breathing disorders in pregnancy. Tuberk Toraks 2009;57(2):237–43.

39. Kessler L, Nedeltcheva A, Imperial J, Penev PD. Changes in serum TSH and free T4 during human sleep restriction. Sleep 2010;33(8):1115–18.

40. Buxton OM, Pavlova M, Reid EW, et al. Sleep restriction for 1 week reduces insulin sensitivity in healthy men. Diabetes 2010;59(9):2126–33.

41. Leproult R, Van Reeth O, Byrne MM, Sturis J, Van Cauter E. Sleepiness, performance, and neuroendocrine function during sleep deprivation: effects of exposure to bright light or exercise. J Biol Rhythms 1997;12(3):245–58.

42. Schwartz MD, Mong JA. Estradiol modulates recovery of REM sleep in a time-of-day-dependent manner. Am J Physiol Regul Integr Comp Physiol 2013;305(3):R271–80.

43. Williams MA, Miller RS, Qiu C, et al. Associations of early pregnancy sleep duration with trimester-specific blood pressures and hypertensive disorders in pregnancy. Sleep 2010;33(10):1363–71.

44. Bonzini M, Palmer KT, Coggon D, et al. Shift work and pregnancy outcomes: a systematic review with meta-analysis of currently available epidemiological studies. BJOG 2011;118(12):1429–37.

45. Poyares D, Guilleminault C, Hachul H, et al. Pre-eclampsia and nasal CPAP: Part 2. Hypertension during pregnancy, chronic snoring, and early nasal CPAP intervention. Sleep Med 2007;9(1):15–21.

46. Young T, Rabago D, Zgierska A, Austin D, Laurel F. Objective and subjective sleep quality in premenopausal, perimenopausal, and postmenopausal women in the Wisconsin Sleep Cohort Study. Sleep 2003;26(6):667–72.

47. Cheng MH, Hsu CY, Wang SJ, et al. The relationship of self-reported sleep disturbance, mood, and menopause in a community study. Menopause 2008;15(5):958–62.

48. Brown JP, Gallicchio L, Flaws JA, Tracy JK. Relations among menopausal symptoms, sleep disturbance and depressive symptoms in midlife. Maturitas 2009;62(2):184–9.

49. Cray L, Woods NF, Mitchell ES. Symptom clusters during the late menopausal transition stage: observations from the Seattle Midlife Women's Health Study. Menopause 2010;17(5):972–7.

50. Constantine GD, Bruyniks N, Princic N, et al. Incidence of genitourinary conditions in women with a diagnosis of vulvar/vaginal atrophy. Curr Med Res Opin 2014;30:143–8.

51. Blümel JE, Cano A, Mezones-Holguín E, et al. Collaborative Group for Research of the Climacteric in Latin America (REDLINC). A multinational study of sleep disorders during female mid-life. Maturitas 2012;72(4):359–66.

52. Dorsey CM, Lee KA, Scharf MB. Effect of zolpidem on sleep in women with perimenopausal and postmenopausal insomnia: a 4-week, randomized, multicenter, double-blind, placebo-controlled study. Clin Ther 2004;26(10):1578–86.

53. Pansini F, Albertazzi P, Bonaccorsi G, et al. Trazodone: a non-hormonal alternative for neurovegetative climacteric symptoms. Clin Exp Obstet Gynecol 1995;22(4):341–4.

54. Silva BH, Martinez D, Wender MC. A randomized, controlled pilot trial of hormone therapy for menopausal insomnia. Arch Womens Ment Health 2011;14(6):505–8.

55. Tranah GJ, Parimi N, Blackwell T, et al. Postmenopausal hormones and sleep quality in the elderly: a population based study. BMC Womens Health 2010;10:15.

56. Anderer P, Semlitsch HV, Saletu B, et al. Effects of hormone replacement therapy on perceptual and cognitive event-related potentials in menopausal insomnia. Psychoneuroendocrinology 2003;28(3):419–45.

57. Caufriez A, Leproult R, L'Hermite-Balériaux M, Kerkhofs M, Copinschi G. Progesterone prevents sleep disturbances and modulates GH, TSH, and melatonin secretion in postmenopausal women. J Clin Endocrinol Metab 2011;96(4):E614–23.

58. Archer DF, Pickar JH, MacAllister DC, Warren MP. Transdermal estradiol gel for the treatment of symptomatic postmenopausal women. Menopause 2012;19(6):622–9.

59. Budhiraja R, Budhiraja P, Quan SF. Sleep-disordered breathing and cardiovascular disorders. Respir Care 2010;55(10):1322–32; discussion 1330–2. PMID: 20875159.

60. Anarte MT, Cuadros JL, Herrera J. Hormonal and psychological treatment: therapeutic alternative for menopausal women? Maturitas 199817;29(3):203–13.

Miscellaneous sleep-related topics

CHAPTER 52

Violent parasomnias and sleep forensics

Michel A. Cramer Bornemann and Mark R. Pressman

Introduction

Parasomnias are defined as unpleasant or undesirable physical events or experiential phenomena that occur during entry into sleep, within sleep, or during arousals from sleep. They were initially thought to represent a unitary phenomenon, often attributed to psychiatric disease. Indeed, the general public and popular media continue to be enamored of the belief that the unconscious mind, in a state of either hypnosis or sleep, may reveal itself in words, mental images, or behaviors although its meaning is kept at a distance from the conscious mind through repression. Various avenues for the interpretation of dreams have evolved based upon the premise that behaviors and/or experiences that arise from the platform of sleep are the result of a breakdown of psychic censorship and may thereby provide insight into the machinations of the unconscious mind. Such "Dream Theory," which may masquerade in subtle forms often involving the principle of "wish fulfillment," has been largely supplanted by testable as well as verifiable neuroscientific constructs to account for parasomnias. Now, careful clinical assessments, polysomnographic (PSG) studies, and refined neurodiagnostic imaging have revealed that parasomnias are not a unitary phenomenon, but rather represent a large number of completely different conditions, most of which are diagnosable and treatable. Furthermore, most are not the manifestation of psychiatric disorders and are far more prevalent than generally appreciated. Many parasomnias have the potential to compromise personal and public safety, particularly those in close proximity to the afflicted, as a result of abrupt outward and potentially injurious behaviors that arise from the platform of sleep.

The parasomnias may conveniently be categorized as "primary parasomnias" (disorders of the sleep states per se) or "secondary" (disorders of other organ systems that interfere with the sleep process). The primary parasomnias can be classified according to the sleep state of origin: rapid eye movement (REM) sleep, non-rapid eye movement (NREM) sleep, or miscellaneous (i.e., those involving but not respecting sleep state). The secondary parasomnias can be further classified by the organ system involved [1].

The concept that sleep and wakefulness are not invariably mutually exclusive states, and that the various state-determining variables of wakefulness, NREM sleep, and REM sleep may occur simultaneously or oscillate rapidly, is the key to understanding primary parasomnias. Recent advances in neurophysiology coupled with refined neurodiagnostic imaging modalities now reveal that the three states are modulated by a host of influences, including the degree of aminergic and cholinergic neurochemical bias, central nervous system (CNS) activation, and the degree of endogenous v exogenous input. Under normal physiological conditions, which include homeostatic drive and circadian rhythmicity, the process of state declaration is maintained in a stable and predictable fashion throughout a 24-hour period. However, as the components of sleep frequently dissociate and oscillate, sleep and wake may be rendered into a state that has not yet fully declared, thereby finding itself in a temporary unstable state of dissociation. Thus, sleep and wake, as well as the associated features of consciousness and unconsciousness, are not dichotomous states, as they occur on a spectrum and are evanescent. The admixture of wakefulness and NREM sleep explains confusional arousals (sleep-drunkenness), automatic behaviors, or microsleeps [2]. The admixture of wakefulness and REM sleep explains cataplexy, wakeful dreaming, hypnagogic hallucinations, lucid dreaming, and the persistence of motor activity during REM sleep (REM sleep behavior disorder, RBD) [3].

The primary parasomnias are clinical phenomena that appear as the brain becomes reorganized across states and therefore are particularly prone to occur during transitions between states. In view of (1) the large number of neural networks involving approximately 100 billion neurons, neurotransmitters, and other state-determining substances that must be recruited synchronously for full state declaration and (2) the frequent transitions among states during the wake–sleep cycle, it is surprising that errors in state declaration do not occur more frequently than they do [2].

This chapter focuses on the acute violent, potentially harmful, and inappropriate, as well as asocial, behaviors associated with sleep triggered by the two most common forms of primary parasomnias (disorders of arousal and RBD), with a subsequent discussion of the forensic issues engendered by these parasomnias.

Disorders of arousal

Disorders of arousal are NREM sleep parasomnias that occur on a broad spectrum and include confusional arousals, sleepwalking, and sleep terrors. The underlying pathophysiology is state dissociation, whereby neither wake nor NREM has been completely declared. Simply stated, the brain is partially awake and partially in NREM sleep. The result of this mixed state of being is that the brain is awake enough to perform potentially very complex behaviors, yet asleep enough to not have conscious awareness.

Disorders of arousal share many common features. They tend to arise from any stage of NREM sleep, most commonly from slow-wave sleep (SWS: stage N3, formerly stages 3 and 4 of NREM sleep), and therefore they usually occur in the first third of the sleep cycle and hence rarely during naps. They are common in childhood, usually decreasing in frequency with increasing age [4].

Disorders of arousal may be associated with prior sleep deprivation, physical activity, or emotional stress. Medication-induced cases have been reported with sedative–hypnotics, neuroleptics, minor tranquilizers, stimulants, and antihistamines, often in combination with each other [4]. Contrary to popular opinion, there is no compelling evidence that overt alcohol intoxication serves to trigger NREM parasomnias [5]. The recently published third edition of the International Classification of Sleep Disorders (ICSD-3: the primary diagnostic, epidemiological, and coding resource for clinicians and researchers in somnology and Sleep Medicine, produced by the American Academy of Sleep Medicine, in association with the European Sleep Research Society, the Japanese Society of Sleep Research, and the Latin American Sleep Society) now states unequivocally that *"Sleepwalking should not be diagnosed in the presence of alcohol intoxication"* [6].

Recently, there have been numerous reports of extremely complex behaviors attributed to sedative–hypnotic agents, often resulting in forensic issues [7–15]. In some women, disorders of arousal may be exacerbated by pregnancy or menstruation, whereas in others, disorders of arousal may be alleviated by pregnancy, suggesting hormonal influences [4]. Underlying predisposing, priming, and precipitating factors have been thoroughly reviewed elsewhere [16].

Numerous other sleep disorders that result in arousals (obstructive sleep apnea (OSA), nocturnal seizures, or periodic limb movements) may provoke these disorders [17]. Sleep disordered breathing (SDB) has been found to be more prevalent in both children and adults with disorders of arousal. One recent study found that sleep fragmentation induced by SDB is more common in adults with disorders of arousal than in normal subjects [18]. The combination of frequent arousals and sleep deprivation seen in these other sleep disorders provides fertile ground for the appearance of disorders of arousal. These represent a sleep disorder within a sleep disorder: the clinical event is a disorder of arousal, but the true culprit is a different, unrelated sleep disorder. This would explain the common clinical experience of improvement of disorders of arousal following identification and treatment of OSA [19]. Conversely, effective treatment of OSA with nasal continuous positive airway pressure (CPAP) may result in disorders of arousal, presumably associated with deep NREM sleep rebound [20, 21].

Numerous studies have dispelled the myth that persistence of these behaviors beyond childhood or appearance in adulthood is suggestive of underlying psychopathology [22–24]. In one study in children, there was an association between disorders of arousal and anxiety [25]. Other studies have noted an elevated frequency of disorders of arousal in individuals diagnosed and treated for severe psychological disorders. However, there is no evidence of causation, and nocturnal wandering may be secondary to the effects of highly sedating medications. These arousals may not be the culmination of ongoing psychologically significant mentation, in that somnambulism can be induced in normal children by standing them up during SWS, and sleep terrors can be precipitously triggered in susceptible individuals by sounding a buzzer during SWS [26–29].

The mechanism of these disorders is not clear, but it is evident both genetic and environmental factors are involved [30]. It has been suggested that sleep terrors may be the manifestation of anomalous REM sleep admixed with NREM sleep [31].

Pathogenesis

In addition to the phenomenon of state dissociation, in which two states of being overlap or occur simultaneously, there are likely additional underlying physiological phenomena that contribute to the appearance of complex motor behaviors during sleep. These include locomotor centers, sleep inertia, and sleep state instability.

Locomotor centers

Locomotor centers (LMCs), present in multiple sites in the CNS, may play a role in the disorders of arousal, which represent motor activity that is dissociated from waking consciousness [32]. These areas project to the central pattern generator of the spinal cord, which itself is able to produce complex stepping movements in the absence of supraspinal influence [33]. This accounts for the fact that decorticate experimental and barnyard animals are capable of performing very complex, integrated motor acts [34]. A biological substrate is further supported by the similarity between spontaneously occurring sleep terrors in humans and "sham rage" induced in animals [35–37]. Indeed, human neuropathology may result in similar behaviors [38–42]. Dissociation of the LMCs from the parent state of NREM sleep would explain the presence of complex motor behavior seen in disorders of arousal. Spontaneous locomotion following decerebration in cats clearly indicates that such centers, if dysfunctional, release motor activity into the sleeping state [43,44]. Single photon emission computed tomography (SPECT) study involving an individual with sleep terrors suggested activation of thalamocingulate pathways with persistent deactivation of other thalamocortical arousal systems, resulting in a dissociation between body sleep and mind sleep [45].

Sleep inertia

Sleep inertia (also termed sleep drunkenness) refers to a period of impaired performance and reduced vigilance following awakening from the regular sleep episode or from a nap. This impairment may be severe, last from minutes to hours, and be accompanied by PSG-recorded microsleep episodes [46]. Support of a gradual disengagement from sleep to wakefulness comes from neurophysiologic studies in animals and cerebral blood flow studies in humans [47–50]. There appears to be great inter-individual variability in the extent and duration of sleep inertia, both following spontaneous awakening after the major sleep period and following naps. Sleep inertia likely plays a role in the susceptibility to disorders of arousal [47].

Sleep state instability

The cyclic alternating pattern (CAP) may also play a role in the etiology of disorders of arousal [51]. CAP is a physiological component of NREM sleep and is functionally correlated with long-lasting arousal oscillations. CAP is a measure of NREM instability with high level of arousal oscillation [52]. More sophisticated monitoring techniques such as topographical EEG mapping suggest that there may be more delta EEG activity prior to the onset of sleep terrors [53]. There is no difference in the macrostructural sleep parameters between patients with disorders of arousal and controls. However, patients with disorders of arousal have been found to have increases in CAP rate, in the number of CAP cycles, and in arousals with EEG synchronization. An increase in sleep instability and in arousal oscillation is a typical microstructural feature of SWS-related parasomnias and may play a role in triggering abnormal motor episodes during sleep in these patients [54,55]. Microarousals preceded by EEG slow-wave synchronization during NREM sleep are more frequent in patients with sleepwalking and sleep terrors than in controls. This supports the existence of an arousal disorder in these individuals [54]. Although some have reported hypersynchronous delta activity on PSGs of young adults with sleepwalking, this has not been the experience of others [56,57]. EEG spectral analysis studies indicate that patients with sleepwalking demonstrate instability of SWS, particularly in the early portion of the sleep period [58]. Impairment of efficiency of inhibitory cortical circuits during wakefulness has also been reported [59].

Clinical features

Disorders of arousal occur on a broad spectrum ranging from confusional arousals, through somnambulism (sleepwalking), to sleep terrors (also termed pavor nocturnus and, erroneously, incubus or succubus). Some take the form of "specialized" behaviors (discussed later) such as sleep-related eating and sleep-related sexual activity, executed without conscious awareness.

Confusional arousals

These are often seen in children and are characterized by movements in bed, occasionally thrashing about, or inconsolable crying [60]. "Sleep drunkenness" is probably a variation on this theme [61]. The prevalence of confusional arousals in adults is approximately 4% [62].

Sleepwalking

Sleepwalking is prevalent in childhood (1–17%), peaking at 11–12 years of age, and is far more common in adults (nearly 4%) than is generally acknowledged [62–65]. Sleepwalking may be either calm or agitated, with varying degrees of complexity and duration.

Sleep terrors

The sleep terror is the most dramatic disorder of arousal. It is frequently initiated by a loud, blood-curdling scream associated with extreme panic, followed by prominent motor activity such as hitting the wall, running around or out of the bedroom, even out of the house, resulting in bodily injury or property damage. A universal feature is inconsolability. Although the victim appears to be awake, he or she usually misperceives the environment, and attempts at consolation are futile and may serve only to prolong or even intensify the confusional state. Some degree of perception may be evident—for example, running for and opening a door or window. Complete amnesia for the activity is typical, but it may be incomplete [26,66,67]. The intense endogenous arousal and exogenous unarousability constitute a curious paradox. As with sleepwalking, sleep terrors are much more prevalent in adults than is generally acknowledged (4–5%) [68]. Although usually benign, these behaviors may be violent, resulting in considerable injury to the victim or others or damage to the environment, occasionally with forensic implications (see the discussion later in this chapter).

Specialized forms of disorders of arousal

Sleep-related eating disorder

Sleep-related eating disorder (SRED) is likely a specialized form of disorder of arousal and consists of recurrent episodes of involuntary eating and drinking during arousals from sleep associated with diminished levels of consciousness and recall. SRED is often not associated with waking eating disorders and needs to be distinguished from the night-eating syndrome (NES), as the latter is characterized by morning anorexia, evening hyperphagia (while awake), and insomnia and is associated with hypothalamic–pituitary axis abnormalities [69–71]. Nocturnal binging may be induced by benzodiazepine-class medications, and sleep-related eating has been associated with the administration of olanzapine and non-benzodiazepine class medications, particularly zolpidem [11,12,72,73].

The episodes of SRED are involuntary and exhibit seemingly "out of control" disinhibited unrestrained behaviors after an interval of sleep, usually associated with partial arousals from sleep. Subsequently, not uncommonly, there is partial recall, though the ability for recall is variable. Some patients cannot be easily brought to full consciousness during an episode of eating, similar to conventional sleepwalking, and may have no recall of having eaten during the night. In contrast, some patients appear to exhibit considerable alertness during an episode, though impulse control remains absent, while maintaining substantial recall the following morning. A majority of individuals with SRED report a nightly frequency of eating, which may occur several times in a given evening and is not partial to any particular time during the sleep cycle. High-caloric foods, often carbohydrates, are preferentially consumed. Food items characteristically consumed during sleep-related eating are not typically consumed with preference during the daytime. Curiously, hunger and thirst are notably absent during episodes of compulsive eating with SRED. The episodes of eating may be experienced as food-related enactment of a dream. Alcoholic beverages are almost never consumed. If an individual is confronted during an episode, the usual response is irritability and agitation.

Recurrent SRED has potential for a broad range of deleterious consequences, which may include (1) consumption of inedible odd combinations of food or toxic substances (eg, buttered cigarettes, cat food, coffee grounds, or ammonia cleaning solutions); (2) sleep-related injury (eg, blunt trauma or lacerations related to manipulation errors of kitchen utensils or heavy dishware; internal or external burns associated with consuming/spilling hot foods or beverages or inadvertent contact with stove burners; or poisoning or internal injuries from ingesting toxic substances); and (3) adverse health consequences (obesity, hypercholesterolemia, hypertriglyceridemia, destabilization of diabetes mellitus type 1 or 2, dental caries, or allergic reactions). Reactive depression may be anticipated as a consequence of personal dejection and sense of failure over the apparent inability to control nocturnal eating. Formal sleep studies are indicated, as SRED may be the manifestation of other sleep disorders such as restless legs syndrome (RLS, also now known as Willis–Ekbom disease), periodic limb movements in sleep (PLMS), or OSA, all of which destabilize sleep and predispose to arousal [66].

Sleep-related abnormal sexual behaviors

Sleep-related abnormal sexual behaviors are now formally recognized by ICSD-3. Sleep-related abnormal sexual behaviors are classified with the disorders of arousal (DOA) from NREM sleep. Of the subtypes of DOA, such sexualized behaviors are most often associated with confusional arousals, but may be associated with other types of parasomnias, such as sleepwalking. This condition has been referred to by many terms in the medical literature and popular media, including "Atypical sexual behavior during sleep," "Sexual behavior in sleep," "Sleep Sex," and "Sexsomnia." Inappropriate sexual behaviors occurring during the sleep state without conscious awareness, presumably the results of an admixture of wakefulness and sleep, have been reported [74]. A broad spectrum of such behaviors exist and may be expressed as sexualized vocalizations or self-stimulatory/autoerotic touching, or may engage those who are in close proximity, such as a bed partner. The persistence of these sexual behaviors may result in feelings of guilt, shame, or depression, and may lead to marital discord in some cases [75].

Despite the increased general awareness and formal clinical recognition, much confusion remains about sleep-related abnormal sexual behaviors, particularly as a multitude of medical, psychiatric, and toxic conditions may have similar features or may mimic this condition [76]. Accurate diagnosis is not only essential as it translates into an effective clinical management strategy with the most favorable benefit-to-risk ratio, but also may have significant legal implications. For instance, the "Sleepwalking Defense" has been well received by defense attorneys and has been successfully applied in the USA in cases of purported "sexsomnia," resulting in a complete acquittal, as in *State of Oregon v. James Kirchner* [77]. Cramer Bornemann presented at the APSS (the Associated Professional Sleep Societies) annual meeting in Minneapolis, Minnesota that over 33% of the more than 260 forensics cases submitted between 2006 and 2013 for formal medico-legal review to a sleep forensics consulting consortium were associated with charges of sexual assault for which a sleep-related abnormal sexual behavior was considered [78]. Despite the broad clinical acceptance of this condition and some success in the court of law, many in the legal community remain skeptical over the legitimacy of "sexsomnia," as demonstrated by a recent update put forth by the National Center for the Prosecution of Child Abuse entitled *Overcoming the Sleep Disorder Defense* [79]. In this regard, in the USA, Daubert or Frye Hearings are not uncommon to attest to the legitimacy of sleep-related abnormal sexual behaviors in the determination of admissibility of potential testimony prior to the formal court room trial.

Diagnosis

Isolated, often bizarre, sleep-related events may be experienced by perfectly normal people, and most do not warrant further extensive or expensive evaluation. The initial approach to the complaint of unusual sleep-related behavior is to determine whether further evaluation is necessary. The patient should be queried regarding the exact nature of the events. Because many of these episodes may be associated with partial or complete amnesia, additional descriptive information from a bed partner or other observer may prove invaluable. Home videotapes of the clinical event may be quite helpful. In general, indications for formal evaluation of parasomnias include behaviors that [1]:

♦ are potentially violent or injurious;

♦ are extremely disruptive to other household members;

♦ result in the complaint of excessive daytime sleepiness;

♦ are associated with medical, psychiatric, or neurological symptoms or findings.

Formal PSG studies, appropriately performed, will provide direct or indirect diagnostic information in the majority of cases. This is of more than academic interest, as most of these conditions are readily treatable. Emphasis must be placed on the types of studies required; routine PSGs performed for conventional sleep disorders are inadequate. In addition to the physiological parameters monitored in the standard PSG, there must be an expanded EEG montage and continuous audiovisual monitoring [56,80].

Observation by an experienced technologist is invaluable. Multiple night studies may be required to capture an event. Interpretation should be made by a polysomnographer experienced in these disorders. Sleep deprivation prior to formal PSG study may increase the likelihood of capturing an event in the sleep laboratory [81]. Unattended studies have no role in the evaluation of parasomnias [82]. Formal sleep studies are indicated to establish a clinical diagnosis, but are of limited utility in forensic cases (discussed later in this chapter). A negative study is not sufficient to rule out a diagnosis of a disorder of arousal, as PSG findings have both low specificity and low sensitivity. The diagnosis of a disorder of arousal remains primarily a clinical diagnosis.

Differential diagnosis

Numerous other conditions may perfectly mimic the disorders of arousal. These include OSA, RBD, nocturnal seizures, psychogenic dissociative disorders, malingering, or psychopathy [83–85]. NREM parasomnias may be particularly difficult to differentiate from nocturnal epileptic phenomena [86]. There may be an association between disorders of arousal and migraine headache [87], neurofibromatosis type 1 [88], or Tourette syndrome [89,90]. In children unable to verbalize, nocturnal cluster or migraine headaches may mimic sleep terrors [91]. OSA may be associated with and even present as disorders of arousal [18,85,92].

Treatment

Given the high prevalence of these disorders in normal individuals, formal sleep center evaluation should be confined to the situations listed above. Treatment is often not necessary. Reassurance of their typically benign nature, lack of psychological significance, and the tendency to diminish over time is often sufficient. Objective studies documenting medication efficacy are lacking. Tricyclic antidepressants and benzodiazepines may be effective and should be administered if the behaviors are dangerous to person or property or extremely disruptive to family members [61]. Paroxetine and trazodone have been reported to be effective in isolated cases of disorders of arousal [93,94]. Nonpharmacological treatment such as psychotherapy [28], progressive relaxation [95], or hypnosis [96] is recommended for long-term management. Anticipatory awakening has been reported to be effective in treating sleepwalking in children [97]. The avoidance of precipitants such as drugs and sleep deprivation is also important. Sleep-related eating may respond to topiramate or dopaminergic agents [66]. Systematic studies of pharmacological treatment of sleep-related abnormal sexual behavior are lacking.

REM sleep behavior disorder

Numerous physiologic phenomena occur during REM sleep and fall into two categories: (1) tonic (appearing throughout a REM period) and (2) phasic (occurring intermittently during a REM period). Tonic elements include electromyographic (EMG) suppression, low voltage desynchronized EEG, high arousal threshold, hippocampal theta rhythm, elevated brain temperature, poikilo-thermia, olfactory bulb activity, and penile tumescence. Phasic elements include REMs, middle ear muscle activity (MEMA), tongue movements, periorbital integrated potentials (PIPs), somatic muscle–limb twitches, variability of autonomic activity (cardiac and respiratory), and pontogeniculo-occipital (PGO) spikes. It is not known whether dreaming occurs tonically or phasically during REM sleep [98].

The tonic and phasic neurophysiological processes underlying each state can be variously dissociated and recombined across states [99]. For REM sleep, the processes that generally occur in concert may also be seen in dissociated form—both experimentally (eg, REM sleep-deprived animals with PGO spikes occurring in NREM sleep and wakefulness) [100] and in human and animal disease (narcolepsy). In narcolepsy, the best-understood dissociated state, the sleep attacks, hypnagogic hallucinations, sleep paralysis, cataplexy, and automatic behavior each represent the intrusion or persistence of one state of being into another—i.e, cataplexy may be the inappropriate isolated intrusion of REM sleep atonia (REM atonia) into wakefulness, usually induced by an emotionally laden event [101,102].

The most common and best-studied REM sleep parasomnia is the RBD. In patients with RBD, somatic muscle atonia, one of the defining features of REM sleep, is absent, permitting the acting out of dream mentation (or the dreaming out of fictive movements), often with violent or injurious results [103].

Ohayon et al. conducted a telephone survey using the Sleep-EVAL expert system on 4972 individuals between the ages of 15 and 100 years of age, which indicated an overall prevalence of violent behaviors in general during sleep of 2%, one-quarter of which were likely due to RBD, giving an overall prevalence of RBD of 0.5% [104]. Another survey estimated the prevalence of REM sleep behavior to be 0.38% in elderly individuals [105].

Pathogenesis

The generalized atonia of REM sleep results from active inhibition of motor activity by pontine centers of the peri-locus coeruleus region that exert an excitatory influence upon the reticularis magnocellularis nucleus of the medulla via the lateral tegmentoreticular tract. The reticularis magnocellularis nucleus, in turn, hyperpolarizes spinal motoneuron postsynaptic membranes via the ventrolateral reticulospinal tract [106,107]. Loss of muscle tone during REM sleep in normal individuals is very complex and has been shown to be due to a combination of activation of brainstem motor inhibitory systems and inactivation of brainstem facilitatory systems [108,109]. Normally, the atonia of REM sleep is briefly interrupted by excitatory inputs that produce the rapid eye movements and the muscle jerks and twitches characteristic of REM sleep [110–112]. REM atonia is felt to be mediated by glycine and may be influenced by medullary enkephalinergic neurons [113,14]. (The prevailing hypothesis that REM atonia is due to glycinergic inhibition has been questioned and modified [115].)

Neuroimaging studies indicate dopaminergic abnormalities in RBD. Various types of neuroimaging studies in patients with idiopathic RBD have been performed. Using proton magnetic resonance spectroscopy (^{1}H-MRS), Miyamoto et al. detected an increase in the choline/creatine ratio in the pons of a 69-year-old man with idiopathic RBD and interpreted these findings as demonstrating functional impairment on the cell membrane level

[116]. However, Iranzo et al. performed ^{1}H-MRS in 15 patients with idiopathic RBD to determine if midbrain or pontine tegmentum abnormalities could be detected compared with matched controls and did not find any significant metabolic disturbances, including the choline/creatine ratio [117]. Despite this discrepancy, neuroimaging studies performed on patients with idiopathic RBD support the relationship between RBD and neurodegenerative disorders. Eisensehr et al. used [^{123}I](N)-(3-iodopropene-2-yl)-2β-carbomethoxy-3β-(4-chlorophenyl)tropane (IPT)-SPECT, which reflects presynaptic dopaminergic transporter integrity, and [^{123}I](S)-2-hydroxy-3-iodo-6-methoxy-([1-ethyl-2-pyrrolidinyl] methyl)benzamide (IBZM)-SPECT, which reflects postsynaptic dopaminergic D_2 receptor integrity, to investigate dopaminergic parameters in patients with RBD, Parkinson disease (PD), and controls [118]. They found that IPT uptake was highest in controls, lower in patients with "subclinical" RBD, even lower in clinically manifest RBD, and lowest yet in patients with PD. Muscle activity during REM sleep was independently associated with reduction of striatal dopamine transporters. There was, however, no significant difference in IBZM uptake between the groups. These findings suggest that there is a continuum of reduced striatal dopamine transporters involved in the pathophysiological mechanisms causing increased muscle activity during REM sleep in patients with "subclinical" RBD [119]. Positron emission tomography (PET) using dihydrotetrabenazine (DTBZ) was utilized by Albin et al. to compare findings in elderly subjects with idiopathic RBD with those in similarly aged controls [120]. As these RBD subjects exhibited a reduction of striatal binding of DTBZ compared with controls, the results suggest a reduction in dopaminergic substantia nigra neurons. This finding appears to be consistent with the hypothesis that RBD reflects an evolving degenerative parkinsonian disorder reflective of the dysfunction of the pedunculopontine nucleus (PPN) that is temporally coupled with basal ganglia dysfunction.

Currently, the most common cause of acute REM sleep without atonia and RBD may be iatrogenic. Acute RBD is almost always induced by medications (most commonly tricyclic antidepressants, monoamine oxidase inhibitors, selective serotonin reuptake inhibitors (SSRIs), or serotonin–norepinephrine reuptake inhibitors (SNRIs)) or associated with withdrawal (alcohol, barbiturate, or meprobamate) [103,121]. Excessive caffeine ingestion has also been implicated [122], as has chocolate ingestion [123]. The chronic form is most often either idiopathic or associated with neurological disorders. Each basic category of neurological disease (vascular, neoplastic, toxic/metabolic, infectious, degenerative, traumatic, congenital, and idiopathic) could be expected to result in RBD. Box 52.1 lists reported associations with RBD [124]. A familial association has been documented [125]. Spontaneously occurring idiopathic RBD has also been reported in dogs and cats [126,127].

The overwhelming male predominance of RBD (not seen in the associated neurodegenerative disorders) raises the intriguing question of hormonal influences, as suggested in male-aggression studies in both animals and humans [128–130]. Another possible explanation for the male predominance is sex differences in brain development and aging [131–133]. There is evidence for a sex difference in the effects of sex steroids on the development of the locus coeruleus in rats [134]. However, serum sex hormone levels are normal in idiopathic RBD or RBD associated with Parkinson disease [135,136]. Recent studies suggest that RBD may be more common in women than previously thought [137,138].

Box 52.1 Conditions associated with RBD

Amyotrophic lateral sclerosis

Autism

Brain stem parainfectious encephalitis (both RBD and narcolepsy)

Cerebrovascular disease

Group A xeroderma pigmentosum

Guillain–Barré syndrome

Implantation of subthalamic stimulator for Parkinson disease (isolated event)

Medication (particularly tricyclic antidepressants and SSRIs)

Möbius syndrome

Machado–Joseph disease (spinocerebellar ataxia type 3)

Multiple sclerosis

Narcolepsy

Paraneoplastic (anti-Ma2) encephalitis (both RBD and narcolepsy)

Parkinson disease associated with parkin mutations

Synucleinopathies (Parkinson disease, multiple system atrophy, dementia with Lewy bodies, pure autonomic failure)

Tauopathies (Alzheimer disease, progressive supranuclear palsy, corticobasal degeneration)

Tourette syndrome

Voltage-gated potassium channel antibody-associated limbic encephalitis

Adapted from Sleep Med Rev, 13(6), Mahowald, M.W. and C.H. Schenck, The REM sleep behavior disorder odyssey, pp. 381–4, Copyright (2009), with permission from Elsevier.

Clinical features

The cases reported to date indicate strikingly similar clinical features [103]. The presenting complaint is often vigorous sleep behaviors, usually accompanying incredibly vivid dreams. These behaviors may result in repeated injury, including ecchymoses, lacerations, and fractures. Some of the self-protection measures taken by patients (tethering themselves to the bed, using sleeping bags or pillow barricades, or sleeping on a mattress in an empty room) reveal the recurrent and serious nature of these episodes [139,140]. The potential for injury to self or bed partner raises interesting and difficult forensic medicine issues [138]. RBD may have serious psychological ramifications for the spouse: one woman threatened suicide because her husband with RBD could not share their bed [141].

Idiopathic RBD is commonly a chronic progressive disorder, with increasing complexity, intensity, and frequency of expressed behaviors, but the symptoms may fluctuate over time [142]. Although irregular jerking of the limbs may occur nightly, the major movement episodes appear intermittently with a frequency minimum of once in 2 weeks to a maximum of four times nightly on 10 consecutive nights. Observed somniloquy runs the spectrum from short and garbled to long-winded and clearly articulated. Angry speech with shouting, but also laughter, can emerge. One patient appeared to have a dissociated RBD-lucid dream state in that he could carry on lengthy and coherent conversations with his wife and family while dreaming and incorporate the conversational material into

his dreams. Most patients complain of sleep injury but rarely of sleep disruption.

In RBD patients, arousal from sleep to alertness and orientation is usually rapid and accompanied by complete dream recall (very unlike the confusional arousals observed in disorders of arousal such as sleepwalking or sleep terrors). After awakening, behavior and social interactions are appropriate, mitigating against a NREM sleep relationship, delirious states, or ictal/postictal phenomena, but rather further supporting a REM sleep phenomenon. It should be emphasized that the behaviors, although complex and violent, are of briefer duration than those seen in disorders of arousal. In some individuals, the clinical features contain elements of both RBD and disorders of arousal (see the section on RBD variations later in this chapter).

A singular feature of the dream-enacted episodes in this group of patients is that customary dreams are generally not being played out; rather, distinctly altered, stereotypical, repetitive, and "action-packed" dreams are put on display. The violence of the sleep-related behavior is often discordant with the waking personality. The increased aggressive dream content experienced by patients with RBD is not associated with increased daytime aggressiveness [143].

RBD and extrapyramidal disease

As more patients with "idiopathic" RBD are carefully followed over time, it is becoming clear that the majority will eventually develop neurodegenerative disorders, most notably the synucleinopathies: PD, multiple system atrophy (including olivopontocerebellar degeneration and the Shy–Drager syndrome), dementia with Lewy bodies, or pure autonomic failure. RBD may be the first manifestation of these conditions and may precede any other manifestation of the underlying neurodegenerative process by more than 10 years [144].

Systematic longitudinal study of patients with such neurological syndromes indicates that RBD and REM sleep without atonia may be far more prevalent than previously suspected. Although the prevalence of RBD in PD is unknown, subjective reports indicate that 25% of patients with PD have behaviors suggestive of RBD or sleep-related injurious behaviors, and PSG studies found RBD in up to 47% of patients with PD with sleep complaints [145–148]. In one large series of patients with multiple system atrophy, 90% were found to have REM sleep without atonia and 69% had clinical RBD [149], and in another, nearly half had RBD [150]. The presence of RBD may differentiate pure autonomic failure from multiple system atrophy with autonomic failure [151]. The finding of incidental Lewy bodies in one patient asymptomatic for PD suggests that this condition may explain idiopathic RBD in some older patients [152]. The presentation of RBD and dementia is suggestive enough of dementia with Lewy bodies that RBD has been proposed as one of the core diagnostic features of the latter [153]. The relationship between neurodegenerative disorders and RBD has been recently thoroughly reviewed [154].

The waking motor impairments of PD may improve or even normalize during REM sleep-related movements in PD–RBD patients. In a study of 53 patients with PD–RBD who slept with bed partners, 100% reported improvement of at least one of the following during RBD episodes: faster, stronger or smoother movements; more intelligible, louder, or better-articulated speech; or normalization of facial expression. Furthermore, 38% of bed partners reported that movements were "much better" even in the most disabled PD patients. The responsible mechanisms for these fascinating observations remain obscure [155].

RBD and narcolepsy

RBD may also be yet another manifestation of narcolepsy: it is present in over half of patients with narcolepsy, may be an early symptom in childhood narcolepsy, and may even be the presenting symptom in narcolepsy [156–160]. Furthermore, tricyclic antidepressants, monoamine oxidase inhibitors (MAOIs), SSRIs, and SNRIs, prescribed to treat cataplexy, can trigger or exacerbate RBD in this population. The demographics (age and sex) of RBD in narcolepsy conform to those of narcolepsy, indicating that RBD in these patients is yet another manifestation of the state boundary dyscontrol seen in narcolepsy [158].

Diagnosis

Routine medical history-taking should include questions that screen for abnormal sleep movements and altered dreams, especially in older adults, patients of any age with acute or chronic CNS disorders (particularly those who have neurological conditions that predispose to RBD such as PD or multiple system atrophy), and patients receiving psychoactive medications known to trigger RBD. The diagnosis of RBD may be suspected on clinical grounds, but PSG confirmation is mandatory. The complaint of sleep-related injurious or violent behaviors should be taken very seriously. Reported injuries in our series include lacerations and fractures to the patient and/or bed partner. RBD has also resulted in subdural hematomas and other serious injuries [161–163].

Detailed PSG data in these patients have been reported elsewhere [98]. The overall sleep architecture is usually normal, with the expected cycling of NREM and REM sleep. Most of the subjects had excessive SWS for age. The conventional scoring parameters of Rechtschaffen and Kales [164] must be modified to allow for the persistence of EMG tone during epochs that are otherwise clearly REM sleep. In addition to the intermittent absence of atonia, there are varying amounts of limb twitching (usually far in excess of that observed in normal REM sleep), gross body movements, and complex, often violent behaviors that correlate with reported dream mentation. A curious feature of the chin EMG and extremity movements seen during the REM period is the variability of involvement and distribution. The submental EMG may be augmented without body movements or may be atonic despite flailing extremities. The arms and legs often move independently, necessitating monitoring of all limbs. Some patients demonstrated persistent (over the span of several years) lateralization of limb EMG activity or also predominant upper or lower extremity movements. Most patients display prominent aperiodic movements of all extremities in every conceivable combination during all stages of NREM sleep. RBD patients may also show conventional periodic movements of sleep usually involving the legs during both NREM and REM sleep, infrequently associated with arousals. Prolonged periods of aperiodic and periodic movements restricted to the arms were noted occasionally.

The PSG marker of RBD is REM sleep without atonia (RWA) (Fig. 52.1). It must be remembered that RWA is a PSG observation and that RBD is a clinical syndrome of dream-enacting behavior

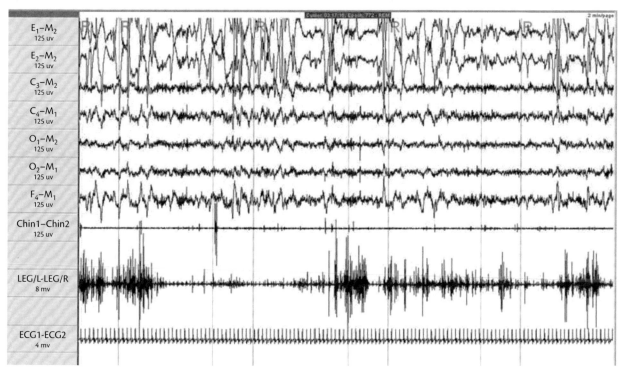

Fig. 52.1 Polysomnographic (PSG) example of REM sleep without atonia. This 2-minute epoch of REM sleep demonstrates prominent phasic anterior tibialis muscle electromyography. Note the persistence of atonia in the submentalis electromyogram. This is the PSG marker of REM sleep without atonia (RWA). This pattern may be seen in patients with or without a history of REM sleep behavior disorder (RBD). RWA in the absence of a history of RBD does not constitute RBD. The diagnosis of RBD depends upon PSG-documented RWA coupled with a clinical history of dream-enacting behaviors. E_1/E_2: left/right outer canthus; M_1/M_2: left/right mastoid; C_3/C_4: left/right central EEG; O_1/O_2: left/right occipital EEG; Chin: submentalis EMG; leg: anterior tibialis EMG; ECG: electrocardiogram.

associated with RWA. RWA often occurs without clinical symptoms and therefore, of itself, does not establish a diagnosis of RBD. The diagnosis of RBD requires both the clinical history of dream-enacting behavior coupled with the PSG finding of RWA. Some cases of RWA may represent "preclinical" RBD, and RWA is most commonly seen in association with medications, particularly SSRIs and SNRIs.

Diagnostic criteria (ICSD-3) [6]

A. Repeated episodes of sleep-related vocalization and/or complex motor behaviors.

B. These behaviors are documented by PSG to occur during REM sleep or, based on clinical history of dream enactment, are presumed to occur during REM sleep.

C. PSG recording demonstrates REM sleep without atonia (RWA).

D. The disturbance is not better explained by another sleep disorder, mental disorder, medication, or substance use.

Notes related to RBD diagnostic criteria

1. This criterion can be fulfilled by observation of repetitive episodes during a single night of video polysomnography.

2. The observed vocalizations or behaviors often correlate with simultaneously occurring dream mentation, leading to the frequent report of "acting out one's dreams."

3. The most current evidence-based data that are in accordance with AASM 30-s epoch scoring guidelines should be utilized.

4. Upon awakening, the individual is typically awake, alert, coherent, and oriented.

5. On occasion, there may be patients with a typical clinical history of RBD with dream-enacting behaviors who also exhibit typical RBD behaviors during video-PSG, but do not demonstrate sufficient RWA, based on the current evidence-based data, to satisfy the PSG criteria for diagnosing RBD. Such patients may be provisionally diagnosed with RBD, based on clinical judgment. The same rule applies when video-PSG is not readily available.

6. Medications may possibly unmask latent RBD with preexisting RWA, according to current expert opinion. Therefore, medication-induced RBD can be diagnosed as RBD, using clinical judgment, pending future longitudinal studies.

The determination of what constitutes either excessive EMG augmentation, EMG twitching, or limb jerking requires both meticulous execution of standard recording techniques and an experienced polysomnographer. Studies remain ongoing to better quantify RWA.

We recommend that any patient suspected of having RBD undergo a systematic evaluation consisting of the following:

1. A review of sleep/wake complaints (from patient and/or bed partner)

2. Neurological and psychiatric examinations

3. A sleep laboratory study that includes continuous videotaping of behavior during standard PSG monitoring of the electro-oculogram (EOG), EEG, EMG (chin, bilateral extensor digitorum, and anterior tibialis muscles), electrocardiogram (ECG), and nasal air flow [164]. An experienced and formally trained technician makes written observations of ongoing behaviors. It is strongly encouraged that such technicians be certified by the American Board of Registered Polysomnographic Technologists (RBPT).

4. As result of the association between RBD and narcolepsy, a multiple sleep latency test (MSLT) is routinely administered the day following the overnight sleep study, particularly in younger patients [165].

More extensive neurological evaluations, including multimodal evoked potentials, brain imaging by magnetic resonance imaging (MRI) or computerized axial tomography (CAT), or comprehensive neuropsychological testing by methods previously reported [166] are indicated only if there is a suggestion of neurological dysfunction by history or neurological examination.

Differential diagnosis

RBD can masquerade as many other conditions. Most conditions in this differential diagnosis represented an initial clinical misdiagnosis in our series, leading to inappropriate and ineffective treatment. The differential diagnosis of these disorders has been reviewed elsewhere [82]. It should be remembered that the clinical event (arousal) may not be primary, but rather triggered by another, underlying sleep disorder (eg, apnea leading to arousal leading to sleep terror). Nocturnal behaviors induced by OSA or sleep-related seizures can perfectly mimic those of RBD [167–169]. "Overlap" parasomnias (discussed later in this chapter) are characterized by a clinical history suggestive of sleepwalking/sleep terrors with PSG features of motor disinhibition during both REM and NREM sleep [170]. Nocturnal panic disorder is poorly understood and requires more study. It is well established that psychogenic dissociative disorders may arise predominately or exclusively from the sleep period [171]. Finally, our group has seen extremely violent sleep-period behavior felt to represent malingering [172].

Treatment

The acute form is self-limited following discontinuation of the offending medication or completion of withdrawal. About 90% of patients with chronic RBD respond well to clonazepam administered a half-hour prior to sleep time. The dose ranges from 0.5 to 2.0 mg, and there has been little, if any, tendency to develop tolerance, dependence, abuse, or adverse sleep effects despite years of continuous administration and efficacy [139,173]. Melatonin at doses up to 12 mg at bedtime or pramipexole may also be effective [174–177]. Although tricyclic antidepressants may sometimes induce or potentiate RBD, imipramine has been reported effective in three clonazepam-resistant cases [178]. Likewise, there are reports of response to an SSRI (paroxetine) [179,180]. Carbamazepine has been effective in one case [181]. Levodopa may be effective, particularly in cases where RBD is the harbinger of PD [182]. There have been anecdotal reports of response to gabapentin, MAOIs, donepezil, and clonidine [183,184]. In RBD associated with narcolepsy, the tricyclic antidepressants or MAOIs administered for cataplexy may be continued and clonazepam added [185]. The treatment of medication-induced or PD-associated RBD is the same as for idiopathic RBD [186]. Pallidotomy has been effective in one case of RBD associated with PD, whereas chronic bilateral subthalamic stimulation was not [187–189]. An isolated episode, however, of

RBD has been reported immediately following left subthalamic electrode implantation for the treatment of PD [190].

Underlying OSA should be ruled out before prescribing clonazepam [191]. Despite the often-dramatic clinical improvement with medications, the effect of clonazepam or melatonin on the PSG features of RBD is unimpressive. (Melatonin may restore some of the tonic REM atonia, and clonazepam may reduce excessive phasic EMG activity during REM sleep—but clearly incompletely [192,193].) This raises the possibility that these medications may act preferentially upon the locomotor systems rather than those affecting REM atonia [194].

The other essential therapeutic intervention concerns environmental safety. Clonazepam is not an absolute guarantee: one patient injured himself during a violent dream 1 year after initiating very satisfactory pharmacotherapy. There was no recurrence during the ensuing 5 months, even though the dose was not increased. Therefore, potentially dangerous objects, particularly firearms, should be removed from the bedroom, cushions positioned around the bed, consideration given to placing the mattress upon the floor, and windows protected. We anticipate some cases in which drug intolerance or ineffectiveness will lead to discontinuation, requiring maximal environmental safety.

RBD variations

Parasomnia overlap syndrome

There is a subgroup of parasomnia patients with both clinical and PSG features of both RBD and disorders of arousal (sleepwalking/sleep terrors). These cases demonstrate motor–behavioral dyscontrol extending across NREM and REM sleep and suggest the possibility of a unifying hypothesis for disorders of arousal and RBD. The primary underlying feature is motor disinhibition during sleep—when predominately during NREM sleep manifesting as disorders of arousal, and when predominately during REM sleep manifesting as RBD—with the parasomnia overlap syndrome occupying an intermediate position, with features of both [170].

Agrypnia excitata

This condition is characterized by generalized overactivity associated with loss of SWS, mental oneirism (inability to initiate and maintain sleep with wakeful dreaming), and marked motor and autonomic sympathetic activation seen in such diverse conditions as delirium tremens, Morvan fibrillary chorea, and fatal familial insomnia [195]. Oneiric dementia is likely a related condition [196]. Agrypnia excitata is similar to "status dissociatus," which may be the most extreme form of RBD, appearing to represent the complete breakdown of state-determining boundaries. Clinically, patients with status dissociatus, by behavioral observation, appear to be either awake or asleep; however, clinically, their outward expression of sleep is very atypical, characterized by frequent muscle twitching, vocalization, and reports of dream-like mentation upon spontaneous or forced awakening. There are no PSG features of either conventional REM or NREM sleep; rather, there is a simultaneous admixture of elements of wakefulness, REM sleep, and NREM sleep. "Sleep" may be perceived as "normal" and restorative by the patient despite the nearly continuous motor and verbal behaviors and absence of PSG-defined REM or NREM sleep. Conditions associated with status dissociatus include protracted withdrawal from alcohol abuse, narcolepsy, olivopontocerebellar degeneration, and prior open heart surgery [197].

Emergent concepts in cognitive neuroscience in understanding parasomnias

The fact that violent or injurious behaviors may arise in the absence of conscious wakefulness raises the crucial question of how such complex behaviors can occur. The widely held concept that the brainstem and other more "primitive" neural structures primarily participate in elemental/vegetative rather than behavioral activities is inaccurate: there is clear evidence that highly complex emotional and motor behaviors may originate from these more primitive structures, without involvement of more rostral neural structures.

Ethology is the study of whole patterns of animal behavior under natural conditions in a manner that highlights the functions and the evolutionary process of those patterns. With an ever-increasing physiological approach through the application of refined and elegant laboratory research techniques to animal behavior, opportunities of cross-fertilization of neurobiology and ethology have coalesced to develop neuroethology [198]. An important behavior type in ethology is the fixed action pattern (FAP), which is an instinctive indivisible behavioral sequence that when initiated will run to full completion. FAPs are invariant and are produced by a neural network known as the innate releasing mechanism in response to an external stimulus known as a sign stimulus. FAPs are ubiquitous in the animal kingdom and are seen from invertebrates to higher primates. Movements resulting in FAPs may be initiated by central pattern generators (CPGs), an anatomical entity well recognized by neurologists.

Tassinari et al., in their neuroethological approach, recognized that motor events related to certain epileptic seizures and parasomnias share very similar features suggestive of stereotyped inborn FAPs perhaps initiated by CPGs [32]. Furthermore, Tassinari recognized CPGs as genetically determined neuronal aggregates in the mesencephalon, pons, and spinal cord that from an evolutionary perspective were linked with innate primal behaviors essential for survival (eg, feeding, locomotion, and reproduction). In higher primates, CPGs are inhibited by the influence of neocortical control. It should be kept in mind that many of the CPGs are located in the brainstem and in proximity to processes that govern the wake, NREM sleep, and REM sleep transitions. Tassinari et al. provide a neuroethological model whereby, despite diurnal neocortical inhibition, both epilepsy and sleep can lead to a temporary loss of control of the neo-mammalian cortex and thereby provide a pathway through a common arousal platform initiated by CPGs, which in turn triggers these FAPs, resulting in the abrupt onset of bizarre motor and/or emotional expressions that are uncharacteristic of the awake neocortical-mediated diurnal behaviors.

In essence, the behaviors of primary sleep parasomnias are FAPs that are mediated through CPGs, which may in turn result in serious injury to self or to others. Important, the victim is almost always someone in proximity: victims are not "sought" out. The behaviors associated with sleepwalking may be protracted, whereas those associated with RBD tend to be very quick and brief. Sleepwalkers have their eyes open, allowing them to navigate complex paths; patients with RBD have their eyes closed, so they tend not to get very far before hitting something, which causes them to awaken. Upon awakening, sleepwalkers tend to be confused, disoriented, and unable to remember complex dream imagery, while those with RBD are immediately awake, alert, and oriented, often with vivid recall of a dream corresponding to the observed behavior.

Prevention of injury with medication and environmental safety measures is most important. Sleeping in a room on the first floor or in the basement and alarming the room or dwelling are prudent actions. It must be remembered that previously benign sleepwalking episodes are no guarantee that a violent event may not occur in the future. Moreover, medication is not failsafe. Last, once the individual has left the bedroom and steps out of the home, the compromise in safety involves not just the individual patient but now the general public, and proactive measures should accordingly be considered.

Individuals seeking medical attention for any type of injury should be queried as to the circumstances of the event. Could the car crash have been related to falling asleep at the wheel or to an episode of sleep-driving? Could the fall down the stairs or out the window have occurred while sleepwalking? Inasmuch as sleep is an anesthetic state, very painful injuries may not be appreciated until awakening after completion of the behavior. Some fatal parasomnias are undoubtedly deemed suicides, rather than correctly attributed to an untoward tragic consequence of sleepwalking [199].

It should be noted that RBD and other parasomnias may appear in the hospital setting. In one series of 20 patients experiencing parasomnias in intensive care units, 17 had RBD (3 developed RBD during admission for neurological disorders, 1 was admitted as a consequence of RBD, and 13 displayed pre-existing RBD during the course of hospitalization for other medical conditions) [200].

Sleep forensics

Definition

"The application of the principles and tools of neuroscience as applied to Somnology and Sleep Medicine that have been widely accepted under international scientific peer-review to the investigation in understanding unusual, irrational, and/or bizarre human behaviors associated with alleged criminal behavior which is to undergo further examination in a conflict resolution legal atmosphere and/or courtroom."

M. A. Cramer Bornemann
WORLDSLEEP 07, Fifth Congress of the WFSRSMS,
Cairns, Australia

Introduction

Sleep disorders, most notably parasomnias, have become increasingly invoked as a legal defense to explain violent, reckless, or asocial behaviors that have resulted in a broad spectrum of criminal allegations. Sleep medicine professionals are often asked to render an opinion as to whether a given alleged criminal act could possibly have been committed during an admixed period of wake/sleep, and therefore have been performed without conscious awareness and hence ultimately without culpability. Alternatively, a prosecutor may request a medical expert opinion to combat an opposing counsel's attempt to use a largely improbable, if not entirely bogus, sleepwalking defense as a means to secure a full acquittal in a criminal case.

Recent advances in neuroscience are providing clues regarding how our brains affect our minds and behaviors. Neuroscience has developed powerful tools to investigate the neural activity underlying elementary aspects of physiology and behavior, which has been extended to encompass research into memory, executive function, and higher levels of cognition. Such innovative tools have also been applied to understanding the pathophysiology, diagnosis, and management of many clinical conditions, including those found in sleep medicine.

Unfortunately, conflicts arise with escalating tension, as law in many ways is the polar opposite of neuroscience. Law usually requires dichotomies with an exacting all-or-none approach, whereas the modern scientist is comfortable describing nonstatic systems in multiple intersecting dimensions. Courts reach decisions savoring the adversarial bipartisan environment, while much of science is consensus-driven and prepared with statistics on groups. Law covets tradition embodying centuries of thought and beliefs that resists change; science values rapidly accelerating innovation. Last, law accepts cultural assumptions and common sense that is largely based upon casual observation and unexamined conjecture.

Advances in cognitive neuroscience have clearly established that consciousness (not unlike wakefulness and sleep) exists on a broad spectrum and certainly is not dichotomous. The element of consciousness is an essential feature addressed in the courtroom of every criminal case, placing neuroscientific principles at the core of criminal law. In many ways, the admixed states resulting from incomplete transitions between sleep and wakefulness are unique experiments in nature, providing the clinician scientist a direct window into the evanescent spectrum of consciousness with its associated expressions of human behavior. Thus, those asked to become engaged in sleep forensics would appear to be well poised at this intersection of law and neuroscience. But to be adequately equipped for the developing field of sleep forensics, a medical expert called upon to investigate criminal allegations should not only be well versed in clinical sleep medicine but also be familiar with (1) the evolution of legal thought, (2) the neuroscience of consciousness, (3) the clinical guidelines to assist in the determination of purported acts of violence arising from sleep, and (4) the guidelines for the role of sleep medicine in expert witness testimony. Such an approach not only will enhance the role of the sleep medicine specialist as a resource to the legal community, but will also begin to develop the framework for further research, particularly in parasomnias, and to facilitate the discourse related to the social implications concerning advances in cognitive neuroscience.

Evolution of legal thought

The first appearance of the "sleepwalking defense" in an American court of law came in *Tirrell v Massachusetts* in 1846 [201]. In the mid- to late-1800s, there were no plausible medical explanations to account for sleepwalking, let alone complex violent behaviors apparently arising from sleep that led to misfortune. Though such tragic circumstances resulting in death appear to be exceedingly rare, when presented to a court of law, as in *HMS Advocate v Fraser* (1878) [202] and *Fain v Commonwealth* (1879) [203], a homicide charge may be acquitted by defense pleas of a temporary "defect of reason" or "disease of mind."

The legal community's perspective toward sleep began to shift in 1968 with Roger Broughton's seminal publication characterizing the relationship between somnambulism, nightmares, confusional states of arousal, and REM sleep [26]. By creating a clear demarcation between sleep disorders and other medical or psychiatric conditions, this appears to be the first scientific sleep-related publication with direct legal implications—as supported by *Regina v Parks* (1992) [204]. It was documented in this criminal case that the defendant drove in the early morning hours to the house of his wife's parents. Apparently while still sleepwalking, he was provoked to attack due to the in-laws' physical contact; he attacked both of them with a kitchen knife, killing the mother and leaving the father seriously injured [205]. The defendant was acquitted in a complete defense of all criminal charges, including homicide, in a courtroom jury trial; the rendering was eventually upheld by a landmark Supreme Court of Canada decision not to characterize sleepwalking as a mental health disorder.

Regina v Park helped to usher the sleepwalking defense into the modern era, but the interface between law and science remains contentious, due in part to conflicting philosophies, methodologies, and goals. Nonetheless, there is now a greater degree of civic responsibility placed upon the field of sleep medicine, given the legal community's growing recognition of sleep's broad implications on behavior (or lack thereof) ranging from parasomnias, to cognitive impairment related to sleep deprivation, to pharmaceutical toxicity, just to name a few. Thus, sleep forensics was born of the need to address civic responsibility while appreciating that advances in neuroscience have social implications. It thereby attempts to facilitate discourse between the two disparate disciplines of law and sleep medicine within currently held rules and regulations of the legal system.

Anglo-American law has traditionally defined criminal offenses as requiring both an *actus reus* (guilty act) and a *mens rea* (guilty mind). The state (or prosecution) must prove both elements to secure a conviction. Regrettably, it has proven exceedingly difficult to establish either the precise meaning of these terms or the relationships connecting them. Criminal law presumes that most human behavior is voluntary and that individuals are consciously aware of their acts. As voluntariness is to *mens rea*, consciousness is to voluntary conduct.

Neuroscience of consciousness

A comprehensive review of the neuroscience of consciousness is well beyond the scope of this chapter. Consciousness is a term that has varied and evolving meanings to neuroscientists, though in the legal realm its definition has held steadfast. In science, for example, consciousness may be used to indicate whether or not an individual is in a conscious state, as in whether it has been altered, reduced, or even lost. On the other hand, consciousness may be a trait or an attribute of a psychological process, as in the ability to think, see, and feel consciously. With trait consciousness, further distinctions may be made between conscious representations, which are usually phenomenal, and required conscious access. Unfortunately, a direct objective marker for the neural basis of state and trait consciousness that is independent of an individual's external expressions or behavior has yet to be determined.

There have been seismic shifts in cognitive neuroscience, which the legal system has yet to appreciate and incorporate into the legal arena. Rather confusingly, the terms "conscious" and "unconscious" are still used in the lexicon of neuroscience, but the ideas and principles behind these terms have been substantially altered and continue to be refined, with one such example being Tononi's information integration theory of consciousness [206,207]. Advances in neuroscience within the past 30 years support the existence of a continuum of conscious and unconscious processes, and it has dispensed with Freudian-influenced psychoanalytic concepts and

theories. The boundaries between our conscious and unconscious, as between wake and sleep, are permeable, dynamic, and interactive, and there is no valid scientific support for the sharp dichotomy that is currently held by the legal community. It is this model of permeability, or state dissociation, that will also assist in the explanation of unusual, irrational, and/or bizarre human behaviors in sleep forensics.

Violent sleep-related behaviors have been reviewed in the context of automatic behavior in general, with many well-documented cases resulting from a wide variety of disorders [208]. Conditions associated with sleep-period-related violence fall into two major categories: neurological and psychiatric. Behaviors arising from a primary neurological condition can be explained by applying conceptual approaches based upon models of evanescent consciousness, the overlapping physiology of clinical disorders, and the platform of CPGs supported by semiotic neuroethology.

Despite considerable attention in the popular media in the United States and the United Kingdom given to the association between alcohol and sleepwalking, there are no compelling scientific research data to support that alcohol intoxication, particularly that beyond legal limits, will either prime or trigger such an admixture of states such as sleepwalking or sleep-related abnormal sexual behaviors or sexsomnia [5,209].

The application of sleep forensics is best based upon an adaptable conceptual approach using the most current neuroscientific and clinical principles, as opposed to a static condition that simply lists or highlights clinical disorders and extrapolates associations with criminal behavior. Such a dynamic approach would apply current neuroscientific concepts of consciousness and sleep–wake state dissociation to sleep medicine. As a result, to effectively translate this information into the courtroom, attention must be given to the controversy between dynamic neuroscientific principles of consciousness that contrast with static definitions put forth by the US Model Penal Code. To assist in the determination of the putative role of an underlying sleep disorder in a specific violent act, guidelines should be proposed that are based upon international clinical experience that have undergone peer-reviewed publication. Last, the role of the sleep medicine specialist and recommendations for expert witness qualifications and testimony should be addressed to ensure that those who practice sleep forensics optimize dialogue and maintain ethical behavior for the process of law to proceed without hindrance.

Tassinari's concept of the role of CPGs and FAPs provides a physiological explanation for parasomnias. As a neuroethological concept, it also sets a framework for future research by promoting a naturalistic approach through behavioral observation, including methodical data collection, to better understand the spectrum of parasomnias for which the duration and complexity of behaviors remain ill defined. Last, this concept is particularly useful in sleep forensics, as parasomnias and epileptic seizures tend to have patterned stereotyped behaviors—without conscious awareness. When addressing criminal allegations and their potential association with sleep-related conditions, behavior pattern recognition applying neuroethological concepts, indicative of process fractionation and neurobehavioral investigative techniques, could be particularly beneficial and would be consistent with the direction of current mainstream science.

Clinical guidelines to assist in the determination of purported violence arising from sleep

The legal implications of automatic behavior have been discussed and debated in both the medical and legal literature [210–213]. As with non-sleep-related automatisms, the identification of a specific underlying organic or psychiatric sleep/violence condition does not establish causality for any given deed. Two questions accompany each case of purported sleep-related violence: (1) directly addressing *mens rea*, is it possible for behavior this complex to have arisen in a mixed state of wakefulness and sleep without consciousness? And, (2) is that what happened at the time of the incident? The answer to the first is usually "yes." The second can never be determined with certainty after the fact.

To assist in the determination of the putative role of an underlying sleep disorder in a specific violent act, the following clinical guidelines have been proposed [104,214,215]:

1. There should be reason by history to suspect a bona fide sleep disorder. Similar episodes, with benign or morbid outcome, should have occurred previously. (It must be remembered that disorders of arousal may begin in adulthood.)

2. The duration of the action is usually brief (seconds), though action of longer duration (minutes) does not necessarily exclude a sleep disorder or a sleep-related behavior.

3. The behavior is usually abrupt, immediate, impulsive, and senseless—without apparent motivation. Although ostensibly purposeful, it is completely inappropriate to the total situation, out of (waking) character for the individual, and without evidence of premeditation.

4. The victim is someone who merely happened to be present, usually in proximity, and who may have been the stimulus for the arousal. Sleepwalkers rarely, if ever, seek out victims [74,216].

5. Immediately following return of consciousness, there is perplexity or horror, without any attempt to escape, conceal, or cover up the action. There is evidence of lack of awareness on the part of the individual during the event.

6. There is usually some degree of amnesia for the event; however, this amnesia need not be complete.

7. Sleep is an analgesic state. The sensory pathway for pain for the most part is considered "off-line" during sleep. Consequently, pain associated with acts committed during disorders of arousal may not be perceived until awakening after the event.

8. In the case of sleep terrors/sleepwalking or sleep inertia, the act:

   A. May occur upon awakening (rarely immediately upon falling asleep)—usually at least 1 hour after sleep onset.

   B. Occurs upon attempts to awaken the subject.

   C. Has been potentiated by sedative–hypnotic administration, or prior sleep deprivation.

9. PSG studies performed "after the fact" are of limited value in determining whether a parasomnia accounted for the remote act in question. Even capturing a parasomnia event during a sleep would indicate behavior at the time of the recording, not remotely. Furthermore, there is no scientific basis for attempting to replicate conditions surrounding the event in question (sleep deprivation, or alcohol or other substance ingestion) during a sleep study. Provocation tests to trigger parasomnias by any intoxicants or mind-altering agents would appear to be ethically challenged until well-controlled validated research studies have been performed.

10. Voluntary intoxication by alcohol, or other illicit mind-altering intoxicants precludes the sleepwalking defense.

It should be emphasized that these guidelines are purely meant to provide direction when beginning the review process to gauge whether or not a medicolegal case has merit for consideration of a sleep disorder to be used as a possible defense. Once determined, the strength of the argument to either support or refute the defendant's claim should be used alongside current neuroscientific models of consciousness and behavior and further sustained with the medical expert's wealth of specialized clinical experience.

Role of the sleep medicine specialist

Recent interest in the forensic aspects of parasomnias provides sleep medicine professionals with an opportunity to educate and assist the legal profession in cases of sleep-related violence. One infrequently used tactic to improve scientific testimony is to use a court-appointed "impartial expert" [217]. When approached to testify, volunteering to serve as a court-appointed expert, rather than one appointed by either the prosecution or defense, may encourage this practice. Other proposed measures include the development of a specific section in scientific journals dedicated to expert witness testimony extracted from public documents with request for opinions and consensus statements from appropriate specialists, or the development of a library of circulating expert testimony that could be used to discredit irresponsible professional witnesses [217]. Good science is not determined by the credentials of the expert witness, but rather by scientific consensus [218], while admissibility in a court of law must also adhere to either the Frye or Daubert standards for cases presented in the USA.

To address the problem of junk science in the courtroom, many professional societies are calling for and some have developed guidelines for expert witness qualifications and testimony. The American Academy of Sleep Medicine's stance on expert witness testimony is to accept those opinions as held by the American Medical Association (AMA) in their 2004 Report of the Council on Ethical and Judicial Affairs [219]. Similarly, influenced by both American Academy of Neurology and the AMA, the following guidelines should serve as a compass [220–222]:

A. Expert witness qualifications

1. Must have a current, valid, unrestricted medical or appropriate psychology license.

2. Must be a Diplomat of the American Board of Sleep Medicine, or have passed the American Board of Internal Medicine specialty examination in sleep medicine.

3. Membership in the Sleep Research Society is strongly encouraged.

4. Must be a recognized resource within the sleep medicine community and should have been actively involved in clinical practice in a manner consistent with the requirement of the criminal case at the time of the event.

5. Given the essential position of *mens rea* in criminal law and the pivotal role of levels of consciousness, must have significant direct experience in either neurology and/or neuroscience.

B. Guidelines for expert testimony

1. Must be impartial: ultimate test for accuracy and impartiality is a willingness to prepare testimony that could be presented unchanged for use by either the plaintiff or the defendant.

2. Fees should relate to time and effort, not contingent upon the outcome of the claim.

3. Practitioner should be willing to submit such testimony for peer review.

4. To establish consistency, the expert witness should make records from his or her previous expert witness testimony available to the attorneys and expert witnesses of both parties.

5. The expert witness must not become a partisan or advocate in the legal proceeding.

It is not the role of the medical expert to win the case for his or her client, though it is not uncommon to use irrelevant disingenuous technicalities in an attempt to deceive to attain an advantage to secure the decision. Instead, the salient ethical decision for those who assume this mantle of medical expert witness is to recognize and value the privileged position given within our society as an educator inside the legal system by promoting current published peer-reviewed science while all along minimizing bias when rendering an opinion. The role of the expert witness is therefore to attempt to succinctly and clearly communicate scientifically valid information to the jury, who in turn determine culpability based upon this information. The weight of the decisions of either guilt or innocence should never rest in the hands of medical experts, whose task is to contribute to the due process of an efficient and functional legal system by ensuring that the jury is educated and well informed [222].

Conclusions

Advances in neuroscience are increasing our understanding of how the brain enables "action" from everything from simple movement, to thought, to the diurnal and nocturnal variability of wake–sleep processing. All this seems to be occurring at a pace never before seen as we appear to be closing in on the idea that humans are a determined system. Such scientific advance certainly comes at a cost, as the societal and cultural implications have yet to be understood—or even conceived [223]. However, the legal community is all too aware of the implications of this "new neuroscience," as it directly challenges its currently held constructs of consciousness as defined by *mens rea* and the voluntary act requirements. To study these problems, the John D. and Catherine T. MacArthur Foundation has established the Research Network on Law and Neuroscience (http://www.lawneuro.org/), omprising 40 neuroscientists, legal specialists, and philosophers, with funding that began in 2007 [224]. One most important concept to be incorporated into the legal community is the fact that consciousness is not all-or-none, but rather occurs on a spectrum, and that consciousness can be dissociated from behavior.

Sleep forensics involves more than providing medical expert testimony in individual legal cases. Here we provide a definition and a conceptual approach for the formal development of the field of sleep forensics so that it not only serves as a resource to the legal community but also so that we can appreciate its complex and important position at the intersection of neuroscience and

law. With this appreciation comes significant social responsibility. Applying process fractionation, much can be learned about consciousness from sleep physiology, particularly in admixed states. The growth of cognitive neuroscience will continue to change our understanding of what it means to be human, and as a result justice will have to change in conformity with it. Last, the conceptual approach to sleep forensics encourages further research to define and characterize admixed states of wake/sleep and parasomnias, all of which are beneficial in understanding the spectrum of complex human behavior. Close collaboration among basic neuroscientists, sleep medicine clinicians, and the legal community will facilitate the development of a commonly shared concept of consciousness and culpability.

References

1. Mahowald MW, Ettinger MG. Things that go bump in the night: the parasomnias revisited. J Clin Neurophysiol 1990;7(1):119–43.
2. Mahowald MW, Schenck CH. Evolving concepts of human state dissociation. Arch Ital Biol 2001;139(3):269–300.
3. Mahowald MW. REM sleep behavior disorder. In: Kryger MH, Roth T, Dement WC, eds. Principles and practice of sleep medicine. Philadelphia: Saunders, 2010.
4. Mahowald MW, Schenck CH. Non-rapid eye movement sleep parasomnias. Neurol Clin 2005;23(4):1077–106, vii.
5. Pressman MR, Mahowald MW, Schenck CH, Cramer Bornemann MA. Alcohol-induced sleepwalking or confusional arousal as a defense to criminal behavior: a review of scientific evidence, methods and forensic considerations. J Sleep Res 2007;16(2):198–212.
6. American Academy of Sleep Medicine. Parasomnias. In: International classification of sleep disorders (ICSD-3). Darien, IL: American Academy of Sleep Medicine, 2014.
7. Zolpidem: sleepwalking and automatic behaviours. Prescrire Int 2007;16(91):200.
8. Canaday BR. Amnesia possibly associated with zolpidem administration. Pharmacotherapy 1996;16(4):687–9.
9. Harazin JT, Berigan R. Zolpidem tartrate and somnambulism. Mil Med 1999;164(9):669–70.
10. Mendelson WB. Sleepwalking associated with zolpidem. J Clin Psychopharmacol 1994;14(2):150.
11. Morgenthaler TI, Silber MH. Amnestic sleep-related eating disorder associated with zolpidem. Sleep Med 2002;3(4):323–7.
12. Najjar M. Zolpidem and amnestic sleep related eating disorder. J Clin Sleep Med 2007;3(6):637–8.
13. Sansone RA, Sansone LA. Zolpidem, somnambulism, and nocturnal eating. Gen Hosp Psychiatry 2008;30(1):90–1.
14. Yang W, Dollear M, Muthukrishnan SR. One rare side effect of zolpidem—sleepwalking: a case report. Arch Phys Med Rehabil 2005;86(6):1265–6.
15. Schenck CH, Connoy DA, Castellanos M, et al. Zolpidem-induced amnestic sleep-related eating disorder (SRED) in 19 patients. Sleep 2005;28(Abstract Suppl):A259.
16. Pressman MR. Factors that predispose, prime and precipitate NREM parasomnias in adults: clinical and forensic implications. Sleep Med Rev 2007;11(1):5–30; discussion 31–3.
17. Guilleminault C, Silvestri R. Disorders of arousal and epilepsy during sleep. In: Sterman MB, Shouse MN, Passouant PP, eds. Sleep and epilepsy. New York: Academic Press, 1982.
18. Guilleminault C, et al. Adult chronic sleepwalking and its treatment based on polysomnography. Brain 2005;128(Pt 5):1062–9.
19. Lateef O, Wyatt J, Cartwright R. A case of violent non-REM parasomnias that resolved with treatment of obstructive sleep apnea. Chest 2005;128:461S (abstract).
20. Millman RP, Kipp GJ, Carskadon MA. Sleepwalking precipitated by treatment of sleep apnea with nasal CPAP. Chest 1991;99(3):750–1.

21. Fietze I, Warmuth R, Witt C. Sleep-related breathing disorder and pavor nocturnus. Sleep Res 1995;24A:301.

22. Schenck CH, et al. A polysomnographic and clinical report on sleep-related injury in 100 adult patients. Am J Psychiatry 1989;146(9):1166–73.

23. Guilleminault C, Kushida C, Leger D. Forensic sleep medicine and nocturnal wandering. Sleep 1995;18(9):721–3.

24. Llorente MD, et al. Night terrors in adults: phenomenology and relationship to psychopathology. J Clin Psychiatry 1992;53(11):392–4.

25. Laberge L, et al. Development of parasomnias from childhood to early adolescence. Pediatrics 2000;106(1 Pt 1):67–74.

26. Broughton RJ. Sleep disorders: disorders of arousal? Enuresis, somnambulism, and nightmares occur in confusional states of arousal, not in "dreaming sleep." Science 1968;159(3819):1070–8.

27. Kales A, et al. Somnambulism: psychophysiological correlates. I. All-night EEG studies. Arch Gen Psychiatry 1966;14(6):586–94.

28. Kales JC, et al. Psychotherapy with night-terror patients. Am J Psychother 1982;36(3):399–407.

29. Fisher C, et al. A psychophysiological study of nightmares and night terrors. I. Physiological aspects of the stage 4 night terror. J Nerv Ment Dis 1973;157(2):75–98.

30. Hori A, Hirose G. Twin studies on parasomnias. Sleep Res 1995;24A:324.

31. Arkin AM. Night-terrors as anomalous REM sleep component manifestation in slow-wave sleep. Waking and Sleeping 1978;2:143–7.

32. Tassinari CA, et al. Central pattern generators for a common semiology in fronto-limbic seizures and in parasomnias. A neuroethologic approach. Neurol Sci 2005;26 Suppl 3:s225–32.

33. Mori S, Nishimura H, Aoki M. Brain stem activation of the spinal stepping generator. In: Hobson JA, Brazier MAB, eds. The reticular formation revisited. New York: Raven Press, 1980.

34. Rossignol S, Dubuc R. Spinal pattern generation. Curr Opin Neurobiol 1994;4(6):894–902.

35. Elliott FA. Neuroanatomy and neurology of aggression. Psychiatric Ann 1987;17:385–8.

36. Siegel A, Pott CB. Neural substrates of aggression and flight in the cat. Prog Neurobiol 1988;31(4):261–83.

37. Bandler R. Brain mechanisms of aggression as revealed by electrical and chemical stimulation: suggestion of a central role for the midbrain periaqueductal region. Progr Psychobiol Physiol Psychol 1988;13:67–154.

38. Kelts KA, Hoehn MM. Hypothalamic atrophy. J Clin Psychiatry 1978;39(4):357–8, 363–5.

39. Kelleffer FA, Stern WE. Chronic effects of hypothalamic injury. Arch Neurol 1970;22:419–29.

40. Reeves AG, Plum F. Hyperphagia, rage, and dementia accompanying a ventromedial hypothalamic neoplasm. Arch Neurol 1969;20(6):616–24.

41. Haugh RM, Markesbery WR. Hypothalamic astrocytoma. Syndrome of hyperphagia, obesity, and disturbances of behavior and endocrine and autonomic function. Arch Neurol 1983;40(9):560–3.

42. Sano K, Mayanagi Y. Posteromedial hypothalamotomy in the treatment of violent, aggressive behaviour. Acta Neurochir Suppl (Wien) 1988;44:145–51.

43. Lai YY, Siegel JM. Brainstem-mediated locomotion and myoclonic jerks. I. Neural substrates. Brain Res 1997;745(1–2):257–64.

44. Lai YY, Siegel JM. Brainstem-mediated locomotion and myoclonic jerks. II Pharmacological effects. Brain Res 1997;745(1–2):265–70.

45. Bassetti C, et al. SPECT during sleepwalking. Lancet 2000;356(9228):484–5.

46. Tassi P, Muzet A. Sleep inertia. Sleep Med Rev 2000;4(4):341–53.

47. Horner RL, et al. Activation of a distinct arousal state immediately after spontaneous awakening from sleep. Brain Res 1997;778(1):127–34.

48. Kuboyama T, et al. Changes in cerebral blood flow velocity in healthy young men during overnight sleep and while awake. Electroencephalogr Clin Neurophysiol 1997;102(2):125–31.

49. Balkin TJ, Wesensten NJ, et al. Shaking out the cobwebs: changes in regional cerebral blood flow (rCBF) across the first 20 minutes of wakefulness. J Sleep Res 1998;21:411A.

50. Balkin TJ, et al. The process of awakening: a PET study of regional brain activity patterns mediating the re-establishment of alertness and consciousness. Brain 2002;125(Pt 10):2308–19.

51. Parrino L, et al. CAP, epilepsy and motor events during sleep: the unifying role of arousal. Sleep Med Rev 2006;10(4):267–85.

52. Terzano MG, Parrino L, Spaggiari MC. The cyclic alternating pattern sequences in the dynamic organization of sleep. Electroencephalogr Clin Neurophysiol 1988;69(5):437–47.

53. Zadra A, Nielsen TA. Topographical EEG mapping in a case of recurrent sleep terrors. Dreaming 1998;8:67–74.

54. Halasz P, Ujszaszi J, Gadoros J. Are microarousals preceded by electroencephalographic slow wave synchronization precursors of confusional awakenings? Sleep 1985;8(3):231–8.

55. Zucconi M, et al. Arousal fluctuations in non-rapid eye movement parasomnias: the role of cyclic alternating pattern as a measure of sleep instability. J Clin Neurophysiol 1995;12(2):147–54.

56. Blatt I, et al. The value of sleep recording in evaluating somnambulism in young adults. Electroencephalogr Clin Neurophysiol 1991;78(6):407–12.

57. Schenck CH, et al. Analysis of polysomnographic events surrounding 252 slow-wave sleep arousals in thirty-eight adults with injurious sleepwalking and sleep terrors. J Clin Neurophysiol 1998;15(2):159–66.

58. Bruni O, et al. NREM sleep instability in children with sleep terrors: the role of slow wave activity interruptions. Clin Neurophysiol 2008;119(5):985–92.

59. Oliviero A, et al. Functional involvement of cerebral cortex in adult sleepwalking. J Neurol 2007;254(8):1066–72.

60. Rosen GM, Mahowald MW, Ferber R. Sleepwalking, confusional arousals, and sleep terrors in the child. In: Ferber R, Kryger M, eds. Principles and practice of sleep medicine in the child. Philadelphia: Saunders, 1995.

61. Nino-Murcia G, Dement WC. Psychophysiological and pharmacological aspects of somnambulism and night terrors in children. In: Meltzer HY, ed. Psychopharmacology: the third generation of progress. New York: Raven Press, 1987.

62. Ohayon MM, Guilleminault C, Priest RG. Night terrors, sleepwalking, and confusional arousals in the general population: their frequency and relationship to other sleep and mental disorders. J Clin Psychiatry 1999;60(4):268–76; quiz 277.

63. Hublin C, et al. Prevalence and genetics of sleepwalking: a population-based twin study. Neurology 1997;48(1):177–81.

64. Klackenberg G. Somnambulism in childhood—prevalence, course and behavioral correlations. A prospective longitudinal study (6-16 years). Acta Paediatr Scand 1982;71(3):495–9.

65. Bixler EO, et al. Prevalence of sleep disorders in the Los Angeles metropolitan area. Am J Psychiatry 1979;136(10):1257–62.

66. Fisher C, et al. A psychophysiological study of nightmares and night terrors. 3. Mental content and recall of stage 4 night terrors. J Nerv Ment Dis 1974;158(3):174–88.

67. Kahn E, Fisher C, Edwards A. Night terrors and anxiety dreams. In: Ellman SD, Antrobus JS, eds. The mind in sleep psychology and psychophysiology. New York: John Wiley & Sons, 1991.

68. Crisp AH. The sleepwalking/night terrors syndrome in adults. Postgrad Med J 1996;72(852):599–604.

69. Birketvedt GS, et al. Behavioral and neuroendocrine characteristics of the night-eating syndrome. JAMA 1999;282(7):657–63.

70. Birketvedt GS, Sundsfjord J, Florholmen JR. Hypothalamic–pituitary–adrenal axis in the night eating syndrome. Am J Physiol Endocrinol Metab 2002;282(2):E366–9.

71. Stunkard AJ, Allison KC. Two forms of disordered eating in obesity: binge eating and night eating. Int J Obes Relat Metab Disord 2003;27(1):1–12.

72. Paquet V, et al. Sleep-related eating disorder induced by olanzapine. J Clin Psychiatry 2002;63(7):597.

73. Menkes DB. Triazolam-induced nocturnal bingeing with amnesia. Aust N Z J Psychiatry 1992;26(2):320–1.

74. Schenck CH, Arnulf I, Mahowald MW. Sleep and sex: what can go wrong? A review of the literature on sleep related disorders and abnormal sexual behaviors and experiences. Sleep 2007;30(6):683–702.

75. Guilleminault C, et al. Atypical sexual behavior during sleep. Psychosom Med 2002;64(2):328–36.

76. Cramer-Bornemann M. Sexsomnia: a medico-legal case-based approach in analyzing potential sleep-related abnormal sexual behaviors. In: Kothare SV, Ivanenko A, eds. Parasomnias—clinical characteristics and treatment. New York: Springer, 2013:431–61.

77. State of Oregon v. Jamers Kirchner, 2008.

78. Cramer-Bornemann M, Mahowald MW, Schenck CS. Sexsomnia and sleep forensics—the interface between sleep-related abnormal sexual behaviors and the law. Sleep 2014;37 (Abstract Suppl):A211.

79. Badawy RS. Sexsomnia: overcoming the sleep disorder defense. In: Update— National Center for Prosecution of Child Abuse, volume 22, numbers 4 and 5. Alexandria, VA: National District Attorneys Association, 2010:1–8.

80. Aldrich MS, Jahnke B. Diagnostic value of video-EEG polysomnography. Neurology 1991;41(7):1060–6.

81. Zadra A, Pilon M, Montplaisir J. Polysomnographic diagnosis of sleepwalking: effects of sleep deprivation. Ann Neurol 2008;63(4):513–19.

82. Mahowald MW, Schenck SC. Parasomnia purgatory: the epileptic/non-epileptic interface. In: Rowan AJ, Gates JR, eds. Non-epileptic seizures. Boston: Butterworth-Heinemann, 1993:123–39.

83. Schenck CH, Mahowald MW. REM sleep parasomnias. Neurol Clin 1996;14(4):697–720.

84. Mahowald MW, Schenck CH. NREM sleep parasomnias. Neurol Clin 1996;14(4):675–96.

85. Goodwin JL, et al. Parasomnias and sleep disordered breathing in Caucasian and Hispanic children—the Tucson children's assessment of sleep apnea study. BMC Med 2004;2:14.

86. Tinuper P, et al. Movement disorders in sleep: guidelines for differentiating epileptic from non-epileptic motor phenomena arising from sleep. Sleep Med Rev 2007;11(4):255–67.

87. Casez O, Dananchet Y, Besson G. Migraine and somnambulism. Neurology 2005;65(8):1334–5.

88. Johnson H, et al. Psychological disturbance and sleep disorders in children with neurofibromatosis type 1. Dev Med Child Neurol 2005;47(4):237–42.

89. Barabas G, Matthews WS, Ferrari M. Disorders of arousal in Gilles de la Tourette's syndrome. Neurology 1984;34(6):815–17.

90. Wand RR, et al. Tourette syndrome: associated symptoms and most disabling features. Neurosci Biobehav Rev 1993;17(3):271–5.

91. Isik U, D'Cruz O. Cluster headaches simulating parasomnias. Pediatr Neurol 2002;27(3):227–9.

92. Espa F, et al. Arousal reactions in sleepwalking and night terrors in adults: the role of respiratory events. Sleep 2002;25(8):871–5.

93. Lillywhite AR, Wilson SJ, Nutt DJ. Successful treatment of night terrors and somnambulism with paroxetine. Br J Psychiatry 1994;164(4):551–4.

94. Balon R. Sleep terror disorder and insomnia treated with trazodone: a case report. Ann Clin Psychiatry 1994;6(3):161–3.

95. Kellerman J. Behavioral treatment of night terrors in a child with acute leukemia. J Nerv Ment Dis 1979;167(3):182–5.

96. Hauri PJ, Silber MH, Boeve BF. The treatment of parasomnias with hypnosis: a 5-year follow-up study. J Clin Sleep Med 2007;3(4):369–73.

97. Tobin JD Jr. Treatment of somnambulism with anticipatory awakening. J Pediatr 1993;122(3):426–7.

98. Schenck CH, Mahowald MW. Rapid eye movement sleep parasomnias. Neurol Clin 2005;23(4):1107–26.

99. Steriade M, Ropert N, Kitsikis A. Ascending activating neuronal networks in midbrain core and related rostral systems. In: Hobson JA, Brazier MAB, eds. The reticular formation revisited. New York: Raven Press, 1980:125–67.

100. Dement WC. The biological role of REM sleep (circa 1968). In: Kales A, ed. Sleep physiology and pathology. Philadelphia: Lippincott, 1969:245–65.

101. Hishikawa Y, et al. The nature of sleep attack and other symptoms of narcolepsy. Electroencephalogr Clin Neurophysiol 1968;24(1):1–10.

102. Guilleminault C, Wilson RA, Dement WC. A study on cataplexy. Arch Neurol 1974;31(4):255–61.

103. Schenck CH, Mahowald MW. REM sleep behavior disorder: clinical, developmental, and neuroscience perspectives 16 years after its formal identification in SLEEP. Sleep 2002;25(2):120–38.

104. Ohayon MM, Caulet M, Priest RG. Violent behavior during sleep. J Clin Psychiatry 1997;58(8):369–76; quiz 377.

105. Chiu HF, Wing YK. REM sleep behaviour disorder: an overview. Int J Clin Pract 1997;51(7):451–4.

106. Sakai K, Sastre JP, Kanamori N, et al. State-specific neurons in the ponto-medullary reticular formation with special reference to the postural atonia during paradoxical sleep in the cat. In: Pompeiano O, Ajmone Marson C, eds. Brain mechanisms and perceptual awareness. New York: Raven Press, 1981:405–29.

107. Webster HH, Friedman L, Jones BE. Modification of paradoxical sleep following transections of the reticular formation at the pontomedullary junction. Sleep 1986;9(1):1–23.

108. Mileykovskiy BY, et al. Activation of pontine and medullary motor inhibitory regions reduces discharge in neurons located in the locus coeruleus and the anatomical equivalent of the midbrain locomotor region. J Neurosci 2000;20(22):8551–8.

109. Mileykovskiy BY, Kiyashchenko LI, Siegel JM. Cessation of activity in red nucleus neurons during stimulation of the medial medulla in decerebrate rats. J Physiol 2002;545(Pt 3):997–1006.

110. Chase MH. The motor functions of the reticular formation are multifaceted and state-determined. In: Hobson JA, Brazier MAB, eds. The reticular formation revisited. New York: Raven Press, 1980:449–72.

111. Chase MH, Morales FR. Subthreshold excitatory activity and motoneuron discharge during REM periods of active sleep. Science 1983;221(4616):1195–8.

112. Askenasy JJ, Weitzman ED, Yahr MD. Rapid eye movements: expression of a general muscular phasic event of the REM state. Sleep Res 1983;12:172.

113. Fort P, et al. Anatomical demonstration of a medullary enkephalinergic pathway potentially implicated in the oro-facial muscle atonia of paradoxical sleep in the cat. Sleep Res Online 1998;1(3):102–8.

114. Lopez-Rodriguez F, et al. State dependency of the effects of microinjection of cholinergic drugs into the nucleus pontis oralis. Brain Res 1994;649(1–2):271–81.

115. Brooks PL, Peever JH. Glycinergic and GABA(A)-mediated inhibition of somatic motoneurons does not mediate rapid eye movement sleep motor atonia. J Neurosci 2008;28(14):3535–45.

116. Miyamoto M, et al. Brainstem function in rapid eye movement sleep behavior disorder: the evaluation of brainstem function by proton MR spectroscopy (1H-MRS). Psychiatry Clin Neurosci 2000;54(3):350–1.

117. Iranzo A, et al. Brainstem proton magnetic resonance spectroscopy in idiopathic REM sleep behavior disorder. Sleep 2002;25(8):867–70.

118. Eisensehr I, et al. Reduced striatal dopamine transporters in idiopathic rapid eye movement sleep behaviour disorder. Comparison with Parkinson's disease and controls. Brain 2000;123 (Pt 6):1155–60.

119. Eisensehr I, et al. Increased muscle activity during rapid eye movement sleep correlates with decrease of striatal presynaptic dopamine transporters. IPT and IBZM SPECT imaging in subclinical and clinically manifest idiopathic REM sleep behavior disorder, Parkinson's disease, and controls. Sleep 2003;26(5):507–12.

120. Albin RL, et al. Decreased striatal dopaminergic innervation in REM sleep behavior disorder. Neurology 2000;55(9):1410–12.

121. Parish JM. Violent dreaming and antidepressant drugs: or how paroxetine made me dream that I was fighting Saddam Hussein. J Clin Sleep Med 2007;3(5):529–31.

122. Stolz SE, Aldrich MS. REM sleep behavior disorder by chocolate ingestion: a case report. Sleep Res 1991;20:341.

123. Vorona RD, Ware JC. Exacerbation of REM sleep behavior disorder by chocolate ingestion: a case report. Sleep Med 2002;3(4):365–7.

124. Mahowald MW, Schenck CH. The REM sleep behavior disorder odyssey. Sleep Med Rev 2009;13(6):381–4.

125. Schenck CH, Bundlie SR, Smith SA, et al. REM behavior disorder in a 10-year old girl and aperiodic REM and NREM sleep movements in an 8-year old brother. Sleep Res 1986;15:162.

126. Hendricks JC, et al. Movement disorders during sleep in cats and dogs. J Am Vet Med Assoc 1989;194(5):686–9.

127. Hendricks JC, et al. A disorder of rapid eye movement sleep in a cat. J Am Vet Med Assoc 1981;178(1):55–7.

128. Goldstein M. Brain research and violent behavior. A summary and evaluation of the status of biomedical research on brain and aggressive violent behavior. Arch Neurol 1974;30(1):1–35.

129. Moyer KE. Kinds of aggression and their physiological basis. Commun Behav Biol 1968;2 (part A):65–87.

130. Ramirez JM. Hormones and aggression in childhood and adolescence. Aggression Violent Behav 2003;8:621–44.

131. Coffey CE, et al. Sex differences in brain aging: a quantitative magnetic resonance imaging study. Arch Neurol 1998;55(2):169–79.

132. Patwardhan AJ, et al. Brain morphology in Klinefelter syndrome: extra X chromosome and testosterone supplementation. Neurology 2000;54(12):2218–23.

133. Cosgrove KP, Mazure CM, Staley JK. Evolving knowledge of sex differences in brain structure, function, and chemistry. Biol Psychiatry 2007;62(8):847–55.

134. Guillamon A, de Blas MR, Segovia S. Effects of sex steroids on the development of the locus coeruleus in the rat. Brain Res 1988;468(2):306–10.

135. Iranzo A, et al. Absence of alterations in serum sex hormone levels in idiopathic REM sleep behavior disorder. Sleep 2007;30(6):803–6.

136. Chou KL, et al. Testosterone not associated with violent dreams or REM sleep behavior disorder in men with Parkinson's. Mov Disord 2007;22(3):411–14.

137. Teman PT, et al. Idiopathic rapid-eye-movement sleep disorder: associations with antidepressants, psychiatric diagnoses, and other factors, in relation to age of onset. Sleep Med 2009;10(1):60–5.

138. Bonakis A, et al. REM sleep behaviour disorder (RBD) and its associations in young patients. Sleep Med 2009;10(6):641–5.

139. Schenck CH, Mahowald MW. Polysomnographic, neurologic, psychiatric, and clinical outcome report on 70 consecutive cases with REM sleep behavior disorder (RBD): sustained clonazepam efficacy in 89.5% of 57 treated patients. Cleveland Clinic J Med 1990;57 (Suppl):S9–23.

140. Mahowald MW, Schenck CH. REM sleep behavior disorder. In: Thorpy MJ, ed. Handbook of sleep disorders. New York: Marcel Dekker, 1990:567–93.

141. Yeh SB, Schenck CH. A case of marital discord and secondary depression with attempted suicide resulting from REM sleep behavior disorder in a 35-year-old woman. Sleep Med 2004;5(2):151–4.

142. Gjerstad MD, et al. Occurrence and clinical correlates of REM sleep behaviour disorder in patients with Parkinson's disease over time. J Neurol Neurosurg Psychiatry 2008;79(4):387–91.

143. Fantini ML, et al. Aggressive dream content without daytime aggressiveness in REM sleep behavior disorder. Neurology 2005;65(7):1010–15.

144. Iranzo A, Santamaria J, Tolosa E. The clinical and pathophysiological relevance of REM sleep behavior disorder in neurodegenerative diseases. Sleep Med Rev 2009;13(6):385–401.

145. Comella CL, et al. Sleep-related violence, injury, and REM sleep behavior disorder in Parkinson's disease. Neurology 1998;51(2):526–9.

146. Eisensehr I, et al. REM sleep behavior disorder in sleep-disordered patients with versus without Parkinson's disease: is there a need for polysomnography? J Neurol Sci 2001;186(1–2):7–11.

147. Gagnon JF, et al. REM sleep behavior disorder and REM sleep without atonia in Parkinson's disease. Neurology 2002;59(4):585–9.

148. Scaglione C, et al. REM sleep behaviour disorder in Parkinson's disease: a questionnaire-based study. Neurol Sci 2005;25(6):316–21.

149. Plazzi G, et al. REM sleep behavior disorders in multiple system atrophy. Neurology 1997;48(4):1094–7.

150. Ghorayeb I, et al. Sleep disorders and their determinants in multiple system atrophy. J Neurol Neurosurg Psychiatry 2002;72(6):798–800.

151. Plazzi G, et al. REM sleep behaviour disorder differentiates pure autonomic failure from multiple system atrophy with autonomic failure. J Neurol Neurosurg Psychiatry 1998;64(5):683–5.

152. Uchiyama M, et al. Incidental Lewy body disease in a patient with REM sleep behavior disorder. Neurology 1995;45(4):709–12.

153. Ferman TJ, et al. Dementia with Lewy bodies may present as dementia and REM sleep behavior disorder without parkinsonism or hallucinations. J Int Neuropsychol Soc 2002;8(7):907–14.

154. Boeve BF. REM sleep behavior disorder: updated review of the core features, the REM sleep behavior disorder–neurodegenerative disease association, evolving concepts, controversies, and future directions. Ann N Y Acad Sci 2010;1184:15–54.

155. De Cock VC, et al. Restoration of normal motor control in Parkinson's disease during REM sleep. Brain 2007;130(Pt 2):450–6.

156. Bonakis A, Howard RS, Williams A. Narcolepsy presenting as REM sleep behaviour disorder. Clin Neurol Neurosurg 2008;110(5):518–20.

157. Mattarozzi K, et al. Clinical, behavioural and polysomnographic correlates of cataplexy in patients with narcolepsy/cataplexy. Sleep Med 2008;9(4):425–33.

158. Nightingale S, et al. The association between narcolepsy and REM behavior disorder (RBD). Sleep Med 2005;6(3):253–8.

159. Dauvilliers Y, et al. REM sleep characteristics in narcolepsy and REM sleep behavior disorder. Sleep 2007;30(7):844–9.

160. Nevsimalova S, et al. REM behavior disorder (RBD) can be one of the first symptoms of childhood narcolepsy. Sleep Med 2007;8(7–8):784–6.

161. Dyken ME, et al. Violent sleep-related behavior leading to subdural hemorrhage. Arch Neurol 1995;52(3):318–21.

162. Morfis L, Schwartz RS, Cistulli PA. REM sleep behaviour disorder: a treatable cause of falls in elderly people. Age Ageing 1997;26(1):43–4.

163. Gross PT. REM sleep behavior disorder causing bilateral subdural hematomas. Sleep Res 1992;21:204 (abstract).

164. Rechtschaffen A, Kales A. A manual of standardized terminology: techniques and scoring system for sleep stages of human subjects. Los Angeles: UCLA Brain Information Service/Brain Research Institute, 1968.

165. Carskadon MA, et al. Guidelines for the multiple sleep latency test (MSLT): a standard measure of sleepiness. Sleep 1986;9(4):519–24.

166. Schenck CH, et al. Rapid eye movement sleep behavior disorder. A treatable parasomnia affecting older adults. JAMA 1987;257(13):1786–9.

167. Nalamalapu U, Goldberg R, DePhillipo M, et al. Behaviors simulating REM behavior disorder in patients with severe obstructive sleep apnea. Sleep Res 1996;25:311.

168. D'Cruz OF, Vaughn BV. Nocturnal seizures mimic REM behavior disorder. Am J END Technol 1997;37:258–64.

169. Iranzo A, Santamaria J. Severe obstructive sleep apnea/hypopnea mimicking REM sleep behavior disorder. Sleep 2005;28(2):203–6.

170. Schenck CH, Boyd JL, Mahowald MW. A parasomnia overlap disorder involving sleepwalking, sleep terrors, and REM sleep behavior disorder in 33 polysomnographically confirmed cases. Sleep 1997;20(11):972–81.

171. Schenck CH, Milner DM, Hurwitz TD, et al. Dissociative disorders presenting as somnambulism: polysomnographic, video, and clinical documentation (8 cases). Dissociation 1989;4:194–204.

172. Mahowald MW, et al. The role of a sleep disorder center in evaluating sleep violence. Arch Neurol 1992;49(6):604–7.

173. Schenck CH, Mahowald MW. Long-term, nightly benzodiazepine treatment of injurious parasomnias and other disorders of disrupted nocturnal sleep in 170 adults. Am J Med 1996;100(3):333–7.

174. Anderson KN, et al. REM sleep behaviour disorder treated with melatonin in a patient with Alzheimer's disease. Clin Neurol Neurosurg 2008;110(5):492–5.

175. Boeve BF, Silber MH, Ferman TJ. Melatonin for treatment of REM sleep behavior disorder in neurologic disorders: results in 14 patients. Sleep Med 2003;4(4):281–4.

176. Fantini ML, et al. The effects of pramipexole in REM sleep behavior disorder. Neurology 2003;61(10):1418–20.

177. Schmidt MH, Koshal VB, Schmidt HS. Use of pramipexole in REM sleep behavior disorder: results from a case series. Sleep Med 2006;7(5):418–23.

178. Matsumoto M, Mutoh F, Naoe H, et al. The effects of imipramine on REM sleep behavior disorder in 3 cases. Sleep Res 1991;20A:351.

179. Takahashi T, et al. Opposite effects of SSRIs and tandospirone in the treatment of REM sleep behavior disorder. Sleep Med 2008;9(3):317–19.

180. Yamamoto K, Uchimura N, Habukawa M, et al. Evaluation of the effects of paroxetine in the treatment of REM sleep behavior disorder. Sleep Biol Rhythm 2006;4:190–2.

181. Bamford CR. Carbamazepine in REM sleep behavior disorder. Sleep 1993;16(1):33–4.

182. Tan A, Salgado M, Fahn S. Rapid eye movement sleep behavior disorder preceding Parkinson's disease with therapeutic response to levodopa. Mov Disord 1996;11(2):214–16.

183. Mike ME, Kranz AJ. MAOI suppression of R.B.D. refractory to clonazepam and other agents. Sleep Res 1996;25:63(abstract).

184. Ringman JM, Simmons JH. Treatment of REM sleep behavior disorder with donepezil: a report of three cases. Neurology 2000;55(6):870–1.

185. Schenck CH, Mahowald MW. Motor dyscontrol in narcolepsy: rapid-eye-movement (REM) sleep without atonia and REM sleep behavior disorder. Ann Neurol 1992;32(1):3–10.

186. Schenck CH, Bundlie SR, Mahowald MW. Delayed emergence of a parkinsonian disorder in 38% of 29 older men initially diagnosed with idiopathic rapid eye movement sleep behaviour disorder. Neurology 1996;46(2):388–93.

187. Rye DB, Dempsay J, Dihenia B, et al. REM-sleep dyscontrol in Parkinson's disease: case report of effects of elective pallidotomy. Sleep Res 1997;26:591(abstract).

188. Iranzo A, et al. Sleep symptoms and polysomnographic architecture in advanced Parkinson's disease after chronic bilateral subthalamic stimulation. J Neurol Neurosurg Psychiatry 2002;72(5):661–4.

189. Arnulf I, et al. Improvement of sleep architecture in PD with subthalamic nucleus stimulation. Neurology 2000;55(11):1732–4.

190. Piette T, et al. A unique episode of REM sleep behavior disorder triggered during surgery for Parkinson's disease. J Neurol Sci 2007;253(1–2):73–6.

191. Schuld A, et al. Obstructive sleep apnea syndrome induced by clonazepam in a narcoleptic patient with REM-sleep-behavior disorder. J Sleep Res 1999;8(4):321–2.

192. Takeuchi N, Uchimura N, Hashizume Y, et al. Melatonin therapy for REM sleep behavior disorder. Psychiatry Clin Neurosciences 2001;55:267–9.

193. Lapierre O, Casademont A, Montplaisir J, et al. Tonic and phasic features of REM sleep behavior disorder. Sleep Res 1991;20:276.

194. Watanabe T, Sugita Y. [REM sleep behavior disorder (RBD) and dissociated REM sleep.] Nihon Rinsho 1998;56(2):433–8.

195. Montagna P, Lugaresi E. Agrypnia excitata: a generalized overactivity syndrome and a useful concept in the neurophysiopathology of sleep. Clin Neurophysiol 2002;113(4):552–60.

196. Cibula JE, et al. Progressive dementia and hypersomnolence with dream-enacting behavior: oneiric dementia. Arch Neurol 2002;59(4):630–4.

197. Mahowald MW, Schenck CH. Status dissociatus--a perspective on states of being. Sleep 1991;14(1):69–79.

198. Lehner PN. Handbook of ethological methods, 2nd ed. New York: Cambridge University Press, 1996.

199. Mahowald MW, et al. Parasomnia pseudo-suicide. J Forensic Sci 2003;48(5):1158–62.

200. Schenck CH, Mahowald MW. Injurious sleep behavior disorders (parasomnias) affecting patients on intensive care units. Intensive Care Med 1991;17(4):219–24.

201. Knappman EW. Great american trials: from Salem witchcraft to Rodney King. Michigan: Gale Group, 1994.

202. Yellowless D. Homicide by somnambulist. J Mental Sci 1878;24:451–8.

203. Fain v. Commonwealth, 1879, 78 Ky. 183.

204. Regina v. Parks, 1992: Canada.

205. Broughton R, et al. Homicidal somnambulism: a case report. Sleep 1994;17(3):253–64.

206. Tononi G, Koch C. The neural correlates of consciousness: an update. Ann N Y Acad Sci 2008;1124:239–61.

207. Tononi G. The information integration theory of consciousness. In: Velmans SSM, ed. The Blackwell companion to consciousness. Oxford: Blackwell, 2007:239–61.

208. Mahowald MW, Schenck CH. Parasomnias: sleepwalking and the law. Sleep Med Rev 2000;4(4):321–39.

209. Pressman MR, Mahowald MW, Schenck CH, et al. No scientific evidence that alcohol causes sleepwalking. J Sleep Res 2008;17:473–4 (letter to editor).

210. Prevezer S. Automatism and involuntary conduct. Criminal Law Rev 1958:361–7.

211. Fitzgerald PJ. Voluntary and involuntary acts. In: Guest AG, ed. Oxford essays in jurisprudence. Oxford: Oxford University Press, 1961:1–28.

212. Shroder RF. Forensic psychiatry. In: Camps FE, ed. Gradwohl's legal medicine. Chicago: John Wiley & Sons, 1976:505.

213. Schopp RF. Automatism, insanity, and the psychology of criminal responsibility. New York: Cambridge University Press, 1991.

214. Bonkalo A. Impulsive acts and confusional states during incomplete arousal from sleep: crinimological and forensic implications. Psychiatr Q 1974;48(3):400–9.

215. Mahowald MW, et al. Sleep violence—forensic science implications: polygraphic and video documentation. J Forensic Sci 1990;35(2):413–32.

216. Pressman MR. Disorders of arousal from sleep and violent behavior: the role of physical contact and proximity. Sleep 2007;30(8):1039–47.

217. Huber PW. Galileo's revenge. Junk science in the courtroom. New York: Basic Books, 1991.

218. Weintraub MI. Expert witness testimony: a time for self-regulation? Neurology 1995;45(5):855–8.

219. Goodrich MS. Report of the council on ethical and judicial affairs. AMA 2004. CEJA Report 12-A-04 (Committee on Constitution and Bylaws). Chicago: American Medical Association.

220. Murray G, Sagsveen JD. American Academy of Neurology policy on expert medical testimony. Neurology 2004;63(9):1555–6.

221. Freeman JM, Nelson KB. Expert medical testimony: responsibilities of medical societies. Neurology 2004;63(9):1557–8.

222. Cramer-Bornemann M. Health law: role of the expert witness in sleep-related violence trial. AMA J Ethics 2008;10:571–7.

223. Churchland PS. The impact of neuroscience on philosophy. Neuron 2008;60(3):409–11.

224. Gazzaniga MS. The law and neuroscience. Neuron 2008;60(3):412–15.

CHAPTER 53

Morbidity, mortality, societal impact, and accident in sleep disorders

Sergio Garbarino

Genetic and environmental factors across the human lifespan: etiology of primary sleep disorders

Sleep problems are common across the human lifespan from childhood to adolescence and then adulthood [1]. Similar types of sleep disorders co-occur in the same family and often in association with emotional, behavioral, and health-related problems, as demonstrated by twin studies, where sample shared environmental factors, rather than genetics, play a role [2]. Moreover, the association between sleep difficulties and depression is largely accounted for by genetics [3].

In addition, a prior sleep problem in a child is a risk factor for the development of depressive symptoms [4], and the genetic background of insomnia seems to be shared with anxiety and depression [5].

In adults, as in children, sleep problems are also often comorbid with emotional, behavioral, anxiety and depression, and other health-related problems [6], owing to genetic and environmental contributions. Genetic factors largely account for an association between sleep disturbance and anxiety (74%) and between sleep disturbance and depression (58%) [7]. However, the genetic correlation between daytime sleepiness and depression decreases after accounting for activities of daily living, snoring, obesity, and history of diabetes. Greater daytime sleepiness is associated with snoring and higher body mass index (BMI) [8]. Obesity is correlated with insomnia and short sleep duration, determined largely by environmental factors and to an extent by some common genetic effects [9,10]. In contrast, genetic factors largely account for evening types and morning types (80% of phenotypic correlations) and for a propensity to externalizing behaviors in those experiencing poor sleep quality. Greater psychopathological symptoms and insomnia seem to be associated with the shorter variant (the short allele instead of the long allele) of the *5HTTLPR* region of the serotonin transporter gene (*SLC6A4*) [11,12], but "long–long" homozygotes experienced poorer sleep quality [13].

Environmental factors (eg, low socioeconomic status, unemployment, low income, and negative life events) and negative lifestyle factors (eg, a lack of exercise, smoking, and alcohol drinking) are associated with sleep problems in adults [14,15] (Fig. 53.1).

Morbidity

Sleep disorders and impairment in daytime functioning attributed to disturbed or poor quality sleep induce consistent decrements in mood and cognitive abilities (concentration, memory, attention, and vigilance), coupled with elevated levels of anxiety, fatigue, and physical pain/discomfort, relative to normal sleepers [16].

Large survey and population-based studies further reveal a number of increased morbidity markers in those suffering from insomnia, increased rates of healthcare utilization (physician visits and medication prescriptions), and chronic health problems [17–19].

Insomnia in older adults is of particular concern because it could increase the risk of injury, impaired quality of life, cognitive impairment, depression, and metabolic syndrome. Insomnia is also associated with a moderately increased risk for cardiovascular disease (CVD) [20].

Snoring, sleep apnea, and obesity–hypoventilation syndrome (OHS) are common disorders that increase the risk of cardiovascular and cerebrovascular morbidity and mortality. Additional effects of sleep disordered breathing (SDB) include reduced social function and quality of life. Because these disorders are chronic, they may also have a deleterious effect on a patient's employment status and ability to work [21].

Many studies have identified a higher rate of comorbid medical conditions associated with narcolepsy; consistently reported comorbidity includes 15% restless legs syndrome (RLS) and 25% sleep apnea [22,23]; obesity, cognitive deficits, and psychiatric disorders, especially depression [24] and anxiety [23,25,26]. Additional medical conditions comorbid with narcolepsy include chronic pain, gastrointestinal disorders, hypercholesterolemia, and hypertension [25,26]. Many of these conditions impart a known increased mortality risk. Excessive daytime sleepiness (EDS) may also be associated with an increased risk of suicidal ideation, especially in the presence of depression.

RLS can significantly impair sleep quality and quantity, with difficulty initiating or maintaining sleep. Patients with moderate to severe RLS reported short sleep times (5.2–5.4 hours per night) and more sleep disturbance [27]. RLS sufferers have also reported an increased frequency (two to five times) of sleep-related complaints: not feeling refreshed upon awakening, headaches upon awakening, and, during daytime, social isolation, depressed mood,

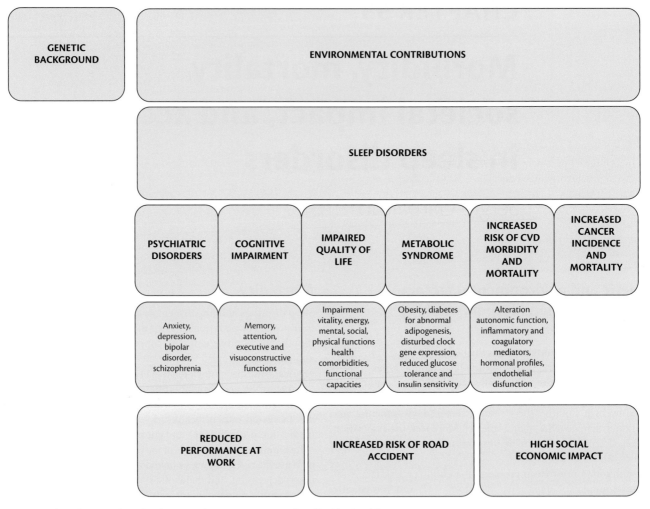

Fig. 53.1 Correlation between sleep disturbances and genetic, environmental, and health-related factors.

difficulty in concentrating, and memory impairment [28]. Severe RLS is known to be associated with sleep fragmentation, depression, anxiety, obesity, obstructive sleep apnea (OSA), CVD, diabetes, erectile dysfunction, and end-stage renal disease (ESRD) [29]. Individuals with RLS may also have difficulties in job performance and participating in social activities [30]. Impacts on next-day functioning attributed to disturbed sleep due to RLS symptoms include activities of daily living (i.e, work and household chores), cognitive functioning (i.e, lack of concentration, forgetfulness, mental tiredness, and decreased alertness), emotional functioning (i.e, irritability and depressed mood), physical functioning (i.e, physical tiredness and decreased ability to perform active leisure activities), energy, daytime sleepiness, and social functioning (i.e, negative effects on relationships and social activities/situations) [31].

Psychiatric disorders and cognitive impairment

Sleep disturbances exert a detrimental influence on the course of psychiatric illness and contribute to impaired function. Even when psychiatric disorders are successfully treated or stabilized, insomnia and other sleep disturbances often fail to remit. Insomnia frequently co-occurs with a wide range of psychiatric disorders. There

appears to be a cyclical relationship between sleep disturbance and medical or psychiatric illness: insomnia predicts the development of a new depressive episode 1–3 years later and future clinical anxiety.

Insomnia is one of the most common prodromal features of depression, with sleep symptoms preceding an episode of depression in 40% of cases and with 90% of patients with major depression reporting sleep disturbances. A history of persistent insomnia is also associated with a significantly increased risk of developing a new depressive episode [32]. In a recent meta-analysis, non-depressed people with insomnia were predicted to have a twofold increased risk of developing depression compared with people with no sleep difficulties [33]. Insomnia treatment improves mood and depressive symptoms.

Sleep problems may also contribute to depressive symptomatology via their effect on brain structure, neurogenesis, and, in particular, hippocampal function. Sleep restriction enhance neuronal sensitivity to subsequent excitotoxic insults [34], increasing the brain's vulnerability to neurotoxic challenges [35], with consequent decreased bilateral hippocampal (bilateral) and gray matter volume in the left orbitofrontal cortex.

Sleep disturbance is a core feature of mood episodes in bipolar disorder. During periods of mania, the majority of patients

(69–99%) experience reduced need for sleep and shortened rapid eye movement (REM) sleep latency [36]. The rate of insomnia in bipolar depression is very high, indeed nearly 100%, and the rate of hypersomnia during the depressive phase of bipolar illness varies between 23% and 78%.

Sleep disturbance is prevalent in schizophrenia, during both psychosis and remission. Sleep complaints include difficulty falling asleep, early morning awakening, awakening during the night, not sleeping soundly, and having increased time in bed. Sleep disturbances have also been associated with exacerbated symptoms in schizophrenia, particularly positive symptoms (eg, delusions, hallucinations, disorganized thinking, and behavior). Moreover, negative symptoms such as anhedonia, social withdrawal, loss of motivation, and poor self-care are unrelated to insomnia symptoms [36].

A recent study suggests clinically significant alterations in attention and episodic memory in individuals with insomnia and supports a role for sleep disturbances (particularly sleep duration, sleep fragmentation, and SDB) in the development of cognitive impairment [37,38].

EDS, mood changes, and cognitive impairments (especially in attention, executive functioning, memory, and visuoconstructive abilities, with consequent reduction in quality of life) are the most common daytime symptoms of OSA syndrome (OSAS) and SDB [39–42].

Continuous positive airway pressure (CPAP) treatment for moderate and severe OSAS generally improves cognitive performance, but some deficits may persist as impairment in executive and visuoconstructive functioning [41,43,44]. Attention and vigilance generally improve, while the effects of CPAP on memory are inconsistent [41,45]. It has been suggested that longer treatment times may be required for specific cognitive changes to take effect [46].

A systematic review [47] of 44 studies showed that OSAS patients' information processing speed was reduced in 50% of studies when compared with healthy controls. CPAP treatment improved the processing speed marginally when compared with placebo or conservative treatment. OSAS severity is associated with delayed information processing speed and induces new deficits in manual dexterity. Higher-level executive dysfunction in OSAS may be caused by impaired lower-level attentional processes, such as slowed information processing and decreased short-term memory span. Motor and processing speed performance was significantly impaired, correlating with oxygen desaturation. Hypoxemia and hypercapnia induced frontally related executive dysfunction. OSAS patients' working memory performance has been shown to be affected by both executive and attentional deficits [48,49].

Sleep disturbance (eg, insomnia) related to RLS has also been found to compromise individuals' ability to focus, memorize, and ultimately to perform optimally at work or school, with alterations in prefrontal cognitive tasks, mainly executive functions [50]. Sleep deprivation also may increase irritability and hyperactivity, resulting in problems in relationships with others and in normal life activities.

In patients with sleepiness due to narcolepsy, depression and psychiatric comorbidity, more than objective cognitive deficits, might play a role in the subjectively perceived attention deficits. When counseling and treating patients with narcolepsy, clinicians should pay attention to potential depression, because subjective cognitive complaints may not relate to objective cognitive impairments [51].

Depressive symptoms have a major impact on quality of life [52]. High levels of depressive symptoms essentially expressed by fatigue affected 25% of children with narcolepsy, with girls older than 10 years being especially vulnerable [53].

Brain function is much more vulnerable to sleep loss in the morning hours than during the wake maintenance zone in the evening hours. Performance at any given time is determined by an interaction of the duration of the preceding wake episode (homeostatic factor), the chronic sleep debt carried by the individual, and the circadian phase (circadian factor) at the time of assessment. Circadian variation in performance is most evident when sleep loss is present [54] (Fig. 53.2).

Cardiovascular disease

Normal sleep continuity is considered to be important for the maintenance of cardiovascular, metabolic, and immune function, physiological homeostasis, and psychological balance. A recent editorial has suggested that it is reasonable to include sleep disturbances among the top 10 potentially modifiable risk factors for CVD [55]. CVD, diabetes, and overweight/obesity are closely linked conditions and are therefore considered together as "cardiometabolic diseases." Many sociocultural and behavioral factors are associated with increased cardiometabolic disease risk, including lower socioeconomic status, deficient diet, and sedentary lifestyle. Evidence from both experimental and epidemiological studies indicates that decreased sleep duration or quality may be risk factors for cardiometabolic diseases.

The association between poor sleep and CVD has been known for decades [56]. The links between insomnia, depression, and CVD show bidirectional associations, as also shown in longitudinal studies [57]. A recent review suggests that extreme sleep duration, either short or long, is a risk factor independent of depression [58], and insomnia is associated with CVD also after adjusting for depression. For women with at least one of the major symptoms (eg, difficulty falling asleep, waking up during the night, waking up too early, or nonrestorative sleep), moderate to severe insomnia is an independent risk factor for subsequent CVD: The fully adjusted hazard ratio (HR) was 1.4 for women and 1.3 for men with a current or former manual occupation [59]. The biological evidence supporting a possible pathway between insomnia and CVD is based partly on alterations in autonomic functioning, inflammatory and coagulatory mediators, and hormonal profiles.

Several epidemiological studies have found significant associations between insomnia and CVD markers, such as carotid intima–media thickness, cardiorespiratory fitness, and Framingham risk score. Difficulty in initiating sleep was associated with myocardial infarction or coronary death among women in the Framingham Study. Furthermore, delayed sleep could also lead to alterations in circadian rhythms, which are important for CVD pathogenesis. Difficulty in initiating sleep and nonrestorative sleep are associated with a modestly higher risk of total mortality and CVD-specific mortality [20].

Other specific sleep disorders, particularly OSA, are also associated with cardiometabolic diseases. Sleep apnea can increase the risk of developing CVD (with an incidence rate of 2 per 100 person-years) through a number of mechanisms: intermittent hypoxia, sleep fragmentation, chronic sympathetic activation, and systemic inflammation [60]. The multivariable models identified

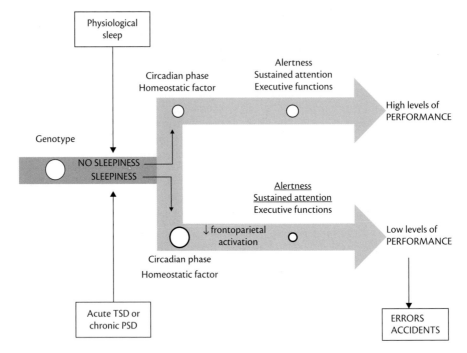

Fig. 53.2 Schematic representation of the performance process: the response to sleepiness is genetically determined and conditioned by other factors. Sleepiness influences our susceptibility to circadian variation (large circle) and reduces our level of alertness, sustained attention, and executive functions (small circle), with increased risk of errors and accidents. TSD: total sleep deprivation.; PSD: partial sleep deprivation.
Reproduced from Garbarino et al [Eds], Sleepiness and Human Impact Assessment, Copyright (2014), with permission from Springer.

OSA-related factors as independent and significant predictors of the occurrence of CV events and all-cause mortality. The strongest OSA-related predictor of CV events was the sleep time spent with arterial oxygen saturation (SaO_2) less than 90%, while the other factors included increased number of awakenings, increased mean heart rate, periodic leg movements, decreased total sleep time (TST), or presence of EDS, which were significantly and independently associated with a 5–50% increased risk of development of CVD by inducing endothelial dysfunction and sympathetic activation. The significant association between apnea–hypopnea index (AHI) and the composite CV outcome was obtained only by univariate analyses [60].

Severe OSA is significantly associated with an increased risk of CVD, stroke, and all-cause mortality. A positive association with CVD was observed for moderate OSA. In contrast, this risk is not significantly increased in patients with mild OSA [61].

After adjustment for potential confounders, OSA severity is associated with higher levels of high-sensitivity troponin T in middle-aged to older individuals, suggesting that subclinical myocardial injury caused by OSA may play a role in the subsequent risk of heart failure [62].

With regard to CPAP therapy, patients with worse oxygen desaturation at night and CPAP adherence of less than 4 hours per night showed a higher rate of hypertension or cardiovascular events than the control group [63].

SDB has been associated with a two- to threefold higher risk of incident stroke. In particular, OSA constitutes a risk factor for cerebrovascular events, and it is frequently seen in patients with both stroke and transient ischemic attack (TIA). OSA increases sympathetic tone, inducing hypertension, which may be a predisposing factor for stroke [64]. The evidence suggests that there is a dose–response relationship between the severity of obstructive SDB and the risk of serious adverse outcomes in stroke and TIA patients. In terms of CPAP treatment, a recent study showed how early nasal CPAP therapy has a positive effect on long-term survival in ischemic stroke patients and moderate–severe OSA [65].

Diabetes

According to the International Diabetes Federation, 382 million people (8.3%) worldwide currently have diabetes. Glucose metabolism is one of numerous physiological functions governed by the circadian apparatus. Nowadays, disruption of circadian timing mechanisms [66] is considered among the factors that play an unequivocal role in increasing the risk of developing type 2 diabetes mellitus (T2DM), promoting pancreatic B-cell dysfunction, abnormal adipogenesis, and absence of adequate insulin responsiveness, with other factors being genetic susceptibility, excessive food consumption or high calorie food intake, and a sedentary lifestyle. Sleep loss/disturbance induces circadian disturbances correlated with the onset of T2DM [67]: abnormal sleep times and poor sleep quality are associated with low levels of glucose tolerance in humans. The distribution of glucose to all parts of the body is organized by the molecular clock present in the liver [68]. Half of the nuclear receptors identified in the liver and in adipocytes exhibit a 24-hour periodicity. Important metabolic processes are dictated by the timing of food intake. Indeed, peripheral oscillator activity, a mechanism by which circadian cycles are regulated in peripheral tissues, closely controls temporal processes in liver and pancreas. Moreover, desynchronization between the circadian period of adipocytes (the peripheral oscillator) and the circadian period of the sleep–wake cycle (the suprachiasmatic nucleus) may play a central role in reduced glucose tolerance. In the absence of circadian regulation, the ensuing desynchrony could induce a metabolic disorder that, if sustained, could ultimately cause T2DM. The misalignment of clock functions may accelerate the development of T2DM. The current evidence thus suggests that these processes have a reciprocal relationship, since an abnormal functioning of metabolism promotes low expression of clock genes, while an impaired clock functioning can disrupt metabolic activity and alter adipogenesis, body mass and obesity. The findings thus underscore the importance of circadian regulation for normal metabolic functioning and the fact that clock gene expression appears to be disturbed in T2DM [69].

Night light exposure, even at low levels, has been reported to alter food timing and body mass accumulation in mice, thus suggesting that artificial lighting may be an important contributing factor to the increased prevalence of metabolic disorders [70].

Shift work, insufficient sunlight exposure, sleep disturbances, late night eating, and nocturnal light exposure are all known to produce circadian clock disruption. Various surveys have documented the increased prevalence of T2DM in night-shift workers. This category of employees, whose work involves irregular schedules and forced exposure to nocturnal lighting, show significant disruptions in sleep architecture and other markers of circadian synchronization [71].

Impairment of clock functions can affect metabolic activities, leading to reduced insulin sensitivity, impaired glucose metabolism, obesity, and altered clock gene expression, and, together with the effects of timing of food, sleep/wake disruption, an impaired melatonin pathway, and exposure of nocturnal light, can cause T2DM, and, by extension, threaten the survival of the organism. This can be seen in the high mortality rate associated with T2DM in the human population [69].

Bed times and sleep restriction have been associated with reduced glucose tolerance and reduced insulin sensitivity, changes in appetite-regulating hormones, including lower levels of leptin and increased levels of ghrelin, increased subjective appetite, increased caloric intake, particularly from fat, increased prevalence of obesity, and higher BMI. Impaired sleep quality (as a consequence of either reduced slow-wave sleep (SWS) or fragmented sleep) is associated with reduced glucose tolerance and reduced insulin sensitivity. Finally, increased blood pressure has been observed after a night of sleep restriction. Taken together, these experimental studies suggest that both sleep duration and reduced sleep quality are associated with over twice the risk of incident hypertension and adverse cardiometabolic effects [72].

Mortality

Sleeping too little or too much impacts severely on health with a U-shaped association between short and long sleep duration, and morbidity and even mortality risks across populations [73]. Typically, short sleep duration is thought to increase mortality risk through adverse endocrinological, immunological, or metabolic effects, through the induction of chronic, low-grade inflammation, or through increases in cortisol secretion or altered growth hormone metabolism. Biological mechanisms proposed for the association between long sleep duration and mortality risk include increased sleep fragmentation, fatigue, changes in immune function, photoperiodic abnormalities, lack of physiological challenge,

depression, or underlying disease processes [74]. Strong evidence exists linking short sleep duration with impairment of memory, reduced immunity, risk to safety, and increased risks of obesity, diabetes, and hypertension or other CVD. There is evidence for an associated between long sleep duration and obesity and depression, but the evidence is unclear regarding a correlation between long sleep duration and diabetes, hypertension or other CVD, and higher mortality [73,75].

Two meta-analyses have reported consistent increases in mortality risk among short and long sleepers of approximately 10% and 20–30%, respectively [76,77]. Conversely, a recent meta-analysis cautions that it is premature to conclude, as previous reviews have, that a robust, U-shaped association between sleep duration and mortality risk exists across populations [74].

It is likely that sleep disturbances characterized by insomnia symptoms represent novel risk factors for mortality especially for men with difficulty initiating sleep and those with nonrestorative sleep. EDS has also been increasingly recognized as a major health hazard and has been linked to an increased risk of all-cause mortality. The increased risk was independent of a variety of risk factors for mortality, including lifestyle factors and presence of several medical morbidities [20]. Insomnia has also been associated with incident depression, a risk factor for cardiovascular morbidity and mortality. Thus, insomnia may increase mortality risk through effects on several biological pathways.

Evidence exists for relationships between OSA and both all-cause mortality and various cardiovascular events, and available data suggest an association between mortality (all-cause and from CVD) and EDS [60]. The strongest OSA-related predictor of cardiovascular events seems to be the sleep time spent with $SaO_2 < 90\%$, but the number of awakenings, mean heart rate, and presence of EDS are significantly and independently associated with a 5–50% increased risk of development of the composite cardiovascular outcome, even after controlling for known CVD risk factors [60].

Moderate–severe OSA is an independent risk factor for all-cause mortality, cancer mortality, cancer incidence, and stroke [78].

In the US population, narcolepsy is associated with 1.5-fold increase in all-cause mortality. Mortality rates increase with age, but there is a peak in the relative mortality risk in the age groups 25–34 and 35–44 years. At least some of the early mortality may be a result of suicide, potentially resulting from the combination of reduced health-related quality of life and comorbid depression [79].

Sleep disorders and quality of life

There is a strong association between sleeping problems and quality-of-life variables (eg, poor economic status, family and social situations like divorce and separation, mental stress, and lifestyle). According to Arber et al. [15], socioeconomic inequalities explain a major part of the gender-related differences in sleep problems. There is a pattern of increasing percentage confirming sleeping problems across worsening categories of economic, social, and family situations in all observed age groups, indicating a general, strong association between socioeconomic status and women's sleep. There is a significant association between perceived mental stress and poor sleep [80].

Chronic insomnia has also been documented as negatively impacting several domains of health-related quality of life (HRQoL), not just the obvious ones, like vitality and energy, but also extending to other aspects of mental, social, and physical functioning [16,81]. Successfully improving sleep, using both pharmacological and nonpharmacological interventions, can lead to significant improvements in domains of HRQoL [16].

Several large surveys have also reported a graded trend with insomnia severity; such associations continue to hold after controlling for both physical and mental health comorbidities [82–84].

Insomnia impacts on quality of life differently according to age: the "young" category (ages 30–49), had significantly lower scores on all domains of the 36-Item Short Form Health Survey (SF-36); the middle category (50–69 years) showed impairment on all but two domains (emotional role limitation and physical role limitation); and the elderly category was significantly impaired in four out of eight domains (pain, vitality, mental health, and physical functioning) relative to reference values [85].

Comparing those with insomnia and normal sleepers under six main domains (energy level, pain, sleep, social isolation, emotional reactions, and physical abilities), individuals with insomnia had significant impairment [86], considering five validated categories: physical role; energy and will to do things; cognitive (concentration, attention, and memory); social (relationships with others); and psychological well-being [87].

RLS impairs HRQoL [88]. In a recent study including a large cohort in the US, RLS symptoms and other sleep complains were longitudinally associated with lower future physical function in elderly population. The authors found a level of disability significantly higher among those with RLS than among those without [30].

The development of specific pathophysiological conditions associated with impaired locomotion or spontaneous locomotor-like movements such as RLS seems to involve the central pattern generator, a network of spinal neurons. Poorer sleep quality, presence of insomnia, or EDS can predict greater disability independent of RLS symptoms and are associated with poorer physical function [30].

EDS and altered circadian rhythms may affect quality of life directly, particularly in relation to functional capacity, health, and sensation of well-being [89]. Sleep apnea is the most common cause of excessive sleepiness, which leads to significant impairments in quality of life and cognitive performance, especially if it is associated with obesity [90,91]. The decrease in vitality, social functioning, and emotional dimensions is significantly related to diurnal sleepiness and impaired alertness [90]. Quality of life scores were reported to be lower in 40–60% of obese populations [92], with an impairment linearly related to BMI and improving after weight loss. Sleepy non-physically active subjects and group with severe apnea had impaired quality of life associated with EDS, a decrease in quality of sleep, a reduction in sleep efficiency, increased stages I and II sleep, and reduced stage III and REM sleep compared with the control group. Nocturnal hypoxemia is a commonly cited causative factor for abnormal sleep patterns with adverse consequences on both physical and mental health [93,94].

Narcolepsy is a chronic disease often requiring lifelong medical treatment, which may have a profound impact on functioning, quality of life, and healthcare costs [95]. Moreover, a recent study on the societal effects of narcolepsy reported a substantial economic burden resulting from high healthcare costs and reduced income observed up to 11 years before diagnosis [79,96]. However, it has also been reported that HRQoL tends to improve over time in patients with narcolepsy [97], perhaps as a result of adaptation

strategies that enable patients to cope with the impact of the disease later in life when they are in their peak productivity [79].

Sleep disorders and performance at work

The relationship between work performance and sleep quality is reciprocal and potentially complex. Occupational injuries are a major problem worldwide. The prevalence of sleep problems varies in the working population, ranging from approximately 18% in Europe to 23% in the US [98]. Thus, work schedules and occupational demands can act as precipitating and perpetuating factors in the development of insomnia [99]. Insomnia-related impaired work performance continues to represent a significant cost burden on the individual worker, healthcare systems and employers (typically, absenteeism). Large survey and population-based studies further reveal a number of increased morbidity markers in those suffering from insomnia, including increased work absenteeism, reduced work productivity, and greater frequency of accidents [101–102]. Such impairments may be compounded by co-occurring illness. However, workplace studies controlling for both mental and physical comorbidities still reveal significant negative effects of insomnia on objective data (eg, absenteeism), self-reported work efficiency [101], work disability pension claims [103], and overall loss in productivity [104]. Workers reporting insomnia symptoms experience a subjective reduction in workplace productivity that appears to be related to symptom severity and may develop incrementally over time [99]. The majority of studies have reported significantly increased absenteeism, the levels of which have also been associated with the severity of the insomnia symptoms [105]). The National Sleep Foundation survey [106] found that the risk of accidents and injuries at work was significantly higher among those reporting a sleep latency of more than 30 minutes.

The prevalence of sleep disorders and of EDS is higher in shift workers than in non-shift workers [107–111]. The association between sleep disorders and shift work is bidirectional. Shift work induces some sleep complaints such as insomnia, poor sleep quality, and daytime sleepiness. On the other hand, underlying sleep disorders decrease workers' capabilities to adapt with shift working and increase the number of accidents at work [107–109,112–114]. Insomnia and low sleep quality had the highest correlation with the incidence of negative occupational impacts [111].

Workers with sleep problems had a 1.62 times greater risk of being injured at work compared with workers without sleep problems. Moreover, each aspect of the sleep problem significantly increased the risk for work injuries, with the largest effects being seen for the use of sleep medication and for breathing-related sleep problems. Approximately 13% of work injuries could be attributed to sleep problems [98].

Sleep disorders and road safety

Every day, more than 3000 people die in motor vehicle crashes around the world—amounting to more than 1.3 million motor-vehicle-related deaths worldwide each year—and between 20 million and 50 million more are injured and often left disabled for life [115]. Human error is found in 90% of accidents [116], with the main human factors being fatigue and sleepiness [113,117,118].

Several reviews have reported that OSA, insomnia, hypersomnias, and sleepiness increased the risk of work-related traffic accidents in commercial drivers. In general, sleep problems cause a two- to sevenfold increased risk of traffic accidents. According to the European statistics on accidents at work (ESAW), road traffic accidents constituted 9.6% of all accidents at work in 2007 [119].

Studies on the relationship between sleep disorders and road accidents are impressive. An Australian study observed that approximately 50% of injured motor drivers surviving a vehicle collision had at least one sleep-related risk factor [120]. In a large cohort of regular highway drivers, 16.9% complained of at least one sleep disorder, with 5.2% reporting OSAS, 9.3% insomnia, and 0.1% narcolepsy and hypersomnia; 8.9% of drivers reported experiencing at least once a month an episode of sleepiness at the wheel so severe that they had to stop driving. One-third of the drivers (31.1%) reported near-miss accidents (50% being sleep-related), 7.2% reported a driving accident in the past year, and 5.8% of these driving accidents were sleep-related [121].

Insomnia is responsible for EDS in 12–15% of adults. EDS as a consequence of insomnia might increase accident risk, but the risk of insomnia symptoms appears to be differentially associated with motor-vehicle and non-motor-vehicle accidents. Moreover, the strong association between hypnotics and road traffic accidents is under debate. Insomnia symptoms significantly elevate accident risk in the workplace, though the extent to which such accident risk is influenced by the concomitant use of hypnotic drugs is less clear [99]. Insomnia and insomnia symptoms can negatively impact the efficiency of daytime psychomotor performance.

OSAS is probably the most studied pathology with respect to traffic and workplace accidents [122]. It results in complaints of severe daytime sleepiness [123], and, most importantly, many sufferers report sleep-related crashes or near-miss incidents. Several studies in the last 20 years have shown a clear positive relationship between OSAS and traffic accidents [124–139].

The most important study regarding driving accidents and OSAS is be the case–control investigation by Teran-Santos et al. [140], which compared apneics with controls to evaluate the accident risk related to nocturnal breathing disorder. Compared with controls, apneics having an AHI ≥10 had an odds ratio of 6.3 (95% confidence interval 2.40–16.02) for experiencing a traffic crash. This relationship remained significant after adjustment for the potential confounders of alcohol consumption, visual-refraction disorders, BMI, years of driving, driver age, traffic accident history, medications causing drowsiness, and sleep schedule. Many other studies have confirmed the increased accident risk associated with OSAS in noncommercial drivers [118,141,142]. Furthermore, many studies have also shown that OSAS plays an important role in road accidents of professional drivers [124,143–145].

From the point of view of legislation, in Europe since 2014, there has been a historic change in the regulation of driving licenses and OSAS: see Box 53.1.

There are too few sufficiently large studies to determine with confidence the actual magnitude of risk posed by narcolepsy for nodding-off driving accidents [128]. The proportion of patients with sleep-related accidents was reported highest in narcoleptics [139]. Other studies showed a significant decrement in the mean level of attention and vigilant scores plus substantial inconsistency of cognitive performance of narcoleptics in simulated driving assessment studies [146,147].

Box 53.1 Commission Directive 2014/85/EU of 1 July 2014 amending Directive 2006/126/EC of the European Parliament and of the Council on Driving Licences

Article 2

- 1. Member States shall adopt and publish, by 31 December 2015 at the latest, the laws, regulations and administrative provisions necessary to comply with this Directive. They shall forthwith communicate to the Commission the text of those provisions.

- They shall apply those provisions from 31 December 2015.

- When Member States adopt those provisions, they shall contain a reference to this Directive or be accompanied by such a reference on the occasion of their official publication. Member States shall determine how such reference is to be made.

Annex

2. In Annex III to Directive 2006/126/EC, Section 11 ("NEUROLOGICAL DISEASES") is replaced by the following:

Obstructive sleep apnoea syndrome

- 11.2. In the following paragraphs, a moderate obstructive sleep apnoea syndrome corresponds to a number of apnoeas and hypopnoeas per hour (Apnoea–Hypopnoea Index) between 15 and 29 and a severe obstructive sleep apnoea syndrome corresponds to an Apnoea–Hypopnoea Index of 30 or more, both associated with excessive daytime sleepiness.

- 11.3. Applicants or drivers in whom a moderate or severe obstructive sleep apnoea syndrome is suspected shall be referred for further authorised medical advice before a driving licence is issued or renewed. They may be advised not to drive until confirmation of the diagnosis.

- 11.4. Driving licences may be issued to applicants or drivers with moderate or severe obstructive sleep apnoea syndrome who show adequate control of their condition and compliance with appropriate treatment and improvement of sleepiness, if any, confirmed by authorised medical opinion.

- 11.5. Applicants or drivers with moderate or severe obstructive sleep apnoea syndrome under treatment shall be subject to a periodic medical review, at intervals not exceeding three years for drivers of group 1 and one year for drivers of group 2, with a view to establish the level of compliance with the treatment, the need for continuing the treatment and continued good vigilance.

http://eur-lex.europa.eu/legal-content/EN/TXT/?uri=uriserv:OJ.L_.2014. 194.01.0010.01.ENG

Even though periodic limb movements of sleep (PLMS) and RLS can give rise to severe excessive daytime sleepiness and fatigue, these disorders have yet to be properly evaluated for the risk each possesses for driving crashes. In a small sample of patients suffering from either PLMS or RLS, about 16% of the subjects had been involved in traffic crashes [139]. Thus, it is impossible to conclude from this quite small sample-sized study the actual risk attributed to each of these sleep disorders.

An example of economic impact

Poor sleep and its consequences result in a significant increase in direct costs of the sleep disorder itself and indirect financial and nonfinancial costs. Other financial costs include non-health costs of work-related injuries, motor vehicle accidents, and productivity losses. Nonfinancial costs derive from loss of quality of life and premature death.

In 2011, in Australia, the Sleep Health Foundation commissioned Deloitte Access Economics, a national economics consultancy with a strong health economics background, to undertake an analysis of the direct and indirect costs associated with sleep disorders for the 2010 calendar year [148]. Deloitte Access Economics examined costs associated with the three most common sleep disorders— OSA, primary insomnia and restless legs syndrome—as the robust data required for analysis were available:

- Total healthcare costs: these were Australian $818 million per year for these conditions, comprising $274 million for the costs of caring for the disorders themselves and $544 million for conditions associated with them. Of these costs, $657 million per year were related to OSA: $248 million for OSA itself and $409 million for the health costs of conditions attributable to OSA. These conditions include hypertension, vascular disease, depression, and motor vehicle and workplace accidents;

- Indirect financial and nonfinancial costs: the indirect financial costs were estimated to be $4.3 billion in 2010. Of these indirect costs, OSA accounted for 61% ($2.6 billion), primary insomnia for 36% ($1.5 billion) and RLS for 3% ($115 million).

- Loss of quality of life cost: a dollar cost was calculated from the product of these years lost (190 000) and the value of a statistical life-year ($165 000). This added a further nonfinancial cost of $31.4 billion to the total economic cost of sleep disorders.

References

1. Barclay NL, Gregory AM. Quantitative genetic research on sleep: a review of normal sleep, sleep disturbances and associated emotional, behavioural, and health-related difficulties. Sleep Med Rev 2013;17(1):29–40.
2. Van den Oord E, Boomsma DI, Verhulst FC. A study of genetic and environmental effects on the co-occurrence of problem behaviors in three-year-old twins. J Abnorm Psychol 2000;109:360e72.
3. Gregory AM, Rijsdijk FV, Dahl RE, McGuffin P, Eley TC. Associations between sleep problems, anxiety, and depression in twins at 8 years of age. Pediatrics 2006;118:1124e32.
4. Gregory AM, Rijsdijk FV, Lau JYF, Dahl RE, Eley TC. The direction of longitudinal associations between sleep problems and depression symptoms: a study of twins aged 8 and 10 years. Sleep 2009;32:189e99.
5. Gehrman P, Meltzer L, Moore M, et al. Heritability of insomnia symptoms in youth and their relationship to depression and anxiety. Sleep 2011;34:1641e6.
6. Ford DE, Kamerow DB. Epidemiologic study of sleep disturbances and psychiatric disorders. An opportunity for prevention. JAMA 1989;262: 1479e84.
7. Gregory AM, Buysse DJ, Willis TA, Rijsdijk FV, Maughan B, Rowe R, et al. Associations between sleep quality and anxiety and depression symptoms in a sample of young adult twins and siblings. J Psychosom Res 2011;71:250e5.
8. Carmelli D, Bliwise DL, Swan GE, Reed T. Genetic factors in self-reported snoring and excessive daytime sleepiness. A twin study. Am J Respir Crit Care Med 2001;164:949e52.
9. Watson NF, Goldberg J, Arguelles L, Buchwald D. Genetic and environmental influences on insomnia, daytime sleepiness, and obesity in twins. Sleep 2006;29:645e9.
10. Watson NF, Buchwald D, Vitiello MV, Noonan C, Goldberg J. A twin study of sleep duration and body mass index. J Clin Sleep Med 2010;6:11e7.
11. Collier DA, Stober G, Li T, et al. A novel functional polymorphism within the promoter of the serotonin transporter gene: possible role in susceptibility to affective disorders. Mol Psychiatry 1996;1:453e60.
12. Lesch KP, Bengel D, Heils A, et al. Association of anxiety-related traits with a polymorphism in the serotonin transporter gene regulatory region. Science 1996;274:1527e31.
13. Barclay NL, Eley TC, Mill J, et al. Sleep quality and diurnal preference in a sample of young adults: associations with *5HTTLPR, PER3* and *CLOCK3111*. Am J Med Genet B Neuropsychiatr Genet 2011;156:681e90.
14. Lavie P. Current concepts: sleep disturbances in the wake of traumatic events. N Engl J Med 2001;345:1825e32.
15. Arber S, Bote M, Meadows R. Gender and socio-economic patterning of self- reported sleep problems in Britain. Soc Sci Med 2009;68:281e9.
16. Kyle SD, Morgan K, Espie CA. Insomnia and health-related quality of life. Sleep Med Rev 2010;14(1):69–82.
17. Leger D, Guilleminault C, Bader G, Levy E, Paillard M. Medical and socio- professional impact of insomnia. Sleep 2002;25:625–9.
18. Simon GE, VonKorff M. Prevalence, burden, and treatment of insomnia in primary care. Am J Psychiatry 1997;154:1417–23.
19. Hatoum HT, Kong SX, Kania CM, Wong JM, Mendelson WB. Insomnia, health-related quality of life and healthcare resource consumption—a study of managed-care organisation enrollees. Pharmacoeconomics 1998;14:629–37.
20. Li Y, Zhang X, Winkelman JW, et al. Association between insomnia symptoms and mortality: a prospective study of US men. Circulation 2014;129:737–46.
21. Jennum P, Kjellberg J. Health, social and economical consequences of sleep-disordered breathing: a controlled national study. Thorax 2011;66(7):560–6.
22. Plazzi G, Ferri R, Franceschini C, et al. Periodic leg movements during sleep in narcoleptic patients with or without restless legs syndrome. J Sleep Res 2012;21:155–62.
23. Sansa G, Iranzo A, Santamaria J. Obstructive sleep apnea in narcolepsy. Sleep Med 2010;11:93–5.
24. Jennum P, Ibsen R, Knudsen S, Kjellberg J. Comorbidity and mortality of narcolepsy: a controlled retro- and prospective national study. Sleep 2013;36:835–40.
25. Fortuyn HA, Mulders PC, Renier WO, et al. Narcolepsy and psychiatry: an evolving association of increasing interest. Sleep Med 2011;12:714–19.
26. Ohayon MM. Narcolepsy is complicated by high medical and psychiatric comorbidities: a comparison with the general population. Sleep Med 2013;14:488–92.
27. Allen RP, Stillman P, Myers AJ. Physician-diagnosed restless legs syndrome in a large sample of primary medical care patients in western Europe: prevalence and characteristics. Sleep Med 2010;11(1):31–7.
28. Ulfberg J, Nystrom B, Carter N, Edling C. Prevalence of restless legs syndrome among men aged 18 to 64 years: an association with somatic disease and neuropsychiatric symptoms. Mov Disord 2001;16(6):1159–63.
29. Broman JE, Mallon L, Hetta J. Restless legs syndrome and its relationship with insomnia symptoms and daytime distress: epidemiological survey in Sweden. Psychiatry Clin Neurosci 2008;62(4):472–5.
30. Zhang C, Li Y, Malhotra A, Ning Y, Gao X. Restless legs syndrome status as a predictor for lower physical function. Neurology 2014;82(14):1212–18.
31. Lasch KE, Abraham L, Patrick J, et al. Development of a next day functioning measure to assess the impact of sleep disturbance due to restless legs syndrome: the restless legs syndrome-next day impact questionnaire. Sleep Med 2011;12(8):754–61.

32. Motivala SJ, Levin MJ, Oxman MN, Irwin MR. Impairments in health functioning and sleep quality in older adults with a history of depression. J Am Geriatr Soc 2006;54:1184–91.

33. Baglioni C, Battagliese G, Feige B, et al. Insomnia as a predictor of depression: a meta-analytic evaluation of longitudinal epidemiological studies. J Affect Disord 2011;135:10–19.

34. Novati A, Hulshof HJ, Granic I, Meerlo P. Chronic partial sleep deprivation reduces brain sensitivity to glutamate N-methyl-D-aspartate receptor-mediated neurotoxicity. J Sleep Res 2012;21:3–9.

35. Lopresti AL, Hood SD, Drummond PD. A review of lifestyle factors that contribute to important pathways associated with major depression: diet, sleep and exercise. J Affect Disord 2013;148(1):12–27.

36. Soehner AM, Kaplan KA, Harvey AG. Insomnia comorbid to severe psychiatric illness. Sleep Med Clin 2013;8(3):361–71.

37. Fortier-Brochu E, Morin CM. Cognitive impairment in individuals with insomnia: clinical significance and correlates. Sleep 2014;37(11):1787–98.

38. Yaffe K, Falvey CM, Hoang T. Connections between sleep and cognition in older adults. Lancet Neurol 2014;13(10):1017–28.

39. Dècary A, Rouleau I, Montplaisir J. Cognitive deficits associated with sleep apnea syndrome: a proposed neuro-psychological test battery. Sleep 2000;23:369–81.

40. Beebe DW, Groesz BA, Wells C, Nichols A, McGee K. The neuropsychological effects of obstructive sleep apnea: a meta-analysis of norm-referenced and case-controlled data. Sleep 2003;26:298–307.

41. Aloia MS, Arnedt T, Davis JD. Neuropsychological sequelae of obstructive sleep apnea–hypopnea syndrome: a critical review. J Int Neuropsychol Soc 2004;10:772–85.

42. Verstraeten E. Neurocognitive effects of obstructive sleep apnea syndrome. Curr Neurol Neurosci Rep 2007;7:161–6.

43. Sanchez AI, Martinez P, Miro E, et al. CPAP and behavioral therapies in patients with obstructive sleep apnea: effects on daytime sleepiness, mood and cognitive function. Sleep Med Rev 2009;13:223–33.

44. Beebe DW, Gozal D. Obstructive sleep apnea and the prefrontal cortex: towards a comprehensive model linking nocturnal upper airway obstruction to daytime cognitive and behavioural deficits. J Sleep Res 2002;11:1–16.

45. McMahon JP, Foresman BH, Chisholm RC. The influence of CPAP on the neurobehavioral performance of patients with obstructive sleep apnea hypopnea syndrome: a systematic review. Wis Med J 2003;102:36–43.

46. Bardwell WA, Ancoli-Israel S, Berry CC. Neuropsychological effects of one-week continuous positive airway pressure treatment in patients with obstructive sleep apnea: a placebo-controlled study. Psychosom Med 2001;63:579–84.

47. Kilpinen R, Saunamäki T, Jehkonen M. Information processing speed in obstructive sleep apnea syndrome: a review. Acta Neurol Scand 2014;129(4):209–18.

48. Lis S, Krieger S, Hennig D, et al. Executive functions and cognitive subprocesses in patients with obstructive sleep apnoea. J Sleep Res 2008;17:271–80.

49. Naegele B, Launois SH, Mazza S, et al. Which memory processes are affected in patients with obstructive sleep apnea? An evaluation of 3 types of memory. Sleep 2006;29:533–44.

50. Ram S, Seirawan H, Kumar SK, Clark GT. Prevalence and impact of sleep disorders and sleep habits in the United States. Sleep Breath 2010;14:63–70.

51. Zamarian L, Högl B, Delazer M, et al. Subjective deficits of attention, cognition and depression in patients with narcolepsy. Sleep Med 2015;16:45–51.

52. Inocente CO, Gustin MP, Lavault S, et al. Quality of life in children with narcolepsy. CNS Neurosci Ther 2014;20(8):763–71.

53. Inocente CO, Gustin MP, Lavault S, et al. Depressive feelings in children with narcolepsy. Sleep Med 2014;15(3):309–14.

54. Philip P, Chaufton C, Nobili L, Garbarino S. Errors and accidents. In: Garbarino S, Nobili L, Costa G, eds. Sleepiness and human impact assessment. Milan: Springer, 2014:81–92.

55. Redline S, Foody J. Sleep disturbances: time to join the top 10 potentially modifiable cardiovascular risk factors? Circulation 2011;124:2049–51.

56. Schwartz S, McDowell Anderson W, et al. Insomnia and heart disease: a review of epidemiologic studies. J Psychosom Res 1999;47:313–33.

57. Sivertsen B, Salo P, Mykletun A, et al. The bidirectional association between depression and insomnia: the HUNT study. Psychosom Med 2012;74:758–65.

58. Mezick EJ, Hall M, Matthews KA. Are sleep and depression independent or overlapping risk factors for cardiometabolic disease? Sleep Med Rev 2011;15:51–63.

59. Canivet C, Nilsson PM, Lindeberg SI, Karasek R, Östergren PO. Insomnia increases risk for cardiovascular events in women and in men with low socioeconomic status: a longitudinal, register-based study. J Psychosom Res 2014;76(4):292–9.

60. Kendzerska T, Gershon AS, Hawker G, Leung RS, Tomlinson G. Obstructive sleep apnea and risk of cardiovascular events and all-cause mortality: a decade-long historical cohort study. PLoS Med 2014;11(2):e1001599.

61. Wang X, Ouyang Y, Wang Z, et al. Obstructive sleep apnea and risk of cardiovascular disease and all-cause mortality: a meta-analysis of prospective cohort studies. Int J Cardiol 2013;169(3):207–14.

62. Querejeta Roca G, Redline S, Punjabi N, et al. Sleep apnea is associated with subclinical myocardial injury in the community. The ARIC-SHHS study. Am J Respir Crit Care Med 2013;188(12):1460–5.

63. Barbe F, Duran-Cantolla J, Sanchez-de-la-Torre M, et al. Effect of continuous positive airway pressure on the incidence of hypertension and cardiovascular events in nonsleepy patients with obstructive sleep apnea: a randomized controlled trial. JAMA 2012;307:2161–8.

64. Johnson KG, Johnson DC. Frequency of sleep apnea in stroke and TIA patients: a meta-analysis. J Clin Sleep Med 2010:6(2):131–7.

65. Parra O, Sánchez-Armengol Á, Capote F, et al. Efficacy of continuous positive airway pressure treatment on 5-year survival in patients with ischaemic stroke and obstructive sleep apnea: a randomized controlled trial. J Sleep Res 2015;24(1):47–53.

66. Shi SQ, Ansari TS, McGuinness OP, Wasserman DH, Johnson CH. Circadian disruption leads to insulin resistance and obesity. Curr Biol 2013;23:372–81.

67. Maury E, Ramsey KM, Bass J. Circadian rhythms and metabolic syndrome: from experimental genetics to human disease. Circ Res 2010;106:447–62.

68. Lamia KA, Storch KF, Weitz CJ. Physiological significance of a peripheral tissue circadian clock. Proc Natl Acad Sci U S A 2008;105:15172–7.

69. Karthikeyan R, Marimuthu G, Spence DW, et al. Should we listen to our clock to prevent type 2 diabetes mellitus? Diabetes Res Clin Pract 2014;106:182–90.

70. Fonken LK, Nelson RJ. The effects of light at night on circadian clocks and metabolism. Endocr Rev 2014;35(4):648–70.

71. Szosland D. Shift work and metabolic syndrome, diabetes mellitus and ischaemic heart disease. Int J Occup Med Environ Health 2010;23:287–91.

72. Orozco-Solis R, Sassone-Corsi P. Epigenetic control and the circadian clock: linking metabolism to neuronal responses. Neuroscience 2014;264:76–87.

73. Léger D, Beck F, Richard JB, Sauvet F, Faraut B. The risks of sleeping "too much." Survey of a national representative sample of 24671 adults (INPES health barometer). PLoS One 2014;9(9):e106950.

74. Kurina LM, McClintock MK, Chen JH, et al. Sleep duration and all-cause mortality: a critical review of measurement and associations. Ann Epidemiol 2013;23(6):361–70.

75. Buxton OM, Marcelli E. Short and long sleep are positively associated with obesity, diabetes, hypertension, and cardiovascular disease among adults in the United States. Soc Sci Med 2010;71:1027–36.

76. Cappuccio FP, D'Elia L, Strazzullo P, Miller MA. Sleep duration and all-cause mortality: a systematic review and meta-analysis of prospective studies. Sleep 2010;33:585e92.

77. Gallicchio L, Kalesan B. Sleep duration and mortality: a systematic review and meta-analysis. J Sleep Res 2009;18:148e58.

78. Marshall NS, Wong KK, Cullen SR, Knuiman MW, Grunstein RR. Sleep apnea and 20-year follow-up for all-cause mortality, stroke, and cancer incidence and mortality in the Busselton Health Study cohort. J Clin Sleep Med 2014;10(4):355–62.

79. Ohayon MM, Black J, Lai C, et al. Increased mortality in narcolepsy. Sleep 2014;37(3):439–44.

80. Rowshan Ravan A, Bengtsson C, Lissner L, Lapidus L, Björkelund C. Thirty-six-year secular trends in sleep duration and sleep satisfaction, and associations with mental stress and socioeconomic factors—results of the Population Study of Women in Gothenburg, Sweden. J Sleep Res 2010;19(3):496–503.

81. Kyle S D, Espie CA. "... Not just a minor thing, it is something major, which stops you from functioning daily": Quality of life and daytime functioning in insomnia. Behavioral Sleep Medicine 2010:8:123–40.

82. Leger D, Scheuermaier K, Philip P, Paillard M, Guilleminault C. SF-36: evaluation of quality of life in severe and mild insomniacs compared with good sleepers. Psychosom Med 2001;63:49–55.

83. Schubert CR, Cruickshanks KJ, Dalton DS, et al. Prevalence of sleep problems and quality of life in an older population. Sleep 2002;25:889–93.

84. Katz DA, McHorney CA. The relationship between insomnia and health-related quality of life in patients with chronic illness. J Fam Pract 2002;51:229–35.

85. Dixon S, Morgan K, Mathers N, Thompson J, Tomeny M. Impact of cognitive behavior therapy on health-related quality of life among adult hypnotic users with chronic insomnia. Behav Sleep Med 2006;4:71–84.

86. Philip P, Leger D, Taillard J, et al. Insomniac complaints interfere with quality of life but not with absenteeism: respective role of depressive and organic comorbidity. Sleep Med 2006;7:585–91.

87. Leger D, Scheuermaier K, Raffray T, et al. HD-16: a new quality of life instrument specifically designed for insomnia. Sleep Med 2005;6:191–8.

88. Happe S, Reese JP, Stiasny-Kolster K, et al. Assessing health-related quality of life in patients with restless legs syndrome. Sleep Med 2009;10:295–305.

89. Jean-Louis G, Kripke DF, Ancoli-Israel S. Sleep and quality of well-being. Sleep 2000; 23:1115–21.

90. Sforza E, Janssens JP, Rochat T, Ibanez V. Determinants of altered quality of life in patients with sleep-related breathing disorders. Eur Respir J 2003;21(4):682–7.

91. Engleman HM, Douglas NJ. Sleep. 4: Sleepiness, cognitive function, and quality of life in obstructive sleep apnoea/hypopnoea syndrome. Thorax 2004;59:618–22.

92. Fontaine KR, Barofsky I. Obesity and health-related quality of life. Obes Rev 2002;2:173–82.

93. Lopes C, Esteves AM, Bittencourt LR, Tufik S, Mello MT. Relationship between the quality of life and the severity of obstructive sleep apnea syndrome. Braz J Med Biol Res 2008;41(10):908–13.

94. Karkoulias K, Lykouras D, Sampsonas F, et al. The impact of obstructive sleep apnea syndrome severity on physical performance and mental health. The use of SF-36 questionnaire in sleep apnea. Eur Rev Med Pharmacol Sci 2013;17(4):531–6.

95. Ozaki A, Inoue Y, Nakajima T, et al. Health-related quality of life among drug-naive patients with narcolepsy with cataplexy, narcolepsy without cataplexy, and idiopathic hypersomnia without long sleep time. J Clin Sleep Med 2008;4:572–8.

96. Jennum P, Ibsen R, Petersen ER, et al. Health, social, and economic consequences of narcolepsy: a controlled national study evaluating the societal effect on patients and their partners. Sleep Med 2012;13:1086–93.

97. Vignatelli L, Plazzi G, Peschechera F, et al. A 5-year prospective cohort study on health-related quality of life in patients with narcolepsy. Sleep Med 2011;12:19–23.

98. Uehli K, Mehta AJ, Miedinger D, et al. Sleep problems and work injuries: a systematic review and meta-analysis. Sleep Med Rev 2014;18(1):61–73.

99. Kucharczyk ER, Morgan K, Hall AP. The occupational impact of sleep quality and insomnia symptoms. Sleep Med Rev 2012;16(6):547–59.

100. Roth T, Ancoli-Israel S. Daytime consequences and correlates of insomnia in the United States: results of the 1991 National Sleep Foundation survey. II. Sleep 1999;22:S354–8.

101. Leger D, Massuel MA, Metlaine A, Sisyphe SG. Professional correlates of insomnia. Sleep 2006;29:171–8.

102. Daley M, Morin CM, LeBlanc M, et al. Insomnia and its relationship to health-care utilization, work absenteeism, productivity and accidents. Sleep Med 2009;10:427–38.

103. Sivertsen B, Overland S, Neckelmann D, et al. The long-term effect of insomnia on work disability—the HUNT-2 historical cohort study. Am J Epidemiol 2006;163:1018–24.

104. Bolge SC, Doan JF, Kannan H, Baran RW. Association of insomnia with quality of life, work productivity, and activity impairment. Qual Life Res 2009;18:415e22.

105. Linton SJ, Bryngelsson IL. Insomnia and its relationship to work and health in a working-age population. J Occup Rehabil 2000;10:169e83.

106. National Sleep Foundation. Gallup poll on sleep, performance and the workplace. Washington, DC: National Sleep Foundation, 2008.

107. Garbarino S, De Carli F, Nobili L, et al. Sleepiness and sleep disorders in shift workers: a study on a group of Italian police officers. Sleep 2002;25(6):648–53.

108. Garbarino S, Nobili L, Beelke M, et al. Sleep disorders and daytime sleepiness in state police shiftworkers. Arch Environ Health 2002;57(2):167–73.

109. Garbarino S, Beelke M, Costa G, et al. Brain function and effects of shift work: implications for clinical neuropharmacology. Neuropsychobiology 2002;45(1):50–6.

110. Fido A, Ghali A. Detrimental effects of variable work shifts on quality of sleep, general health and work performance. Med Princ Pract 2008;17(6):453–7.

111. Yazdi Z, Sadeghniiat-Haghighi K, Loukzadeh Z, Elmizadeh K, Abbasi M. Prevalence of sleep disorders and their impacts on occupational performance: a comparison between shift workers and nonshift workers. Sleep Disord 2014;2014:870320.

112. Garbarino S, De Carli F, Mascialino B, et al. Sleepiness in a population of Italian shiftwork policemen. J Hum Ergol (Tokyo) 2001;30(1–2):211–16.

113. Garbarino S, Nobili L, Beelke M, De Carli F, Ferrillo F. The contributing role of sleepiness in highway vehicle accidents. Sleep 2001;24:203–6.

114. Akerstedt T. Shift work and disturbed sleep/wakefulness. Occup Med 2003;53(2):89–94.

115. World Health Organization. Global status report on road safety 2013. Available from: http://www.who.int/violence_injury_prevention/road_safety_status/2013/en/

116. Bilincoe LJ, Secy AG, Zaloshnja E, et al. The economic impact of motor vehicle crashes 2000. Washington, DC: National Highway Traffic Safety Administration, 2002.

117. Kaneita Y, Ohida T, Uchiyama M, et al. Excessive daytime sleepiness among the Japanese general population. J Epidemiol 2005;15:1–8.

118. Masa JF, Rubio M, Findley LJ. Habitually sleepy drivers have a high frequency of automobile crashes associated with respiratory disorders during sleep. Am J Respir Crit Care Med 2000;162(4):1407–12.

119. Eurostat. Health and safety at work in Europe (1999–2007): a statistical portrait. Luxembourg: Eurostat Statistical Books, 2010.

120. Crummy F, Cameron PA, Swann P, Kossmann T, Naughton MT. Prevalence of sleepiness in surviving drivers of motor vehicle collisions. Intern Med J 2008;38:769–75.

121. Philip P, Sagaspe P, Lagarde E, et al. Sleep disorders and accidental risk in a large group of regular registered highway drivers. Sleep Med 2010;11:973–9.

122. Garbarino S, Magnavita N. Obstructive sleep apnea syndrome (OSAS), metabolic syndrome and mental health in small enterprise workers. Feasibility of an action for health. PLoS One 2014; 9(5):e97188.

123. Young T, Blustein J, Finn L, Palta M. Sleep-disordered breathing and motor vehicle accidents in a population-based sample of employed adults. Sleep 1997;20:608–13.

124. Stevenson MR, Elkington J, Sharwood L, et al. The role of sleepiness, sleep disorders, and the work environment on heavy-vehicle crashes in 2 Australian states. Am J Epidemiol 2014;179(5):594–601.

125. Chu HC. Assessing factors causing severe injuries in crashes of high-deck buses in long-distance driving on freeways. Accid Anal Prev 2014;62:130–6.

126. Catarino R, Spratley J, Catarino I, Lunet N, Pais-Clemente M. Sleepiness and sleep-disordered breathing in truck drivers: risk analysis of road accidents. Sleep Breath 2014;18(1):59–68.

127. Philip P, Sagaspe P. [Sleep and accidents.] Bull Acad Natl Med 2011;195(7):1635–43.

128. Smolensky MH, Di Milia L, Ohayon MM, Philip P. Sleep disorders, medical conditions, and road accident risk. Accid Anal Prev 2011;43(2):533–48.

129. Swanson LM, Arnedt JT, Rosekind MR, et al. Sleep disorders and work performance: findings from the 2008 National Sleep Foundation Sleep in America poll. J Sleep Res 2011;20(3):487–94.

130. Garbarino S. [Sleep disorders and road accidents in truck drivers.] G Ital Med Lav Ergon 2008;30(3):291–6.

131. Mazza S, Pépin JL, Naëgelé B, et al. Driving ability in sleep apnoea patients before and after CPAP treatment: evaluation on a road safety platform. Eur Respir J 2006;28(5):1020–8.

132. Barbé F, Sunyer J, de la Peña A, et al. Effect of continuous positive airway pressure on the risk of road accidents in sleep apnea patients. Respiration 2007;74(1):44–9.

133. Philip P. Sleepiness of occupational drivers. Ind Health 2005;43(1):30–3.

134. George CF. Sleep. 5: Driving and automobile crashes in patients with obstructive sleep apnoea/hypopnoea syndrome. Thorax 2004;59(9):804–7.

135. Turkington PM, Sircar M, Allgar V, Elliott MW. Relationship between obstructive sleep apnoea, driving simulator performance, and risk of road traffic accidents. Thorax 2001;56(10):800–5.

136. Akerstedt T, Haraldsson PO. [International consensus meeting on fatigue and the risk of traffic accidents. The significance of fatigue for transportation safety is underestimated.] Lakartidningen 2001;98(25):3014–17.

137. Semple SJ, London DR. Obstructive sleep apnoea. Treatment prevents road accidents, injury, and death caused by daytime sleepiness. BMJ 1997;315(7104):368–9.

138. Wright J, Johns R, Watt I, Melville A, Sheldon T. Health effects of obstructive sleep apnoea and the effectiveness of continuous positive airways pressure: a systematic review of the research evidence. BMJ 1997;314(7084):851–60.

139. Aldrich MS. Automobile accidents in patients with sleep disorders. Sleep 1989;12(6):487–94.

140. Teran-Santos J, Jimenez-Gomez A, Cordero-Guevara J. The association between sleep apnea and the risk of traffic accidents. N Engl J Med 1999;340:847–51.

141. Lloberes P, Levy G, Descals C, et al. Self-reported sleepiness while driving as a risk factor for traffic accidents in patients with obstructive sleep apnoea syndrome and in non-apnoeic snorers. Respir Med 2000;94:971–6.

142. Vakulin A, Catcheside PG, Baulk SD, et al. Individual variability and predictors of driving simulator impairment in patients with obstructive sleep apnea. J Clin Sleep Med 2014;10(6):647–55.

143. Stoohs RA, Bingham L, Itoi A, Guilleminault C, Dement WC. Sleep and sleep-disordered breathing in commercial long-haul truck drivers. Chest 1995;107:1275–82.

144. Pack AI, Maislin G, Staley B, et al. Impaired performance in commercial drivers: role of sleep apnea and short sleep duration. Am J Respir Crit Care Med 2006;174:446–54.

145. Ellen RL, Marshall SC, Palayew M, Molnar FJ, Wilson KG. Systematic review of motor vehicle crash risk in persons with sleep apnea. J Clin Sleep Med 2006;2:193–200.

146. Findley LJ, Suratt PM, Dinges DF. Time-on-task decrements in "steerclear" performance of patients with sleep apnea and narcolepsy. Sleep 1999;15:804–9.

147. Kotterba S, Mueller N, Leidag M, et al. Comparison of driving simulator performance of neuropsychological testing in narcolepsy. Clin Neurol Neurosurg 2004;106:275–9.

148. Hillman DR, Lack LC. Public health implications of sleep loss: the community burden. Med J Aust 2013;199(8):S7–10.

CHAPTER 54

Sleep at high altitude and during space travel

Yvonne Nussbaumer-Ochsner and Konrad E. Bloch

Introduction

Both at high altitude and during space travel, humans are exposed to unusual environmental conditions like hypobaric hypoxia and microgravity, respectively, that may directly or indirectly affect sleep and wakefulness functions. Exposures to altitude and space exert quite dissimilar physical stimuli that elicit distinct physiological responses. Nevertheless, a mountaineer climbing in remote highlands and an astronaut travelling through space may experience sleep difficulties through similar mechanisms. The challenge of prolonged physical exertion, disruption of the regular sleep–wake rhythm, noise, uncomfortable temperature and sleeping conditions, the excitement of participating in an extraordinary mission, hope of great achievements, and fear of life-threatening failure may all contribute to sleep difficulties in mountain climbing and space travel. Illnesses specific to hypoxia at high altitude or to microgravity in space may additionally interfere with refreshing sleep and performance during wakefulness. Both healthy persons and subjects with a particular susceptibility or a pre-existing disease may be affected.

In this chapter, the effects of high altitude and space travel on sleep will be reviewed. While conclusions on sleep at high altitude are supported by data from an increasing number of observational and randomized, controlled studies, the few case reports on sleep in space published to date provide only limited insights.

Sleep at high altitude

With increasing altitude, barometric pressure falls exponentially (Fig. 54.1). As a consequence, the inspired and arterial partial pressures of oxygen decrease. This has a profound influence on virtually all organ systems [1]. With prolonged exposure to altitude, compensatory mechanisms, termed acclimatization, take place that mitigate some of the adverse effects. For example, the hypoxic stimulation of ventilation at altitude and the increased ventilatory sensitivity to hypoxia and hypercapnia increase the arterial oxygen partial pressure. In addition, erythropoiesis and a shift in the hemoglobin–oxygen dissociation curve related to respiratory alkalosis enhance the oxygen-carrying capacity of arterial blood. However, depending on individual susceptibility, speed of ascent, and altitude reached, the adaptation may be inappropriate, leading to excessive instability of respiratory control with pronounced periodic breathing and high-altitude-related illness that induce sleep disturbances. These conditions will be discussed later in this chapter, after a review of studies on the effect of altitude on sleep.

Sleep at high altitude in healthy subjects

According to a common belief, sleep in newcomers at high altitude is not as refreshing as near sea level. This assumption has, however, only recently been corroborated by scientific evidence. For example, a study using the Groeningen Sleep Quality Questionnaire in 100 tourists arriving in a ski resort at 3500 m revealed that 46 perceived poor sleep quality in their first night at altitude [2]. As subjective perception of sleep quality correlates poorly with objective measures of sleep duration and structure, it is important to consider studies using objective measurement methods when assessing the effect of altitude on sleep [3]. Few studies have used polysomnography (PSG), the gold standard for objectively recording sleep at altitude. This limitation is most likely due to logistic difficulties and the lack of electricity in remote mountain facilities. A systematic literature search on studies evaluating the effect of altitude on sleep based on objective measurements (either PSG or actimetry) revealed only three randomized, controlled studies

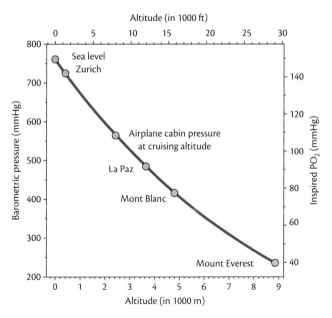

Fig. 54.1 Nonlinear fall of barometric pressure and the estimated inspiratory oxygen partial pressure with increasing altitude.

Reproduced from Nussbaumer-Ochsner Y, Bloch KE, Air travel and altitude. In: Ayres JG, Harrison RM, Nichols GL, Maynard RL, [eds], Environmental Medicine, pp. 547–561, Copyright (2010), with permission from CRC Press.

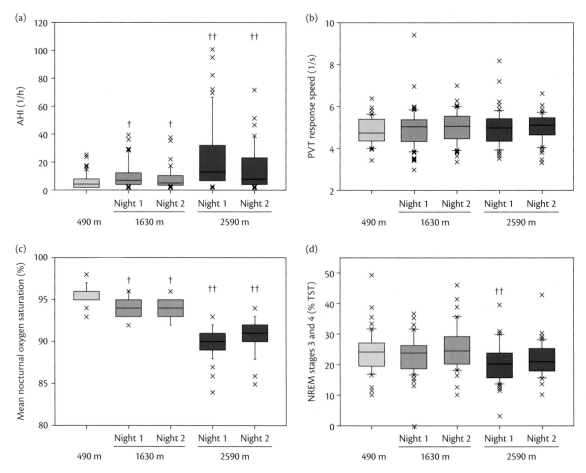

Fig. 54.2 Results of sleep and vigilance studies obtained in 51 healthy men living below 800 m during a sojourn at 1630 and 2590 m for 2 days each: (a) apnea–hypopnea index (AHI); (b) psychomotor vigilance test response speed; (c) mean nocturnal oxygen saturation; (d) slow-wave sleep (NREM sleep stages 3 and 4 as percentage of total sleep time). Horizontal lines, boxes, and whiskers represent the median, quartiles, and 10th and 90th percentiles, respectively; individual values beyond this range are displayed by asterisks. † indicates $p < 0.05$ versus 490 m; †† indicates $p < 0.05$ versus 490 and 1630 m.

Reproduced from Sleep, 36(12), Latshang TD, Lo Cascio CM, Stowhas AC et al., Are nocturnal breathing, sleep, and cognitive performance impaired at moderate altitude (1,630–2,590 m)?, pp. 1969–1976, Copyright (2013), with permission from Associated Professional Sleep Societies, LLC.

[4–6], including a total of 76 subjects, of these 51 participated in one of these studies [4]. In addition, five case–control studies [7–11] (including a total of 135 subjects) and 28 uncontrolled observational studies [3,5,12–37] (including a total of 302 subjects) were identified and analyzed in detail. Field studies performed in the mountains [4,7–9,14,18,22,23,28,30,34,35] were differentiated from studies simulating altitude by use of normobaric hypoxia (low inspired oxygen fraction) [21,31] or by hypobaric hypoxia (using a decompression chamber) [5,6,19,20,24,27]. Studies were further classified according to the range of altitudes at which they were conducted: $n = 8$ at moderate altitude (1500–2500 m) [4–6,15,26,28,31,34], $n = 27$ at high altitude (2501–4500 m) [4,5,8–14,16–18,21,23–29,33,34,37–41], and $n = 12$ at very high altitude (> 4500 m) [3,7,9,15,19,20,22,28,32,34–36]. This classification was chosen based on the prevalence of acute mountain sickness. Very limited information on sleep of highlanders living permanently at high altitude is available [42–46].

In a randomized crossover trial in 51 healthy young men, we found that sleep structure was significantly altered already at an altitude of 1630 m and even more so at 2590 m [4]. The main changes consisted of a slight reduction in deep sleep (NREM stages

3 and 4) (Fig. 54.2) [4]. This was corroborated by quantitative EEG analyses demonstrating a reduction in slow-wave activity correlating with periodic breathing that emerged at 1630 and 2590 m (Fig. 54.3) [47,48]. The alterations in sleep structure were not associated with impaired performance in a battery of cognitive and psychomotor tests applied to the subjects in the morning after sleeping at altitude (Fig. 54.2) [4]. In studies performed in healthy mountaineers at higher altitude (4559 m), the reduction in slow wave-sleep (SWS) was more pronounced than in the cited study at 2590 m, and subjects experienced a reduced sleep efficiency and more frequent arousals compared with baseline measurements at 490 m (Fig. 54.4) [49]. While other studies performed at altitudes of 4500 m or more [19,20,22,50] confirmed an increased sleep fragmentation, no trend of increasing arousals was observed in studies performed at altitudes below 3200 m [7,23,31]. Notably, there was a major discrepancy between subjective and objective assessment of sleep at high altitude, as shown by a comparison of subjective estimates of sleep latency with corresponding PSG measurements (Fig. 54.5) [3]. Whether acclimatization improves sleep quality at altitude has not been conclusively studied, although one report suggests that this is indeed the case [50]. We have identified only two reports on sleep

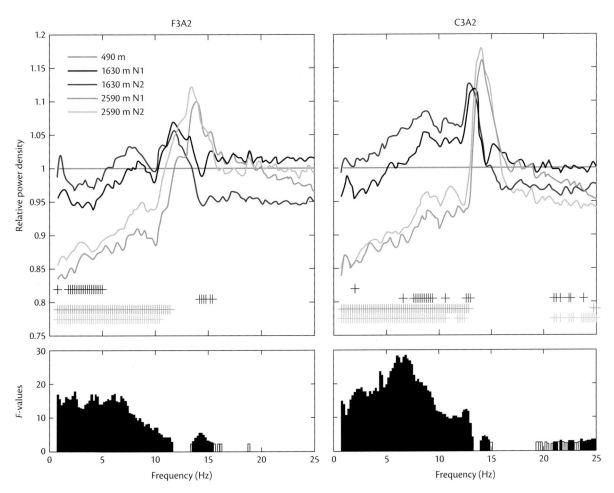

Fig. 54.3 (See colour plate section) Relative NREM sleep EEG power density spectra at moderate altitude recorded in healthy subjects. Upper panels: Spectra at altitude (1630 and 2590 m, N1 (first night) and N2 (second night)) are plotted relative to baseline sleep (490 m; line at 1). Significant differences ($p < 0.05$) between baseline and altitude are indicated by "+" ($n = 44$). Frequency resolution: 0.2 Hz. Lower panels: F-values of the frequency bins with significant p-values for factor Condition (490 m N1, 1630 m N1, 1630 m N2, 2590 m N1 and 2590 m N2) of mixed model ANOVA with factors Condition and Order. F3A2: frontal derivation; C3A2: central derivation. Reproduced from PLoS One, 8(10), Stadelmann K, Latshang TD, Lo Cascio CM et al., Quantitative changes in the sleep EEG at moderate altitude (1630 m and 2590 m), pp. e76945 Copyright (2013), with permission from PLoS under Creative Commons License 4.0.

in children at altitude. In these studies, actigraphic recordings suggested a more restless sleep in unacclimatized prepubertal children aged 11–12 years at 3560 m [8] and in preverbal children aged 3–33 months at 3109 m [26] compared with sea level.

When evaluating the available literature on sleep at altitude, it becomes evident that the studies are heterogeneous, encompassing different study protocols and settings that do not always allow a generalization of the results to the vast number of tourists travelling to altitude. Subjects are mostly selected from among healthy, highly trained mountaineers, athletes, or soldiers. The study settings vary greatly even within the same investigation, and the sample size is often inadequate. With these limitations and taking the more robust evidence from a few recent randomized or controlled studies into particular consideration, one may cautiously conclude that with increasing altitude, there is a trend for reduced SWS and sleep efficiency and increasing sleep fragmentation (Fig. 54.4).

High-altitude periodic breathing during sleep

High-altitude sleep disturbances are linked to periodic breathing, an oscillating pattern of waxing and waning of ventilation with periods of hyperventilation alternating with central apneas or hypopneas (Fig. 54.6). Exposure to hypoxia induces an immediate increase in ventilation (hypoxic ventilatory response) and ventilatory sensitivity to hypoxia and hypercapnia increases with acclimatization [51]. Hyperventilation with hypocapnia is therefore typically observed in newcomers at altitude. Once the arterial partial pressure of carbon dioxide ($PaCO_2$) falls below a certain level, called the apneic threshold, ventilation ceases until $PaCO_2$ rises again owing to metabolic activity. The resulting breathing pattern, characterized by waxing and waning of ventilation with periods of apnea/hypopnea alternating with hyperpnea, is called periodic breathing. It is a prominent characteristic of sleep at high altitude, but it may even occur during wakefulness and exercise at altitude [52]. The apneic phases of periodic breathing may be perceived as a distressing sense of suffocation followed by gasping for air in a few deep breaths.

Propensity for periodic breathing is increased during NREM sleep compared with wakefulness because of the absence of the stabilizing effect of the tonic "wakefulness drive" [53]. Furthermore, the reduced background drive to breathe during NREM sleep

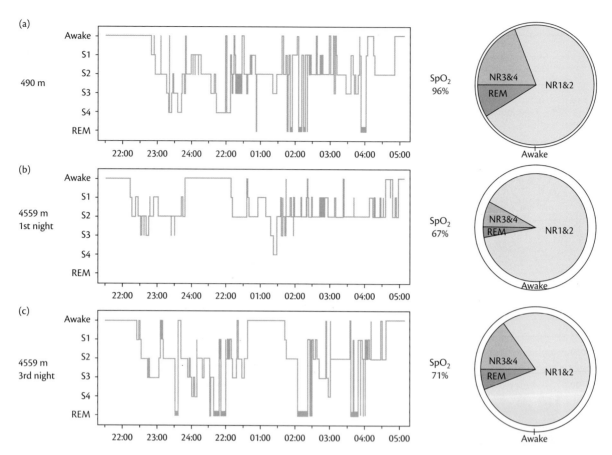

Fig. 54.4 Effects of short-term acclimatization to high altitude on sleep in healthy subjects. The hypnogram obtained in a subject during a night at 490 m (a) shows a normal distribution of sleep stages and several NREM/REM sleep cycles. In contrast, the hypnogram recorded during the 1st night at 4559 m (b) reveals predominantly superficial sleep stages with frequent awakenings, very rare deep sleep stages 3 and 4, and no REM sleep. The hypnogram from the 3rd night at 4559 m (c) reveals a partial restoration of normal sleep architecture. The right panels qualitatively summarize the trends of alterations in sleep structure at high altitude. The mean nocturnal oxygen saturation (SpO_2) and the distribution of sleep stages are represented in the pie charts. The outer circles of each panel represent the time in bed, the white area is the time spent awake and the pie chart area reflects total sleep time comprising NREM stages 1–4 (NR1&2: superficial stages; NR3&4: slow-wave or deep sleep stages) and REM sleep.
Adapted from High Alt Med Biol, 12(3), Nussbaumer-Ochsner Y, Schuepfer N, Siebenmann C, Maggiorini M, Bloch KE, High altitude sleep disturbances monitored by actigraphy and polysomnography, pp. 229–236, Copyright (2011), Mary Ann Liebert, Inc. publishers; Nussbaumer-Ochsner Y, Bloch KE, Sleep, In: Swenson ER, Bärtsch P [eds], High Altitude: Human Adaptation to Hypoxia, pp. 325–339, Copyright (2014), Springer.

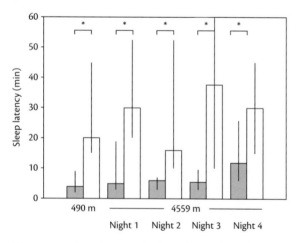

Fig. 54.5 Sleep latencies estimated subjectively (white bars) significantly exceed the corresponding values measured by PSG (green bars) in mountaineers studied at 4559 m (*$p < 0.05$). Bars and vertical lines represent medians and quartile ranges; the upper quartile in night 3 was 120 minutes.
Reproduced from High Alt Med Biol, 12(3), Nussbaumer-Ochsner Y, Schuepfer N, Siebenmann C, Maggiorini M, Bloch KE, High altitude sleep disturbances monitored by actigraphy and polysomnography, pp. 229–236, Copyright (2011), Mary Ann Liebert, Inc. publishers.

related to a reduced hypercapnic and hypoxic ventilatory response compared with wakefulness is associated with hypercapnia [54,55]. This reduces the amount of hyperventilation required to cross the apneic threshold because of the hyperbolic shape of the isometabolic line reflecting the relationship between alveolar ventilation and alveolar partial pressure of carbon dioxide ($PaCO_2$) relationship (Fig. 54.7) [56].

Most studies reveal an increasing prevalence of periodic breathing with increasing altitude and hypoxemia. It is observed already at 1630 m with great inter-individual variation in prevalence (Fig. 54.2) [4]. The reported number of periodic breathing cycles with central apnea/hypopnea is associated with an altitude-dependent decrease in oxygen saturation and ranges from 10 events/h at a simulated altitude of 2650 m [57] to as much as 254 events/h at 7620 m [20]. Correspondingly, with increasing altitude, the fraction of the night spent with periodic breathing increased from 34–58% at 4559 m [8,9] to 68% at 5050 m [22,58], to 73–75% at 7620–8050 m [21,59]. Periodic breathing may be associated with short awakenings or brief arousals that result in fragmented, non-restorative sleep. In one study, up to 52% of nocturnal arousals were associated with periodic breathing cycles, suggesting an important

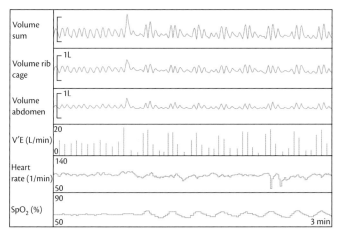

Fig. 54.6 Nocturnal polygraphic recording obtained at 6850 m in a 29-year-old woman. The channels are the respiratory inductive plethysmographic sum, rib cage and abdominal volumes, minute ventilation (V'E), heart rate, and oxygen saturation (SpO$_2$). In the first part of the 3-minute recording, breathing is regular. Subsequently, periodic breathing is triggered by a large breath (sigh or gasp). This results in oscillations of oxygen saturation from 64% to 71%.

Reproduced from Am J Respir Crit Care Med, 182(4), Bloch KE, Latshang TD, Turk AJ et al., Nocturnal periodic breathing during acclimatization at very high altitude at Mount Muztagh Ata (7,546 m), pp. 562–568, Copyright (2010), with permission from American Thoracic Society.

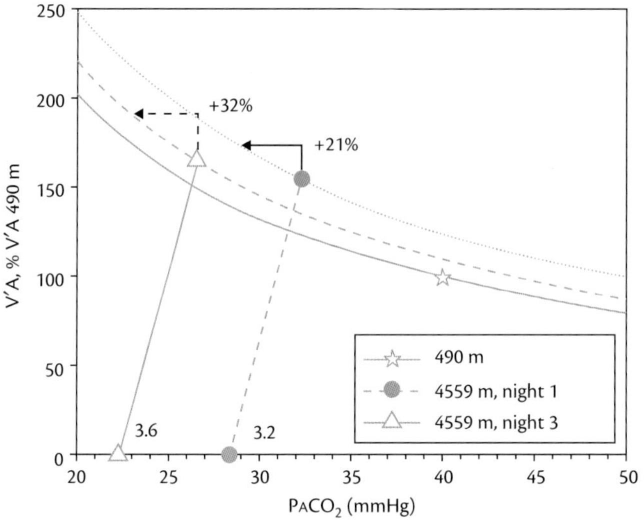

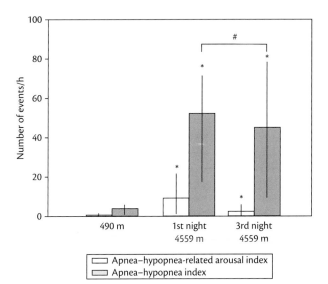

Fig. 54.7 Based on recordings in healthy mountaineers at 4559 m, determinants of periodic breathing are illustrated here in a diagram of alveolar ventilation (V'A) versus alveolar partial pressure of carbon dioxide (PACO$_2$, which is represented by the end-tidal PCO$_2$ as a surrogate). Assuming an increase in the metabolic rate on the 1st and 3rd night at 4559 m compared with the low-altitude baseline at 490 m, the corresponding isometabolic lines are displaced by 25% and 10%, respectively. The eupneic PCO$_2$ during stable breathing dropped from 40 mmHg at 490 m to 32 and 26 mmHg, respectively, on the 1st and 3rd nights at 4559 m. This was associated with a decrease in the corresponding apnea threshold from 28 to 22 mmHg (PACO$_2$ at V'A = 0). The increase in the slope of the line connecting the eupneic PCO$_2$ with the apnea threshold suggested an increase in the ventilatory sensitivity to hypocapnia in the 3rd compared with the 1st night (from 3.2 to 3.6 L/mmHg). Correspondingly, the displacement of the eupneic PCO$_2$ to the left on the isometabolic line increased the overshoot in V'A required to drive the PCO$_2$ from the eupneic level to the apnea threshold (from +21 to +32%). These changes were associated with a reduction in the AHI on the 3rd compared with the 1st night at 4559 m.

Reproduced from Sleep, 35(10), Nussbaumer-Ochsner Y, Schuepfer N, Ursprung J, Siebenmann C, Maggiorini M, Bloch KE, Sleep and breathing in high altitude pulmonary edema susceptible subjects at 4,559 meters, pp. 1413–1421, Copyright (2012), with permission from Associated Professional Sleep Societies, LLC.

but not exclusive role of periodic breathing in causing sleep disruption at altitude [19]. In more recent field studies [3,4,34,50], the correlation of arousals and periodic breathing during exposure to hypoxia was less consistent (Fig. 54.8) than in the cited hypobaric chamber study [19]. Of note, there may be a mutual interaction among arousals and periodic breathing, since periodic breathing may induce arousals, and they may in turn promote periodic breathing due to changes in ventilatory control during the sleep–wakefulness transition.

Research on ventilatory adaptation to high altitude has been nearly exclusively focused on adults. Only one study investigated the nocturnal breathing pattern in prepubertal children aged 10–11 years in comparison with adults [8]. Pairs of children with their fathers underwent PSG studies at the Jungfrau Joch (3450 m) in Switzerland after rapid ascent by train. It was found that despite a similar degree of nocturnal hypoxemia (mean nocturnal oxygen saturation of 85% versus 84%) and hypocapnia (mean of 32 versus 32 mmHg), children had less periodic breathing than adults (32.5 versus 54.1 periodic breathing cycles/h in the first night at 3450 m, $p < 0.05$). This was related to a lower apneic threshold for CO$_2$, a greater CO$_2$ reserve, and a shorter circulation time in children promoting a more stable control of breathing compared to adults [8].

There is only little information on the effect of ventilatory acclimatization on periodic breathing at altitude. In a field study performed at 4559 m in 16 mountaineers, ventilation initially increased to almost one and a half of the value at lowland owing to an increase in both tidal volume and breath rate [49]. Over the course of 4 days, minute ventilation slightly decreased, and this was associated with a gradual increase in arterial oxygen saturation (SpO$_2$) while end-tidal partial pressure of carbon dioxide (P$_{ET}$CO$_2$)

Fig. 54.8 Data from sleep studies performed in healthy mountaineers at 4559 m. Medians and quartile ranges (bars, vertical lines) of the apnea–hypopnea index (AHI) and the apnea–hypopnea-related arousals index at 490 m and on the 1st and the 3rd night at 4559 m are shown. Only 11% and 4% of apneas/hypopneas were followed by an arousal during the 1st and 3rd night, respectively. *$p < 0.05$ versus 490 m, #$p < 0.05$ versus 1st night at 4559 m.

Source data from Sleep, 35(10), Nussbaumer-Ochsner Y, Schuepfer N, Siebenmann C, Maggiorini M, Bloch KE, Sleep and breathing in high altitude pulmonary edema susceptible subjects at 4,559 meters, pp. 1413–1421, Copyright (2012), Associated Professional Sleep Societies, LLC.

remained stable. However, the apnea–hypopnea index (AHI) further increased from 60.9/h to 86.5/h. In a hypobaric chamber study simulating an altitude of 4200 m in 7 healthy men, ventilation increased over the course of 4 days, associated with progressive hypocapnia and gradually improved arterial oxygen saturation [17]. Changes were similar in wakefulness, NREM sleep, and REM sleep, suggesting that suprapontine influences were not essential for the acclimatization to chronic hypoxia, despite the marked influence of the sleep/wakefulness state on the stability of ventilatory control. Periodic breathing was not reported in the cited study [17], but other investigations have revealed variable results in this regard during acclimatization. While some authors reported a decrease in the prevalence of periodic breathing over the course of 7 days at 4300 m [51], others found no significant change during 6 days at 3200 m [23] or even an increase during 28 days at 5050 m [22]. In 34 mountaineers ascending Mount Muztagh Ata, periodic breathing increased during acclimatization over the course of more than 2 weeks at altitudes between 3730 and 6850 m, despite improving arterial oxygen saturation consistent with a progressive increase in the loop gain of the respiratory control system [58].

Sleep in subjects affected by altitude-related illness

Altitude-related illnesses may exert a major impact on sleep through the associated symptoms and excessive hypoxemia. A summary of the different forms is provided in Table 54.1. Acute forms include acute mountain sickness (AMS), high-altitude cerebral edema (HACE), and high-altitude pulmonary edema (HAPE). Chronic forms include chronic mountain sickness (CMS, Monge disease), and high-altitude pulmonary hypertension (HAPH). AMS is the most common form of high-altitude-related illness, affecting 10–40% of lowlanders ascending rapidly to moderate altitudes (3000 m) and 40–60% ascending to altitudes between 4000 and 5000 m [60,61]. The diagnosis relies on the presence of headache, sleep disturbance, and other typical symptoms in the appropriate setting (Table 54.2). Obviously, headache, the cardinal symptom of AMS, and other AMS symptoms, including stomach upset, might affect sleep quality at altitude. Insomnia is therefore commonly reported by mountaineers suffering from AMS, and it is one of the symptoms evaluated by the Lake Louise AMS Questionnaire (Table 54.2). As already mentioned, lowlanders arriving at 3500 m commonly reported sleep disturbances during their first night at altitude, and this was most prominent in those suffering from symptoms of AMS [2]. Correspondingly, unacclimatized mountaineers suffering from AMS at 4590 m (Capanna Regina Margherita, Mt. Rosa) perceived their sleep quality as poor, and actigraphy confirmed pronounced nocturnal restlessness [49]. These symptoms were partially relieved with acclimatization for 2 days. Untreated AMS may progress to HACE, a life-threatening condition characterized by severe headache (often resistant to painkillers), ataxia and progressive impairment of consciousness. Evacuation to a lower altitude, supplemental oxygen, and dexamethasone may be lifesaving.

HAPE is a noncardiogenic form of pulmonary edema developing in otherwise healthy, susceptible subjects within 2–5 days after rapid ascent to altitudes over 3000 m [62]. With an estimated prevalence of 3–5% at 4559 m, HAPE is much less common than AMS [63]. The main clinical manifestations of HAPE are dyspnea, cough, and reduced exercise tolerance associated with severe hypoxemia, a restrictive pattern of pulmonary function, and an

Table 54.1 Altitude-related illnesses

Condition	Time of exposure	Main manifestations and diagnostic criteria
Acute mountain sickness (AMS)	Hours to days	Headache, loss of appetite, insomnia, fatigue
High-altitude cerebral edema (HACE)	Hours to days	Severe headache, ataxia, confusion, loss of consciousness
High-altitude pulmonary edema (HAPE)	Days	Dyspnea, cough with eventually blood-tinged sputum, cyanosis, exercise intolerance, pulmonary hypertension
High-altitude pulmonary hypertension (HAPH), or cardiac chronic mountain sickness	Years	Dyspnea, exercise intolerance, right heart failure. Mean pulmonary artery pressure (mPAP) >30 mmHg or systolic pulmonary artery pressure (sPAP) >50 mmHg at altitude of residence; absence of excessive erythrocytosis (hemoglobin concentration <19 g/dL in women, <21 g/dL in men)
Chronic mountain sickness, Monge disease (CMS)	Years	Headache, dizziness, dyspnea, sleep disturbances, fatigue. Excessive erythrocytosis (hemoglobin concentration ≥19 g/dL in women, ≥21 g/dL in men). In some patients, pulmonary hypertension, right heart failure, hypoventilation
Subacute mountain sickness, or adult and infantile forms of cardiac subacute mountain sickness (CSMS)	Weeks to months	Dyspnea, exercise intolerance, pulmonary hypertension, right heart failure

Source data from N Engl J Med, 369(17), Bartsch P, Swenson ER, Acute high-altitude illnesses, pp. 1666–67, Copyright (2013), Massachusetts Medical Society.

impaired diffusing capacity [64]. Subjects affected by HAPE experience severe sleep disruption and pronounced periodic breathing [3]. Nifedipine or dexamethasone administered prophylactically may prevent HAPE.

Only a few studies have investigated sleep disturbances in highlanders affected by chronic altitude-related illness [42,46]. Among Kyrgyz highlanders with HAPH studied at their altitude of residence (3250 m), SWS was reduced compared with healthy highlanders and the prevalence of sleep apnea was increased. This suggested a potential role of sleep apnea in predisposing to elevated pulmonary artery pressure [42].

Effect of altitude in lowlanders with pre-existing sleep and breathing disorders

In lowlanders suffering from the obstructive sleep apnea (OSA) syndrome who discontinued their continuous positive airway pressure (CPAP) therapy during a sojourn at 1860 and 2590 m, we observed pronounced hypoxemia and exacerbated sleep-related breathing disturbances due to frequent central apneas/hypopneas (Fig. 54.9) [65]. This was associated with sleep-related cerebral hypoxia as monitored by near-infrared spectroscopy (Fig. 54.10) [66]. During

Table 54.2 Lake Louise Score Questions and Rating

Self-report (by mountaineer)	1. Headache	0	None
		1	Mild
		2	Moderate
		3	Severe, incapacitating
	2. Gastrointestinal symptoms	0	None
		1	Poor appetite or nausea
		2	Moderate nausea or vomiting
		3	Severe nausea or vomiting, incapacitating
	3. Fatigue and/or weakness	0	None
		1	Mild
		2	Moderate
		3	Severe, incapacitating
	4. Dizziness/ lightheadedness	0	None
		1	Mild
		2	Moderate
		3	Severe, incapacitating
	5. Difficulty sleeping	0	Slept as usual
		1	Did not sleep as well as usual
		2	Woke up many times, poor night sleep
		3	Could not sleep at all
Clinical assessment (by investigator)	6. Change in mental status	0	None
		1	Lethargy lassitude
		2	Disoriented/confused
		3	Stupor/semi-consciousness
		4	Coma
	7. Ataxia (heel-to-toe walking)	0	None
		1	Maneuvers to maintain balance
		2	Steps off line
		3	Falls down
		4	Cannot stand
	8. Peripheral edema	0	None
		1	Peripheral edema at one location
		2	Peripheral edema at two or more locations

The sum of the scores of self-rating (questions 1–5) and clinical assessment (questions 6–8) is the Lake Louise Score. A score > 3 points on the AMS Self-Reported Questionnaire in the presence of headache—while at an altitude > 2500 m—constitutes AMS. A sum score > 4 indicates clinically relevant acute mountain sickness (AMS)

Source data from Sutton JR, Coates G, Huston CS, [eds], The Lake Louise acute mountain sickness scoring system. Hypoxia and molecular medicine: proceedings of the 8th international hypoxia symposium, Copyright (1993), Queen City Press.

daytime, driving simulator tests revealed impaired performance at 2590 m compared with 490 m baseline, and patients showed an increase in blood pressure, cardiac arrhythmias, and weight gain associated with leg edema [65]. Subsequent randomized placebo-controlled trials revealed that combined treatment with CPAP using computer-controlled variable mask pressure and acetazolamide provided improved oxygenation and optimal control of breathing disturbances in sleep apnea patients at altitude [67,68].

In patients with chronic obstructive pulmonary disease (COPD), sleep is commonly disturbed near sea level [69] owing to dyspnea, cough, coexistent sleep-related breathing disorders, and other factors that are yet incompletely understood. In a randomized controlled study, we observed that COPD patients with moderate to severe impairment in pulmonary function at 490 m (i.e, GOLD grade 2–3) developed considerable nocturnal hypoxemia and severe high-altitude periodic breathing associated with sleep disturbances during the first night at 2590 m [70].

Prevention and treatment of sleep disturbances at altitude

Sleep disturbances at altitude can be mitigated by following a few basic rules. By selecting a gradual ascent to altitude, acclimatization may improve oxygenation and hence altitude tolerance. In addition, the risk of altitude-related illness is reduced. According to recommendations for healthy subjects, the ascent rate at altitudes above 3000 m should not exceed 300 m/24 h, and sleeping altitude should be selected as low as possible to avoid excessive nocturnal hypoxemia [71]. The use of drugs might also improve altitude tolerance. However, the potential advantages and disadvantages of pharmacological therapy should be carefully considered, and its use should be restricted to mountaineers who suffer from altitude-related illness or severe sleep problems. Several drugs used to prevent and treat high-altitude-related illness (AMS, HACE, or HAPE), including acetazolamide, dexamethasone, and nifedipine, may also improve sleep. In the following subsections, several treatment options are discussed.

Oxygen

Using supplemental oxygen counteracts the effect of hypobaric hypoxia and is a rational way to treat altitude-related illnesses and thereby improve sleep quality. Raising the oxygen concentration at a given high altitude by 1% increases the inspired oxygen partial pressure to a degree corresponding to an altitude reduction of approximately 300 m [72]. Raising the fraction of inspired oxygen (FiO_2) in the sleeping room at 3800 m by 3% using oxygen concentrators increased nocturnal oxygen saturation, reduced the amount of periodic breathing, and improved subjective sleep quality and some tests of cognitive daytime performance [73,74]. Unfortunately, oxygen is often not available in remote mountain areas.

Carbonic anhydrase inhibitors

The carbonic anhydrase inhibitor acetazolamide has been extensively tested and found to be an effective drug for the prevention and treatment of AMS [75]. Acetazolamide stimulates renal bicarbonate excretion, thereby inducing metabolic acidosis. This counteracts the hypoxia-induced respiratory alkalosis and stimulates ventilation through augmenting the hypercapnic ventilatory response. Acetazolamide improves nocturnal oxygen saturation and reduces high-altitude periodic breathing [76–78]. In a randomized comparison with theophylline, acetazolamide was equally effective in normalizing periodic breathing at 3454 m but provided a higher nocturnal oxygen saturation [25]. In another study performed in mountaineers suffering from sleep disturbances at 3450 m, there

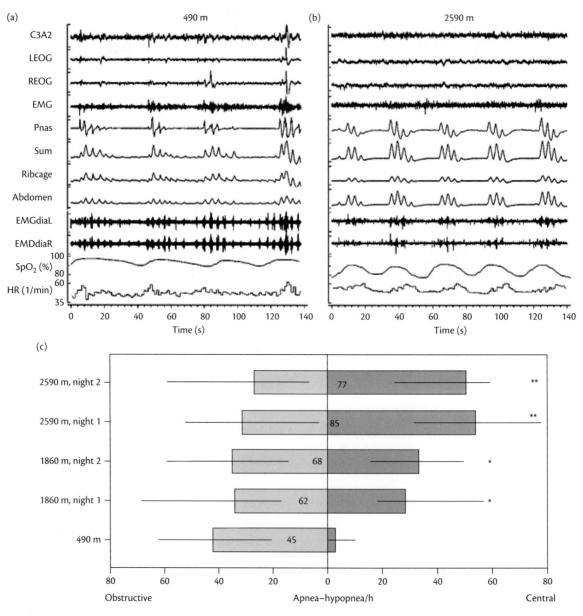

Fig. 54.9 The effect of altitude travel in patients with untreated obstructive sleep apnea syndrome was investigated in a randomized study [65]. (a, b) Polysomnographic recordings in one patient with predominantly obstructive apneas at 490 m (a) and central apneas at 2590 m (b). (c) Sleep-related breathing disturbances at 490 m and on the 1st and 2nd night at 1860 and 2590 m, respectively, in the entire group of 34 untreated patients with obstructive sleep apnea syndrome. The bars and horizontal lines represent median values and quartile ranges of obstructive and central apnea–hypopnea indices. At higher altitudes, the total apnea–hypopnea index increased significantly, related to the emergence of central apnea/hypopnea during NREM sleep. *$p < 0.01$ versus 490 m; **$p < 0.01$ versus 490 m and versus 1860 m.

was no difference between acetazolamide (125 mg) and temazepam (7.5 mg) concerning oxygen saturation, percent periodic breathing, and actigraphic measures of sleep [79]. However, subjective sleep quality was significantly better in the group receiving temazepam. Because acetazolamide acts as a diuretic, subjects on acetazolamide complained significantly more about nightly awakenings due to urination. Apart from polyuria (8–55%), other frequent side effects of acetazolamide comprise acral paresthesias (35–90%) and unpleasant taste (4–14%) [80]. In otherwise-untreated OSA patients travelling to 1680 and 2590 m, we found that acetazolamide (250 mg bid) improved oxygenation, nocturnal breathing disturbances, and sleep quality, and it prevented an excessive blood pressure rise [68]. Even though the amount of residual breathing

disturbances was considerable, acetazolamide was superior to no therapy at all and may therefore be recommended for OSA patients at altitude if CPAP therapy is not feasible. An even better and nearly optimal control of breathing disturbances was achieved in another randomized trial with combined treatment by acetazolamide and auto-adjusting CPAP [67].

Dexamethasone

Dexamethasone is a potent drug that prevents and effectively treats AMS and prevents HAPE in susceptible subjects [81]. Moreover, in a recent study in HAPE-susceptible subjects ascending from lowlands to 4559 m within 24 hours, we found that dexamethasone (4 mg bid) taken before ascent improved nocturnal oxygen

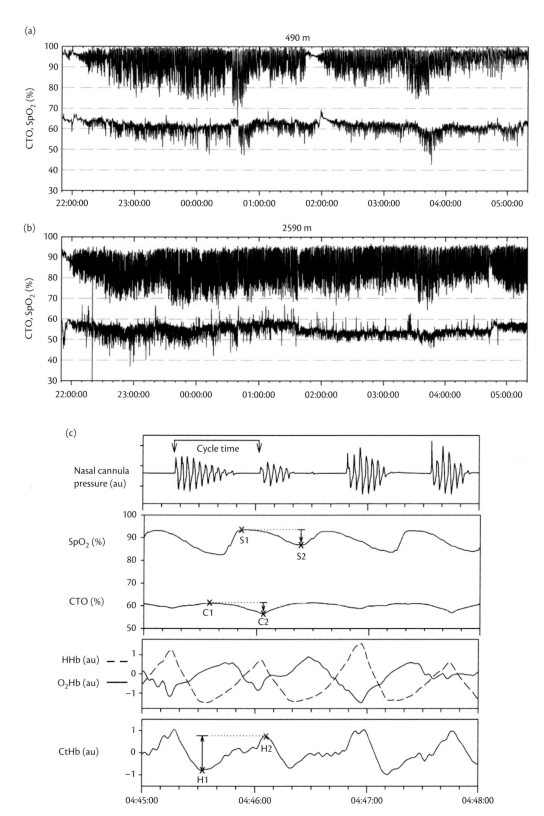

Fig. 54.10 Recordings of cerebral oxygenation by near-infrared spectroscopy (NIRS) in a patient with untreated obstructive sleep apnea syndrome at 490 m and on the 1st night at 2590 m. (a, b) Entire nights (7.5 hours) with large swings of finger pulse oximetry (SpO_2), and more moderate swings of cerebral tissue oxygen saturation (CTO) that depart from lower baseline levels. (c) A 3-minute episode of the recording at 2590 m. Nasal cannula pressure swings show several apnea/hyperpnea cycles and corresponding changes in SpO_2, CTO, oxygenated hemoglobin (O_2Hb), deoxygenated hemoglobin (HHb), and total cerebral hemoglobin (CtHb). Variables listed in Table 54.2 are marked: SpO_2 baseline (S1); SpO_2 nadir (S2); SpO_2 desaturation amplitude = difference in amplitude S1 − S2; SpO_2 desaturation time to nadir = difference in time S2 − S1; CTO baseline (C1); CTO nadir (C2); CTO desaturation amplitude = difference in amplitude C1 − C2; CTO desaturation time to nadir = difference in time C2 − C1; CtHb rise in amplitude = H2-H1; CtHb time from CTO drop to CtHb peak = difference in time H2 − C1.

Reproduced from Chest, 146(2), Ulrich S, Nussbaumer-Ochsner Y, Vasic I et al., Cerebral oxygenation in patients with obstructive sleep apnea. Effects of hypoxia at altitude and of acetzolamide, pp. 299–308, Copyright (2014), with permission from Elsevier.

saturation and increased the amount of SWS at 4559 m [50]. The powerful action of the drug in the prevention and the treatment of AMS—and thereby also improving sleep—seems to outweigh by far the potential sleep-disturbing effects, which are not well established [82].

Theophylline

Theophylline reduces nocturnal periodic breathing [25], but does not show any beneficial effects on oxygen saturation and sleep structure [83]. It may exert its action by an increase in ventilatory drive and in cardiac output, but the mechanisms have not been studied in detail. Theophylline has a narrow therapeutic window, shows interactions with many other drugs, and promotes cardiac arrhythmia. It is therefore not recommended as a standard treatment of high-altitude periodic breathing.

Hypnotics

Several randomized placebo-controlled trials have evaluated the effect of benzodiazepines and non-benzodiazepine hypnotics in subjects at simulated or real altitude [15,24,27,30,84,85]. Contrary to some negative expectations, neither the benzodiazepine temazepam nor the non-benzodiazepine hypnotics zolpidem and zaleplon had adverse effects on oxygen saturation and ventilation, but they were effective in improving sleep quality at altitude and, in some studies, even next-day performance [24,27,30,84,85]. Therefore, the cited hypnotics may be used cautiously to treat insomnia in mountaineers at moderate altitude (up to 4000 m) in a safe setting where resting in a state of reduced arousability is not considered to represent an unacceptable risk. Since zaleplon has a relatively short half-life (1 h) compared with zolpidem (2.4 h), it might be particularly suitable for use in the mountains. In mountaineers sleeping in exposed camps, the use of hypnotics is discouraged because of the potential danger associated with a potential paradoxical reaction or impaired arousability. Further studies on sleep and treatment of its disturbances at altitude have been systematically reviewed [86].

Sleep in space travel

Given the necessity and opportunity of performing interplanetary spaceflights, the effects of microgravity and other associated physical effects on human sleep have become of increasing interest. Restorative sleep is essential for maintaining optimal alertness and neurobehavioral functioning over the course of long-lasting, demanding space missions. Reduction of the gravitational force to less than 1g (microgravity) may induce space motion sickness. The symptoms are similar to those of terrestrial motion sickness and comprise headache, malaise, disorientation, nausea, and vomiting usually lasting for not more than 2–3 days [87]. Space missions are associated with sleep restriction and disruption and with disturbances of the circadian rhythm, especially if the mission requires very long and irregular shifts. Various physiological functions (eg, hormone secretion, body temperature, and sleep rhythm) exhibit a circadian periodicity with a cycle length of approximately 24 hours. Space flight may alter this circadian rhythm, causing profound disturbances in physiological functions. Thus, during a 520-day ground simulation of a Mars mission in six subjects, disturbances of sleep quality, sleep–wake periodicity, and timing recorded by actigraphy suggested inadequate circadian entrainment [88]. Sleeping in an unusual, noisy, and uncomfortably warm environment, confined to a sleeping bag, and the excitement and stress of the flight

may further impair sleep quality. The relevance of sleep problems during space missions is highlighted by common in-flight use of sleep medication. During 79 US Space Shuttle missions, involving 219 person-flights, the use of any medication was recorded in 94% [89]. Of these medications, 47% were for space motion sickness and 45% for sleep disturbances, with smaller percentages of analgesics or anti-inflammatory agents. The most commonly used hypnotics were temazepam (67% of all sleep medications), followed by zolpidem (10%), triazolam (10%) and flurazepam (7.5%). In contrast to medication against space motion sickness, which was mainly used at the beginning of the mission, sleep medications were taken throughout the mission duration.

A detailed analysis of the effects of space flight on sleep is hampered by the lack of conclusive studies. Most of what is currently known about sleep, circadian rhythms, and work–rest schedules in space is based on anecdotal reports originating from log books and interviews with astronauts, plus a few observational studies. The first experiments were performed in monkeys and revealed that sleep was remarkably fragmented and unusually brief in duration [90–92]. In the following discussion, only human studies performed during real space travel are considered [93–96], since simulations (water immersion and head-down rest) may not appropriately reflect the complex physical, physiological, and psychological effects of real space flight [97–99]. We identified seven observational studies including a total of 21 astronauts evaluating sleep in space using electrophysiological monitoring [93–96,100–102]. In one of these studies, the effect of microgravity on breathing during sleep was evaluated in five astronauts [103].

In 1974, Frost et al. reported on sleep studies in 2 astronauts living in space for 28 (Skaylab II) and 59 days (Skylab III) [93]. Data from 9 of 12 and from 18 of 20 attempted sleep recordings during Skylab II and III missions, respectively, were available for analysis. During the Skylab II mission, the mean in-flight sleep duration was shorter (6.04 h) than the sleep duration before departure (6.9 h), which was related to a shorter resting time. During the Skylab III mission, sleep times did not differ significantly from preflight baseline. No major changes in sleep stages were noted. Post-flight changes concerned mostly REM sleep, with an increase from 18.5% to 25% in Skylab II and from 13% to 22% in Skylab III. Gundel and colleagues performed PSG together with body temperature recordings as a marker of the circadian rhythm in four astronauts aboard the Russian Mir station [95]. Analysis of recordings did not reveal significant changes in any of the sleep parameters. Monk et al. studied four astronauts during a 17-days Space Shuttle mission [96]. For operational reasons, there were changes in bedtime and wake time throughout the flight, but these were distributed equally throughout the mission, leading to a phase advance of 25 minutes per day with a strict schedule of a 23.58-hour day and an 8-hour sleep opportunity. No hypnotics were used during the whole mission. Sleep time was reduced from an average of 392 minutes to 353 minutes in early flight and to 375 minutes in late flight, with a marked reduction in SWS. No difference in sleep architecture in late flight compared with early flight periods was found. Similar results were obtained on board the Mir orbiting station in four subjects living up to 241 days in space. The durations of SWS and REM sleep did not change, and the cyclic structure of sleep persisted [101].

The only randomized trial performed in space was conducted during Space Shuttle missions STS-90 and STS-95 [100,103]. In a double-blind placebo-controlled crossover design [100], 0.3 mg melatonin was administered on alternate nights in five subjects during a 16-day space mission. No significant effect of melatonin was observed apart from increased awakenings after melatonin administration. In-flight sleep was similar to pre-flight sleep for all sleep variables. Sleep efficiency varied between 83.8% and 84.5%. In the same mission, assessments included breathing pattern and oxygenation during sleep. The pre-flight mean AHI was 8.3/h, and recordings during space flight revealed an AHI of 3.4/h ($p < 0.05$) [103]. This was accompanied by a reduction in snoring and respiratory-related arousals. Microgravity thus seemed to have reduced the tendency for obstructive apnea/hypopnea and snoring. A potential explanation of this finding relates to the absence of gravitational forces during space flight. On Earth, gravity reduces upper airway size, thereby increasing upper airway resistance in supine position [104,105], whereas such gravitational impairments of upper airway patency do not occur in space, although this requires further study [103].

In summary, based on the limited available data from only a small number of subjects, taking differences in mission times, sleep–wake schedules, and various other confounding factors into account, it is not possible to draw firm conclusions on the effect of microgravity on sleep. Nevertheless, the reduction of sleep time during space travel compared with pre- and post-flight measurements is a common observation made in all studies. The reduction in sleep time is most likely related to the combined influences of physiological effects associated with microgravity, including motion sickness, disturbances of circadian rhythm, challenges of work schedules, environmental disturbances, and psychological factors. Further studies are required to elucidate the contribution of the various potential influences on sleep in space and to identify measures that may contribute to promote restorative sleep.

References

1. West JB, Schoene RB, Milledge JS. High altitude medicine and physiology, 4th ed. London: Hodder Arnold, 2007.
2. Jafarian S, Gorouhi F, Taghva A, Lotfi J. High-altitude sleep disturbance: results of the Groningen Sleep Quality Questionnaire survey. Sleep Med 2008;9(4):446–9.
3. Nussbaumer-Ochsner Y, Schuepfer N, Siebenmann C, Maggiorini M, Bloch KE. High altitude sleep disturbances monitored by actigraphy and polysomnography. High Alt Med Biol 2011;12(3):229–36.
4. Latshang TD, Lo Cascio CM, Stowhas AC, et al. Are nocturnal breathing, sleep, and cognitive performance impaired at moderate altitude (1,630–2,590 m)? Sleep 2013;36(12):1969–76.
5. Mizuno K, Asano K, Okudaira N. Sleep and respiration under acute hypobaric hypoxia. Jpn J Physiol 1993;43(2):161–75.
6. Muhm JM, Signal TL, Rock PB, et al. Sleep at simulated 2438 m: effects on oxygenation, sleep quality, and postsleep performance. Aviat Space Environ Med 2009;80(8):691–7.
7. Eichenberger U, Weiss E, Riemann D, Oelz O, Bartsch P. Nocturnal periodic breathing and the development of acute high altitude illness. Am J Respir Crit Care Med 1996;154:1748–54.
8. Kohler M, Kriemler S, Wilhelm EM, et al. Children at high altitude have less nocturnal periodic breathing than adults. Eur Respir J 2008;32(1):189–97.
9. Erba P, Anastasi S, Senn O, Maggiorini M, Bloch KE. Acute mountain sickness is related to nocturnal hypoxemia but not to hypoventilation. Eur Respir J 2004;24(2):303–8.
10. Kinsman TA, Townsend NE, Gore CJ, et al. Sleep disturbance at simulated altitude indicated by stratified respiratory disturbance index but not hypoxic ventilatory response. Eur J Appl Physiol 2005;94(5-6):569–75.
11. Julian CG, Vargas E, Gonzales M, et al. Sleep-disordered breathing and oxidative stress in preclinical chronic mountain sickness (excessive erythrocytosis). Respir Physiol Neurobiol 2013;186(2):188–96.
12. Natani K, Shurley JT, Pierce CM, Brooks RE. Long-term changes in sleep patterns in men on the South Polar Plateau. Arch Intern Med 1970;125(4):655–9.
13. Miller JC, Horvath SM. Sleep at altitude. Aviat Space Environ Med 1977;48(7):615–20.
14. Reite M, Jackson D, Cahoon RL, Weil JV. Sleep physiology at high altitude. Electroencephalogr Clin Neurophysiol 1975;38(5):463–71.
15. Nicholson AN, Smith PA, Stone BM, Bradwell AR, Coote JH. Altitude insomnia: studies during an expedition to the Himalayas. Sleep 1988;11(4):354–61.
16. Berssenbrugge A, Dempsey J, Iber C, Skatrud J, Wilson P. Mechanisms of hypoxia-induced periodic breathing during sleep in humans. J Physiol 1983;343:507–24.
17. Berssenbrugge AD, Dempsey JA, Skatrud JB. Effects of sleep state on ventilatory acclimatization to hypoxia in humans. J Appl Physiol 1984;57(4):1089–96.
18. Normand H, Barragan M, Benoit O, Bailliart O, Raynaud J. Periodic breathing and O_2 saturation in relation to sleep stages at high altitude. Aviat Space Environ Med 1990;61(3):229–35.
19. Khoo MC, Anholm JD, Ko SW, et al. Dynamics of periodic breathing and arousal during sleep at extreme altitude. Respir Physiol 1996;103(1):33–43.
20. Anholm JD, Powles AC, Downey R III, et al. Operation Everest II: arterial oxygen saturation and sleep at extreme simulated altitude. Am Rev Respir Dis 1992;145(4 Pt 1):817–26.
21. Matsuzawa Y, Kobayshi T, Fujimoto YS, et al. Nocturnal periodic breathing and arterial oxygen saturation in acute montain sickness. J Wilderness Med 1994;5:269–81.
22. Salvaggio A, Insalaco G, Marrone O, et al. Effects of high-altitude periodic breathing on sleep and arterial oxyhaemoglobin saturation. Eur Respir J 1998;12(2):408–13.
23. Zielinski J, Koziej M, Mankowski M, et al. The quality of sleep and periodic breathing in healthy subjects at an altitude of 3,200 m. High Alt Med Biol 2000;1(4):331–6.
24. Beaumont M, Goldenberg F, Lejeune D, et al. Effect of zolpidem on sleep and ventilatory patterns at simulated altitude of 4,000 meters. Am J Respir Crit Care Med 1996;153(6 Pt 1):1864–9.
25. Fischer R, Lang SM, Leitl M, et al. Theophylline and acetazolamide reduce sleep-disordered breathing at high altitude. Eur Respir J 2004;23(1):47–52.
26. Yaron M, Lindgren K, Halbower AC, et al. Sleep disturbance after rapid ascent to moderate altitude among infants and preverbal young children. High Alt Med Biol 2004;5(3):314–20.
27. Beaumont M, Batejat D, Coste O, et al. Effects of zolpidem and zaleplon on sleep, respiratory patterns and performance at a simulated altitude of 4,000 m. Neuropsychobiology 2004;49(3):154–62.
28. Burgess KR, Johnson P, Edwards N, Cooper J. Acute mountain sickness is associated with sleep desaturation at high altitude. Respirology 2004;9(4):485–92.
29. Mizuno K, Asano K, Inoue Y, Shirakawa S. Consecutive monitoring of sleep disturbance for four nights at the top of Mt Fuji (3776 m). Psychiatry Clin Neurosci 2005;59(2):223–5.
30. Beaumont M, Batejat D, Pierard C, et al. Zaleplon and zolpidem objectively alleviate sleep disturbances in mountaineers at a 3,613 meter altitude. Sleep 2007;30(11):1527–33.
31. Hoshikawa M, Uchida S, Sugo T, et al. Changes in sleep quality of athletes under normobaric hypoxia equivalent to 2,000-m altitude: a polysomnographic study. J Appl Physiol 2007;103(6):2005–11.
32. Szymczak RK, Sitek EJ, Slawek JW, et al. Subjective sleep quality alterations at high altitude. Wilderness Environ Med 2009;20(4):305–10.
33. Weiss MD, Tamisier R, Boucher J, et al. A pilot study of sleep, cognition, and respiration under 4 weeks of intermittent nocturnal hypoxia in adult humans. Sleep Med 2009;10(7):739–45.

34. Johnson PL, Edwards N, Burgess KR, Sullivan CE. Sleep architecture changes during a trek from 1400 to 5000 m in the Nepal Himalaya. J Sleep Res 2010;19(1 Pt 2):148–56.

35. Nussbaumer-Ochsner Y, Ursprung J, Siebenmann C, Maggiorini M, Bloch KE. Effect of short-term acclimatization to high altitude on sleep and nocturnal breathing. Sleep 2012;35(3):419–23.

36. Burgess KR, Lucas SJ, Shepherd K, et al. Worsening of central sleep apnea at high altitude—a role for cerebrovascular function. J Appl Physiol 2013;114(8):1021–8.

37. Selvamurthy W, Raju VR, Ranganathan S, Hegde KS, Ray US. Sleep patterns at an altitude of 3500 metres. Int J Biometeorol 1986;30(2):123–35.

38. Nespoulet H, Wuyam B, Tamisier R, et al. Altitude illness is related to low hypoxic chemoresponse and low oxygenation during sleep. Eur Respir J 2012;40(3):673–80.

39. Jones JE, Muza SR, Fulco CS, et al. Intermittent hypoxic exposure does not improve sleep at 4300 m. High Alt Med Biol 2008;9(4):281–7.

40. Fulco CS, Muza SR, Beidleman BA, et al. Effect of repeated normobaric hypoxia exposures during sleep on acute mountain sickness, exercise performance, and sleep during exposure to terrestrial altitude. Am J Physiol Regul Integr Comp Physiol 2011;300(2):R428–36.

41. Fujimoto K, Matsuzawa Y, Hirai K, et al. Irregular nocturnal breathing patterns high altitude in subjects susceptible to high-altitude pulmonary edema (HAPE): a preliminary study. Aviat Space Environ Med 1989;60(8):786–91.

42. Latshang TD, Furian M, Aeschbacher S, et al. Association between sleep apnoea and pulmonary hypertension in Kyrgyz highlanders. Eur Respir J 2016. doi: 10.1183/13993003.01530-2016.

43. Coote JH, Stone BM, Tsang G. Sleep of Andean high altitude natives. Eur J Appl Physiol Occup Physiol 1992;64(2):178–81.

44. Coote JH, Tsang G, Baker A, Stone B. Respiratory changes and structure of sleep in young high-altitude dwellers in the Andes of Peru. Eur J Appl Physiol Occup Physiol 1993;66(3):249–53.

45. Plywaczewski R, Wu TY, Wang XQ, et al. Sleep structure and periodic breathing in Tibetans and Han at simulated altitude of 5000 m. Respir Physiol Neurobiol 2003;136(2-3):187–97.

46. Kryger M, Glas R, Jackson D, et al. Impaired oxygenation during sleep in excessive polycythemia of high altitude: improvement with respiratory stimulation. Sleep 1978;1(1):3–17.

47. Stadelmann K, Latshang TD, Lo Cascio CM, et al. Quantitative changes in the sleep EEG at moderate altitude (1630 m and 2590 m). PLoS One 2013;8(10):e76945.

48. Stadelmann K, Latshang TD, Tarokh L, et al. Sleep respiratory disturbances and arousals at moderate altitude have overlapping electroencephalogram spectral signatures. J Sleep Res 2014;23:463–8.

49. Nussbaumer-Ochsner Y, Ursprung J, Siebenmann C, Maggiorini M, Bloch KE. Effect of short-term acclimatization to high altitude on sleep and nocturnal breathing. Sleep 2012;35(3):419–23.

50. Nussbaumer-Ochsner Y, Schuepfer N, Ursprung J, et al. Sleep and breathing in high altitude pulmonary edema susceptible subjects at 4,559 meters. Sleep 2012;35(10):1413–21.

51. White DP, Gleeson K, Pickett CK, et al. Altitude acclimatization: influence on periodic breathing and chemoresponsiveness during sleep. J Appl Physiol 1987;63(1):401–12.

52. Latshang TD, Turk AJ, Hess T, et al. Acclimatization improves submaximal exercise economy at 5533 m. Scand J Med Sci Sports 2013;23(4):458–67.

53. White DP. Pathogenesis of obstructive and central sleep apnea. Am J Respir Crit Care Med 2005;172(11):1363–70.

54. Douglas NJ, White DP, Weil JV, et al. Hypoxic ventilatory response decreases during sleep in normal men. Am Rev Respir Dis 1982;125(3):286–9.

55. Douglas NJ, White DP, Weil JV, Pickett CK, Zwillich CW. Hypercapnic ventilatory response in sleeping adults. Am Rev Respir Dis 1982;126(5):758–62.

56. Dempsey JA, Smith CA, Przybylowski T, et al. The ventilatory responsiveness to CO_2 below eupnoea as a determinant of ventilatory stability in sleep. J Physiol 2004;560(Pt 1):1–11.

57. Kinsman TA, Hahn AG, Gore CJ, et al. Respiratory events and periodic breathing in cyclists sleeping at 2,650-m simulated altitude. J Appl Physiol 2002;92(5):2114–18.

58. Bloch KE, Latshang TD, Turk AJ, et al. Nocturnal periodic breathing during acclimatization at very high altitude at Mount Muztagh Ata (7,546 m). Am J Respir Crit Care Med 2010;182(4):562–8.

59. West JB, Peters RM Jr, Aksnes G, et al. Nocturnal periodic breathing at altitudes of 6,300 and 8,050 m. J Appl Physiol 1986;61(1):280–7.

60. Basnyat B, Murdoch DR. High-altitude illness. Lancet 2003;361(9373):1967–74.

61. Maggiorini M, Muller A, Hofstetter D, Bartsch P, Oelz O. Assessment of acute mountain sickness by different score protocols in the Swiss Alps. Aviat Space Environ Med 1998;69(12):1186–92.

62. Maggiorini M, Melot C, Pierre S, et al. High-altitude pulmonary edema is initially caused by an increase in capillary pressure. Circulation 2001;103(16):2078–83.

63. Maggiorini M, Buhler B, Walter M, Oelz O. Prevalence of acute mountain sickness in the Swiss Alps. BMJ 1990;301(6756):853–5.

64. Clarenbach CF, Senn O, Christ AL, et al. Lung function and breathing pattern in subjects developing high altitude pulmonary edema. PLoS One 2012;7(7):e41188.

65. Nussbaumer-Ochsner Y, Schuepfer N, Ulrich S, Bloch KE. Exacerbation of sleep apnoea by frequent central events in patients with the obstructive sleep apnoea syndrome at altitude: a randomised trial. Thorax 2010;65(5):429–35.

66. Ulrich S, Nussbaumer-Ochsner Y, Vasic I, et al. Cerebral oxygenation in patients with obstructive sleep apnea: effects of hypoxia at altitude and of acetazolamide. Chest 2014;146(2):299–308.

67. Latshang TD, Nussbaumer-Ochsner Y, Henn RM, et al. Effect of acetazolamide and autoCPAP therapy on breathing disturbances among patients with obstructive sleep apnea syndrome who travel to altitude: a randomized controlled trial. JAMA 2012;308(22):2390–8.

68. Nussbaumer-Ochsner Y, Latshang TD, Ulrich S, et al. Patients with obstructive sleep apnea syndrome benefit from acetazolamide during an altitude sojourn: a randomized, placebo-controlled, double-blind trial. Chest 2012;141(1):131–8.

69. Collop N. Sleep and sleep disorders in chronic obstructive pulmonary disease. Respiration 2010;80(1):78–86.

70. Latshang TD, Furian M, Flueck D, et al. Breathing and sleep disturbanes in lowlanders with COPD staying at moderate altitude (1650 m and 2590 m). Respiration 2015;89(5) (abstract).

71. Nussbaumer-Ochsner Y, Bloch KE. Lessons from high-altitude physiology. Breathe 2007;4:123–32.

72. West JB. Oxygen enrichment of room air to relieve the hypoxia of high altitude. Respir Physiol 1995;99(2):225–32.

73. Luks AM, van MH, Batarse RR, et al. Room oxygen enrichment improves sleep and subsequent day-time performance at high altitude. Respir Physiol 1998;113(3):247–58.

74. McElroy MK, Gerard A, Powell FL, et al. Nocturnal O_2 enrichment of room air at high altitude increases daytime O_2 saturation without changing control of ventilation. High Alt Med Biol 2000;1(3):197–206.

75. Bartsch P, Swenson ER. Acute high-altitude illnesses. N Engl J Med 2013;369(17):1666–7.

76. Hackett PH, Roach RC, Harrison GL, Schoene RB, Mills WJ Jr. Respiratory stimulants and sleep periodic breathing at high altitude. Almitrine versus acetazolamide. Am Rev Respir Dis 1987;135(4):896–8.

77. Sutton JR, Houston CS, Mansell AL, et al. Effect of acetazolamide on hypoxemia during sleep at high altitude. N Engl J Med 1979;301(24):1329–31.

78. Swenson ER, Leatham KL, Roach RC, et al. Renal carbonic anhydrase inhibition reduces high altitude sleep periodic breathing. Respir Physiol 1991;86(3):333–43.

79. Tanner JB, Tanner SM, Thapa GB, et al. A randomized trial of temazepam versus acetazolamide in high altitude sleep disturbance. High Alt Med Biol 2013;14(3):234–9.

80. Low EV, Avery AJ, Gupta V, Schedlbauer A, Grocott MP. Identifying the lowest effective dose of acetazolamide for the prophylaxis of acute mountain sickness: systematic review and meta-analysis. BMJ 2012;345:e6779.

81. Maggiorini M, Brunner-La Rocca HP, Peth S, et al. Both tadalafil and dexamethasone may reduce the incidence of high-altitude pulmonary edema: a randomized trial. Ann Intern Med 2006;145(7):497–506.

82. Born J, DeKloet ER, Wenz H, Kern W, Fehm HL. Gluco- and antimineralocorticoid effects on human sleep: a role of central corticosteroid receptors. Am J Physiol 1991;260(2 Pt 1):E183–8.

83. Kupper TE, Strohl KP, Hoefer M, et al. Low-dose theophylline reduces symptoms of acute mountain sickness. J Travel Med 2008;15(5):307–14.

84. Dubowitz G. Effect of temazepam on oxygen saturation and sleep quality at high altitude: randomised placebo controlled crossover trial. BMJ 1998;316(7131):587–9.

85. Nickol AH, Leverment J, Richards P, et al. Temazepam at high altitude reduces periodic breathing without impairing next-day performance: a randomized cross-over double-blind study. J Sleep Res 2006;15(4):445–54.

86. Bloch KE, Buenzli JC, Latshang TD, Ulrich S. Sleep at high altitude: guesses and facts. J Appl Physiol 2015;119(12):1466–80.

87. Shupak A, Gordon CR. Motion sickness: advances in pathogenesis, prediction, prevention, and treatment. Aviat Space Environ Med 2006;77(12):1213–23.

88. Basner M, Dinges DF, Mollicone D, et al. Mars 520-d mission simulation reveals protracted crew hypokinesis and alterations of sleep duration and timing. Proc Natl Acad Sci U S A 2013;110(7):2635–40.

89. Putcha L, Berens KL, Marshburn TH, Ortega HJ, Billica RD. Pharmaceutical use by U.S. astronauts on space shuttle missions. Aviat Space Environ Med 1999;70(7):705–8.

90. Hanley J, Adey WR. Sleep and wake states in the Biosatellite 3 monkey: visual and computer analysis of telemetered electroencephalographic data from earth orbital flight. Aerosp Med 1971;42(3):304–13.

91. Hoshizaki T, Durham R, Adey WR. Sleep–wake activity patterns of a *Macaca nemestrina* monkey during nine days of weightlessness. Aerosp Med 1971;42(3):288–95.

92. Balzamo E. Evolution of sleep and wakefulness organization in *Macaca mulatta* during Spacelab flight simulation. J Gravit Physiol 1997;4(3):35–41.

93. Frost JD Jr, Shumate WH, Booher CR, DeLucchi MR. The Skylab sleep monitoring experiment: methodology and initial results. Acta Astronaut 1975;2(3–4):319–36.

94. Quadens O, Green H. Eye movements during sleep in weightlessness. Science 1984;225(4658):221–2.

95. Gundel A, Polyakov VV, Zulley J. The alteration of human sleep and circadian rhythms during spaceflight. J Sleep Res 1997;6(1):1–8.

96. Monk TH, Buysse DJ, Billy BD, Kennedy KS, Willrich LM. Sleep and circadian rhythms in four orbiting astronauts. J Biol Rhythms 1998;13(3):188–201.

97. Myasnikov VI. Characteristics of the sleep of men in simulated space flights. Aviat Space Environ Med 1975;46(4 Sec 1):401–8.

98. Komada Y, Inoue Y, Mizuno K, et al. Effects of acute simulated microgravity on nocturnal sleep, daytime vigilance, and psychomotor performance: comparison of horizontal and 6 degrees head-down bed rest. Percept Mot Skills 2006;103(2):307–17.

99. Saiki H, Nakaya M. Dynamics of sleep patterns during prolonged simulated weightlessness. Life Sci Space Res 1977;15:225–31.

100. Dijk DJ, Neri DF, Wyatt JK, et al. Sleep, performance, circadian rhythms, and light–dark cycles during two space shuttle flights. Am J Physiol Regul Integr Comp Physiol 2001;281(5):R1647–64.

101. Stoilova IM, Zdravev TK, Yanev TK. How human sleep in space—investigations during space flights. Adv Space Res 2003;31(6):1611–15.

102. Quadens O, Green H. Eye movements during sleep in weightlessness. Science 1984;225(4658):221–2.

103. Elliott AR, Shea SA, Dijk DJ, et al. Microgravity reduces sleep-disordered breathing in humans. Am J Respir Crit Care Med 2001;164(3):478–85.

104. Yildirim N, Fitzpatrick MF, Whyte KF, et al. The effect of posture on upper airway dimensions in normal subjects and in patients with the sleep apnea/hypopnea syndrome. Am Rev Respir Dis 1991;144(4):845–7.

105. Brown IB, McClean PA, Boucher R, Zamel N, Hoffstein V. Changes in pharyngeal cross-sectional area with posture and application of continuous positive airway pressure in patients with obstructive sleep apnea. Am Rev Respir Dis 1987;136(3):628–32.

Index